Dental Management

of the Medically Compromised Patient

Dental Management
of the Medically Compromised Patient

SEVENTH EDITION

James W. Little, DMD, MS

Professor Emeritus
University of Minnesota
School of Dentistry
Minneapolis, Minnesota; Naples, Florida

Donald A. Falace, DMD

Professor and Division Chief

Oral Diagnosis and Oral Medicine
Department of Oral Health Practice
The University of Kentucky
College of Dentistry
Lexington, Kentucky

Craig S. Miller, DMD, MS

Professor
Department of Oral Health Practice
Department of Microbiology, Immunology, and Genetics
The University of Kentucky
College of Dentistry and College of Medicine
Lexington, Kentucky

Nelson L. Rhodus, DMD, MPH

Morse Distinguished Professor and Director
Division of Oral Medicine, Oral Diagnosis and Oral Radiology
University of Minnesota
School of Dentistry and College of Medicine
Minneapolis, Minnesota

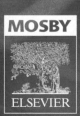

11830 Westline Industrial Drive
St. Louis, Missouri 63146

DENTAL MANAGEMENT OF THE MEDICALLY
COMPROMISED PATIENT, 7TH EDITION

ISBN 13: 978-0-323-04535-3

Notice

Knowledge and best practice in this field are constantly changing. As new research and experience broaden our knowledge, changes in practice, treatment, and drug therapy may become necessary or appropriate. Readers are advised to check the most current information provided (i) on procedures featured or (ii) by the manufacturer of each product to be administered, to verify the recommended dose or formula, the method and duration of administration, and contraindications. It is the responsibility of practitioners, relying on their own experience and knowledge of the patient, to make diagnoses, to determine dosages and the best treatment for each individual patient, and to take all appropriate safety precautions. To the fullest extent of the law, neither the Publisher nor the Authors assumes any liability for any injury and/or damage to persons or property arising out of or related to any use of the material contained in this book.

The Publisher

Library of Congress Control Number 2007928086

Publisher: Linda Duncan
Senior Editor: John Dolan
Developmental Editor: Courtney Sprehe
Managing Editor: Jaime Pendill
Publishing Services Manager: Pat Joiner-Myers
Senior Project Manager: Karen M. Rehwinkel
Design Direction: Julia Dummitt
Cover Designer: Julia Dummitt

Printed in Canada

Last digit is the print number: 9 8 7 6 5 4 3 2 1

Five individuals brought the professional triad of technically capable,
biologically oriented, and socially sensitive to life in 1962 as the first class
was admitted to the University of Kentucky College of Dentistry.
We would like to dedicate this edition to
Dean Alvin Morris
and his planning group of Harry Bohannon, Stephen Dachi,
Michael Romano, and Roy Durocher,
whose efforts have dramatically influenced our professional lives.

James W. Little

FOREWORD

It is now 5 years since the sixth edition of *Dental Management of the Medically Compromised Patient* was published. The number of patients in this critically complex area of healthcare delivery continues to expand along with the scientific advances in diagnosis and treatment. The number of Americans over age 65, which now approximates 14% of the population, is expected to increase to more than 20% within the next few decades. Thus the pool for such patients seeking and needing dental care grows. Furthermore, as longevity increases, so do the number of diseases and conditions that disable individuals, converting them to compromised patients.

Along with increasing longevity, other factors such as obesity, new infections, and widespread use and abuse of drugs, the rising number of medically compromised patients will continue to grow. As a consequence, an ever-enlarging number of individuals with oral health problems will create demands and responsibilities on dental professionals regarding standards of care. Education and readily available resource material is essential to providing these services in an optimal and safe manner, and the thoroughly revised seventh edition fills this role perfectly.

A multitude of diseases have an impact on oral healthcare services. Some examples follow. Cancer is an age-related disease that afflicts more than 1.4 million new patients each year in the United States. This in turn accounts for almost 25% of all deaths, and is the second leading cause of death. Because of the ever-increasing number of new malignancies and the complications caused by aggressive therapy to increase survival rates, dental services and information—for example, oral complications of cancer treatments and rehabilitation—take on significant importance.

Other examples of conditions that commonly affect dental-oral care are cardiovascular diseases, the number one killer of Americans, and diabetes, which affects an estimated 20 million Americans. The list goes on endlessly. Again, this underscores the need for current, reliable, and practical information to minimize or prevent potential problems related to general health and ongoing oral-dental care. Knowledge of the pathophysiology of the common medical diseases and conditions, along with the potential risks of dental procedures and services, is essential.

Interrelationships between oral and general health involve most organ systems. Some examples of medical-dental interaction relate to hematologic, autoimmune, and infectious diseases that strike both the young and the elderly. These include blood dyscrasias, vesiculoerosive inflammatory diseases, and many bacterial, viral, and fungal infections. Thus a very common problem calls upon recognition and management of oral manifesta-tions, control of blood-borne pathogens, and avoiding complications when providing dental treatment. Again, to appropriately meet this challenge, updated information in a concise and understandable format is essential.

Because the majority of medically compromised patients need and/or want oral healthcare, a working knowledge of the multitude of medically complex conditions is critical for dental professionals. This information will support and enable high standards for dental-oral healthcare delivery. This knowledge includes an understanding of medical conditions and compromised states and is necessary to help prevent, minimize, and alert clinicians to possible adverse side effects potentially associated with procedures and drugs used in dentistry. An understanding will assist in formulating treatment plans that are safe and compatible with a patient's medical status.

Care of the medically compromised patient often is complicated, requiring specialists. However, occurrence of compromised patients is so common that practitioners and students must know how to recognize and prevent problems associated with dental management, and to use consultations and referrals appropriately. This updated, revised, and expanded text recognizes and supplies this type of information with practical and organized overviews of diagnosis and management. This is accomplished in 30 well-organized and revised chapters by comprehensively covering diseases and conditions that lead to compromised states that affect a person's well-being. The 30 chapters, now in color, are presented in 9 logical parts that enhance user-friendly utility. The material is supported by summary tables for easy access to information, figures and graphs to supplement text, and appendices that allow the reader to recognize disease states, be aware of potential complications, and select an approach to drug management. An appendix on alternative and complementary medicine has also been added.

Although the main focus is on the management of medically compromised patients having dental procedures, the text effectively includes a medical overview of each disease entity, including etiology, signs and symptoms, pathophysiology, diagnoses, treatment, and prognosis. Therefore it also serves as a mini-text on common medical diseases and conditions. Because tobacco use is the most common cause of preventable deaths in the United States (more than 440,000 each year), a chapter on this topic has been added. In its present format, it serves as both a quick reference and a somewhat in-depth resource for this critical interface of medicine and dentistry. It will help ensure high standards of care and help reduce the occurrence of adverse reactions by improving knowledge and encouraging judgment in the management of at-risk patients.

In summary, treating the medically compromised patient is a complex part of dentistry, requiring competent practitioners with many attributes: sound technical skills, insight into medicine, familiarity with pharmacotherapeutics, and the capability of analyzing findings from patient histories and signs and symptoms. Therefore the usefulness of this excellent updated, comprehensive text as a reference for students and practitioners is evident.

Sol Silverman, Jr.
Professor of Oral Medicine
University of California, San Francisco

PREFACE

As the flow of new knowledge and changing concepts in medicine and dentistry continues to expand, the need for a seventh edition of *Dental Management of the Medically Compromised Patient* became apparent.

A number of major changes have been made in the seventh edition. The chapters have been reorganized and placed under topic headings to streamline the text. For example, the following chapters are placed under the topic heading of Cardiovascular Disease—Chapter 2: *Infective Endocarditis Prophylaxis;* Chapter 3: *Hypertension;* Chapter 4: *Ischemic Heart Disease;* Chapter 5: *Cardiac Arrhythmias;* and Chapter 6: *Heart Failure.*

Three new chapters have been added—Chapter 8: *Smoking and Tobacco Use Cessation;* Chapter 9: *Tuberculosis;* and Chapter 10: *Sleep-Related Breathing Disorders.* Chapters that had previously been one combined chapter have been split into two separate chapters for better readability. This includes Chapter 23: *Disorders of Red Blood Cells* and Chapter 24: *Disorders of White Blood Cells,* and Chapter 28: *Behavioral and Psychiatric Disorders (Anxiety, Delirium, and Eating Disorders),* and Chapter 29: *Psychiatric Disorders.* A new appendix devoted to the use of alternative and complementary drugs in dentistry has been added—Appendix E: *Alternative and Complementary Drugs.*

Chapters 2 and 3 (*Infective Endocarditis* and *Cardiac Conditions Associated With Endocarditis*) from the sixth edition have been combined into one new chapter, Chapter 2: *Infective Endocarditis Prophylaxis,* which incorporates the latest guidelines for the prevention of bacterial endocarditis from the American Heart Association. Alzheimer's disease now appears in Chapter 27: *Neurologic Disorders,* and the use of bisphosphonates and its complications are discussed in Chapter 26: *Cancer and Oral Care of the Patient.* Appendix C has been updated and now includes the sixth edition of the American Academy of Oral Medicine's *Clinician's Guide to Treatment of Common Oral Conditions.*

All of the chapters have been updated where necessary, and many have been provided with new figures and tables. The majority of the figures in the book are now in full color.

The purpose of the book remains the same—to give the dental provider an up-to-date, concise, factual reference describing the dental management of patients with selected medical problems. The more common medical disorders that may be encountered in a dental practice continue to be the focus. This book is not a comprehensive medical reference, but rather a book containing enough core information about each of the medical conditions covered to enable the reader to recognize the basis for various dental management recommendations.

Medical problems are organized to provide a brief overview of the basic disease process, epidemiology, pathophysiology, signs and symptoms, laboratory findings, and currently accepted medical therapy of each disorder. This is followed by a detailed explanation and recommendations for specific dental management. The accumulation of evidence-based research over the years has allowed us to make more specific dental management guidelines that will benefit the audience of this text, which includes practicing dentists and dental hygienists, dental graduate students in specialty or general practice programs, and dental and dental hygiene students. In particular, the text is intended to give the dental provider an understanding of how to ascertain the severity and stability of common medical disorders and make dental management decisions that afford the patient the utmost health and safety.

Continued emphasis has been placed on the medications used to treat the medical conditions covered in this seventh edition. Dosages, side effects, and drug interactions with agents used in dentistry—including those used during pregnancy—are discussed in greater detail. Emphasis also has been placed on having contemporary equipment and diagnostic information to assess and monitor patients with moderate to severe medical disease.

Our sincere thanks and appreciation are extended to those many individuals who have contributed their time and expertise to the writing and revision of this text.

James W. Little
Donald A. Falace
Craig S. Miller
Nelson L. Rhodus

CONTENTS

Dental Management: A Summary

This table presents the more important factors to be considered in the dental management of medically compromised patients. Each medical problem is outlined according to potential problems related to dental treatment, oral manifestations, prevention of these problems, and effects of complications on dental treatment planning.

This table has been designed for use by dentists, dental students, graduate students, dental hygienists, and dental assistants as a convenient reference work for the dental management of patients who have medical diseases discussed in this book.

Dental Management: A Summary

Potential Problems Related to Dental Care | **Oral Manifestations**

INFECTIVE ENDOCARDITIS
Chapter 2

1. Dental procedures that involve the manipulation of gingival tissues or the periapical region of teeth or perforation of the oral mucosa can produce a bacteremia. Bacteremias can also be produced on a daily basis as the result of toothbrushing, flossing, chewing, or the use of toothpicks or irrigating devices. Although it is unlikely that a single dental procedure–induced bacteremia will result in infective endocarditis (IE), it is remotely possible that it can occur.

2. Patients with mechanical prosthetic heart valves may have excessive bleeding following invasive dental procedures as the result of anticoagulant therapy.

- Oral petechiae may be found in patients with IE.

HYPERTENSION
Chapter 3

1. Routine delivery of dental care to a patient with severe uncontrolled hypertension could result in a serious outcome such as angina, myocardial infarction, or stroke.

2. Stress and anxiety related to the dental visit may cause an increase in blood pressure, leading to angina, myocardial infarction, or stroke.

3. In patients taking nonselective beta blockers, excessive use of vasoconstrictors can potentially cause an acute elevation in blood pressure.

4. Some antihypertensive drugs can cause oral lesions or oral dryness and can predispose patients to orthostatic hypotension.

- No oral complications are due to hypertension itself; however, adverse effects such as dry mouth, taste changes, and oral lesions may be drug related.

Prevention of Problems	Treatment Planning Modifications

- Referral for medical diagnosis and treatment
- Drug considerations—Some antibiotics (macrolides, penicillins, and cephalosporins) used for oral infections have a higher incidence of agranulocytosis. Avoid these antibiotics if possible.

- During periods of low blood count, provide emergency care only. Treatment should include the use of antimicrobial agents and supportive therapy for oral lesions (see Appendix C for specific treatment regimens).

- Antibiotics should be given to prevent infection.
- Serial white blood cell count (WBC) should be performed to identify the safest period for dental treatment (i.e., when the WBC is closest to normal level).

- Modifications not required when the WBC is normal.
- If the WBC is depressed severely, antibiotics should be provided to prevent postoperative infection.

- Referral for medical diagnosis, treatment, and consultation
- Complete blood count to determine risk for anemia, bleeding, and infection
- Antibiotics, antivirals, and antifungals provided during chemotherapy to prevent opportunistic oral infection
- Chlorhexidine rinse/bland rinses to manage mucositis

- Inspect head, neck, and radiographs for undiagnosed or latent disease (e.g., retained root tips, impacted teeth) and infections that require acute attention prior to chemotherapy.
- Eliminate infections prior to chemotherapy.
- Extractions should be performed at least 10 days before initiation of chemotherapy.
- Implement plaque control measures and chlorhexidine during chemotherapy.
- Use prophylactic antibiotics if WBC count is less than 2000, or neutrophil count is less than 500 (or 1000 at some institutions).
- Platelet replacement may be required (if platelet count is <50,000) when invasive dental procedures are performed.

- Patients with oral soft tissue lesions and/or osseous lesions should have them biopsied by the dentist or should be referred for diagnosis and treatment as indicated.
- Medical history should identify patients with diagnosed disease; medical consultation is needed to establish current status. (See sections on chemotherapy and radiation therapy on prevention and management of medical complications.)
- Be aware of and take precautions for bisphosphonate-induced osteonecrosis.

- Provide supportive dental care only for patients in terminal stage.
- Long-term prognosis is poor, so complex dental procedures may not be indicated.
- If thrombocytopenia or leukopenia is present, special precautions (platelet replacement, antibiotic therapy) are needed to prevent bleeding and infection when invasive dental procedures are performed.
- Patients may be bleeders because of the presence of abnormal immunoglobulin M macroglobulins, which form complexes with clotting factors, thus inactivating the clotting factors. (See sections on chemotherapy and radiation therapy for treatment plan modifications.)

- Patients with generalized lymphadenopathy, extranodal tumors, and osseous lesions must be identified and referred for medical evaluation and treatment.
- The dentist can biopsy extranodal or osseous lesions to establish a diagnosis; patients with lesions involving the lymph nodes should be referred for excisional biopsy.

- Patients in terminal phase should receive only supportive dental treatment.
- Patients under "control" may receive any indicated treatment; however, complex restorative treatment may not be indicated in cases with a poor prognosis.
- Platelet replacement may be needed for patients with thrombocytopenia. (See sections on radiation therapy and chemotherapy for treatment plan modifications.)

Dental Management: A Summary—cont'd

Potential Problems Related to Dental Care	Oral Manifestations

LYMPHOMAS: HODGKIN'S DISEASE, NON-HODGKIN'S LYMPHOMA, BURKITT'S LYMPHOMA (cont'd)

4. Xerostomia may occur in patients treated by radiation to the head and neck region.
5. Non-Hodgkin's lymphoma may be found in patients with AIDS; hence, transmission of infections agents may be a problem.

- Mucositis in patients treated by radiation therapy or chemotherapy

BLEEDING PROBLEM SUGGESTED BY EXAMINATION AND HISTORY FINDINGS BUT NO CLUES AS TO UNDERLYING CAUSE
Chapter 25

1. Excessive blood loss following surgical procedures, scaling, etc.

- Excessive bleeding after dental procedures

THROMBOCYTOPENIA (PRIMARY OR SECONDARY) CAUSED BY CHEMICALS, RADIATION, OR LEUKEMIA
Chapter 25

1. Prolonged bleeding
2. Infection in patients with bone marrow replacement or destruction
3. In patients being treated with steroids, a serious medical emergency resulting from stress

- Spontaneous bleeding
- Prolonged bleeding following certain dental procedures
- Petechiae
- Ecchymoses
- Hematomas

VASCULAR WALL ALTERATIONS (SCURVY, INFECTION, CHEMICAL, ALLERGIC, AUTOIMMUNE, OTHER)
Chapter 25

1. Prolonged bleeding after surgical procedures or any insult to integrity of oral mucosa

- Excessive bleeding after scaling and surgical procedures
- Petechiae
- Ecchymoses
- Hematomas

Prevention of Problems	**Treatment Planning Modifications**
• Medical history should identify patients with diagnosed disease; medical consultation will be needed to establish current status. (See sections on chemotherapy and radiation therapy on management and prevention of medical complications.) • Prior to invasive procedures, a complete blood count should be obtained to determine risks for bleeding and infection.	• Use prophylactic antibiotics if the WBC count is less than 2000, or the neutrophil count is less than 500 (or 1000 at some institutions).

• Screen patients with the following (if one or more are abnormal, refer for diagnosis and medical treatment):
  • Prothrombin time
  • Activated partial thromboplastin time
  • Thrombin time
  • Platelet count
  • PFA-100
• Avoid use of aspirin and related drugs.
	• None, unless test(s) abnormal; then, manage on the basis of the nature of the underlying problem once diagnosis has been established by the physician.

• Identification of patients to include the following:
  • History
  • Examination findings
  • Screening tests—PFA-100, platelet count
• Referral and consultation with hematologist
• Correction of underlying problem or replacement therapy before surgery
• Local measures to control blood loss—Splint, gelfoam, thrombin, etc.
• Prophylactic antibiotics may be considered in surgical cases to prevent postoperative infection.
• Additional steroids should be used for patients being treated with steroids, if indicated (see section on adrenal insufficiency).
• Aspirin, aspirin-containing compounds, and NSAIDs are not to be used; acetaminophen (Tylenol) with or without codeine may be used.
	• In general dental procedures can be performed if the platelet count is 30,000/mm^3 or higher.
	• Extractions and minor surgery can be performed if the platelet count is 50,000/mm^3 or higher.
	• Major oral surgery can be performed if the platelet count is 80,000/mm^3 to 100,000/mm^3 or higher.
	• Platelet transfusion will be needed for patients with platelet counts below the above values.
	• Patients with severe neutropenia (500/mm^3 or less) may require antibiotics for certain surgical procedures.
	• In children with primary thrombocytopenia, many will respond to steroids with platelet levels increasing to levels allowing dental procedures to be performed.

• Identification of patients should include the following:
  • History
  • Clinical findings
  • Screening test, bleeding time (not reliable)
• Consultation with the hematologist should be obtained.
• Local measures should be used to control blood loss. Splints, gelfoam, Oxycel, and surgical thrombin (see Table 25-5).
• Prevention of allergy is causative, and the antigen is identified.
	• Surgical procedures must be avoided in these patients unless the underlying problem has been corrected, or the patient has been prepared for surgery by the hematologist, and the dentist is prepared to control excessive loss of blood through local measures; splints, thrombin, microfibrillar collagen, gelfoam, Oxycel, Amicar (see Table 25-5).

Dental Management: A Summary—cont'd

Potential Problems Related to Dental Care	Oral Manifestations

CONGENITAL DISORDERS OF COAGULATION (HEMOPHILIA)
Chapter 25

1. Excessive bleeding following dental procedures
2. HIV-, HBV-, and HCV—infected patients are potentially infectious (see Appendix B)

- Spontaneous bleeding
- Prolonged bleeding after dental procedures that injure soft tissue or bone
- Hematomas
- Oral lesions associated with HIV infection in patients who receive infected replacement products (most occurred before 1986)

Prevention of Problems	**Treatment Planning Modifications**

Prevention of Problems

- Identification of patients includes the following:
  - History—Bleeding problems in relatives, excessive bleeding following trauma or surgery
  - Examination findings:
    1. Ecchymoses
    2. Hemarthrosis
    3. Dissecting hematomas
  - Screening tests—Prothrombin time (normal), activated partial thromboplastin time (prolonged), thrombin time (normal), platelet count (normal), PFA-100 (normal)
- Consultation and referral should be provided for diagnosis and treatment and for preparation before dental procedures are performed.
- Replacement options include the following:
  - Cryoprecipitate (used rarely)
  - Fresh frozen plasma (used rarely)
  - Factor VIII concentrates, including:
    1. Heat-treated concentrate
    2. Purified factor VIII
    3. Recombinant factor VIII
    4. Porcine factor VIII
- Mild and moderate factor VIII deficiency, consider using:
  1. 1-desamino-8-D-arginine vasopressin (oral or nasal)
  2. Epsilon aminocaproic acid (Amicar) rinse or orally
  3. Tranexamic acid (Cyklokapron); not available in the United States
  4. Factor VIII replacement for some cases
  5. Often treated on an outpatient basis.
- For severe factor VIII deficiency, alleviate by such measures as:
  - Agents used above for mild to moderate deficiency
  - Higher dose(s) of factor VIII
- Patients who are low responders:
  - Agents used for mild to moderate deficiency
  - Very high dose(s) of factor VIII
- Patients who are high responders:
  - No elective surgery
  - Agents used for mild to moderate deficiency
  - High doses of porcine factor VIII concentrate
  - Nonactivated prothrombin/complex concentrate
  - Activated prothrombin/complex concentrate
  - Plasmapheresis
  - Factor VIIA
  - Steroids
  - In rare cases plasmapheresis
- Treatment is provided on an outpatient basis in accordance with results of the consultation (mild to moderate deficiency, no inhibitors).
- Local measures (splints, thrombin, microfibrillar collagen, etc.) are used for control of bleeding (see Table 25-5).
- Aspirin, aspirin-containing compounds, and NSAIDs should be avoided.

Treatment Planning Modifications

- No dental procedures unless the patient has been prepared on the basis of consultation with the hematologist
- Avoid aspirin, aspirin-containing compounds, and NSAIDs—Use acetaminophen (Tylenol) with or without codeine.

Dental Management: A Summary—cont'd

Potential Problems Related to Dental Care	Oral Manifestations

VON WILLEBRAND'S DISEASE
Chapter 25
1. Excessive bleeding after invasive dental procedures

- Spontaneous bleeding
- Prolonged bleeding following dental procedures that injure soft tissue or bone
- Petechiae
- Hematomas

ACQUIRED DISORDERS OF COAGULATION (LIVER DISEASE, BROAD-SPECTRUM ANTIBIOTICS, MALABSORPTION SYNDROME, BILIARY TRACT OBSTRUCTION, HEPARIN, AND OTHERS)
Chapter 25
1. Excessive bleeding following dental procedures that result in soft tissue or osseous injury

- Excessive bleeding
- Spontaneous bleeding
- Petechiae
- Hematomas

Prevention of Problems	**Treatment Planning Modifications**

- Identification of patients should include:
  - History of bleeding problems in relatives and of excessive bleeding after surgery or trauma, etc.
  - Examination findings to include:
    1. Petechiae
    2. Hematomas
  - Screening laboratory tests—Prolonged platelet function analyzer (PFA)-100; possible prolonged partial thromboplastin time, platelet count may be low
- Consultation and referral should be provided for diagnosis and treatment and preparation before dental procedures.
- Type I and many type II cases require the following:
  - I-desamino-8-D-arginine vasopressin
  - Local measures (see Table 25-5)
  - May be treated on an outpatient basis
- Type III and some type II patients require the following:
  - Fresh frozen plasma
  - Cryoprecipitate
  - Special factor VIII concentrates (retain vWF)
    1. Humate-P
    2. Koate HS
  - Local measures (see Table 25-5)
- Outpatient treatment is possible on the basis of results of consultation.
- Local measures for control of bleeding include:
  - Splints
  - Gelfoam with thrombin
  - Oxycel, Surgicel
- Avoid aspirin, aspirin-containing compounds, and NSAIDs.

- No invasive dental procedures unless the patient has been prepared on the basis of consultation with the hematologist.
- Most dental procedures including complex restorations can be offered to these patients.
- Emphasis on maintaining good oral hygiene, topical fluorides, and diet.
- Acetaminophen with or without codeine may be used for postoperative pain control

- Identification of patients with disorder should include:
  - History
  - Examination findings
  - Screening laboratory tests—Prothrombin time (prolonged), PFA-100 (in liver disease prolonged if hypersplenism present)
- Consultation and referral should be provided.
- Preparation before the dental procedure may include vitamin K injection by the physician and platelet replacement if indicated.
- Local measures are used to control blood loss (see Table 25-5)
- For patients with liver disease, avoid or reduce dosage of drugs metabolized by the liver.
- Do not use aspirin, aspirin-containing compounds, and NSAIDs.

- No dental procedures unless the patient is prepared on the basis of a consultation with the hematologist.

Dental Management: A Summary—cont'd

Potential Problems Related to Dental Care	Oral Manifestations

ANTICOAGULATION WITH COUMARIN DRUGS
Chapter 25

1. Excessive bleeding after dental procedures that result in soft tissue or osseous injury

- Excessive bleeding
- Hematomas
- Petechiae
- In rare cases, spontaneous bleeding

DISSEMINATED INTRAVASCULAR COAGULATION (DIC)
Chapter 25

1. Excessive bleeding after invasive dental procedures; in chronic form of disease, widespread thrombosis may occur

- Spontaneous gingival bleeding
- Petechiae
- Ecchymoses
- Prolonged bleeding following invasive dental procedures

Prevention of Problems	**Treatment Planning Modifications**

- Identify patients who are taking anticoagulants/Coumarin in the following ways:
  - History
  - Screening laboratory test—International normalized ratio (INR), prothrombin time (PT) (prolonged), PFA-100 (may be prolonged)
- Consultation should be obtained regarding level of anticoagulation:
  - If international normalized ratio (INR) is 3.5 or less, most surgical procedures can be performed.
  - Dosage of anticoagulant should be reduced if INR is greater than 3.5 (it takes several days for the INR to fall to the desired level; confirmation should be attained by new tests before surgery is completed).
  - Patients having major oral surgery should be managed on an individual basis; in most cases the INR should be below 3.0 at the time of surgery.
- Amicar rinses, just before surgery and every how for 6-8 hours, will aid in control of bleeding. Local measures should be instituted to control blood loss after surgery (see Table 25-5).

- No dental procedures should be performed unless medical consult has been obtained and level of anticoagulation is at an acceptable range; the procedure may have to be delayed by 2 to 3 days if the dosage of anticoagulant has to be reduced.
- Avoid aspirin or aspirin-containing compounds. Use Tylenol for postoperative pain control.

- Identification of patients includes the following:
  - History—Excessive bleeding after minor trauma; spontaneous bleeding from the nose, gingiva, gastrointestinal tract, or urinary tract; recent infection, burns, shock and acidosis, or autoimmune disease; history of cancer most often associated with chronic form of DIC, in which thrombosis rather than bleeding is usually the major clinical problem
  - Examination findings include the following:
    1. Petechiae
    2. Ecchymoses
    3. Spontaneous gingival bleeding; bleeding from nose, ears, etc.
  - Screening laboratory findings include the following:
    1. Acute DIC—Prothrombin time (prolonged), partial thromboplastin time (prolonged), thrombin time (prolonged), PFA-100 (prolonged), platelet count (decreased)
    2. Chronic DIC—Most tests may be normal, but fibrin-split products are present (positive D-Dimer test).
- Obtain referral and consultation with physician if invasive dental procedures must be performed, and include information on:
  - Acute DIC—Cryoprecipitate, fresh frozen plasma, and platelets
  - Chronic DIC—Anticoagulants such as heparin or vitamin K antagonists
- Aspirin or aspirin-containing products are prohibited.
- Local measures are used to control bleeding (see Table 25-5).
- Antibiotic therapy may be considered to prevent postoperative infection.

- Depending on the cause of DIC, the treatment plan should be altered in the following ways:
  - Cases of acute DIC—No routine dental care until medical evaluation and correction of cause
  - Cases of chronic DIC—No routine dental care until medical evaluation and correction of cause when possible; if prognosis is poor on the basis of underlying cause (advanced cancer), limited dental care is indicated
- Avoid aspirin, aspirin-containing compounds, NSAIDS
- Acetaminophen with or without codeine can be used for postoperative pain

Dental Management: A Summary—cont'd

Potential Problems Related to Dental Care	Oral Manifestations

DISORDERS OF PLATELET RELEASE
Chapter 25
1. Excessive bleeding after invasive dental procedures

- Excessive bleeding may occur following surgery.
- Petechiae, ecchymoses, and hematomas may be found when other platelet or coagulation disorders are present.

PRIMARY FIBRINOGENOLYSIS
Chapter 25
1. Excessive bleeding after invasive dental procedures

- Prolonged bleeding following invasive dental procedures
- Jaundice of mucosa
- Ecchymoses

LOW MOLECULAR WEIGHT HEPARIN THERAPY: ENOXAPARIN (LOVENOX), ARDEPARIN (NORMIFLO), DALTEPARIN (FRAGMIN), NADROPARIN (FRAXIPARINE), REVIPARIN (CLIVARIN), TINZAPARIN (INNOHEP)
Chapter 25
1. Used in patients who have received prosthetic knee or hip replacement; patient takes medication for approximately 2 weeks after getting out of the hospital
2. Complications include the following:
   a. Excessive bleeding
   b. Anemia
   c. Fever
   d. Thrombocytopenia
   e. Peripheral edema

- Gingival bleeding
- Petechiae
- Ecchymoses
- In rare cases, excessive bleeding after dental procedures

Prevention of Problems	Treatment Planning Modifications

- Identification of patient should include the following:
  - History—Recent use of aspirin, indomethacin, phenylbutazone, ibuprofen, or sulfinpyrazone; presence of other platelet or coagulation disorders
  - Examination—Often negative unless signs related to other platelet or coagulation disorders are present
  - Screening laboratory tests—PFA-100 (prolonged), partial thromboplastin time (prolonged)
- Most patients on drugs noted above without an additional platelet or coagulation problem will not bleed excessively following surgery.
- Patients with prolonged PFA-100 and/or partial thromboplastin time should be referred for evaluation prior to performance of any surgical procedures.
- Elective surgery can be performed after withdrawal of drug for at least 3 days and management of other platelet or coagulation disorders by appropriate means.

- Usually, no modifications are indicated for patients who have no other platelet or coagulation disorders.

- Identification of patients should include the following:
  - History—Liver disease, cancer of lung, cancer of prostate, and heatstroke may cause this condition.
  - Examination findings to consider:
    1. Jaundice
    2. Spider angiomas
    3. Ecchymoses
    4. Hematomas
  - Screening laboratory tests
    1. Platelet count (often normal)
    2. Prothrombin time (prolonged)
    3. PFA-100 (usually normal)
    4. Partial thromboplastin time (prolonged)
    5. Thrombin time (prolonged)
- Consultation and referral prior to any invasive dental procedure; epsilon-aminocaproic acid therapy will inhibit plasmin and plasmin activators.

- Patients with advanced cancer should have treatment limited to emergency dental procedures and preventive measures; complex dental restorations in general are not indicated; in other patients, once preparation to avoid excessive bleeding has occurred (epsilon-aminocaproic acid), most dental treatment can be rendered.

- Delay procedure until patient is off the medication.
- Have physician stop medication and perform surgery the next day; once hemostasis is obtained, have the physician resume medication.
- Perform surgery, and manage any excessive bleeding through local means (preferred if excessive bleeding is not anticipated).

- Usually none needed

Dental Management: A Summary—cont'd

Potential Problems Related to Dental Care	Oral Manifestations

ANTIPLATELET DRUG THERAPY: ASPIRIN, ASPIRIN PLUS DIPYRIDAMOLE (AGGRENOX), IBUPROFEN (ADVIL, MOTRIN)

Chapter 25

1. Used for prevention of initial or recurrent myocardial infarction and stroke prevention
2. Complications include:
   a. Excessive bleeding
   b. Gastrointestinal bleeding
   c. Tinnitus
   d. Bronchospasm

- Gingival bleeding
- Petechiae
- Ecchymoses
- In rare cases, excessive bleeding following dental procedures

FIBRINOGEN RECEPTOR THERAPY (GLYCOPROTEIN [GP] IIB/IIIA INHIBITORS: CLOPIDOGREL [PLAVIX], TICLOPIDINE [TICLID])

Chapter 25

1. Used for prevention of recurrent myocardial infarction and stroke
2. Complications include:
   a. Excessive bleeding
   b. Gastrointestinal bleeding
   c. Neutropenia
   d. Thrombocytopenia

- Gingival bleeding
- Petechiae
- Ecchymoses
- In rare cases, excessive bleeding following dental procedures
- Adverse reactions increase risk for infection (neutropenia) and bleeding (thrombocytopenia).

RADIATION-TREATED PATIENTS (RADIATION TO HEAD AND NECK)

Chapter 26

1. Patients treated by radiation tend to develop the following problems during and just after completion of therapy:
   a. Mucositis
   b. Xerostomia
   c. Loss of taste
   d. Constricture of muscles (trismus)
   e. Secondary infections—Viral, bacterial, fungal (candidiasis)
   f. Tooth sensitivity
2. Chronic problems caused by radiation therapy include the following:
   a. Xerostomia
   b. Cervical caries
   c. Osteonecrosis
   d. Muscle trismus
   e. Tooth sensitivity
   f. Loss of taste

- Mucositis
- Candidiasis
- Xerostomia
- Loss of taste
- Trismus
- Sensitivity of teeth
- Cervical caries
- Osteonecrosis

Prevention of Problems

- Before starting chemotherapy, the dentist should:
- Eliminate gross infection in the following areas:
  - Periapical
  - Periodontal
  - Soft tissue
- Treat advanced carious lesions.
- Tooth edges are smooth and not sharp.
- Remove appliances.
- Provide oral hygiene instructions.
- Ensure that in children and young adults, the following occur:
  - Mobile primary teeth are removed.
  - Gingival operculum is removed.
  - Adequate time is allowed for healing before induction.
- During chemotherapy, the dentist should:
  - Consult with oncologist prior to any invasive dental procedures.
  - Perform the following if invasive procedures are required:
    1. Consider antibiotic prophylaxis if granulocyte count is less than 2000/mm^3 or absolute neutrophil count is less than 500/mm^3.
    2. Consider platelet replacement if platelet count is less than 50,000/mm^3.
  - Perform culture and antibiotic sensitivity testing of exudate from areas of infection.
  - Control spontaneous bleeding with gauze, periodontal packing, and soft mouth guard.
  - Use topical fluoride for caries control.
  - Apply chlorhexidine rinses for plaque and candidiasis control (see Appendix C).
  - Provide symptomatic relief of mucositis and xerostomia (see Appendix C).
  - Be aware of and take precautions for bisphosphonate-induced osteonecrosis.
  - If severe anemia is present, avoid general anesthesia.
  - Consider modifying home care instructions on the basis of oral status, reduce or stop flossing and brushing if excessive bleeding or tissue irritation results; damp gauze can be used to wipe the gingiva and teeth; solution of water and baking soda can be used to rinse the mouth to clean ulcerated tissues.
  - Minimize food aversion during chemotherapy—Fast before treatment (4 hours), eat novel nonimportant food just before treatment, and avoid nutritionally important foods during posttreatment nausea.
- Following completion of chemotherapy:
  - Monitor patient until all adverse effects of therapy have cleared.
  - Place patient on dental recall program.
  - Antibiotic prophylaxis is not indicated for these patients on the basis of available evidence; however, need should be decided on an individual patient basis following medical consultation.
  - Be aware of and take precautions for bisphosphonate-induced osteonecrosis.

Treatment Planning Modifications

- Perform only emergency dental treatment during chemotherapy.
- On the basis of the prognosis of underlying disease, consider limiting dental treatment to only immediate care needs for patients who are being treated in a palliative sense; however, children and adults who are being treated for leukemia may have a very good prognosis, and any indicated dental treatment may be performed; also, many patients with lymphoma may have a good prognosis.

Dental Management: A Summary—cont'd

Potential Problems Related to Dental Care	Oral Manifestations
SEIZURE DISORDER (Epilepsy)	
Chapter 27	
1. Occurrence of generalized tonic-clonic seizure in dental office	• Gingival overgrowth caused by phenytoin (Dilantin)
2. Drug-induced leukopenia and thrombocytopenia (phenytoin, carbamazepine, valproic acid)	• Traumatic oral injuries
3. Drug-induced gingival overgrowth that affects periodontal health.	• Drug-induced erythema multiforme
STROKE	
Chapter 27	
1. Dental treatment could precipitate or coincide with a stroke.	• May have unilateral atrophy and one-sided neglect
2. Bleeding is caused by drug therapy used to prevent clots.	
PARKINSON'S DISEASE	
Chapter 27	
1. Patient may be unable to perform oral hygiene procedures.	• Excess salivation and drooling
2. Patient may have a tremor or may be unable to cooperate during dental treatment.	• Muscle rigidity and repetitive muscle movements contribute to poor oral hygiene
	• Antiparkisonian drugs may cause xerostomia, nausea, and tardive dyskinesia

Prevention of Problems

- Identify epileptic patient by history, including:
  - Type of seizure
  - Age at time of onset
  - Cause of seizures
  - Medications
  - Regularity of physician visits
  - Degree of control
  - Frequency of seizures, last seizure
  - Precipitating factors
  - History of seizure-related injuries
- Well controlled—Normal care provided
- Poorly controlled—Consultation with physician; medication change may be required
- Awareness of adverse effects of anticonvulsants
- Patients taking valproic acid—perform PFA-100 test; avoid aspirin and NSAIDs
- Avoid propoxyphene and erythromycin in patients taking carbamazepine
- Seizure managed with the use of a ligated mouth prop at beginning of the appointment

- Identify stroke-prone patient from history (hypertension, congestive heart failure, diabetes, transient ischemic attacks, age >75 years, etc.).
- Reduce patient's risk factors for stroke (smoking, elevated cholesterol, hypertension).
- For past history of stroke:
  - For current transient ischemic attacks—No elective care
  - Delay elective care for 6 months.
  - Drug considerations include the following:
    1. Aspirin and dipyridamole—Order pretreatment PFA-100; if grossly abnormal, consult with physician.
    2. Warfarin (Coumadin)—Order INR; should be 3.5 or less before invasive procedures are performed.
  - Schedule short, morning appointments.
  - Monitor blood pressure.
  - Use minimal amount of vasoconstrictor in local anesthetic.
  - Advoid epinephrine-containing retraction cord.

- Provide frequent dental recall and specialized toothbrushes (e.g., Collis curve toothbrush, mechanical brushes) to maintain adequate oral hygiene.
- Salivary substitutes and topical fluoride are beneficial.
- Personal care providers should be educated about their role in assisting and maintaining the oral hygiene of these patients (also applies to stroke victims).

Treatment Planning Modifications

- Maintenance of optimal oral hygiene
- Surgical reduction of gingival hyperplasia, if indicated
- Replacement of missing teeth with fixed prosthesis as opposed to removable
- Metal prosthodontic devices used instead of porcelain when possible
- Protect patient during a seizure, manage airway, and discontinue treatment afterward.

- Consider periodic panoramic film to assess carotid patency.
- Plan is dependent on physical impairment.
- All restorations should be made easily cleansable— Porcelain occlusals should be prevented.
- Modified oral hygiene aids may be needed.

- Sedation may be required to overcome muscle rigidity.

Dental Management: A Summary—cont'd	
Potential Problems Related to Dental Care	**Oral Manifestations**

ANXIETY
Chapter 28
1. Extreme apprehension
2. Avoidance of dental care
3. Elevation of blood pressure
4. Precipitation of arrhythmia
5. Adverse effects and drug interactions with agents used in dentistry

- Usually none
- Oral lesions associated with adverse effects of medications

EATING DISORDER: ANOREXIA NERVOSA AND BULIMIA NERVOSA
Chapter 28
1. Patients with anorexia are in a state of self-starvation (severe weight loss) and may be subject to hypotension, bradycardia, severe arrhythmia, and death.
2. Bulimic patients are at risk for serum electrolyte disturbances, esophageal or gastric rupture, cardiac arrhythmia, and death.
3. Patients with bulimia may induce vomiting through the use of physical means (finger in throat) or the use of ipecac (may cause myopathy or cardiomyopathy); laxatives and diuretics also are used by bulimics to purge.
4. Some patients may show signs and symptoms of both anorexia and bulimia.

- In bulimia, the following may be noted:
  - Dental erosion of the lingual surfaces of teeth (usually maxillary teeth)
  - Patients with poor oral hygiene may have increased risk for caries and periodontal disease.
  - Extensive dental caries (associated with diet—Lots of carbohydrates)
  - Tooth sensitivity to thermal changes
- In anorexia, the following may be noted:
  - Usually, no oral findings
  - Patients with poor oral hygiene may have increased risk for caries and periodontal disease.

DELIRIUM
Chapter 28
1. Consists of an acute disorder of attention and cognitive function
2. Inability of patient to interact and follow directions
3. A number of problems associated with underlying cause(s):
   a. Cardiovascular—Heart failure, myocardial infarction, embolism
   b. Endocrine—Diabetes, hypothyroidism, hyperthyroidism
   c. Gastrointestinal disorders—Hepatic failure, pancreatitis
   d. Intoxications—Alcohol, prescribed drugs, illicit drugs
   e. Neurologic disorders—Tumors, meningitis, encephalitis
4. Refer to specific disorder in summary table for details.

- No specific oral manifestations
- Oral manifestations may be found on the basis of cause(s) of delirium in specific patient.
- Refer to specific disorder in summary table for listing of oral changes.

Prevention of Problems	Treatment Planning Modifications

- Behavioral aspects—The dentist should do the following:
  - Provide effective communication (be open and honest).
  - Explain what is going to happen.
  - Make procedures as "pain free" as possible.
  - Encourage patient to ask questions at any time.
  - Use relaxation techniques such as hypnosis, music, etc.
- Pharmacologic aspects—The dentist should provide the following as indicated:
  - Oral sedation—Alprazolam, diazepam, triazolam
  - Inhalation sedation—Nitrous oxide
  - Intramuscular sedation—Midazolam, meperidine
  - Intravenous sedation—Diazepam, midazolam, fentanyl
  - Analgesics for pain control—Salicylates, NSAIDs, acetaminophen, codeine, oxycodone, fentanyl
  - Adjunctive medications—Antidepressants, muscle relaxants, steroids, anticonvulsants, antibiotics

- Postpone complex dental procedures until patient is more comfortable in the dental environment.
- It is important to develop trust and establish communication with patients with posttraumatic stress disorder.
- May need to refer for diagnosis and treatment patients with panic attack or phobic symptoms related to dentistry.

- Patients with severe weight loss and no history of cancer or other illnesses, and who are hypotensive should be referred for medical evaluation and management.
- Attempts should be made to ascertain the cause of dental erosion involving the lingual surfaces of teeth. Consider referral for medical evaluation
- For the patient to act on these recommendations, the dentist must point out to the patient the serious complications of anorexia (hypotension, severe arrhythmia, and death) and of bulimia (gastric and esophageal tears, cardiac arrhythmia, and death).

- Avoid elective dental procedures until the patient is stable from a cardiac standpoint.
- In general, for both anorexic and bulimic patients, the emphasis should be on oral hygiene maintenance and noncomplex repair, until significant improvement of their condition has occurred from a medical standpoint.
- Complex restorative procedures should be avoided in bulimic patients until the purging has been corrected. However, crowns may have to be placed to stabilize a tooth or to protect it from thermal symptoms in patients who are still actively purging.

- Elective dental treatment is usually not indicated for patients with delirium.
- Once the cause(s) of delirium has been identified and managed, the patient can receive routine dental treatment.
- Management will have to involve underlying causes such as heart failure, myocardial infarction, diabetes, etc.

- Emergency dental treatment during the acute phase of delirium
- Once the acute phase has been managed, the treatment plan may be influenced by the underlying disorder(s).

Dental Management: A Summary—cont'd	
Potential Problems Related to Dental Care	**Oral Manifestations**

ANXIOLYTIC DRUGS (anxiety control): Benzodiazepines, Librium (chlordiazepoxide), Valium (diazepam), Ativan (Lorazepam), Serax (oxazepam), Xanax (alprazolam)
Chapter 28

1. Drug adverse effects include the following:
   a. Daytime sedation
   b. Aggressive behavior
   c. Amnesia (older adults)
2. Drug interactions (central nervous system [CNS] depression):
   a. Antipsychotic agents
   b. Antidepressants
   c. Narcotics
   d. Sedative agents
   e. Antihistamines
   f. H2 histamine receptor blockers

- Usually no significant oral findings

DEPRESSION AND BIPOLAR DISORDERS
Chapter 29

1. Little or no interest in oral health
2. Factors increasing risk of suicide:
   a. Age—Adolescent and elderly at greatest risk
   b. Chronic illness, alcoholism, drug abuse, and depression
   c. Recent diagnosis of serious condition such as AIDS and cancer
   d. Previous suicide attempts
   e. Recent psychiatric hospitalization
   f. Loss of a loved one
   g. Living alone or little social contact
3. Taking medications that have significant adverse effects and that may interact with agents used by the dentist

- Depression—Poor oral hygiene and xerostomia associated with agents used to treat depression increase risks for caries and periodontal disease; facial pain syndromes and glossodynia
- Manic disorder—Injury to soft tissue and abrasion of teeth from overflossing and overbrushing
- Oral lesions associated with the adverse effects of medications used to treat depression and mania

SCHIZOPHRENIA
Chapter 29

1. Patient may be difficult to communicate with and uncooperative during dental care.
2. Significant drug adverse effects are common, and agents used by the dentist may interact with medications the patient is taking [see section below regarding antipsychotic (neuroleptic) drugs].

- Usually none
- Oral lesions may be self-inflicted or may develop as adverse effects of medications used to treat the patient (see section below on antipsychotic drugs).

ANTIDEPRESSANT DRUGS
Chapter 29

1. Drug adverse effects include the following:
   a. Xerostomia
   b. Hypotension
   c. Orthostatic hypotension
   d. Arrhythmia
   e. Nausea and vomiting
   f. Leukopenia, anemia, thrombocytopenia, agranulocytosis
   g. Mania, seizures
   h. Hypertension (venlafaxine)
   i. Loss of libido
2. Drug interactions (**CAVEAT:** Do not mix the different classes of antidepressant drugs.) include the following:
   a. Epinephrine
      - Hypertensive crisis
      - Myocardial infarction

- Usually, no significant oral findings associated with medications, unless the following drug adverse effects are present:
  - Xerostomia—Increases risk for caries, periodontal disease, and mucositis
  - Leukopenia—Infection
  - Thrombocytopenia—Bleeding

Prevention of Problems | **Treatment Planning Modifications**

- Look up specific medication the patient is taking to explore significant adverse effects associated with the drug and possible drug interactions with agents used in dentistry.

- Identify by medical and drug histories that patients are taking these medications.
- Refer to physician when significant drug adverse effects occur.
- Avoid the use of NSAIDs and erythromycin, or use in reduced dosage in patients on lithium.
- Avoid the use of erythromycin, or use in reduced dosage in patients who are taking valproic acid or carbamazepine.

- No special modifications are needed in the treatment plan of patients whose condition is well controlled with lithium or anticonvulsant drugs.
- Patients with signs or symptoms of lithium toxicity should be referred to their physician for evaluation.
- NSAIDs should be avoided or used in reduced dosage for pain control in patients who are taking lithium, to prevent lithium toxicity.
- Erythromycin should not be used for infection because lithium toxicity may result.
- Patients on the anticonvulsant drugs (valproic acid or carbamazepine) who develop oral ulcerations, infection, or bleeding should be referred for medical evaluation.
- Erythromycin should be avoided in patients who are taking valproic acid or carbamazepine.

- Identification of patients:
  - Obtain history of mental disorder (patient may be taking antipsychotic medication).
  - Ask patients to list all drugs that they are taking.
  - Identify patients with recent onset of adverse effects.
- Refer patients with significant adverse effects.
- Obtain consultation with patient's physician to confirm current status and medications.
- Reduce dosage or avoid:
  - Epinephrine
  - Sedatives, hypnotics, opioids, antihistamines
  - Erythromycin should also be avoided.

- Local anesthetic guidelines include the following:
  - Use without vasoconstrictor for most dental procedures, if possible.
  - For surgical or complex restorative procedures, epinephrine is the vasoconstrictor of choice:
    1. Use 1:100,000 concentration.
    2. Aspirate before injecting.
    3. In general, do not use more than two cartridges.
- Do not use topical epinephrine to control bleeding or in the retraction cord.
- On the basis of patient needs and wants, any dental procedure can be provided.
- Provide treatment to deal with xerostomia, if present (see Appendix C).
- Patients with tardive dyskinesia may be difficult to manage; if this adverse effect has just started, refer patients to their physician for evaluation and possible change in medication.

Dental Management: A Summary—cont'd

Potential Problems Related to Dental Care	Oral Manifestations

SOMATOFORM DISORDERS—CONVERSION DISORDER, PAIN DISORDER, FACTITIOUS DISORDER AND OTHERS

Chapter 29

1. Somatoform disorders:
   a. Isolated symptoms with no physical cause that do not conform to known anatomic pathways
   b. Psychological factors involved in the origin
   c. May serve as a defense to reduce anxiety (primary gain)
   d. Secondary gain reason for not working, attention from family
   e. When these patients are followed over time, in 10% to 50%, a physical disease process will become apparent.
2. Factitious disorders:
   a. Intentional production of physical or psychological signs
   b. Voluntary production of symptoms without external incentive
   c. More often seen in men and health care workers

- Examples of oral symptoms that can be related to somatoform disorders:
  - Burning tongue
  - Painful tongue
  - Numbness of soft tissues
  - Tingling sensations in oral tissues
  - Pain in the facial region
- Oral examples of factitious injuries:
  - Self-extraction of teeth
  - Picking gingival with fingernails
  - Nail file gingival injury
  - Chemical burning of the lips and oral mucosa
  - Thermal burning of lips and oral mucosa

SUBSTANCE ABUSE

Chapter 29

1. Dilated pupils, elevated blood pressure, and cardiac arrhythmias may indicate recent use.
2. Extreme anxiety and aggressive behavior may also be related to recent use.
3. Stroke is a risk during the "high" with these drugs.
4. Myocardial ischemia may occur, and myocardial infarction is a risk.
5. Cardiac arrhythmias may be severe and life threatening.
6. Vasopressors such as epinephrine and levonordefrin can precipitate hypertensive crisis, myocardial infarction, arrhythmia, or stroke.
7. Patients with rash caused by cocaine use may react to ester-type local anesthetics.
8. If the drugs are abused by injecting the agents, a risk of infection with hepatitis B virus, hepatitis C virus, and HIV is present (examine for needle tracks on the arm, if exposed).
9. Xerostomia, particularly with methamphetamine
10. Gastrointestinal regurgitation, bulimia, or vomiting in methamphetamine abusers
11. High intake of refined carbohydrates and sucrose

- Oral hygiene is usually better in cocaine and amphetamine abusers.
- Oral findings in methamphetamine abusers may include the following (when severe, these are referred to as "Meth" mouths):
  - Xerostomia
  - Rampant caries
  - Periodontal disease
  - Enamel erosion
- Other oral findings, particularly in methamphetamine abusers, include the following:
  - Bad taste
  - Bruxism
  - Muscle trismus (jaw clenching)

OLDER ADULTS: FALLS

Chapter 30

1. Falling in dental reception area or in operatory
2. Patient who is taking multiple medications may be at increased risk for falls.
3. Patient with dementia, musculoskeletal disorders, proprioceptive dysfunction, or peripheral neuropathy also may be at increased risk for falls.

- Tooth fracture
- Jaw fracture
- Soft tissue lacerations
- Bleeding

Prevention of Problems	Treatment Planning Modifications

- Refer patients found to have psychological disorders for diagnosis and management, but stay involved from a dental standpoint.
- Discuss with patient the possible causes of symptoms, and rule out underlying systemic conditions that could account for the symptoms.
- Continue to examine for signs and symptoms that may be related to an underlying systemic or local condition.

- Do not perform dental treatment on the basis of the patient's symptoms, unless a dental cause can be established.
- Maintain good oral hygiene and dental repair for the patient, but avoid complex dental procedures until somatoform symptoms have been managed.
- Patients may insist that the dentist do something to "cure" the symptom such as extraction or endodontic therapy; the dentist must avoid this.
- A diagnosis of an oral somatoform disorder should not be made until after a thorough search over time has failed to uncover pathologic findings that could explain the symptoms.
- Antidepressants and pain medication may be used to comfort the patient.

- Do not treat patients who are "high" on these drugs or who show evidence of recent use.
- Wait at least 6 hours after administration of these drugs before providing any dental treatment. (Cocaine and methamphetamine effects take several hours to wear off.)
- Avoid ester-type local anesthetics in patients who have skin rash associated with cocaine use.
- Use standard infection control procedures for all patients.
- Avoid additive drugs for pain control.
- Monitor blood pressure and pulse rate in these patients during dental procedures when possible.

- Patients found to be abusing these drugs should be encouraged to seek professional help in dealing with their addiction; the dentist can attempt to make an appointment for this purpose.
- If the patient presents with evidence of being "high" on these drugs, the dental appointment must be rescheduled for another day.
- Emphasis should be placed on attempting to improve the patient's oral hygiene, which in the case of many methamphetamine abusers will be difficult at best until they deal with their addiction.
- Cocaine and methamphetamine abusers may be using other drugs and may try to get prescriptions for strong pain medications or may steal prescription pads or drugs.
- Care must be taken in selection of medications used for sedation and pain control.
- Tolerance may be present for sedative drugs and local anesthetics, requiring increased dosage; this increases the risk for toxic adverse effects.
- The dentist should not prescribe addictive substances for these patients.
- Anxiety control can be provided with the use of propranolol, if needed.
- Pain control can be attained with the use of acetaminophen or NSAIDs.

- Move chair position slowly, aid patient in getting out of the chair, and support patient for the first few steps.
- For patients taking multiple medications whose balance is impaired, the dentist may consult with the physician to see whether the number of medications can be reduced, or if the dosage of any of the drugs can be reduced.
- Plan for short appointments in late morning or early afternoon.
- May have to transfer patient from wheelchair to the dental chair, and then back to the wheelchair

- Usually none

Dental Management: A Summary—cont'd

Potential Problems Related to Dental Care	Oral Manifestations

OLDER ADULTS: POOR EYESIGHT, LOSS OF HEARING, DEMENTIA, OR ADVANCED ILLNESS

Chapter 30

1. Difficult to fill out health and dental history questionnaire
2. Unable to hear questions or directions
3. Difficult to follow directions during dental treatment
4. Unable to sit still during appointments
5. Difficult or impossible to render effective oral hygiene procedures

- Usually none
- Periodontal disease, recurrent caries, mucositis, xerostomia, fractured restorations, infections, and others, depending on the medical illness and medications used to treat it

OLDER ADULTS: ORGAN SYSTEM CHANGES WITH AGING

Chapter 30

1. General—Increase in fat, decrease in body water:
   a. Less initial and more prolonged effects of fat-soluble drugs
   b. Increased effects of water-soluble drugs
2. Immune system—Decrease in numbers of lymphocytes and their response to antigens with increased risk for infection and cancer
3. Musculoskeletal—Decrease in muscle mass and bone density with increased risk for fracture of bones and functional impairment
4. Cardiovascular—Increased risk for syncope, heart failure, and heart block
5. Respiratory—Decreased lung elasticity and increased chest wall stiffness, decreasing ventilation and perfusion and causing a decrease in pO_2. May lead to breathing difficulty during some dental procedures
6. Endocrine—Blood glucose increase in response to illness, decreased vitamin D absorption and activation, and decreased T_4 clearance. These changes can complicate diabetes, increase risk for osteomalacia and fracture, or cause thyroid dysfunction. Decrease in testosterone levels in males leads to impotency.
7. Nervous system—Brain atrophy, decrease in catechol synthesis, dopaminergic synthesis, and righting reflexes. These changes may result in benign forgetfulness, stiffer gait, and increased body sway (increasing the risk for falls). Impaired thermal regulation, leading to hypothermia
8. Gastrointestinal—Loss of liver mass, which can affect drugs metabolized in the liver; decreased gastric acidity, which can cause decreased absorption of calcium; decreased colonic motility, which can cause constipation

- Usually none, but in severe cases, increased risk of fracture of mandible and loss of masticatory muscle function. Increased incidence of periodontal disease
- Oral complications associated with diabetes, hypothyroidism, liver failure, dementia, and major depression—See respective topics in summary table.

Prevention of Problems	Treatment Planning Modifications

- Have spouse of relative help fill out questionnaire, or take history orally.
- Speak slowly and directly to the patient while increasing the volume of your voice.
- Use nonverbal communication to show what you want the patient to do (pressure on side of head—turn head).
- Schedule short appointments, usually in the late morning.
- Instruct spouse, relative, or care provider on how to provide basic oral hygiene procedures for the patient.

- None for patients with loss of hearing and poor eyesight who are in good general health.
- Patients with significant dementia or advanced illness are usually not candidates for complex dental procedures; emphasis should be placed on maintaining oral and dental health as well as possible.

- Use lowest effective dosage for fat-soluble drugs and decreased dosage for water-soluble drugs—"Start low and go slow."
- Avoid oral infection; if it occurs, treat by local and systemic means, and search for early signs of oral cancer.
- Avoid falls in the dental office by escorting older adults to the operatory, changing dental chair position slowly, supporting patients when they are getting out of the dental chair, and escorting patients back to the reception area.
- Do not treat patients with symptomatic congestive heart failure (refer for medical treatment); avoid epinephrine in patients with severe arrhythmia, unstable angina, or recent myocardial infarction.
- Do not use rubber dam or give bilateral mandibular blocks in patients with breathing difficulties. Avoid drugs that will suppress the respiratory center, such as barbiturates and narcotics. Treat patient in upright chair position if breathing difficulty is severe.
- Refer patients with signs and symptoms of diabetes mellitus and hypothyroidism or history of fracture. Patients should ask their physician about possible vitamin D and calcium supplementation.
- Refer to rule out dementia, depression, and Parkinson's disease; take actions listed above to avoid falls in the dental office.
- Avoid or use lowest effective dose of drugs metabolized by the liver.

- Minimize the use of medications, and use in the lowest possible dosage.
- Changes in body composition seen with advancing age do not affect the selection of treatment options for the older adult, except in cases with extreme loss of muscle mass and bone density. In these cases, certain complex oral surgical procedures or periodontal surgery may not be indicated.
- Complex or elective dental procedures are not indicated for patients with heart failure that is nonresponsive to medical treatment.
- Avoid complex dental procedures for patients with severe pulmonary dysfunction.
- Changes seen in the endocrine system in general will not affect the selection of dental treatment procedures, unless complicated by diabetes, hypothyroidism, or renal failure.
- Changes seen in the nervous system in general will not affect the selection of dental procedures, unless complicated by dementia, major depression, Parkinson's disease, or severe peripheral neuropathy.
- Changes seen in the gastrointestinal tract usually will not affect the selection of dental procedures, unless complicated by severe liver disease, cancer, or complications of cancer therapy.

PART ONE

Evaluation and Risk Assessment

Physical Evaluation and Risk Assessment

CHAPTER

1

Dentistry today is far different from what was practiced only a decade or two ago, not only in techniques and procedures but also in the types of patients seen. As a result of advances in medical science, people are living longer and are receiving medical treatment for disorders that were fatal only a few years ago. For example, damaged heart valves are surgically replaced, occluded coronary arteries are surgically bypassed or opened by balloons, organs are transplanted, severe hypertension is medically controlled, and many types of malignancies and immune deficiencies are managed or controlled.

Because of the increasing numbers of dental patients, especially among the elderly, who may have chronic medical problems, the dentist must remain knowledgeable about patients' medical conditions. Many chronic disorders or their treatments necessitate alterations in the provision of dental treatment. Failure to make appropriate treatment modifications may result in serious consequences.

The key to successful dental management of a medically compromised patient is a thorough evaluation and assessment of risk to determine whether a patient can safely tolerate a planned procedure. Risk assessment involves the evaluation of at least four components: (1) the nature, severity, and stability of the patient's medical condition; (2) the functional capacity of the patient; (3) the emotional status of the patient; and (4) the type and magnitude of the planned procedure (invasive or noninvasive). All factors must be carefully weighed for each patient.

Risk assessment cannot be approached as a cookbook exercise. Each situation requires thoughtful consideration to determine whether the benefits of having dental treatment outweigh the potential risks to the patient (Figure 1-1). For example, a patient may have symptomatic heart failure, but the risk is minimal if the planned dental procedure is limited to taking radiographs

(noninvasive) and the patient is not anxious or fearful. Conversely, in the same patient, the risk may be significant if the planned procedure is a full mouth extraction (invasive), and the patient is very anxious. Therefore, the dentist must carefully weigh the physical and emotional state of the patient against the invasiveness and trauma of the planned procedure. The cornerstone of patient evaluation and risk assessment is the medical history, supplemented by physical examination, laboratory tests, and medical consultation.

MEDICAL HISTORY

A medical history must be taken on every patient who is to receive dental treatment. The two basic techniques used to obtain a medical history consist of the interview (medical model), in which the interviewer questions the patient and then records the patient's verbal responses on a blank sheet, and a printed questionnaire that the patient fills out. The latter is most commonly used in dental practice and is very convenient and efficient. However, it is important that follow-up questioning occur so the dentist can gain additional information about the positive responses given by the patient, to determine their significance and effects on dental treatment.

Many questionnaires are commercially available today, including one from the American Dental Association. Dentists also may develop or modify questionnaires to meet the specific needs of their individual practice. Although medical history questionnaires differ in organization and content detail, most attempt to elicit information about the same basic medical problems. The following information provides a brief rationale for why certain questions are asked and the significance of positive responses. Detailed information concerning most of these medical problems is found in the specific subsequent chapters.

Risk Assessment

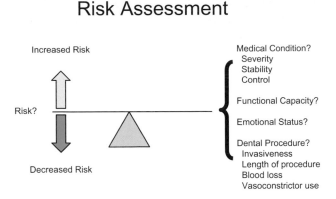

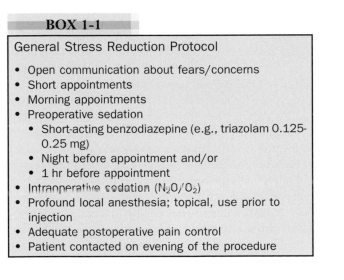

Figure 1-1. Risk assessment by weighing of key determining factors.

BOX 1-1

General Stress Reduction Protocol

- Open communication about fears/concerns
- Short appointments
- Morning appointments
- Preoperative sedation
  - Short-acting benzodiazepine (e.g., triazolam 0.125-0.25 mg)
  - Night before appointment and/or
  - 1 hr before appointment
- Intraoperative sedation (N_2O/O_2)
- Profound local anesthesia; topical, use prior to injection
- Adequate postoperative pain control
- Patient contacted on evening of the procedure

Cardiovascular Disease

Patients with various forms of cardiovascular disease are especially vulnerable to physical or emotional challenges that may be encountered during dental treatment.

Heart Failure. Heart failure is not a disease per se but rather a clinical syndrome complex that results from an underlying cardiovascular problem such as coronary heart disease or hypertension. The underlying cause of heart failure should be identified and its potential significance assessed. Patients with untreated or symptomatic heart failure are at increased risk for myocardial infarction (MI), arrhythmias, acute heart failure, or sudden death and generally are not candidates for elective dental treatment. Chair position may influence a patient's ability to breathe, with some patients unable to tolerate a supine position. Vasoconstrictors should be avoided, if possible, in patients taking digitalis glycosides (digoxin) because the combination can precipitate arrhythmias (see Chapter 6). Stress reduction measures also may be advisable (Box 1-1).

Heart Attack. A history of a heart attack (MI) within the very recent past may preclude elective dental care because during the immediate postinfarction period,

patients have increased risk for reinfarctions, arrhythmias, and heart failure. Patients may be taking medications such as antianginals, anticoagulants, adrenergic blocking agents, calcium channel blockers, antiarrhythmic agents, and digitalis. Some of these drugs may alter the dental management of patients because of potential interactions with vasoconstrictors in the local anesthetic, drug adverse effects, or other considerations (see Chapter 4). Stress and anxiety reduction measures may be advisable (see Box 1-1).

Angina Pectoris. Brief substernal pain resulting from myocardial ischemia, commonly provoked by physical activity or emotional stress, is a common and significant symptom of coronary heart disease. Patients with angina, especially unstable angina, are at increased risk for arrhythmias, MI, and sudden death. A variety of vasoactive medications, such as nitroglycerin, beta-blocking agents, and calcium channel blockers, are used to treat angina. Vasoconstrictors should be used cautiously. Patients with unstable or progressive angina are not candidates for elective dental care (see Chapter 4). Stress and anxiety reduction measures may be appropriate (see Box 1-1).

High Blood Pressure. Patients with hypertension (blood pressure greater than 140/90 mm Hg) should be identified by history and confirmed by blood pressure measurement. Patients with a history of hypertension should be asked if they are taking or are supposed to be taking antihypertensive medication. Failure to take medication is often the cause of elevated blood pressure in a patient who reports being under treatment for high blood pressure. Current blood pressure readings and any symptoms that may be associated with hypertension, such as visual changes, dizziness, and headaches, should be noted. Some antihypertensive medications, such as the nonselective beta-blocking agents, may require cautious use of vasoconstrictors (see Chapter 3). Stress and anxiety reduction measures also may be appropriate (see Box 1-1). Elective dental care should be deferred for patients with blood pressure ≥180/110.

Heart Murmur. A heart murmur is caused by turbulence of blood flow that produces vibratory sounds during the beating of the heart. Turbulence may result from physiologic (normal) factors or pathologic abnormalities of the heart valves, vessels, or both. The presence of a heart murmur may be of significance in the dental patient in that it may be an indication of underlying heart disease. The primary goal is to determine the nature of the heart murmur; consultation with the patient's physician is often necessary to make this determination. Previously, the American Heart Association recommended antibiotic prophylaxis for many patients with heart murmurs caused by valvular disease (e.g., mitral valve prolapse, rheumatic heart disease); however, on the basis of accumulated scientific evidence, recently revised guidelines have omitted this recommendation. If a murmur is due to a specific cardiac condition (e.g., previous endocarditis, prosthetic heart valve, complex congenital cyanotic heart disease), the American Heart Association recommends antibiotic prophylaxis for most dental procedures (see Chapter 2).

Mitral Valve Prolapse. In mitral valve prolapse (MVP), the leaflets of the mitral valve are thickened and redundant and "prolapse" or balloon back into the left atrium during systole. As a result, tight closure of the leaflets may not occur, which may result in leakage or backflow of blood (regurgitation) from the ventricle to the atrium. Previously, the American Heart Association recommended that patients with MVP with regurgitation receive antibiotic prophylaxis for invasive dental procedures to prevent bacterial endocarditis. However, on the basis of accumulated scientific evidence, recently revised guidelines have omitted this recommendation (see Chapter 2).

Rheumatic Fever. Rheumatic fever is an autoimmune condition that can follow an upper respiratory beta-hemolytic streptococcal infection and may lead to damage of the heart valves (rheumatic heart disease). Previously, the American Heart Association recommended that patients with rheumatic heart disease receive antibiotic prophylaxis for invasive dental procedures to prevent bacterial endocarditis. However, on the basis of accumulated scientific evidence, recently revised guidelines have omitted this recommendation (see Chapter 2).

Congenital Heart Disease. Patients with some forms of severe congenital heart disease are at risk for bacterial endocarditis. The American Heart Association recommends that patients with certain conditions be given prophylactic antibiotics for most dental procedures. These are primarily patients with complex cyanotic heart disease (e.g., tetralogy of Fallot), and those who have had surgical repair of a congenital defect with residual leak. These patients have a high risk for bacterial endocarditis and require antibiotic prophylaxis for certain dental procedures. Patients with most other types of congenital heart disease are not considered at risk for bacterial endocarditis from invasive dental procedures, and the American Heart Association does not recommend antibiotic prophylaxis (see Chapter 2).

Artificial Heart Valve. Patients with prosthetic heart valves are considered to be at high risk for bacterial endocarditis with significant morbidity and mortality. As a result, the American Heart Association recommends that all patients with a prosthetic heart valve be given prophylactic antibiotics for most dental procedures (see Chapter 2).

Arrhythmias. Arrhythmias are frequently related to heart failure or ischemic heart disease. Stress, anxiety, physical activity, drugs, and hypoxia are some elements that can precipitate arrhythmias. Vasoconstrictors in local anesthetics should be used cautiously in patients prone to arrhythmias because they can be precipitated by excessive quantities or inadvertent intravascular injections. Stress reduction measures may be appropriate (see Box 1-1). Some of these patients take antiarrhythmic drugs; certain agents may cause oral manifestations or other effects. Patients with arrhythmias may require a pacemaker or a defibrillator to artificially regulate or pace heart rhythm. These patients do not require antibiotic prophylaxis. Caution is advised with the use of certain electrical equipment (e.g., electrosurgery, ultrasonic scalers) in these patients because of the possibility of electromagnetic interference with the function of the pacemaker (see Chapter 5). Elective dental care is not recommended in patients with serious, symptomatic arrhythmias.

Coronary Artery Bypass Graft/Angioplasty/Stent. These procedures are performed on patients with coronary heart disease to restore patency to blocked coronary arteries. One of the most common forms of cardiac surgery performed today is the coronary artery bypass graft (CABG). The grafted artery bypasses the occluded portion of the artery. These patients do not require antibiotic prophylaxis. Another method of restoring patency is via a balloon catheter, which is inserted into the partially blocked artery; the balloon is then inflated, which compresses the atheromatous plaque against the vessel wall. A metallic mesh stent is often placed to aid in the maintenance of patency. Patients who have had balloon angioplasty with or without placement of a stent do not require prophylaxis (see Chapter 4).

Hematologic Disorders

Hemophilia or Inherited Bleeding Disorder. Patients with an inherited bleeding disorder such as hemophilia A or B, or von Willebrand's disease, are at risk for severe bleeding following any type of dental treatment that causes bleeding, including scaling and root planing. These patients must be identified and managed in cooperation with their physician or hematologist. Patients with severe factor deficiency may require factor replacement prior to invasive treatment, as well as aggressive postoperative measures to maintain hemostasis (see Chapter 25).

Blood Transfusion. Patients with a history of blood transfusions are of concern from at least two aspects. The underlying problem that necessitated a blood transfusion, such as an inherited or acquired bleeding disorder, must be identified, and alterations in the delivery of dental treatment may have to be made. Patients may also be at risk to be carriers of hepatitis B or C or may become infected with the human immunodeficiency virus (HIV) and must be identified. Laboratory screening or medical consultation may be appropriate to determine the status of liver function, and, as always, standard infection control procedures are mandatory (see Chapters 11 and 25).

Anemia. A significant reduction in the oxygen-carrying capacity of the red blood cells may result from an underlying pathologic process such as acute or chronic blood loss, decreased production of red blood cells, or hemolysis. Some anemias, such as glucose-6-phosphate dehydrogenase deficiency and sickle cell disease, require dental management modifications. Oral lesions, infections, delayed wound healing, and adverse responses to hypoxia are all potential matters of concern (see Chapter 23).

Leukemia. Depending on the type of leukemia, status of the disease, and type of treatment, some patients may have bleeding problems or delayed healing, or may be prone to infection. Gingival enlargement can be a sign of leukemia. Some adverse effects can result from the use of chemotherapeutic agents and may require dental management modifications (see Chapter 24).

Taking a "Blood Thinner"/Tendency to Bleed Longer Than Normal. A potentially significant problem is that of a patient with a history of abnormal bleeding, or who is taking an anticoagulant or an antiplatelet drug. This is of obvious concern, especially if surgical treatment is planned. Information about an episode of unexplained bleeding should be attained and evaluated. Many reports of abnormal bleeding are more apparent than real; additional questioning or screening laboratory tests may allow the dentist to make this distinction. Patients taking anticoagulant or antiplatelet medication will need to be evaluated to determine the risk for postoperative bleeding. Many patients can be treated without alteration of their medications; however, laboratory testing may be required to make this determination (see Chapter 25).

Neurologic Disorders

Stroke. Disorders that predispose to stroke such as hypertension and diabetes must be identified so that appropriate management alterations can be made. Elective dental care should be avoided in the immediate post-stroke period because of increased risk for subsequent strokes. Vasoconstrictors should be used cautiously. Anticoagulant medications and antiplatelet medications can result in prolonged bleeding. Stress and anxiety reduction measures may be necessary (see Box 1-1). Some stroke victims may have hemiplegia, speech impairment, and other physical handicaps. Occasionally, calcified atheromatous plaques may be seen in the carotid arteries on panoramic films; these may be a risk factor for stroke (see Chapter 27).

Epilepsy, Seizures, and Convulsions. A history of epilepsy or grand mal seizures should be identified, and the degree of seizure control that is needed should be determined. Specific triggers of seizures (e.g., odors, bright lights) should be identified and avoided. Some medications used to control seizures may affect dental treatment because of drug actions or adverse effects. For example,

gingival hyperplasia is a well-known adverse effect of diphenylhydantoin. Patients may discontinue use of anti-seizure medication without their doctors' knowledge and thus may be susceptible to seizures during dental treatment. Therefore, verification of patients' adherence to their medication schedule is important (see Chapter 27).

Behavioral Disorders/Psychiatric Treatment. Patients with a history of a behavioral disorder or psychiatric illness and the nature of the problem need to be identified. This information may help explain patients' behavioral patterns, problems, or complaints such as unexplainable or unusual conditions or pain. Additionally, some psychiatric drugs have the potential to interact adversely with vasoconstrictors in local anesthetics and produce oral adverse effects such as xerostomia. Other adverse effects such as dystonia, akathisia, or tardive dyskinesia may complicate dental treatment. Some patients may be excessively anxious or apprehensive about dental treatment, requiring stress-reduction measures (see Box 1-1 and Chapters 28 and 29).

Gastrointestinal Diseases

Stomach or Intestinal Ulcers, Gastritis, and Colitis. Patients with gastric or intestinal disease should not be given drugs that are directly irritating to the gastrointestinal tract, such as aspirin or nonsteroidal antiinflammatory drugs. Patients with colitis or a history of colitis may not be able to take certain antibiotics. Many antibiotics can cause a particularly severe form of colitis (i.e., pseudomembranous colitis). Some drugs used to treat ulcers may cause dry mouth (see Chapter 12).

Hepatitis, Liver Disease, Jaundice, and Cirrhosis. Patients who have a history of viral hepatitis are of concern in dentistry because they may be asymptomatic carriers of the disease and can transmit it unknowingly to dental personnel or other patients. Of the several types of viral hepatitis, only B, C, and D have carrier stages. Fortunately, laboratory tests are available to identify these patients. Patients also may have chronic hepatitis (B or C) or cirrhosis and, as a result, have impaired liver function. This may result in prolonged bleeding and an impaired ability to efficiently metabolize certain drugs, including local anesthetics and analgesics (see Chapter 11).

Respiratory Tract Disease

Allergies or Hives. Patients may be allergic to some drugs or materials used in dentistry. Common drug allergens include antibiotics and analgesics. Latex allergy also is common. For these patients, alternative materials such as vinyl or powderless gloves can be used to prevent an adverse reaction. True allergy to amide local anesthetics is uncommon. Dentists should procure an allergic history by specifically asking patients how they react to a particular substance. This will help to establish a diagnosis of allergy rather than an intolerance or adverse effect that has been incorrectly identified as an allergy. Symptoms consistent with allergy include itching, urticaria (hives), rash, swelling, wheezing, angioedema, runny nose, and tearing eyes. Isolated symptoms such as nausea, vomiting, palpitations, and fainting are generally not of an allergic origin but rather are manifestations of drug intolerance, adverse effects, or psychogenic reactions (see Chapter 20).

Asthma. The type of asthma should be identified, as should the drugs taken and any precipitating factors or triggers. Stress may be a precipitating factor and should be minimized when possible (see Box 1-1). It is often helpful to ask whether the patient has had to go to an emergency room for acute treatment of asthma, as this would indicate more significant disease. If patients use an inhaler for acute attacks, they should bring it to the dental appointment with them (see Chapter 7).

Emphysema/Chronic Bronchitis. Patients with chronic pulmonary diseases such as emphysema and chronic bronchitis must be identified. The use of medications or procedures that might further depress respiratory function or dry or irritate the airway should be avoided. Chair position may be a factor; some patients may not be able to tolerate a supine position. Use of a rubber dam may not be tolerated because of a choking or smothering feeling. The use of high-flow oxygen may be contraindicated in patients with severe disease because it can decrease the respiratory drive (see Chapter 7).

Tuberculosis. Patients with a history of tuberculosis (TB) must be identified, and information about the treatment received must be sought. A positive skin test means that the person has been infected with TB but not that the patient has active disease. A diagnosis of active TB is made by chest x-ray, sputum culture, and clinical examination. Positive skin testers who do not have active disease and are not infectious may be placed on chemophylaxis (e.g., isoniazid) to prevent the development of active disease. Medical treatment for active disease includes the use of multiple medications taken for several months. A history of follow-up medical evaluation is important to detect reactivation of the disease or inadequate treatment. Patients with AIDS have a high incidence of tuberculosis; this relationship should be explored (see Chapter 9).

Sleep Apnea/Snoring. Patients with obstructive sleep apnea are at increased risk for hypertension, MI, and stroke and should receive treatment for the disorder. Patients who report snoring, daytime sleepiness, and breathing cessation during sleep should be referred to a sleep physician specialist for evaluation. Obesity and large neck circumference are common risk factors for the disease. The gold standard for treatment is positive airway pressure; however, many patients cannot tolerate this.

Other treatment options include oral appliances and various forms of upper airway surgery (see Chapter 10).

Musculoskeletal Disease

Arthritis. Many types of arthritis have been identified; the most common of these are osteoarthritis and rheumatoid arthritis. Patients with arthritis may be taking a variety of medications that could influence dental care. Nonsteroidal antiinflammatory drugs, aspirin, corticosteroids, and cytotoxic and immunosuppressive drugs are examples. Tendencies for bleeding and infection should be considered. Chair position may be a factor in physical comfort. Patients may have problems with manual dexterity and oral hygiene. In addition, patients with arthritis may have involvement of the temporomandibular joints (see Chapter 21).

Prosthetic Joints. Some patients with artificial joints are at increased risk for infection of the prosthesis and may need to be provided with prophylactic antibiotics prior to any dental treatment that is likely to produce bacteremia. Patients included in this category are those with rheumatoid arthritis, type 1 diabetes, recent joint placement, and hemophilia, as well as those who are immunosuppressed. Patients with joint prostheses who do not fall into these risk categories do not require antibiotic prophylaxis (see Chapter 21).

Endocrine Disease

Diabetes. Patients with diabetes mellitus must be identified in terms of type of diabetes diagnosed and control measures taken. Patients with type 1 diabetes require insulin, whereas type 2 diabetes is usually controlled through diet and/or oral hypoglycemic agents. Some patients with type 2 diabetes may also require insulin. Those with type 1 diabetes have a greater number of complications and are of greater concern regarding management than are those with type 2 diabetes. Symptoms suggestive of diabetes include excessive thirst and hunger, frequent urination, weight loss, and frequent infections. Complications include blindness, hypertension, and kidney failure, which may affect dental management. Patients with diabetes typically do not handle infection very well and may have exaggerated periodontal disease. Patients who take insulin are potentially prone to episodes of hypoglycemia in the dental office if meals are skipped (see Chapter 15).

Thyroid Disease. Patients with uncontrolled hyperthyroidism are potentially hypersensitive to stress and sympathomimetics; the use of vasoconstrictors is generally contraindicated. In rare cases, infection or surgery can initiate a thyroid crisis—a serious medical emergency. Patients with uncontrolled hyperthyroidism may be easily upset emotionally and intolerant of heat, and they may exhibit tremors. Exophthalmos may be present. Patients with known hypothyroidism usually are taking a thyroid supplement and generally pose minimal concern as long as the thyroid hormone level is not excessive (see Chapter 17).

Genitourinary Tract Disease

Kidney Failure. Patients with end-stage kidney failure or a kidney transplant must be identified. The potential for abnormal drug metabolism, immunosuppressive drug therapy, bleeding problems, hepatitis, infection, high blood pressure, and heart failure must be considered in management (see Chapter 13). Patients on hemodialysis do not require antibiotic prophylaxis.

Sexually Transmitted Diseases. A variety of sexually transmitted diseases such as syphilis, gonorrhea, human immunodeficiency virus (HIV) infection, and AIDS can have manifestations in the oral cavity because of oral/genital contact or hematogenous dissemination in the blood. The dentist may be the first to identify these conditions. In addition, some sexually transmitted diseases, including HIV, hepatitis B and C, and syphilis, can be transmitted to the dentist via direct contact with oral lesions or infectious blood (see Chapters 11, 14, and 19).

Other Conditions

Tobacco and Alcohol Use. The use of tobacco products is a risk factor that is associated with cancer, cardiovascular disease, pulmonary disease, and periodontal disease. Patients who use tobacco products should be asked whether they would like to quit and should be encouraged to do so (see Chapter 8). Excessive use of alcohol is a risk factor for malignancy and heart disease and may cause liver disease (see Chapter 11).

Drug Addiction and Substance Abuse. Patients who have a history of intravenous drug use are at risk for infectious diseases such as hepatitis B or C, AIDS, and infective endocarditis. Narcotic and sedative medications should be prescribed cautiously, if at all, for these patients, because of the risk of triggering a relapse. Vasoconstrictors should be avoided in active cocaine or methamphetamine users because they may precipitate arrhythmias or severe hypertension (see Chapter 29).

Tumor and Cancer. Patients who have had cancer are at risk for recurrent disease; additional lesions and recurrences are always possible. Also, chemotherapeutic agents and radiation therapy may pose significant management considerations, possibly resulting in infection, gingival bleeding, oral ulcerations, mucositis, and impaired healing after invasive dental treatment. Patients with a history of intravenous bisphosphonate therapy for metastatic bone disease are at risk for osteonecrosis of the jaw and should be managed cautiously (see Chapter 26).

Radiation Therapy and Chemotherapy. Patients with previous radiation treatment of the head, neck, or jaw must be carefully evaluated because radiation can permanently destroy the blood supply to the jaws, leading to osteoradionecrosis after extraction or trauma. Radiation treatment in the head and neck can destroy the salivary glands, resulting in decreased saliva, increased dental caries, and mucositis. Fibrosis of masticatory muscles also may occur. Chemotherapy can produce many undesirable adverse effects, most commonly a severe mucositis (see Chapter 26).

Steroids. Corticosteroid usage is important because it can result in adrenal insufficiency and may render a patient unable to adequately respond to the stress of a dental procedure such as an extraction or periodontal surgery. Cortisone and prednisone are examples of steroids that are used in the treatment of many diseases. Generally, however, most routine dental procedures, other than extraction or other surgery, do not require supplemental steroids (see Chapter 16).

Operations or Hospitalizations. A history of hospitalizations can provide a record of past serious illnesses that may have current significance. For example, a patient may have been hospitalized for cardiac catheterization for ischemic heart disease. Another example is a patient who is hospitalized for hepatitis C. Both types of patients may not have received medical follow-up care for these problems, and the response to this question is the only indication of there past problems. Information about hospitalizations should include diagnosis, treatment, and complications. If a patient has undergone any operation, the reason for the procedure and any untoward events associated with it such as anesthetic emergencies, unusual postoperative bleeding, infection, and drug allergy should be addressed.

Pregnancy. Women who are or may be pregnant may need special consideration in the taking of radiographs, administration of drugs, or timing of dental treatment (see Chapter 18).

Current Physician

As part of the medical history, information should be sought regarding the patient's physician, why the patient is under medical care, diagnoses, and treatment received. If the reason for seeing a physician was the need for a routine physical examination only, the patient should be asked whether any abnormalities were discovered and the date of the examination. The name, address, and phone number of the patient's physician should be recorded for future reference. The patient who does not have a physician may need a more cautious approach than the patient who sees one regularly. This is especially true for the patient who has not seen a physician in several years because of the possibility of undiagnosed problems. The response to this question also may provide insight into the priorities that a person assigns to health care.

Drugs, Medicines, or Pills

All of the drugs, medicines, or pills that a patient is taking, or is supposed to be taking, should be identified and investigated for actions, adverse effects, and potential drug interactions. The interviewer should stress drugs, medicines, or pills "of any kind" when questioning patients because frequently patients do not list over-the-counter drugs or herbal medicines. The dentist should have a reliable, up-to-date, comprehensive source for drug information, which may be available in print format or through an on-line database. Medication listings may provide the only clues to a patient's medical disorder. The patient may not have believed that mentioning a problem was important or may just have omitted the information inadvertently. However, the patient may report taking medication typically prescribed for a disease. An example might be a patient with hypertension who fails to report a history of that problem but lists medications used to treat hypertension such as an angiotensin-converting enzyme (ACE) inhibitor or a diuretic.

Functional Capacity

In addition to asking patients about specific diagnoses, it is also important to ask some screening questions regarding the ability of the patient to engage in normal physical activity (functional capacity). A patient's ability to perform common daily tasks can be expressed in metabolic equivalent levels (METs), which provide a way of quantifying a patient's general physical status. A MET is a unit of oxygen consumption; 1 MET equals 3.5 mL/kg/min at rest.[1] It has been shown that the risk for occurrence of a serious perioperative event (e.g., MI, heart failure) is increased in patients who are unable to meet a 4 MET demand during normal daily activity.[2] Daily activities requiring 4 METs include level walking at 4 miles/hr or climbing a flight of stairs. Activities requiring >10 METs include swimming and singles tennis. An exercise capacity of 13 METs indicates excellent physical conditioning.[1] Thus a patient who reports an inability to walk up a flight of stairs without shortness of breath, fatigue, or chest pain may be at increased risk for problems during dental treatment.

PHYSICAL EXAMINATION

In addition to a medical history, the dental patient should be afforded the benefits of a simple, abbreviated physical examination. This should include assessment of general appearance, measurement of vital signs, and an examination of the head and neck.

General Appearance

Much can be learned about a patient and the state of health from a purposeful but tactful visual inspection. Careful observation can lead to awareness and recognition of abnormal or unusual features or medical conditions that may exist and may influence the provision of dental care. This survey consists of an assessment of the general appearance of the patient and inspection of exposed body areas, including skin, nails, face, eyes, nose,

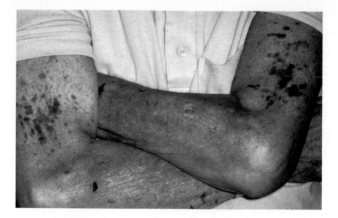

Figure 1-2. Petechiae and ecchymosis in a patient that may signal a bleeding disorder. (Courtesy Robert Henry, DMD, Lexington, Ky.)

ears, and neck. Each visually accessible area may demonstrate peculiarities that can signal underlying systemic disease or abnormalities.

The outward appearance of a patient can give an indication of the patient's general state of health and well-being. Examples of possible trouble include a wasted, cachectic appearance; a lethargic demeanor; ill-kept, dirty clothing and hair; body odors; a staggering or halting gait; extreme thinness or obesity; bent posture; and difficulty breathing. The dentist should remain sensitive to breath odors such as acetone associated with diabetes, ammonia associated with renal failure, putrefaction of pulmonary infections, and alcohol, possibly associated with alcohol abuse or subsequent liver disease.

Skin and Nails. The skin is the largest organ of the body; usually, large areas are exposed and accessible for inspection. Changes in the skin and nails frequently are associated with systemic disease. For example, cyanosis can indicate cardiac or pulmonary insufficiency, yellowing may be caused by liver disease, pigmentation may be associated with hormonal abnormalities, and petechiae or ecchymoses can be signs of a blood dyscrasia or a bleeding disorder (Figure 1-2). Alterations in the fingernails, such as clubbing (seen in cardiopulmonary insufficiency) (Figure 1-3), white nails (seen in cirrhosis), yellowing of nails (from malignancy), and splinter hemorrhages (from bacterial endocarditis), are usually caused by chronic disorders. The dorsal surfaces of the hands are common sites for actinic keratosis and basal cell carcinomas, as are the bridge of the nose, infraorbital regions, and the ears (Figure 1-4).

Face. The shape and symmetry of the face are abnormal in a variety of syndromes and conditions. Well-known examples include the coarse features of acromegaly (Figure 1-5); the pale, edematous features of nephrotic syndrome; moon facies in Cushing's syndrome (Figure 1-6); the dull, puffy facies of myxedema; and the unilateral paralysis of Bell's palsy (Figure 1-7).

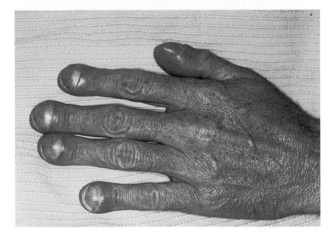

Figure 1-3. Clubbing of digits and nails may be associated with cardiopulmonary insufficiency.

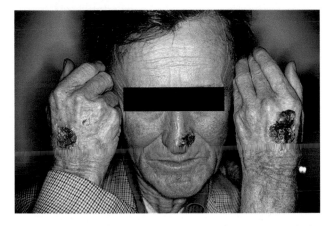

Figure 1-4. Basal cell carcinomas of the dorsum of the hands and the bridge of the nose.

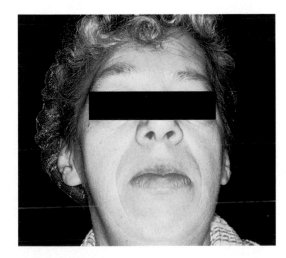

Figure 1-5. Patient with acromegaly.

Eyes and Nose. The eyes can be sensitive indicators of systemic disease and therefore should be closely inspected. Patients who wear glasses should be requested to remove them during examination of the head and neck. Hyperthyroidism may produce a characteristic lid retraction,

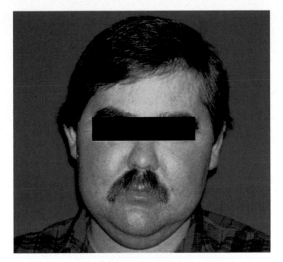

Figure 1-6. Patient with cushingoid facies after several weeks of prednisone administration. (From Bricker SL, Langlais RP, Miller CS. Oral Diagnosis, Oral Medicine, and Treatment Planning, ed 2. Hamilton, Ontario, BC Decker, 2002.)

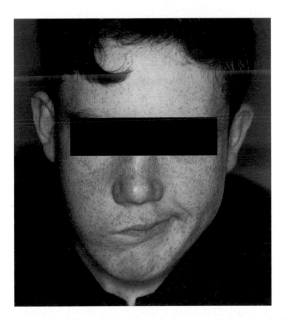

Figure 1-7. Unilateral facial paralysis in a patient with Bell's palsy.

resulting in a wide-eyed stare (Figure 1-8). Xanthomas of the eyelids are frequently associated with hypercholesterolemia (Figure 1-9), as is arcus senilis in an older individual. Scleral yellowing may be caused by hepatitis. Reddened conjunctiva can result from the sicca syndrome, allergy, or iritis.

Ears. The ears should be inspected for gouty tophi in the helix or antihelix. An earlobe crease occurs more frequently in patients with coronary artery disease than in those without this condition.[3] Malignant or premalignant lesions (i.e., skin cancer) may be found on and around the ears (Figure 1-10).

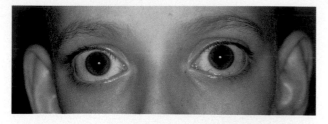

Figure 1-8. Lid retraction from hyperthyroidism.

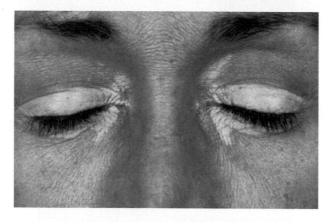

Figure 1-9. Xanthomas of the eyelids may signal hypercholesterolemia.

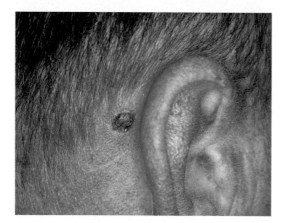

Figure 1-10. Malignant melanoma posterior to the ear.

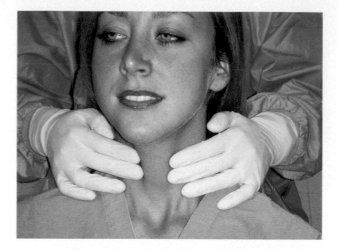

Figure 1-11. Bimanual palpation of the anterior neck.

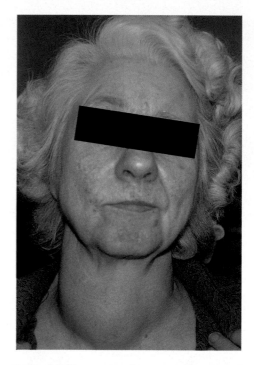

Figure 1-12. Midline neck enlargement from a goiter.

Neck. The neck should be inspected for enlargement and asymmetry. Bilateral palpation of the thyroid gland should be performed (Figure 1-11). Depending on location and consistency, enlargement may be caused by goiter (Figure 1-12), infection, cysts (Figure 1-13), enlarged lymph nodes (Figure 1-14), or vascular deformities.

Vital Signs

Vital signs consist of blood pressure, pulse, respiratory rate, temperature, height, and weight. In the dental setting, usually only blood pressure and pulse are measured directly. Respiratory rate is determined by observation. Temperature is usually measured only when indicated, such as with infection or suspected systemic involvement. Height and weight can be determined by questioning of the patient. Abnormal readings may require further investigation or referral.

The benefits of vital sign measurement during an initial examination are twofold. First, the establishment of baseline normal values ensures a standard of comparison in the event that an emergency occurs during treatment. If an emergency occurs, knowledge of a patient's normal values is essential in determination of the severity of the problem. For example, if a patient lost consciousness unexpectedly and blood pressure was 90/50 mm Hg, the concern would be entirely different for a patient whose blood pressure was normally 110/65 mm Hg than for the patient with hypertension whose blood pressure was normally 180/110 mm Hg. In the second example, the patient may well be in a shock state.

Prevention of Problems

- Identify patients at greatest risk for adverse outcomes of IE, including patients with:
  - Prosthetic cardiac valves
  - A history of previous IE
  - Certain types of congenital heart disease (i.e., unrepaired cyanotic congenital heart disease, including patients with palliative shunts and conduits, completely repaired congenital heart disease for the first 6 months after a procedure, or repaired congenital heart disease with residual defect)
  - Cardiac transplantation recipients who develop cardiac valvulopathy
- Prescribe antibiotic prophylaxis for only those patients above who undergo dental procedures that involve manipulation of gingival tissue or the periapical region of teeth or perforation of the oral mucosa.
- If prophylaxis is required for an adult, take a single dose 30 minutes to 1 hour before the procedure:
  - Standard (oral amoxicillin, 2 g)
  - Allergic to penicillin (oral *cephalexin 2 g, oral clindamycin 600 mg, or azithromycin or clarithromycin 500 mg) *NOTE: Cephalexin should not be used in individuals with a history of anaphylaxis, angioedema, or urticaria with penicillins.
  - Unable to take oral medications (intravenous [IV] or intramuscular [IM] ampicillin, cefazolin, or ceftriaxone)
  - Allergic to penicillin and unable to take oral medications (IV or IM clindamycin phosphate, cefazolin, or ceftriaxone)
- See Chapter 25 for management of potential bleeding problems associated with anticoagulant therapy.

- Detection of patients with hypertension and referral to a physician if poorly controlled or uncontrolled. Defer elective dental treatment if blood pressure (BP) is ≥180/110.
- For patients who are being treated for hypertension, consider the following:
  - Take measures to reduce stress and anxiety.
  - Provide oral sedative premedication and/or inhalation sedation.
  - Provide local anesthesia of excellent quality.
  - For patients who are taking a nonselective beta blocker, limit epinephrine to ≤2 cartridges of 1:100,000 epinephrine.
  - Avoid epinephrine-containing gingival retraction cord.
  - For patients with upper level stage 2 hypertension, consider intraoperative monitoring of BP, and terminate appointment if BP reaches 180/110.
  - Make slow changes in chair position to avoid orthostatic hypotension.

Treatment Planning Modifications

- Encourage the maintenance of optimal oral hygiene in all patients at increased risk for IE.
- Provide antibiotic prophylaxis for only those patients with the highest risk for adverse outcomes of IE.
- Provide antibiotic prophylaxis for all dental procedures, except
  - Routine anesthetic injections
  - Taking of radiographs
  - Placement of removable prosthodontic or orthodontic appliances
  - Adjustment of orthodontic appliances
  - Shedding of deciduous teeth or bleeding from trauma to the lips or oral mucosa.
- For patients selected for prophylaxis, perform as much dental treatment as possible during each coverage period.
- A second antibiotic dose may be indicated if the appointment lasts longer than 4 to 6 hours, or if multiple appointments occur on the same day.
- For multiple appointments, allow at least 9 days between treatment sessions so that penicillin-resistant organisms can clear from the oral flora. If treatment becomes necessary before 9 days have passed, select one of the alternative antibiotics for prophylaxis.
- For patients with prosthetic heart valves who are taking anticoagulants, the dosage may have to be reduced on the basis of international normalized ratio (INR) level and the degree of invasiveness of the planned procedure (see Chapter 25).

- For patients with BP <180/110, and no evidence of target organ involvement, any treatment may be provided
- For patients with BP ≥ 180/110, defer elective dental care
- For patients with target organ involvement, refer to appropriate chapter for management recommendations

---

Dental Management: A Summary—cont'd

Potential Problems Related to Dental Care	**Oral Manifestations**

ANGINA PECTORIS

Chapter 4

1. The stress and anxiety of a dental visit could precipitate an anginal attack, myocardial infarction, or sudden death.
2. For patients who are taking a nonselective beta blocker, the use of excessive amounts of epinephrine could precipitate a dangerous elevation in blood pressure.
3. Patients who are taking aspirin or other platelet aggregation inhibitor may experience excessive bleeding.
4. Questions may arise as to the necessity of antibiotic prophylaxis for patients with a history of coronary artery bypass graft, balloon angioplasty, or stent.

- No oral complications are due to angina; however, adverse effects such as dry mouth, taste changes, and oral lesions may be drug related.
- Excessive bleeding may occur as the result of the use of aspirin or other platelet aggregation inhibitors.

PREVIOUS MYOCARDIAL INFARCTION

Chapter 4

1. The stress and anxiety of a dental visit could precipitate an anginal attack, myocardial infarction, or sudden death in the office.
2. Patients may have some degree of heart failure.
3. If the patient has a pacemaker, some dental equipment may potentially cause electromagnetic interference.
4. In patients who are taking a nonselective beta blocker, excessive amounts of epinephrine may cause a dangerous elevation in blood pressure.
5. Patients who are taking aspirin or another platelet aggregation inhibitor or Coumadin may experience excessive postoperative bleeding.
6. Questions may arise as to the necessity of antibiotic prophylaxis for patients with a history of CABG, balloon angioplasty, or stent.

- No oral complications are due to myocardial infarction; however, adverse effects such as dry mouth, taste changes, and oral lesions may be drug related. Also, bleeding may be excessive because of the use of aspirin, other platelet aggregation inhibitors, or Coumadin.

Prevention of Problems	**Treatment Planning Modifications**

Unstable Angina (major risk)
- Elective dental care should be deferred; if care becomes necessary, it should be provided in consultation with the physician. Management may include establishment of an IV line; sedation; monitoring of electrocardiogram, pulse oximeter, and blood pressure; oxygen; cautious use of vasoconstrictors; and prophylactic nitroglycerin.

Stable Angina (intermediate risk)
- Elective dental care may be provided with the following management considerations:

  - For stress/anxiety reduction: Provide oral sedative premedication and/or inhalation sedation if indicated, assess pretreatment vital signs and availability of nitroglycerin, and limit the quantity of vasoconstrictor used.
  - For patients who are taking a nonselective beta blocker: Limit epinephrine to ≤2 cartridges of 1:100,000 epinephrine.
  - Avoid the use of epinephrine-impregnated gingival retraction cord.
  - Avoid anticholinergics
  - Provide local anesthesia of excellent quality and postoperative pain control.
  - If the patient is taking aspirin or another platelet aggregation inhibitor: Excess bleeding is usually manageable through local measures only; discontinuation of medication is not recommended.
  - Antibiotic prophylaxis is *not* recommended for patients with a history of coronary artery bypass graft (CABG), angioplasty, or stent.

Unstable Angina
- Dental treatment should be limited to urgent care only such as treatment of acute infection, bleeding, or pain.

Stable Angina
- Any indicated dental treatment may be provided if appropriate management issues are considered.

Recent Myocardial Infarction (<1 month) (major risk)
- Elective dental care should be deferred; if care becomes necessary, it should be provided in consultation with the physician.
- Management may include establishment of an IV line; sedation; monitoring of electrocardiogram, pulse oximeter, and blood pressure; oxygen; cautious use of vasoconstrictors; and prophylactic nitroglycerin.

Past Myocardial Infarction (>1 month without symptoms) (intermediate risk)
- Elective dental care may be provided with the following management considerations:
  - For stress/anxiety reduction: Provide oral sedative premedication and/or inhalation sedation if indicated, assess pretreatment vital signs and availability of nitroglycerin, and limit the quantity of vasoconstrictor used.
  - For patients who are taking a nonselective beta blocker: Limit epinephrine to ≤2 cartridges of 1:100,000 epinephrine.
  - Avoid the use of epinephrine-impregnated gingival retraction cord.
  - Avoid anticholinergics
  - Provide local anesthesia of excellent quality and postoperative pain control.

Recent Myocardial Infarction
- Dental treatment should be limited to urgent care only such as treatment of acute infection, bleeding, or pain

Past Myocardial Infarction
- Any indicated dental treatment may be provided taking into consideration appropriate management considerations

Dental Management: A Summary—cont'd

Potential Problems Related to Dental Care	Oral Manifestations

PREVIOUS MYOCARDIAL INFARCTION (cont'd)

ARRHYTHMIAS
Chapter 5

1. The stress and anxiety of dental treatment or excessive amounts of epinephrine may induce life-threatening arrhythmias in susceptible patients.
2. Patients with existing arrhythmia are at increased risk for serious complications such as angina, myocardial infarction, stroke, heart failure, or cardiac arrest.
3. Patients with a pacemaker or a defibrillator are at risk for possible malfunction caused by electromagnetic interference from some dental equipment; some question about the need for prophylactic antibiotics may arise.
4. In patients who are taking a nonselective beta blocker, excessive amounts of epinephrine may cause a dangerous elevation in blood pressure.
5. Patients with atrial fibrillation who are taking Coumadin are at risk for excessive postoperative bleeding.
6. Patients who are taking digoxin are at risk for arrhythmia if epinephrine is used; digoxin toxicity is also a potential problem.

- No oral complications are due to arrhythmia; however, adverse effects such as dry mouth, taste changes, and oral lesions may be drug related.
- Excessive bleeding may occur as the result of use of Coumadin.

HEART FAILURE
Chapter 6

1. Providing dental treatment to a patient with symptomatic or uncontrolled heart failure may result in worsening of symptoms, acute failure, arrhythmia, myocardial infarction, or stroke.

- No oral complications are caused by heart failure; however, adverse effects such as dry mouth, taste changes, and oral lesions may be drug related.
- Digoxin can cause an enhanced gag reflex.

Prevention of Problems	**Treatment Planning Modifications**

Prevention of Problems

- If the patient is taking aspirin or another platelet aggregation inhibitor, excessive bleeding is usually manageable by local measures only; discontinuation of medication is not recommended.
- If the patient has a pacemaker or implanted defibrillator, avoid the use of electrosurgery and ultrasonic scalers; antibiotic prophylaxis is not recommended for these patients.
- If the patient is taking Coumadin, the INR should be 3.5 or less prior to performance of invasive procedures.
- Antibiotic prophylaxis is *not* recommended for patients with a history of CABG, angioplasty, or stent.

- Determine the nature, severity, and appropriate treatment of arrhythmia through history and clinical findings; if unclear, obtain medical consultation to confirm the following:
  - For high-risk arrhythmia (high-grade atrioventricular [AV] block, symptomatic ventricular arrhythmia, supraventricular arrhythmia with uncontrolled ventricular rate):
    1. Elective dental care should be deferred; if care becomes necessary, it should be provided in consultation with the physician.
    2. Management may include establishment of an IV line; sedation; monitoring of electrocardiogram, pulse oximeter, and blood pressure; oxygen; and cautious use of vasoconstrictors.
  - For intermediate- and low-risk arrhythmia (essentially all others):
    1. Elective dental care may be provided with the following management considerations for stress/anxiety reduction: Provide oral sedative premedication and/or inhalation sedation if indicated; assess pretreatment vital signs; avoid excessive use of epiephrine (for patients who are taking a nonselective beta blocker, limit epinephrine to ≤2 cartridges of 1:100,000 epinephrine, avoid the use of epinephrine-impregnated gingival retraction cord, and provide local anesthesia of excellent quality and postoperative pain control)
    2. For patients who are taking Coumadin, the INR should be 3.5 or less prior to any invasive dental procedure; provide local measures for hemostasis.
    3. For patients with a pacemaker or an implanted defibrillator, avoid the use of electrosurgery and ultrasonic scalers; antibiotic prophylaxis is *not* recommended for these patients.
    4. For patients who are taking digoxin, avoid the use of epinephrine because of the increased risk of inducing arrhythmia; be observant for signs of digoxin toxicity (e.g., hypersalivation).

Treatment Planning Modifications

High-Risk Arrhythmias
- Dental treatment should be limited to urgent care only such treatment of acute infection, bleeding, or pain

All Other Arrhythmias
- Any indicated dental treatment may be provided as long as appropriate management issues are considered.

Symptomatic Heart Failure (NYHA Class III or IV)
- Elective dental care should be deferred and medical consultation obtained; if care becomes necessary, it should be provided in consultation with the physician.

Symptomatic Heart Failure (NYHA Class III or IV)
- Dental treatment should be limited to urgent care only such as treatment of acute infection, bleeding, or pain.

Dental Management: A Summary—cont'd

Potential Problems Related to Dental Care	Oral Manifestations

HEART FAILURE (cont'd)

2. Patients with heart failure may have difficulty breathing and may not tolerate a supine chair position.
3. Heart failure is due to an underlying condition such as coronary artery disease or hypertension that may require management considerations.
4. In patients who are taking a nonselective beta blocker, excessive amounts of epinephrine may cause a dangerous elevation in blood pressure.
5. The use of epinephrine in patients who are taking digoxin may cause arrhythmia.

CHRONIC OBSTRUCTIVE PULMONARY DISEASE

Chapter 7

1. Aggravation or worsening of compromised respiratory function

- Leukoplakia, erythroplakia, or squamous cell carcinoma in chronic smokers of tabacco

ASTHMA

Chapter 7

1. Precipitation of an acute asthma attack

- Oral candidiasis is reported with the use of an inhaler without a "spacer," but it occurs rarely.
- Maxillofacial growth is altered when asthma is severe during childhood.

Prevention of Problems	Treatment Planning Modifications

Management may include establishment of an IV line; sedation; monitoring of electrocardiogram, pulse oximeter, and blood pressure; oxygen; cautious use of vasoconstrictors; and possibly, prophylactic nitroglycerin.

Asymptomatic/Mild Heart Failure (NYHA Class I and II and possibly III)
- Elective dental care may be provided with the following management considerations:
  - For stress/anxiety reduction: Provide oral sedative premedication and/or inhalation sedation if indicated, and assess pretreatment vital signs.
  - For patients who are taking a nonselective beta blocker, limit epinephrine to ≤2 cartridges of 1:100,000 epinephrine, avoid the use of epinephrine-impregnated gingival retraction cord, and provide local anesthesia of excellent quality and postoperative pain control.
  - Ensure a comfortable chair position; supine position may not be tolerated.
  - If patient is taking digoxin, avoid the use of epinephrine.
  - Avoid the use of nonsteroidal anti-inflammatory drugs (NSAIDs).

Asymptomatic/Mild Heart Failure (NYHA Class I and II)
- Any necessary dental treatment may be provided.

- Avoid treating if upper respiratory infection is present.
- Use an upright chair position.
- Use of local anesthesia is okay; minimize the use of bilateral mandibular or palatal blocks.
- Do not use a rubber dam in severe disease.
- Use pulse oximetry to monitor oxygen saturation.
- Use of low-flow oxygen is helpful.
- Do not use nitrous oxide–oxygen sedation in cases of severe emphysema.
- Low-dose oral diazepam is acceptable.
- Avoid barbiturates, narcotics, antihistamines, and anticholinergics.
- An additional steroid dose may be needed in patients who are taking systemic steroids for surgical procedures.
- Avoid macrolide antibiotics (erythromycin, clarithromycin) and ciprofloxacin for patients who are taking theophylline.
- Outpatient general anesthesia is contraindicated.

- None

- Identify asthmatic patient by history.
- Determine character of asthma:
  - Type (allergic or nonallergic)
  - Precipitating factors
  - Age at onset
  - Level of control (frequency, severity of attacks [mild, moderate, severe])
  - How usually managed

- None required

Dental Management: A Summary—cont'd

Potential Problems Related to Dental Care	**Oral Manifestations**

ASTHMA (cont'd)

TUBERCULOSIS

Chapter 9

1. Tuberculosis may be contracted by the dental health care worker from an actively infectious patient.
2. Patients and staff may be infected by a dentist who is actively infectious.

- Oral ulceration (rare); tongue most common
- Tuberculous involvement of cervical and submandibular lymph nodes (scrofula)

Prevention of Problems   **Treatment Planning Modifications**

- Medications being taken
- Necessity for past emergency care
- Baseline forced expiratory volume at 1 second (FEV_1) stable (not decreasing)
- Avoid known precipitating factors.
- Consult with physician for severe persistent asthma.
- Reduce the risk of an attack: Have the patient bring medication inhaler to each appointment, and prophylax with an inhaler prior to each appointment for persons with moderate to severe persistent asthma.
- Drugs to avoid:
  - Aspirin-containing medications
  - NSAIDs
  - Narcotics and barbiturates
  - Macrolide antibiotics (e.g., erythromycin), if the patient is taking theophylline
  - Discontinue cimetidine 24 hours before IV sedation in patients who are taking theophylline.
- Sulfite-containing local anesthetic solutions may need to be avoided.
- An additional steroid dose may be needed for surgical procedures in patients who are taking systemic steroids.
- Premedication (nitrous oxide or diazepam) may be needed for anxious patients.
- Provide a stress-free environment.
- Use a pulse oximeter.
- Recognize signs and symptoms of a severe or worsening asthma attack (e.g., difficulty breathing, tachypnea).

CAVEAT: Many patients with infectious disease cannot be identified by history or examination; therefore, all patients should be approached with the use of standard precautions (see Appendix B).
- Patient with active sputum-positive tuberculosis:
  - Consult with physician before treatment.
  - Treatment is limited to emergency care (older than 6 years of age)
  - Treatment is provided in the hospital setting with proper isolation, sterilization, mask, gloves, gown, and ventilation.
  - For patients younger than 6 years of age, treat as a normal (noninfectious) patient after consulting with the physician.
  - For patients producing consistently negative sputum after undergoing at least 2 to 3 weeks of chemotherapy, treat as a normal patient.
- Patients with a past history of tuberculosis:
  - Patients should be approached with caution; obtain good history of disease and its treatment, and conduct appropriate review of systems.
  - Obtain history of adequate treatment, periodic chest radiographs, and examination findings to rule out reactivation.
  - Dental treatment should be postponed if:
    1. Questionable history of adequate treatment
    2. Lack of appropriate medical supervision since recovery
    3. Signs or symptoms of relapse

- None required

Dental Management: A Summary—cont'd	
Potential Problems Related to Dental Care	**Oral Manifestations**

TUBERCULOSIS (cont'd)

OBSTRUCTIVE SLEEP APNEA
Chapter 10

1. Patients with untreated obstructive sleep apnea are at increased risk for hypertension, stroke, arrhythmia, myocardial infarction, and diabetes.

- Large tongue, long soft palate, long uvula, redundant parapharyngeal tissues, large tonsils, retrusive mandible

VIRAL HEPATITIS, TYPES B, C, D, AND E
Chapter 11

1. Hepatitis may be contracted by the dentist from an infectious patient.
2. Patients or staff may be infected by the dentist with active hepatitis or who is a carrier.
3. With chronic active hepatitis, the patient may have chronic liver dysfunction, which may be associated with a bleeding tendency or altered drug metabolism.

- Bleeding
- Lichenoid eruptions

Prevention of Problems	**Treatment Planning Modifications**
<ul><li>If present status is free of clinical disease, patient should be treated as a normal patient.</li><li>Patients with recent conversion to a positive tuberculin skin test (purified protein derivative [PPD]):<ul><li>Should have been evaluated by the physician to rule out clinical disease</li><li>May be receiving isoniazid (INH) prophylactically for 6 months to 1 year</li><li>Should be treated as a normal patient when the physician approves health status</li></ul></li><li>Patients with signs or symptoms of tuberculosis:<ul><li>Should be referred to the physician and should have treatment postponed</li><li>If treatment is necessary, provide treatment as for patient with active sputum-positive tuberculosis (above).</li></ul></li></ul>	
<ul><li>Patients should be identified by history and clinical examination and referred to a sleep medicine specialist for diagnosis and treatment planning.</li><li>Signs and symptoms suggestive of obstructive sleep apnea include heavy snoring, witnessed apnea episodes during sleep, excessive daytime sleepiness, obesity, and large neck circumference.</li><li>Depending upon the diagnosis and severity of the disease, treatment may include positive airway pressure, oral appliances, or various forms of upper airway surgery.</li></ul>	<ul><li>Patients with obstructive sleep apnea may undergo any necessary dental treatment.</li></ul>
CAVEAT: Because most carriers are undetectable by history, all patients should be treated with the use of standard precautions (see Appendix B); risk may be decreased by the use of hepatitis B vaccine.<ul><li>For patient with active hepatitis, use the following procedures:<ul><li>Consult with the physician (to determine status).</li><li>Treat on an emergency basis only.</li></ul></li><li>For patients with a history of hepatitis, use the following procedures:<ul><li>Consult with the physician (to determine status).</li><li>Probable type determination:<ol><li>Age at time of infection (type B uncommon at younger than 15 years of age)</li><li>Source of infection (if food or water, usually type A or E)</li><li>If blood transfusion related, probably type C</li><li>If type is indeterminate, assay for hepatitis B surface antigen (HBsAg) may be considered.</li></ol></li></ul></li><li>With patients in high-risk categories, consider screening for HBsAg or anti–hepatitis C virus.</li><li>If HBsAg or hepatitis C virus positive (carrier):<ul><li>Consult with the physician to determine the status of liver dysfunction and/or recommendations for early treatment.</li><li>Minimize the use of drugs metabolized by the liver.</li><li>Monitor preoperative prothrombin time and bleeding time in chronic active hepatitis.</li></ul></li></ul>	<ul><li>None required</li></ul>

Dental Management: A Summary—cont'd

Potential Problems Related to Dental Care	**Oral Manifestations**

VIRAL HEPATITIS, TYPES B, C, D, AND E (cont'd)

ALCOHOLIC LIVER DISEASE (CIRRHOSIS)
Chapter 11

1. Bleeding tendencies; unpredictable drug metabolism

- Neglect
- Bleeding
- Ecchymoses
- Petechiae
- Glossitis
- Angular cheilosis
- Impaired healing
- Parotid enlargement
- Candidiasis
- Oral cancer
- Alcohol breath odor
- Bruxism
- Dental attrition
- Xerostomia

PEPTIC ULCER DISEASE
Chapter 12

1. Further injury to the intestinal mucosa caused by aspirin and NSAIDs
2. Fungal overgrowth during or after systemic antibiotic use

- Rare—Enamel dissolution associated with persistent regurgitation
- Fungal overgrowth
- Rare—Vitamin B deficiency (glossopyrosis) with omeprazole use

INFLAMMATORY BOWEL DISEASE
Chapter 12

1. In patients who are being treated with steroids, stress may lead to serious medical problems.

- Cobblestoned—Aphthous lesions
- Pyostomatitis vegetans

PSEUDOMEMBRANOUS COLITIS
Chapter 12

1. Fungal overgrowth during or after course of antibiotics

- Rare—Fungal overgrowth

END-STAGE RENAL DISEASE
Chapter 13

1. Bleeding tendency
2. Hypertension
3. Anemia
4. Intolerance to nephrotoxic drugs metabolized by the kidney
5. Enhanced susceptibility to infection

- Mucosal pallor
- Xerostomia
- Metallic taste
- Ammonia breath odor
- Stomatitis
- Loss of lamina dura
- Bone radiolucencies
- Bleeding tendency

Prevention of Problems	**Treatment Planning Modifications**

- Needle stick:
  - Consult the physician.
  - Consider hepatitis B immunoglobulin.

- Identify alcoholic patients through the following methods:
  - History
  - Clinical examination
  - Detection of odor on breath
  - Information from friends or relatives
- Consult with the physician to determine the status of liver dysfunction.
- Perform clinical screening with the CAGE questionnaire, and attempt to guide patients during treatment.
- Laboratory screening should include the following:
  - Complete blood count with differential
  - Aspartate aminotransferase, alanine aminotransferase
  - Platelet count
  - Thrombin time
  - Prothrombin time
- Minimize the use of drugs metabolized by the liver.
- If screening tests are abnormal for surgery, consider antifibrinolytic agents, fresh frozen plasma, vitamin K, and platelets.
- Defer routine care if ascites (encephalopathy), if present.

Treatment Planning Modifications:
- Because oral neglect is commonly seen in alcoholic individuals, patients should be required to demonstrate interest in and ability to care for dentition before any significant treatment is rendered.

- Avoid aspirin and NSAIDs.
- Avoid corticosteroids.
- Examine oral cavity for signs of fungal overgrowth.

Treatment Planning Modifications:
- Provide as stress free an environment as possible.

- Additional steroids may be needed for surgical procedures.
- Complete blood count is needed to monitor toxic hematologic effects of drugs.

Treatment Planning Modifications:
- Schedule appointments during remissions.

- Select appropriate antibiotic, dosage, and duration.
- Take precautions with prolonged antibiotic use in the elderly and those previously affected.

Treatment Planning Modifications:
- Schedule appointments when the patient is free of disease.

- Consult with physician (to determine status).
- Provide pretreatment screening (i.e., PFA-100, prothrombin time, partial thromboplastin time, hematocrit, hemoglobin) for hematologic disorder.
- Closely monitor blood pressure before and during treatment.
- Avoid drugs excreted by the kidney and nephrotoxic drugs.
- Meticulous attention should be paid to good surgical technique to minimize the risk of abnormal bleeding or infection.
- Provide aggressive management of infection.

Treatment Planning Modifications:
- Major emphasis on oral hygiene and optimal maintenance care to eliminate possible sources of infection
- No contraindications for routine dental care, but extensive reconstructive crown and bridge procedures not recommended

Dental Management: A Summary—cont'd

Potential Problems Related to Dental Care	Oral Manifestations

HEMODIALYSIS

Chapter 13

1. Bleeding tendency
2. Hypertension
3. Anemia
4. Intolerance to nephrotoxic drugs metabolized by the kidney
5. Bacterial endarteritis of arteriovenous fistula secondary to bacteremia
6. Hepatitis (active or carrier)
7. Bacterial endocarditis
8. Collapse of shunt

- Bleeding
- Lichenoid eruptions

GONORRHEA

Chapter 14

1. Remote possibility of transmission from oral or pharyngeal lesions of an infected patient

- Rare but varied expression, including generalized stomatitis, ulceration, and formation of pseudomembranous coating of oropharynx

SYPHILIS

Chapter 14

1. Syphilis may be contracted by the dentist from an actively infectious patient.
2. Patients or staff may be infected by the dentist who has syphilis.

- Chancre
- Mucous patch
- Gumma
- Interstitial glossitis
- Congenital syphilis (associated with Hutchinson's incisors and mulberry molars)

Prevention of Problems	Treatment Planning Modifications
1. Consultation with physician. 2. Delay dental treatment for at least 4 hours following dialysis to avoid heparin effects (potential for excessive bleeding); best to perform dental treatment on the day following dialysis. 3. Avoid drugs metabolized by kidney or nephrotoxic drugs. 4. AHA does not recommend antibiotic prophylaxis for invasive dental procedures. 5. Avoid placing blood pressure cuff on the arm containing the shunt used for dialysis.	• None required

CAVEAT: Many patients with sexually transmitted disease cannot be identified by history or examination; therefore, all patients must be approached with the use of standard precautions (see Appendix B).
• For patients currently receiving treatment for gonorrhea, provide necessary care.
• For patients with past history of gonorrhea, perform the following:
  • Obtain a good history of disease and its treatment.
  • Provide necessary care.
• For patients with signs or symptoms suggestive of gonorrhea, perform the following:
  • Refer to physician for evaluation.
  • Provide necessary care after disease treatment has been initiated.
	• None required

• For patients receiving treatment for syphilis:
  • Consult with physician before treatment.
  • Provide necessary care.
  • Be aware that oral lesions of primary and secondary syphilis are infectious prior to initiation of antibiotic therapy.
	• None required

Dental Management: A Summary—cont'd	
Potential Problems Related to Dental Care	**Oral Manifestations**

SYPHILIS (cont'd)

GENITAL HERPES
Chapter 14
1. Inoculation of oral cavity and potential transmission to dentist (fingers, eyes)

- Autoinoculation of type 2 herpes to oral cavity

HUMAN PAPILLOMAVIRUS (HPV) INFECTION
Chapter 14
1. Inoculation of oral cavity and potential transmission to fingers

- Autoinoculation of HPV to oral cavity
- Specific genotypes associated with risk for development of carcinoma

DIABETES MELLITUS
Chapter 15
1. In uncontrolled diabetic patients:
   a. Infection
   b. Poor wound healing
2. Insulin reaction in patients treated with insulin
3. In diabetic patients, early onset of complications relating to cardiovascular system, eyes, kidneys, and nervous system (angina, myocardial infarction, cerebrovascular accident, renal failure, peripheral neuropathy blindness, hypertension, congestive heart failure)

- Accelerated periodontal disease
- Gingival proliferations
- Periodontal abscesses
- Xerostomia
- Poor healing
- Infection
- Oral ulcerations
- Candidiasis
- Mucormycosis
- Numbness, burning, or pain in oral tissues

Prevention of Problems	**Treatment Planning Modifications**

Prevention of Problems

- For patients with a past history of syphilis:
  - Approach with caution; obtain good history of disease, its treatment, and negative serologic tests for syphilis test following completion of therapy.
  - Treat as normal patient if free of disease.
- For patients showing signs or symptoms suggestive of syphilis:
  - Refer to physician, and postpone treatment.
  - The dentist may elect to order serologic tests for syphilis before referral.
  - Defer treatment until diagnosis established and medical treatment provided.

CAVEAT: Many patients with sexually transmitted disease cannot be identified by history or examination; therefore, all patients must be approached with the use of standard precautions (see Appendix B).
- Localized genital infection poses no problem; however, be aware of the possibility of autoinoculation to dermal sites and the oral cavity by the patient.
- For oral infection with HSV-1 or HSV-2 postpone elective dental care until lesion is healing (in scab phase or when it disappears).

CAVEAT: Many patients with sexually transmitted disease cannot be identified by history or examination; therefore, all patients must be approached with the use of standard precautions (see Appendix B).
- Localized genital infection poses no problem; however, be aware of the possibility of autoinoculation to the oral cavity by the patient.
- Oral lesions should be excised and submitted for histologic examination.

- Detection by the following methods:
  - History
  - Clinical findings
  - Screening for blood glucose
- Referral for diagnosis and treatment
- Monitoring and control of hyperglycemia by assessment of blood glucose
- Monitoring of hemoglobin A1c (HbA)1c status
- For patients receiving insulin, an insulin reaction is prevented by the following methods:
  - Eating of normal meals before appointments
  - Scheduling of appointments in morning or midmorning
  - Informing the dentist of any symptoms of insulin reaction when they first occur
  - Having sugar available in some form in cases of insulin reaction

Treatment Planning Modifications

- None is usually required; patients prone to recurrence after dental treatment should be provided a short-term systemic antiviral drug for prophylactic use.

- Discuss risks of transmission and the potential for development of carcinoma with high-risk types (HPV 16, 18, 31, 33, 35). Appropriate treatment and follow-up care should be provided.

- In well-controlled diabetic patients, no alteration of treatment plan is indicated unless complications of diabetes present, such as:
  - Hypertension
  - Congestive heart failure
  - Myocardial infarction
  - Angina
  - Renal failure
- Defer prosthodontic care until periodontal disease is well controlled.

Dental Management: A Summary—cont'd

Potential Problems Related to Dental Care | **Oral Manifestations**

DIABETES MELLITUS (cont'd)

ADRENAL INSUFFICIENCY
Chapter 16
1. Inability to tolerate stress
2. Delayed healing
3. Susceptibility to infection
4. Hypertension (with steroid use)

- Primary pigmentation of oral mucous membranes
- Delayed healing
- Possible oral infection

HYPERTHYROIDISM (THYROTOXICOSIS)
Chapter 17
1. Thyrotoxic crisis (thyroid storm) may be precipitated in untreated or incompletely treated patients with thyrotoxicosis by:
   a. Infection
   b. Trauma
   c. Surgical procedures
   d. Stress
2. Patients with untreated or incompletely treated thyrotoxicosis may be very sensitive to actions of epinephrine and other pressor amines; thus, these agents must not be used; once the patient is well managed from a medical standpoint, these agents may be administered.
3. Thyrotoxicosis increases the risk for hypertension, angina, MI, congestive heart failure, and severe arrhythmias.

- Osteoporosis may occur.
- Periodontal disease may be more progressive.
- Dental caries may be more extensive.
- Premature loss of deciduous teeth and early eruption of permanent teeth may occur.
- Early jaw development may be noted.
- Tumors found at the midline of the posterior dorsum of the tongue must not be surgically removed until the possibility of functional thyroid tissue has been ruled out by ^{131}I uptake tests.

Prevention of Problems	Treatment Planning Modifications

Prevention of Problems

- Treatment with insulin of diabetic patients who develop oral infection may require increased insulin dosage and consultation with the physician, in addition to aggressive local and systemic management of infection (including antibiotic sensitivity testing).
- Drug considerations include the following:
  - Insulin—Insulin reaction
  - Hypoglycemic agents—On rare occasions, aplastic anemia, etc.
  - Avoidance of general anesthesia in patients with severe diabetes

- For routine dental procedures (excluding extractions):
  - Patients currently taking corticosteroids—no additional supplementation generally required; be sure to obtain good local anesthesia and good postoperative pain control
  - Patients with past history of regular corticosteroid usage; none generally required
  - Patients using topical or inhalational steroids— generally no supplementation required
- For extractions or other surgery, extensive procedures, or extreme patient anxiety, with local anesthetic include the following:
  - Discontinue drugs that decrease cortisol levels (e.g., ketoconazole) at least 24 hours before surgery with the consent of the patient's physician.
  - Target dose of 25 mg hydrocortisone per day for minor oral and periodontal surgery, administered prior to procedure.
  - Target dose of 50 to 100 mg hydrocortisone within first hour of major oral surgery or procedures involving general anesthesia. Give 25 mg hydrocortisone every 8 hours for 24 to 48 hours postoperatively.
  - Monitor blood pressure throughout procedure and initial postoperative phase.
  - Provide good pain control.

- Detection of patients with thyrotoxicosis by history and examination findings
- Referral for medical evaluation and treatment
- Avoidance of any dental treatment for patient with thyrotoxicosis until good medical control is attained; however, any acute oral infection will have to be dealt with by antibiotic therapy and other conservative measures to prevent development of thyrotoxic crisis; suggest consultation with patient's physician during management of acute oral infection
- Avoidance of epinephrine and other pressor amines in untreated or incompletely treated patient
- Recognition of early stages of thyrotoxic crisis:
  - Severe symptoms of thyrotoxicosis
  - Fever
  - Abdominal pain
  - Delirious, obtunded, or psychotic

Treatment Planning Modifications

- None required

- Once under good medical management, the patient may receive any indicated dental treatment.
- If acute infection occurs, the physician should be consulted regarding management.

Dental Management: A Summary—cont'd

Potential Problems Related to Dental Care	**Oral Manifestations**

HYPERTHYROIDISM (THYROTOXICOSIS) (cont'd)

HYPOTHYROIDISM
Chapter 17

1. Untreated patients with severe hypothyroidism exposed to stressful situations such as trauma, surgical procedures, or infection may develop hypothyroid (myxedema) coma.
2. Untreated hypothyroid patients may be highly sensitive to actions of narcotics, barbiturates, and tranquilizers.

- Increase in tongue size
- Delayed eruption of teeth
- Malocclusion
- Gingival edema

THYROIDITIS
Chapter 17

1. Acute suppurative—Patient has acute infection, antibiotics
2. Subacute painful—Period of hyperthyroidism
3. Subacute painless—Up to 6-month period of hyperthyroidism
4. Hashimoto's—Leads to severe hypothyroidism
5. Chronic fibrosing (Riedel's)—Usually euthyroid

- Usually none

- Pain may be referred to mandible
- None

- Tongue may enlarge
- None

THYROID CANCER
Chapter 17

1. Usually none
2. Levothyroxine suppression following surgery and radioiodine ablation is usual treatment for follicular carcinomas. Patient may have mild hyperthyroidism. May be sensitive to actions of pressor amines.
3. Patients with multiple endocrine neoplasia-2 (MEN-2) may have symptoms of hypertension and/or hypercalcemia.
4. Anaplastic carcinomas may be treated by external radiation and/or chemotherapy. See problems listed in summary for Chapter 26

- Usually none; metastasis to the oral cavity is rare
- Usually none

- Patients with MEN-2 can develop cystic lesions of the jaws related to hyperparathyroidism

- See oral complications listed in summary for Chapter 26

Prevention of Problems	Treatment Planning Modifications

• Initiation of immediate emergency treatment procedures:
  • Seek immediate medical aid.
  • Cool with cold towels, ice packs.
  • Hydrocortisone (100 to 300 mg)
  • Monitor vital signs
  • Start CPR if needed	

• Detection and referral of patients suspected of being hypothyroid for medical evaluation and treatment
• Avoidance of narcotics, barbiturates, and tranquilizers in untreated hypothyroid patients
• Recognition of initial stage of hypothyroid (myxedema) coma
  • Hypothermia
  • Bradycardia
  • Hypotension
  • Epileptic seizures
• Initiation of immediate treatment for myxedema coma
  • Seek immediate medical aid.
  • Administer hydrocortisone (100 to 300 mg).
  • Provide cardiopulmonary resuscitation (CPR) as indicated.
	• In hypothyroid patients under good medical management, indicated dental treatment may be performed.
	• In patients with a congenital form of disease and severe mental retardation, assistance with hygienic procedures may be needed.

• None • Include in differential diagnosis of jaw pain, see above under hyperthyroidism • See above under hyperthyroidism • See above under hypothyroidism • None	• Postpone elective dental care until infection has been treated. • Avoid elective dental care if possible until symptoms of hyperthyroidism have cleared. • Avoid elective dental care if possible until symptoms of hyperthyroidism have cleared. • In hypothyroid patients under good medical management, any indicated dental treatment can be performed. See above for uncontrolled disease. • None

• Examine for signs and symptoms of thyroid cancer:
  a. Hard, painless lump in thyroid
  b. Dominant nodule in multinodular goiter
  c. Hoarseness, dysphagia, dyspnea
  d. Cervical lymphadenopathy
  e. Nodule that is fixed to underlying tissues
  f. Patient is usually euthyroid
• Patients found to have thyroid nodule(s) should be referred for fine-needle aspiration biopsy.
• Consult with patient's physician regarding degree of hyperthyroidism for patients treated with thyroid hormone.
• Manage complications of radiation and chemotherapy as described in summary of Chapter 26.
	• For most patients the dental treatment plan is not affected unless patient has been treated by external radiation or chemotherapy. See summary of Chapter 26. Patients with anaplastic carcinoma have a poor prognosis and complex dental procedures are usually not indicated.
	
	• May have to take care in the use of epinephrine in patients treated with thyroid hormone.
	
	• Prognosis is poor with anaplastic carcinoma.

Dental Management: A Summary—cont'd

Potential Problems Related to Dental Care	Oral Manifestations

PREGNANCY AND LACTATION
Chapter 18
1. Dental procedures could harm the developing fetus via:
   a. Radiation
   b. Drugs
   c. Stress
2. Supine hypotension in late pregnancy
3. Poor nutrition and diet can affect oral health.
4. Transmission of drugs to infant via breast milk
5. Lack of proper oral health care during pregnancy could harm the development of the fetus and time of delivery

- Exaggeration of periodontal disease, "pregnancy gingivitis"
- "Pregnancy tumor"
- Tooth mobility

ANTIBODY POSITIVE FOR HIV (AIDS) BUT ASYMPTOMATIC
Chapter 19
1. Transmission of infectious agents to dental personnel and patients includes:
   a. Acquired immunodeficiency syndrome (AIDS) virus (human immunodeficiency virus [HIV])
   b. Hepatitis B virus (HBV)
   c. Hepatitis C virus (HCV)
   d. Epstein-Barr virus (EBV)
   e. Cytomegalovirus (CMV)
2. To date, no dental health care workers have been infected with HIV through occupational exposure; six patients may have been infected by an HIV-infected dentist; thus, risk of HIV transmission in the dental setting is very low, but the potential exists.
3. Individuals who are hepatitis carriers may transmit HBV or HCV infection.

- None in the early stage; however, increased incidence of certain oral lesions associated with AIDS is found when compared with noninfected individuals (i.e., candidiasis).

Prevention of Problems	**Treatment Planning Modifications**

- Women of childbearing age:
  - Always use contemporary radiographic techniques, including lead apron, when performing radiographic examination.
  - Do not prescribe drugs that are known to be harmful to the fetus, or whose effects are as yet unknown (see Table 18-3).
  - Encourage patients to maintain a balanced, nutritious diet.
- For pregnant women:
  - Contact the patient's physician to verify physical status and present management plan; ask for suggestions regarding patient's treatment, especially as it relates to drug administration.
  - Maintain optimal oral hygiene, including prophylaxis, throughout pregnancy.
  - Minimize oral microbial load (consider chlorhexidine and/or fluoride).
  - Avoid elective dental care during the first trimester. The second trimester and most of the third trimester are the best times for elective treatment.
  - Do not schedule radiographs during the first trimester; thereafter, take only those necessary for treatment, always with the use of a lead apron.
  - Avoid drugs known to be harmful to the fetus, or whose effects are unknown (see Table 18-3).
  - In advanced stages of pregnancy (late third trimester), do not place the patient in the supine position for prolonged periods; avoid aspirin, NSAIDs.
- For lactating mothers:
  - Most drugs are of little pharmacologic significance to lactation.
  - Do not prescribe drugs known to be harmful (see Table 18-3).
  - Administer drugs just after breast feeding.

- None, except that major reconstructive procedures, crown and bridge fabrication, and significant operations are best delayed until after delivery.

- Identification of HIV-infected patient is difficult; interview questions should address promiscuous sexual behavior; infectious disease control procedures must be used for *all* patients.
- Extreme care must be taken to avoid needle stick and instrument wounding.
- All dental personnel should be vaccinated to be protected from HBV infection.
- All asymptomatic antibody-positive (HIV) individuals may go on to develop AIDS; however, it may take as long as 15 years before a diagnosis of AIDS is made.
- The HIV-infected patient's CD4 count and HIV titer must be monitored.
- Patients' immune status, medications, and potential for opportunistic infections must be determined and monitored.

- None indicated

Dental Management: A Summary—cont'd

Potential Problems Related to Dental Care	Oral Manifestations

HIV-INFECTED, ASYMPTOMATIC PATIENT (CD4 LYMPHOCYTE COUNT LESS THAN 500, MORE THAN 200)
Chapter 19

1. Transmission of infectious agents to dental personnel and patients includes the following:
   a. HIV
   b. Hepatitis B virus
   c. Hepatitis C virus
   d. Epstein-Barr virus
   e. Cytomegalovirus
2. To date, with the exception of possible transmission by a Florida dentist:
   a. HIV has not been found to be transmitted to patients in the dental setting.
   b. No dental health care workers have been HIV infected through occupational exposure.
   c. However, transmission of HBV and HCV has been well documented on numerous occasions.
3. Patients with decreasing CD4 lymphocytes may have significant immune suppression and be at increased risk for infection.
4. Patients with decreasing CD4 lymphocytes may be thrombocytopenic and hence potential bleeders.

- Oral candidiasis
- Hairy leukoplakia
- Persistent lymphadenopathy
- With the exception of Kaposi's sarcoma and non-Hodgkin's lymphoma, other lesions listed under AIDS may be found with increased frequency.

AIDS (CD4 LYMPHOCYTE COUNT LESS THAN 200)
Chapter 19

1. Transmission of infectious agents to dental personnel and patients:
   a. HIV
   b. Hepatitis B virus
   c. Hepatitis C virus
   d. Epstein-Barr virus
   e. Cytomegalovirus
2. To date, HIV has not been found to be transmitted to patients in the dental setting (possible exception of six patients who may have been infected by a Florida dentist); no dental health care workers have been HIV infected through occupational exposure; however, HBV and HCV have been transmitted to patients or dental health care workers on a number of occasions in the dental setting.
3. Patients with advanced disease have significant suppression of their immune system and may be at risk for infection resulting from invasive dental procedures.
4. Patients may be bleeders because of thrombocytopenia.

- Kaposi's sarcoma
- Non-Hodgkin's lymphoma
- Oral candidiasis
- Lymphadenopathy
- Hairy leukoplakia
- Xerostomia
- Salivary gland enlargement
- Venereal warts
- Linear gingivitis erythema
- Necrotizing ulcerative periodontitis
- Necrotizing stomatitis
- Herpes zoster
- Primary or recurrent herpes simplex lesions
- Major aphthous lesions
- Herpetiform aphthous lesions
- Petechiae, ecchymoses
- Others (see Table 19-8)

ANAPHYLAXIS
Chapter 20

1. Severe reaction following administration of agent to patient who is allergic to agents such as:
   a. Drugs
   b. Local anesthctic
   c. Latex gloves or other rubber products (rubber dam, gutta percha)

- Usually none

Prevention of Problems	**Treatment Planning Modifications**
<ul><li>Use infectious disease control procedures for *all* patients.</li><li>Vaccinate dental personnel for protection from HBV infection.</li><li>Identify patients by the presence of signs and symptoms associated with decreasing CD4 lymphocytes; refer for medical evaluation, counseling, and management.</li><li>Establish platelet status and immune status of patients with decreasing CD4 lymphocytes before performing invasive dental procedures (see AIDS, next page).</li><li>Inform patients of various support groups available to help in terms of education and emotional, financial, legal, and other issues.</li></ul>	<ul><li>None indicated</li></ul>
<ul><li>Use infectious disease control procedures for *all* patients.</li><li>Vaccinate dental personnel for protection from HBV.</li><li>Through medical history and examination findings, identify undiagnosed cases and refer for medical evaluation, counseling, and management.</li><li>Give patients with significant immune suppression antibiotic prophylaxis for surgical or invasive dental procedures, if neutrophil count is less than 500 cu/m.</li><li>Platelet count should be ordered before any surgical procedure is performed; if significant thrombocytopenia is present, platelet replacement may be needed.</li><li>The patient's immune status, medications (highly active antiretroviral therapy [HAART]), and potential for opportunistic infections must be determined and monitored.</li></ul>	<ul><li>None for cases in "remission"; however, complex restorative procedures usually are not indicated because of poor prognosis (death occurs most often within 2 years after diagnosis).</li><li>Patients in advanced stages of disease should receive emergency and preventive dental care; elective dental treatment usually is not indicated at this stage.</li></ul>
<ul><li>Take careful history and identify patients who are allergic to agents used in dentistry, and who have a history of atopic reactions (e.g., asthma, hay fever, urticaria, angioneurotic edema).</li><li>Do not use agents to which the patient is allergic, as identified in the medical history.</li><li>For patients with a history of atopic reactions, use care when giving drugs and materials with a high incidence of allergy such as penicillin; be prepared to deal with severe allergic reaction in the following ways:<ul><li>Identify anaphylactic reaction.</li><li>Call for medical help.</li></ul></li></ul>	<ul><li>Do not use agents to which the patient is allergic, as identified in the medical history.</li></ul>

Dental Management: A Summary—cont'd

Potential Problems Related to Dental Care	Oral Manifestations
ANAPHYLAXIS (cont'd)	
URTICARIA (ANGIONEUROTIC EDEMA) *Chapter 20* 1. Nonemergency; edematous swelling of lips, cheek, etc., after contact with antigen 2. Emergency; edematous swelling of tongue, pharynx, and larynx with obstruction of airway	• Soft tissue swelling

Prevention of Problems	**Treatment Planning Modifications**

Prevention of Problems

- Place patient in the supine position.
- Check for open airway.
- Administer oxygen.
- Check vital signs—Respiration, blood pressure, pulse rate, and rhythm.
- If vital signs depressed or absent, inject 0.3 to 0.5 mL of epinephrine 1:1000 IM into the tongue.
- Provide CPR as indicated.
- Repeat injection of epinephrine, if no response.
- When prescribing drugs, inform the patient regarding signs and symptoms of allergic reactions; advise the patient to call the dentist if such a reaction occurs, or to report to the nearest hospital emergency room.

- Identify patients who have had allergic reactions through the history and what drug or materials caused the reaction.
- Avoid the use of antigen in allergic persons.
- If patients develop allergic reaction to drug or material to which they gave no indication of being allergic, consider the following:
  - Nonemergency reaction, no further contact with agent—Administer diphenhydramine 50 mg up to 4 times a day, orally or IM.
  - Emergency reaction—Put patient in the supine position; with patent airway and oxygen, inject 0.3 to 0.5 mL epinephrine 1:1000 IM; support respiration if necessary; check pulse; obtain medical assistance.
- Before administering local anesthetics, consider the following:
  - Obtain from the patient information about being allergic to a local anesthetic. (Most patients who say they are allergic will describe a fainting episode or a toxic reaction.) If an allergic reaction has occurred, identify the type of anesthetic used, and select one from various chemical groups.
    1. Inject 1 drop (aspirate first) of alternate anesthetic, and wait 5 minutes; if no reaction occurs, proceed with injection of remaining anesthetic.
    2. If anesthetic that patient has reacted to cannot be identified, consider the following procedures:
       a. Refer to allergist for provocative dose testing, or
       b. Use diphenhydramine (Benadryl) with epinephrine 1:100,000 as local anesthetic (1% solution, 1 to 4 mL).
- Allergy to penicillin
  - Administer erythromycin or another macrolide antibiotic.
  - In nonallergic person, administer by the oral route whenever possible—Lowest incidence of sensitization.
  - Do not use in topical form.

Treatment Planning Modifications

- Do not use agents to which the patient is allergic, as identified in the medical history.

Dental Management: A Summary—cont'd

Potential Problems Related to Dental Care	Oral Manifestations
INTRAVASCULAR ACCESS DEVICES (ULDALL CATHETER, CENTRAL IV LINE, BROVIAC-HICKMAN DEVICE) *Chapter 21* 1. High rate of infection, but the role of transient dental bacteremias that cause these infections has not been established.	• None

SOLID ORGAN TRANSPLANTATION
Chapter 22
1. Infection from suppression of immune response by the following:
  a. Cyclosporine
  b. Azathioprine
  c. Prednisone
  d. Antithymocyte globulin
  e. Antilymphocyte globulin
  f. Orthoclone (monoclonal antibody)
2. Acute rejection, reversible
3. Chronic rejection, nonreversible, includes the following:
  a. Graft failure—End-stage organ failure
  b. Bleeding—Liver, kidney
  c. Drug overdosage—Liver, kidney
  d. Death or need for transplantation of heart, liver
  e. Osteoporosis
  f. Psychoses
  g. Anemia
  h. Leukopenia
  i. Thrombocytopenia
  j. Gingival hyperplasia
  k. Adrenocortical suppression
  l. Tumors (listed above)
  m. Poor healing
  n. Bleeding
  o. Infection
	• Usually none
	• Excessive immune suppression includes the following:
	  • Candidiasis
	  • Herpes simplex
	  • Herpes zoster
	  • Hairy leukoplakia
	  • Lymphoma
	  • Kaposi's sarcoma
	  • Aphthous stomatitis
	  • Squamous cell carcinoma of lip
	• Adverse effects of immunosuppressant drugs include the following:
	  • Bleeding (spontaneous)
	  • Infection
	  • Ulceration
	  • Petechiae
	  • Ecchymoses
	  • Gingival hyperplasia
	  • Salivary gland dysfunction
	• Graft failure includes the following:
	  • Uremic stomatitis (kidney)
	  • Bleeding (liver)
	  • Petechiae (liver, kidney)
	  • Ecchymoses (liver)

Prevention of Problems

Treatment Planning Modifications

- The CDC does not recommend antibiotic prophylaxis for invasive dental procedures.

- Dental evaluation and treatment before transplantation includes the following:
  - Establish stable oral and dental status free of active dental disease.
  - Initiate aggressive oral hygiene program to maintain oral health.
  - Arrange medical consultation for patients with organ failure before performing needed dental treatment to establish the following:
    1. Degree of failure
    2. Current status of patient
    3. Need for antibiotic prophylaxis
    4. Need to modify drug selection or dosage
    5. Need to take special precautions to avoid bleeding
    6. If surgery is indicated, access to recent prothrombin time, partial thromboplastin time, bleeding time, and white cell count or differential may be needed.
- Dental treatment after transplantation includes the following:
  - Immediate posttransplant period (6 months):
    1. Provide emergency dental care only.
    2. Continue oral hygiene procedures.
  - Stable graft period.
    1. Maintain oral hygiene.
    2. Recall every 3 months.
    3. Use universal precautions.
    4. Vaccinate dental staff against HBV infection.
    5. Schedule medical consultation on the following topics:
       a. Need for antibiotic prophylaxis
       b. Need for precautions to avoid excessive bleeding
       c. Need for supplemental steroids
       d. Selection of drugs and dosage
    6. Examine for clinical evidence of the following:
       a. Organ failure or rejection
       b. Overimmunosuppression (tumors, infection, etc.)
    7. Monitor blood pressure at every appointment.
    8. If evidence of drug adverse effects, graft rejection, or overimmunosuppression is found, refer patient to physician
  - Chronic rejection period
    1. Perform immediate or emergency dental care only.
    2. Follow guidelines for stable graft when treatment is performed.

- Depends on the reason for the intravascular device

- Before transplantation, consider the following:
  - For patients with poor dental status, consider extractions and full dentures.
  - For patients with good dental status, perform the following:
    1. Maintain dentition.
    2. Establish aggressive oral hygiene program in the following areas:
       a. Toothbrushing, flossing
       b. Diet modification, if indicated
       c. Topical fluorides
       d. Plaque control, calculus removal
       e. Chlorhexidine or Listerine mouth rinse
    3. Treat all active dental disease in the following areas:
       a. Extraction—Nonrestorable teeth
       b. Endodontics—Nonvital teeth
       c. Restoration of carious teeth
       d. Complex dental prostheses, etc., deferred until after transplantation
  - For patients with dental status between the above extremes:
    1. Decision to maintain natural dentition must be made on an individual patient basis.
    2. Factors to be considered:
       a. Extent and severity of dental disease
       b. Importance of teeth to patient
       c. Cost of maintaining natural dentition
       d. Systemic status of patient and prognosis
       e. Physical ability to maintain good oral hygiene
- Following transplantation:
  - Immediate posttransplantation period—Limit dental care to emergency needs.
  - Stable graft period—Base treatment plan on needs and desires of the patient; recall every 3 to 6 months.
  - Chronic rejection period—Limit dental care to immediate or emergency needs.
  - Maintain aggressive oral hygiene program throughout all periods.
  - Consult with physician to confirm patient's current status and the need for special precautions.

Dental Management: A Summary—cont'd

Potential Problems Related to Dental Care	Oral Manifestations

HEART TRANSPLANTATION, SPECIAL CONSIDERATIONS
Chapter 22

1. Patient may be on long-term anticoagulation therapy; excessive bleeding may occur with surgical procedures.
2. Graft atherosclerosis may occur, increasing the risk for myocardial infarction.
3. No nerve supply exists to the transplanted heart; thus, pain will not be symptom of myocardial infarction.
4. Some patients require cardiac pacing; electrical equipment may interfere with the pacemaker.
5. Cardiac valvular disease may develop.

- Usually none
- See Chapter 25

LIVER TRANSPLANTATION, SPECIAL CONSIDERATIONS
Chapter 22

1. Drugs that may be toxic to the liver must not be prescribed.
2. Some patients may be on anticoagulation medication.
3. Excessive bleeding may occur with surgical procedures.

- See Solid Organ Transplantation (previous pages).

KIDNEY TRANSPLANTATION, SPECIAL CONSIDERATIONS
Chapter 22

1. Drugs that may be toxic to the kidney must not be prescribed.

- See Solid Organ Transplantation (previous pages).

PANCREAS TRANSPLANTATION
Chapter 22

1. No special considerations

- See Solid Organ Transplantation (previous pages).

BONE MARROW TRANSPLANTATION
Chapter 22

1. Immune suppression and pancytopenia resulting from conditioning therapy, including:
   a. Total body irradiation
   b. Cyclophosphamide
   c. Busulfan
2. Problems during conditioning phase and critical phase (until transplanted marrow becomes functional) include:
   a. Infection
   b. Bleeding
   c. Poor healing
3. Immune suppression resulting from maintenance medications used to prevent graft-versus-host disease and
   a. Cyclosporine
   b. Prednisone
   c. Methotrexate
4. Problems during maintenance phase include:
   a. Infection
   b. Others listed above under solid organ transplantation related to medication(s) being used
5. Graft-versus-host disease and chronic rejection:
   a. Infection
   b. Bleeding

- Mucositis
- Gingivitis
- Xerostomia
- Candidiasis
- Herpes simplex infections
- Osteoradionecrosis
- Gingival hyperplasia (with cyclosporine)

Prevention of Problems	**Treatment Planning Modifications**
• Have physician modify degree of anticoagulation to 2.5 normal prothrombin time or less (INR, 3.5 or less), if surgical procedures are planned. • Consult with physician to establish status of coronary vessels of transplanted heart; if advanced graft atherosclerosis is present, manage as described under section on coronary atherosclerotic heart disease. • Be aware of signs and symptoms of myocardial infarction, other than pain; if these occur, obtain immediate medical assistance for patient. • Do not use Cavitron or electrosurgery in patients with a pacemaker.	• The American Heart Association has stated that evidence regarding the need for antibiotic prophylaxis for prevention of endocarditis in patients with heart transplantation is inconclusive. • The American Heart Association recommends that prophylaxis be considered for cardiac transplant patients who develop cardiac valvular disease. • If prophylaxis is planned, the standard amoxicillin regimen of the American Heart Association would be appropriate.
• Avoid drugs that are toxic to the liver. • Have the physician modify the degree of anticoagulant to an INR of 3.5 or less.	• The need for prophylactic antibiotics for invasive dental procedures in patients with stable liver transplants should be determined on an individual patient basis through medical consultation.
• Avoid drugs that are toxic to the kidney.	• The need for prophylactic antibiotics for invasive dental procedures in patients with stable kidney transplants should be determined on an individual patient basis through medical consultation.
	• The need for prophylactic antibiotics for invasive dental procedures in patients with stable pancreas transplants should be determined on an individual patient basis through medical consultation.

• Avoid dental treatment during conditioning and critical phases of bone marrow transplantation.
• Treat all active dental disease prior to bone marrow transplantation.
• Observe requirements for antibiotic prophylaxis for invasive dental procedures:
  • Prophylaxis is indicated if procedures must be performed on an emergency basis during conditioning or critical phases of bone marrow transplantation.
  • Need should be determined through medical consultation. (See Solid Organ Transplantation [previous pages] for details of hygiene program and dental management.)
	• If possible, treat active dental disease before transplantation.
	• Prognosis varies according to reason for transplantation, source of marrow to be transplanted, and techniques used to condition and maintain the patient; other factors that may affect prognosis include age and general health status; complex dental prostheses may not be indicated for many patients.
	• (See Solid Organ Transplantation [previous pages] for other suggested treatment planning considerations.) (For management of soft tissue complications, see Appendix C.)

Dental Management: A Summary—cont'd

Potential Problems Related to Dental Care	Oral Manifestations
IRON DEFICIENCY ANEMIA *Chapter 23* 1. Usually none 2. In rare cases, severe leukopenia and thrombocytopenia may result in problems with infection and excessive loss of blood.	• Paresthesias • Loss of papillae on dorsum of tongue • In rare cases, infection and bleeding complications • In patients with dysphagia, increased incidence of carcinoma of oral and pharyngeal areas (Plummer-Vinson syndrome)
G-6-PD DEFICIENCY *Chapter 23* 1. Accelerated hemolysis of red blood cells	• Usually none
PERNICIOUS ANEMIA *Chapter 23* 1. Infection 2. Bleeding 3. Delayed healing	• Paresthesias of oral tissues (burning, tingling, numbness) • Delayed healing (severe cases), infection, bald red tongue, angular cheilosis • Petechial hemorrhages
SICKLE CELL ANEMIA *Chapter 23* 1. Sickle cell crisis	• Loss of trabecular pattern • Delayed eruption of teeth, growth abnormalities • Hypoplasia of teeth • Pallor of oral mucosa • Jaundice of oral mucosa • Bone pain • Osteoporosis

Prevention of Problems	Treatment Planning Modifications
• Detection and referral for diagnosis and treatment • Recognition that in women most cases are caused by physiologic process—Menstruation or pregnancy • Recognition that in men most cases are the result of underlying disease—Peptic ulcer, carcinoma of colon, etc.—requiring referral to the patient's physician	• Usually none
• Control infection. • Avoid drugs that contain certain antibiotics, aspirin, or acetaminophen, which may increase risk for hemolytic anemia. • Be aware that these patients also often have increased sensitivity to sulfa drugs and chloramphenicol.	• Usually none unless anemia is severe; then, perform only urgent dental needs
• Detection and medical treatment (early detection and treatment can prevent permanent neurologic damage)	• None, once the patient is under medical care

• Consult with patient's physician to ensure that condition is stable.
• Institute aggressive preventive dental care.
• Avoid any procedure that may produce acidosis or hypoxia (avoid long, complicated procedures).
• Consideration of the following drug situations:
  • Avoid excessive use of barbiturates and narcotics because suppression of the respiratory center may occur, leading to acidosis, which can precipitate acute crisis. Use benzodiazepine instead.
  • Avoid excessive use of salicylates because "acidosis" may result, again leading to possible acute crisis; codeine and acetaminophen in moderate dosage can be used for pain control.
  • Avoid the use of general anesthesia because hypoxia can lead to precipitation of acute crisis.
  • Nitrous oxide may be used, provided that 50% oxygen is supplied at all times; it is critical to avoid diffusion hypoxia at the termination of nitrous oxide administration. For nonsurgical procedures, use local without vasoconstrictor; for surgical procedures, use 1:100,000 epinephrine in anesthetic solution.
1. Aspirate before injecting.
2. Inject slowly.
3. Use no more than two cartridges.
4. It is necessary to prevent infection. Use prophylactic antibiotics for major surgical procedures.
5. If infection occurs, manage aggressively, with the use of:
  a. Heat
  b. Incision and drainage
  c. Antibiotics
  d. Corrective treatment—Extraction, pulpectomy, etc.
6. Avoid dehydration in patients with infection and in patients who are receiving surgical treatment.
	• Usually none, unless symptoms of severe anemia are present; then, only urgent dental needs should be met

Dental Management: A Summary—cont'd

| **Potential Problems Related to Dental Care** | **Oral Manifestations** |

AGRANULOCYTOSIS
Chapter 24
1. Infection

- Oral ulcerations
- Periodontitis
- Necrotic tissue

CYCLIC NEUTROPENIA
Chapter 24
1. Infection

- Periodontal disease
- Oral infection
- Oral ulceration similar to aphthous stomatitis

LEUKEMIA
Chapter 24
1. Infection
2. Bleeding
3. Delayed healing
4. Mucositis

- Gingival swelling/enlargement
- Mucosal or gingival bleeding
- Oral infection

MULTIPLE MYELOMA
Chapter 24
1. Excessive bleeding after invasive dental procedures
2. Risk of infection because of decrease in normal immunoglobulins
3. Risks of infection and bleeding in patients who are being treated by radiation or chemotherapy
4. Risk of osteonecrosis in patients who are taking bisphosphonates (especially intravenously).

- Soft tissue tumors
- Osteolytic lesions
- Amyloid deposits in soft tissues
- Unexplained mobility of teeth
- Exposed bone

LYMPHOMAS: HODGKIN'S DISEASE, NON-HODGKIN'S LYMPHOMA, BURKITT'S LYMPHOMA
Chapter 24
1. Increased risk for infection
2. Risks of infection and excessive bleeding in patients receiving chemotherapy
3. Minor risk of osteonecrosis in patients treated by radiation to the head and neck region (this usually does not occur because radiation dosage seldom exceeds 50 Gy)

- Extranodal oral tumors in Waldeyer's ring or osseous soft tissues
- Xerostomia in patients treated by radiation; some of these patients prone to osteonecrosis
- Burning mouth or tongue symptoms
- Petechiae or ecchymoses if thrombocytopenia present because of tumor invasion of bone marrow
- Cervical lymphadenopathy

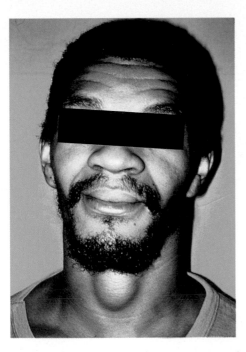

Figure 1-13. Midline neck enlargement caused by a thyroglossal duct cyst.

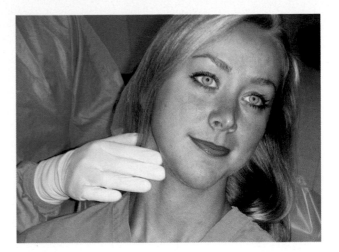

Figure 1-15. Palpation of the carotid pulse.

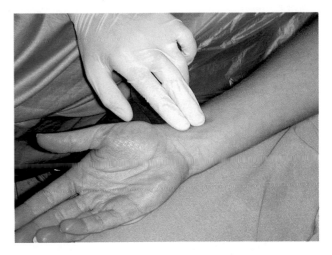

Figure 1-16. Palpation of the radial pulse.

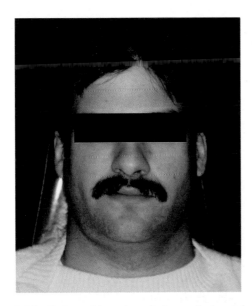

Figure 1-14. Enlarged lymph node beneath the right body of the mandible, resulting from a salivary gland infection.

A second benefit of vital sign measurement during an examination involves screening to identify abnormalities, either diagnosed or undiagnosed. For example, if a person with severe, uncontrolled hypertension was not identified and was treated with no management alteration, the consequences could be serious. The purpose of this examination is merely detection of an abnormality and not diagnosis. This is the responsibility of the physician. If an abnormal finding is deemed significant, the patient should be referred to a physician for further evaluation.

Pulse. The standard procedure for assessing the pulse rate is to palpate the carotid artery at the side of the trachea (Figure 1-15) or the radial artery on the thumb side of the wrist (Figure 1-16). The pulse should be palpated for 1 minute so that rhythm abnormalities can be detected. Alternatively, it may be palpated for 30 seconds and multiplied by 2. Use of the carotid artery for pulse determination has some advantages. First, the carotid pulse is familiar because of cardiopulmonary resuscitation (CPR) training provided to the dentist. Second, it is reliable because it is a central artery that supplies the brain; therefore, in emergency situations, it may remain palpable when peripheral arteries are not. Finally, it is easily located and palpated because of its size.

The carotid pulse can best be palpated along the anterior border of the sternocleidomastoid muscle at approximately the level of the thyroid cartilage. Displacement of the sternocleidomastoid muscle slightly posteriorly allows palpation of the pulse with the first and middle finger of the examiner. It is best to monitor the pulse for a full minute to detect irregular rhythm patterns.

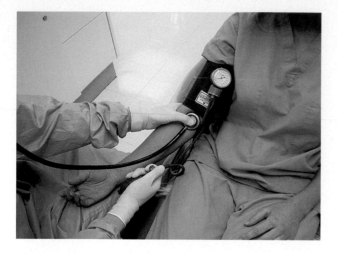

Figure 1-17. Blood pressure cuff and stethoscope in place.

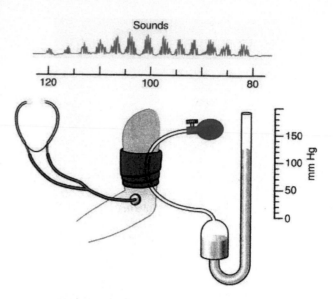

Figure 1-18. Diagrammatic representation of the typical sound pattern obtained when blood pressure in a normotensive adult is recorded. (From Guyton AC, Hall JE. Textbook of medical physiology, ed 11, Philadelphia, 2006, Elsevier Saunders.)

Rate. The average pulse rate in normal adults is 60 to 100 beats per minute. A pulse rate greater than 100 beats per minute is called *tachycardia*, whereas a slow pulse rate of less than 60 beats per minute is called *bradycardia*. An abnormal pulse rate may be a sign of a cardiovascular disorder but also may be influenced by exercise, conditioning, anxiety, drugs, or fever.

Rhythm. The normal pulse is a series of rhythmic beats that occur at regular intervals. When the beats occur at irregular intervals, the pulse is called *irregular, dysrhythmic,* or *arrhythmic.*

Blood Pressure. Blood pressure is determined by indirect measurement in the upper extremities with a blood pressure cuff and stethoscope (Figure 1-17). The cuff should be of the correct width to give an accurate recording. Ideally, the bladder within the cuff should encompass 80% of the circumference of the arm, with the center of the bladder positioned over the brachial artery. The standard cuff width for an average adult arm is 12 to 14 cm. A cuff that is too small yields falsely elevated values, whereas a cuff that is too large yields falsely low values. Narrower cuffs are available for use with children, and wider cuffs or thigh cuffs are available for use with obese or larger patients. As an alternative for an obese patient, a standard-size cuff can be placed on the forearm below the antecubital fossa, and the radial artery may be palpated so that only the approximate systolic pressure can be determined.[4] Instruments that measure blood pressure at the wrist or fingers have become popular; however, their use is not recommended because of potential inaccuracies.[4] The stethoscope should be of good standard quality. The bell end (cup) is preferred for auscultation of the brachial artery; however, use of the diaphragm (flat) is common in practice and is acceptable.

The auscultation method of blood pressure measurement has gained universal acceptance. This technique, advocated by the American Heart Association, is described as follows.[4] The patient should be comfortably seated without the legs crossed. Prior to placement of the cuff, the brachial artery is located. The cuff is then placed snugly on the bared upper arm, with the lower border appearing approximately an inch above the antecubital fossa. The standard cuff typically has a mark or arrow that designates the midpoint of the cuff, which is centered above the previously palpated brachial artery (at the medial aspect of the tendon of the biceps). Then, while the radial pulse is palpated, the cuff is inflated until the radial pulse disappears; it is then inflated an additional 20-30 mm Hg. The stethoscope is placed over the previously palpated brachial artery at the bend of the elbow in the antecubital fossa (not touching the cuff), and no sounds should be heard. The pressure release valve is then slowly turned, allowing the needle to fall at a rate of 2 to 3 mm Hg per second. As the needle falls, a point is noted at which beating sounds (Korotkoff sounds) first become audible. This is recorded as the systolic pressure.

As the needle continues to fall, the sound of the beats becomes louder, then gradually diminishes until a point is reached at which a sudden, marked diminution in intensity occurs. The weakened beats are heard for a few moments longer and then disappear altogether (Figure 1-18). The most reliable index of diastolic pressure is the point at which sound completely disappears. Occasionally, muffled sounds can be heard continuously far below the true diastolic pressure. When this occurs, the initial point of muffling is used as the diastolic pressure. In older patients with a wide pulse pressure, Korotkoff sounds may become inaudible between systolic and diastolic pressure, and then may reappear as cuff deflation is continued. This phenomenon is known as the *auscultatory gap.*[4]

In the average healthy adult, normal systolic pressure ranges between 90 and 140 mm Hg and generally

Unfortunately, the physician is often not available to take a phone call, and a nurse or receptionist must relay the response of the physician. It is imperative that the conversation be recorded in the progress notes to ensure a permanent record. It is also recommended that a follow-up fax or letter should be sent to the physician that summarizes the conversation and asks that any corrections be faxed to the office. This should be attached to the patient's chart. The advantage of a letter or fax is that it provides a written statement of the physician's reply that can become a permanent part of the patient record.

RISK ASSESSMENT

Once collection of the patient's health data (history, clinical examination, laboratory test results, consultations) is complete, the data must be assessed to determine whether the patient can safely undergo dental treatment and what, if any, modifications in the delivery of dental care are required. One widely used method of expressing medical risk is the American Society of Anesthesiologists (ASA) Physical Classification System. This system was originally developed to classify patients according to their risk for general anesthesia; however, it has been adapted for outpatient medical and dental use and for all types of surgical and nonsurgical procedures, regardless of the type of anesthesia used. Briefly, the system is as follows:

ASA I   Normal healthy patient
ASA II   Patient with mild systemic disease that does
          not interfere with daily activity, or patient
          with a significant health risk factor (e.g.,
          smoking, alcohol abuse, gross obesity)
ASA III   Patient with moderate to severe systemic
          disease that is not incapacitating but that
          may alter daily activity
ASA IV   Patient with severe systemic disease that is
          incapacitating and is a constant threat to life

The implication is that as the classification level increases (ASA II through IV), so does the risk.

Although it is generally helpful to classify patients according to the ASA system, the practical usefulness of this system is limited in that it does not provide specific information about how treatment may need to be modified; thus, further consideration is necessary. This can be done by considering the ABCs of risk assessment (Box 1-2).

A:

Antibiotics. Will the patient need antibiotics, prophylactically or therapeutically?
Anesthesia. Are any potential problems or concerns associated with the use of local anesthetics or with vasoconstrictors found in the local anesthetic?
Anxiety. Will the patient need a sedative/anxiolytic?
Allergy. Is the patient allergic to anything that the dentist may prescribe or with which he or she may come into contact in the dental office?

B:

Bleeding. Is abnormal hemostasis a possibility?

BOX 1-2

Possible Issues or Concerns in Risk Assessment

A:
Antibiotics (prophylactic or therapeutic)
Anesthesia (type, vasoconstrictor)
Anxiety
Allergy

B:
Bleeding

C:
Chair position

D:
Drugs (interactions, adverse effects, side effects, allergies)
Devices (prosthetic valves, prosthetic joints, stents, pacemakers, A-V fistulas)

E:
Equipment (x-rays, ultrasonic scaler, electrosurgery, oxygen)
Emergencies (potential for occurrence)

AV, Arteriovenous.

C:

Chair position. Can the patient tolerate a supine chair position?

D:

Drugs. Have any potential drug interactions, adverse effects, or allergies been associated with any of the drugs being taken by the patient or with drugs that the dentist may prescribe?
Devices. Does the patient have prosthetic or therapeutic devices such as a prosthetic heart valve, prosthetic joint, coronary artery stent, pacemaker, or arteriovenous (AV) fistula that may require consideration?

E:

Equipment. Have any potential problems or concerns been associated with the use of dental equipment such as x-ray, ultrasonic cleaners, electrosurgery, or oxygen?
Emergencies. Can any medical emergencies be encountered with this patient?

TREATMENT MODIFICATIONS

On the basis of this assessment, modifications may need to be made in the delivery of dental treatment; these can be divided into preoperative, intraoperative, and postoperative modifications.

Examples include the following:
Preoperative:
• Prophylactic antibiotics given prior to certain dental procedures in a patient at risk for bacterial endocarditis

- Determination of the international normalized ratio (INR) prior to surgery in a patient taking Coumadin
- Ensuring food intake prior to dental treatment in a diabetic patient on insulin
- Prescribing an anxiolytic drug for an anxious patient with stable angina

Intraoperative:
- Limiting the amount of vasoconstrictor in a patient who takes a nonselective beta blocker
- Administering nitrous oxide/oxygen to an anxious patient with poorly controlled hypertension
- Using an upright chair position for a patient with heart failure
- Avoiding the use of electrosurgery in a patient with a pacemaker
- Avoiding elective radiographs in a pregnant patient

Postoperative:
- Use of extra local measures for hemostasis in a patient taking Coumadin
- Prescribing antibiotics for a poorly controlled diabetic following surgery
- Prescribing adequate post-operative analgesia for a patient on chronic steroids

Thus, through systematic assessment of risk and identification of potential problems, simple modifications in the delivery of dental treatment can be made in an effort to reduce risk to the patient. It should be remembered that risk is always increased when a medically compromised patient is treated; however, the goal is to reduce that risk as much as possible.

STRESS AND ANXIETY REDUCTION

In all patients, especially those with medical problems, stress and anxiety control is important and helps to reduce risk (see Box 1-1). Establishment of good rapport and trust is of paramount importance. Allowing the patient to ask questions and frank and open discussions are equally important. Explaining what is to be done before treatment is initiated often helps put a patient at ease. Short morning appointments may be better tolerated than appointments later in the day. In patients with pronounced anxiety or fear about a planned dental procedure, oral premedication with an anxiolytic/sedative drug 1 hour prior to an appointment is recommended. In addition, an anxiolytic/sedative can be prescribed the night before the appointment to ensure a good night's rest. One of the most commonly used drugs for this purpose is triazolam, a short-acting benzodiazepine. Other drugs such as diazepam, oxazepam, lorazepam, or hydroxyzine may also be used. If an anxiolytic or a sedative is prescribed, patients should be cautioned not to drive or operate machinery while under the influence of the drug. Intraoperative monitoring by pulse oximetry is recommended

for those who are sedated with oral medication. In addition to oral premedication, intraoperative inhalation sedation with nitrous oxide/oxygen may be considered for additional anxiolysis and sedation. This may be especially beneficial for patients with cardiovascular disease because oxygen is continuously administered during the procedure.

Injection of local anesthetic is the procedure that most patients fear; therefore, every effort should be made to avoid pain during administration. Keeping the needle and syringe out of the patient's sight until it is ready to use is important. Topical anesthetic should be applied, followed by slow advancement of the needle and slow injection of the solution after aspiration. Adequate time should then be allowed after injection to ensure adequate anesthesia prior to the start of work. It is imperative to ensure profound local anesthesia to prevent intraoperative pain.

At the completion of the appointment, it should be determined whether postoperative pain is likely; if so, appropriate analgesia should be prescribed. Instructions should be provided to the patient, along with a phone number to call if the patient needs to contact the dentist. An especially helpful tactic is to call the patient on the evening of the appointment to see how he or she is doing.

REFERENCES

1. Fletcher GF, Balady G, Froelicher VF, Hartley LH, Haskell WL, Pollock ML. Exercise standards: A statement for healthcare professionals from the American Heart Association. Circulation 1995;91:580-615.
2. Eagle KA, Berger PB, Calkins H, et al. ACC/AHA guideline update for perioperative cardiovascular evaluation for noncardiac surgery—Executive summary: A report of the American College of Cardiology/American Heart Association Task Force on Practice Guidelines (Committee to Update the 1996 Guidelines on Perioperative Cardiovascular Evaluation for Noncardiac Surgery). Circulation 2002;105:1257-1267.
3. Moraes D, McCormack P, Tyrrell J, Feely J. Ear lobe crease and coronary heart disease. Ir Med J 1992;85:131-132.
4. Pickering TG, Hall JE, Appel LJ, et al. Recommendations for blood pressure measurement in humans and experimental animals. Part 1: Blood pressure measurement in humans: A statement for professionals from the Subcommittee of Professional and Public Education of the American Heart Association Council on High Blood Pressure Research. Circulation 2005;111:697-716.
5. Chobanian AV, Bakris GL, Black HR, et al. The Seventh Report of the Joint National Committee on Prevention, Detection, Evaluation, and Treatment of High Blood Pressure: The JNC 7 report. JAMA 2003;289:2560-2572.

TABLE **1-2**
Clinical Laboratory Tests and Normal Values

Test	Range of Normal Values
COMPLETE BLOOD COUNT	
White blood cells	4400-11,000/mL
Red blood cells (male)	4.5-5.9 $10^6/\mu$L
Red blood cells (female)	4.5-5.1 $10^6/\mu$L
Platelets	150,000-450,000/μL
Hematocrit (male)	41.5%-50.4%
Hematocrit (female)	35.9%-44.6%
Hemoglobin (male)	13.5-17.5 g/dL
Hemoglobin (female)	12.3-15.3 g/dL
Mean corpuscular volume (MCV)	80-96 μm^3
Mean corpuscular hemoglobin (MCH)	27.5-33.2 pg
Mean corpuscular hemoglobin concentration (MCHC)	33.4%-35.5%
DIFFERENTIAL WHITE BLOOD CELL COUNT	MEAN %
Segmented neutrophils	56
Bands	3
Eosinophils	2.7
Basophils	0.3
Lymphocytes	34
Monocytes	4
HEMOSTASIS	
Bleeding time (BT)	2-8 minutes
Platelet function analyzer (PFA) 100	Closure time <175 seconds
Prothrombin time (PT)	10-13 seconds
Activated partial thromboplastin time (aPTT)	25-35 seconds
SERUM CHEMISTRY	
Glucose, fasting	70-110 mg/dL
Blood urea nitrogen (BUN)	8-23 mg/dL
Creatinine	0.6-1.2 mg/dL
Bilirubin, indirect (unconjugated)	0.1-1.0 mg/dL
Bilirubin, direct (conjugated)	<0.3 mg/dL
Calcium, total	9.2-11 mg/dL
Magnesium	1.8-3.0 mg/dL
Phosphorus, inorganic	2.3-4.7 mg/dL
SERUM ELECTROLYTES	
Sodium	136-142 mEq/L
Potassium	3.8-5.0 mEq/L
Chloride	95-103 mEq/L
Bicarbonate	21-28 mmol/L
SERUM ENZYMES	
Alkaline phosphatase	20-130 IU/L
Alanine aminotransferase	4-36 μ/L
Aspartate aminotransferase	8-33 μ/L
Amylase	16-120 Somogyi units/dL
Creatine kinase (male)	55-170 U/L
Creatine kinase (female)	30-135 U/L

Data compiled from McPherson RA, Pincus MR. Henry's Clinical Diagnosis and Management by Laboratory Methods, ed 21. Philadelphia, Saunders Elsevier, 2007, pp 1404-1418.

TABLE **1-1**
Classification of Blood Pressure in Adults and Recommendations for Follow-up

BP Classification	Systolic BP (mm Hg)	Diastolic BP (mm Hg)	Follow-up Recommended
Normal	<120	*and* <80	Recheck in 2 years
Prehypertension	120-139	*or* 80-89	Recheck in 1 year
Stage 1 hypertension	140-159	*or* 90-99	Confirm within 2 months
Stage 2 hypertension	≥160	*or* ≥100	Evaluate or refer to source of care within 1 month. For those with higher pressures (e.g., >180/110 mm Hg), evaluate and treat immediately or within 1 week, depending on the clinical situation and complications

From Chobanian AV et al: Seventh Report of the Joint National Committee on Prevention, Detection, Evaluation, and Treatment of High Blood Pressure. Hypertension 2003;42:1206-1252.

---

increases with age. Normal diastolic pressure ranges between 60 and 90 mm Hg. Pulse pressure is the difference between systolic and diastolic pressures. Hypertension in adults is defined as blood pressure that is equal to or greater than 140/90 mm Hg[5] (Table 1-1). It is recommended that blood pressure be measured twice during the appointment, separated by several minutes, and the average taken as the final measurement.

Respiration. The rate and depth of respiration should be noted through careful observation of the movement of the chest and abdomen in the quietly breathing patient. The respiratory rate in a normal resting adult is approximately 12 to 16 breaths per minute. The respiratory rate in small children is higher than that of an adult. Notice should be made of patients with labored breathing, rapid breathing, or irregular breathing patterns because all may be signs of systemic problems, especially cardiopulmonary disease. A common finding in apprehensive patients is hyperventilation (rapid, prolonged, deep breathing or sighing), which may result in lowered carbon dioxide levels and may cause disturbing symptoms, including perioral numbness, tingling in the fingers and toes, nausea, a "sick" feeling, and carpopedal spasms.

Temperature. Temperature is not usually recorded during a routine dental examination but rather when a patient has febrile signs or symptoms such as might be found with an abscessed tooth or a mucosal/gingival infection. Normal oral temperature is 98.6°F (37°C) but may vary by as much as plus or minus 1°F over 24 hours and is usually highest in the afternoon. Rectal temperature is about 1°F higher than oral, and axillary temperature is about 1°F lower than oral.

Weight. Patients should be questioned about any recent unintentional gain or loss of weight. A rapid loss of weight may be a sign of malignancy, diabetes, tuberculosis, or other wasting disease, whereas a rapid weight gain can be a sign of heart failure, edema, hypothyroidism, or neoplasm.

Head and Neck Examination

Examination of the head and neck may vary in its comprehensiveness but should include inspection and palpation of the soft tissues of the oral cavity, maxillofacial region, and neck, as well as evaluation of cranial nerve function. (See standard texts on physical diagnosis for additional descriptions.)

CLINICAL LABORATORY TESTS

Laboratory evaluation can be an important part of the evaluation of a patient's health status. Whether the dentist orders tests personally or refers the patient to a physician for testing, the dentist should be familiar with indications for clinical laboratory testing, what tests measure, and what abnormal results mean. Some indications for clinical laboratory testing in dentistry include the following:

1. Aiding in the detection of suspected disease (e.g., diabetes, infection, bleeding disorders, malignancy)
2. Screening high-risk patients for undetected disease (e.g., diabetes, AIDS)
3. Establishing normal baseline values before treatment (e.g., anticoagulant status, white blood cells, platelets)
4. Addressing medicolegal considerations (e.g., possible bleeding disorders, hepatitis B infection)

A comprehensive discussion of laboratory tests is beyond the scope of this chapter; however, Table 1-2 lists several common laboratory tests and ranges of normal values.

PHYSICIAN REFERRAL AND CONSULTATION

On the basis of medical history, physical examination, and laboratory screening, contact with the patient's physician for consultation or referral purposes may be warranted. Requests for information should be made in writing by letter or fax if possible; however, a phone call may be more expedient or convenient. The principal advantages of a phone call are the opportunity to obtain immediate information and the chance to ask follow-up questions.

Prevention of Problems	Treatment Planning Modifications
• If no other complications occur, dental procedures and surgery can usually be performed. • Screening with PFA-100 can be done, and, if less than 175 seconds, most surgeries can be performed.	• Usually none needed unless these are other medical problems, such as recent MI or stroke
• If no other complications occur, dental procedures and surgery may be performed.	• Usually none needed unless these are other medical problems such as recent MI or stroke

• Before radiation therapy is started, the dentist should be involved; after a complete examination, the following procedures should be done:
  • Extract teeth that cannot be repaired.
  • Extract teeth with advanced periodontal disease.
  • Perform preprosthetic surgery.
  • Restore large carious lesions.
  • Perform surgeries with adequate time for healing, or consider hyperbaric oxygen therapy.
  • Establish good oral hygiene.
  • Start daily fluoride treatment with the use of a flexible tray and gel.
  • Start sialogogue (pilocaprine HCl) therapy.
  • Treat endodontically, or extract nonvital teeth.
  • Treat chronic infection in jaw bones.
• During radiation treatment, the dentist can be involved with the following:
  • Symptomatic treatment of mucositis (see Appendix C)
  • Management of xerostomia (see Appendix C)
  • Prevention of trismus by having the patient use (several) tongue blades in the mouth as daily exercise
  • Chlorhexidine rinses for plaque and candidiasis control (see Appendix C)
  • Diagnosis and treatment of secondary infection—Candidiasis, etc. (see Appendix C)
  • Continue daily fluoride treatment.
• Following radiation treatment, the dentist should ensure the following:
  • Have patient back for frequent recall appointments (every 3 to 4 months).
  • Continue emphasis on good oral hygiene.
  • Treat carious lesions when first detected.
  • Make every effort to avoid oral infection.
  • Manage xerostomia (see Appendix C).
  • Manage chronic loss of taste (see Appendix C).
	• Once radiation treatment has been completed and more than 6000 cGy used, every effort must be made to avoid osteonecrosis:
	  • Teeth should not be extracted.
	  • Diseased teeth should be endodontically treated, if indicated.
	• Aggressive preventive measures are needed to prevent periodontal disease and cervical caries.
	• Most dental procedures other than extractions and surgical procedures can be done if performed atraumatically and without vascular compromise.

Dental Management: A Summary—cont'd

Potential Problems Related to Dental Care	Oral Manifestations
PATIENTS RECEIVING CHEMOTHERAPY FOR CANCER	
Chapter 26	
1. Excessive bleeding because of bone marrow suppression (thrombocytopenia)	• Mucositis
2. Prone to infection because of bone marrow suppression (leukopenia)	• Excessive bleeding following minor trauma
3. Severe anemia from bone marrow suppression	• Spontaneous gingival bleeding
4. Thrombocytopenia, leukopenia, and anemia are possible complications of underlying cancer.	• Xerostomia
	• Infection
	• Poor healing

Dental Management: A Summary—cont'd	
Potential Problems Related to Dental Care	**Oral Manifestations**

ANTIDEPRESSANT DRUGS (cont'd)

    b. Sedative, hypnotics, narcotics, and barbiturates may cause respiratory depression.

    c. Atropine: Increase intraocular pressure.

    d. Warfarin metabolism may be inhibited, thus causing bleeding.

3. Patients taking monoamine oxidase inhibitors (MOIs) must avoid foods that contain tyramine (may cause severe hypertension).

ANTIMANIC DRUGS

Chapter 29

1. Lithium

    a. Adverse effects include the following:

      • Nausea, vomiting, diarrhea

      • Metallic taste

      • Hypothyroidism

      • Diabetes insipidus

      • Arrhythmia

      • Sedation

      • Seizures

    b. Drug interactions (toxicity) include the following:

      • NSAIDs

      • Diuretics

      • Erythromycin

2. Valproic acid and carbamazepine

    a. Adverse effects include the following:

      • Nausea, ataxia, blurred vision

      • Tremor

      • Agranulocytosis (infection)

      • Platelet dysfunction (bleeding)

      • Seizures, if abruptly stopped

    b. Drug interactions (toxicity) include the following:

      • Erythromycin

      • Isoniazid

      • Cimetidine

Oral Manifestations:

• Lithium (metallic taste)

• Valproic acid and carbamazepine

    • Oral ulcerations

    • Bleeding

    • Infection

    • Tremor of the tongue

ANTIPSYCHOTIC (Neuroleptic) DRUGS

Chapter 29

1. Drug adverse effects include the following:

    a. Hypotension

    b. Acute dystonia, akathisia

    c. Parkinsonism

    d. Tardive dyskinesia

    e. Xerostomia, dry eyes

    f. Dizziness, postural hypotension

    g. Sexual dysfunction

    h. Seizures

    i. Neuroleptic malignant syndrome

    j. Agranulocytosis

2. Drug interactions include the following:

    a. Prolong or intensify the actions of the following:

      • Alcohol

      • Sedatives, hypnotics, opioids, antihistamines

      • Anesthetics (general)

    b. Antiarrhythmics—Increase risk of arrhythmia

    c. Anticonvulsants—Reduce effects of neuroleptic drugs

    d. Antihypertensives—Increase risk of hypotension

    e. Erythromycin—Increase serum level of neuroleptic drugs

    f. Sympathomimetics (epinephrine)—Risk for hypotension

Oral Manifestations:

• No significant oral findings are associated with these medications, unless the following drug adverse effects are present:

    • Agranulocytosis—Ulceration, infection

    • Xerostomia—Mucositis, caries, periodontal disease

    • Leukopenia—Infection

    • Thrombocytopenia—Bleeding

    • Tardive dyskinesia—Uncontrolled movement of the lips and tongue

- concentrations.
- Use epinephrine with caution and only in small concentrations.
- Avoid atropine in patients with glaucoma.
- Support patients as they get out of the dental chair.
- Change chair position slowly.
- Minimize effects of orthostatic hypotension:
- Consult with patient's physician to confirm current status and medications.
- Refer patients with significant drug adverse effects.
- Examination—Blood pressure, pulse rate, bleeding, soft tissue lesions, infection
- History
- Identify patients with significant drug adverse effects:
- Identify by medical and drug history patients who are taking any of these medications.

- Consider sedation with diazepam or oxazepam.
- Perform elective dental care only if patient is under good medical management.
- Avoid confrontational and authoritative attitudes.
- Schedule morning appointments.
- Have family member or attendant accompany the patient.

- If history and examination findings suggest presence of significant drug adverse effects, refer patients to their physician.
- Obtain good history, including medications (prescription, herbal, over-the-counter), and avoid using agents that may have significant interactions (see Table 29-6).
- If possible, involve family member or relative.
- Immediately refer patient who is suicidal for medical intervention.
  - 2. Do they have the means to carry out their plan?
  - 1. Do they have a plan?
- Ask if they have thoughts of suicide:
- If patients appear very depressed:

- Do not dispense to patients with narrow angle glaucoma.
  - Erythromycin
  - Ranitidine
  - Cimetidine
- Use in reduced dosage in patients taking:
- CNS depressant drugs.
- Do not dispense or reduce dosage for patients on other
- Use reduced dosage in older adults.
- Advise patient not to drive when using these medications.

- Provide treatment to deal with xerostomia (see Appendix C).
- Do not use topical epinephrine to control bleeding or in retraction cord.
  - 4. In general, do not use more than two cartridges.
  - 3. Aspirate before injecting.
  - 2. Use 1:100,000 concentration of epinephrine.
  - 1. Epinephrine is the vasoconstrictor of choice.
- For surgical or complex restorative procedures:
- Use without vasoconstrictor for most dental procedures.
- Local anesthetic:
- Avoid elective dental procedures until depression has been managed by medication or behavioral means.

- Complex dental procedures are usually not indicated.
- Family member or attendant may have to assist patient with home care procedures.
- Emphasis is on maintaining oral health and comfort by preventing and controlling dental disease.

- Dental treatment should be directed toward immediate needs with elective and complex procedures put off until effective medical management of depression and mania is obtained.
- Emphasis should be on maintaining the best possible oral health during depressive episodes.
- Patients often have little interest in dental health or home care procedures, and poor dental repair is common.

- Use anxiolytic drugs in dentistry for short durations to avoid tolerance and dependency.
- All dental procedures can be provided to patients on these medications.
- When using sedative agents, narcotics or antihistamines, reduce dosage or do not use these agents.

PART TWO

Cardiovascular Disease

Infective Endocarditis Prophylaxis

CHAPTER 2

Infective endocarditis (IE) is a microbial infection of the endothelial surface of the heart or heart valves that most often occurs in proximity to congenital or acquired cardiac defects.[1] A clinically and pathologically similar infection that may occur in the endothelial lining of an artery, usually adjacent to a vascular defect (e.g., coarctation of the aorta) or a prosthetic device (e.g., arteriovenous [AV] shunt), is called *infective endarteritis*.[1] Although bacteria most often cause these diseases, fungi and other microorganisms may also cause infection; thus, the term *infective endocarditis (IE)* is used to reflect this multimicrobial origin. The term *bacterial endocarditis (BE)* commonly is used, reflecting the fact that most cases of IE are due to bacteria; however, *IE* has become the preferred term and thus will be used in this chapter.

Previously, IE was classified as acute and subacute, to reflect the rapidity of onset and duration of symptoms prior to diagnosis; however, this classification was found to be somewhat arbitrary. It has now largely been replaced by a classification that is based on the causative microorganism (e.g., streptococcal endocarditis, staphylococcal endocarditis, candidal endocarditis) and the type of valve that is infected (e.g., native valve endocarditis [NVE], prosthetic valve endocarditis [PVE]). IE is also classified according to the source of infection, that is, whether community acquired or hospital acquired, or whether the patient is an intravenous (IV) drug user.

IE is a disease of significant morbidity and mortality that is difficult to treat; therefore, emphasis has long been directed toward prevention. Historically, various dental procedures have been implicated as a significant cause of IE because the oral flora is frequently found to be the causative agent. Furthermore, whenever a patient is given a diagnosis of IE caused by oral flora, dental procedures performed at any point within the previous several months have typically been blamed for the infection. As a result, antibiotics have been administered prior to certain invasive dental procedures in an attempt to prevent infection. It is of note, however, that the effectiveness of this practice in humans has never been substantiated, and that accumulating evidence questions the validity of this practice.

EPIDEMIOLOGY

IE is a serious, life-threatening disease that affects more than 15,000 patients each year in the United States; the overall mortality rate approaches 40%.[2] IE is a relatively rare disease that is most common in middle-aged and elderly persons, and is more common in men than in women. The incidence rate varies with the population under study. In the general population, it has remained relatively stable over the past 4 or 5 decades, ranging between 1.7 and 4.9 cases per 100,000 person-years.[1,3] A somewhat higher incidence has been reported, however, in more recent studies. A community study in Minnesota reported an incidence of 5 to 7 cases per 100,000 person-years, and a study in the metropolitan Philadelphia area reported an overall incidence of 11.6 per 100,000 person-years.[4,5] In the Philadelphia study, the rate of community-acquired IE was found to be 4.45 per 100,000 person-years, which is comparable to that reported in previous studies; however, the higher overall incidence was attributed to a high prevalence of intravenous drug users (IVDUs) in the population under study.

When populations at enhanced risk are considered, the incidence rate is increased. One study reported the lifetime risk of acquiring IE with various conditions.[6] In that study, the risk ranged from 5 per 100,000 person-years in the general population to 2160 per 100,000 person-years in patients who underwent surgical replacement of an infected prosthetic valve (Table 2-1). Previously, the most common underlying condition predisposing to endocarditis was rheumatic heart disease (RHD) (Figure 2-1); however, in developed countries, the frequency of RHD has markedly declined over the past

TABLE 2-1
Lifetime Risk of Acquiring Infective Endocarditis

Predisposing Condition	No. of Patients/100,000 Patient-Years
General population	5
MVP without audible cardiac murmur	4.6
MVP with audible murmur of mitral regurgitation	52
RHD	380-440
Mechanical or bioprosthetic valve	308-383
Cardiac valve replacement surgery for native valve	630
Previous endocarditis	740
Prosthetic valve replacement in patients with PVE	2160

Data compiled from Steckelberg JM, Wilson WR. Risk factors for infective endocarditis. Infect Dis Clin North Am 1993;7:9-19. MVP, Mitral valve prolapse; PVE, prosthetic valve endocarditis; RHD, rheumatic heart disease.

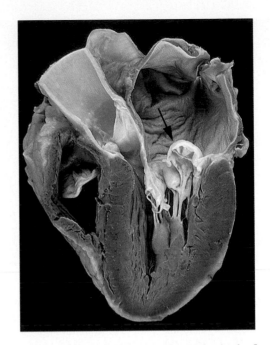

Figure 2-2. Prolapse of the posterior mitral valve leaflet into the left atrium. (Courtesy of William D. Edwards, MD, Mayo Clinic, Rochester, Minn. From Kumar V, Abbas AK, Fausto N. Robbins and Cotran Pathologic Basis of Disease, 7th ed. Philadelphia, Saunders, 2005.)

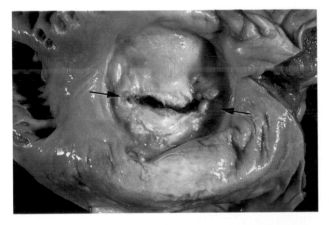

Figure 2-1. Mitral stenosis with diffuse fibrous thickening and distortion of the valve leaflets in chronic rheumatic heart disease. (From Kumar V, Abbas AK, Fausto N. Robbins and Cotran Pathologic Basis of Disease, 7th ed. Philadelphia, Saunders, 2005.)

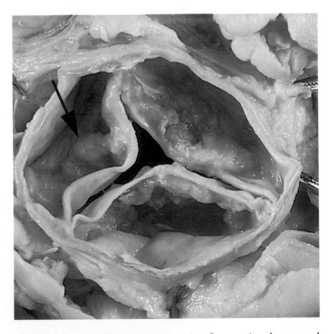

Figure 2-3. Calcific aortic stenosis of a previously normal valve. Nodular masses of calcium are heaped up within the sinuses of Valsalva. (From Kumar V, Abbas AK, Fausto N. Robbins and Cotran Pathologic Basis of Disease, 7th ed. Philadelphia, Saunders, 2005.)

several decades, and this disorder has become a much less significant factor. Mitral valve prolapse (MVP) (Figure 2-2), which accounts for 25% to 30% of cases of adults with NVE, is now the most common underlying condition among patients who develop IE.[5,7] Aortic valve disease (either stenosis or regurgitation or both) (Figure 2-3) appears to account for 12% to 30% of cases.[8] Congenital heart disease (e.g., patent ductus arteriosus, ventricular septal defect, bicuspid aortic valve) (Figure 2-4) is the substrate for IE in 10% to 20% of younger adults and 8% of older adults.[1,9] Tetralogy of Fallot, the most common type of congenital cyanotic heart disease, generally requires extensive reconstructive surgery for survival (Figure 2-5). PVE (Figure 2-6) accounts for 10% to 30% of all cases of IE.[1,9] It should be noted that in 25% to

47% of patients with IE, a predisposing cardiac condition cannot be identified[1] (Table 2-2).

The incidence of IE in IVDUs ranges from 150 to 2000 per 100,000 person-years.[7] Conversely, in patients with IE, the concomitant rate of IVDU ranges from 5% to 20%.[10] Several unique features of IE are seen in

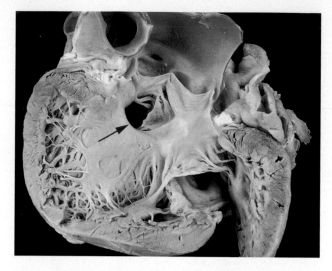

Figure 2-4. Gross photograph of a ventricular septal defect (defect denoted by arrow). (Courtesy of William D. Edwards, MD, Mayo Clinic, Rochester, Minn. From Kumar V, Abbas AK, Fausto N. Robbins and Cotran Pathologic Basis of Disease, 7th ed. Philadelphia, Saunders, 2005.)

IVDUs. In 75% to 93% of cases, the cardiac valves are normal prior to infection.[11,12] Also, in contrast to most other cases of IE, infection usually affects the right heart valves (tricuspid), and *Staphylococcus aureus* is the most common pathogen.[1] Thus, because of these unique characteristics, IE in IVDUs historically has not been linked to dental treatment.

ETIOLOGY

A total of 80% to 90% of cases of identified IE are due to streptococci and staphylococci.[2] This variation depends on the type of valve infected (i.e., native or prosthetic), whether the infection is community acquired or hospital acquired (nosocomial), and whether or not the patient is an IVDU. Streptococci continue to be the most common cause of IE, but staphylococci have been gaining increasing importance. Viridans streptococci (alpha-hemolytic streptococci), constituents of the normal oral flora and gastrointestinal tract, remain the most common cause of community-acquired NVE, without regard for IV drug

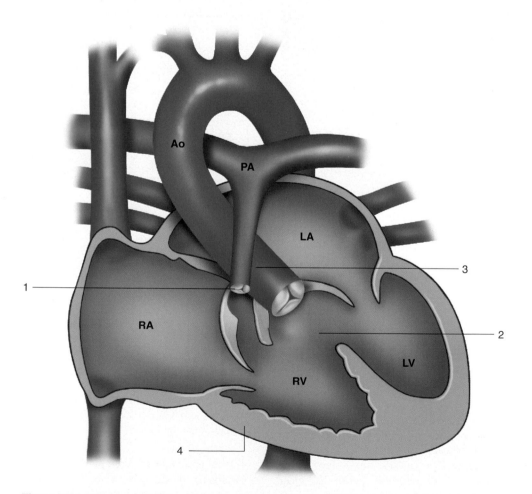

Figure 2-5. Tetralogy of Fallot. **1,** Pulmonary stenosis. **2,** Ventricular septal defect. **3,** Overriding aorta. **4,** Right ventricular hypertrophy. RA, Right atrium; RV, right ventricle; LA, left atrium; LV, left ventricle; Ao, aorta; PA, pulmonary artery. (From Mullins CE, Mayer DC. Congenital Heart Disease: A Diagrammatic Atlas. New York, Wiley-Liss, 1988.)

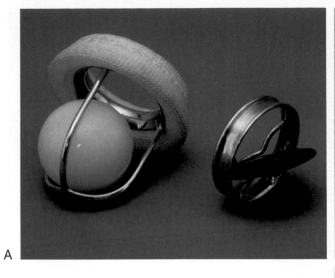

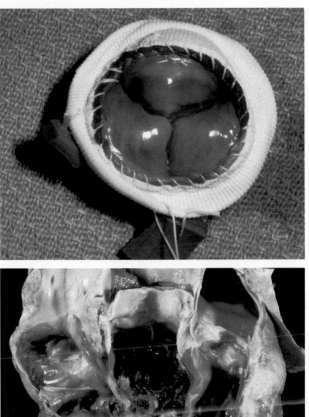

Figure 2-6. Prosthetic cardiac valves. **A,** Starr-Edwards caged ball mechanical valve. **B,** Hancock porcine bioprosthetic valve. **C,** Prosthetic valve endocarditis.

TABLE **2-2**

Predisposing Conditions Attributed to Infective Endocarditis (IE)

Underlying Condition	Percentage of Cases of IE
Mitral valve prolapse	25%-30%
Aortic valve disease	12%-30%
Congenital heart disease	10%-20%
Prosthetic valve	10%-30%
Intravenous drug abuse	5%-20%
No identifiable condition	25%-47%

abuse, and they cause 30% to 65% of cases of IE.[1] The species that most commonly cause endocarditis are *Streptococcus sanguis, Streptococcus oralis (mitis), Streptococcus salivarius, Streptococcus mutans,* and *Gemella morbillorum* (formerly called *Streptococcus morbillorum*).[13] Group D streptococci, which include *Streptococcus bovis* and the enterococci *(Enterococcus faecalis),* are normal inhabitants of the gastrointestinal (GI) tract and account for 5% to 18% of cases of IE.[14] *Streptococcus pneumoniae* has decreased in incidence and now accounts for only 1% to 3% of cases of IE.[2] Group A beta-hemolytic streptococci rarely cause IE.[1]

Staphylococci are the cause of at least 30% to 40% of cases of IE; of these, 80% to 90% are due to coagulase-

positive *S aureus.*[7] *S aureus,* the cause of most cases of acute IE, is the most common pathogen in IE associated with IV drug abuse. It is also the most common pathogen in nonvalvular cardiovascular device infections.[15] It should be noted that *S aureus* is not a normal constituent of the oral flora. In PVE, staphylococci are the most common pathogens in early and intermediate infections; however, streptococci predominate in late PVE.[7] The proportion of cases of IE due to *S aureus* appears to be increasing at community and university hospitals. This increase in the proportion of IE due to *S aureus* appears to be due in large part to increasing health care contact, such as through surgical procedures or the use of indwelling catheters.

Other microbial agents that less commonly cause IE include the HACEK group *(Haemophilus, Actinobacillus, Cardiobacterium, Eikenella, Kingella), Pseudomonas aeruginosa, Corynebacterium pseudodiphtheriticum, Listeria monocytogenes, Bacteroides fragilis,* and fungi.

PATHOPHYSIOLOGY AND COMPLICATIONS

Although the precise mechanism whereby IE occurs has not been fully elucidated, it is thought to be the result of a series of complex interactions of several factors involving endothelium, bacteria, and the host immune response. The sequence of events leading to infection usually begins

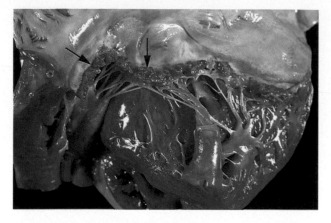

Figure 2-7. Nonbacterial thrombotic endocarditis (NBTE). (From Kumar V, Abbas AK, Fausto N. Robbins and Cotran Pathologic Basis of Disease, 7th ed. Philadelphia, Saunders, 2005.)

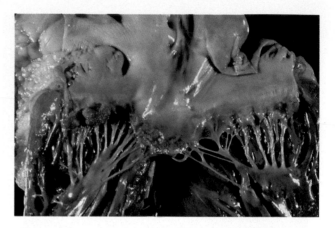

Figure 2-8. Viridans streptococcal endocarditis of mitral valve. (Courtesy W. O'Conner, MD, Lexington, Ky.)

with injury or damage to an endothelial surface, most often of a cardiac valve leaflet. Although IE can occur on normal endothelium, most cases begin with a damaged surface, usually in proximity to an anatomic defect or prosthesis. Endothelial damage can result from any one of a variety of events, including the following[1]:

- A high-velocity jet striking endothelium
- Flow from a high- to a low-pressure chamber
- Flow across a narrowed orifice at high velocity

Fibrin and platelets then adhere to the roughened endothelial surface and form small clusters or masses called *nonbacterial thrombotic endocarditis (NBTE)* (Figure 2-7). A similar and frequently indistinguishable condition is found in some patients with systemic lupus erythematosus and is called *Libman-Sacks verrucous endocarditis.* Initially, these masses are sterile and do not contain microorganisms. With the occurrence of a transient bacteremia, however, bacteria can be seeded into and adhere to the mass. Additional platelets and fibrin are then deposited onto the surface of the mass, which serves to sequester and protect the bacteria that undergo rapid multiplication within the protection of the vegetative mass (Figure 2-8). Once established, the metabolic activity and cellular division of the bacteria are reduced, which decreases the effectiveness of antibiotics. Bacteria are slowly and continually released from the vegetations and shed into the bloodstream, resulting in a continuous bacteremia; fragments of the friable vegetations break off and embolize. A variety of host immune responses to bacteria may occur. This sequence of events results in the clinical manifestations of IE.

The clinical outcome of IE depends upon several factors, including the following[1]:

- Local destructive effects of intracardiac (valvular) lesions
- Embolization of vegetative fragments to distant sites, resulting in infarction or infection
- Hematogenous seeding of remote sites during continuous bacteremia

- Antibody response to the infecting organism with subsequent tissue injury caused by deposition of preformed immune complexes or antibody/complement interaction with antigens deposited in tissues

Although combination antibiotic and surgical treatment is effective for many patients, complications are common.

The most common complication of IE, and the leading cause of death, is heart failure that results from severe valvular dysfunction. This most commonly occurs as a problem with aortic valve involvement followed by mitral and then tricuspid valve infection. Embolization of vegetation fragments leads to complications in up to 35% of cases of IE, with stroke being the most common.[3] In fact, stroke is the presenting sign of IE in up to 14% of cases.[16] Myocardial infarction can occur as the result of embolism of the coronary arteries, and distal emboli can produce peripheral metastatic abscesses. Pulmonary emboli, usually septic in nature, occur in 66% to 75% of IVDUs who have tricuspid valve endocarditis.[17] Emboli also may involve other systemic organs, including the liver, spleen, kidney, and abdominal mesenteric vessels. The incidence of embolic events is markedly reduced by the initiation of antibiotic therapy.[18] Renal dysfunction is also common and may be due to immune complex glomerulonephritis or infarction.[19]

SIGNS AND SYMPTOMS

The classic findings of IE include fever, heart murmur, and positive blood culture, although the clinical presentation may be varied. It is of particular significance that the interval between the presumed initiating bacteremia and the onset of symptoms of IE is estimated to be less than 2 weeks in more than 80% of patients with IE.[1,20] In many cases of IE that have been purported to be due to dentally induced bacteremia, the interval between the dental appointment and the diagnosis of IE has been much longer than 2 weeks (sometimes months), and thus it is

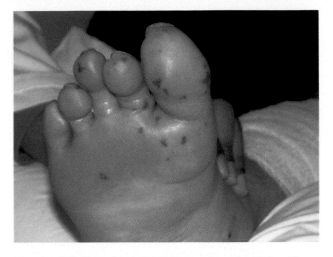

Figure 2-9. Petechiae in infective endocarditis. (From Goldman L, Ausiello D. Cecil Textbook of Medicine, 22nd ed. Philadelphia, Saunders, 2004.)

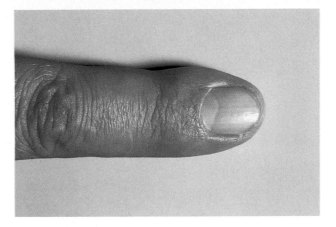

Figure 2-11. Splinter hemorrhages of the nail beds in infective endocarditis. (From Porter SR, Scully C, Welsby P, Gleeson M. Medicine and Surgery for Dentistry, 2nd ed. London, Churchill Livingstone, 1999.)

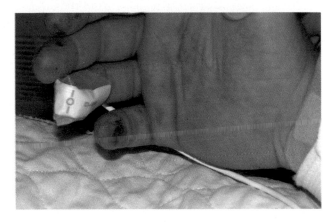

Figure 2-10. Osler's node in intective endocarditis. (From Goldman L, Ausiello D. Cecil Textbook of Medicine, 22nd ed. Philadelphia, Saunders, 2004.)

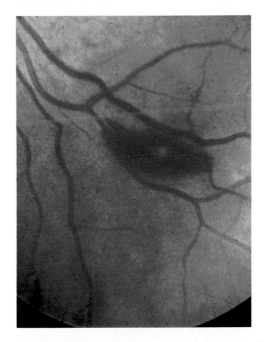

Figure 2-12. A Roth spot in the retina in infective endocarditis. (From Forbes CD, Jackson WF. Color Atlas and Text of Clinical Medicine, 3rd ed. Edinburgh, Mosby Ltd., 2003.)

very unlikely that the initiating bacteremia was associated with dental treatment.

Fever, the most common sign of IE, occurs in up to 95% of patients.[3] It may be absent, however, in the elderly or in patients with heart failure or renal failure. New or changing heart murmurs, systolic or diastolic, are found in 80% to 85% of patients.[1] Heart murmurs are often not heard initially in patients who are IVDUs but appear later in the course of the disease. This is characteristic of tricuspid valve IE caused by *S aureus*. Peripheral manifestations of IE due to emboli and/or immunologic responses are less frequently seen since the advent of antibiotics. These include petechiae of the palpebral conjunctiva, the buccal and palatal mucosa, and extremities (Figure 2-9), Osler's nodes (small, tender, subcutaneous nodules that develop in the pulp of the digits) (Figure 2-10), Janeway lesions (small, erythematous or hemorrhagic, macular nontender lesions on the palms and soles), splinter hemorrhages in the nail beds (Figure 2-11), and Roth spots (oval retinal hemorrhages with pale centers) (Figure 2-12).[1] Other signs include splenomegaly and clubbing of

the digits (Figure 2-13). Sustained bacteremia is typical of IE, and blood cultures are positive in most cases. Although up to 30% of cases of IE are initially found to be "culture negative," when strict diagnostic criteria are used, only 5% of patients are negative.[21] Many patients with negative blood cultures have taken antibiotics prior to the diagnosis of IE. Three separate sets of blood cultures obtained over a 24-hour period are recommended in the evaluation of a patient for suspected IE.[22]

The diagnosis of IE should be considered for a patient with fever with one or more of the following cardinal elements of IE: a predisposing cardiac lesion or behavior pattern, bacteremia, embolic phenomena, and evidence

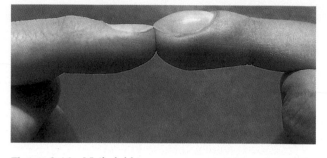

Figure 2-13. Nail clubbing may appear within a few weeks of development of IE. (From Zipes DP, Libby P, Bonow RO, Braunwald E. Braunwald's Heart Disease: A Textbook of Cardiovascular Medicine, 7th ed. Philadelphia, Saunders, 2005.)

of an active endocardial process.[1] The clinical presentation of IE is variable, and other conditions can cause similar signs and symptoms. The Duke criteria were developed and later modified to facilitate the definitive diagnosis of IE.[23,24] This set of diagnostic criteria assesses the presence or absence of major and minor criteria.

Major criteria include the following:
- Positive blood cultures
- Evidence of endocardial involvement (e.g., positive echocardiography, presence of new valvular regurgitation)

Minor criteria include those listed here:
- Predisposing heart condition or IV drug use
- Fever
- Vascular phenomena
- Immunologic phenomena
- Microbiologic evidence other than positive blood culture

Definitive diagnosis of IE requires the presence of two major criteria, one major and three minor criteria, or five minor criteria.

LABORATORY FINDINGS

Other than blood culturing, laboratory tests used for the diagnosis and treatment of IE are basic and nonspecific and may include a complete blood count with differential, electrolytes, renal function tests, urinalysis, chest x-ray, and electrocardiogram (ECG).[1,3] Patients with IE frequently have a normocytic, normochromic anemia that tends to worsen as the disease progresses. The white blood cell count may or may not be elevated. Urinalysis often reveals microscopic hematuria and proteinuria. Chest x-ray may be abnormal with evidence of heart failure. ECG may show evidence of conduction block with myocardial involvement or infarction. Other abnormal findings may include an elevated erythrocyte sedimentation rate, increased immune globulins, circulating immune complexes, and positive rheumatoid factor.

Echocardiography, transthoracic or transesophageal, is used to confirm the presence of vegetation in patients suspected of having IE; it has become a cornerstone in the diagnostic process. Positive echocardiographic evidence of vegetation is one of the major findings included in the Duke criteria.

MEDICAL MANAGEMENT

Prior to the advent of antibiotics, IE was almost always fatal. This has changed dramatically with early diagnosis and the institution of antibiotic therapy and/or surgery. Although the survival rate has greatly improved, the overall mortality rate still hovers around 40%.[2] However, the mortality rate varies significantly among different groups. For example, patients with viridans group streptococcal PVE have a mortality of approximately 20%, but the mortality of viridans group streptococcal NVE is 5% or less.[13,25] For nonaddicted patients with S aureus endocarditis, the mortality rate ranges between 25% and 40%, and for fungal endocarditis, the mortality rate exceeds 80%. For patients who are IV drug abusers with IE of the tricuspid valve, the mortality rate is between 2% and 4%.[11] The management of patients with IE requires effective antibiotic therapy and, for cases with significant structural damage, cardiac or surgical intervention.

Recently, guidelines for the diagnosis, antimicrobial therapy, and management of infective endocarditis have been revised as an American Heart Association (AHA) Scientific Statement.[13] Most strains of viridans streptococci, "other" streptococci (including *Streptococcus pyogenes*), and nonenterococcal group D streptococci (primarily *S bovis*) are exquisitely sensitive to penicillins, with a minimal inhibitory concentration (MIC) of less than 0.2 μg/mL.[2] Bacteriologic cure rates ≥98% may be anticipated in patients who complete 4 weeks of therapy with parenteral penicillin or ceftriaxone for NVE caused by highly penicillin-susceptible viridans group streptococci or *S bovis*. The addition of gentamicin sulfate to penicillin exerts a synergistic killing effect in vitro on viridans group streptococci and *S bovis*. A 2-week regimen of penicillin or ceftriaxone combined with single daily-dose gentamicin is appropriate for uncomplicated cases of endocarditis caused by highly penicillin-susceptible viridans group streptococci or *S bovis* in patients at low risk for adverse events caused by gentamicin therapy. For patients who are unable to tolerate penicillin or ceftriaxone, vancomycin is the most effective alternative.

Patients with endocarditis that is complicating prosthetic valves or other prosthetic material caused by a highly penicillin-susceptible strain (MIC ≤0.12 μg/mL) should receive 6 weeks of therapy with penicillin or ceftriaxone, with or without gentamicin for the first 2 weeks. Those with endocarditis caused by a strain that is relatively or highly resistant to penicillin (MIC >0.12 μg/mL) should receive 6 weeks of therapy with penicillin or ceftriaxone combined with gentamicin. Vancomycin therapy is recommended only for patients who are unable to tolerate penicillin or ceftriaxone.

Regardless of whether IE is community or hospital acquired, most *S aureus* organisms produce beta-lactamase; therefore, the condition is highly resistant to penicillin G. In this case, the drugs of choice for treatment of IE caused by methicillin-susceptible *S aureus* (MSSA) are the semisynthetic, penicillinase-resistant penicillins such as nafcillin or oxacillin sodium. For patients with native valve *S aureus* endocarditis, a 6-week course of oxacillin or nafcillin with the optional addition of gentamicin for 3 to 5 days is recommended. Staphylococcal PVE is treated similarly to NVE, except that treatment is given for a longer period. For strains resistant to oxacillin, vancomycin is combined with rifampin and gentamicin.

Surgical intervention may be necessary to facilitate a cure for IE or to repair damage caused by the infection. Indications for surgery include moderate to severe heart failure caused by valvular dysfunction, unstable or obstructed prosthesis, infection uncontrollable by antibiotics alone, fungal endocarditis, and intracardiac complications with PVE.[1]

DENTAL MANAGEMENT
Antibiotic Prophylaxis

Dental treatment has long been implicated as a significant cause of IE. Conventional wisdom has taught that in a patient with a predisposing cardiovascular disorder, IE was most often due to a bacteremia that resulted from an invasive dental procedure, and that through the administration of antibiotics prior to those procedures, IE could be prevented. Based on these assumptions, over the past 50 years, the AHA published nine sets of recommendations for antibiotic prophylaxis for dental patients at risk for IE.[20,26-33] (Table 2-3). These recommendations,

first put forth in 1955 and revised every few years, varied in terms of identification of risk conditions, selection of antibiotics, timing of antibiotic administration, and route of administration of antibiotics. It is important to recognize that although these recommendations were a rational and prudent attempt to prevent life-threatening infection, they were largely based on circumstantial evidence, expert opinion, clinical experience, and descriptive studies in which surrogate measures of risk were used.[34] Furthermore, the effectiveness of these recommendations has never been proved in humans. Recently, accumulating evidence suggests that many of the widely held assumptions on which these previous recommendations were made may not be accurate.

Source and Frequency of Bacteremia

The primary assumption that has driven the previous recommendations was that dental procedures were the source of most of the bacteremias that led to IE; therefore, antibiotics given just prior to dental procedures would prevent IE. Although it is undisputed that many dental procedures can cause bacteremia,[35-40] is also clear that bacteremia can result from many normal daily activities such as toothbrushing, flossing, using toothpicks, using oral water irrigation devices, and chewing[35,36,38,40-47] (Table 2-4). Given that the average person living in the United States has less than two dental visits per year, the frequency of and exposure to bacteremia is far greater through routine daily activities.[34] It is thus likely that the frequency and cumulative duration of exposure to bacte-

TABLE 2-3
Summary of Nine Previous Iterations of American Heart Association–Recommended Antibiotic Regimens (from 1955-1997) for Dental/Respiratory Tract Procedures (for adults)

Year	Primary Regimens for Dental Procedures
1955	600,000 U of aqueous penicillin and 600,000 U of procaine penicillin in oil containing 2% aluminum monostearate administered intramuscularly 30 minutes before the operative procedure
1957	For 2 days prior to surgery, 200,000 to 250,000 U of penicillin by mouth 4 times a day. On day of surgery, 200,000 to 250,000 U by mouth 4 times a day and 600,000 U aqueous penicillin with 600,000 units procaine penicillin IM 30 minutes before surgery. For 2 days after, 200,000 to 250,000 U by mouth 4 times a day
1960	Step 1: Prophylaxis 2 days before surgery with 600,000 U of procaine penicillin intramuscularly on each day Step 2: Day of surgery: 600,000 U procaine penicillin intramuscularly, supplemented by 600,000 U of crystalline penicillin intramuscularly 1 hour before surgical procedure Step 3: For 2 days after surgery: 600,000 U procaine penicillin intramuscularly each day
1965	Day of procedure: Procaine penicillin 600,000 U, supplemented by 600,000 U of crystalline penicillin intramuscularly 1 to 2 hours before the procedure For 2 days after procedure: Procaine penicillin 600,000 U intramuscularly each day
1972	600,000 U of procaine penicillin G with 200,000 U of crystalline penicillin G intramuscularly 1 hour prior to procedure and once daily for 2 days after the procedure
1977	Aqueous crystalline penicillin G (1,000,000 U intramuscularly) mixed with procaine penicillin G (600,000 U intramuscularly). Give 30 minutes to 1 hour prior to procedure, and then give penicillin V 500 mg orally every 6 hours for 2 doses
1984	Penicillin V 2 g orally 1 hour before procedure; then, give 1 g 6 hours after initial dose
1990	Amoxicillin 3 g orally 1 hour before procedure; then, 1.5 g 6 hours after initial dose
1997	Amoxicillin 2 g orally 1 hour before procedure

From Prevention of Infective Endocarditis. Guidelines From the American Heart Association. A Guideline From the American Heart Association Rheumatic Fever, Endocarditis, and Kawasaki Disease Committee, Council on Cardiovascular Disease in the Young, and the Council on Clinical Cardiology, Council on Cardiovascular Surgery and Anesthesia, and the Quality of Care and Outcomes Research Interdisciplinary Working Group. Copyright © 2007, American Heart Association, Inc.

TABLE 2-4
Reported Frequency of Bacteremia Associated With Various Dental Procedures and Oral Manipulation

Dental Procedure/Oral Manipulation	Reported Frequency of Bacteremia
Tooth extraction	10%-100%
Periodontal surgery	36%-88%
Scaling and root planing	8%-80%
Teeth cleaning	≤40%
Rubber dam matrix/wedge placement	9%-32%
Endodontic procedures	≤20%
Toothbrushing and flossing	20%-68%
Use of wooden toothpicks	20%-40%
Use of water irrigation devices	7%-50%
Chewing food	7%-51%

Data compiled from Wilson W, Taubert KA, Gewitz M, Lockhart PB, Baddour LM, Levison M, et al. Prevention of Infective Endocarditis: Guidelines From The American Heart Association. Circulation 2007;115:1-17. Available at http://www.circulationaha.org, DOI: 10.1116/circulationAHA.106.183095. Accessed April 19, 2007.

remia from routine daily events over 1 year are much higher than those resulting from dental procedures. It has been estimated that the risk of IE is many magnitudes greater with bacteremias resulting from normal daily activities than with those produced by a single dental procedure.[48,49] Accordingly, it is inconsistent to recommend antibiotic prophylaxis for dental procedures (which can be done) but not for these same patients during routine daily activities (which would be impractical and/or impossible).[34]

Magnitude of Bacteremia

Another assumption made is that the magnitude of bacteremia resulting from dental procedures is more likely to cause IE than that seen with bacteremia resulting from normal daily activities. No published data support this contention. Furthermore, the magnitude of bacteremia resulting from dental procedures is relatively low (fewer than 10^4 colony-forming units of bacteria per milliliter), is similar to that of bacteremia resulting from normal daily activities, and is far less than that (10^6 to 10^8 colony-forming units of bacteria per milliliter) needed to cause experimental BE in animals.[50-52] Thus, although the infective dose required to cause IE in humans is unknown, the number of microorganisms in blood after a dental procedure or associated with daily activities is similarly low, and cases of IE caused by oral bacteria probably result from frequent exposure to low inocula of bacteria in the bloodstream, resulting from routine daily activities and not from a dental procedure.[34] It also is noteworthy that most patients with IE have not undergone a dental procedure within the 2 weeks prior to the onset of symptoms.[53-55]

With this in mind, it would appear that emphasis on maintaining good oral hygiene and eradicating dental/oral disease would be important for decreasing the frequency of bacteremia produced by normal daily activities, although no controlled studies support this contention. It has been shown, however, that in patients with poor oral hygiene, the frequency of positive blood cultures just prior to dental extraction was similar to that following extraction.[49,56]

BLEEDING AND BACTEREMIA

Previous AHA recommendations have suggested that, on the basis of the likelihood that significant bleeding will be encountered during the procedure, prophylaxis should be provided for some dental procedures but not for others.[20] This has often been confusing for the practitioner and has resulted in conflicting and arbitrary decisions, because it is impossible to accurately predict the likelihood that significant bleeding will be encountered during a given dental procedure. Subsequently, it has been shown that visible bleeding during a dental procedure is not a reliable predictor of bacteremia.[49] Collective published data suggest that the vast majority of dental office visits result in some degree of bacteremia, and that it is not clear which dental procedures are more or less likely to cause transient bacteremia or to result in a greater magnitude of bacteremia than is caused by bacteremia produced by routine daily activities such as chewing food, toothbrushing, or flossing.[34]

Efficacy of Antibiotic Prophylaxis

The assumption that antibiotics given to at-risk patients prior to a dental procedure will prevent or reduce a bacteremia that can lead to IE is controversial. Some studies report that antibiotics administered prior to a dental procedure reduced the frequency, nature, and/or duration of bacteremia,[57-59] although others did not.[37,60-62] Recent studies suggest that amoxicillin therapy has a statistically significant impact on reducing the incidence, nature, and duration of bacteria associated with dental procedures, but it does not eliminate bacteremia.[57,58,63,64] However, no data show that such a reduction caused by antibiotic therapy reduces the risk of or prevents IE.[4]

No prospective, randomized, placebo-controlled trials have examined the efficacy of antibiotic prophylaxis for preventing IE in patients who undergo a dental procedure; it is highly unlikely that any such studies will ever be done because of the complex logistical and medicolegal issues that are involved. Some retrospective studies, however, have suggested that prophylaxis is beneficial, but these studies are small in size and report insufficient clinical data.[34] Also, in many of the cases cited in retrospective studies, the time interval between purported occurrence of bacteremia and onset of symptoms was longer than 2 weeks.

A study from the Netherlands by van der Meer and colleagues[65] investigated the efficacy of antibiotic prophylaxis for preventing IE in patients with native or prosthetic cardiac valves. Investigators concluded that dental or other procedures probably caused only a small fraction of cases of IE, and that prophylaxis would prevent only a small number of cases, even if it were 100% effective. In a case control study undertaken by the same authors,[66] among patients for whom prophylaxis was provided, 5 of 20 cases of IE occurred despite administration of antibiotics (75% efficacy rate at best), leading to the conclusion that prophylaxis was not effective. A more recent large, multicenter, case control study was undertaken in the Philadelphia area by Strom and colleagues[55] to evaluate the relationship between antibiotic prophylaxis and cardiac risk factors. The authors concluded that dental treatment was not a risk factor for IE even in patients with valvular heart disease, and that few cases of IE could be prevented with prophylaxis even if it were 100% effective. Finally, a recent French study[67] estimated that only about 2.6% of cases of IE occurred annually because patients were undergoing unprotected procedures, and that a "huge number of prophylaxis doses would be necessary to prevent a very low number of IE cases."

Risk of Bacterial Endocarditis Due to Dental Procedures

Although the absolute risk for IE caused by a dental procedure is impossible to measure precisely, the best available estimates are as follows: If dental treatment causes 1% of all cases of viridans group streptococcal IE annually in the United States, the overall risk in the general population is estimated to be as low as 1 case of IE per 14 million dental procedures.[34] The estimated absolute risk rates for IE caused by a dental procedure in patients with underlying cardiac conditions are as follows: mitral valve prolapse, 1 per 1.1 million procedures; congenital heart disease, 1 per 475,000; rheumatic heart disease, 1 per 142,000; presence of a prosthetic cardiac valve, 1 per 114,000; and previous IE, 1 per 95,000 dental procedures.[34]

Thus, although it has long been assumed that dental procedures may cause IE in patients with underlying cardiac risk factors, and that antibiotic prophylaxis is effective, scientific proof to support these assumptions is lacking. The AHA[34] has concluded that "of the total number of cases of IE that occur annually, it is likely that an exceedingly small number of these cases are caused by bacteremia-producing dental procedures. Accordingly, only an extremely small number of cases of IE might be prevented by antibiotic prophylaxis, even if it were 100% effective. The vast majority of cases of IE caused by oral microflora most likely result from random bacteremias caused by routine daily activities." Thus, on the basis of accumulated available evidence, the AHA has recently revised the 1997 recommendations.

CURRENT AMERICAN HEART ASSOCIATION RECOMMENDATIONS (2007)[34]

In summarizing the above data, the AHA cites the following reasons for revision of the previous recommendations:

- IE is much more likely to result from frequent exposure to random bacteremia associated with daily activities than from bacteremia caused by a dental procedure
- Prophylaxis may prevent an exceedingly small number, if any, of cases of IE in individuals who undergo a dental procedure
- The risk of antibiotic-associated adverse events exceeds the benefit, if any, from prophylactic antibiotic therapy
- Maintenance of optimal oral health and hygiene may reduce the incidence of bacteremia from daily activities and is more important than prophylactic antibiotics for reducing the risk of IE resulting from a dental procedure

Patients Recommended to Receive Antibiotic Prophylaxis[34]

Because no published data demonstrate convincingly that the administration of prophylactic antibiotics prevents bacteremia from an invasive procedure, it would seem logical that antibiotic prophylaxis should no longer be recommended prior to dental procedures for any patient. Indeed, a recent Cochrane review[68] concluded that no evidence supports the use of prophylactic penicillin to prevent endocarditis related to dental procedures. However, the AHA states the following:

> "We cannot exclude the possibility that there may be an exceedingly small number of cases of IE that could be prevented by prophylactic antibiotics in patients who undergo an invasive procedure. However, if prophylaxis is effective, such therapy should be restricted to those patients with the highest risk of adverse outcome from IE who would derive the greatest benefit from prevention of IE. In patients with underlying cardiac conditions associated with the highest risk for adverse outcome from IE, IE prophylaxis for dental procedures may be reasonable, even though we acknowledge that the effectiveness is unknown."

A similar approach is advocated in recently revised Guidelines for the Prevention of Endocarditis by the Working Party of the British Society for Antimicrobial Chemotherapy,[69] as well as in a recent update of the 1992 French guidelines.[70] The British document states that, in view of the lack of evidence of benefit, the most logical step is to withhold antibiotic prophylaxis for dental procedures. However, it was acknowledged that many clinicians would be reluctant to accept these "radical, but logical" changes, and therefore a compromise was accepted in which prophylaxis would be indicated only for those high-risk patients with the most serious outcome of IE.

Prior AHA recommendations used the lifetime risk for acquiring IE due to underlying cardiac disorders in the selection of patients who would receive antibiotic prophylaxis when undergoing dental procedures (see Table 2-1). Current guidelines, however, recommend antibiotic prophylaxis on the basis of risk of adverse outcomes from IE. Consequently, prophylaxis is recommended only for those patients with the most serious outcomes of IE. For

---

BOX 2-1

Cardiac Conditions Associated With the Highest Risk of Adverse Outcome From Endocarditis for Which Prophylaxis With Dental Procedures Is Recommended

- Prosthetic cardiac valve
- Previous infective endocarditis
- Congenital heart disease (CHD)[†]
  - Unrepaired cyanotic CHD, including those with palliative shunts and conduits
  - Completely repaired CHD with prosthetic material or device by surgery or catheter intervention during the first 6 months after the procedure[*]
  - Repaired CHD with residual defects at the site or adjacent to the site of a prosthetic patch or prosthetic device, which inhibits endothelialization
- Cardiac transplantation recipients who develop cardiac valvulopathy

From Prevention of Infective Endocarditis. Guidelines From the American Heart Association. A Guideline From the American Heart Association Rheumatic Fever, Endocarditis, and Kawasaki Disease Committee, Council on Cardiovascular Disease in the Young, and the Council on Clinical Cardiology, Council on Cardiovascular Surgery and Anesthesia, and the Quality of Care and Outcomes Research Interdisciplinary Working Group. Copyright © 2007, American Heart Association, Inc.
*Prophylaxis is recommended because endothelialization of prosthetic material occurs within 6 months after the procedure.
†Except for the conditions listed above, antibiotic prophylaxis is no longer recommended for any other form of CHD.

BOX 2-2

Dental Procedures for Which Endocarditis Prophylaxis Is Recommended for Patients in Box 2-1

- All dental procedures that involve manipulation of gingival tissue or the periapical region of teeth or perforation of the oral mucosa
- This includes all dental procedures except the following procedures and events:
  - Routine anesthetic injections through noninfected tissue
  - Taking of dental radiographs
  - Placement of removable prosthodontic or orthodontic appliances
  - Adjustment of orthodontic appliances
  - Shedding of deciduous teeth and bleeding from trauma to the lips or oral mucosa

From Prevention of Infective Endocarditis. Guidelines From the American Heart Association. A Guideline From the American Heart Association Rheumatic Fever, Endocarditis, and Kawasaki Disease Committee, Council on Cardiovascular Disease in the Young, and the Council on Clinical Cardiology, Council on Cardiovascular Surgery and Anesthesia, and the Quality of Care and Outcomes Research Interdisciplinary Working Group. Copyright © 2007, American Heart Association, Inc.

---

example, with viridans group streptococcal or enterococcal IE, outcomes of disease can vary widely between a relatively benign infection and death, with a mortality rate of less than 5% reported for streptococcal NVE.[13] However, patients with those underlying conditions listed in Box 2-1 virtually always have an adverse outcome, and thus, they are recommended for prophylaxis.

Dental Procedures for Which Antibiotic Prophylaxis Is Recommended[34]

Previous AHA recommendations[20] listed specific dental procedures for which antibiotic prophylaxis was recommended on the basis of the likelihood that significant bleeding would be encountered. However, a review of the published data suggests that transient viridans group streptococcal bacteremia may result from *any* dental procedure that involves manipulation of the gingival or periapical region of the teeth or perforation of the oral mucosa. Therefore, antibiotic prophylaxis is recommended only for patients listed in Box 2-1 who undergo any dental procedure that involves the manipulation of gingival tissues or the periapical region of a tooth, and for those procedures that perforate the oral mucosa (Box 2-2). This does not include routine local anesthetic injections through noninfected tissue, taking of dental radiographs, placement of removable prosthodontic or orthodontic appliances, adjustment of orthodontic appli-

ances, or the shedding of deciduous teeth and bleeding from trauma to the lips or oral mucosa.

Antibiotic Prophylaxis Regimens[34]

In the limited patient population for which antibiotic prophylaxis is recommended, prophylaxis should be directed against viridans group streptococci. Unfortunately, over the past 2 decades, a significant increase has been noted in the percentages of strains of viridans group streptococci resistant to the antibiotics recommended in previous AHA recommendations. In many studies, typical resistance rates of viridans group streptococci to penicillin range from 17% to 50%, for ceftriaxone from 22% to 42%, for macrolides from 22% to 58%, and for clindamycin from 13% to 27%.[34] Although this is indeed alarming, the effect on selection of prophylactic antibiotics is unclear. The AHA states the following:

"The impact of viridans group streptococcal resistance on antibiotic prevention of IE is unknown. If resistance in vitro is predictive of lack of clinical efficacy, the high resistance rates of viridans group streptococci provide additional support for the assertion that prophylactic therapy for a dental procedure is of little, if any, value. It is impractical to recommend prophylaxis with only those antibiotics, such as vancomycin or a fluoroquinolone, that are highly active in vitro against viridans group streptococci. There is no evidence that such therapy is effective for prophylaxis of IE, and their use might result in the development of resistance of viridans group streptococci and other microorganisms to these and other antibiotics."

Antibiotic prophylaxis should be administered in a single dose prior to the procedure. If the antibiotic is *inadvertently* not administered prior to the procedure, the dosage may be administered up to 2 hours after the pro-

TABLE **2-5**
Antibiotic Regimens for a Dental Procedure

Situation	Agent	Regimen: Single Dose 30-60 Minutes before Procedure	
		Adults	Children
Oral	Amoxicillin	2 g	50 mg/kg
Unable to take oral medication	Ampicillin or Cefazolin or Ceftriaxone	2 g IM or IV 1 g IM or IV	50 mg/kg IM or IV 50 mg/kg IM or IV
Allergic to penicillins or ampicillin (oral)	Cephalexin*† or Clindamycin	2 g 600 mg	50 mg/kg 20 mg/kg
	Azithromycin or Clarithromycin	500 mg	15 mg/kg
Allergic to penicillins or ampicillin and unable to take oral medication	Cefazolin or Ceftriaxone† Clindamycin phosphate	1 g IM or IV 600 mg IM or IV	50 mg/kg 20 mg/kg IM or IV

From Prevention of Infective Endocarditis. Guidelines From the American Heart Association. A Guideline From the American Heart Association Rheumatic Fever, Endocarditis, and Kawasaki Disease Committee, Council on Cardiovascular Disease in the Young, and the Council on Clinical Cardiology, Council on Cardiovascular Surgery and Anesthesia, and the Quality of Care and Outcomes Research Interdisciplinary Working Group. Copyright © 2007, American Heart Association, Inc.
IM, Intramuscularly; IV, intravenously.
*Or other first- or second-generation oral cephalosporin in equivalent adult or pediatric dosage.
†Cephalosporins should not be used in an individual with a history of anaphylaxis, angioedema, or urticaria following penicillins or ampicillin.

cedure. Table 2-5 lists the recommended antibiotic regimens for use for dental procedures in patients from Box 2-1. It should be noted that, because of the possibility of cross-allergenicity, the use of cephalosporins is not recommended for patients who have a history of anaphylaxis, angioedema, or urticaria (immediate onset IgE mediated hypersensitivity) caused by the administration of penicillin. It also is important to recognize that the use of antibiotics is not risk free and is associated with allergic reactions, adverse drug effects, and promotion of antibiotic resistance.

Study results are contradictory regarding the efficacy of using oral antimicrobial mouth rinses (e.g., chlorhexidine, povidone-iodine) to reduce the frequency of bacteremia associated with dental procedures; however, the preponderance of evidence suggests that no clear benefit is associated with their use. It is interesting to note, however, that British guidelines do recommend the preoperative use of chlorhexidine (0.2%) mouthwash.[69]

It is important that the dentist continue to identify from history taking those patients with cardiac conditions that increase risk for IE, such as mitral valve prolapse, rheumatic heart disease, or SLE. Patients with these conditions should be under the care of a physician for monitoring of the status of their valvular heart disease and potential complications. Also, when treating a patient with a cardiac condition that conveys an increased risk for IE, the dentist should remain alert and refer the patient with signs or symptoms of IE to his or her physician. This would apply whether or not the patient has received prophylactic antibiotics for dental procedures.

Special Situations[34]

Patients Already Taking Antibiotics. Patients who are already taking penicillin or amoxicillin for eradication of an infection (e.g., sinus infection) or for long-term secondary prevention of rheumatic fever are likely to have viridans group streptococci that are relatively resistant to penicillin or amoxicillin. Therefore, clindamycin, azithromycin, or clarithromycin should be selected for prophylaxis if treatment is immediately necessary. Because of cross resistance with cephalosporins, this class of antibiotics should be avoided. An alternative approach is to wait for at least 10 days after completion of antibiotic therapy before administering prophylactic antibiotics. In this case, the usual regimen can be used.

Patients Who Undergo Cardiac Surgery. It is recommended that a preoperative dental evaluation be performed and necessary dental treatment provided whenever possible prior to cardiac valve surgery or replacement or repair of congenital heart disease, in an effort to decrease the incidence of late PVE caused by viridans group streptococci.

Prolonged Dental Appointment. The length of a dental appointment in relation to the effective plasma concentration of an administered antibiotic is not addressed in these recommendations; however, for a lengthy appointment, this may be a matter of concern. With amoxicillin, which has a half-life of approximately 80 minutes, the average peak plasma concentration of 4 μg/mL is reached about 2 hours after oral administration of a 250-mg dose.[71] Most of the penicillin-sensitive viridans group streptococci have an MIC requirement of 0.2 μg/mL.[13] Thus, it would appear that a 2-g dose of amoxicillin would produce an acceptable MIC for at least 6 hours. If a procedure lasts longer than 6 hours, it may be prudent to administer an additional 2-g dose.

Other Considerations[34]

No evidence suggests that coronary artery bypass graft surgery is associated with long-term risk for infection; thus, antibiotic prophylaxis is not recommended for these

---

TABLE 2-6
Nonvalvular Cardiovascular Device–Related Infections

Type of Device	Incidence of Infection, %
INTRACARDIAC	
Pacemakers (temporary and permanent)	0.13-19.9
Defibrillators	0.00-3.2
Left ventricular assist devices	25-70
Total artificial hearts	To be determined
Ventriculoatrial shunts	2.4-9.4
Pledgets	Rare
Patent ductus arteriosus occlusion devices	Rare
Atrial septal defect and ventriculoseptal defect occlusion devices	Rare
Conduits	Rare
Patches	Rare
ARTERIAL	
Peripheral vascular stents	Rare
Vascular grafts, including hemodialysis	1.0-6
Intra-aortic balloon pumps	≤5-26
Angioplasty/angiography-related bacteremias	<1
Coronary artery stents	Rare
Patches	1.8
VENOUS	
Vena caval filters	Rare

From Baddour LM, Bettmann MA, Bolger AF, et al. Nonvalvular cardiovascular device–related infections. Circulation 2003;108: 2015-2031.

---

individuals. Patients who have had a heart transplant are at increased risk for acquired valvular dysfunction, especially during episodes of rejection. Endocarditis that occurs in this instance is associated with a high risk of adverse outcome; therefore, IE prophylaxis may be reasonable in these patients, although its usefulness has not been established. Patients with mechanical or tissue prosthetic valves will often be taking long-term anticoagulant medication (e.g., warfarin) to prevent valve-associated thrombosis. These patients are at risk for excessive bleeding during and after surgical procedures (see Chapter 25).

Implementation of the Recommendations

In view of the significant changes that have been made since previous AHA recommendations for antibiotic prophylaxis were put forth, it can be anticipated that patients may have questions and may be concerned about the implementation of these new recommendations. Patients with various valvular disorders (e.g., mitral valve prolapse, rheumatic heart disease) who have been told for many years that they needed antibiotics because of the risk for IE caused by dental treatment are now suddenly told that they no longer require antibiotics when they go to the dentist. Additionally, patients who were previously told that they required antibiotic prophylaxis only for invasive dental procedures (only those patients in Box 2-1) are now told that antibiotic prophylaxis is recommended for essentially all dental treatment. The AHA recommends dis-

cussing the reasons for the revision cited on p. 27 with the patient in an effort to alleviate concern. It is interesting to note, however, that the British guidelines do provide an appendix that can be given to patients to explain the rationale for changes.

It would seem that a reasonable approach is to share the new recommendations document with the patient and explain the rationale for changes, emphasizing that they are based on an extensive review of current scientific evidence. It is also recommended that the dentist consult with the patient's physician to ensure that he or she is aware of the new AHA recommendations, and to discuss their implementation in treatment of the individual patient. These conversations should be documented in the patient's progress notes.

Nonvalvular Cardiovascular Devices

In a recent AHA scientific statement, guidelines are provided regarding antibiotic prophylaxis for patients with various types of nonvalvular cardiovascular devices (e.g., coronary artery stents, hemodialysis grafts) who are undergoing dental procedures.[15] Table 2-6 provides a list of various devices, along with reported incidences of infection. After performing an extensive review of available data, the committee concluded that no convincing evidence suggests that microorganisms associated with dental procedures cause infection of nonvalvular vascular devices at any time after implantation. Indeed, infections of these devices most often are due to staphylococci,

TABLE **2-7**
Catheters Used for Venous and Arterial Access

Catheter Type	Entry Site	Comments
Peripheral venous catheters (short)	Usually inserted into veins of forearm or hand	Phlebitis with prolonged use; rarely associated with bloodstream infection
Peripheral arterial catheters	Usually inserted into radial artery; can be placed in femoral, axillary, brachial, posterior tibial arteries	Low infection risk; rarely associated with bloodstream infection
Midline catheters	Inserted via the antecubital fossa into the proximal basilica or cephalic veins; does not enter central veins, peripheral catheters	Anaphylactoid reactions have been reported with catheters made of elastomeric hydrogel; lower rates of phlebitis than with short peripheral catheters
Nontunneled central venous catheters	Percutaneously inserted into central veins (subclavian, internal jugular, or femoral)	Account for most catheter-related bloodstream infections
Pulmonary artery catheters	Inserted through a Teflon introducer into a central vein (subclavian, internal jugular, or femoral)	Usually heparin bonded; similar rates of bloodstream infection as central venous catheters
Peripherally inserted central venous catheters (PICCs)	Inserted into basilica, cephalic, or brachial veins and enter into superior vena cava	Lower rate of infection than nontunneled central venous catheters
Tunneled central venous catheters	Implanted into subclavian, internal jugular, or femoral veins	Cuff inhibits migration of organisms into catheter tract; lower rate of infection than with nontunneled central venous catheters
Totally implantable	Tunneled beneath skin with subcutaneous port access with a needle; implanted in subclavian or internal jugular vein	Lowest risk for catheter-related bloodstream infections; improved patient self-image, no need for local catheter site care; surgery required for catheter removal
Umbilical catheters	Inserted into umbilical vein or umbilical artery	Risk for catheter-related bloodstream infection similar with catheters placed in umbilical vein vs artery

From Centers for Disease Control and Prevention. Guidelines for the prevention of intravascular catheter-related infections. MMWR 2002;51:1-29.

Gram-negative bacteria, or other microorganisms in association with implantation of the device or resulting from wound or other active infections. Accordingly, the committee does not recommend routine antibiotic prophylaxis for patients with any of these devices who undergo dental procedures. Prophylaxis is recommended, however, for selected patients with these devices, including the following:

- Those undergoing incision and drainage of infection (abscesses)
- Those patients with residual leak after device placement for attempted closure of leaks associated with patent ductus arteriosus, atrial septal defect, or ventricular septal defect

Intravascular Catheters

Concerns often arise about the need for antibiotic prophylaxis to prevent infection in patients with various types of intravenous or intra-arterial catheters. Examples include peripheral venous catheters, peripheral arterial catheters, midline catheters, nontunneled central venous catheters, pulmonary artery catheters, peripherally inserted central venous catheters (PICCs), tunneled central venous catheters, totally implantable catheters, and umbilical catheters (Table 2-7). The causative micro-

organisms of these infections include coagulase-negative staphylococci, *S aureus*, enterococci, Gram-negative rods, *Escherichia coli*, *Enterobacter* and *Candida* species, *P aeruginosa*, and *Klebsiella pneumoniae*. None of these, with the exception of *Candida*, are normal inhabitants of the oral cavity; thus, they do not introduce risk for infection due to viridans group streptococci. The Centers for Disease Control and Prevention in its published Guidelines for the Prevention of Intravascular Catheter-Related Infections[72] does not include any recommendation for antibiotic prophylaxis for patients with any of these devices who are undergoing dental procedures.

REFERENCES

1. Karchmer AW. Infective endocarditis. In Zipes D, Libby P, Bonow RO, Braunwald E (eds). Braunwald's Heart Disease: A Textbook of Cardiovascular Medicine, 7th ed. Philadelphia, Elsevier Saunders, 2005, pp 1633-1658.
2. Bashore TM, Cabell C, Fowler V Jr. Update on infective endocarditis. Curr Probl Cardiol 2006;31:274-352.
3. Chambers H. Infective endocarditis. In Goldman L, Ausiello D (eds). Cecil Textbook of Medicine, 22nd ed. Philadelphia, Saunders, 2004, pp 1794-1803.

4. Berlin JA, Abrutyn E, Strom BL, et al. Incidence of infective endocarditis in the Delaware Valley, 1988-1990. Am J Cardiol 1995;76:933-936.
5. Tieyjeh I, Steckelberg J, Murad H, et al. Temporal trends in infective endocarditis: A population based study in Olmsted County, Minnesota. J Am Med Assoc 2005;293:3022-3028.
6. Steckelberg JM, Wilson WR. Risk factors for infective endocarditis. Infect Dis Clin North Am 1993;7:9-19.
7. Mylonakis E, Calderwood SB. Infective endocarditis in adults. N Engl J Med 2001;345:1318-1330.
8. Michel PL, Acar J. Native cardiac disease predisposing to infective endocarditis. Eur Heart J 1995;16(suppl B):2-6.
9. Hoen B, Alla F, Selton-Suty C, et al. Changing profile of infective endocarditis: Results of a 1-year survey in France. JAMA 2002;288:75-81.
10. Miro JM, del Rio A, Mestres CA. Infective endocarditis in intravenous drug abusers and HIV-1 infected patients. Infect Dis Clin North Am 2002;16:273-295.
11. Mathew J, Addai T, Anand A, et al. Clinical features, site of involvement, bacteriologic findings, and outcome of infective endocarditis in intravenous drug users. Arch Intern Med 1995;155:1641-1648.
12. Sande M, Lee B, Mills J, et al. Endocarditis in intravenous drug users. In Kaye D (ed). Infective Endocarditis, 2nd ed. New York, Raven Press, 1992, pp 345-359.
13. Baddour LM, Wilson WR, Bayer AS, et al. Infective endocarditis: Diagnosis, antimicrobial therapy, and management of complications. A statement for healthcare professionals from the Committee on Rheumatic Fever, Endocarditis, and Kawasaki Disease, Council on Cardiovascular Disease in the Young, and Councils on Clinical Cardiology, Stroke, and Cardiovascular Surgery and Anesthesia, American Heart Association— Executive Summary. Circulation 2005;111:3167-3184.
14. Megran DW. Enterococcal endocarditis. Clin Infect Dis 1992;15:63-71.
15. Baddour LM, Bettmann MA, Bolger AF, et al. Nonvalvular cardiovascular device–related infections. Circulation 2003;108:2015-2031.
16. Jones HR Jr, Siekert RG. Neurological manifestations of infective endocarditis: Review of clinical and therapeutic challenges. Brain 1989;112(Pt 5):1295-1315.
17. Mathew J, Addai T, Anand A, et al. Clinical features, site of involvement, bacteriologic findings, and outcome of infective endocarditis in intravenous drug users. Arch Intern Med 1995;155:1641-1648.
18. Heiro M, Nikoskelainen J, Engblom E, et al. Neurologic manifestations of infective endocarditis: A 17-year experience in a teaching hospital in Finland. Arch Intern Med 2000;160:2781-2787.
19. Majumdar A, Chowdhary S, Ferreira MA, et al. Renal pathological findings in infective endocarditis. Nephrol Dial Transplant 2000;15:1782-1787.
20. Dajani AS, Taubert KA, Wilson W, et al. Prevention of bacterial endocarditis: Recommendations by the American Heart Association. J Am Dent Assoc 1997;128: 1142-1151.
21. Hoen B, Selton-Suty C, Lacassin F, et al. Infective endocarditis in patients with negative blood cultures: Analysis of 88 cases from a one-year nationwide survey in France. Clin Infect Dis 1995;20:501-506.
22. Bayer AS, Bolger AF, Taubert KA, et al. Diagnosis and management of infective endocarditis and its complications. Circulation 1998;98:2936-2948.
23. Durack DT, Lukes AS, Bright DK. New criteria for diagnosis of infective endocarditis: Utilization of specific echocardiographic findings. Duke Endocarditis Service. Am J Med 1994;96:200-209.
24. Li JS, Sexton DJ, Mick N, et al. Proposed modifications to the Duke criteria for the diagnosis of infective endocarditis. Clin Infect Dis 2000;30:633-638.
25. Baddour LM, Wilson WR. Infections of prosthetic valves and other cardiovascular devices. In Mandell GL, Bennett JE, Dolin R (eds). Mandell, Douglas, and Bennett's Principles and Practice of Infectious Diseases. Philadelphia, Elsevier Churchill Livingstone, 2005, pp 1022-1044.
26. Dajani AS, Bisno AL, Chung KJ, et al. Prevention of bacterial endocarditis: Recommendations by the American Heart Association. JAMA 1990;264:2919-2922.
27. Shulman ST, Amren DP, Bisno AL, et al. Prevention of bacterial endocarditis: A statement for health professionals by the Committee on Rheumatic Fever and Infective Endocarditis of the Council on Cardiovascular Disease in the Young. Circulation 1984;70:1123A-1127A.
28. Kaplan EL. Prevention of bacterial endocarditis. Circulation 1977;56:139A-143A.
29. American Heart Association. Prevention of bacterial endocarditis. J Am Dent Assoc 1972;85:1377-1379.
30. Prevention of rheumatic fever and bacterial endocarditis through control of streptococcal infections. Circulation 1960;21:151-155.
31. Committee on Prevention of Rheumatic Fever, Bacterial Endocarditis, Rammelkamp CH. Prevention of rheumatic fever and bacterial endocarditis through control of streptococcal infections. Circulation 1957;15: 154-158.
32. Jones T, Baumgartner L, Bellows M, et al. Prevention of rheumatic fever and bacterial endocarditis through control of streptococcal infections. Circulation 1955;11: 317-320.
33. Prevention of bacterial endocarditis. Circulation 1965; 31:953-954.
34. Wilson W, Taubert KA, Gewitz M, Lockhart PB, Baddour LM, Levison M, et al. Prevention of Infective Endocarditis: Guidelines From The American Heart Association. Circulation 2007;115:1-17. Available at http://www.circulationaha.org, DOI: 10.1116/circulation AHA.106.183095. Accessed April 19, 2007.
35. Cobe HM. Transitory bacteremia. Oral Surg Oral Med Oral Pathol 1954;7:609-615.
36. Lockhart PB. The risk for endocarditis in dental practice. Periodontology 2000;23:127-135.
37. Lockhart PB, Durack DT. Oral microflora as a cause of endocarditis and other distant site infections. Infect Dis Clin North Am 1999;13:833-850, vi.
38. Pallasch TJ, Slots J. Antibiotic prophylaxis and the medically compromised patient. Periodontology 1996; 10:107-138.
39. Roberts GJ, Holzel HS, Sury MR, et al. Dental bacteremia in children. Pediatr Cardiol 1997;18:24-27.
40. Sconyers JR, Crawford JJ, Moriarty JD. Relationship of bacteremia to toothbrushing in patients with periodontitis. J Am Dent Assoc 1973;87:616-622.

41. Faden HS. Letter: Dental procedures and bacteremia. Ann Intern Med 1974;81:274.

42. Felix JE, Rosen S, App GR. Detection of bacteremia after the use of an oral irrigation device in subjects with periodontitis. J Periodontol 1971;42:785-787.

43. O'Leary TJ, Shafer WG, Swenson HM, Nesler DC. Possible penetration of crevicular tissue from oral hygiene procedures. II. Use of the toothbrush. J Periodontol 1970;41:163-164.

44. O'Leary TJ, Shafer WG, Swenson HM, et al. Possible penetration of crevicular tissue from oral hygiene procedures. I. Use of oral irrigating devices. J Periodontol 1970;41:158-162.

45. Rise E, Smith JF, Bell J. Reduction of bacteremia after oral manipulations. Arch Otolaryngol 1969;90:198-201.

46. Round H, Kirkpatrick HJR, Hails CG. Further investigations on bacteriological infections of the mouth. Proc R Soc Med 1936;29:1552-1556.

47. Schlein RA, Kudlick EM, Reindorf CA, et al. Toothbrushing and transient bacteremia in patients undergoing orthodontic treatment. Am J Orthod Dentofacial Orthop 1991;99:466-472.

48. Guntheroth WG. How important are dental procedures as a cause of infective endocarditis? Am J Cardiol 1984;54:797-801.

49. Roberts GJ. Dentists are innocent! "Everyday" bacteremia is the real culprit: A review and assessment of the evidence that dental surgical procedures are a principal cause of bacterial endocarditis in children. Pediatr Cardiol 1999;20:317-325.

50. Durack DT, Beeson PB. Experimental bacterial endocarditis. II. Survival of bacteria in endocardial vegetations. Br J Exp Pathol 1972;53:50-53.

51. Lucas VS, Lytra V, Hassan T, et al. Comparison of lysis filtration and an automated blood culture system (BACTEC) for detection, quantification, and identification of odontogenic bacteremia in children. J Clin Microbiol 2002;40:3416-3420.

52. Roberts GJ, Jaffray EC, Spratt DA, et al. Duration, prevalence and intensity of bacteraemia after dental extractions in children. Heart 2006;92:1274-1277.

53. Durack DT. Prevention of infective endocarditis. N Engl J Med 1995;332:38-44.

54. Durack DT. Antibiotics for prevention of endocarditis during dentistry: Time to scale back? Ann Intern Med 1998;129:829-831.

55. Strom BL, Abrutyn E, Berlin JA, et al. Dental and cardiac risk factors for infective endocarditis: A population-based, case-control study. Ann Intern Med 1998;129:761-769.

56. Hockett RN, Loesche WJ, Sodeman TM. Bacteraemia in asymptomatic human subjects. Arch Oral Biol 1977;22:91-98.

57. Lockhart PB, Brennan MT, Kent ML, et al. Impact of amoxicillin prophylaxis on the incidence, nature, and duration of bacteremia in children after intubation and dental procedures. Circulation 2004;109:2878-2884.

58. Roberts GJ, Radford P, Holt R. Prophylaxis of dental bacteraemia with oral amoxicillin in children. Br Dent J 1987;162:179-182.

59. Shanson DC, Akash S, Harris M, Tadayon M. Erythromycin stearate, 1.5 g, for the oral prophylaxis of streptococcal bacteraemia in patients undergoing dental extraction: Efficacy and tolerance. J Antimicrob Chemother 1985;15:83-90.

60. Hall G, Hedstrom SA, Heimdahl A, Nord CE. Prophylactic administration of penicillins for endocarditis does not reduce the incidence of postextraction bacteremia. Clin Infect Dis 1993;17:188-194.

61. Hall G, Heimdahl A, Nord CE. Effects of prophylactic administration of cefaclor on transient bacteremia after dental extraction. Eur J Clin Microbiol Infect Dis 1996;15:646-649.

62. Hall G, Heimdahl A, Nord CE. Bacteremia after oral surgery and antibiotic prophylaxis for endocarditis. Clin Infect Dis 1999;29:1-8; quiz 9-10.

63. Lockhart PB. An analysis of bacteremias during dental extractions: A double-blind, placebo-controlled study of chlorhexidine. Arch Intern Med 1996;156:513-520.

64. Brennan MT, Kent ML, Fox PC, et al. The impact of oral disease and nonsurgical treatment on bacteremia in children. J Am Dent Assoc 2007;138:80-85.

65. van der Meer JT, Thompson J, Valkenburg HA, Michel MF. Epidemiology of bacterial endocarditis in The Netherlands. II. Antecedent procedures and use of prophylaxis. Arch Intern Med 1992;152:1869-1873.

66. van der Meer JT, Van Wijk W, Thompson J, et al. Efficacy of antibiotic prophylaxis for prevention of native-valve endocarditis. Lancet 1992;339:135-139.

67. Duval X, Alla F, Hoen B, et al. Estimated risk of endocarditis in adults with predisposing cardiac conditions undergoing dental procedures with or without antibiotic prophylaxis. Clin Infect Dis 2006;42:e102-e107.

68. Oliver R, Roberts GJ, Hooper L. Penicillins for the prophylaxis of bacterial endocarditis in dentistry. Cochrane Database Syst Rev 2004(2):CD003813.

69. Gould FK, Elliott TS, Foweraker J, et al. Guidelines for the prevention of endocarditis: Report of the Working Party of the British Society for Antimicrobial Chemotherapy. J Antimicrob Chemother 2006;57:1035-1042.

70. Danchin N, Duval X, Leport C. Prophylaxis of infective endocarditis: French recommendations 2002. Heart 2005;91:715-718.

71. Petri WA. Penicillins, cephalosporins, and other β-lactam antibiotics. In Brunton LL, Lazo JS, Parker KL (eds). Goodman and Gilman's The Pharmacological Basis of Therapeutics, 11th ed. New York, McGraw-Hill, 2006, pp 1127-1154.

72. O'Grady NP, Alexander M, Dellinger EP, et al. Guidelines for the prevention of intravascular catheter–related infections. Centers for Disease Control and Prevention. MMWR Recomm Rep 2002;51:1-29.

Hypertension

CHAPTER 3

Hypertension is an abnormal elevation in arterial pressure that can be fatal if sustained and untreated. People with hypertension may not display symptoms for many years but eventually can experience symptomatic damage to several target organs, including kidneys, heart, brain, and eyes. In adults, a sustained systolic blood pressure of 140 mm Hg or greater and/or a sustained diastolic blood pressure of 90 mm Hg or greater is defined as hypertension. The Seventh Report of the Joint National Committee on Prevention, Detection, Evaluation, and Treatment of High Blood Pressure (JNC 7) provided several revisions to the previous 1997 guidelines[1] (Table 3-1). These new guidelines include an updated classification that redefines "normal" blood pressure as <120/80 mm Hg and introduces a new category of "prehypertension" (120-139/80-89 mm Hg), which encompasses the previously designated categories of "normal" and "borderline" hypertension. This reflects the findings that health risks are increased with blood pressures as low as 115/75 mm Hg and that lowering blood pressure in patients with what was formerly considered "normal" or "borderline" blood pressure can result in decreased adverse vascular events such as stroke and myocardial infarction (MI). In addition, the previously designated stages 2 and 3 of hypertension were combined into a single stage 2 category because treatment for both groups is essentially the same. Table 3-1 also includes recommendations for follow-up care based on initial blood pressure measurements. A separate publication provides similar information on the classification, detection, diagnosis, and management of hypertension in children and adolescents, while updating 1996 guidelines.[2] In children and adolescents, hypertension is defined as elevated blood pressure that persists on repeated measurement at the 95th percentile or greater for age, height, and gender (Table 3-2 and Table 3-3). For example, according to Table 3-3, a 6-year-old girl who is at the 50th percentile in height would be considered to have

hypertension if her blood pressure was persistently ≥111/74 mm Hg.

The dental health professional can play a significant role in the detection and control of hypertension and may well be the first to detect a patient with an elevation in blood pressure or with symptoms of hypertensive disease. Along with detection, monitoring is an equally valuable service because patients who are receiving treatment for hypertension but may not be adequately controlled because of poor compliance or inappropriate drug selection or dosing. The JNC 7 specifically encourages the active participation of all health care professionals in the detection of hypertension and the surveillance of treatment compliance.[3] Only a physician can make the diagnosis of hypertension and decide upon its treatment. The dentist, however, should detect abnormal blood pressure measurements, which then become the basis for referral to or consultation with a physician.

The dental patient with hypertension poses several potentially significant management considerations. These include identification of disease, monitoring, stress and anxiety reduction, prevention of drug interactions, and awareness and management of drug adverse effects.

GENERAL DESCRIPTION
Prevalence

With 35 million office visits annually, hypertension is the most common primary diagnosis in America.[3] Prior to 1990, the prevalence of hypertension was steadily declining; however, recent evidence indicates that the trend has reversed, and hypertension is once again on the rise.[4] According to National Health and Nutrition Examination Survey (NHANES) data for the period 1999 to 2000, at least 65 million adults in the United States have high blood pressure (HBP) or are taking antihypertensive medication.[5] This is about one third of the population and represents a 30% increase from the period 1988 to

TABLE 3-1

Classification of Blood Pressure in Adults and Recommendations for Follow-up

BP Classification	Systolic BP (mm Hg)	Diastolic BP (mm Hg)	Recommended Follow-up
Normal	<120	*and* <80	Recheck in 2 years
Prehypertension	120-139	*or* 80-89	Recheck in 1 year
Stage 1 hypertension	140-159	*or* 90-99	Confirm within 2 months
Stage 2 hypertension	≥160	*or* ≥100	Evaluate or refer to source of care within 1 month. For those with higher pressures (e.g., >180/110 mm Hg), evaluate and treat immediately or within 1 week, depending on the clinical situation and complications

From Chobanian AV et al: Seventh Report of the Joint National Committee on Prevention, Detection, Evaluation, and Treatment of High Blood Pressure. Hypertension 2003;42:1206-1252.
BP, Blood pressure.

TABLE 3-2

Classification of Blood Pressure in Children and Adolescents

BP Classification	SBP or DBP Percentile*
Normal	<90th
Prehypertension	90th to <95th, or BP exceeds 120/80 even if <90th percentile up to <95th percentile
Stage 1 hypertension	95th-99th percentile plus 5 mm Hg
Stage 2 hypertension	>99th percentile plus 5 mm Hg

Modified from The Fourth Report on the Diagnosis, Evaluation, and Treatment of High Blood Pressure in Children and Adolescents. Pediatrics 2004;114:555-576.
BP, Blood pressure; DBP, diastolic blood pressure; SBP, systolic blood pressure.
*For gender, age, and height, as measured on at least three separate occasions.

1994.[6] This marked increase is attributed to aging of the population and to the epidemic increase in obesity. The National High Blood Pressure Education Program was begun in 1972, and in a little more than 3 decades, it has had significant success.[3] The number of people with HBP who are aware of their condition has increased from 51% to 70%, and the percentage of those receiving treatment for HBP has increased from 31% to 59%. The percentage of patients taking medication whose blood pressure is controlled to <140/90 increased from 10% to 34% during the same time period. Concomitant with increased awareness and treatment has been a significant decline in mortality from coronary heart disease (50%) and from stroke (57%), although this decline has slowed in recent years.[3] Although these trends are encouraging, 30% of patients with HBP remain unaware of their disease, 40% of patients with HBP are not being treated, and more than 60% of hypertensive patients are taking medications but are not being adequately controlled.

Diagnosis and treatment of hypertension once were largely based on diastolic blood pressure; however, with growing recognition of the importance of systolic blood pressure, this is no longer the case. Isolated systolic hypertension gradually increases with age such that among patients over the age of 50, it is the most prevalent form of hypertension.

The prevalence of high blood pressure increases with aging, such that more than half of all Americans aged 65 and older have hypertension.[7] Systolic blood pressure continues to rise throughout life, but diastolic blood pressure rises until around age 50 and then levels off or falls. After the age of 50, isolated systolic hypertension becomes the more prevalent pattern.[8] In one study, isolated systolic hypertension was identified in 87% of inadequately controlled patients older than 60 years of age.[9] Isolated diastolic hypertension is most commonly seen before age 50. Diastolic blood pressure is a more potent cardiovascular risk factor than is systolic blood pressure until age 50; thereafter, systolic blood pressure is more important.[10]

Prevalence varies with race as well and is highest among African Americans. In general, it is lower among Hispanics than among whites; however, variation has been noted among racial subgroups. For example, the prevalence of hypertension among Mexican Americans is lower than among non-Hispanic whites, although among Puerto Rican Americans, it is higher.[11,12] Prevalence is generally higher in Asian Americans, Native Americans, and Native Alaskans than in whites; however, again, variation is seen among subgroups.[13]

Etiology

About 90% of patients have no identifiable cause for their disease, which is referred to as *essential, primary,* or *idiopathic* hypertension. For the remaining 10% of patients, an underlying cause or condition may be identified; for these patients, the term *secondary* hypertension is applied. The most common cause of secondary hypertension is renal parenchymal disease, followed by renovascular disease and various adrenal disorders.[8] Most conditions that cause secondary hypertension lead to an elevation in diastolic and systolic blood pressure. Box 3-1 is a listing of the most common identifiable causes of hypertension. Lifestyle can play an important role in the severity and

TABLE **3-3**

95th Percentile of Blood Pressure by Selected Ages, by the 50th and 75th Height Percentiles, and by Gender in Children and Adolescents

Age, yr	Girls' SBP/DBP		Boys' SBP/DBP	
	50th Percentile for Height	75th Percentile for Height	50th Percentile for Height	75th Percentile for Height
1	104/58	105/59	103/56	104/57
6	111/74	113/74	114/74	115/75
12	123/80	124/81	123/81	125/82
17	129/84	130/85	136/87	138/87

Compiled from the Fourth Report on the Diagnosis, Evaluation, and Treatment of High Blood Pressure in Children and Adolescents. Pediatrics 2004;114:555-576.
DBP, Diastolic blood pressure; SBP, systolic blood pressure.

BOX **3-1**

Identifiable Causes of Hypertension

- Chronic kidney disease
- Coarctation of the aorta
- Cushing's syndrome and other glucocorticoid excess states, including chronic long-term steroid therapy
- Drug-induced or drug-related (e.g., NSAIDs, oral contraceptives, decongestants)
- Obstructive uropathy
- Pheochromocytoma
- Primary aldosteronism and other mineralocorticoid excess states
- Renovascular hypertension
- Sleep apnea
- Thyroid or parathyroid disease

From Chobanian AV et al: Seventh Report of the Joint National Committee on Prevention, Detection, Evaluation, and Treatment of High Blood Pressure. Hypertension 2003;42:1206-1252.
NSAIDs, Nonsteroidal antiinflammatory drugs.

progression of hypertension; obesity, excessive alcohol intake, excessive dietary sodium, and physical inactivity are significant contributing factors.

Many patients with secondary hypertension may be cured with treatment of the underlying condition. Patients with secondary hypertension caused by unilateral renal disease such as renal artery obstruction or pyelonephritis may be cured by surgical correction of the defect or removal of the diseased kidney. In a few patients with secondary hypertension, a pheochromocytoma of the adrenal medulla has been found to be responsible. This lesion is surgically treatable. Hyperfunction of the adrenal gland caused by a tumor of the adrenal cortex or cortical hyperplasia may cause secondary hypertension in a few cases. These conditions also are amenable to surgery. Recently, obstructive sleep apnea has been recognized as an independent cause of hypertension; it is correctable with successful treatment (see Chapter 10).

Pathophysiology and Complications

In sustained essential hypertension, the basic underlying defect is a failure in the regulation of vascular resistance.

The pulsating force is modified by the degree of elasticity of the walls of larger arteries and the resistance of the arteriolar bed. Control of vascular resistance is multifactorial, and abnormalities may exist in one or more areas. Mechanisms of control include neural reflexes and ongoing maintenance of sympathetic vasomotor tone; neurotransmitters such as norepinephrine, extracellular fluid, and sodium stores; the renin-angiotensin-aldosterone pressor system; and locally active hormones and autacoids such as prostaglandins, kinins, adenosine, and hydrogen ions (H^+). In isolated systolic hypertension, which is commonly seen in the elderly, the problem is one of central arterial stiffness and loss of elasticity.[8]

Many physiologic factors may have an effect on blood pressure. Increased viscosity of the blood (e.g., polycythemia) may cause an elevation in blood pressure that results from an increase in resistance to flow. A decrease in blood volume or tissue fluid volume (e.g., anemia, hemorrhage) reduces blood pressure. Conversely, an increase in blood volume or tissue fluid volume (e.g., sodium/fluid retention) increases blood pressure. Increases in cardiac output associated with exercise, fever, and thyrotoxicosis also may increase blood pressure.

A linear relationship exists between blood pressures at any level above normal and an increase in morbidity and mortality rates from stroke and coronary heart disease. Blood pressures as low as 115 mm Hg systolic and 75 mm Hg diastolic and upward are associated with increased risk of cardiovascular disease.[14] It is estimated that about 15% of all blood pressure–related deaths from coronary heart disease occur in individuals with blood pressure in the prehypertensive range.[15] However, the higher the blood pressure, the greater the chances of heart attack, heart failure, stroke, and kidney disease. For every 20 mm Hg systolic and 10 mm Hg diastolic increase in blood pressure, a doubling of mortality from ischemic heart disease and stroke occurs.[3] Hypertension precedes the onset of vascular changes in the kidney, heart, brain, and retina that lead to such clinical complications as renal failure, cerebrovascular accident, coronary insufficiency, MI, congestive heart failure, dementia, encephalopathy, and blindness. If untreated, about 50% of hypertensive

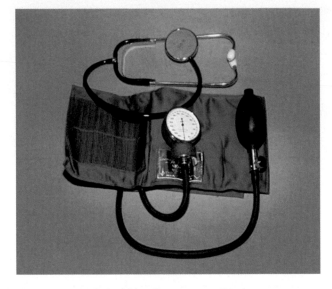

Figure 3-1. Standard blood pressure cuff (sphygmomanometer) and stethoscope.

patients die of coronary heart disease or congestive heart failure, about 33% of stroke, and 10% to 15% of renal failure.[8]

CLINICAL PRESENTATION
Signs and Symptoms

Hypertension may remain an asymptomatic disease for many years, with the only sign being elevated blood pressure. Blood pressure is measured with the use of a sphygmomanometer (Figure 3-1). Pressure at the peak of ventricular contraction is *systolic pressure. Diastolic pressure* represents the total resting resistance in the arterial system after passage of the pulsating force produced by contraction of the left ventricle. The difference between diastolic and systolic pressures is called *pulse pressure. Mean arterial pressure* is roughly defined as the sum of the diastolic pressure plus one-third the pulse pressure. Patients are commonly found to have significant variability in blood pressures. *Labile* hypertension is the term that was previously used to describe a subgroup of patients with wide variability in blood pressures; however, this term has fallen into disuse because it is now recognized that variability in blood pressure is the norm rather than the exception.[7] About 15% to 20% of patients with untreated stage 1 hypertension have what is called *white coat hypertension*, which is defined as persistently elevated blood pressure only in the presence of a health care worker but not elsewhere.[7] In these patients, accurate blood pressure readings may require self-measurement at home or 24-hour ambulatory monitoring. These individuals are at lower risk for hypertensive complications than are those with sustained hypertension.

Before the age of 50, hypertension is typically characterized by an elevation in both diastolic and systolic pressures. Isolated diastolic hypertension, defined as a systolic pressure <140 and a diastolic pressure ≥90, is uncommon

and is most often found in younger adults. Although the prognostic significance of this condition remains unclear and controversial, it appears that it may be relatively benign.[16] Isolated systolic hypertension is defined as a systolic pressure ≥140 and a diastolic blood pressure <90; it is generally found in older patients and constitutes an important risk factor for cardiovascular disease. Occasionally, isolated systolic blood pressure is found in older children and young adults, often male. This is due to the combination of rapid growth in height and very elastic arteries, which accentuate the normal amplification of the pressure wave between the aorta and the brachial artery, resulting in high systolic pressure in the brachial artery but normal systolic pressure in the aorta.[7]

The earliest sign of hypertension is an elevated blood pressure reading; however, funduscopic examination of the eyes may show early changes of hypertension consisting of narrowed arterioles with sclerosis. As indicated earlier, hypertension may remain an asymptomatic disease for many years, but when symptoms do occur, they include headache, tinnitus, and dizziness. These symptoms are not specific for hypertension, however, and may be seen just as commonly in normotensive individuals.[8]

Late signs and symptoms are related to involvement of various target organs, including kidney, brain, heart, or eye (Box 3-2). In advanced cases, retinal vessel hemorrhage, exudate, and papilledema may occur and are indicative of accelerated-malignant hypertension, which is a medical emergency and requires immediate intervention. Hypertensive encephalopathy is characterized by headache, irritability, alterations in consciousness, and other signs of central nervous system (CNS) dysfunction.[8] Also, in advanced cases, the left ventricle may be enlarged and cardiac function may be impaired, leading to congestive heart failure. Renal involvement can result in hematuria, proteinuria, and renal failure. Persons with hypertension may report fatigue and coldness in the legs that result from peripheral arterial changes that may occur in advanced hypertension. Patients with hypertension often have an accelerated cognitive decline with aging.[17] Although these findings may be seen in patients with both essential and secondary hypertension, additional signs or symptoms may be present in secondary hypertension associated with underlying disease.

Laboratory Findings

The JNC 7 recommends that patients who have sustained hypertension should be screened through routine laboratory tests, including 12-lead electrocardiogram, urinalysis, blood glucose, hematocrit, and a serum potassium, creatinine, calcium, and lipid profile. These tests serve as baseline laboratory values that the physician should obtain before initiating therapy. Additional tests should be ordered if clinical and laboratory findings suggest the presence of an underlying cause for hypertension.

MEDICAL MANAGEMENT

Evaluation of a patient with hypertension includes a thorough medical history, a complete physical examination, and routine laboratory tests as described earlier. Additional diagnostic tests or procedures may be performed to detect secondary causes of hypertension or to make a definitive diagnosis. Patients found to have an identifiable cause for their hypertension should be treated for that disorder. Those without an identifiable cause are diagnosed with essential hypertension.

Classification and diagnosis of blood pressure (see Table 3-1) are based on an average of two or more properly measured, seated blood pressure readings on each of two or more office visits.[3] Measurement of blood pressure is most commonly achieved through the auscultatory method with a mercury, aneroid, or hybrid sphygmomanometer (see Fig. 3-1). Mercury sphygmomanometers have long been considered the most accurate of devices and the gold standard; however, because of increasing concern about mercury and the risk of breakage and spill, their use may be limited in the future. Aneroid devices are the type most commonly used in dental offices. They are easy to use; however, they require regular calibration. Automatic digital devices for the arm, wrist, or finger have become popular for use both in the office and at home. They are very convenient and easy to use; however, it is critical that they be regularly calibrated to ensure their accuracy.

Patients given a diagnosis of prehypertension are not candidates for drug therapy but rather are encouraged to adopt lifestyle modifications to decrease their risk of developing the disease. Prehypertension is not a disease but rather a designation that reflects the fact that these patients are at increased risk of developing hypertension. Lifestyle modifications include losing weight; adopting a diet rich in vegetables, fruits, and low-fat dairy products; reducing cholesterol and saturated fats; decreasing sodium intake; limiting alcohol intake; and engaging in daily

---

BOX 3-3

Lifestyle Modifications for the Prevention and Reduction of High Blood Pressure

- Weight loss
- DASH (Dietary Approaches to Stop Hypertension) Diet
  - Fruits
  - Vegetables
  - Low-fat dairy products
- Reduce cholesterol
- Reduce saturated and total fat
- Reduce sodium to <2.4 g/day
- Regular aerobic physical activity on most days (30 minutes of brisk walking)
- Limited alcohol intake to no more than 1 oz/day (2 drinks for men and 1 drink for women)

From Chobanian AV et al: Seventh Report of the Joint National Committee on Prevention, Detection, Evaluation, and Treatment of High Blood Pressure. Hypertension 2003;42:1206-1252.

---

aerobic physical activity (Box 3-3). It is considered essential that patients with prehypertension as well as those with diagnosed hypertension follow these recommendations because lifestyle modifications have been shown to effectively reduce blood pressure, prevent or delay the incidence of hypertension, enhance antihypertensive drug therapy, and decrease cardiovascular risk.[3] If lifestyle modifications are found to be inadequate for achieving desired blood pressure reduction, drug therapy is initiated.

The JNC 7 suggests that all people with hypertension—stages 1 and 2—should be treated. The treatment goal for most patients with hypertension is to reduce blood pressure to <140/90 mm Hg. However, for hypertensive patients with diabetes or kidney disease, the goal is <130/80 mm Hg. Evidence demonstrates the clear benefits of aggressive treatment of hypertension. In clinical trials, antihypertensive therapy resulted in an average reduction in stroke incidence of 35% to 40%; MI, 20% to 25%; and heart failure, >50%.[18]

Many drugs are currently available to treat hypertension (Table 3-4). Those most commonly used include thiazide diuretics, angiotensin-converting enzyme inhibitors (ACEIs), angiotensive receptor blockers (ARBs), beta blockers (BBs), and calcium channel blockers (CCBs). Other drugs that are less frequently used include alpha$_1$ blockers, central alpha$_2$ agonists and other centrally acting drugs, and direct vasodilators. Figure 3-2 depicts the algorithm suggested by the JNC 7 for the treatment of hypertension. If lifestyle modification is ineffective at lowering blood pressure adequately, then thiazide diuretics are most often the first drugs of choice, given either alone or in combination with ACEIs, ARBs, BBs, or CCBs, depending on the degree of elevation of blood pressure. For stage 1 hypertension, single-drug therapy may be effective; however, for stage 2 hypertension, two-drug combinations are recommended. Additional drugs

TABLE 3-4
Drugs Used in the Management of Hypertension

Drug	Vasoconstrictor Interactions	Oral Manifestations	Other Considerations
DIURETICS			
Thiazide Diuretics	None	Dry mouth, lichenoid reactions	Orthostatic hypotension; avoid prolonged use of NSAIDs—May reduce antihypertensive effects
Chlorothiazide (Diuril)			
Chlorthalidone (generic)			
Hydrochlorothiazide (HCTZ, HydroDIURIL, Microzide)			
Polythiazide (Renese)			
Indapamide (Lozol)			
Metolazone (Mykrox)			
Metolazone (Zaroxolyn)			
Loop Diuretics			
Bumetanide (Bumex)			
Furosemide (Lasix)			
Torsemide (Demadex)			
Potassium-Sparing Diuretics			
Amiloride (Midamor)			
Triamterene (Dyrenium)			
Aldosterone Receptor Blockers			
Eplerenone (Inspra)			
Spironolactone (Aldactone)			
Combination			
Aldactazide, Dyazide			
BETA BLOCKERS (BBs)			
Nonselective	Nonselective— Potential increase in blood pressure (use maximum of 0.036 mg epinephrine or 0.20 mg levonordefrin)	Taste changes, lichenoid reactions	Avoid prolonged use of NSAIDs—May reduce antihypertensive effects
Propranolol (Inderal)			
Timolol (Blocadren)			
Nadolol (Corgard)			
Pindolol (Visken)			
Penbutolol (Levatol)			
Carteolol (Cartrol)			
Cardioselective	Cardioselective—Normal use		
Metoprolol (Lopressor)			
Acebutolol (Sectral)			
Atenolol (Tenormin)			
Betaxolol (Kerlone)			
Bisoprolol (Zebeta)			
COMBINED ALPHA AND BETA BLOCKERS			
Carvedilol (Coreg)	Because both $beta_1$ and $beta_2$ receptor sites are blocked, the potential for an adverse interaction is present; however, it is unlikely to occur because of compensatory alpha receptor blockade	Taste changes	Orthostatic hypotension; avoid prolonged use of NSAIDs—May reduce antihypertensive effects
Labetalol (Normodyne, Trandate)			
ANGIOTENSIN-CONVERTING ENZYME INHIBITORS (ACEIs)			
Benazepril (Lotensin)	None	Angioedema of lips, face, tongue; taste changes	Orthostatic hypotension; avoid prolonged use of NSAIDs—May reduce antihypertensive effects
Captopril (Capoten)			
Enalapril (Vasotec)			
Fosinopril (Monopril)			
Lisinopril (Prinivil; Zestril)			

TABLE **3-4**
Drugs Used in the Management of Hypertension—cont'd

Drug	Vasoconstrictor Interactions	Oral Manifestations	Other Considerations
Moexipril (Univasc) Perindopril (Aceon) Quinapril (Accupril) Ramipril (Altace)			
ANGIOTENSIN RECEPTOR BLOCKERS (ARBs)			
Candesartan (Atacand) Eprosartan (Teveten) Irbesartan (Cozaar) Olmesartan (Benicar) Telmisartan (Micardis) Valsartan (Diovan)	None	Angioedema of the lips, face, tongue	Orthostatic hypotension
CALCIUM CHANNEL BLOCKERS (CCBs)			
Diltiazem (Cardizem) Verapamil (Calan) Amlodipine (Norvasc) Felodipine (Plendil) Isradipine (DynaCirc) Nicardipine (Cardene) Nifedipine (Procardia) Nisoldipine (Sular)	None	Gingival hyperplasia	
ALPHA$_1$ BLOCKERS			
Doxazosin (Catapres) Prazosin (Minipress) Terazosin (Hytrin)	None	Dry mouth, taste changes	Orthostatic hypotension, avoid prolonged use of NSAIDs—May reduce antihypertensive effects
CENTRAL ALPHA$_2$ AGONISTS AND OTHER CENTRALLY ACTING DRUGS			
Clonidine (Catapres) Methyldopa (Aldomet) Reserpine (generic) Guanfacine (Tenex)	None	Dry mouth, taste changes	Orthostatic hypotension
DIRECT VASODILATORS			
Hydralazine (Apresoline) Minoxidil (Loniten)	None	Lupuslike oral and skin lesions, lymphadenopathy	Orthostatic hypotension; avoid prolonged use of NSAIDs—May reduce antihypertensive effects

NSAIDs, Nonsteroidal antiinflammatory drugs.

may be added as needed. Most people require more than one drug to effectively lower their blood pressure. The presence of certain comorbid conditions such as heart failure, post MI, diabetes, or kidney disease may be a compelling reason to select specific drugs or classes of drugs that have been found beneficial in clinical trials.

Severe hypertension, defined as blood pressure ≥180/120, may be classified as an emergency or urgency.[3] Hypertensive emergencies are characterized by a severe elevation in blood pressure *with* evidence of impending or progressive target organ dysfunction such as hypertensive encephalopathy, intracerebral hemorrhage, acute

MI, left ventricular failure with pulmonary edema, or unstable angina pectoris. Patients require immediate blood pressure reduction (within 1 hour) and should be admitted to an intensive care unit (ICU).[8]

Patients with severe hypertension but with less ominous symptoms such as headache, shortness of breath, nosebleeds, or severe anxiety require urgent treatment but do not constitute an emergency. These patients are most often found to be noncompliant or are inadequately medicated. They should receive timely treatment to reduce blood pressure but without the immediacy of concern associated with evidence of progressive target

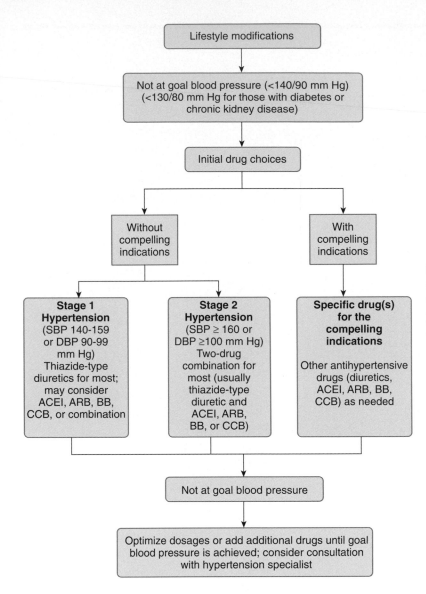

Lifestyle modifications

Not at goal blood pressure (<140/90 mm Hg)
(<130/80 mm Hg for those with diabetes or
chronic kidney disease)

Initial drug choices

Without compelling indications

With compelling indications

Stage 1 Hypertension
(SBP 140-159 or DBP 90-99 mm Hg)
Thiazide-type diuretics for most; may consider ACEI, ARB, BB, CCB, or combination

Stage 2 Hypertension
(SBP ≥ 160 or DBP ≥100 mm Hg)
Two-drug combination for most (usually thiazide-type diuretic and ACEI, ARB, BB, or CCB)

Specific drug(s) for the compelling indications

Other antihypertensive drugs (diuretics, ACEI, ARB, BB, CCB) as needed

Not at goal blood pressure

Optimize dosages or add additional drugs until goal blood pressure is achieved; consider consultation with hypertension specialist

Figure 3-2. The treatment of hypertension. (From the Seventh Report of the Joint National Committee on Prevention, Detection, Evaluation, and Treatment of High Blood Pressure. Hypertension 2003;42:1206-1252.)

organ damage. Treatment may include the administration of a short-acting oral antihypertensive agent followed by several hours of observation and subsequent adjustments in medications. Patients typically do not require admission to the ICU. It is interesting to note that failure to aggressively lower the blood pressure of these patients in the emergency room has not been shown to increase short-term risks to the patient.[3] This further supports the fact that emergency treatment is not critical for these patients. It should be noted that in another group of patients, severe or uncontrolled hypertension occurs with complete absence of symptoms. These patients should likewise receive timely medical treatment, but this is not considered an emergent or urgent situation.

DENTAL MANAGEMENT
Medical Considerations

The first task of the dentist is to identify patients with hypertension, both diagnosed and undiagnosed. A medical history, including the diagnosis of hypertension, how it is being treated, identification of antihypertensive drugs, compliance of the patient, the presence of symptoms associated with hypertension, and the level of stability of the disease, should be obtained. On occasion, patients may fail to report that they have been given a diagnosis of hypertension; however, they may report taking medications, including herbal medications, that are typically used to treat high blood pressure. This may be the only way for the clinician to uncover information revealing that the patient has hypertension. Patients also may be receiving treatment for complications of hypertensive disease, such as congestive heart failure, cerebrovascular disease, MI, renal disease, peripheral vascular disease, and diabetes mellitus. These problems should be identified as well because they may necessitate modification of the dental management plan.

In addition to a medical history, all patients should undergo blood pressure measurement (see Chapter 1). Blood pressure measurements should be routinely performed for all new patients and at recall appointments.

More frequent blood pressure measurements are indicated for patients who are not compliant with treatment, who are poorly controlled, or who have comorbid conditions such as heart failure, previous MI, or stroke. Patients who are being treated for hypertension but who have blood pressures above normal are most often noncompliant or inadequately treated; they should be encouraged to return to their physician. The patient who has not been given a diagnosis of hypertension but who has an abnormally elevated blood pressure should also be encouraged to see his or her physician. When a patient with upper level stage 2 blood pressure is treated, consideration should be given to leaving the blood pressure cuff on the patient's arm and periodically checking pressure during the appointment. The dentist should not make a diagnosis of hypertension but rather should tell the patient that his or her blood pressure reading is elevated, and that a physician should evaluate the condition.

The primary concern when one is providing dental treatment for a patient with hypertension is that during the course of treatment, the patient might experience an acute elevation in blood pressure that could lead to a serious outcome such as stroke or MI. This acute elevation in blood pressure could result from the release of endogenous catecholamines in response to stress and anxiety, from injection of exogenous catecholamines in the form of vasoconstrictors in the local anesthetic, or from absorption of a vasoconstrictor from the gingival retraction cord. Other concerns include potential drug interactions between the patient's antihypertensive medications and the drugs prescribed and oral adverse effects that might be caused by antihypertensive medications.

The following two questions should be answered before dental treatment is provided for a patient with hypertension:

1. What is the risk if a patient with high blood pressure is treated?
2. At what level of blood pressure is it unsafe to treat a patient?

The American College of Cardiology and the American Heart Association have published practice guidelines for the preoperative evaluation of patients with various types of cardiovascular disease who are undergoing noncardiac surgery that can be used to help answer these questions.[19] These guidelines assess the risk of occurrence of a serious event such as stroke, MI, acute heart failure, or sudden death if a patient with cardiovascular disease undergoes some form of noncardiac surgery. Oral and maxillofacial surgery and periodontal surgery are both forms of noncardiac surgery; thus these guidelines are directly applicable. In addition, the guidelines may be applied to nonsurgical dental treatment. Determination of risk includes the evaluation of three factors: the risk imposed by the patient's cardiovascular disease, the risk imposed by the surgery or procedure, and the risk imposed by the functional reserve or capacity of the patient.

BOX 3-4

Clinical Predictors of Increased Perioperative Cardiovascular Risk (myocardial infarction, heart failure, death)

MAJOR
- Unstable coronary syndromes
- Acute or recent myocardial infarction (*) with evidence of important ischemic risk in clinical symptoms or noninvasive study
- Unstable or severe angina (Canadian Class III or IV)[†‡]
- Decompensated heart failure
- Significant arrhythmias
- High-grade atrioventricular block
- Symptomatic ventricular arrhythmias in the presence of underlying heart disease
- Supraventricular arrhythmias with uncontrolled ventricular rate
- Severe valvular disease

INTERMEDIATE
- Mild angina pectoris (Canadian Class I or II)[†]
- Previous myocardial infarction by history or pathological Q waves
- Compensated or prior heart failure
- Diabetes mellitus (particularly insulin-dependent)
- Renal insufficiency

MINOR
- Advanced age
- Abnormal ECG (left ventricular hypertrophy, left bundle-branch block, ST-T abnormalities)
- Rhythm other than sinus (e.g., atrial fibrillation)
- Low functional capacity (e.g., inability to climb one flight of stairs with a bag of groceries)
- History of stroke
- Uncontrolled systemic hypertension (≥180/110 mm Hg)

From ACC/AHA Guideline Update for Perioperative Cardiovascular Evaluation for Noncardiac Surgery—Executive Summary. Copyright © 2002, American Heart Association.
ECG, Electrocardiogram.
*The American College of Cardiology National Database Library defines *recent MI* as greater than 7 days but less than or equal to 1 month (30 days); acute MI occurs within 7 days.
†May include "stable" angina in patients who are unusually sedentary.
‡Campeau L. Grading of angina pectoris. Circulation 1976;54: 522-523. the Canadian Classification is a system of grading angina severity (grade I-IV), with grade I angina occurring only with strenuous exertion and grade IV angina occurring with any physical activity or at rest.

The risk imposed by the presence of a specific cardiovascular condition or disease is stratified into major, intermediate, and minor risks for the intraoperative occurrence of an untoward event (Box 3-4). Uncontrolled blood pressure, defined as ≥180/110 mm Hg, is classified as a *minor* risk condition, but a statement is included that blood pressure should be brought under control before any surgery is performed. It should be recalled that the

JNC 7 classification recommends immediate treatment for patients with blood pressures ≥180/110 (see Table 3-1). The JNC 7 further identifies *severe* hypertension as blood pressure ≥180/120 mm Hg and bases the need for emergency treatment on the presence of progressive target organ dysfunction.

Risk imposed by the type of surgery (or procedure) is also stratified into high (>5% risk), intermediate (<5% risk), and low (<1% risk). In general, risk is greatest with elderly patients, emergency surgery, lengthy procedures, and excessive blood loss (Box 3-5). Head and neck surgery, which may include major oral and maxillofacial procedures and extensive periodontal procedures, is classified as *intermediate* risk. Superficial surgical procedures, which include minor oral and periodontal surgery and nonsurgical dental procedures, are classified as *low* risk.

The third factor involved in risk assessment is determination of the functional capacity or cardiopulmonary reserve of the patient, defined as metabolic equivalents (METs) (see Chapter 1). Perioperative cardiac risk is increased in patients who are unable to meet a 4-MET demand during most normal daily activities, which is equivalent to climbing a flight of stairs. Thus a patient who reports an inability to climb a flight of stairs while carrying a bag of groceries without chest pain, shortness of breath, or fatigue would be at increased, but *minor*, risk during a procedure (see Box 3-4).

Thus it is apparent that the risk of providing routine dental treatment for most patients with high blood pressure is very low. Table 3-5 provides dental management recommendations for patients with various levels of blood pressure. In summary, patients with blood pressure less than 180/110 can undergo any necessary dental treatment, both surgical and nonsurgical, with very little risk of an adverse outcome. For patients found to have asymptomatic blood pressure ≥180/110 mm Hg (uncontrolled hypertension), elective dental care should be deferred and the patient referred to a physician as soon as possible for evaluation and treatment. Patients with elevated blood pressure with symptoms such as headache, shortness of breath, chest pain, nosebleeds, or severe anxiety (severe hypertension) may require more urgent medical attention. In patients with uncontrolled or severe hypertension, the need for urgent dental treatment (pain, infection, or bleeding) may necessitate treatment. In this instance, the patient should be managed in consultation with the physician, and measures such as intraoperative blood pressure monitoring, electrocardiogram monitoring, establishment of an intravenous line, and sedation may be used. The decision must always be made as to whether the benefit of proposed treatment outweighs the potential risks.

Once it has been determined that the hypertensive patient can be safely treated, a management plan should be developed (Box 3-6). For all patients, the dentist should make every effort to reduce as much as possible

---

BOX 3-5

Cardiac Risk* Stratification for Noncardiac Surgical Procedures

HIGH (REPORTED CARDIAC RISK OFTEN GREATER THAN 5%)
- Emergent major operations, particularly in the elderly
- Aortic and other major vascular surgery
- Peripheral vascular surgery
- Anticipated prolonged surgical procedures associated with large fluid shifts and/or blood loss

INTERMEDIATE (REPORTED CARDIAC RISK GENERALLY LESS THAN 5%)
- Carotid endarterectomy
- Head and neck surgery
- Intraperitoneal and intrathoracic surgery
- Orthopaedic surgery
- Prostate surgery

LOW (REPORTED CARDIAC RISK GENERALLY LESS THAN 1%)
- Endoscopic procedures
- Superficial procedures
- Cataract surgery
- Breast surgery

From ACC/AHA Guideline Update for Perioperative Cardiovascular Evaluation for Noncardiac Surgery—Executive Summary. Copyright © 2002, American Heart Association.
*Combined incidence of cardiac death and nonfatal myocardial infarction.

TABLE 3-5

Dental Management and Follow-up Recommendations Based on Blood Pressure

Blood Pressure	Dental Treatment Recommendation	Referral to Physician
≤120/80	Any required	No
≥120/80 but <140/90	Any required	Encourage patient to see physician
≥140/90 but <160/100	Any required	Encourage patient to see physician
≥160/100 but <180/110	Any required; consider intraoperative monitoring of blood pressure for upper level stage 2	Refer patient to physician promptly (within 1 month)
≥180/110	Defer elective treatment	Refer to physician as soon as possible; if patient is symptomatic, refer immediately

BOX 3-6

Dental Management Recommendations for Patients With Hypertension

- Stress/anxiety reduction
- Establishment of good rapport
- Short, morning appointments
- Consider premedication with sedative/anxiolytic
- Consider intraoperative use of nitrous oxide/oxygen
- Obtain excellent local anesthesia; OK to use epinephrine in modest amounts
- Cautious use of epinephrine in local anesthetic in patients taking non-selective β-beta blockers or peripheral adrenergic antagonists
- Avoid the use of epinephrine-impregnated gingival retraction cord
- Consider periodic intraoperative BP monitoring for patients with upper level stage 2 hypertension; terminate appointment if BP rises above 179/109
- Slow position changes to prevent orthostatic hypotension

BP, Blood pressure.

the stress and anxiety associated with dental treatment. This is of particular importance when treating the patient with hypertension. A critical factor in providing an anxiety-free situation is the relationship established among the dentist, office staff, and patient. Patients should be encouraged to express and discuss their fears, concerns, and questions about dental treatment.

Stress management is important for patients with hypertension to lessen the chances of endogenous release of catecholamines during the appointment (see Chapter 1). Long or stressful appointments are best avoided. Short morning appointments seem best tolerated. If the patient becomes anxious or apprehensive during the appointment, the appointment may be terminated and rescheduled for another day. Anxiety can be reduced for many patients by oral premedication with a short-acting benzodiazepine such as triazolam (Halcion; Pharmacia & Upjohn, Kalamazoo, Mich). An effective approach is to prescribe a dose at bedtime the night before and another dose 1 hour before the dental appointment. Dose is dictated by the age and size of the patient and by prescribing guidelines for the agent selected. Nitrous oxide plus oxygen inhalation sedation is an excellent intraoperative anxiolytic for use in patients with hypertension. Care should be used to ensure adequate oxygenation at all times, especially at the termination of administration. Hypoxia is to be avoided because of the resultant elevation in blood pressure that may occur. When patients with upper level stage 2 hypertension are treated, it may be advisable to leave the blood pressure cuff on the patient's arm, and to periodically check the pressure during treatment. If the blood pressure rises above 179/109, the appointment should be terminated and the patient rescheduled.

Because some antihypertensive agents tend to produce orthostatic hypotension, sudden changes in chair position during dental treatment should be avoided. When treatment has concluded for that appointment, the dental chair should be returned slowly to an upright position. After patients have had time to adjust to the change in posture, they should be physically supported while slowly getting out of the chair and should have obtained good balance and stability. If they complain of dizziness or lightheadedness, they should sit back down until they recover equilibrium.

Ambulatory (outpatient) general anesthesia in the dental office is generally recommended only for patients with classification by the American Society of Anesthesiologists (ASA) as ASA I (healthy, normal patient) or ASA II (mild to moderate systemic disease). Some patients with severe hypertension may be excluded.

Use of Vasoconstrictors. Profound local anesthesia is critical for pain and anxiety control and is especially important in patients with hypertension or other cardiovascular disease to decrease endogenous catecholamine release. The effectiveness of local anesthesia is enhanced by the inclusion of a vasoconstrictor in the local anesthetic solution that delays systemic absorption, increases the duration of anesthesia, and provides local hemostasis. These properties allow for enhanced quality and duration of pain control and markedly facilitate performance of the technical procedures. Thus the advantages of including a vasoconstrictor in the local anesthetic are obvious. Concerns, however, have been associated with the use of a vasoconstrictor. The potential danger in administering a local anesthetic containing epinephrine or another vasoconstrictor to a patient with hypertension or other cardiovascular disease lies in the potential to cause an acute increase in blood pressure or an arrhythmia.

To make rational decisions regarding the use of vasoconstrictors in patients who are hypertensive or otherwise medically compromised, the dentist should first understand the physiology of adrenergic receptors. The two basic types of adrenergic receptors are alpha and beta, which are further divided into $alpha_1$ and $alpha_2$, and $beta_1$ and $beta_2$. These receptors are found throughout the body in most tissues and organs; however, usually one type predominates. Of particular interest are their effects on blood vessels and the heart. $Alpha_1$ receptors predominate in peripheral arterioles and cause vasoconstriction, $beta_1$ receptors predominate in the heart and cause an increase in cardiac output and heart rate, and $beta_2$ receptors predominate in arterioles in skeletal muscle, causing vasodilatation. $Alpha_2$ receptors act in concert with $alpha_1$ receptors.

Drugs that stimulate adrenergic receptors are called *sympathomimetic* or *adrenergic* drugs. Vasoconstrictors, which are examples of these drugs, include epinephrine, norepinephrine, and levonordefrin. These drugs stimulate adrenergic receptors to varying degrees, and their effects are dose dependent (Table 3-6). Epinephrine is a

TABLE 3-6
Adrenergic Receptor Activity of Vasoconstrictors*

Drug	Alpha$_1$	Alpha$_2$	Beta$_1$	Beta$_2$
Epinephrine	+++	+++	+++	+++
Norepinephrine	++	++	++	+
Levonordefrin	+	++	++	+

From Jastak JT, Yagiela JA, Donaldson D: Local Anesthesia of the Oral Cavity. Philadelphia, Saunders, 1995.
*Symbols indicate relative potency: +++, high; ++, intermediate; +, low.

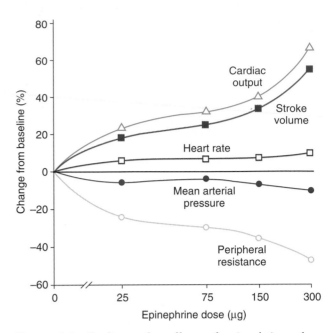

Figure 3-3. Cardiovascular effects of epinephrine when used in regional anesthesia. (Redrawn from Jastak JT, Yagiela JA, Donaldson D. Local Anesthesia of the Oral Cavity. Philadelphia, Saunders, 1995.)

potent stimulator of alpha and beta receptors, with a predominance of beta$_2$ activation. Norepinephrine is a potent stimulator of alpha$_1$ and beta$_1$ receptors but has little effect on beta$_2$. As a result, norepinephrine may cause a significant rise in systolic and diastolic blood pressures. Levonordefrin is similar to norepinephrine in action but has somewhat less alpha$_1$ potency and slightly more beta$_2$ potency. Norepinephrine is not available for use as a vasoconstrictor in the United States.

The cardiovascular response to conventional doses of injected epinephrine in patients who are healthy and in those with hypertension is usually of little concern. A meta-analysis of several clinical studies determined that the mean resting venous plasma epinephrine concentration is 39 pg/mL; this is approximately doubled by the intraoral injection of a single cartridge of 2% lidocaine with 1:100;000 epinephrine.[20] This elevation in plasma epinephrine is linear and dose dependent. Although large doses of epinephrine may cause a significant rise in blood pressure and heart rate, small doses such as those contained in one or two cartridges of lidocaine with 1:100,000 epinephrine may cause minimal pharmacologic change (Figure 3-3). This fact is due to a preponderance of action among beta$_2$ receptors and a decrease in diastolic pressure; thus, mean arterial pressure is essentially unchanged with only a minimal increase in heart rate.

Several clinical investigations have evaluated changes in plasma epinephrine concentration and hemodynamic parameters in healthy patients after dental injections of 2% lidocaine with 1:100,000 epinephrine. After injection of 1.8 mL (one cartridge), plasma levels increased twofold to threefold, but no significant changes were observed in heart rate or blood pressure.[21-23] With 5.4 mL of solution (three cartridges), however, plasma levels increased fivefold to sixfold; these changes were accompanied by a significant increase in heart rate and systolic blood pressure with no adverse symptoms or sequelae.[24,25] The critical question is how does a patient with hypertension or other cardiovascular disease react to these dose challenges of epinephrine?

This question was addressed empirically in 1955 by the New York Heart Association, which recommended that a maximum of 0.2 mg of epinephrine (11 cartridges of 1:100,000 epinephrine with procaine) be used during a single session in dental patients with heart disease.[26] In 1964, a Working Conference of the American Dental Association and the American Heart Association[27] concluded, "Concentrations of vasoconstrictors normally used in dental local anesthetic solutions are not contraindicated in patients with cardiovascular disease when administered carefully and with preliminary aspiration." Contrary to these recommendations, Abraham-Inpijn et al[28] found that patients with hypertension undergoing dental extractions had a greater increase in blood pressure than did patients thought to be normotensive after injection of 2% lidocaine with 1:80,000 epinephrine. In addition, 7.5% of patients with hypertension developed significant arrhythmias. In a similar study, however, in which the responses of patients who were normotensive and hypertensive were compared using lidocaine plain, with 1:100,000 epinephrine, and 1:20,000 norepinephrine during extractions, no significant differences were noted in heart rate or blood pressure between plain lidocaine and lidocaine with epinephrine. However, lidocaine with norepinephrine produced a significant increase in blood pressure and decreased heart rate.[29] Another study of dental patients who were undergoing oral surgery found no difference in the blood pressures of patients with hypertension who received 2% lidocaine with 1:80,000 epinephrine.[30]

Of particular interest is a study that evaluated epinephrine infusion used as a stress test in 39 patients suspected of having coronary artery disease in whom epinephrine was injected intravenously in progressively increasing doses from 2.1 to 21.0 μg per minute over a 30-minute period.[31] (A total of 18 μg of epinephrine is found in one cartridge of 1:100,000 epinephrine.) Of 24 patients who were subsequently found not to have coronary artery disease, none developed electrocardiographic changes, and none had symptoms over the course of 30 minutes. Of 15 patients in whom coronary artery disease was diagnosed, however, 7 developed significant arrhythmias, 7 had chest pain, and 4 had shortness of breath or other symptoms. In spite of the symptoms and hemodynamic changes, no test had to be terminated, and all symptoms subsided after the test without sequelae.

A systematic review of the literature on the cardiovascular effects of epinephrine on hypertensive dental patients[32] concluded that although the quantity and quality of pertinent articles were problematic, the increased risk for adverse events among uncontrolled hypertensive patients was low, and the reported occurrence of adverse events associated with the use of epinephrine in local anesthetics was minimal. This review was cited by the JNC 7 report and supported its conclusions. Another recent review of the subject noted an absence of adverse case reports involving epinephrine in local anesthetics and cited the numerous studies that demonstrated the safety and efficacy of these preparations.[33]

Thus, from the existing evidence, it would appear that one or two cartridges of 2% lidocaine with 1:100,000 epinephrine are of little clinical significance in most patients with hypertension; the benefits of its use far outweigh any potential disadvantages or risks. Use of more than this amount may well be tolerated but with increasing risk for adverse hemodynamic changes. Norepinephrine and levonordefrin should be avoided in patients with hypertension because of their comparative excessive alpha$_1$ stimulation. The use of epinephrine is generally not advised in patients with uncontrolled or severe hypertension, and indeed, elective dental care should be deferred. However, if urgent treatment becomes necessary, a decision must be made about the use of epinephrine, which will be dictated by the situation. From all available evidence, it would seem that the benefits of its use outweigh the increased risks, as long as modest doses are used and care is taken to avoid inadvertent intravascular injections. It is advisable to consult with the patient's physician prior to making a decision.

An additional concern when patients with hypertension are treated is the potential for adverse drug interactions between vasoconstrictors and antihypertensive drugs, specifically, the adrenergic blocking agents. The basis for concern with nonselective beta-adrenergic blocking agents (e.g., propranolol) is that the normal compensatory vasodilatation of skeletal muscle vasculature mediated by beta$_2$ receptors is inhibited by these drugs, and injection of epinephrine, levonordefrin, or any other pressor agent may result in uncompensated peripheral vasoconstriction because of unopposed stimulation of alpha$_1$ receptors. This may cause a significant elevation in blood pressure and a compensatory bradycardia.[34,35] Several cases of this interaction have been reported in the

literature, but it appears to be dose dependent.[36-38] Adverse interactions are less likely to occur in patients who take cardioselective beta blockers.[25] Peripheral adrenergic antagonists, such as reserpine and guanethidine, also present the potential for adverse interaction with vasoconstrictors because of enhanced receptor sensitivity to direct-acting sympathomimetics, resulting in reports of enhanced systemic response to vasoconstrictors.[39] Although the potential exists for adverse interactions between vasoconstrictors and the nonselective beta-blocking agents or peripheral adrenergic antagonists, available reports and clinical experience suggest that epinephrine in small doses of one to two cartridges containing 1:100,000 epinephrine can be used safely in most patients. Jastak et al[25] suggest that a small test dose (1 mL of the 1:100,000 epinephrine solution) should be given to patients taking these drugs and that blood pressure should be monitored every minute for at least 5 minutes. If no significant change in blood pressure is noted during this period, epinephrine can be safely used in modest amounts.

Topical vasoconstrictors generally should not be used for local hemostasis in patients with hypertension. When performing crown and bridge procedures for patients with hypertension, the dentist should avoid using gingival retraction cord that contains epinephrine because these cords contain highly concentrated epinephrine, which can be quickly absorbed through the gingival sulcular tissues, resulting in tachycardia and elevated blood pressure. As an alternative, one study reported that tetrahydrozoline (Visine; Pfizer Inc, New York, NY), oxymetazoline (Afrin; Schering-Plough, Summit, NJ), and phenylephrine (Neo-Synephrine; Bayer, Morristown, NJ) may be used to soak the cord, providing similar hemostatic effects as epinephrine but with minimal cardiovascular effects.[40]

Several other effects are of concern with antihypertensive agents and dentistry. Some antihypertensive agents, especially alpha blockers, alpha/beta blockers, and diuretics, may predispose patients to orthostatic hypotension and potentiate the actions of anxiolytic and sedative drugs. Anxiolytics and sedatives may be used for patients who take these antihypertensive medications; however, their usual dosage may have to be reduced. The efficacy of antihypertensive drugs may be decreased by the prolonged use of nonsteroidal antiinflammatory drugs, which should be considered if these drugs are used for analgesia, although the use of nonsteroidal antiinflammatory drugs for a few days is of little practical concern.[41] Some antihypertensive agents may produce a tendency for nausea and vomiting, and excessive stimulation of the gag reflex during dental treatment may precipitate nausea or vomiting. Another concern is the patient, with or without hypertension, who may be using cocaine. Cocaine may cause hypertension and tachycardia, and this effect can be magnified if epinephrine-containing local anesthetic is inadvertently injected intravascularly (see Chapter 29). Therefore, whenever possible, local anesthetics that

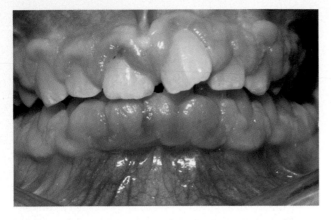

Figure 3-4. Gingival hyperplasia in a patient taking a calcium channel blocker. (Courtesy Dr. Terry Wright.)

contain vasopressors should not be administered to patients who have used cocaine on the day of their dental appointment.[42,43]

Treatment Planning Modifications

Patients whose blood pressures are <180/110 can receive any indicated dental treatment; however, those with elevated blood pressures (upper levels of stage 2) should be referred to their physician. No elective dental procedures should be performed for the patient who has uncontrolled or severe hypertension (≥180/110) (see Table 3-5).

Oral Manifestations. No oral complications have been associated with hypertension itself. Patients with malignant hypertension have been reported to occasionally develop facial palsy.[44] Patients with severe hypertension have been reported to bleed excessively after surgical procedures or trauma; however, excessive bleeding in patients with hypertension is not common and is controversial. Patients who take antihypertensive drugs, especially diuretics, may report dry mouth. Mercurial diuretics may cause oral lesions on an allergic or toxic basis. Lichenoid reactions have been reported with thiazides, methyldopa, propranolol, and labetalol. ACE inhibitors may cause neutropenia, resulting in delayed healing or gingival bleeding. Nonallergic angioedema may be caused by ACE inhibitors. Burning mouth has also been reported to be caused by ACE inhibitors. All calcium channel blockers may cause gingival hyperplasia (Figure 3-4; see Table 3-4).

REFERENCES

1. Chobanian AV, Bakris GL, Black HR, et al. Seventh Report of the Joint National Committee on Prevention, Detection, Evaluation, and Treatment of High Blood Pressure. Hypertension 2003;42:1206-1252.
2. The Fourth Report on the Diagnosis, Evaluation, and Treatment of High Blood Pressure in Children and Adolescents. Pediatrics 2004;114:555-576.
3. Chobanian AV, Bakris GL, Black HR, et al. The Seventh Report of the Joint National Committee on Prevention, Detection, Evaluation, and Treatment of High Blood Pressure: The JNC 7 report. JAMA 2003;289:2560-2572.
4. Hajjar I, Kotchen JM, Kotchen TA. Hypertension: Trends in prevalence, incidence, and control. Annu Rev Public Health 2006;27:465-490.
5. Fields LE, Burt VL, Cutler JA, Hughes J, Roccella EJ, Sorlie P. The burden of adult hypertension in the United States 1999 to 2000: A rising tide. Hypertension 44:398-404, 2004.
6. Burt VL, Whelton P, Roccella EJ, et al. Prevalence of hypertension in the US adult population: Results from the Third National Health and Nutrition Examination Survey, 1988-1991. Hypertension 1995;25:305-313.
7. Pickering TG, Hall JE, Appel LJ, et al. Recommendations for blood pressure measurement in humans and experimental animals. Part 1: Blood pressure measurement in humans: A statement for professionals from the Subcommittee of Professional and Public Education of the American Heart Association Council on High Blood Pressure Research. Circulation 2005;111:697-716.
8. Kaplan N. Systemic hypertension: Mechanisms and diagnosis. In Zipes D, Libby P, Bonow R, Braunwald E (eds). Braunwald's Heart Disease: A Textbook of Cardiovascular Medicine, 7th ed. Philadelphia, Elsevier, 2005.
9. Franklin SS, Jacobs MJ, Wong ND, L'Italien GJ, Lapuerta P. Predominance of isolated systolic hypertension among middle-aged and elderly US hypertensives: Analysis based on National Health and Nutrition Examination Survey (NHANES) III. Hypertension 2001; 37:869-874.
10. Franklin SS. Hypertension in older people: Part 1. J Clin Hypertens (Greenwich) 2006;8:444-449.
11. Lorenzo C, Serrano-Rios M, Martinez-Larrad MT, et al. Prevalence of hypertension in Hispanic and non-Hispanic white populations. Hypertension 2002;39: 203-208.
12. Hypertension-related mortality among Hispanic subpopulations—United States, 1995-2002. MMWR Morb Mortal Wkly Rep 2006;55:177-180.
13. Smith SC Jr, Clark LT, Cooper RS, et al. Discovering the full spectrum of cardiovascular disease: Minority Health Summit 2003: Report of the Obesity, Metabolic Syndrome, and Hypertension Writing Group. Circulation 2005;111:e134-e139.
14. Lewington S, Clarke R, Qizilbash N, Peto R, Collins R. Age-specific relevance of usual blood pressure to vascular mortality: A meta-analysis of individual data for one million adults in 61 prospective studies. Lancet 2002; 360:1903-1913.
15. Miura K, Daviglus ML, Dyer AR, et al. Relationship of blood pressure to 25-year mortality due to coronary heart disease, cardiovascular diseases, and all causes in young adult men: The Chicago Heart Association Detection Project in Industry. Arch Intern Med 2001; 161:1501-1508.
16. Pickering TG. Isolated diastolic hypertension. J Clin Hypertens (Greenwich) 2003;5:411-413.
17. Reinprecht F, Elmstahl S, Janzon L, Andre-Petersson L. Hypertension and changes of cognitive function in 81-

year-old men: A 13-year follow-up of the population study "Men born in 1914," Sweden. J Hypertens 2003; 21:57-66.

18. Neal B, MacMahon S, Chapman N. Effects of ACE inhibitors, calcium antagonists, and other blood-pressure–lowering drugs: Results of prospectively designed overviews of randomised trials. Blood Pressure Lowering Treatment Trialists' Collaboration. Lancet 2000;356:1955-1964.

19. Eagle KA, Berger PB, Calkins H, et al. ACC/AHA guideline update for perioperative cardiovascular evaluation for noncardiac surgery—Executive summary: A report of the American College of Cardiology/American Heart Association Task Force on Practice Guidelines (Committee to Update the 1996 Guidelines on Perioperative Cardiovascular Evaluation for Noncardiac Surgery). Circulation 2002;105:1257-1267.

20. Yagiela J. Local anesthetics. In Dionne R, Phero J (eds). Management of Pain and Anxiety in Dental Practice. New York, Elsevier Science, 1991.

21. Cioffi GA, Chernow B, Glahn RP, Terezhalmy GT, Lake CR. The hemodynamic and plasma catecholamine responses to routine restorative dental care. J Am Dent Assoc 1985;111:67-70.

22. McInnes GT. Integrated approaches to management of hypertension: Promoting treatment acceptance. Am Heart J 1999;138:252-255.

23. Tolas AG, Pflug AE, Halter JB. Arterial plasma epinephrine concentrations and hemodynamic responses after dental injection of local anesthetic with epinephrine. J Am Dent Assoc 1982;104:41-43.

24. Beilin LJ, Puddey IB, Burke V. Lifestyle and hypertension. Am J Hypertens 1999;12:934-945.

25. Jastak J, Yagiela J, Donaldson D. Local Anesthesia of the Oral Cavity. Philadelphia, WB Saunders, 1995.

26. Use of epinephrine in connection with procaine in dental procedures. J Am Med Assoc 1955;157:854.

27. Akutsu A, Chiba T, Takahashi H, Shimoda M, Suematsu T. Management of dental problems in patients with cardiovascular disease. J Am Dent Assoc 1964;68: 333-342.

28. Abraham-Inpijn L, Borgmeijer-Hoelen A, Gortzak RA. Changes in blood pressure, heart rate, and electrocardiogram during dental treatment with use of local anesthesia. J Am Dent Assoc 1988;116:531-536.

29. Meyer FU. Hemodynamic changes of local dental anesthesia in normotensive and hypertensive subjects. Int J Clin Pharmacol Ther Toxicol 1986;24:477-481.

30. Meechan JG. Plasma potassium changes in hypertensive patients undergoing oral surgery with local anesthetics containing epinephrine. Anesth Prog 1997;44:106-109.

31. Schechter E, Wilson MF, Kong YS. Physiologic responses to epinephrine infusion: The basis for a new stress test for coronary artery disease. Am Heart J 1983;105:554-560.

32. Bader JD, Bonito AJ, Shugars DA. A systematic review of cardiovascular effects of epinephrine on hypertensive dental patients. Oral Surg Oral Med Oral Pathol Oral Radiol Endod 2002;93:647-653.

33. Brown RS, Rhodus NL. Epinephrine and local anesthesia revisited. Oral Surg Oral Med Oral Pathol Oral Radiol Endod 2005;100:401-408.

34. Houben H, Thien T, van't Laar A. Effect of low-dose epinephrine infusion on hemodynamics after selective and nonselective beta-blockade in hypertension. Clin Pharmacol Ther 1982;31:685-690.

35. Reeves RA, Boer WH, DeLeve L, Leenen FH. Nonselective beta-blockade enhances pressor responsiveness to epinephrine, norepinephrine, and angiotensin II in normal man. Clin Pharmacol Ther 1984;35:461-466.

36. Foster CA, Aston SJ. Propranolol–epinephrine interaction: A potential disaster. Plast Reconstr Surg 1983;72: 74-78.

37. Kram J, Bourne HR, Melmon KL, Maibach H. Letter: Propranolol. Ann Intern Med 1974;80:282.

38. Mito RS, Yagiela JA. Hypertensive response to levonordefrin in a patient receiving propranolol: Report of case. J Am Dent Assoc 1988;116:55-57.

39. Jinks MJ, Hansten PD, Hirschman JL. Drug interaction exposures in an ambulatory Medicaid population. Am J Hosp Pharm 1979;36.923-927.

40. Bowles WH, Tardy SJ, Vahadi A. Evaluation of new gingival retraction agents. J Dent Res 1991;70:1447-1449.

41. Oates JA, FitzGerald GA, Branch RA, Jackson EK, Knapp HR, Roberts LJ 2nd. Clinical implications of prostaglandin and thromboxane A2 formation. N Engl J Med 1988;319:689-698.

42. Van Dyke C, Barash PG, Jatlow P, Byck R. Cocaine: Plasma concentrations after intranasal application in man. Science 1976;191:859-861.

43. Malamed S. Handbook of Local Anesthesia, 5th ed. St. Louis, Elsevier Mosby, 2004.

44. Scully C, Cawson R. Medical Problems in Dentistry, 5th ed. Edinburgh, Elsevier Churchill Livingstone, 2005.

Ischemic Heart Disease

Coronary atherosclerotic heart disease is a major health problem in the United States and in other industrialized nations. Atherosclerosis is the thickening of the intimal layer of the arterial wall caused by the accumulation of lipid plaques. The atherosclerotic process results in a narrowed arterial lumen with diminished blood flow and oxygen supply. Atherosclerosis is the most common underlying cause of not only coronary heart disease (angina and myocardial infarction [MI]) but also cerebrovascular disease (stroke) and peripheral arterial disease (intermittent claudication).

Symptomatic coronary atherosclerotic heart disease is often referred to as *ischemic heart disease*. Ischemic symptoms are the result of oxygen deprivation caused by reduced blood flow to a portion of the myocardium. Other conditions such as embolism, coronary ostial stenosis, coronary artery spasm, and congenital abnormalities also may cause ischemic heart disease.

GENERAL DESCRIPTION

Incidence and Prevalence

More than 70 million Americans (about 25% of the population) are estimated to have some form of cardiovascular disease, with about 13 million having coronary heart disease.[1] The mortality rate per year from cardiovascular diseases as a group has been declining since 1940. From 1970 to 2000, mortality from coronary heart disease decreased by 50% and from stroke by 60%.[2] In spite of this decline, cardiovascular diseases continue to pose the most serious threat to health in America, accounting for about 40% of all deaths.[3] Coronary heart disease is the leading cause of death in the United States after age 65, and it is responsible for 1.1 million new or recurrent heart attacks annually, of which 40% are fatal.[4] Autopsy studies in the United States have shown that cardiovascular disease begins at an early age, and that one in six American teenagers already has pathologic intimal thick-

ening of the coronary arteries.[5] Autopsy studies of soldiers killed during the Korean and Vietnam Wars and of trauma victims have shown that atherosclerosis begins early in life, although its symptoms and complications typically manifest later, in midlife.[6,7]

Etiology

The cause of coronary atherosclerosis is not known; however, research indicates that the disease is related to a variety of risk factors. These risk factors include male gender, older age, a family history of cardiovascular disease, hyperlipidemia, hypertension, cigarette smoking, physical inactivity, obesity, insulin resistance and diabetes mellitus, mental stress, and depression. In addition to these conventional risk factors, markers of inflammation such as C-reactive protein, homocysteine, fibrinogen, and lipoprotein(a) have been found to be associated with atherosclerosis.[8]

Between the ages of 35 and 44 years, the risk is 5 times greater for men than for women.[3] MI and sudden death are rare in premenopausal women; however, after menopause, a rapid reduction occurs in this gender difference. The fact that men are more prone to the clinical manifestations of coronary atherosclerosis is accentuated in nonwhite populations (e.g., African Americans, Native Americans, Hispanics). Studies have confirmed that individuals with parents or siblings affected by coronary atherosclerotic heart disease have a greater risk of developing the disease at a younger age than do those without such a history.[9-11] This risk may be as high as 5 times greater.

Elevation in serum lipid levels is a major risk factor for atherosclerosis. Increased levels of low-density lipoprotein cholesterol pose the greatest risk for coronary atherosclerosis, whereas increased levels of high-density lipoprotein cholesterol have been shown to reduce the risk.[12] Individuals with elevated triglyceride or beta-lipoprotein levels have an increased risk for the disease.

A diet rich in total calories, saturated fats, cholesterol, sugars, and salts also enhances the risk.

Increased blood pressure appears to be one of the most significant risk factors for coronary atherosclerotic heart disease. The Framingham Study showed that angina, MI, and nonsudden death were all significantly correlated with elevated blood pressure (140/90 mm Hg or greater).[13] Sudden death in men was related only to elevation in systolic blood pressure (SBP), and no correlation of sudden death in women was found with increased blood pressure. In general, systolic blood pressure is more strongly related to the incidence of cardiovascular disease than is diastolic blood pressure, especially in the elderly.[4] SBP rises throughout life, and diastolic blood pressure (DBP) tends to level off or decrease after the age of 50. Most epidemiologic studies, however, recognize the importance of both DBP and SBP in the assessment of cardiovascular risk.[8] In the Framingham Study, even prehypertension (SBP, 130-139; DBP, 85-89) was associated with a twofold risk of cardiovascular disease when compared with lower pressures.[14]

Cigarette smoking is the single most important modifiable risk factor for coronary heart disease (see Chapter 8). Multiple prospective studies have clearly documented that, compared with nonsmokers, persons who smoke 20 or more cigarettes daily have a two- to threefold increase in coronary heart disease.[8] This increased risk appears to be proportionate to the number of cigarettes smoked per day. In a 5-year study of 4165 smokers with coronary atherosclerotic heart disease, the death rate was reduced for individuals who stopped smoking.[15] The death rate was 22% for 2675 individuals who continued smoking and 15% for 1490 who stopped. In the Framingham Study, participants who discontinued smoking lowered their risk of MI within 2 years.[16] Pipe and cigar smoking apparently convey little risk for development of heart disease.

Patients with diabetes mellitus have a greater incidence of coronary atherosclerotic heart disease and more extensive lesions. They develop the condition at an earlier age than do persons who do not have diabetes. Almost 35 million Americans have some degree of abnormal glucose tolerance—a condition along with obesity that markedly increases the risk for type 2 diabetes and premature atherosclerosis.[17] Patients with diabetes have two- to eightfold higher rates of future cardiovascular events as compared with age-matched and ethnically matched nondiabetic individuals.[18] Three fourths of all deaths among diabetic patients result from coronary heart disease.[19] Compared with unaffected individuals, diabetic patients have a greater atherosclerotic burden in the major arteries and in the microvascular circulation.[8] Although hyperglycemia is associated with microvascular disease, insulin resistance itself promotes atherosclerosis even before it produces frank diabetes, and available data corroborate the role of insulin resistance as an independent risk factor for atherothrombosis.[8] *Metabolic syndrome* is the term used to describe a clustering of conditions in an individual consisting of hyperinsulinemia, centrally distributed adiposity, mild glucose intolerance, dyslipidemia, and hypertension, all of which are risk factors for atherosclerosis.[20] The clustering of these conditions reflects the combined importance of multiple risk factors that act synergistically on the development of atherosclerosis.[21] The prevalence of metabolic syndrome in the United States is estimated to be almost 25%, or nearly 50 million people.[22]

Other risk factors for the development of atherosclerosis have emerged and include elevated levels of C-reactive protein (inflammatory marker), fibrinogen (procoagulant), and plasminogen activator inhibitor (antifibrinolytic). Elevated levels of homocysteine also may promote thrombosis, but the exact mechanism of this is unclear.[8]

Numerous studies have reported an association between periodontal disease and cardiovascular disease, raising the question of whether periodontal disease is a risk factor for cardiovascular disease.[23] Although the mechanism to explain this relationship is unclear, it is hypothesized that the chronic inflammatory burden of periodontal disease may lead to impaired functioning of the vascular endothelium.[24] It should be emphasized, however, that at this point, this is merely an association, and causation has not been proved. Additional interventional studies will be required to further elucidate this relationship.

No single risk factor is responsible for the development of coronary atherosclerosis, but many factors act synergistically. Evidence suggests that modification of those risk factors that can be controlled such as cigarette smoking, hypertension, hyperlipidemia, and diabetes may reduce or modify the clinical effects of the disease.

Pathophysiology and Complications

Our understanding of the pathophysiology of atherosclerosis has evolved significantly over the past 2 or 3 decades. In essence, it has gone from the concept of a cholesterol storage disease with a buildup of plaques on the surface of an artery, analogous to rust buildup in a pipe, to one of an inflammatory disorder of the cellular lining of the arteries, with inflammation playing a fundamental role at all stages of the disease.[6,25] Furthermore, it is now clear that narrowing of the arteries does not necessarily presage MI, and that simply treating narrowed blood vessels does not prolong life. In fact, vascular events rarely result from inexorable plaque growth but more often follow the rupture of a less prominent plaque, resulting in clot formation or thrombus.[6]

Libby and Theroux[25] have elegantly described the formation of atheromatous plaques. The first steps in the formation of an atheromatous plaque remain largely conjectural; however, they involve an inflammatory repair response of the injured arterial intima. Chronic minimal injury to the arterial endothelium is common and results from both physiologic and pathologic processes.[26] Physiologic injury often occurs as the result of disturbed blood flow at bending points or bifurcations in the artery. Endothelial injury or dysfunction may also be caused by hypercholesterolemia, glycation end products in diabetes, irritants in tobacco smoke, circulating vasoactive amines, immune complexes, and infection.

An atheroma is initiated by adherence of monocytes to an area of injured or altered endothelium. Usually, monocytes do not adhere to intact endothelium; however, triggers of atherosclerosis such as a high saturated fat diet, smoking, hypertension, hyperglycemia, obesity, and insulin resistance initiate the expression of adhesion molecules by the endothelial cells, thus promoting attachment. The attached monocytes then migrate into the intima of the vessel and become macrophages. Lipids derived from plasma low-density lipoproteins (LDLs) also enter through the injured or dysfunctional endothelium, forming extracellular deposits or small pools. Macrophages then engulf lipid molecules to become "foam cells," which are characteristic features of the "fatty streak." Foam cells are joined by T lymphocytes and produce a variety of inflammatory cytokines, which promote the migration and proliferation of smooth muscle cells and collagen to surround the foam cells, thereby forming a fibrous covering or cap. The appearance of the smooth muscle cells triggers a coalescence of the foam cells and small extracellular pools of lipid into a larger pool or lipid core. The T lymphocytes secrete cytokines that inhibit the further production of collagen, possibly leading to weakening and thinning of the fibrous cap and rendering it susceptible to rupture. With rupture or disruption of the plaque surface, tissue factor comes into contact with blood, and a thrombus is subsequently formed (Figure 4-1).

Plaques may grow and proliferate outwardly, away from the lumen of the artery, or inwardly, into the lumen. Coronary arteries may enlarge and compensate for the developing plaque, thus preserving blood flow to the myocardium, becoming overwhelmed only when the stenosis occupies >40% of the arterial lumen.[27] With inward proliferation, the size of the lumen is progressively reduced (stenosis). Thus, blood flow may be chronically decreased, and when demand exceeds supply, the outcome is ischemic pain. Ischemic symptoms may be produced when occlusion reaches 75% of the cross-sectional area of the artery[28] (Figure 4-2). It is interesting to note that serial angiogram data show that extreme narrowing of the artery leads to MI in only about 15% of cases.[29]

Most acute coronary syndromes (unstable angina; myocardial infarction) are caused by physical disruption or fracture of the atheromatous plaque, most commonly of a plaque that did not cause extreme stenosis.[6] In plaque rupture, the fibrous cap tears, allowing arterial blood to enter the lipid core, where contact with tissue factor and collagen induces platelet adhesion, aggregation, and activation of the coagulation cascade. This results in thrombus formation and sudden expansion of the lesion. Blood flow through the affected artery may become compromised or completely blocked.

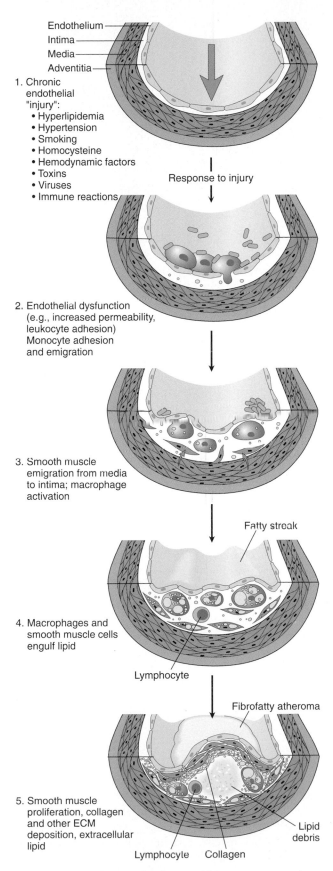

Figure 4-1. Evolution of a plaque within a coronary artery. (Schoen FJ. Blood vessels. In Kumar V, Abbas AK, Fausto N [eds]. Robbins and Cotran Pathologic Basis of Disease, 7th ed. Philadelphia, Saunders, 2005.)

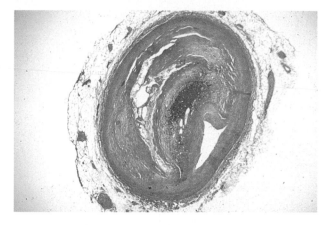

Figure 4-2. Photomicrograph of a cross section of a coronary artery with severe stenosis and narrowing. (Courtesy W. O'Conner, MD, Lexington, Ky.)

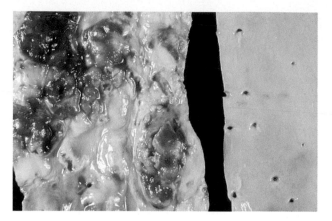

Figure 4-3. The segment of aorta on the left demonstrates advanced atheromatous plaques, and the specimen on the right side is unaffected. (Courtesy W. O'Conner, MD, Lexington, Ky.)

Atherosclerosis is usually a focal disease that commonly occurs in certain areas or regions of arteries while sparing others.[30] For example, the proximal left anterior descending coronary artery is a common area of atherosclerosis, as are the proximal portions of the renal arteries; however, the internal mammary artery is rarely involved. The lumen of an affected artery may be circumferentially narrowed evenly or eccentrically, depending on the location and extent of the plaque.

The outcome of the atherosclerotic process is extremely variable. Some lesions never progress past the fatty streak phase; however, in most Western societies, the presence of frank plaques is the norm. Even so, most atheromatous plaques produce no symptoms and may never cause clinical manifestations.[30] Several factors may be responsible, including arterial remodeling, in which the plaque grows outward away from the lumen with a compensatory increase in the diameter of the vessel. In addition, collateral circulation may develop to compensate for diminished blood flow. For those lesions that do produce symptoms, flow-limiting intact plaques usually produce symptoms such as chest pain (angina) when oxygen need exceeds demand, as during exercise. However, plaque rupture produces acute or unstable symptoms such as angina at rest, MI, or sudden death. Not all plaques have the same propensity to rupture, and risk depends on the physical and biochemical characteristics of the plaque.

Intra-arterial complications of coronary atherosclerosis consist of luminal narrowing, intramural hemorrhage, thrombosis, embolism, and aneurysm. Intramural hemorrhage, which occurs because of weakening of the intimal tissues, may lead to thrombosis. It also may serve as an irritant and may cause a reflex reaction, resulting in spasm of the collateral vessels. Once formed, a thrombus may become encapsulated and may undergo fibrous organization and recanalization. The atherosclerotic process is not limited to the coronary arteries but is found throughout other arteries of the body (Figure 4-3).

If the degree of ischemia that results from coronary atherosclerosis is significant and prolonged, the area of myocardium supplied by that vessel may undergo necrosis. Reduced blood flow may result from thrombosis of the affected artery, a hypotensive episode, an increased demand for blood, or emotional stress. The infarction, or area of necrosis, may be subendocardial or transmural (Figure 4-4), the latter involving the entire thickness of the myocardium. This is reflected in the electrocardiogram (ECG), on which the ST segment is not elevated with partial obstruction to blood flow and limited myocardial necrosis, but the ST segment is elevated with more profound ischemia and a larger area of necrosis. Complications of MI include weakened heart muscle, resulting in acute congestive heart failure, postinfarction angina, infarct extension, cardiogenic shock, pericarditis, and arrhythmias. Causes of death in patients who have had an acute MI (AMI) include ventricular fibrillation, cardiac standstill, congestive heart failure, embolism, and rupture of the heart wall or septum.[31]

CLINICAL PRESENTATION
Symptoms

Chest pain is the most important symptom of coronary atherosclerotic heart disease. The pain may be brief, as in angina pectoris resulting from temporary ischemia of the myocardium, or it may be prolonged, as in unstable angina or AMI. Ischemic myocardial pain results from an imbalance between the oxygen supply and the oxygen demand of the muscle. Atherosclerotic narrowing of the coronary arteries is an important cause of this imbalance. The exact mechanism or agents involved in producing the cardiac pain are not known.

Angina pectoris usually is described as an aching, heavy, squeezing pressure or tightness in the midchest region.[28] The area of discomfort often is described to be approximately the size of the fist and may radiate into the left or right arm to the neck or lower jaw. In rare cases,

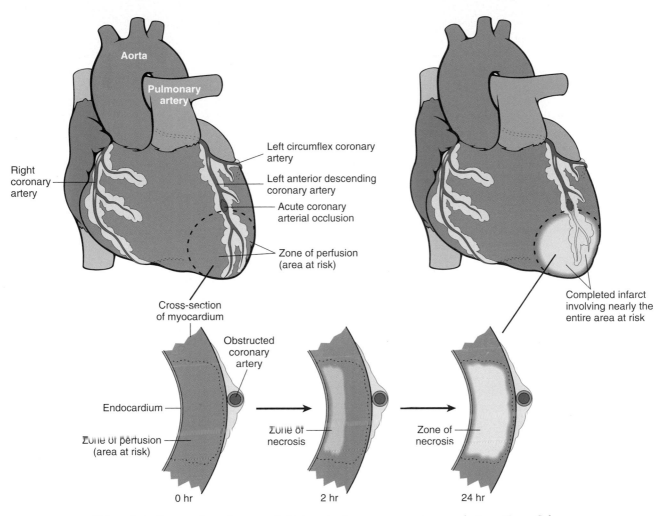

Figure 4-4. Progression of myocardial necrosis after coronary artery occlusion. (From Schoen FJ. The heart. In Kumar V, Abbas AK, Fausto N [eds]. Robbins and Cotran Pathologic Basis of Disease, 7th ed. Philadelphia, Saunders, 2005.)

it may be present in only one of these distant sites, and the patient is free of central chest pain. The pain is brief, lasting 5 to 15 minutes if the provoking stimulus is stopped or for a shorter time if nitroglycerin is used. Angina is defined in terms of its pattern of symptom stability. *Stable angina* is pain that is predictably reproducible and consistent over time. This pain typically is precipitated by physical effort such as walking or climbing stairs but may also occur with eating or stress. Pain is relieved by cessation of the precipitating activity, by rest, or by the use of nitroglycerin. *Unstable angina* is defined as new onset of pain, pain that is increasing in frequency, more intense pain than before, pain that is precipitated by less effort than before, or pain that occurs at rest. This pain is not readily relieved by nitroglycerin. The key feature is the changing character or pattern of the pain. Patients with stable angina have a relatively good prognosis. Patients with unstable angina have a poorer prognosis and often develop MI within a short time. The term *acute coronary syndrome* describes a continuum of myocardial ischemia that ranges from unstable angina at one end of the spectrum to non–ST segment

MI at the other. Differentiation requires diagnostic and laboratory testing. A relatively uncommon form of angina, *Prinzmetal's variant angina*, occurs at rest and is caused by focal spasm of a coronary artery, usually with varying amounts of atherosclerosis.[28] Angina also may occur in individuals with normal coronary vessels.

Patients with coronary atherosclerosis who develop prolonged pain as a result of myocardial ischemia usually have unstable angina or are having an AMI. This pain usually is more severe and lasts longer than 15 minutes but has the same general character as that described for stable angina. Its location is the same and it may radiate in the same pattern as the brief pain that results from temporary myocardial ischemia. Vasodilators or cessation of activity does not relieve the pain caused by infarction. Neither brief nor prolonged pain resulting from myocardial ischemia is aggravated by deep breathing.

Sudden cardiac death accounts for 300,000 deaths annually in the United States and is often, but not always, due to cardiac arrhythmia.[32] Most cardiac arrest survivors have structural heart disease; nearly 75% have coronary artery disease. Predominant symptoms that most often precede sudden death include chest pain, cough, shortness of breath, fainting, dizziness, palpitations, and fatigue. The most common cause of sudden death is ventricular fibrillation, a form of abnormal electrical activity resulting from interruption of the electrical conduction system.[32]

Palpitations of the heart (disagreeable awareness of the heartbeat) may be present in patients with coronary atherosclerotic heart disease with normal or abnormal rhythm. The complaint is not directly related to the seriousness of the underlying cardiac problem. Syncope, a transient loss of consciousness resulting from inadequate cerebral blood flow, also may occur in patients with coronary atherosclerotic heart disease.

Symptoms of congestive heart failure experienced as a complication of coronary atherosclerotic heart disease include dyspnea, orthopnea, paroxysmal nocturnal dyspnea, edema, hemoptysis, fatigue, weakness, and cyanosis. Fatigue and weakness may be present early in the course of the disease before the onset of congestive failure (see Chapter 6).

Signs

Clinical signs of coronary atherosclerotic heart disease are few, and the patient may appear entirely normal. Most clinical signs relate to other underlying cardiovascular disease or conditions such as congestive failure. Conditions such as corneal arcus and xanthoma of the skin are related to hyperlipidemia and hypercholesterolemia. Blood pressure may become elevated, and abnormalities in the rate and/or rhythm of the pulse may occur. Diminished peripheral pulses in the lower extremities may be seen, along with bruits in the carotid arteries. Panoramic radiographs of the jaws may occasionally demonstrate carotid calcifications in the areas of C_3 and C_4, consistent with atherosclerotic plaques in the carotid arteries (see Chapter 27). Retinal changes are common in hypertensive disease and diabetes mellitus. Signs associated with advanced coronary atherosclerotic heart disease usually reflect the presence of congestive heart failure. Distention of neck veins, peripheral edema, cyanosis, ascites, and enlarged liver may be found.

Laboratory Findings

Blood tests are used in the evaluation of patients with symptoms of angina pectoris to screen for abnormalities that may contribute to or worsen coronary heart disease. These include complete blood count to rule out anemia, thyroid function tests to exclude hyperthyroidism, renal function testing to exclude renal insufficiency, lipid screening for hypercholesterolemia, glucose for diabetes, homocysteine levels, and levels of C-reactive protein. Other diagnostic tests that are specific for coronary heart disease include resting ECG, chest x-ray, exercise stress testing, ambulatory (Holter) electrocardiography, stress thallium-201 perfusion scintigraphy, exercise echocardiography, ambulatory ventricular function monitoring, and cardiac catheterization and angiography.[28]

Along with physical examination and diagnostic testing, serum enzyme determinations are necessary to establish the diagnosis of acute MI and determine the extent of infarction. Serum markers of acute MI most commonly used in practice include troponin I, troponin T, and creatine kinase isoenzyme (CK-MB).[33] These enzymes are released only when cell death (infarction) or injury occurs. Troponins are proteins that are derived from the breakdown of myocardial sarcomeres; they have largely replaced creatine kinase (CK) and CK-MB because they are more specific in differentiating trauma from skeletal muscle or other organs.[31] Very little difference has been noted between the two troponins. Plasma troponins are virtually absent in normal individuals and are found only after cardiac injury. Troponins are first detectable 3 to 6 hours after the onset of an acute MI; they reach peak values at 18 to 24 hours and persist for 5 to 14 days.[34]

CK-MB is another enzymatic marker of cardiac cell injury with similar characteristics as the troponins; however, in addition to its presence in the heart, CK-MB is found following injury to skeletal muscle and other tissues. In spite of this, elevated levels of CK-MB are usually considered to be the result of an MI.[33] CK-MB is detectable within 3 to 6 hours after infarction; it reaches peak values at 10 to 12 hours and persists for 2 to 3 days.[34] In many centers, troponin has replaced CK-MB as the diagnostic test of choice for MI because of its sensitivity and specificity, and as a result of cost issues. In any case, definitive diagnosis of MI requires serial testing over several days rather than reliance on single test results. In the past, CK and CK-MB were the standard tests; however, with the presence of CK in skeletal muscle and its elevation even with minor skeletal muscle trauma, it is no longer relied upon for diagnosis. Myoglobin is another enzymatic marker that may be used, but it is not specific for cardiac injury. It is detectable within 2 to 3 hours following infarct, peaks at around 6 to 8 hours, and persists for 18 to 24 hours.[34]

MEDICAL MANAGEMENT
Angina Pectoris

Medical management of a patient with chronic stable angina involves five aspects:

1. Identification and treatment of associated diseases that can precipitate or worsen angina
2. Reduction in coronary risk factors
3. Application of general and nonpharmacologic methods, with particular attention toward adjustments in lifestyle
4. Pharmacologic management
5. Revascularization by percutaneous catheter–based techniques or by coronary bypass surgery[35] (Box 4-1)

Management may include general lifestyle measures such as an exercise program; weight control; restriction of salt, cholesterol, and saturated fatty acids; cessation of smoking; and control of exacerbating conditions such as

Medical Management of Patients With Stable Angina Pectoris

- Identification and treatment of associated diseases that can precipitate or worsen angina (anemia, obesity, hyperthyroidism)
- Reduction in coronary risk factors (hypertension, smoking, hyperlipidemia)
- Application of general and nonpharmacologic methods (lifestyle modifications)
- Pharmacologic management
  - Nitrates
  - Beta blockers
  - Calcium channel blockers
  - Antiplatelet agents
- Revascularization
  - Percutaneous transluminal coronary angioplasty with stenting
  - Coronary artery bypass grafting

anemia, hypertension, and hyperthyroidism. Patients who have significant angina are encouraged to avoid long hours of work, take rest periods during the working day, obtain adequate rest at night, use mild sedatives, take frequent vacations, and, in some cases, change their occupation or retire. Patients should avoid precipitating factors that may bring on cardiac pain such as cold weather, hot and humid weather, big meals, emotional upset, cigarette smoking, and drugs (e.g., amphetamines, caffeine, ephedrine, cyclamates, alcohol).

Drug therapy consists of nitrates (nitroglycerin or long-acting nitrates), antiplatelet agents, beta-adrenergic blockers, and calcium channel blockers (Table 4-1). Although it is not currently recommended for the routine treatment of patients with stable angina, significant benefit appears to be associated with the use of angiotensin-converting enzyme (ACE) inhibitors. Studies are currently being conducted to determine their effectiveness and to define their role in the treatment of angina.

Nitrates are vasodilators, predominantly venodilators, and are the cornerstone in the pharmacologic management of angina. Their mechanism of action is unknown; however, researchers believe their effect may be caused by a decrease in cardiac load, resulting in decreased oxygen demand. Nitrates also may alleviate coronary artery spasm. Nitroglycerin may be used acutely for the relief of anginal pain and prophylactically to prevent angina. It comes in a variety of forms, including tablet, lingual spray, ointment, and transdermal patch. Nitroglycerin tablets are placed under the tongue to dissolve; the spray can be administered beneath the tongue or onto the oral mucosa. Nitrates are taken orally to prevent anginal symptoms and are supplied in tablet form, as an ointment that may be applied to the skin, or as long-acting transdermal nitrate patches that are applied to the skin. Nitrates are used to reduce symptoms of angina, but they do not slow, alter, or reverse the progression of coronary artery disease.

Beta blockers, which are effective in the treatment of many patients with angina, compete with catecholamines for beta-adrenergic receptor sites, resulting in decreased heart rate and myocardial contractility and reducing myocardial oxygen demand. Nonselective beta blockers block the $beta_1$ and $beta_2$ receptors, whereas cardioselective beta blockers preferentially block the $beta_1$ receptors at normal therapeutic doses. Nonselective beta blockers may cause unwanted effects, such as increasing the tone of vascular smooth muscle and causing both vasoconstriction of peripheral vessels and contraction of bronchial smooth muscle. Thus, nonselective beta blockers are not prescribed for patients with a history of asthma. Injections of sympathomimetic drugs such as epinephrine or levonordefrin may result in elevation of blood pressure in patients taking nonselective beta blockers; therefore, they should be used cautiously.

Calcium channel blockers are effective in the treatment of chronic stable angina when given alone or in combination with beta blockers and nitrates. These drugs decrease intracellular calcium, resulting in vasodilatation of coronary, peripheral, and pulmonary vasculature, along with decreased myocardial contractility and heart rate.

Aspirin used as antiplatelet therapy is another cornerstone of treatment in patients with angina.[36] The use of aspirin in patients with stable angina is associated with a 33% reduction in fatal events.[37] In patients with unstable angina, aspirin decreases the chances of fatal and nonfatal MI.[38] Aspirin, in daily doses of 75 to 325 mg, is recommended for all patients with acute and chronic ischemic heart disease, regardless of the presence or absence of symptoms.[36] Clopidogrel, another antiplatelet agent, has been shown to have effects equivalent to those of aspirin; it is used in place of or in combination with aspirin. Ticlopidine and dipyridamole have not been shown to have any beneficial effects and are not recommended for use.

Revascularization is an option for patients with stable or unstable angina. Available procedures for revascularization include percutaneous transluminal coronary angioplasty, stents, and coronary artery bypass grafting. Percutaneous transluminal coronary angioplasty, also known as *balloon angioplasty*, involves the use of a small, inflatable balloon catheter over a thin guidewire that is threaded through the occluded segment of the artery. Once in place, the balloon is inflated and compresses the plaque and thrombus against the arterial wall, thus enlarging the lumen of the vessel (Figure 4-5). This results in an immediate increase in blood flow and provides symptomatic relief for ischemia. However, restenosis recurs within 6 months in approximately 30% to 40% of patients, along with a return of symptoms.[39]

One method of decreasing the occurrence of restenosis with percutaneous transluminal coronary angioplasty involves the use of a thin, expandable, metallic mesh stent positioned by the balloon and expanded against the plaque and vessel wall, then left in place. This stent functions as a permanent scaffold to help maintain vessel

TABLE 4-1
Drugs Used in the Management of Angina

Drug	Vasoconstrictor Interactions	Oral Manifestations	Other Considerations
NITRATES			
Nitroglycerin	None	Dry mouth	Orthostatic hypotension, headache
Nitrogard			
Nitrolingual			
Nitro-Bid			
Nitrek			
Nitrostat			
Nitro-Time			
Nitrol			
Nitro-Tab			
Nitrogard			
Nitro-Dur			
Minitran			
Isosorbide dinitrate			
Dilatrate-SR			
Isordil			
Isosorbide 5-mononitrate			
Monoket			
Imdur			
Ismo			
BETA BLOCKERS (NS, BLOCKADE OF BETA$_1$ AND BETA$_2$ RECEPTORS; CS, BLOCKADE OF BETA$_1$ RECEPTORS ONLY)			
Propranolol/LA (Inderal) (NS)	NS, increase in blood pressure possible with sympathomimetics, cautious use recommended (maximum 0.036 mg epinephrine; 0.20 mg levonordefrin)	Taste changes, lichenoid reactions	Orthostatic hypotension
Nadolol (Corgard) (NS)			
Carteolol (Cartrol) (NS)			
Timolol (Blocadren) (NS)			
Penbutolol (Levatol) (NS)			
Pindolol (Visken) (NS)			
Sotalol (Betapace) (NS)			
Metoprolol/XL (Lopressor) (CS)	CS, minimal effect with sympathomimetics, normal use		
Atenolol (Tenormin) (CS)			
Acebutolol (Sectral) (CS)			
Labetalol (Normodyne, Trandate) (CS)			
CALCIUM CHANNEL BLOCKERS			
Bepridil (Vascor)	None	Gingival hyperplasia, dry mouth, lichenoid eruptions (rare)	None
Diltiazem/CD (Cardizem, Cartia, Dilacor, Diltia, Taztia, Tiazac)			
Felodipine (Plendil)			
Isradipine (DynaCirc)			
Nifedipine/PA/XL (Adalat, Nifedical, Procardia)			
Verapamil/SR (Calan, Isoptin, Verelan, Covera)			
Amlodipine (Norvasc)			
Nicardipine/SR (Cardene)			
Nisoldipine (Sular)			
Nitrendipine			
PLATELET AGGREGATION INHIBITORS			
Aspirin	None	None	Increased bleeding but not clinically significant with daily doses ≤325 mg
Clopidogrel (Plavix)	None	None	Increased bleeding time

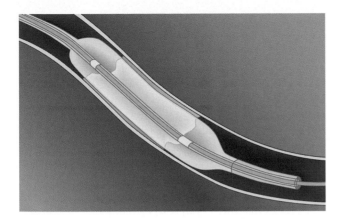

Figure 4-5. Balloon angioplasty catheter. (From Teirstein PS. Percutaneous coronary interventions. In Goldman L, Ausiello D [eds]. Cecil Textbook of Medicine, 22nd ed. Philadelphia, Saunders, 2004.)

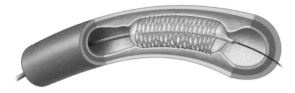

Figure 4-6. Expandable metallic stent that is left in place after deflation and withdrawal of the balloon catheter.

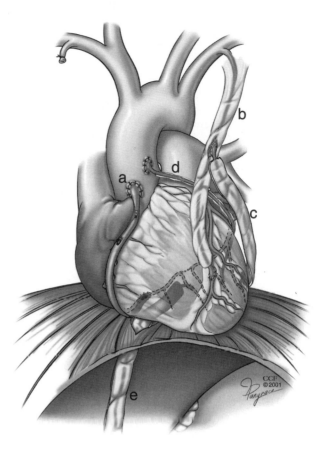

Figure 4-7. Types of bypass grafts: **a,** Saphenous vein graft from aorta to right coronary artery. **b,** In situ left internal mammary artery graft to anterior descending coronary artery. **c,** Y-graft of right internal mammary artery from left internal mammary artery to circumflex coronary artery. **d,** Radial artery graft from aorta to circumflex coronary artery. **e,** In situ gastroepiploic graft to posterior descending branch of the right coronary artery. (From Lytle BW. Surgical treatment of coronary artery disease. In Goldman L, Ausiello D [eds]. Cecil Textbook of Medicine, 22nd ed. Philadelphia, Saunders, 2004.)

patency (Figure 4-6). Stents become covered by endothelium within 2 weeks after placement. The use of stents has decreased the incidence of restenosis to about 20% to 30%; however, it has not prevented restenosis from occurring.[39] Recently, greater success has been achieved with the use of stents that are coated with various bioactive medications to decrease endothelial proliferation and the use of intravascular radiation therapy. Other non–balloon angioplasty methods include rotational atherectomy and the use of lasers. With percutaneous intervention, symptomatic and angiographic improvement is expected in more than 90% of patients, and the complication rate is less than 10%.[28]

Coronary artery bypass graft (CABG) surgery is an effective means of controlling symptoms in the management of unstable angina; it can improve the long-term survival rate in certain subsets of patients. It also is effective in controlling symptoms in patients whose pain persists despite medical control. With CABG, a segment of artery or vein is harvested or released from a donor site; it is then grafted to the affected segment of coronary artery, thus bypassing the area of occlusion (Figure 4-7). Two primary graft donor sites are used: the saphenous vein and the internal mammary artery. Of the two, the internal mammary artery graft is sturdier and much less susceptible to graft atherosclerosis and occlusion than are vein grafts. Within 10 years postoperatively, 30% to 50% of saphenous vein grafts become occluded, and internal mammary grafts become resistant to occlusion. The latter are preferred for the first bypass procedures when possi-

ble. Reoperation is difficult because of surgical site scarring and the limited supply of graft donor material. The perioperative morality rate for elective CABG is 0.2%.[28]

Myocardial Infarction

Patients who have experienced an AMI should be hospitalized or should receive emergency treatment as soon as possible (Box 4-2). The basic management goal is to minimize the size of the infarction and prevent death from lethal arrhythmias. The size and extent of the infarct are critical in the determination of outcome. Early administration of aspirin is recommended, with 160 to 325 mg being chewed and swallowed to decrease platelet aggregation and limit thrombus formation. The definitive treatment of patients with AMI depends on the extent of ischemia as reflected on the ECG by the presence or absence of ST segment elevation. MI *without* ST segment elevation is due to partial blockage of coronary blood flow; MI *with* ST segment elevation is due to complete

BOX 4-2

Medical Management of Patients With Acute Myocardial Infarction

- Rapid hospitalization and determination of ST segment changes
- Aspirin administration
- Early thrombolytic therapy (for ST segment elevation only)
  - Streptokinase
  - Urokinase
  - Alteplase
  - Reteplase
- Early revascularization
  - Thrombolysis (for ST segment elevation only)
  - Percutaneous transluminal coronary angioplasty with stenting
  - Coronary artery bypass grafting
- Pharmacologic therapy
  - Antiplatelet drugs (glycoprotein IIa/IIIb inhibitor,[61] aspirin, clopidogrel)
  - Nitrates
  - Beta-adrenergic blockers
  - Calcium channel blockers
  - Angiotensin-converting enzyme (ACE) inhibitors
  - Lipid-lowering drugs
  - Anticoagulants (unfractionated heparin, low molecular weight heparin)
  - Morphine
  - Sedatives/hypnotics
- Oxygen

---

blockage of coronary blood flow and more profound ischemia involving a relatively large area of myocardium (Figure 4-8). This distinction is clinically important because early fibrinolytic therapy improves outcomes in ST segment elevation MI but not in non–ST segment elevation MI.[40]

The management of AMI has undergone significant change over the past several years with the recognition that thrombolytic therapy can result in significant reduction of morbidity and mortality in ST segment elevation MI. The greatest benefit is realized when patients receive thrombolytic drugs within the first 3 hours after infarction; however, modest benefit is possible even up to 12 hours after the event.[33] The early use of thrombolytic drugs may decrease the extent of necrosis and myocardial damage and dramatically improve outcome and prognosis. Thrombolytic (or fibrinolytic) drugs used in the treatment of AMI include streptokinase, urokinase, alteplase (rt-PA), and reteplase. For most patients with ST segment elevation MI, the preferred method for revascularization is fibrinolysis or percutaneous coronary angioplasty. Percutaneous transluminal coronary angioplasty with stenting is an alternative to thrombolytic therapy that yields better outcomes.

In patients with ST segment elevation MI, non–ST segment elevation MI, or unstable angina (acute coronary syndrome), anticoagulation is often applied in the form of unfractionated heparin or low molecular weight heparin; in addition, glycoprotein IIa/IIIb inhibitors (abciximab, eptifibatide, tirofiban) are administered intravenously for their antiplatelet effects. Cardiac catheterization and revascularization with percutaneous intervention or bypass is indicated within the first 2 hours in non–ST segment elevation MI.[41]

General pharmacologic measures for patients with AMI include the use of nitrates, beta blockers, calcium channel blockers, ACE inhibitors, and lipid-lowering agents. Antiplatelet drugs are significant in decreasing morbidity and mortality, and aspirin is the drug of choice. Daily doses of 81 to 325 mg are recommended. Clopidogrel (Plavix; Bristol-Myers Squibb/Sanofi Pharmaceuticals, New York, NY) and ticlopidine (Ticlid; Roche Laboratories, Inc., Nutley, NJ) are other antiplatelet drugs that may be used, although the use of ticlopidine has been supplanted by the administration of clopidogrel because of superior outcomes reported with the latter. For pain relief, morphine sulfate is the drug of choice. Sedatives and anxiolytic medications also may be used. Oxygen may be administered by nasal cannula during the acute period to enhance oxygen saturation of the blood and keep the heart workload at a minimum level. The development of arrhythmias in patients who have had an AMI constitutes an emergency that must be treated aggressively with antiarrhythmic drugs. During the first several weeks after an infarction, the conduction system of the heart may be unstable, and patients are prone to serious arrhythmias and reinfarction. A pacemaker may be used with severe myocardial damage and resultant heart failure.

DENTAL MANAGEMENT
Medical Considerations

Risk assessment for the dental management of patients with ischemic heart disease involves three determinants:
1. Severity of the disease
2. Type and magnitude of the dental procedure
3. Stability and reserve of the patient

All must be factored into a dental management plan so that a rational and safe decision can be made, specifically, to determine whether a patient can safely tolerate a planned procedure. The American College of Cardiology and the American Heart Association[42] published risk stratification guidelines for patients with various types of heart disease who are undergoing various noncardiac surgical procedures. These guidelines can provide significant value in the determination of risk for surgical and nonsurgical dental procedures (Boxes 4-3 and 4-4).

Recent MI (within the past 7 to 30 days) and unstable angina are classified as clinical predictors of major risk for perioperative complications. Stable (mild) angina and past history of MI are identified as clinical predictors of intermediate risk for perioperative complications. The type and magnitude of the planned procedure also must

Figure 4-8. A, Waves and intervals of a normal electrocardiogram (ECG). Note the normal ST segment. **B,** Electrocardiographic tracing shows an acute anterior/lateral MI. Note ST elevation in leads I, aVL, and V$_{1-6}$. (**A** from Goldberger AL. Clinical Electrocardiography: A Simplified Approach, 6th ed. St. Louis, Mosby, 1999. **B** courtesy of Dr. Thomas Evans. From Anderson JL. ST-elevation acute myocardial infarction and complications of myocardial infarction. In Goldman L, Ausiello D [eds]. Cecil Textbook of Medicine, 22nd ed. Philadelphia, Saunders, 2004.)

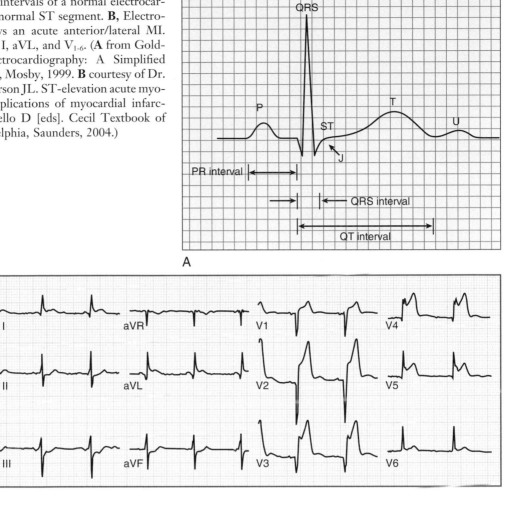

be considered, as well as the perioperative risk conveyed by the diseases themselves. Based on these guidelines, most dental procedures, including minor oral surgery and periodontal surgery, would fall within the low-risk, "superficial procedures" category, with less than 1% risk. Nonsurgical dental procedures are likely to pose even less of a risk than is incurred by surgical procedures. More extensive oral and maxillofacial surgical procedures, and perhaps some of the more extensive periodontal surgical procedures, would fall in the intermediate cardiac risk category under "head and neck procedures." These procedures carry a risk lower than 5%. Procedures that present the highest risk include emergency major surgery in the elderly, aortic or vascular surgery, and peripheral vascular surgery. These procedures are performed with the patient under general anesthesia and have the potential for significant blood and fluid loss with resultant adverse hemodynamic effects.

These risk stratification guidelines may be applied to various dental management scenarios. For example, a patient with unstable angina or recent MI is classified as a major cardiac risk. However, if the planned dental procedure is limited to routine clinical examination with x-rays (considered at extremely low risk), and the patient is stable and not anxious, the risk for an adverse occurrence is not significant; thus, alterations needed in the dental management approach would be minimal. Conversely, a patient with stable angina or a past history of MI (intermediate risk) with minimal cardiac reserve, who is scheduled for multiple extractions and implant placement (low to intermediate risk), poses a more significant risk and may require a more complex dental management plan.

Angina Pectoris. A determination should be made about the severity and stability of angina. A patient with stable angina characteristically describes the occurrence of chest pain in a consistent, recurring, and predictable pattern. Pain is precipitated by typical physical activity such as exercising, mowing the lawn, or climbing stairs and subsides within 5 to 15 minutes with rest or the use of nitroglycerin. Pain occurs in a chronic, unchanging pattern over time. These patients pose an intermediate cardiac risk.

A patient with unstable angina conversely may describe the recent onset of chest pain, or progressively worsening chest pain that occurs with physical exertion or at rest. Typically, a pattern of increasing severity, frequency, or duration of pain occurs. Pain occurring at rest or during

---

BOX 4-3

Clinical Predictors of Increased Perioperative Cardiovascular Risk (myocardial infarction [MI], heart failure, death)

MAJOR
- Unstable coronary syndromes
  - Acute or recent myocardial infarction (*) with evidence of important ischemic risk seen by clinical symptoms or noninvasive study
  - Unstable or severe angina (Canadian Class III or IV)[†‡]
- Decompensated heart failure
- Significant arrhythmias
  - High-grade atrioventricular block
  - Symptomatic ventricular arrhythmias in the presence of underlying heart disease
  - Supraventricular arrhythmias with uncontrolled ventricular rate
- Severe valvular disease

INTERMEDIATE
- Mild angina pectoris (Canadian Class I or II)[†]
- Previous myocardial infarction by history or pathological Q waves
- Compensated or prior heart failure
- Diabetes mellitus (particularly insulin-dependent)
- Renal insufficiency

MINOR
- Advanced age
- Abnormal ECG electrocardiogram (left ventricular hypertrophy, left bundle-branch block, ST-T abnormalities)
- Rhythm other than sinus (e.g., atrial fibrillation)
- Low functional capacity (e.g., inability to climb one flight of stairs with a bag of groceries)
- History of stroke
- Uncontrolled systemic hypertension (≥180/110 mm Hg)

From ACC/AHA Guideline Update for Perioperative Cardiovascular Evaluation for Noncardiac Surgery—Executive Summary. Copyright © 2002, American Heart Association.
ECG, Electrocardiogram.
*The American College of Cardiology National Database Library defines *recent MI* as greater than 7 days but less than or equal to 1 month (30 days); *acute MI* occurs within 7 days.
†May include "stable" angina in patients who are unusually sedentary.
†Campeau L. Grading of angina pectoris. Circulation 1976;54:522-523; the Canadian Classification is a system of grading angina severity (grade I-IV), with grade I angina occurring only with strenuous exertion and grade IV angina occurring with any physical activity or at rest.

BOX 4-4

Cardiac Risk* Stratification for Noncardiac Surgical Procedures

HIGH (REPORTED CARDIAC RISK OFTEN GREATER THAN 5%)
- Emergent major operations, particularly in the elderly
- Aortic and other major vascular surgery
- Peripheral vascular surgery
- Anticipated prolonged surgical procedures associated with large fluid shifts and/or blood loss

INTERMEDIATE (REPORTED CARDIAC RISK GENERALLY LESS THAN 5%)
- Carotid endarterectomy
- Head and neck surgery
- Intraperitoneal and intrathoracic surgery
- Orthopaedic surgery
- Prostate surgery

LOW (REPORTED CARDIAC RISK GENERALLY LESS THAN 1%)
- Endoscopic procedures
- Superficial procedures
- Cataract surgery

From ACC/AHA Guideline Update for Perioperative Cardiovascular Evaluation for Noncardiac Surgery—Executive Summary. Copyright © 2002, American Heart Association.
*Combined incidence of cardiac death and nonfatal myocardial infarction.

---

ischemic symptoms (intermediate risk) may include the following: short appointments in the morning, comfortable chair position, pretreatment vital signs, availability of nitroglycerin, oral sedation, nitrous oxide/oxygen sedation, excellent local anesthesia, limited amount of vasoconstrictor, avoidance of epinephrine-impregnated retraction cord, avoidance of anticholinergics, and effective postoperative pain control. For patients who have had balloon angioplasty with placement of a coronary artery stent, or for those who have undergone a CABG procedure, antibiotic prophylaxis is not recommended[43,44] (Box 4-5).

For patients with symptoms of unstable angina or those who have had an MI within the past 30 days (major risk), elective care should be postponed (Box 4-6). If treatment becomes necessary, it should be performed as conservatively as possible and directed primarily toward pain relief, infection control, or the control of bleeding. Consultation with the physician is advised. Additional management recommendations may include establishing and maintaining an intravenous line, continuously monitoring the ECG and vital signs, using a pulse oximeter, and administering nitroglycerin prophylactically just before the initiation of treatment. These measures may require the patient be treated in a special patient care facility or hospital dental clinic.

The use of vasoconstrictors in local anesthetics poses potential problems for patients with ischemic heart disease because of the possibilities of precipitating cardiac

sleep is particularly ominous. Patients with unstable angina should be considered a major cardiac risk.

Based on the assessment of medical risk, the type of planned dental procedure, and the stability and anxiety level of the patient, general management strategies for patients with stable angina or a past history of MI without

BOX 4-5

Dental Management Considerations for Patients With Stable Angina or Past History of Myocardial Infarction*

- Morning appointments
- Short appointments
- Comfortable chair position
- Pretreatment vital signs
- Nitroglycerin readily available
- Stress-reduction measures:
  - Good communication
  - Oral sedation (e.g., triazolam 0.125- to 0.25 mg on the night before and 1 hour before the appointment)
  - Intraoperative N_2O/O_2
  - Excellent local anesthesia
- Limited use of vasoconstrictor (maximum 0.036 mg epinephrine, 0.20 mg levonordefrin); also applicable if patient is taking a nonselective beta-blocker
- Avoidance of epinephrine-impregnated retraction cord
- Antibiotic prophylaxis *not* recommended for patients with coronary artery stents
- Antibiotic prophylaxis *not* recommended for history of coronary artery bypass graft (CABG)
- Avoidance of anticholinergics (e.g., scopolamine, and atropine)
- Adequate postoperative pain control

*Defined as longer than 1 month since myocardial infarction (MI), with no ischemic symptoms. It is recommended that at least 4 to 6 weeks should elapse after an uncomplicated MI before elective procedures are performed.

BOX 4-6

Dental Management Considerations for Patients With Unstable Angina or Recent Myocardial Infarction*

- Avoid elective care
- If treatment is necessary, consult with physician and limit treatment to pain relief, treatment of acute infection, or control of bleeding
- Consider including the following:
  - Prophylactic nitroglycerin
  - Placement of intravenous line
  - Sedation
  - Oxygen
  - Continuous electrocardiographic monitoring
  - Pulse oximeter
  - Frequent monitoring of blood pressure
  - Cautious use of epinephrine in local anesthetic, combined with above measures

*Myocardial infarction within the past 30 days.

effects equivalent to those of epinephrine without adverse cardiovascular effects.[48]

Patients who take daily aspirin (160 to 325 mg) can expect some increase in surgical and postoperative bleeding, but this is generally not clinically significant and can be controlled with local measures only. Discontinuation of these agents before dental treatment generally is unnecessary.[49,50]

Myocardial Infarction. The dentist should determine whether the patient has had an MI or any symptoms of ischemia (e.g., chest pain, shortness of breath, easy fatigue) for the purpose of quantifying risk. Patients who have had an MI have some degree of permanent damage to the heart. The outcome depends on the extent and location of the damage and its effect on the function of the heart. Damage may be minimal, with little effect on the patient's daily activity. Patients who have had an MI within the previous month with residual ischemic symptoms are classified as a *major cardiac risk* and are not candidates for elective dental care. Patients with a past history of an MI longer than 1 month ago who are clinically stable are classified as being an *intermediate cardiac risk* and, in most cases, are at minimal risk for routine dental treatment. However, myocardial damage may be extensive, resulting in cardiac instability and an inability of the heart to function properly (i.e., heart failure) (see Chapter 6). These patients are classified as a *major cardiac risk* and pose a significant risk for the provision of routine dental care. Management recommendations for stable angina are also applicable to patients with an uneventful past history of an MI (see Box 4-6).

For several weeks after an MI has occurred, risks of cardiac instability, arrhythmias, and reinfarction may be increased. These effects decrease with time, assuming that the electrical conduction system of the heart has not been seriously damaged. In the past, most authorities

tachycardias, arrhythmias, and increases in blood pressure. Local anesthetics without vasoconstrictors may be used as needed. If a vasoconstrictor is necessary, patients with intermediate risk and those taking nonselective beta blockers can safely be given up to 0.036 mg epinephrine (2 cartridges containing 1:100,000 epi) or 0.20 mg levonordefrin (2 cartridges containing 1:20,000 levo); intravascular injections are avoided. Greater quantities of vasoconstrictor may well be tolerated, but increasing quantities increase the risk of adverse cardiovascular effects. For patients at higher risk, the use of vasoconstrictors should be discussed with the physician. Studies have shown, however, that modest quantities of vasoconstrictors may be used safely even in high-risk patients when accompanied by oxygen, sedation, nitroglycerin, and excellent pain control measures.[45-47]

For patients at all levels of cardiac risk, the use of gingival retraction cord impregnated with epinephrine should be avoided because of the rapid absorption of a high concentration of epinephrine and the potential for adverse cardiovascular effects. As an alternative, plain cord saturated with tetrahydrozoline HCl 0.05% (Visine; Pfizer Inc, New York, NY) or oxymetazoline HCl 0.05% (Afrin; Schering-Plough, Summit, NJ) provides gingival suggested that the dentist not provide elective dental care for the first 6 months after an MI because of the risks cited earlier. This recommendation stems from studies conducted during the late 1960s and 1970s that examined the reinfarction rates of patients who had had an MI and were undergoing emergency or elective surgery while under general anesthesia.[51-53] These studies reported reinfarction rates of 27% to 37% during the first 3 months after an MI, 11% to 26% during the next 3 to 6 months, and 4% to 5% for 6 months or longer. These cases involved general surgery, including abdominal and thoracic procedures, performed with the patient under general anesthesia. Subsequent studies[54] of similar patients under similar conditions have reported much lower reinfarction rates of approximately 4% to 6% for the first 3 months, 0% to 2% for 3 to 6 months, and 2% to 6% for 6 months or longer. Contributing to this improvement is the early institution of fibrinolysis and revascularization that is commonplace today.

An examination of the reinfarction rate when only local anesthesia is used finds the risk reduced further. Backer and associates[55] reported on 195 patients with past MIs at various times who underwent ophthalmic surgery while under local anesthesia. None of these patients was reported to have developed perioperative or postoperative reinfarction. Three studies have described the performance of a variety of dental procedures in which local anesthesia was used in 129 patients with recent MI or unstable angina; no significant adverse effects were reported.[45-47] Local anesthesia with vasoconstrictor was used in conjunction with sedation and close monitoring in all cases. Thus, it is apparent that many patients recovering from a recent MI can undergo dental treatment safely if such treatment should become necessary. Delaying elective treatment for at least 4 to 6 weeks after an uncomplicated MI is recommended, prior to the provision of elective care.[42] Again, risk assessment must be undertaken as a precursor to decision making. Consultation with the physician is advisable. Patients with postinfarction disability or heart failure face significant risk and should delay elective care.

Patients who take aspirin or another platelet aggregation antagonist can expect some increase in bleeding. This effect generally is not clinically significant, and bleeding may be controlled through local measures. Discontinuation of these agents before dental treatment is provided generally is unnecessary. Laboratory assessment of platelet function is problematic in that no currently available test accurately and predictably reflects the ability of platelets to perform their normal function.[56] Bleeding time can be assessed before invasive procedures if desired; however, it has been shown that bleeding time does not correlate with clinical bleeding outcomes.[57] The platelet function analyzer (PFA)-100 is another laboratory test that may have some usefulness; however, a recent review concluded that the test does not have adequate sensitivity and specificity to be used as a routine screening tool for platelet disorders.[58]

Patients who take warfarin (Coumadin; Bristol-Myers Squibb Co., Princeton, NJ) for anticoagulation must have a current international normalized ratio (INR) determined before any invasive procedure can be performed. Most dental procedures, including minor surgery, may be performed safely without discontinuation or alteration of the Coumadin dosage, as long as the INR is within the therapeutic range (3.5 or less).[59,60] Local hemostatic measures generally are adequate to control bleeding and include the use of hemostatic agents in the sockets, suturing, gauze pressure packs, and tranexamic acid or ε-aminocaproic acid mouth rinses. More extensive surgical procedures associated with anticipated significant blood loss should be discussed with the patient's physician.

Oral Manifestations

No lesions or oral complications are the direct result of coronary atherosclerotic heart disease. Drugs used in the treatment of this disease and its complications, however, may produce oral changes such as dry mouth, taste changes, and stomatitis. Patients who take warfarin or aspirin may have increased bleeding after trauma or surgical procedures. In rare cases, patients with coronary atherosclerotic heart disease with angina may have pain referred to the lower jaw or teeth. The pattern of onset of pain caused by physical activity and its disappearance with rest usually serves as a clue to its cardiac origin.

REFERENCES

1. Thom T, Haase N, Rosamond W, et al. Heart disease and stroke statistics—2006 update: A report from the American Heart Association Statistics Committee and Stroke Statistics Subcommittee. Circulation 2006;113: e85-e151.
2. Chobanian AV, Bakris GL, Black HR, et al. The Seventh Report of the Joint National Committee on Prevention, Detection, Evaluation, and Treatment of High Blood Pressure: The JNC 7 report. JAMA 2003;289:2560-2572.
3. National Heart Lung and Blood Institute. Morbidity and Mortality Chartbook on Cardiovascular, Lung, and Blood Diseases. Bethesda, Md, NHLBI, 2004.
4. Criqui MH. Epidemiology of cardiovascular disease. In Goldman L, Ausiello D (eds). Cecil Textbook of Medicine. Philadelphia, WB Saunders, 2004.
5. Tuzcu EM, Kapadia SR, Tutar E, et al. High prevalence of coronary atherosclerosis in asymptomatic teenagers and young adults: Evidence from intravascular ultrasound. Circulation 2001;103:2705-2710.
6. Libby P. Inflammation and cardiovascular disease mechanisms. Am J Clin Nutr 2006;83:456S-460S.
7. Virmani R, Robinowitz M, Geer JC, Breslin PP, Beyer JC, McAllister HA. Coronary artery atherosclerosis revisited in Korean War combat casualties. Arch Pathol Lab Med 1987;111:972-976.
8. Ridker PM, Libby P. Risk factors for atherothrombotic disease. In Zipes D, Libby P, Bonow R, Braunwald E (eds). Braunwald's Heart Disease. Philadelphia, Elsevier, 2005.

9. Becker DM, Becker LC, Pearson TA, Fintel DJ, Levine DM, Kwiterovich PO. Risk factors in siblings of people with premature coronary heart disease. J Am Coll Cardiol 1988;12:1273-1280.

10. Jorde LB, Williams RR. Relation between family history of coronary artery disease and coronary risk variables. Am J Cardiol 1988;62:708-713.

11. Nasir K, Michos ED, Rumberger JA, et al. Coronary artery calcification and family history of premature coronary heart disease: Sibling history is more strongly associated than parental history. Circulation 2004;110: 2150-2156.

12. Genest J, Libby P, Gotto AM. Lipoprotein disorders and cardiovascular disease. In Zipes D, Libby P, Bonow R, Braunwald E (eds). Braunwald's Heart Disease: A Textbook of Cardiovascular Medicine, 7th ed. Philadelphia, Elsevier, 2005.

13. Gordon T, Kannel WB. Premature mortality from coronary heart disease: The Framingham study. JAMA 1971;215:1617-1625.

14. Vasan RS, Larson MG, Lcip EP, et al. Impact of high-normal blood pressure on the risk of cardiovascular disease. N Engl J Med 2001;345:1291-1297.

15. Vlietstra RE, Kronmal RA, Oberman A, Frye RL, Killip T 3rd. Effect of cigarette smoking on survival of patients with angiographically documented coronary artery disease: Report from the CASS registry. JAMA 1986; 255:1023-1027.

16. Kannel WB. Hypertension, blood lipids, and cigarette smoking as co-risk factors for coronary heart disease. Ann N Y Acad Sci 1978;304:128-139.

17. Grundy SM, Howard B, Smith S Jr, Eckel R, Redberg R, Bonow RO. Prevention Conference VI: Diabetes and Cardiovascular Disease: Executive summary: Conference proceeding for healthcare professionals from a special writing group of the American Heart Association. Circulation 2002;105:2231-2239.

18. Howard BV, Rodriguez BL, Bennett PH, et al. Prevention Conference VI: Diabetes and Cardiovascular Disease: Writing Group I: Epidemiology. Circulation 2002;105:e132-e137.

19. Gu K, Cowie CC, Harris MI. Mortality in adults with and without diabetes in a national cohort of the U.S. population, 1971-1993. Diabetes Care 1998;21:1138-1145.

20. Sherwin RS. Diabetes mellitus. In Goldman L, Ausiello D (eds). Cecil Textbook of Medicine, 22nd ed. Philadelphia, WB Saunders, 2004.

21. Semenkovich CF. Insulin resistance and atherosclerosis. J Clin Invest 2006;116:1813-1822.

22. Ford ES, Giles WH, Dietz WH. Prevalence of the metabolic syndrome among US adults: Findings from the Third National Health and Nutrition Examination Survey. JAMA 2002;287:356-359.

23. Beck JD, Offenbacher S. Systemic effects of periodontitis: Epidemiology of periodontal disease and cardiovascular disease. J Periodontol 2005;76(11 suppl):2089-2100.

24. Elter JR, Hinderliter AL, Offenbacher S, et al. The effects of periodontal therapy on vascular endothelial function: A pilot trial. Am Heart J 2006;151:47.

25. Libby P, Theroux P. Pathophysiology of coronary artery disease. Circulation 2005;111:3481-3488.

26. Fuster V. Atherosclerosis, thrombosis, and vascular biology. In Goldman L, Ausiello D (eds). Cecil Textbook of Medicine, 22nd ed. Philadelphia, WB Saunders, 2004.

27. Glagov S, Weisenberg E, Zarins CK, Stankunavicius R, Kolettis GJ. Compensatory enlargement of human atherosclerotic coronary arteries. N Engl J Med 1987;316: 1371-1375.

28. Theroux P. Angina pectoris. In Goldman L, Ausiello D (eds). Cecil Textbook of Medicine, 22nd ed. Philadelphia, WB Saunders, 2004.

29. Hackett D, Davies G, Maseri A. Pre-existing coronary stenoses in patients with first myocardial infarction are not necessarily severe. Eur Heart J 1988;9:1317-1323.

30. Libby P. The vascular biology of atherosclerosis. In Zipes D, Libby P, Bonow RO, Braunwald E (eds). Braunwald's Heart Disease: A Textbook of Cardiovascular Medicine, 7th ed. Philadelphia, Elsevier, 2005.

31. Anderson JL. ST-elevation acute myocardial infarction and complications of myocardial infarction. In Goldman L, Ausiello D (eds). Cecil Textbook of Medicine, 22nd ed. Philadelphia, WB Saunders, 2004.

32. Lerman BB. Ventricular arrhythmias and sudden death. In Goldman L, Ausiello D (eds). Cecil Textbook of Medicine, 22nd ed. Philadelphia, WB Saunders, 2004.

33. Antman EM, Braunwald E. ST-elevation myocardial infarction: Pathology, pathophysiology, and clinical features. In Zipes D, Libby P, Bonow RO, Braunwald E (eds). Braunwald's Heart Disease: A Textbook of Cardiovascular Medicine, 7th ed. Philadelphia, Elsevier Saunders, 2005.

34. Dufour DR, Lott JA, Henry JB. Clinical enzymology. In Henry JB (ed). Clinical Diagnosis and Management by Laboratory Methods, 20th ed. Philadelphia, WB Saunders, 2001.

35. Morrow DA, Gersh BJ, Braunwald E. Chronic coronary artery disease. In Zipes D, Libby P, Bonow RO, Braunwald E (eds). Braunwald's Heart Disease: A Textbook of Cardiovascular Medicine, 7th ed. Philadelphia, Elsevier Saunders, 2005.

36. Gibbons RJ, Abrams J, Chatterjee K, et al. ACC/AHA 2002 guideline update for the management of patients with chronic stable angina—Summary article: A report of the American College of Cardiology/American Heart Association Task Force on Practice Guidelines (Committee on the Management of Patients With Chronic Stable Angina). Circulation 2003;107:149-158.

37. Collaborative overview of randomised trials of antiplatelet therapy—I: Prevention of death, myocardial infarction, and stroke by prolonged antiplatelet therapy in various categories of patients. Antiplatelet Trialists' Collaboration. BMJ 1994;308:81-106.

38. Lewis HD Jr, Davis JW, Archibald DG, et al. Protective effects of aspirin against acute myocardial infarction and death in men with unstable angina: Results of a Veterans Administration Cooperative Study. N Engl J Med 1983; 309:396-403.

39. Teirstein PS. Percutaneous coronary interventions. In Goldman L, Ausiello D (eds). Cecil Textbook of Medicine, 22nd ed. Philadelphia, WB Saunders, 2004.

40. Waters DD. Acute coronary syndrome: Unstable angina and non–ST segment elevation myocardial infarction.

In Goldman L, Ausiello D (eds). Cecil Textbook of Medicine, 22nd ed. Philadelphia, WB Saunders, 2004.

41. Cannon CP, Braunwald E. Unstable angina and non–ST elevation myocardial infarction. In Zipes D, Libby P, Bonow RO, Braunwald E (eds). Braunwald's Heart Disease: A Textbook of Cardiovascular Medicine, 7th ed. Philadelphia, Elsevier Saunders, 2005.

42. Eagle KA, Berger PB, Calkins H, et al. ACC/AHA guideline update for perioperative cardiovascular evaluation for noncardiac surgery—Executive summary: A report of the American College of Cardiology/American Heart Association Task Force on Practice Guidelines (Committee to Update the 1996 Guidelines on Perioperative Cardiovascular Evaluation for Noncardiac Surgery). Anesth Analg 2002;94:1052-1064.

43. Baddour LM, Bettmann MA, Bolger AF, et al. Nonvalvular cardiovascular device–related infections. Circulation 2003;108:2015-2031.

44. Dajani AS, Taubert KA, Wilson W, et al. Prevention of bacterial endocarditis: Recommendations by the American Heart Association. J Am Dent Assoc 1997;128:1142-1151.

45. Cintron G, Medina R, Reyes AA, Lyman G. Cardiovascular effects and safety of dental anesthesia and dental interventions in patients with recent uncomplicated myocardial infarction. Arch Intern Med 1986;146:2203-2204.

46. Findler M, Galili D, Meidan Z, Yakirevitch V, Garfunkel AA. Dental treatment in very high risk patients with active ischemic heart disease. Oral Surg Oral Med Oral Pathol 1993;76:298-300.

47. Niwa H, Sato Y, Matsuura H. Safety of dental treatment in patients with previously diagnosed acute myocardial infarction or unstable angina pectoris. Oral Surg Oral Med Oral Pathol Oral Radiol Endod 2000;89:35-41.

48. Bowles WH, Tardy SJ, Vahadi A. Evaluation of new gingival retraction agents. J Dent Res 1991;70:1447-1449.

49. Ardekian L, Gaspar R, Peled M, Brener B, Laufer D. Does low-dose aspirin therapy complicate oral surgical procedures? J Am Dent Assoc 2000;131:331-335.

50. Madan GA, Madan SG, Madan G, Madan AD. Minor oral surgery without stopping daily low-dose aspirin therapy: A study of 51 patients. J Oral Maxillofac Surg 2005;63:1262-1265.

51. Rao TL, Jacobs KH, El-Etr AA. Reinfarction following anesthesia in patients with myocardial infarction. Anesthesiology 1983;59:499-505.

52. Steen PA, Tinker JH, Tarhan S. Myocardial reinfarction after anesthesia and surgery. JAMA 1978;239:2566-2570.

53. Tarhan S, Moffitt EA, Taylor WF, Giuliani ER. Myocardial infarction after general anesthesia. JAMA 1972;220:1451-1454.

54. Shah KB, Kleinman BS, Sami H, Patel J, Rao TL. Reevaluation of perioperative myocardial infarction in patients with prior myocardial infarction undergoing noncardiac operations. Anesth Analg 1990;71:231-235.

55. Backer CL, Tinker JH, Robertson DM, Vlietstra RE. Myocardial reinfarction following local anesthesia for ophthalmic surgery. Anesth Analg 1980;59:257-262.

56. Miller JL. Blood platelets. In Henry JB (ed). Clinical Diagnosis and Management by Laboratory Methods, 20th ed. Philadelphia, WB Saunders, 2001.

57. Brennan MT, Shariff G, Kent ML, Fox PC, Lockhart PB. Relationship between bleeding time test and postextraction bleeding in a healthy control population. Oral Surg Oral Med Oral Pathol Oral Radiol Endod 2002;94:439-443.

58. Hayward CP, Harrison P, Cattaneo M, Ortel TL, Rao AK. Platelet function analyzer (PFA)-100 closure time in the evaluation of platelet disorders and platelet function. J Thromb Haemost 2006;4:312-319.

59. Wahl MJ. Dental surgery in anticoagulated patients. Arch Intern Med 1998;158:1610-1616.

60. Wahl MJ. Myths of dental surgery in patients receiving anticoagulant therapy. J Am Dent Assoc 2000;131:77-81.

Cardiac Arrhythmias

Cardiac arrhythmia, which refers to any variation in the normal heartbeat, includes disturbances of rhythm, rate, or the conduction pattern of the heart. Cardiac arrhythmias are present in a significant percentage of the population, many of whom will seek dental treatment. Most arrhythmias are of little concern to the patient or the dentist; however, some can produce symptoms, and a few may be life threatening. It has been shown that potentially fatal arrhythmias can be precipitated by strong emotion such as anxiety or anger,[1,2] as well as by various drugs,[3] both of which can be experienced in the dental setting. Therefore, patients with significant arrhythmias must be identified before undergoing dental treatment.

GENERAL DESCRIPTION

Incidence and Prevalence

Cardiac arrhythmias are relatively common in the general population; however, their prevalence increases with age. They are frequently found in patients taking certain drugs or with various systemic diseases. In the United States, arrhythmias are present in 12.6% of patients over the age of 65 years,[4] with a rate of 13.6 per 100,000 reported in the general population.[5] Arrhythmias directly account for more than 38,000 deaths annually and are the underlying or contributing cause in almost 480,000 cases.[6] The most common type of persistent arrhythmia is atrial fibrillation, which affects approximately 2.2 million people.[6]

Little and associates[7,8] found the prevalence of cardiac arrhythmias in a large population of over 10,000 general dental patients to be 17.2%; more than 4% of those were serious, potentially life-threatening cardiac arrhythmias. In a study of more than 2300 dental health care professionals, Simmons and colleagues[9] reported a prevalence of arrhythmias of 15.6%, with more than 4% considered potentially serious. In a study of dental and dental hygiene students, Rhodus and Little[10] found similar results, with disorder prevalence of 15.3%, 1.7% of whom had serious, potentially life-threatening cardiac arrhythmias.

Etiology

Cardiac contractions are controlled by a complex system of specialized excitatory and conductive neuronal circuitry (Figure 5-1). The normal pattern of sequential depolarization consists of (1) sinoatrial (SA) node, (2) atrioventricular (AV) node, (3) bundle of His, (4) right and left bundle branches, and finally (5) subendocardial Purkinje network.[11] The electrocardiogram is a recording of this electrical activity. The primary pacemaker for the heart is the SA node, a crescent-shaped structure 9 to 15 mm long that is located at the junction of the superior vena cava and the right atrium. The SA node regulates the functions of the atria and is responsible for production of the P wave (atrial depolarization) on the electrocardiogram (ECG) (Figure 5-2). The ends of the sinus nodal fibers connect with atrial muscle fibers. The generated action potential travels along the muscle fibers (internodal pathways) and eventually arrives at and excites the AV node, which serves as a gate that regulates the entry of atrial impulses into the ventricles. It also slows the conduction rate of impulses generated within the SA node. From the AV node, impulses travel along the AV bundle (His bundle) within the ventricular septum, which divides into right and left bundle branches. The bundle branches then terminate in the small Purkinje fibers, which course throughout the ventricles and become continuous with cardiac muscle fibers. Simultaneous depolarization of the ventricles produces the QRS complex on ECG. The T wave is formed by repolarization of the ventricles. Repolarization of the atria occurs at about the same time as depolarization of the ventricles and thus is usually obscured by the QRS wave.[11]

Normal cardiac function depends on cellular automaticity (impulse formation), conductivity, excitability, and contractility. Disorders in automaticity and conductivity form the basis of the vast majority of cardiac arrhythmias. Under normal conditions, the SA node is responsible for impulse formation, resulting in a sinus rhythm with a normal rate of 60 to 100 beats per minute.[12] However,

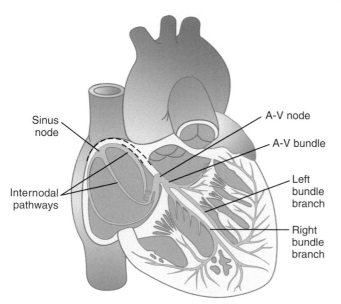

Figure 5-1. The electrical conduction system of the heart. (From Guyton AC, Hall JE. Textbook of Medical Physiology, 11th ed. Philadelphia, Saunders, 2006.)

other cells or groups of cells also are capable of generating impulses (ectopic pacemakers), and under certain conditions, these may emerge outside of the normal conduction system. After a normal impulse is generated (depolarization), cells of the SA node need time for recovery and repolarization and are refractory; during this time, they cannot conduct an impulse. Complete refractoriness results in a block and partial refractoriness in delay of conductivity.

Disorders of conductivity (block or delay) paradoxically may lead to rapid cardiac rhythm through the mechanisms of reentry. Reentry arrhythmias occur when accessory or ectopic pacemakers reexcite previously depolarized fibers before they would become depolarized in the normal sequential impulse pathway, typically producing tachyarrhythmias. The type of arrhythmia may suggest the nature of its cause. For example, paroxysmal atrial tachycardia with block suggests digitalis toxicity.[12] However, many cardiac arrhythmias are not specific for a given cause. In these patients, a careful search is undertaken to identify the cause of the arrhythmia. The most common causes include primary cardiovascular disorders, pulmonary disorders (embolism, hypoxia), autonomic disorders, systemic disorders (thyroid disease), drug-related adverse effects, and electrolyte imbalances (Box 5-1). Cardiac arrhythmias may be associated with many systemic diseases

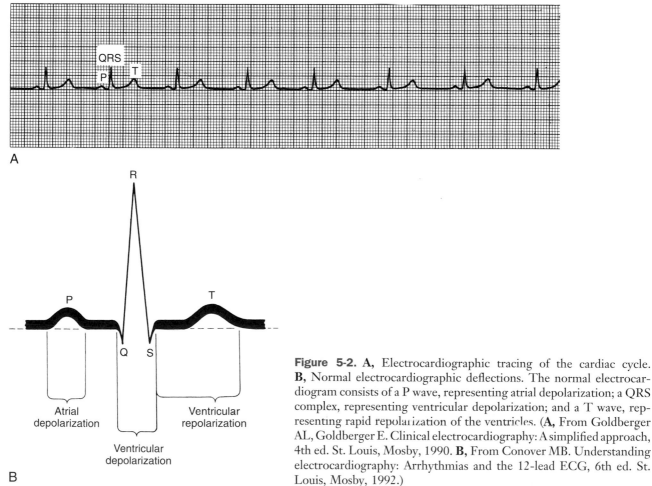

Figure 5-2. A, Electrocardiographic tracing of the cardiac cycle. **B,** Normal electrocardiographic deflections. The normal electrocardiogram consists of a P wave, representing atrial depolarization; a QRS complex, representing ventricular depolarization; and a T wave, representing rapid repolarization of the ventricles. (**A,** From Goldberger AL, Goldberger E. Clinical electrocardiography: A simplified approach, 4th ed. St. Louis, Mosby, 1990. **B,** From Conover MB. Understanding electrocardiography: Arrhythmias and the 12-lead ECG, 6th ed. St. Louis, Mosby, 1992.)

(Table 5-1).[3,12-14] Various drugs or foods also may induce cardiac arrhythmias (Table 5-2).[3,14]

Pathophysiology and Complications

The outcome of an arrhythmia often depends on the nature of the arrhythmia and the physical condition of the patient. For example, a young healthy person with paroxysmal atrial tachycardia may have minimal symptoms, whereas an elderly patient who has heart disease with the same arrhythmia may develop shock, congestive heart failure, or myocardial ischemia. Furthermore, evidence suggests that patients with certain types of cardiac arrhythmias (e.g., atrial fibrillation) are susceptible to ischemic events within the dental office.[15]

Arrhythmias are classified by site of origin (Box 5-2). Any arrhythmia that arises above the bifurcation of the His bundle into right and left bundle branches is classified as supraventricular.[16] Supraventricular cardiac arrhythmias may be broadly categorized into tachyarrhythmias and bradyarrhythmias. Following are brief descriptions of some of the more common arrhythmias likely to be encountered in dental patients.

Supraventricular Arrhythmias
Sinus nodal disturbances.
- Sinus Arrhythmia—Sinus arrhythmia is characterized by phasic variation in sinus cycle length.[12] In the respiratory type, heart rate increases with inhalation and decreases with exhalation. It is predominantly seen in the young and reflects variations in parasympathetic and sympathetic signals to the heart and is considered a normal event. Nonrespiratory sinus arrhythmia is unrelated to respiratory effort and is seen in digitalis intoxication.
- Sinus Tachycardia—Tachycardia in an adult is defined as a heart rate greater than 100 beats per minute, with an otherwise normal ECG.[12] The rate is usually between 100 and 180 beats per minute. This condition is most often a physiologic response to exercise, anxiety, stress, or emotion. Pathophysiologic causes include fever, hypotension, hypoxia, infection, anemia, hyperthyroidism, and heart failure. Drugs that may cause sinus tachycardia include atropine, epinephrine, alcohol, nicotine, and caffeine.

BOX 5-1

Major Causes of Cardiac Arrhythmias

- Primary cardiovascular disease
- Pulmonary disorders
- Autonomic disorders
- Systemic diseases
- Drug-related adverse effects
- Electrolyte imbalances

BOX 5-2

Classification of Common Cardiac Arrhythmias

- Supraventricular arrhythmias
  - Sinus nodal disturbances
    - Sinus arrhythmia
    - Sinus tachycardia
    - Sinus bradycardia
  - Disturbances of atrial rhythm
    - Premature atrial complexes
    - Atrial flutter
    - Atrial fibrillation
    - Atrial tachycardias
  - Tachycardias involving the atrioventricular (AV) junction
    - Pre-excitation syndrome (Wolff-Parkinson-White)
  - Heart block
    - AV block/Complete AV block
- Ventricular arrhythmias
  - Premature ventricular complexes
  - Ventricular tachycardia
  - Ventricular fibrillation

TABLE 5-1

Cardiac Arrhythmias Associated With Various Systemic Diseases

Arrhythmia	Systemic Condition
Sinus bradycardia	Infectious diseases, hypothermia, myxedema, obstructive jaundice, increased intracranial pressure, myocardial infarction
Atrial extrasystoles	Congestive heart failure, coronary insufficiency, myocardial infarction
Sinoatrial block	Rheumatic heart disease, myocardial infarction, acute infection
Sinus tachycardia	Febrile illness, infection, anemia, hyperthyroidism
Atrial tachycardia	Obstructive lung disease, pneumonia, myocardial infarction
Atrial flutter	Ischemic heart disease, mitral stenosis, myocardial infarction, open heart surgery
Atrial fibrillation	Myocardial infarction, mitral stenosis, ischemic heart disease, thyrotoxicosis, hypertension
Atrioventricular block	Rheumatic heart disease, ischemic heart disease, myocardial infarction, hyperthyroidism, Hodgkin's disease, myeloma, open heart surgery
Ventricular extrasystole	Ischemic heart disease, congestive heart failure, mitral valve prolapse
Ventricular tachycardia	Mitral valve prolapse, myocardial infarction, coronary atherosclerotic heart disease
Ventricular fibrillation	Blunt cardiac trauma, mitral valve prolapse, anaphylaxis, cardiac surgery, rheumatic heart disease, cardiomyopathy, coronary atherosclerotic heart disease

TABLE 5-2
Drugs/Foods That Can Induce Cardiac Arrhythmias

Cardiac Arrhythmias	Drug/Food
Bradycardia	Digitalis
	Morphine
	Beta blockers
	Calcium channel blockers
Tachycardia	Atropine
	Epinephrine
	Nicotine
	Ephedrine
	Caffeine
Premature Atrial Beats	Alcohol
	Nicotine
	Tricyclic antidepressants
	Caffeine
Ventricular Extrasystoles	Digitalis
	Alcohol
	Epinephrine
	Amphetamines
Ventricular Tachycardia	Digitalis
	Quinidine
	Procainamide
	Potassium
	Sympathetic amines

- Sinus Bradycardia—Bradycardia is defined as a heart rate less than 60 beats per minute, with an otherwise normal ECG.[12] It often coexists with a sinus arrhythmia. It is often seen in well-conditioned athletes and healthy young adults and decreases in prevalence with advancing age. Pathophysiologic causes of bradycardia include intracranial tumor, increased intracranial pressure, myxedema, hypothermia, and Gram-negative sepsis. Bradycardia may occur during vomiting and vasovagal syncope and as the result of carotid sinus stimulation. Drugs that may cause bradycardia include lithium, amiodarone, beta blockers, clonidine, and calcium channel blockers.

Disturbances of atrial rhythm.
- Premature atrial complexes—Impulses arising from ectopic foci anywhere in the atrium may result in premature atrial beats. Premature atrial contractions occur frequently in otherwise healthy people but often occur during infection, inflammation, or myocardial ischemia.[12] They may be provoked by smoking, lack of sleep, excessive caffeine, and alcohol.[11] They are common in conditions associated with dysfunction of the atria such as congestive heart failure.
- Atrial flutter—Atrial flutter is characterized by a rapid, regular atrial rate of 250 to 350 beats per minute. It is rare in healthy individuals and most often occurs along with septal defects, pulmonary emboli, mitral or tricuspid valve stenosis or regurgitation, or chronic ventricular failure.[12] It is also noted in patients with hyperthyroidism, alcoholism, and pericarditis.

- Atrial fibrillation—Atrial fibrillation (AF) is the most common sustained arrhythmia in adults.[16] It is characterized by rapid, disorganized, and ineffective atrial contractions that occur at a rate of 350 to 600 beats per minute. The ventricular response is highly irregular. The atria do not contract effectively; therefore, intra-arterial clot formation is promoted along with subsequent embolism and stroke. Thus, patients with AF who are at risk for stroke (e.g., history of previous stroke, valvular heart disease, hypertension, diabetes, coronary heart disease, congestive failure) should be placed on warfarin for antithrombotic therapy, with a target international normalized ratio (INR) of 2.0 to 3.0.[12] Patients who cannot take warfarin, as well as those who do not have risk factors for stroke, may be placed on aspirin therapy. AF is associated with a history of congestive heart failure, valvular heart disease and stroke, left atrial enlargement, abnormal mitral or aortic valve function, or treated systemic hypertension, as well as with advanced age.[12] It may occur intermittently or may be chronic. Symptoms are variable and depend on underlying cardiac status, ventricular rate, and loss of atrial contraction. Treatment consists of medication or cardioversion.
- Atrial tachycardias—Any tachycardia arising above the AV junction, which has a P wave configuration different from sinus rhythm, is called atrial tachycardia.[16] Atrial tachycardia is characterized by an atrial rate of between 150 and 200 beats per minute[12] and may result from enhanced normal automaticity, abnormal automaticity, triggered activity, or reentry. It is commonly seen in patients with coronary artery disease, myocardial infarction, cor pulmonale (right ventricular hypertrophy and pulmonary hypertension), or digitalis intoxication.

Tachycardias involving the AV junction.
- Preexcitation syndrome (Wolff-Parkinson-White syndrome)—The atria and ventricles are electrically insulated by each other through fibrous tissue that forms the anatomic AV junction. Normally, impulses are transmitted from atria to ventricles via this electrical bridge; however, in some individuals, additional electrical bridges connect the atria and ventricles, bypassing the normal pathways and forming the basis for preexcitation syndromes such as Wolff-Parkinson-White syndrome.[16] The basic defect in this disorder involves premature activation (preexcitation) of the ventricles by way of an accessory AV pathway that allows the normal SA/AV pathway to be bypassed. This accessory pathway allows rapid conduction and short refractoriness,

with impulses passed rapidly between atria and ventricles, and it provides a route for reentrant (backflow) tachyarrhythmias. Resultant paroxysmal tachycardia is characterized by a normal QRS, a regular rhythm, and ventricular rates of 150 to 250 beats per minute, along with sudden onset and termination.[12] Wolff-Parkinson-White syndrome is found in all ages but is more prevalent among men and decreases with age. Most adults have normal hearts. For most patients with recurrent tachycardia, the prognosis is good, but sudden death occurs rarely, with a frequency of 0.1%.[12]

Heart block.

- AV block—Heart block is a disturbance of impulse conduction that may be permanent or transient, depending on the type of anatomic or functional impairment that has occurred. Conduction impairment in heart block is classified by severity into three categories.[12] During first-degree heart block, conduction time is prolonged, but all impulses are conducted. Second-degree heart block occurs in two forms: Mobitz types I (Wenckebach) and II. Type I heart block is characterized by progressive lengthening of conduction time until an impulse is not conducted. Type II heart block denotes occasional or repetitive sudden block of conduction of an impulse without prior lengthening of conduction time. When no impulses are conducted, complete or third-degree block is present. AV block occurs when the atrial impulse is conducted with delay or is not conducted at all to the ventricles at a time when the AV junction is not physiologically refractory.[12] Conduction delay may occur at the AV node, within the His-Purkinje system (bundle branches), or at both sites. AV block may be first-degree or second-degree block, or it may be complete. AV block may be caused by a multitude of conditions such as surgery, electrolyte disturbance, myoendocarditis, tumor, myxedema, rheumatoid nodules, Chagas' disease, calcific aortic stenosis, polymyositis, and amyloidosis. In children, the most common cause is congenital. Drugs (digitalis, propranolol, potassium, quinidine) also may cause AV heart block. Symptoms increase with severity of the block.

Ventricular arrhythmias.

- Premature ventricular complexes—Premature ventricular complexes (PVCs) (or contractions) are very common arrhythmias that are characterized by the premature occurrence of an abnormally shaped QRS wave (ventricular contraction), followed by a pause. PVCs may occur alone, as bigeminy (every other beat is a PVC), as trigeminy (every third beat is a PVC), or with higher periodicity. The combination of two consecutive PVCs is called a couplet; three or more in a row at a rate of 100 beats per minute are referred to as ventricular tachycardia.[17] In patients without structural heart disease, PVCs have no prognostic significance and no impact on longevity or limitation of activity.[18] The prevalence of PVCs increases with age; they are associated with male sex and are related to serum potassium concentration. PVCs may be provoked by a variety of medications, by electrolyte imbalance, by tension states, and by excessive use of tobacco, caffeine, and alcohol. Among patients with prior myocardial infarction or valvular heart disease, however, frequent PVCs are associated with an increased risk of death.[12]

- Ventricular tachycardia—The occurrence of three or more ectopic ventricular beats (PVCs) at a rate of 100 or more per minute is defined as ventricular tachycardia (VT). VT may be sustained or episodic. Sustained VT that persists for 30 seconds or longer may require termination because of hemodynamic instability. VT can quickly degenerate into ventricular fibrillation. A variant of VT, called *torsades de pointes*, is characterized by QRS complexes of changing amplitude that appear to twist around the isoelectrical line; this occurs at rates of 200 to 250 beats per minute.[19] VT almost always occurs in patients with heart disease, most commonly ischemic heart disease and cardiomyopathy.[12] Certain drugs such as digitalis, sympathetic amines (epinephrine), potassium, quinidine, and procainamide may induce ventricular tachycardia.

- Ventricular flutter and fibrillation—Ventricular flutter and ventricular fibrillation (VF) are lethal arrhythmias characterized by chaotic, disorganized electrical activity that results in failure of sequential cardiac contraction and inability to maintain cardiac output.[17] The distinction between flutter and fibrillation can be difficult and is of academic interest only; therefore, the two can be discussed together. If not rapidly treated within 3 to 5 minutes, death will ensue. VF occurs most commonly as a sequela of ischemic heart disease.

CLINICAL PRESENTATION

Signs and Symptoms

Arrhythmias may be symptomatic or asymptomatic; however, symptoms alone cannot be relied upon to determine the seriousness of an arrhythmia. Some arrhythmias such as PVCs may be highly symptomatic, yet are not associated with an adverse outcome, whereas some patients with atrial fibrillation have no symptoms at all but may be at significant risk of stroke.[20] The symptoms most commonly associated with cardiac arrhythmias include palpitations, syncope, presyncope, and those associated with congestive heart failure (e.g., shortness of breath, orthopnea). The only clinical sign of an arrhythmia is a pulse that is too fast, too slow, or irregular (Box 5-3).

Signs and Symptoms of Cardiac Arrhythmias

SIGNS
- Slow heart rate (<60 beats/min)
- Fast heart rate (>100 beats/min)
- Irregular rhythm

SYMPTOMS
- Palpitations
- Fatigue
- Dizziness
- Syncope
- Angina
- Congestive heart failure
  - Shortness of breath
  - Orthopnea
  - Peripheral edema

Laboratory Findings

The electrocardiogram (ECG) is the primary tool used in the identification and diagnosis of cardiac arrhythmias. Additional tests that may be used include exercise or stress testing, long-term or ambulatory ECG (Holter) recording, baroreceptor reflex sensitivity testing, body surface mapping, and upright tilt-table testing. Electrode catheter techniques allow for intracavitary recordings of the specialized conducting systems, which aid greatly in the diagnosis of arrhythmias.[20]

MEDICAL MANAGEMENT

Management of cardiac arrhythmias involves medications, cardioversion, pacemakers, implanted cardioverter-defibrillators, radiofrequency catheter ablation, and surgery. Patients with asymptomatic arrhythmias usually require no therapy; those with symptomatic arrhythmias usually are treated first with medications. Patients who do not respond to medications may be treated by cardioversion, ablation, implanted pacemaker, or a cardioverter-defibrillator. Surgery may be necessary for the treatment of patients with certain arrhythmias. Cardioversion is indicated for any tachyarrhythmias that compromise hemodynamics or life. Cardiac arrest also is treated by cardioversion.

Antiarrhythmic Drugs

Generally, molecular targets for optimal action of these drugs involve channels within the cellular membranes through which ions are diffused rapidly. Antiarrhythmic drugs, therefore, are classified on the basis of their effect on sodium, potassium, or calcium channels and whether they block beta receptors (Table 5-3).[21] Class I drugs have "local anesthetic" properties or "membrane stabilizing" effects and work by primarily blocking the fast sodium channels. Class II drugs are beta-blocking agents. Class III drugs prolong the duration of the cardiac action potential and enhance refractoriness through their effects on potassium channels. Class IV drugs are calcium channel blockers. Although this classification implies a single action for each class, the reality is that they typically have multiple sites of action across different classification categories. For example, procainamide blocks both sodium and potassium channels, and amiodarone blocks sodium, potassium, and calcium channels.[22] Many of the antiarrhythmic drugs have very narrow therapeutic ranges; therefore, overtreatment or undertreatment may occur. As a result, undermedicated patients may be at increased risk during dental treatment, and drug toxicity may occur. Patients with atrial fibrillation often are prescribed warfarin sodium (Coumadin; Bristol-Myers Squibb, Princeton, NJ) to prevent atrial thrombosis and embolism; the target INR (therapeutic range) is between 2.0 and 3.0.

Implanted Permanent Pacemakers

A permanent, implanted pacemaker consists of a lithium battery–powered generator implanted subcutaneously in the left infraclavicular area that produces an electrical impulse that is transmitted by a lead inserted into the heart via the subclavian vein to an electrode in contact with endocardial or myocardial tissue (Figure 5-3). The leads are unipolar (stimulating only one chamber) or, more commonly, bipolar (stimulating two chambers). With a bipolar pacemaker, one lead is usually inserted into the right atrium, and the second lead is positioned within the right ventricle.[23]

Pacemakers are capable of very specific individualized pacing programs or modes, depending upon the individual's needs. A classification code is used to describe pacing modes of a pacemaker, which include the chamber that is paced, the chamber that is sensed, inhibitory or tracking function capability, rate modulation capability, and whether the unit is capable of antitachycardia pacing and/or the delivery of a shock.[23] Most pacemakers are of the demand variety, which can detect the patient's natural heartbeat and prevent competitive pacemaker firing; they are rate adaptive. Newer units contain pacing circuits that allow for programming, memory, and telemetry. In general, pacemakers are indicated to treat bradycardias in patients with acquired AV block, congenital AV block, chronic bifascicular and trifascicular block, AV block associated with acute myocardial infarction (MI), sinus node dysfunction, hypersensitive carotid sinus and neurocardiogenic syncope, and certain forms of cardiomyopathy; they are also indicated for the prevention and termination of certain tachyarrhythmias.[24]

Complications are infrequent but may occur as a result of pacemaker placement. These include pneumothorax, perforation of the atrium or ventricle, dislodgment of the leads, infection, and erosion of the pacemaker pocket.[23] Infective endocarditis rarely may occur; however, antibiotic prophylaxis for dental treatment is not recommended.[25,26] ECG abnormalities can be broadly grouped into failure to capture, failure to output, sensing abnormalities, and inappropriate rate changes.[27]

TABLE 5-3
Drugs Used to Treat Arrhythmias

Drug	Vasoconstrictor Interactions	Oral Manifestations	Other Considerations
CLASS I (SODIUM CHANNEL BLOCKERS)			
Quinidine	None	Bitter taste, dry mouth, petechiae, gingival bleeding	Syncope, hypotension, nausea, vomiting, thrombocytopenia
Procainamide	None	Bitter taste, oral ulcerations	Worsening of arrhythmias, lupus-like syndrome, rash, myalgia, fever, agranulocytosis
Disopyramide (Norpace)	None	Dry mouth	Urinary hesitancy, constipation
Mexiletine (Mexitil)	None	Dry mouth	Tremor, dizziness, diplopia, nausea, vomiting
Propafenone (Rythmol)	None	Taste aberration, dry mouth	Worsening of arrhythmias, dizziness, nausea, vomiting
Flecainide (Tambocor)	None	Metallic taste	Worsening of arrhythmias, confusion, irritability
CLASS II (BETA BLOCKERS)			
Propranolol (Inderal) (nonselective beta blocker) Also, acebutolol, esmolol, metoprolol, atenolol, timolol	Possible increase in blood pressure (BP) is possible with nonselective (NS) beta blockers; cautious use of vasoconstrictors is recommended (maximum, 0.036 mg epinephrine, 0.20 mg levonordefrin) With cardioselective (CS) beta blockers, use vasoconstrictors normally	Taste changes; lichenoid reactions	Hypotension, bradycardia, fatigue; avoid long-term use of nonsteroidal anti-inflammatory drugs (NSAIDs)
CLASS III (PROLONGED ACTION POTENTIAL AND REFRACTORINESS)			
Amiodarone (Cordarone)	None	Taste aberration	Interstitial pneumonitis, hyper- or hypothyroidism, elevated liver enzymes, bluish skin discoloration
Sotalol (Betapace) (nonselective beta blocker)	Possible increase in BP is possible with NS beta blockers; cautious use of vasoconstrictors is recommended (maximum, 0.036 mg epinephrine, 0.20 mg levonordefrin)	Taste changes; lichenoid reactions	Hypotension, bradycardia, torsades de pointes, fatigue; avoid long-term use of NSAIDs
CLASS IV (CALCIUM CHANNEL BLOCKERS)			
Verapamil (Calan) Also diltiazem	None	Gingival hyperplasia	Hypotension, bradycardia
MISCELLANEOUS			
Digoxin (Lanoxin)	Increased risk for arrhythmias; avoid if possible	Hypersalivation (toxicity)	Precipitation of arrhythmias, toxicity (headache, nausea, vomiting, altered color perception, malaise)

Implantable Cardioverter-Defibrillators

An implantable cardioverter-defibrillator (ICD) is a device that is similar to a pacemaker and is implanted in the same way as a pacemaker. ICDs are capable not only of delivering a shock but of providing antitachycardia pacing (ATP) and ventricular bradycardia pacing. Most ICDs have a single lead that is inserted into the right ventricle and function by continuously monitoring a patient's cardiac rate and delivering ATP or a shock when

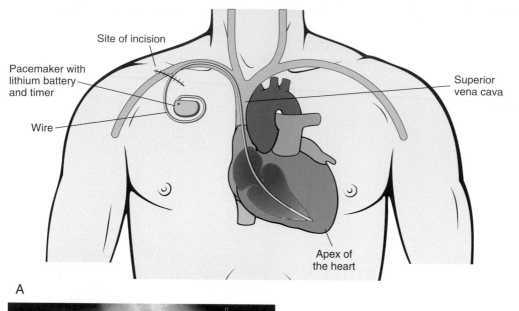

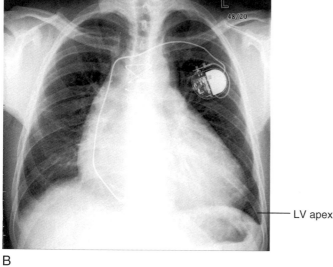

Figure 5-3. **A,** The site of implantation of a permanent pacemaker. **B,** A chest x-ray showing a pacemaker in a patient. (**A** from Chabner DA. The Language of Medicine, 6th ed. Philadelphia, Saunders, 2001. **B** from Zipes DP, et al [eds]. Braunwald's Heart Disease: A Textbook of Cardiovascular Medicine, 7th ed. Philadelphia, Saunders, 2005.)

the rate exceeds a predetermined cutoff point, such as in VT or VF.[27] ATP has the advantage of terminating a rhythm disturbance without delivering a shock. ICDs are generally larger than pacemakers, and their batteries do not last as long as those of a pacemaker.

Electromagnetic Interference. Electromagnetic interference (EMI) from nonintrinsic electrical activity can temporarily interfere with the function of a pacemaker or ICD. The pacemaker or ICD senses these extraneous signals and misinterprets them, which may cause rate alterations, sensing abnormalities, asynchronous pacing, noise reversion, or reprogramming.[28] Numerous sources of EMI are present in daily life, industry, and medical or dental settings (Box 5-4). Examples of EMI in daily life include cell phones, metal detectors, high-voltage power lines, and some home appliances (e.g., electric razor). EMI sources in the workplace include welders and induction furnaces. In the medical setting, magnetic resonance imaging scanners, electrosurgery, neurostimulators, defi-

brillators, TENS (transcutaneous electrical nerve stimulation) units, radiofrequency catheter ablation, therapeutic diathermy, therapeutic ionizing radiotherapy, and lithotripsy are all documented sources of potentially harmful EMI.[29] The effects of EMI on pacemakers and ICDs vary with the intensity of the electromagnetic field, the frequency of the spectrum of the signal, the distance and positioning of the device relative to the source, the electrode configuration, nonprogrammable device characteristics, programmed settings, and patient characteristics.[28] Electrical and magnetic fields are reduced inversely with the square of the distance from the source. It has also been demonstrated that devices from different manufacturers differ in their susceptibility to various sources of EMI.[28]

In a study by Miller and associates,[30] the only devices that caused significant EMI with a pacemaker in the dental office setting were electrosurgery units, ultrasonic bath cleaners, and ultrasonic scaling devices. Amalgamators, electrical pulp testers, curing lights, handpieces,

BOX 5-4

Sources of Electromagnetic Interference for Pacemakers/ICDs

DAILY LIVING
- Cell phones
- Metal detectors
- High-voltage power lines
- Household appliances (e.g., electric razors)

INDUSTRIAL
- Arc welders
- Induction furnaces

MEDICAL
- Magnetic resonance imaging scanners
- Electrosurgery
- Neurostimulators
- Defibrillators
- Transcutaneous electrical nerve stimulators (TENS units)
- Radiofrequency catheter ablation
- Therapeutic diathermy
- Therapeutic ionizing radiotherapy
- Lithotripsy

DENTAL
- Electrosurgery
- Ultrasonic bath cleaners
- Ultrasonic scalers

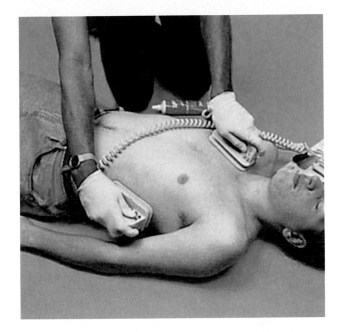

Figure 5-4. Cardioversion/defibrillation paddles in place on a patient. (From Sanders MJ. Mosby's Paramedic Textbook, 3rd ed. St. Louis, Mosby, 2005.)

electric toothbrushes, microwave ovens, x-ray units, and sonic scalers did not cause any significant EMI with the pacemakers tested. Internal shielding has been increased on newer generators to minimize the adverse effects of electromagnetic interference. These units now are protected against adverse effects from microwave oven signals.

Radiofrequency Catheter Ablation

Radiofrequency catheter ablation is a technique whereby a catheter (electrode) is introduced percutaneously into a vein and is threaded into the heart. The catheter is positioned in contact with the area determined by electrophysiologic testing to be the anatomic source of an arrhythmia. Radiofrequency energy is then delivered through the electrode catheter whose tip is in contact with the target tissue, which results in resistive heating of the tissue and irreversible tissue destruction of an area 5 to 6 mm in diameter and 2 to 3 mm deep, destroying the ectopic pacemaker. This technique can eliminate a variety of supraventricular and ventricular tachycardias that previously required long-term pharmacologic treatment for suppression or surgery for cure.[23]

Surgery

Surgery is another therapeutic approach that is used to treat patients with tachycardia. Direct surgical approaches designed to interrupt accessory pathways consist of resec-

tion of tissue and ablation. In addition to direct surgical approaches, indirect approaches such as aneurysmectomy, coronary artery bypass grafting, and relief of valvular regurgitation or stenosis may be useful in selected patients.[21]

Cardioversion and Defibrillation

Transthoracic delivery of a shock can be performed electively (cardioversion) to terminate persistent or refractory arrhythmias, or on an emergent basis (defibrillation) to terminate a lethal arrhythmia. Direct current defibrillators deliver an electrical charge by way of two paddles (electrodes) placed on the chest wall. One electrode is placed on the left chest over the region of the apex, and the other on the right side of the chest just to the right of the sternum and below the clavicle (Figure 5-4). The shock terminates arrhythmias caused by reentry by simultaneously depolarizing large portions of the atria and ventricles, thereby causing reentry circuits to disappear.[23] Defibrillation usually is instantaneous, and cardiac pumping resumes within a few seconds. It may have to be repeated if defibrillation is unsuccessful (i.e., a regular heartbeat is not occurring). The most common arrhythmias treated by cardioversion/defibrillation are VF, VT, atrial fibrillation, and atrial flutter. Treatment of patients with VF is always emergent; treatment of patients with VT may be elective or emergent, depending on the patient's hemodynamic status. Treatment of those with atrial flutter and atrial fibrillation is usually elective.

Several types of automated external defibrillators (AEDs) are available for use in the dental office for emergency defibrillation; these should be considered for inclusion in the dentist's emergency medical kit. The use of

AEDs is now taught as part of basic and advanced cardiopulmonary resuscitation courses, and their use is encouraged by the public. These devices, which are commonly found in public areas such as theaters, shopping centers, sports arenas, and airplanes, are simple and easy to use and are a critical part of successful resuscitation for a victim of cardiac arrest.

DENTAL MANAGEMENT

Medical Considerations

Stress associated with dental treatment or excessive amounts of injected epinephrine may lead to life-threatening cardiac arrhythmias in susceptible dental patients. Patients with an existing arrhythmia, diagnosed or undiagnosed, are at increased risk in the dental environment. In addition, patients at risk for developing an arrhythmia may be in danger in the dental office if they are not identified and measures are not taken to minimize stressful situations that can precipitate an arrhythmia. Other patients may have their arrhythmias under control with the use of drugs or a pacemaker but require special consideration when receiving dental treatment. The keys to successful dental management of patients prone to developing a cardiac arrhythmia and those with an existing arrhythmia are identification and prevention. Even under the best of circumstances, however, a patient may develop a cardiac arrhythmia that requires immediate emergency measures.

Identification of patients with a history of an arrhythmia, those with an undiagnosed arrhythmia, and those prone to developing one is the first step in risk assessment and in avoiding an untoward event (Box 5-5). This is accomplished by obtaining a thorough medical history, including a pertinent review of systems, and taking and evaluating vital signs (pulse rate and rhythm, blood pressure, respiratory rate). In a review of systems, patients should be asked about the presence of signs or symptoms related to the cardiovascular and pulmonary systems. Patients who report palpitations, dizziness, chest pain, shortness of breath, or syncope may have a cardiac arrhythmia or other cardiovascular disease, and should be evaluated by a physician. Patients with an irregular cardiac rhythm (even without symptoms) also may require consultation with the physician to determine its significance.

Patients with a known history of arrhythmia should be questioned as to the type of arrhythmia (if known), how it is being treated, medications being taken, presence of a pacemaker or defibrillator, effects on their activity, and stability of their disease. Because the classification and diagnosis of arrhythmia are often complex, patients often do not know the specific diagnosis that has been assigned to their disorder; thus, the physician must be relied upon to provide this information. It is important to identify any known triggers, such as stress, anxiety, or medications. Patients with a history of other heart, thyroid, or chronic pulmonary disease should be identified, as these may be a cause of or contributor to the arrhythmia, and they may require special management as well. If any questions or uncertainties arise, a medical consultation should be sought regarding patient diagnosis and current status, and to aid the dentist in assessing risk for aggravating or precipitating a cardiac arrhythmia, stroke, or MI during or in relation to dental treatment.

The dentist must make a determination of the risk involved in providing dental treatment to a patient with a history of arrhythmia and must decide whether the benefits of treatment outweigh any risk. This often requires consultation with the physician. The American College of Cardiology and the American Heart Association[31] have published guidelines that can help to make this determination. These guidelines are intended for use by physicians who are evaluating patients with cardiovascular disease to determine whether they can safely undergo surgical procedures. They also may be applied to the provision of dental care and may be of significant value to the dentist in making a determination of risk.

Box 5-6 provides an estimate of the risk that a serious event (acute MI, unstable angina, or sudden death) may occur during noncardiac surgery in patients with various arrhythmias. Patients with a significant arrhythmia (i.e., high-grade AV block, symptomatic ventricular arrhythmias in the presence of cardiovascular disease, and supraventricular arrhythmias with an uncontrolled ventricular rate) are at major risk for complications and are not candidates for elective dental care. Dental care should be deferred until a consultation with the physician has occurred. The presence of other types of arrhythmias poses significantly less risk. The presence of pathologic

---

BOX 5-5

Identifying Patients With Cardiac Arrhythmias

Patients with cardiac arrhythmias may be identified by the following

- Medical history to identify: (may need to consult with physician to obtain or verify this information)
  - Type of arrhythmia
  - How treated
  - Presence of pacemaker or defibrillator
  - Stability
- Risk for arrhythmia is increased in the presence of other cardiovascular or pulmonary disease
- Patient does not report an arrhythmia, but may be taking one or more of the antiarrhythmic drugs
- Pertinent review of systems asks about the presence of symptoms that could be caused by arrhythmias (palpitations, dizziness, chest pain, shortness of breath, syncope)
- Vital signs are suggestive of arrhythmia (rapid pulse rate, slow pulse rate, irregular pulse)
- Refer patient to physician if signs or symptoms are present that are suggestive of a cardiac arrhythmia or other cardiovascular disease

BOX 5-6	**BOX 5-7**

BOX 5-6

Perioperative Risk and Dental Treatment for Patients With Cardiac Arrhythmias

ARRHYTHMIAS ASSOCIATED WITH MAJOR PERIOPERATIVE RISK
- High-grade atrioventricular (AV) block
- Symptomatic ventricular arrhythmias in the presence of underlying heart disease
- Supraventricular arrhythmias with uncontrolled ventricular rate
  Dental Management: Avoid elective dental care.

ARRHYTHMIAS ASSOCIATED WITH INTERMEDIATE PERIOPERATIVE RISK
- Pathological Q waves on electrocardiogram (ECG) (markers of previous myocardial infarction)
  Dental Management: Elective dental care OK.

ARRHYTHMIAS ASSOCIATED WITH MINOR PERIOPERATIVE RISK
- ECG abnormalities consistent with:
  - Left ventricular hypertrophy
  - Left bundle-branch block
  - ST-T abnormalities
  - Any rhythm other than sinus (e.g., atrial fibrillation)
  Dental Management: Elective dental care OK.

(Modified from ACC/AHA guideline update for perioperative cardiovascular evaluation for noncardiac surgery, American Heart Association, 2002.)

BOX 5-7

Cardiac Risk* Stratification for Noncardiac Surgical Procedures

HIGH (REPORTED CARDIAC RISK OFTEN GREATER THAN 5%)
- Emergent major operations, particularly in the elderly
- Aortic and other major vascular surgery
- Peripheral vascular surgery
- Anticipated prolonged surgical procedures associated with large fluid shifts and/or blood loss

INTERMEDIATE (REPORTED CARDIAC RISK GENERALLY LESS THAN 5%)
- Carotid endarterectomy
- Head and neck surgery
- Intraperitoneal and intrathoracic surgery
- Orthopaedic surgery
- Prostate surgery

LOW (REPORTED CARDIAC RISK GENERALLY LESS THAN 1%)
- Endoscopic procedures
- Superficial procedures
- Cataract surgery
- Breast surgery

Data from ACC/AHA guideline update for perioperative cardiovascular evaluation for noncardiac surgery. American Heart Association, 2002.
*Combined incidence of cardiac death and nonfatal myocardial infarction.

Q waves (marker of a previous MI) is a clinical predictor of intermediate risk for perioperative complications; other ECG abnormalities, including left ventricular hypertrophy, left bundle branch block, and ST-T abnormalities, as well as any rhythm other than sinus rhythm, constitute minor perioperative risk. Patients with these types of arrhythmias can undergo elective dental treatment with only minimally increased risk.

The type and magnitude of the planned dental procedure also must be considered in determination of risk. Again, the guidelines provide help to the dentist in making this determination. Box 5-7 provides an estimate of risk for specific surgical procedures in patients with cardiovascular disease. Although dental procedures are not specifically listed, they would certainly be included in the low-risk, "superficial procedures" category with a risk of less than 1%; nonsurgical dental procedures are likely to pose even less risk than is introduced with the use of surgical procedures. More extensive oral and maxillofacial surgical procedures, and perhaps some of the more extensive periodontal surgical procedures, would likely be included in the intermediate cardiac risk category under "head and neck procedures," with a risk of less than 5%. Procedures associated with the highest risk (>5%) include emergency major surgery in the elderly, aortic or vascular surgery, and peripheral vascular surgery. These procedures are performed with the patient under general anesthesia and have the potential for significant blood and fluid loss with resultant adverse hemodynamic effects. Therefore, it seems clear that the vast majority of dental procedures, whether surgical or nonsurgical, convey low to very low risk in patients with arrhythmias and other cardiovascular diseases.

Stress and Anxiety Reduction. Based on the assessment of medical risk, the type of planned dental procedure, and the stability and anxiety level of the patient, stress reduction strategies for patients with arrhythmias of low to intermediate risk may include the following: establishment of good rapport, short appointments in the morning, comfortable chair position, pretreatment vital signs, oral sedation, nitrous oxide/oxygen sedation, excellent local anesthesia, and effective postoperative pain control (see Chapter 1). On occasion, it may be considered necessary to provide urgent dental care to a patient with a significant arrhythmia. If treatment becomes necessary, it should be performed as conservatively as possible and should be directed primarily toward pain relief, infection control, or the control of bleeding. Consultation with the physician is advised. Additional management recommendations may include establishing and maintaining an intravenous line, continuously monitoring the ECG and vital signs, and using a pulse oximeter. These measures may require that the patient be treated in a special patient care facility or hospital dental clinic (Box 5-8).

BOX 5-8

Dental Management Recommendations for Patients With Cardiac Arrhythmias

STRESS AND ANXIETY REDUCTION
- Establish good rapport
- Schedule short, morning appointments
- Ensure comfortable chair position
- Provide preoperative sedation (short-acting benzodiazepine night before and/or 1 hour before appointment)
- Administer intraoperative sedation (nitrous oxide/oxygen)
- Obtain pretreatment vital signs
- Ensure profound local anesthesia
- Provide adequate postoperative analgesia

VASOCONSTRICTORS
- Epinephrine-containing local anesthetic can be used with minimal risk if the dose is limited to 0.036 mg epinephrine (2 capsules containing 1:100,000 concentration). Higher doses may be tolerated, but the risk of complications increases with dose. Avoid the use of epinephrine in retraction cord.

FOR PATIENTS WITH ATRIAL FIBRILLATION WHO ARE TAKING WARFARIN (COUMADIN)
- Should have current international normalized ratio (INR) (within 24 hours of surgical procedure)
- If INR is within the therapeutic range (INR, 2.0-3.5), dental treatment, including minor oral surgery, can be performed without stopping or altering the Coumadin

- Local measures include gelatin sponge or oxidized cellulose in sockets, suturing, gauze pressure packs, preoperative stents, and tranexamic acid or ε-aminocaproic acid mouth rinse and/or to soak gauze

FOR PATIENTS WITH PACEMAKERS
- Antibiotic prophylaxis to prevent bacterial endocarditis is *not* recommended
- Avoid the use of electrosurgery and ultrasonic scalers

FOR PATIENTS TAKING DIGOXIN
- Watch for signs or symptoms of toxicity (e.g., hypersalivation)
- Avoid epinephrine or levonordefrine

FOR THE HIGH-RISK PATIENT WHO REQUIRES URGENT CARE, CONSIDER TREATING IN SPECIAL CARE CLINIC OR HOSPITAL
- Consult with physician
- Provide limited care only for pain control, treatment of acute infection, or control of bleeding
  - Intravenous line
  - Sedation
  - Electrocardiogram (ECG) monitoring
  - Pulse oximeter
  - Blood pressure monitoring
  - Avoid or limit epinephrine

Use of Vasoconstrictors. The use of vasoconstrictors in local anesthetics poses potential problems for patients with arrhythmias because of the possibility of precipitating cardiac tachycardia or another arrhythmia. A local anesthetic without vasoconstrictor may be used as needed. If a vasoconstrictor is deemed necessary, patients at low to intermediate risk and those taking nonselective beta blockers can safely be given up to 0.036 mg epinephrine (2 cartridges containing 1:100,000 epinephrine) or 0.20 mg levonordefrin (2 cartridges containing 1:20,000 levonordefrin); intravascular injections are to be avoided. Greater quantities of vasoconstrictor may well be tolerated, but increasing quantities increase the risk of adverse cardiovascular effects. Vasoconstrictors should be avoided in patients taking digoxin because of the potential for inducing arrhythmias. For patients at major risk for arrhythmias, the use of vasoconstrictors should be avoided, but if their use is considered essential, it should be discussed with the physician (see Box 5-8). Studies have shown that modest amounts of vasoconstrictor can be used safely in high-risk cardiac patients when accompanied by oxygen, sedation, nitroglycerin, and excellent pain control measures.[32-34]

For patients at all levels of cardiac risk, the use of gingival retraction cord impregnated with epinephrine should be avoided because of the rapid absorption of a high concentration of epinephrine and the potential for adverse cardiovascular effects. As an alternative, plain cord saturated with tetrahydrozoline HCl 0.05% (Visine;

Pfizer, New York, NY), or oxymetazoline HCl 0.05% (Afrin; Schering-Plough, Summit, NJ), provides gingival effects equivalent to those of epinephrine without the adverse cardiovascular effects.[35]

Warfarin (Coumadin). Patients with atrial fibrillation often are given anticoagulant therapy (warfarin) to prevent thrombus formation, embolism, and stroke; thus, they are at risk for increased bleeding. The target range for anticoagulation in patients with atrial fibrillation is usually an INR of between 2 and 3 times the normal value.[36] Studies have shown that minor oral surgery, such as simple extractions, can be performed without alteration or stopping of warfarin, provided that the INR is within the therapeutic range. (Depending upon the reason for the anticoagulant, the therapeutic range of the INR is between 2.0 and 3.5.[37-40]) This also includes the use of local measures such as placing of gelatin sponges or oxidized cellulose in the sockets, suturing, gauze sponges for pressure pack, preoperative fabrication of stents, and the topical use of tranexamic acid or ε-aminocaproic acid used postoperatively as a mouthrinse and/or to soak sponges (see Box 5-8). For more significant surgery, consultation with the physician should be obtained.

Pacemakers/ICDs and Antibiotic Prophylaxis. Patients with pacemakers or ICDs are not at risk for bacterial endocarditis related to dental procedures; thus, antibiotic prophylaxis is not indicated.[25,26]

Pacemakers/ICDs and Electromagnetic Interference.
The risk of encountering significant EMI with a pacemaker in the dental office is low. Box 5-4 lists the known sources of EMI. In the dental setting, only electrosurgery, ultrasonic bath cleaners, and ultrasonic scalers have been shown to produce potential interference.[30] Therefore, these devices should not be used on or around a patient with a pacemaker (see Box 5-8).

Digoxin Toxicity. Because the therapeutic range for digoxin is very narrow, toxicity can easily occur (see Box 5-8). This is a special concern in elderly patients and in those with hypothyroidism, renal insufficiency, dehydration, hypokalemia, hypomagnesemia, or hypocalcemia. Patients with electrolyte disturbances are generally more susceptible to digoxin toxicity. Signs of toxicity include hypersalivation, nausea and vomiting, headache, drowsiness, and visual distortions, with objects appearing yellow or green.[41] Thus, the dentist should be alert to these changes and should refer the patient to the physician should they occur.

Treatment Planning Considerations

A patient who is susceptible to cardiac arrhythmias can receive virtually any indicated dental procedure once it has been identified and the steps just described are taken. Complex dental procedures should be spread over several appointments to avoid overstressing the patient (see Box 5-8).

Oral Manifestations

The only significant oral complications found in patients with arrhythmias are those that occur as adverse effects of the medications used to control arrhythmia. Table 5-3 lists the oral manifestations of antiarrhythmic drugs.

REFERENCES

1. Lampert R, Joska T, Burg MM, Batsford WP, McPherson CA, Jain D. Emotional and physical precipitants of ventricular arrhythmia. Circulation 2002;106:1800-1805.
2. Culic V, Eterovic D, Miric D, Giunio L, Lukin A, Fabijanic D. Triggering of ventricular tachycardia by meteorologic and emotional stress: Protective effect of beta-blockers and anxiolytics in men and elderly. Am J Epidemiol 2004;160:1047-1058.
3. Mirvis DM, Goldberger AL. Electrocardiography. In Zipes D, Libby P, Bonow RO, Braunwald E (eds). Braunwald's Heart Disease: A Textbook of Cardiovascular Medicine, 7th ed. Philadelphia, Elsevier Saunders, 2005.
4. Lok NS, Lau CP. Prevalence of palpitations, cardiac arrhythmias and their associated risk factors in ambulant elderly. Int J Cardiol 1996;54:231-236.
5. Gaziano JM. Global burden of cardiovascular disease. In: Zipes D, Libby P, Bonow R, Braunwald E (eds). Braunwald's Heart Disease: A Textbook of Cardiovascular Medicine. Philadelphia, Elsevier Saunders, 2005.
6. Thom T, Haase N, Rosamond W, et al. Heart disease and stroke statistics—2006 update: A report from the American Heart Association Statistics Committee and Stroke Statistics Subcommittee. Circulation 2006;113: e85-e151.
7. Little JW, Simmons MS, Rhodus NL, Merry JW, Kunik RL. Dental patient reaction to electrocardiogram screening. Oral Surg Oral Med Oral Pathol 1990; 70:433-439.
8. Little JW, Simmons MS, Kunik RL, Rhodus NL, Merry JW. Evaluation of an EKG system for the dental office. Gen Dent 1990;38:278-281.
9. Simmons MS, Little JW, Rhodus NL, Verrusio AC, Kunik RL, Merry JW. Screening dentists for risk factors associated with cardiovascular disease. Gen Dent 1994; 42:440-445.
10. Rhodus NL, Little JW. The prevalence of cardiac arrhythmias in dental and dental hygiene students. California Institute of Continuing Education in Dentistry 1998;5:23-26.
11. Guyton AC, Hall JE. Textbook of Medical Physiology, 11th ed. Philadelphia, Elsevier Saunders, 2006.
12. Olgin JE, Zipes D. Specific arrhythmias: Diagnosis and treatment. In Zipes D, Libby P, Bonow RO, Braunwald E (eds). Braunwald's Heart Disease: A Textbook of Cardiovascular Medicine, 7th ed. Philadelphia, Elsevier Saunders, 2005.
13. Calkins H. Principles of electrophysiology. In Goldman L, Ausiello D (eds). Cecil Textbook of Medicine, 22nd ed. Philadelphia, Saunders, 2004.
14. Rubart M, Zipes D. Genesis of cardiac arrhythmias: Electrophysiological considerations. In Zipes D, Libby P, Bonow RO, Braunwald E (eds). Braunwald's Heart Disease: A Textbook of Cardiovascular Medicine, 7th ed. Philadelphia, Elsevier Saunders, 2005.
15. Matsuura H. The systemic management of cardiovascular risk patients in dental practice. Anesth Pain Control Dent 1999 winter;2(1):49-61.
16. Akhtar M. Cardiac arrhythmias with supraventricular origin. In Goldman L, Ausiello D (eds). Cecil Textbook of Medicine, 22nd ed. Philadelphia, Saunders, 2004.
17. Lerman BB. Ventricular arrhythmias and sudden death. In Goldman L, Ausiello D (ed). Cecil Textbook of Medicine, 22nd ed. Philadelphia, Saunders, 2004.
18. Kennedy HL. Use of long-term (Holter) electrocardiographic recordings. In Zipes D, Jalife J (eds). Cardiac Electrophysiology: From Cell to Bedside, 3rd ed. Philadelphia, WB Saunders, 2000.
19. Schwartz PL, Locati EH, Napolitano C. The long QT syndrome. In Zipes D, Jalife J (eds). Cardiac Electrophysiology: From Cell to Bedside, 3rd ed. Philadelphia, WB Saunders, 2000, p 788-811.
20. Miller JM, Zipes D. Diagnosis of cardiac arrhythmias. In Zipes D, Libby P, Bonow RO, Braunwald E (eds). Braunwald's Heart Disease: A Textbook of Cardiovascular Medicine, 7th ed. Philadelphia, Elsevier Saunders, 2005.
21. Miller JL, Zipes D. Therapy for cardiac arrhythmias. In Zipes D, Libby P, Bonow RO, Braunwald E (eds). Braunwald's Heart Disease: A Textbook of Cardiovascular Medicine, 7th ed. Philadelphia, Elsevier Saunders, 2005.

22. Woolsey RL. Antiarrhythmic drugs. In Goldman L, Ausiello D (eds). Cecil Textbook of Medicine, 22nd ed. Philadelphia, Saunders, 2004.

23. Morady F. Electrophysiologic interventional procedures and surgery. In Goldman L, Ausiello D (eds). Cecil Textbook of Medicine, 22nd ed. Philadelphia, Saunders, 2004.

24. Gregoratos G, Abrams J, Epstein AE, et al. ACC/AHA/NASPE 2002 guideline update for implantation of cardiac pacemakers and antiarrhythmia devices—Summary article: A report of the American College of Cardiology/American Heart Association Task Force on Practice Guidelines (ACC/AHA/NASPE Committee to Update the 1998 Pacemaker Guidelines). J Am Coll Cardiol 2002;40:1703-1719.

25. Baddour LM, Bettmann MA, Bolger AF, et al. Nonvalvular cardiovascular device–related infections. Circulation 2003;108:2015-2031.

26. Dajani AS, Taubert KA, Wilson W, et al. Prevention of bacterial endocarditis: Recommendations by the American Heart Association. J Am Dent Assoc 1997;128:1142-1151.

27. Hayes DL, Zipes D. Cardiac pacemakers and cardioverter-defibrillators. In Zipes D, Libby P, Bonow RO, Braunwald E (eds). Braunwald's Heart Disease: A Textbook of Cardiovascular Medicine, 7th ed. Philadelphia, Elsevier Saunders, 2005.

28. Pinski SL, Trohman RG. Interference in implanted cardiac devices. Part I. Pacing. Clin Electrophysiol 2002;25:1367-1381.

29. Pinski SL, Trohman RG. Interference in implanted cardiac devices. Part II. Pacing. Clin Electrophysiol 2002;25:1496-1509.

30. Miller CS, Leonelli FM, Latham E. Selective interference with pacemaker activity by electrical dental devices. Oral Surg Oral Med Oral Pathol Oral Radiol Endod 1998;85:33-36.

31. Eagle KA, Berger PB, Calkins H, et al. ACC/AHA guideline update for perioperative cardiovascular evaluation for noncardiac surgery—Executive summary: A report of the American College of Cardiology/American Heart Association Task Force on Practice Guidelines (Committee to Update the 1996 Guidelines on Perioperative Cardiovascular Evaluation for Noncardiac Surgery). Anesth Analg 2002;94:1052-1064.

32. Cintron G, Medina R, Reyes AA, Lyman G. Cardiovascular effects and safety of dental anesthesia and dental interventions in patients with recent uncomplicated myocardial infarction. Arch Intern Med 1986;146:2203-2204.

33. Findler M, Galili D, Meidan Z, Yakirevitch V, Garfunkel AA. Dental treatment in very high risk patients with active ischemic heart disease. Oral Surg Oral Med Oral Pathol 1993;76:298-300.

34. Niwa H, Sato Y, Matsuura H. Safety of dental treatment in patients with previously diagnosed acute myocardial infarction or unstable angina pectoris. Oral Surg Oral Med Oral Pathol Oral Radiol Endod 2000;89:35-41.

35. Bowles WH, Tardy SJ, Vahadi A. Evaluation of new gingival retraction agents. J Dent Res 1991;70:1447-1449.

36. Fuster V, Ryden LE, Asinger RW, et al. ACC/AHA/ESC guidelines for the management of patients with atrial fibrillation: Executive summary. A report of the American College of Cardiology/American Heart Association Task Force on Practice Guidelines and the European Society of Cardiology Committee for Practice Guidelines and Policy Conferences (Committee to Develop Guidelines for the Management of Patients With Atrial Fibrillation) developed in collaboration with the North American Society of Pacing and Electrophysiology. Circulation 2001;104:2118-2150.

37. Jafri SM. Periprocedural thromboprophylaxis in patients receiving chronic anticoagulation therapy. Am Heart J 2004;147:3-15.

38. Jeske AH, Suchko GD. Lack of a scientific basis for routine discontinuation of oral anticoagulation therapy before dental treatment. J Am Dent Assoc 2003;134:1492-1497.

39. Wahl MJ. Myths of dental surgery in patients receiving anticoagulant therapy. J Am Dent Assoc 2000;131:77-81.

40. Ansell J, Hirsh J, Poller L, Bussey H, Jacobson A, Hylek E. The pharmacology and management of the vitamin K antagonists: The Seventh ACCP Conference on Antithrombotic and Thrombolytic Therapy. Chest 2004;126(3 suppl):204S-233S.

41. Dowd FJ. Cardiac glycosides and other drugs used in heart failure. In Yagiela JA, Dowd FJ, Neidle EA (eds). Pharmacology and Therapeutics for Dentistry, 5th ed. St. Louis, Elsevier Mosby, 2004.

Heart Failure

CHAPTER

6

Heart failure (HF) is much like anemia in that it represents a symptom complex that may be caused by a number of specific diseases (Box 6-1). HF represents the end stage of many of the cardiovascular diseases. The American College of Cardiology/American Heart Association 2005 Guideline Update for the Diagnosis and Management of Chronic Heart Failure in the Adult[1] defines HF as a complex clinical syndrome that may result from any structural or functional cardiac disorder that impairs the ability of the ventricle to fill with or eject blood. Patients with untreated or poorly managed HF are at high risk during dental treatment for complications such as cardiac arrest, cerebrovascular accident, and myocardial infarction. The dentist must be able to identify these patients on the basis of history and clinical findings, refer them for medical diagnosis and management, and work closely with the physician to develop a dental management plan that will be effective and safe for the patient.

GENERAL DESCRIPTION

Incidence and Prevalence

Approximately 5 million people in the United States have HF, and more than 550,000 patients each year are given this diagnosis for the first time.[2] HF is the most common Medicare diagnosis-related group (i.e., hospital discharge diagnosis), and more Medicare dollars are spent on the diagnosis and treatment of HF than on any other diagnosis.[3] HF is primarily a condition of the elderly. The annual incidence rate of new cases of HF rises from less than 1 per 1000 patient-years younger than age 45 to 10 per 1000 patient-years older than age 65 to 30 per 1000 patient-years older than age 80.[4] Approximately 80% of patients hospitalized with heart failure are older than 65 years of age.[5]

Any condition that causes myocardial necrosis or produces chronic pressure or volume overload can induce myocardial dysfunction and HF. The most common underlying causes of HF in the United States are coronary heart disease, hypertension, cardiomyopathy, and valvular heart disease, with coronary heart disease accounting for 60% to 75% of cases.[4] The second most common cause of HF, accounting for about one fourth of all cases, is dilated cardiomyopathy (DCM). DCM is a syndrome characterized by cardiac enlargement with impaired systolic function of one or both ventricles, often accompanied by signs and symptoms of HF.[6] About half of all cases of DCM have no identifiable cause; it is therefore considered idiopathic.[6] Known causes of cardiomyopathy include alcohol abuse, hereditary cardiomyopathy, and viral infection.[6] Although hypertension is often not a primary cause of HF, it is a major contributor to HF, with more than 75% of patients with HF having a long-standing history of hypertension.[4] Valvular heart disease used to be a significant cause of HF; however, with rates of rheumatic heart disease and congenital heart disease declining in the United States, a subsequent decline has occurred in HF caused by valvular disease.

Although the mortality rates from myocardial infarction and stroke are declining, HF continues to be a major cause of morbidity and mortality. Between 1979 and 2000, the number of HF hospitalizations rose from 377,000 to 999,000—an increase of 165%.[2] In the United States, approximately 56,000 deaths each year are primarily caused by HF, and it is listed as a contributing cause in 262,000 deaths.[2] The prognosis for patients with HF is poor. Of patients who survive an acute onset of HF, only 35% of men and 50% of women are alive 5 years after diagnosis.[4]

Pathophysiology and Complications

Heart failure is caused by the inability of the heart to function efficiently as a pump, which results in inadequate emptying of the ventricles during systole or incomplete filling of the ventricles during diastole. This in turn

BOX 6-1

Most Common Causes of Heart Failure

- Coronary heart disease
- Hypertension
- Cardiomyopathy
- Valvular heart disease
- Myocarditis
- Infective endocarditis
- Congenital heart disease
- Pulmonary hypertension
- Pulmonary embolism
- Endocrine disease

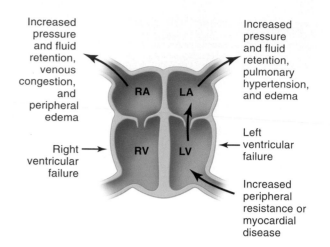

Figure 6-1. Effects of right- and left-sided heart failure.

results in a decrease in cardiac output, with an inadequate volume of blood supplied to the tissues or in a backup of blood, causing systemic congestion. HF may involve one or both ventricles. Most acquired disorders that lead to HF result in initial failure of the left ventricle. Left ventricular failure often is followed by failure of the right ventricle. By the time most patients are seen for medical treatment, failure of both sides of the heart usually has occurred. The cardinal manifestations of HF are dyspnea and fatigue.[1]

HF may result from acute injury to the heart, such as from myocardial infarction, or more commonly, from a chronic process, such as hypertension or cardiomyopathy. Failure of the heart most often begins with left ventricular failure brought on by an increased workload or disease of the heart muscle.[7] Determination of left ventricular failure is often based on a finding of an abnormal ejection fraction, which is the percentage of blood that is ejected from the left ventricle during systole. Normal values for ejection fraction, at rest, vary between 55% and 70%.[8] Although arbitrary, a left ventricular ejection fraction of 45% to 50% is often used as a threshold by which to diagnose left ventricular failure.[4] The outstanding symptom of left ventricular failure is dyspnea, which results from accumulation or congestion of blood within the pulmonary vessels—thus, the term *congestive heart failure*. Acute pulmonary edema is often the result of left ventricular failure. Left-sided heart failure leads to pulmonary hypertension, which increases the work of the right ventricle as it pumps against increased pressure and often leads to right-sided heart failure.

The most common cause of right-sided heart failure is preceding failure of the left ventricle. Outcomes of right ventricular failure consist of systemic venous congestion and peripheral edema (Figure 6-1). Failure of the right side of the heart alone is uncommon. The most common cause of pure right-sided heart failure is emphysema.[7] Ventricular failure leads to dilation and hypertrophy of the ventricle as it attempts to compensate for its inability to keep up with the workload. Venous pressure and myocardial tone increase, as does blood volume. The net effect is diastolic dilation, which increases the force and volume of the subsequent systolic contraction. This leads to dyspnea, orthopnea, and pulmonary edema.[7]

When right-sided ventricular enlargement occurs as the result of a lung disorder (e.g., emphysema), pulmonary hypertension is produced; this condition is called *cor pulmonale*.

Signs and symptoms of HF appear when the heart no longer functions properly as a pump. As cardiac output falls, an increase occurs in the disproportion between required hemodynamic load and the capacity of the heart to handle the load. With decreasing cardiac output, stimulation of the renin-angiotensin system and the sympathetic nervous system (neurohumoral responses) occurs in an attempt to compensate for loss of function.[9] The effects of these responses include increased heart rate and myocardial contractility, increased peripheral resistance, sodium and water retention, redistribution of blood flow to the heart and brain, and increased efficiency of oxygen utilization by the tissues.[10] If these responses result in improved cardiac output along with elimination of symptoms, the condition is called *compensated HF*. Symptomatic HF is called *decompensated HF*.

The American Heart Association/American College of Cardiology (AHA/ACC) classifies HF into four stages, reflecting the fact that HF is a progressive disease, whose outcome may be modified by early identification and treatment.[1] Stages A and B denote patients with risk factors that predispose to the development of HF, such as coronary artery disease, hypertension, and diabetes, but who do not have any symptoms of HF. The difference between stages A and B is that in stage A, patients do not demonstrate left ventricular hypertrophy (LVH) or dysfunction; those in stage B do have LVH and/or dysfunction (structural heart disease). Stage C denotes patients with past or present symptoms of HF associated with underlying structural heart disease (the bulk of patients), and stage D designates patients with refractory HF who might be eligible for specialized, advanced treatment or for end of life care. This classification system complements the New York Heart Association classification system, which is discussed in the subsequent section of this chapter on signs and symptoms.

BOX 6-2

Symptoms of Heart Failure

- Dyspnea (perceived shortness of breath)
- Fatigue and weakness
- Orthopnea (dyspnea in recumbent position)
- Paroxysmal nocturnal dyspnea (dyspnea that awakens patient from sleep)
- Acute pulmonary edema (cough or progressive dyspnea)
- Exercise intolerance (inability to climb a flight of stairs)
- Fatigue (especially muscular)
- Dependent edema (swelling of feet and ankles after standing or walking)
- Report of weight gain or increased abdominal girth (fluid accumulation; ascites)
- Right upper quadrant pain (liver congestion)
- Anorexia, nausea, vomiting, constipation (bowel edema)
- Hyperventilation followed by apnea during sleep (Cheyne-Stokes respiration)

BOX 6-3

Signs of Heart Failure

- Rapid, shallow breathing
- Cheyne-Stokes respiration (hyperventilation alternating with apnea during sleep)
- Inspiratory rales (crackles)
- Heart murmur
- Gallop rhythm
- Increased venous pressure
- Enlargement of cardiac silhouette on chest radiograph
- Pulsus alternans
- Distended neck veins
- Large, tender liver
- Jaundice
- Peripheral edema
- Ascites
- Cyanosis
- Weight gain
- Clubbing of fingers

HF is a progressive disease, and symptoms worsen over time because of ongoing deterioration of cardiac structure and function. The prognosis is better if the underlying cause can be treated. One year after HF has been diagnosed, 20% of patients succumb to the disease. In people given a diagnosis of HF, sudden death occurs at 6 to 9 times the rate seen in the general population.[11]

CLINICAL PRESENTATION

Signs and Symptoms

The symptoms and signs of HF (Boxes 6-2 and 6-3) reflect respective ventricular dysfunction. Left ventricular failure produces pulmonary vascular congestion with resultant pulmonary edema and dyspnea. Dyspnea is the most common symptom of HF and usually is present only with exertion or physical activity. Dyspnea at rest is an indication of severe HF.[4,12] Orthopnea is positional dyspnea, which is precipitated or worsened by a recumbent or semirecumbent position. Most patients with mild to moderate HF do not exhibit orthopnea when treated adequately.[4] Paroxysmal nocturnal dyspnea (PND) is an attack of sudden, severe shortness of breath that awakens the patient from sleep, usually within 1 to 3 hours after the patient goes to bed, and resolves within 10 to 30 minutes after the patient arises, often gasping for air.[4] The occurrence of PND is uncommon. Both orthopnea and PND are relatively specific indicators of HF and are due to increased venous return encouraged by the recumbent position, with resultant increases in pulmonary venous pressure and alveolar edema. Central regulation of respiration also may be impaired in patients with advanced HF, resulting in alternating cycles of rapid, deep breathing (hyperventilation) and periods of central apnea, called *Cheyne-Stokes respiration.*[10] PND is a common clinical feature associated with Cheyne-Stokes respiration in patients with HF.[12] Exercise intolerance (e.g., inability to climb a flight of stairs) is one of the hallmark symptoms of HF and is due to a combination of dyspnea and reduced blood and oxygen supply to the skeletal muscles.[4] Fatigue (especially muscle fatigue) is a common, nonspecific symptom of HF. The pulmonary examination of patients with HF is usually unremarkable. However, rales (or crackles), representing alveolar fluid, are a hallmark of HF when present.[4] Chest radiographs may reveal enlargement and displacement of the cardiac silhouette or abnormalities of the pulmonary vasculature. Evidence of interstitial fluid or pleural effusion also may be seen (Figure 6-2).

Right ventricular failure results in systemic venous congestion and peripheral edema. Evidence of systemic venous congestion may be detected by the presence of distended neck veins (Figure 6-3), a large tender liver, peripheral edema (Figure 6-4), and ascites (Figure 6-5). Retention of fluid results in weight gain and may increase body girth owing to accumulation of fluid within the peritoneal cavity. On occasion, patients with chronic HF may have clubbing of the fingers (Figure 6-6).

Cardiac examination usually reveals evidence of the underlying cardiac abnormality, as well as compensatory or degenerative changes in cardiac structure.[4,12] Auscultation often reveals a laterally displaced apical impulse caused by left ventricular hypertrophy. A murmur of mitral regurgitation may be heard, as well as an S_3 or S_4 gallop. Pulsus alternans, a regular rhythm with alternating strong and weak ventricular contractions, is pathognomonic of left ventricular failure but is not present in most patients with heart failure.[12] Central venous pressure increases.

The New York Heart Association (NYHA) has developed a widely used classification system of HF that is based on severity of symptoms and the amount of effort

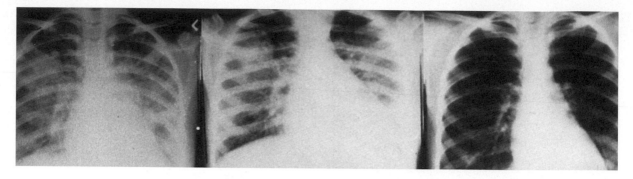

Figure 6-2. Serial chest radiographs demonstrating resolution of pulmonary edema (*left* to *right*). Note the enlargement of the cardiac silhouette. (Courtesy J. Noonan, MD, Lexington, Ky.)

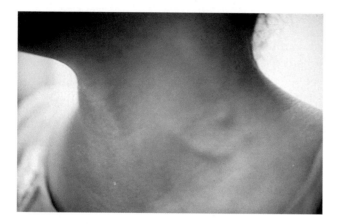

Figure 6-3. Distended jugular vein in patient with heart failure.

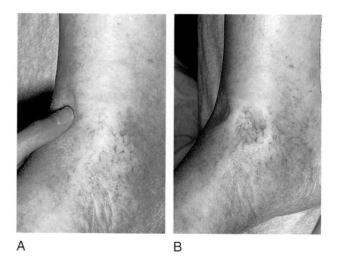

A   B

Figure 6-4. Pitting edema in a patient with heart failure. A depression ("pit") remains in the edematous tissue for some minutes after firm fingertip pressure is applied. (From Forbes CD, Jackson WF. Color Atlas and Text of Clinical Medicine. Edinburgh, Mosby, 2004.)

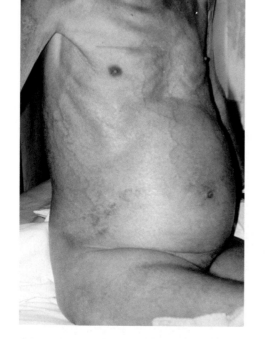

Figure 6-5. Ascites. (Courtesy P. Akers, MD, Evanston, Ill.)

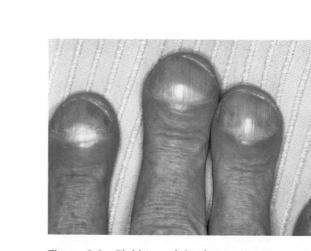

Figure 6-6. Clubbing of the fingers in a patient with congestive heart failure.

NYHA Classification of Heart Failure

- **Class I:** No limitation of physical activity. No dyspnea, fatigue, or palpitations with ordinary physical activity.
- **Class II:** Slight limitation of physical activity. These patients have fatigue, palpitations, and dyspnea with ordinary physical activity but are comfortable at rest.
- **Class III:** Marked limitation of activity. Less than ordinary physical activity results in symptoms, but patients are comfortable at rest.
- **Class IV:** Symptoms are present at rest, and any physical exertion exacerbates the symptoms.

NYHA, New York Heart Association.

needed to elicit symptoms (Box 6-4).[1] It is complementary to the AHA/ACC staging system described earlier and essentially is a subclassification of stage C.

Laboratory Findings

A variety of specialized tests are used to diagnose and monitor heart failure, depending on the cause. Among these are chest radiography, electrocardiography, echocardiography, radionuclide angiography or ventriculography, exercise stress testing, ambulatory electrocardiography (Holter) monitoring, and cardiac catheterization. Measurement of plasma hormone levels of norepinephrine, plasma atrial natriuretic peptide, and plasma renin has possible prognostic value and may be helpful clinically.[4,12] Routine testing may include complete blood count, renal function testing and electrolytes, liver function testing, blood glucose, lipids, and thyroid function testing.

MEDICAL MANAGEMENT

The medical management of HF is applied with a graduated approach, depending on the stage of the disease (Box 6-5).[1] For stages A and B, management begins with risk reduction and includes the identification and treatment of underlying medical problems such as hypertension, atherosclerotic disease, diabetes, obesity, and metabolic syndrome (abdominal obesity, elevated blood glucose, dyslipidemia, hypertension). In addition, behavioral modification is promoted for smoking cessation, weight loss for the obese patient, reduction of risk factors for cardiovascular disease, mild aerobic exercise, adequate rest, and avoidance of alcohol and illicit drugs. Drug therapy may be indicated for the treatment of patients with vascular disease or diabetes in stage A, as well as for those with ventricular dysfunction in stage B.

In stage C, all measures from stage A and B apply, in addition to salt restriction and drug therapy (Table 6-1). Drug therapy begins with diuretics to control fluid retention. Several types of diuretics, including loop diuretics, thiazide diuretics, and potassium-sparing diuretics, are used. Diuretics are used for three purposes: (1) they are

Medical Management of Patients With Heart Failure[1]

STAGE A (PATIENTS AT HIGH RISK FOR HEART FAILURE [HF] BUT WITHOUT STRUCTURAL HEART DISEASE OR SYMPTOMS OF HF)
- Treat hypertension, encourage smoking cessation, treat lipid disorders, encourage regular exercise, discourage alcohol intake and illicit drug use, and control metabolic syndrome.
- Use angiotensin-converting enzyme (ACE) inhibitors or angiotensin receptor blockers (ARBs) in appropriate patients for treatment of vascular disease or diabetes.

STAGE B (PATIENTS WITH STRUCTURAL HEART DISEASE BUT WITHOUT SIGNS OR SYMPTOMS OF HF)
Provide all measures for stage A, *plus*
- ACE inhibitors (or ARBs) in appropriate patients
- Beta-blockers in appropriate patients

STAGE C (PATIENTS WITH STRUCTURAL HEART DISEASE WITH PRIOR OR CURRENT SYMPTOMS OF HF)
Provide all measures for stages A and B, dietary salt restriction, *plus*
- Drugs for routine use: diuretics, ACE inhibitors, beta-blockers
- Drugs in selected patients: aldosterone antagonists, ARBs, digitalis, hydralazine/nitrates
- Devices in selected patients: biventricular pacing, implantable defibrillators

STAGE D (PATIENTS WITH REFRACTORY HF REQUIRING SPECIAL INTERVENTIONS)
- Provide appropriate measures from stages A, B, and C.
- Use heart transplant, chronic inotropes, permanent mechanical support, experimental drugs, or surgery.
- Provide compassionate end-of-life care/hospice.

the only drugs that can adequately control fluid retention, (2) they produce more rapid symptomatic relief than other drugs, and (3) they modulate other drugs used to treat HF.[9] Although diuretics are effective in decreasing the signs and symptoms of fluid retention, they cannot maintain the clinical stability of patients with HF when used alone. Spironolactone, a potassium-sparing diuretic, also blocks the action of aldosterone (aldosterone antagonist) and, when used in patients with class IV symptoms, has been shown to reduce the risk of death by 25% to 30%.[9] Other than spironolactone, diuretics do not influence the natural history of chronic HF.[13]

In addition to diuretics, drugs that modulate or decrease neurohormonal activity have become the foundation of treatment for HF. These drugs decrease the morbidity and mortality of HF by inhibiting the cardiotoxic effects of the neurohormonal system, thereby retarding the progression of HF.[9] Several types of neurohormonal antagonists, including angiotensin-converting enzyme inhibitors (ACEIs), beta-adrenergic blockers,

TABLE 6-1
Drugs Used in the Treatment of Patients With Heart Failure

Drug	Vasoconstrictor Interactions	Oral Manifestations	Other Considerations
DIURETICS			
Loop Diuretics Bumetanide (Bumex) Furosemide (Lasix) Torsemide (Demadex)	None	Dry mouth	Orthostatic hypotension
Thiazide Diuretics Chlorothiazide (Diuril) Chlorthalidone (Thalitone) Hydrochlorothiazide (HCTZ) Indapamide (Lozol) Metolazone (Mykrox)	None	Dry mouth	Orthostatic hypotension
Potassium-Sparing Diuretics Amiloride (Midamor) Spironolactone (Aldactone) Triamterene (Dyrenium)	None	Dry mouth	Orthostatic hypotension
ACE Inhibitors Benazepril (Lotensin) Captopril (Capoten) Enalapril (Vasotec) Fosinopril (Monopril) Lisinopril (Prinivil) Moexapril (Univasc) Perindopril (Coversyl) Quinapril (Accupril) Ramipril (Altace) Trandolapril (Mavik)	None	Angioedema of lip, face, or tongue; taste changes; burning mouth; lichenoid reactions	Orthostatic hypotension; avoid prolonged use of NSAIDs
Angiotensin Receptor Blockers Candesartan (Atacand) Eprosartan (Teveten) Irbesartan (Avapro) Losartan (Cozaar) Olmesartan (Benicar) Telmisartan (Micardis) Valsartan (Diovan)	None		Orthostatic hypotension
Aldosterone Inhibitors Eplerenone (Inspra) Spironolactone (Aldactone)	None		Orthostatic hypotension
Beta Blockers Acebutolol (Sectral) (CS) Atenolol (Tenormin) (CS) Betaxolol (Kerlone) (CS) Bisoprolol (Zebeta) (CS) Carteolol (Cartrol) (NS) Carvedilol (Coreg) (NS/alpha blocker) Labetalol (Normodyne) (CS) Metoprolol (Lopressor) (CS) Nadolol (Corgard) (NS) Penbutolol (Levatol) (NS) Pindolol (Visken) (NS) Propranolol (Inderal) (NS) Timolol (Blocadren) (NS)	Increase in BP is possible with nonselective (NS) beta blockers; cautious use of vasoconstrictors is recommended (maximum 0.036 mg epinephrine; 0.20 mg levonordefrin) With cardioselective (CS) beta blockers, use vasoconstrictors normally	Lichenoid reactions	Orthostatic hypotension; avoid long-term use of NSAIDs
Digitalis Digoxin (Lanoxin)	Increased risk for arrhythmias; avoid if possible	Increased gag reflex; hypersalivation (sign of toxicity)	Erythromycin and clarithromycin may increase the toxic effects of digoxin; avoid
Vasodilators Hydralazine (Apresoline) Isosorbide dinitrate (Isordil)	None	Lupuslike oral lesions, lymphadenopathy, dry mouth	Orthostatic hypotension

ACE, Angiotensin-converting enzyme; NSAID, nonsteroidal antiinflammatory drug.

Clinical Manifestations of Digitalis Toxicity

- Headache, nausea, vomiting
- Hypersalivation
- Altered vision and color perception
- Fatigue, malaise, drowsiness
- Arrhythmias (tachycardias or bradycardias)

and angiotensin receptor blockers (ARBs), are used to treat HF. ACEIs are first-line drugs used to treat patients with HF; they have been shown to reduce risks of death and hospitalization by 20% to 30%.[9] They are typically prescribed along with or following diuretic therapy, and they decrease the need for large doses of diuretics, as well as some of the adverse metabolic effects of diuretics.[9] In addition to ACEIs, beta-adrenergic blockers are advocated; when used in combination with ACEIs, beta blockers appear to reduce the risk of death or hospitalization for heart failure by 30% to 40%.[9]

Digitalis glycosides have been used for many years for the treatment of patients with HF; digoxin is most commonly prescribed. However, with the advent of ACEIs, their use has declined. Digoxin has not been shown to decrease the risk of death or of hospitalization, as opposed to ACEIs and beta blockers, both of which do decrease these risks. Digoxin is, however, effective in alleviating symptoms; therefore, it is principally used to treat residual symptoms not controlled by other drugs. Digoxin is the preferred agent in patients with HF who have atrial fibrillation and a rapid ventricular response.[9] A significant problem with digitalis glycosides is their narrow therapeutic range and the resultant toxicity that easily may occur (Box 6-6). Other drugs used to treat HF that is unresponsive to ACEIs include angiotensin receptor blockers and direct-acting vasodilators (hydralazine, isosorbide dinitrate). For all patients with HF, drugs that are known to worsen clinical status should be avoided. These include nonsteroidal anti-inflammatory drugs (NSAIDs), most antiarrhythmic drugs, and calcium channel blockers. In selected patients, other nonpharmacologic measures, such as biventricular pacing or the use of an implantable defibrillator, may be indicated.

If drug therapy is found to be inadequate to control the disorder in patients with severe, refractory HF (stage D), mechanical and surgical intervention may be provided. These measures may include intra-aortic balloon counterpulsation, a left ventricular assist device, and heart transplantation. The final measure is end of life hospice care.

DENTAL MANAGEMENT
Medical Considerations

The risk of treating a patient with symptomatic HF is that symptoms could abruptly worsen and result in acute failure, a fatal arrhythmia, stroke, or myocardial infarc-

tion. Identification of patients with a history of HF, those with undiagnosed HF, or those prone to developing HF is the first step in risk assessment and in avoiding an untoward event. It should be recalled that HF is a symptom complex that is the end result of an underlying disease such as coronary heart disease, hypertension, or cardiomyopathy; therefore, the cause of HF must be identified and steps taken toward appropriate dental management. Identification is accomplished by obtaining a thorough medical history, including a pertinent review of systems, and measuring and evaluating vital signs (i.e., pulse rate and rhythm, blood pressure, respiratory rate). All medications that are being taken should be identified as well. In a review of systems, patients should be asked about the presence of signs or symptoms related to the cardiovascular and pulmonary systems. Patients who report shortness of breath, orthopnea, PND, fatigue, or exercise intolerance may have HF or another cardiovascular disease. A report of an inability to climb a flight of stairs without shortness of breath or fatigue may reflect poor functional capacity or diminished cardiopulmonary reserve, with increased risk for an adverse outcome. Patients with a previous history of HF and those who are asymptomatic have compensated HF (NYHA class I). Those who are symptomatic have decompensated HF (NYHA classes II, III, and IV).

The dentist must make a determination of the risk involved in providing dental treatment to a patient with HF and must decide whether the benefits of treatment outweigh the risks. This often requires consultation with the physician. The American College of Cardiology and the American Heart Association[14] have published guidelines that can help the clinician to make this determination. These guidelines are intended for use by physicians who are evaluating patients with cardiovascular disease to determine whether they can safely undergo surgical procedures. They also can be applied to the provision of dental care and are of significant value to the dentist who must make a determination of risk.

These guidelines suggest that patients with decompensated HF constitute a major risk for the occurrence of a serious event (acute MI, unstable angina, or sudden death) during treatment. Thus, patients with symptoms of HF (decompensated; NYHA class II, III, or IV) generally are not candidates for elective dental care, and treatment should be deferred until medical consultation can be obtained (Box 6-7). Patients who have a history of HF but who are asymptomatic (compensated; NYHA class I) constitute an intermediate risk for occurrence of a serious event. With good functional capacity and reserve (i.e., can climb a flight of stairs), however, they generally can undergo any required treatment with little likelihood of problems. Thus, patients who are NYHA class I may receive routine outpatient dental care. Many patients who are NYHA class II and some who are class III also may undergo routine treatment in an outpatient setting after approval from the physician. Remaining NYHA class III patients and all class IV patients are best treated

---

Dental Management of the Patient With Heart Failure

- Evaluate patient for history, signs, or symptoms of heart failure (HF).
- For patients with symptoms of untreated or uncontrolled HF, defer elective dental care and refer to physician.
- For patients diagnosed and treated for HF:
  - Confirm status with patient or physician
  - New York Heart Association (NYHA) class I patients (asymptomatic)—Provide routine care.
  - NYHA class II (and some class III patients)—Obtain consultation with physician for medical clearance and provide routine care.
  - NYHA (some class III and class IV) patients—Obtain consultation with physician; consider treatment in a special care or hospital setting.
  - Identify underlying cardiovascular disease (i.e., coronary artery disease, hypertension, cardiomyopathy, valvular disease), and manage appropriately.
- Drug considerations:
  - For patients taking digitalis, avoid epinephrine; if considered essential, use cautiously (maximum 0.036 mg epinephrine or 0.20 mg levonordefrin); avoid gag reflex; avoid erythromycin and clarithromycin, which may increase the absorption of digitalis and lead to toxicity.
  - For patients with NYHA class III and IV congestive heart failure, avoid use of vasoconstrictors; if use is considered essential, discuss with physician.
  - Avoid epinephrine-impregnated retraction cord.
- See Table 6-1 for drug considerations and adverse effects.
- Schedule short, stress-free appointments.
- Use semisupine or upright chair position.
- Watch for orthostatic hypotension, make position or chair changes slowly, and assist patient into and out of chair.
- Avoid the use of nonsteroidal antiinflammatory drugs (NSAIDs).
- Watch for signs of digitalis toxicity (i.e., tachycardia, hypersalivation, visual disturbances, etc.).
- Nitrous oxide/oxygen sedation may be used with a minimum of 30% oxygen.

---

in a special care facility, such as a hospital dental clinic with continuous monitoring.

Recommendations for management include short, stress-free appointments. Patients with HF may not tolerate a supine chair position because of pulmonary edema and will need a semisupine or upright chair position. For patients taking a digitalis glycoside (digoxin), epinephrine should be avoided, if possible, as the combination can potentially precipitate arrhythmias. If it is considered essential to use epinephrine, it should be used cautiously. A maximum of 0.036 mg epinephrine (two cartridges of 2% lidocaine with 1:100,000 epinephrine) is recom-

mended, with care taken to avoid inadvertent intravascular injection. Epinephrine-impregnated gingival retraction cord should be avoided. Patients should be observed for signs of digitalis toxicity, such as hypersalivation. If toxicity is suspected, patients should promptly be referred to their physician. For patients who are NYHA class III or IV, vasoconstrictors should be avoided; however, if their use is considered essential, it should be discussed with the physician. NSAIDs should be avoided because they can exacerbate symptoms of HF. Nitrous oxide plus oxygen sedation may be used if adequate O_2 flow (at least 30%) is maintained.

Treatment Planning Modifications

In general, patients with HF who are under good medical management can receive any indicated dental treatment as long as the dental management plan deals effectively with the problems presented by HF, its underlying cause, and the effects of medications. Patients with symptomatic HF present a definite challenge that mandates specific management considerations.

Oral Manifestations

No oral manifestations are related to HF per se; however, many of the drugs used to manage HF can cause dry mouth and oral lesions (see Table 6-1). Digitalis may exaggerate the patient's gag reflex.

REFERENCES

1. Hunt SA, Abraham WT, Chin MH, et al. ACC/AHA 2005 Guideline Update for the Diagnosis and Management of Chronic Heart Failure in the Adult—Summary Article: A report of the American College of Cardiology/American Heart Association Task Force on Practice Guidelines (Writing Committee to Update the 2001 Guidelines for the Evaluation and Management of Heart Failure): Developed in collaboration with the American College of Chest Physicians and the International Society for Heart and Lung Transplantation. Endorsed by the Heart Rhythm Society. Circulation 2005;112:1825-1852.
2. American Heart Association. Heart Disease and Stroke Statistics. Dallas, Tex, American Heart Association, 2005.
3. Massie BM, Shah NB. Evolving trends in the epidemiologic factors of heart failure: Rationale for preventive strategies and comprehensive disease management. Am Heart J 1997;133:703-712.
4. Massie BM. Heart failure: pathophysiology and diagnosis. In Goldman L, Ausiello D (eds). Cecil Textbook of Medicine, 22nd ed. Philadelphia, Saunders, 2004.
5. Masoudi FA, Havranek EP, Krumholz HM. The burden of chronic congestive heart failure in older persons: Magnitude and implications for policy and research. Heart Fail Rev 2002;7:9-16.
6. Wynn J, Braunwald E. The cardiomyopathies. In Zipes D, Libby P, Bonow RO, Braunwald E (eds). Braunwald's Heart Disease: A Textbook of Cardiovascular Medicine, 7th ed. Philadelphia, Saunders, 2005.

7. Colucci WS, Braunwald E. Pathophysiology of heart failure. In Zipes D, Libby P, Bonow RO, Braunwald E (eds). Braunwald's Heart Disease: A Textbook of Cardiovascular Medicine, 7th ed. Philadelphia, Saunders, 2005.

8. Burkoff D, Weisfeldt ML. Cardiac function and circulatory control. In Goldman L, Ausiello D (eds). Cecil Textbook of Medicine, 22nd ed. Philadelphia, Saunders, 2004.

9. Packer M. Heart failure: Management and prognosis. In Goldman L, Ausiello D (eds). Cecil Textbook of Medicine, 22nd ed. Philadelphia, Saunders, 2004.

10. Guyton AC, Hall JE. Textbook of Medical Physiology, 11th ed. Philadelphia, Saunders, 2006.

11. Thom T, Haase N, Rosamond W, et al. Heart Disease and Stroke Statistics—2006 Update: A report from the American Heart Association Statistics Committee and Stroke Statistics Subcommittee. Circulation 2006;113: e85-e151.

12. Givertz MM, Colucci WS, Braunwald E. Clinical aspects of heart failure: Pulmonary edema, high-output failure. In Zipes D, Libby P, Bonow RO, Braunwald E (eds). Braunwald's Heart Disease: A Textbook of Cardiovascular Medicine, 7th ed. Philadelphia, Saunders, 2005.

13. Bristow MR, Linas S, Port JD. Drugs in the treatment of heart failure. In Zipes D, Libby P, Bonow RO, Braunwald E (eds). Braunwald's Heart Disease: A Textbook of Cardiovascular Medicine, 7th ed. Philadelphia, Saunders, 2005.

14. Eagle KA, Berger PB, Calkins H, et al. ACC/AHA Guideline Update for Perioperative Cardiovascular Evaluation for Noncardiac Surgery—Executive Summary: A report of the American College of Cardiology/American Heart Association Task Force on Practice Guidelines (Committee to Update the 1996 Guidelines on Perioperative Cardiovascular Evaluation for Noncardiac Surgery). Anesth Analg 2002;94:1052-1064.

PART THREE

Pulmonary Disease

Pulmonary Disease

CHAPTER

7

Chronic obstructive pulmonary disease (bronchitis and emphysema) and asthma, common pulmonary diseases that cause obstruction in airflow, are discussed in this chapter.

CHRONIC OBSTRUCTIVE PULMONARY DISEASE

DEFINITION

Chronic obstructive pulmonary disease (COPD) is a general term for pulmonary disorders characterized by chronic airflow limitation from the lungs that is not fully reversible. The two most common diseases classified as COPD are chronic bronchitis and emphysema. The basis for obstructed airflow in these two diseases is different. Chronic bronchitis is a condition associated with excessive tracheobronchial mucous production (at the bronchial level) sufficient to cause a chronic cough with sputum production for at least 3 months in at least 2 consecutive years. *Emphysema* is defined as distention of the air spaces distal to the terminal bronchioles because of destruction of alveolar walls/septa (at the acinar level).[1] These diseases are described as individual entities but often represent the progression of disease. Thus, patients may have overlapping symptoms, making differentiation difficult. Because of the potential overlap in clinical symptoms, experts have recently recommended measurement of lung function to aid clinicians in diagnosing and categorizing these disorders.[2]

EPIDEMIOLOGY

COPD is the fourth leading cause of death in the United States and is estimated to affect more than 20 million people—about 17 million with chronic bronchitis and 3 million with emphysema.[3,4] COPD affects approximately 6% of adults in the United States.[1,3,5] In the past, the disease was more common in men; however, in 2000, for the first time, more women than men died of COPD. COPD is disabling, second only to arthritis as the leading cause of long-term disability and functional impairment. Prevalence, incidence, and hospitalization rates increase with age and are now similar between men and women.[1,3,5] Emphysema, which can be definitively diagnosed only through autopsy, is found to some degree in two thirds of men and one fourth of women. Most of those affected, however, have no recognized dysfunction. On the basis of current figures, the average dental practice is estimated to have 133 patients who experience features of COPD.

Etiology

The most important cause of COPD is cigarette smoking. Approximately 12.5% of current smokers and 9% of former smokers have COPD.[6] Smoking also accounts for 80% to 90% of COPD mortality in both men and women. The risk of COPD is dose related and increases as the number of cigarettes smoked per day and the duration of smoking increase.[7] The risk of death from COPD is 13 times higher in female smokers and 12 times higher in male smokers compared with nonsmokers of the same gender.[8] Despite the increased risk, only about one in five chronic smokers develops COPD. This suggests that genetic susceptibility to the production of inflammatory mediators (i.e., cytokines) in response to smoke plays an important role. In addition to cigarette smoking, long-term exposure to occupational and environmental pollutants and the absence of alpha$_1$-antitrypsin are causative factors that contribute to COPD.

Pathophysiology and Complications

Although chronic bronchitis and emphysema both lead to obstruction of airflow, the pathophysiologic responses of each are distinct. In chronic bronchitis, pathologic changes consist of thickened bronchial walls with inflammatory cell infiltrate, increased size of the mucous glands,

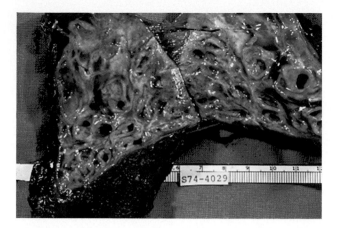

Figure 7-1. Gross pathologic specimen shows lung changes (thickened bronchial walls, narrowing of small airways) due to chronic bronchitis. (Courtesy R. N. McLay, J. H. Harrison, C. D. Fermin, H. Johnson, Tulane Gross Pathology Tutorial. Last modified July 15, 1997, Tulane University School of Medicine. Available at: http://www.som.tulane. edu/classware/pathology/medical_pathology/mcpath. Accessed August 22, 2006.)

and goblet cell hyperplasia. Obstruction is caused by narrowing of small airways, increased sputum production, mucous plugging, and collapse of peripheral airways resulting from loss of surfactant (Figure 7-1).[1] Obstruction is present on inspiration and expiration.

In emphysema, by contrast, smoke injures alveolar epithelium and causes release of inflammatory mediators that attract activated neutrophils. These neutrophils release enzymes (elastase) that destroy the alveolar walls, resulting in enlarged air spaces distal to the terminal bronchioles and loss of elastic recoil of the lungs (Figure 7-2). Obstruction is caused by the collapse of these unsupported and enlarged air spaces on expiration—not inspiration.[1] Increased susceptibility for developing emphysema occurs in smokers and patients who have a deficiency in alpha$_1$-antitrypsin. This enzyme, which is made in the liver, neutralizes neutrophil elastase.

The course of COPD is one of deterioration and periodic exacerbations unless intervention is provided early in its onset. The types of complications that develop vary depending on the predominance of chronic bronchitis or

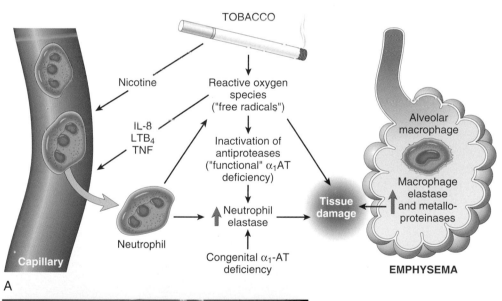

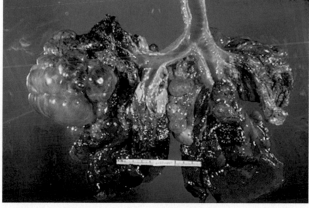

Figure 7-2. A, Pathogenesis of emphysema involving imbalance in proteases/antiproteases that results in tissue damage and collapse of alveoli. (From Kumar V, Abbas A, Fausto N. Robbins & Cotran Pathologic Basis of Disease, 7th ed. Philadelphia, Saunders, 2005.) **B,** Gross pathologic specimen of an emphysemic lung. (Courtesy R. N. McLay, J. H. Harrison, C. D. Fermin, H. Johnson, Tulane Gross Pathology Tutorial. Last modified July 15, 1997, Tulane University School of Medicine. Available at: http://www.som.tulane.edu/classware/pathology/medical_pathology/mcpath. Accessed August 22, 2006.)

emphysema. With continued exposure to primary etiologic factors (cigarette smoking, environmental pollutants), COPD usually results in progressive dyspnea and hypercapnia to the point of severe debilitation. Recurrent pulmonary infections with *Haemophilus influenzae*, *Moraxella catarrhalis*, and *Streptococcus pneumoniae* are especially common with bronchitis. These acute exacerbations are managed with antibiotics. Pulmonary hypertension can develop, leading to cor pulmonale (right-sided heart failure) in chronic bronchitis, whereas patients with emphysema more frequently experience enlarged air space, thoracic bullae, and pneumothorax. Poor quality of sleep because of nocturnal hypoxemia is common with both types of COPD. Although emphysema and chronic bronchitis are irreversible processes for which no cure exists, avoidance of pulmonary irritants can be of significant benefit in decreasing the morbidity and mortality rates of both diseases.

CLINICAL PRESENTATION

Signs and Symptoms

The onset phase of COPD takes many years in most patients. Individuals who have chronic bronchitis often have a chronic cough with copious sputum production. Patients tend to be sedentary, overweight, cyanotic, edematous, and breathless—leading to the term "blue bloaters."

Patients with emphysema exhibit severe exertional dyspnea with a minimal, nonproductive cough. Their chest walls enlarge and they become "barrel chested" while losing weight as the disease progresses. Cyanosis usually is not seen, and these patients are labeled "pink puffers." Expiration often is accompanied by pursing of the lips to forcibly exhale air from the lungs. The clinical presentation of chronic bronchitis is distinct from that of emphysema until progression to emphysema occurs (Box 7-1). However, many patients have elements of both diseases.

Laboratory Findings

Diagnosing COPD in its early stages can be difficult. The hallmark feature of COPD is reduced maximal expiratory flow rate. Clinical symptoms of dyspnea, cough, and sputum production, and blood gas and chest radiographic abnormalities are additional features of COPD.[9]

Measures of expiratory airflow are key to the diagnosis of obstructive pulmonary disease. Forced expiratory volume in 1 second (FEV_1) on spirometry is the measure of choice for determining pulmonary function. The term *COPD* is used when patients have pulmonary symptoms and an FEV_1 of less than 70% of predicted volume (forced vital capacity [FVC]) in the absence of any other pulmonary disease. Mild COPD is defined by an FEV_1/FVC ratio of <70% and an FEV_1 >80% of that predicted. Moderate COPD has an FEV_1/FVC ratio of <70% and an FEV_1 ≤80% predicted.[2] The term *end-stage COPD* is used when the FEV_1/FVC ratio is less than 50%.

BOX 7-1

Predominant Features of Patients With Chronic Bronchitis or Emphysema

CHRONIC BRONCHITIS (BLUE BLOATER)
- Onset ≈50 years
- Frequently overweight
- Chronic productive cough
- Copious mucopurulent sputum
- Mild dyspnea
- Frequent respiratory infections
- Elevated pCO_2
- Decreased pO_2 (hypoxia)
- Elevated hematocrit value
- Cor pulmonale common
- Chest radiograph shows prominent blood vessels and large heart

EMPHYSEMA (PINK PUFFER)
- Onset ≈60 years
- Thin, barrel-chested
- Cough not prominent
- Scanty sputum
- Severe dyspnea
- Few respiratory infections
- Normal pCO_2
- Decreased pO_2 (hypoxia)
- Normal hematocrit value
- Cor pulmonale rare
- Chest radiograph shows hyperinflation and small heart

In addition, patients with chronic bronchitis have an elevated partial pressure of carbon dioxide (pCO_2) and decreased partial pressure of oxygen (pO_2) (as measured by arterial blood gases), leading to secondary erythrocytosis, an elevated hematocrit value, and compensated respiratory acidosis. Total lung capacity usually is normal, with a moderate elevation in residual volume. Patients with emphysema have a relatively normal pCO_2 and a decreased pO_2, which maintain normal hemoglobin saturation, thus avoiding erythrocytosis. These patients have normal hematocrit values. Total lung capacity and residual volume are markedly increased. The ventilatory drive of hypoxia also is reduced in both types of patients with COPD.

Chest radiographs of patients with chronic bronchitis demonstrate increased bronchovascular markings at the base of the lungs (Figure 7-3). In emphysema, films demonstrate persistent and marked overdistention of the lungs, flattening of the diaphragm, and emphysematous bullae.

MEDICAL MANAGEMENT

No cure is known for COPD. However, much can be done to improve the quality of life of these patients and to prevent progression of the disease. The cornerstone of management is early intervention. Smoking cessation and elimination of exposure to environmental pollutants and irritants are critical in limiting progression of the disease. Other recommended palliative measures include regular exercise, good nutrition, prevention of respiratory infection with annual pneumococcal and influenza vaccinations, aggressive treatment of pulmonary infection with antibiotics, adequate daily hydration, and low-flow oxygen therapy.[10,11]

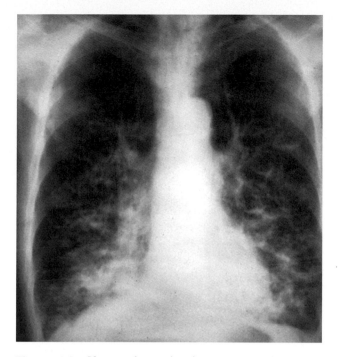

Figure 7-3. Chest radiograph of a patient with chronic bronchitis and prominent vascular markings.

Agents used in the management of COPD are listed in Table 7-1. Anticholinergics (e.g., ipratropium, tiotropium) that block acetylcholine and bronchoconstriction and beta$_2$-adrenergic bronchodilators are preferred therapy for relieving symptoms in COPD. Second-line drugs include inhaled corticosteroids combined with a long-acting beta$_2$ agonist in a single inhaler. Theophylline, a methylxanthine medication, has been relegated to third-line therapy in COPD.[12] Theophylline is usually added to inhaled bronchodilators for patients with more severe disease and provides clinical improvement when added to a long-acting beta$_2$ agonist. Theophylline relaxes bronchial smooth muscle cells weakly by blocking adenosine receptors and inhibiting the formation of cyclic adenosine monophosphate, as well as through its immunomodulating effects.[13] Theophylline has a narrow therapeutic range. Numerous factors and medications can displace the protein-bound fraction of the drug within the bloodstream, causing toxicity. Because of the likelihood of occurrence of its adverse effects (especially in the elderly), a low dose of theophylline is recommended. Low-flow oxygen therapy may be used for severe COPD.[14]

DENTAL MANAGEMENT

Prevention of Potential Problems

Most patients with COPD have a history of smoking tobacco. Dental health providers can take an important step in the management of patients with COPD by encouraging those who smoke to quit. By providing knowledge of the diseases associated with smoking, dental health providers may help patients to start thinking seri-

---

BOX 7-2

Dental Management of the Patient With COPD

Review history for evidence of concurrent heart disease; take appropriate precautions if heart disease is present.
- Avoid treating if upper respiratory infection is present.
- Treat in upright chair position.
- Use local anesthetic as usual.
- Avoid use of rubber dam in severe disease.
- Use pulse oximetry to monitor oxygen saturation.
- Use low-flow (2 to 3 L/min) supplemental oxygen when oxygen saturation drops below 95%; it may become necessary when oxygen saturation drops below 91%.
- Avoid nitrous oxide/oxygen inhalation sedation with severe COPD and emphysema.
- Consider low-dose oral diazepam or other benzodiazepine; these may cause oral dryness.
- Avoid use of barbiturates, narcotics, antihistamines, and anticholinergics.
- Supplemental steroids may be needed if patient is taking steroids and an invasive procedure is planned.
- Avoid erythromycin, macrolide antibiotics, and ciprofloxacin for patients taking theophylline.
- Do not use outpatient general anesthesia.

COPD, Chronic obstructive pulmonary disease.

---

ously about giving up the habit. Many interventional approaches (e.g., nicotine replacement, bupropion) are available, and providers should use the method with which they feel most comfortable[15] (see Chapter 8).

Before initiating dental care, clinicians should assess the severity of the patient's disease and the degree to which is has been controlled. A patient coming to the office for routine dental care who displays shortness of breath at rest, a productive cough, upper respiratory infection, or an oxygen saturation level less than 91% (as determined by pulse oximetry) is unstable, and staff should reschedule the appointment. If the patient is stable and the breathing is adequate, efforts should be directed toward the avoidance of anything that could further depress respiration (Box 7-2). Patients should be placed in a semisupine or upright chair position for treatment, rather than in the supine position, to prevent orthopnea and a feeling of respiratory discomfort. Pulse oximetry monitoring is advised. Humidified low-flow oxygen—generally between 2 and 3 L per minute—may be provided and should be considered for use when the oxygen saturation level is less than 95%.

No contraindication to the use of local anesthetic has been identified. However, the use of bilateral mandibular blocks or bilateral palatal blocks can cause an unpleasant airway constriction sensation in some patients. This may be more important in the management of a patient with severe COPD with a rubber dam, or when medications

TABLE 7-1
Drugs Used in the Outpatient Management of COPD and Asthma

Category and Generic Names	Product Name	Dental Considerations
ANTIINFLAMMATORY DRUGS		
Corticosteroids—Inhaled		Not intended for acute asthma attack; may contribute to the development of oral candidiasis if used improperly or excessively
Beclomethasone dipropionate	Vanceril, Beclovent	
Budesonide	Pulmicort	
Dexamethasone	Decadron	
Flunisolide	AeroBid	
Fluticasone propionate	Flonase	
Triamcinolone acetonide	Azmacort	
Corticosteroids—Systemic		Not intended for acute asthma attack; possible adrenal suppression, cushingoid features with long-term use
Prednisone	Deltasone or generic	
Prednisolone	Delta-Cortef	
Methylprednisolone	Solu-Medrol	
Antileukotrienes		Not intended for acute asthma attack
5-Lipoxygenase inhibitor:		
Zileuton	Zyflo	
Leukotriene D_4 receptor antagonists:		
Zafirlukast		
Montelukast	Accolate	
	Singulair	
Nonsteroidal—Chromones		Not intended for acute asthma attack
Cromolyn sodium	Intal inhaler	
Nedocromil	Tilade inhaler	
BETA-ADRENERGIC BRONCHODILATORS		
Fast-acting nonselective beta agonist inhalers		Drugs for use during acute asthma attack
Epinephrine*	Primatene Mist, Bronkaid (available parenteral also)	
Ephedrine†	Eted II	
Intermediate-acting nonselective beta agonist inhalers (3 to 6 hours)		Not best choice for use during acute asthma attack
Isoproterenol‡	Isuprel	
Isoetharine	Bronkosol	
Metaproterenol§	Alupent, Metaprel, and others	
Beta₂ selective agonist inhalers		Drugs for use during acute asthma attack
Albuterol‡	Proventil, Ventolin	
Bitolterol mesylate	Tornalate	
Pirbuterol	Maxair, Maxair Autohaler	
Terbutaline‡	Brethaire, Bricanyl	
Fenoterol	Not available in United States, restricted availability in New Zealand	
Long-acting beta₂ selective agonist inhalers (>12 hours)		Not intended for acute asthma attack
Salmeterol (slow onset, long duration)	Serevent	
Formoterol (rapid onset, long duration)	Foradil	
METHYLXANTHINES		Adverse drug interaction with erythromycin and azithromycin
Theophylline	Theo-Dur	
QUATERNARY AMMONIUM DERIVATIVE OF ATROPINE (ANTICHOLINERGIC BRONCHODILATOR)		Not intended for acute asthma attack; generally used in combination with other antiasthma drugs
Ipratropium bromide	Atrovent	
Tiotropium	Spiriva	

COPD, Chronic obstructive pulmonary disease.
*Inhalation and parenteral.
†Oral and parenteral.
‡Inhalation, oral, and parenteral.
§Inhalation and oral.

are administered that dry mucous secretions. Humidified low-flow oxygen can be provided to alleviate the unpleasant airway feeling produced by nerve blocks, use of a rubber dam, and/or medications.

If sedative medication is required, low-dose oral diazepam (Valium) may be used. Nitrous oxide (N_2O)/oxygen inhalation sedation should be used with caution in patients with mild to moderate chronic bronchitis. It should not be used in patients with severe COPD and emphysema because gas may accumulate in air spaces of the diseased lung. If used in the patient with chronic bronchitis, flow rates should be reduced to an overall rate of no greater than 3 L per minute, and the clinician should anticipate induction and recovery times approximately twice as long with N_2O as they are with healthy patients.[16] Narcotics and barbiturates should not be used because of their respiratory depressant properties. Anticholinergics and antihistamines generally should be used with caution in patients with COPD because of their drying properties and the resultant increase in mucous tenacity, and because patients with chronic bronchitis may already be taking these types of medications; concurrent administration could result in additive effects.

Patients with COPD often have hypertension and coronary heart disease (see Chapters 3 and 4). Patients taking systemic corticosteroids may require supplementation for major surgical procedures because of adrenal suppression (see Chapter 16). Macrolide antibiotics (e.g., erythromycin, azithromycin) and ciprofloxacin hydrochloride should be avoided in patients taking theophylline because these antibiotics can retard the metabolism of theophylline, resulting in theophylline toxicity. The dentist should be aware of the manifestations of theophylline toxicity. Symptoms include anorexia, nausea, nervousness, insomnia, agitation, thirst, vomiting, headache, cardiac arrhythmias, and convulsions. Outpatient general anesthesia is contraindicated for most patients with COPD.

Treatment Planning Modifications

No technical treatment planning modifications are required in patients with COPD.

Oral Complications and Manifestations

Patients with COPD who are chronic smokers have an increased likelihood of developing halitosis, extrinsic tooth stains, nicotine stomatitis, periodontal disease, and oral cancer. In rare instances, theophylline has been associated with the development of Stevens-Johnson syndrome.

ASTHMA

DEFINITION

Asthma is a chronic inflammatory respiratory disease that is associated with increased airway hyperresponsiveness, resulting in recurrent episodes of dyspnea, coughing, and wheezing.[17] The bronchiolar lung tissue of patients with asthma is particularly sensitive to a variety of stimuli. Overt attacks may be provoked by allergens, upper respiratory tract infection, exercise, cold air, certain medications (salicylates, nonsteroidal anti-inflammatory drugs, cholinergic drugs, and beta-adrenergic blocking drugs), chemicals, smoke, and highly emotional states such as anxiety, stress, and nervousness.

EPIDEMIOLOGY

Incidence and Prevalence

Asthma affects 300 million persons worldwide and accounts for 1 of every 250 deaths worldwide. In the United States, its prevalence has more than doubled since the 1960s, from about 2% to ≥5% (20 million).[17,18] Asthma is a disease primarily of children, with 10% of children affected.[19] Young persons with asthma most often are male, whereas adults who contract the disease more frequently are women. Increased body mass index (BMI) increases the risk for asthma in women.[20] The disease occurs in all races, with a slightly higher prevalence in African Americans and a lower prevalence in Hispanics than in other races or ethnic groups.[19,21] On the basis of current figures, the average dental practice is estimated to have at least 100 patients who have asthma.

Etiology

Asthma is a multifactorial and heterogeneous disease whose exact cause is not completely understood. Five types of asthma have been described on the basis of pathophysiology: extrinsic (allergic or atopic), intrinsic (idiosyncratic, nonallergic, or nonatopic), drug induced, exercise induced, and infectious. These categories are discussed in the following paragraphs.

Allergic or extrinsic asthma is the most common form and accounts for approximately 35% of all adult cases. It is an exaggerated inflammatory response that is triggered by inhaled seasonal allergens such as pollens, dust, house mites, and animal danders. Allergic asthma is usually seen in children and young adults.[22] In these patients, a dose-response relationship exists between allergen exposure and immunoglobulin E (IgE)-mediated sensitization, positive skin testing to various allergens, and associated family history of allergic disease. Inflammatory responses are mediated primarily by type 2 helper T (T_H2) cells that secrete interleukins and stimulate B cells to produce IgE (Figure 7-4). During an attack, allergens interact with IgE antibodies affixed to mast cells, basophils, and eosinophils along the tracheobronchial tree. The complex of antigen with antibody causes leukocytes to degranulate and secrete vasoactive autocoids and cytokines such as bradykinins, histamine, leukotrienes, and prostaglandins.[13] Histamine and leukotrienes cause smooth muscle contraction (bronchoconstriction) and increased vascular permeability, and they attract eosinophils into the airway.[23] The release of platelet-activating factor sustains

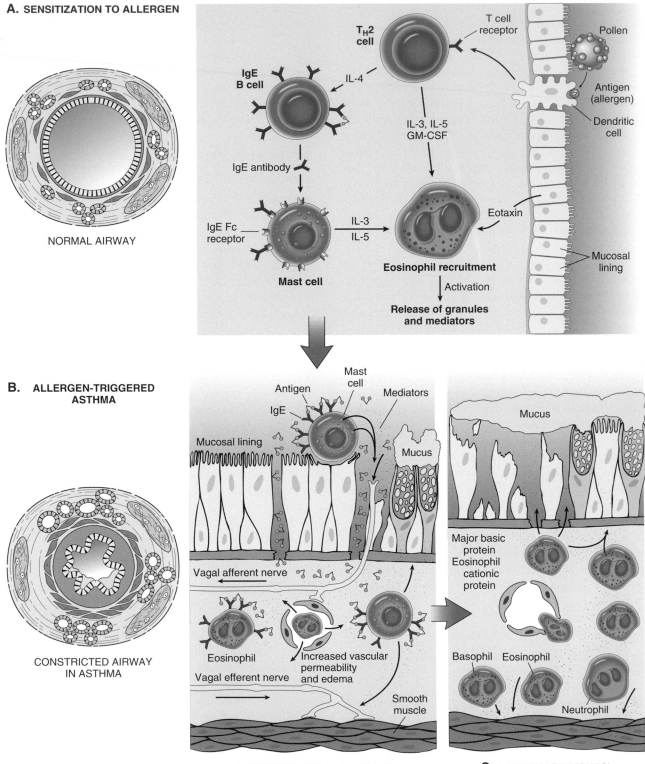

A. SENSITIZATION TO ALLERGEN

NORMAL AIRWAY

TH2 cell

T cell receptor

Pollen

IgE B cell

IL-4

Antigen (allergen)

Dendritic cell

IL-3, IL-5 GM-CSF

IgE antibody

IgE Fc receptor

IL-3 IL-5

Eotaxin

Mast cell

Eosinophil recruitment

Mucosal lining

Activation

Release of granules and mediators

B. ALLERGEN-TRIGGERED ASTHMA

CONSTRICTED AIRWAY IN ASTHMA

Mast cell

Antigen

Mediators

IgE

Mucus

Mucosal lining

Mucus

Vagal afferent nerve

Major basic protein Eosinophil cationic protein

Eosinophil

Increased vascular permeability and edema

Vagal efferent nerve

Basophil   Eosinophil

Smooth muscle

Neutrophil

IMMEDIATE PHASE (MINUTES)

C. LATE PHASE (HOURS)

Figure 7-4. Processes involved in allergic (extrinsic) asthma. (From Kumar V, Abbas A, Fausto N. Robbins & Cotran Pathologic Basis of Disease, 7th ed. Philadelphia, Saunders, 2005.)

bronchial hyperresponsiveness. Release of E-selectin and endothelial cell adhesion molecules, neutrophil chemotactic factor, and eosinophilic chemotactic factor of anaphylaxis are responsible for recruitment of leukocytes to the airway wall, which increases tissue edema and mucous secretion. T lymphocytes prolong the inflammatory

response (late phase response), and imbalances in matrix metalloproteinases and tissue inhibitor metalloproteinases may contribute to fibrotic changes.

Intrinsic asthma accounts for about 30% of asthma cases and seldom is associated with a family history of allergy or with a known cause. Patients usually are nonresponsive to skin testing and demonstrate normal IgE levels. This form of asthma generally is seen in middle-aged adults, and its onset is associated with endogenous causes such as emotional stress (implicated in at least 50% of persons with asthma), gastroesophageal acid reflux, or vagally mediated responses.[22,24]

Ingestion of drugs (e.g., aspirin, nonsteroidal antiinflammatory drugs, beta blockers, angiotensin-converting enzyme inhibitors) and some food substances (e.g., nuts, shellfish, strawberries, milk, tartrazine food dye yellow color no. 5) can trigger asthma. Aspirin causes bronchoconstriction in about 10% of patients with asthma, and sensitivity to aspirin occurs in 30% to 40% of people with asthma who have pansinusitis and nasal polyps (triad asthmaticus).[25] The ability of aspirin to block the cyclo-oxygenase pathway appears causative. The buildup of arachidonic acid and leukotrienes via the lipoxygenase pathway results in bronchial spasm.[26]

Metabisulfite preservatives of foods and drugs (local anesthetics containing epinephrine) may cause wheezing when metabolic levels of the enzyme sulfite oxidase are low.[27] Sulfur dioxide is produced in the absence of sulfite oxidase.[28] The buildup of sulfur dioxide in the bronchial tree precipitates an acute asthma attack.[28]

Exercise-induced asthma is stimulated by exertional activity. Although the pathogenesis of this form of asthma is unknown, thermal changes during inhalation of cold air provoke mucosal irritation and airway hyperactivity. Children and young adults are more severely affected because of their high level of physical activity.

Patients with infectious asthma develop bronchial constriction and increased airway resistance because of the inflammatory response of the bronchi to infection. Causative agents often include viruses, bacteria, dermatologic fungi *(Trichophyton)*, and *Mycoplasma* organisms. Treatment of the infection usually improves control of pulmonary constriction.

Pathophysiology and Complications

In asthma, obstruction of airflow occurs as the result of bronchial smooth muscle spasm, inflammation of bronchial mucosa, mucous hypersecretion, and sputum plugging. The most striking macroscopic finding in the asthmatic lung is occlusion of the bronchi and bronchioles by thick, tenacious mucous plugs (Figure 7-5). Characteristic histologic findings include (1) thickened basement membrane (because of collagen deposition) of the bronchial epithelium, (2) edema, (3) mucous gland hypertrophy and goblet cell hyperplasia, (4) hypertrophy of the bronchial wall muscle, (5) mast cell and inflammatory cell infiltrate, and (6) epithelial damage and detachment.[29,30] These changes contribute to decreased diameter of the airway, increased airway resistance, and difficulty in expiration.

Asthma is relatively benign in terms of morbidity. Most patients can expect a reasonably good prognosis, especially those in whom the disease develops during childhood. In many young children, the condition resolves

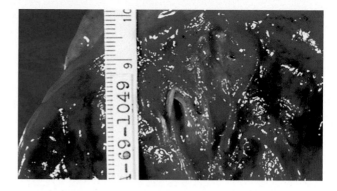

Figure 7-5. Section of a lung with the bronchioles occluded by mucous plugs. (Courtesy R. N. McLay, J. H. Harrison, C. D. Fermin, H. Johnson, Tulane Gross Pathology Tutorial. Last modified July 15, 1997, Tulane University School of Medicine. Available at: http://www.som.tulane.edu/classware/pathology/medical_pathology/mcpath. Accessed August 22, 2006.)

spontaneously after puberty. However, a recent report indicates that two thirds of asthmatic children still have symptoms at age 21 years.[31] Also, a small percentage of patients can progress to emphysema and respiratory failure or may develop status asthmaticus, the most serious manifestation of asthma. Status asthmaticus is a particularly severe and prolonged asthmatic attack (one lasting longer than 24 hours) that is refractory to usual therapy. Signs include increased and progressive dyspnea, jugular venous pulsation, cyanosis, and pulsus paradoxus (a fall in systolic pressure with inspiration). Status asthmaticus often is associated with a respiratory infection and can cause exhaustion, severe dehydration, peripheral vascular collapse, and death. Although death directly attributable to asthma is relatively uncommon, the disease causes more than 5000 deaths per year in the United States. Asthma deaths occur more often in persons over age 45 years, are largely preventable, and often relate to delays in delivery of appropriate medical care.[31]

CLINICAL PRESENTATION

Signs and Symptoms

Asthma is a disease of episodic attacks of airway hyperresponsiveness. For reasons that are unclear, attacks occur often at night but also may follow exposure to an allergen, exercise, respiratory infection, or emotional upset and excitement. Typical symptoms of asthma consist of reversible episodes of breathlessness (dyspnea), wheezing, cough that is worse at night, chest tightness, and flushing. Onset usually is sudden, with peak symptoms occurring within 10 to 15 minutes. Inadequate treatment results in emergency department visits for about 25% of patients.[31] Respirations become difficult and are accompanied by expiratory wheezing. Tachypnea and prolonged expiration are characteristic. Termination of an attack is commonly accompanied by a productive cough with thick, stringy mucus. Episodes usually are self-limiting,

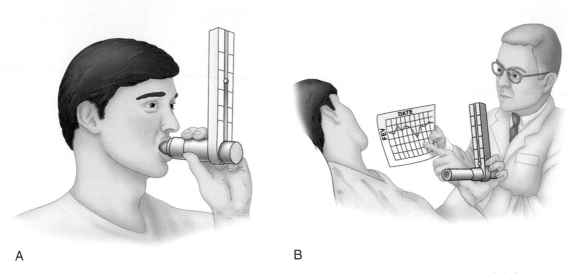

Figure 7-6. A, Measure of forced expiratory volume by spirometry. **B,** Discussion of daily spirometry results with physician.

although severe episodes may require medical assistance.[32]

Laboratory Findings

Diagnostic testing by a physician is important in the differentiation of asthma from COPD. Clinical judgment is required because laboratory tests for asthma are relatively nonspecific, and any test alone is not diagnostic. Commonly ordered tests include chest radiographs (for hyperinflation), skin testing (for specific allergens), histamine or methacholine chloride challenge testing, sputum smears and blood counts (for eosinophilia), arterial blood gases, antibody-based enzyme-linked immunosorbent assay (ELISA) for measurement of environmental allergen exposure, and spirometry (a peak expiratory flowmeter that measures pulmonary function) before and after administration of a short-acting bronchodilator.[33] Spirometry is widely applied in diagnosing asthma because this disease requires that airflow obstruction must be episodic and at least partially reversible. Accordingly, decreased pulmonary function (i.e., FEV_1) as measured by spirometry is a feature of the disease. A recent drop in FEV_1 can be interpreted as a prediction of an asthma attack (Figure 7-6), and a drop of more than 10% during exercise fulfills the diagnosis of exercise-induced asthma.

Classification

Patients with chronic asthma are clinically classified as mild (intermittent or persistent), moderate, or severe. Severity is based on the frequency of acute attacks and level of lung function (Box 7-3). Persons with mild asthma have symptoms only when exposed to a condition that triggers asthma, and their FEV_1 is greater than 80%. Symptoms last less than an hour and do not occur daily. Patients with moderate asthma have FEV_1 greater than 60% but less than 80% and daily symptoms that affect sleep and activity level, and on occasion, require emer-

gency care. Asthma is severe when patients have less than 60% FEV_1, which results in ongoing symptoms that limit normal activity. Attacks are frequent or continuous, occur at night, and result in emergency hospitalization.

MEDICAL MANAGEMENT

The goals of asthma therapy are to limit exposure to triggering agents, allow normal activities, restore and maintain normal pulmonary function, minimize frequency and severity of attacks, control chronic and nocturnal symptoms, and avoid adverse effects of medications.[34] Experts agree that this is best accomplished by educating patients and involving them in the prevention or elimination of precipitating factors, establishment of an intervention plan for regular self-monitoring and management, and provision of regular follow-up care.[35] Specifically, it is recommended that a written action plan should be given to each patient, and patients should be instructed to use it. Inexpensive peak expiratory flowmeters should be used regularly at home and levels recorded daily in diaries. For patients with known allergies, the importance of avoidance of allergens to prevent attacks should be explained. This can be emphasized by monitoring of allergen levels (tobacco smoke and pollutants) in the patient's home, provision of desensitization intradermal injections, and monitoring of the pulmonary function zone on the basis of daily peak flowmeter results (spirometry). Unfortunately, poor control of asthma often is related to low socioeconomic status (e.g., the patient cannot afford medication), increased anxiety, poor compliance, and poor home environment.

Antiasthmatic drug selection is based on the type and severity of asthma and whether the drug is to be used as a prophylactic or as therapy.[29] Chronic asthma once was controlled with the use of beta₂-adrenergic agonists and theophylline. However, current guidelines recommend a "step care" approach with the use of inhaled anti-

BOX 7-3

Classification of Asthma and Drug Management

MILD INTERMITTENT

Intermittent wheezing on less than 2 days per week, exacerbations that are brief, asymptomatic between exacerbations, nocturnal symptoms less than 2 times a month, relatively good exercise tolerance, FEV_1 more than 80% predicted, less than 20% variability	No daily medication or short-acting beta$_2$ agonist as needed

MILD PERSISTENT

Wheezing 2 to 5 days per week (occurs over several days), exacerbations that affect activity and sleep, nocturnal asthma attacks more than 2 times a month, limited exercise tolerance; rare ER visit, FEV_1 more than 80% predicted, 20% to 30% variability	Low-dose inhaled corticosteroids or other antiinflammatory, as needed; short-acting beta$_2$ agonist

MODERATE PERSISTENT

Daily symptoms of wheezing (occur over several days), daily use of short-acting beta agonist, exacerbations that affect activity and sleep and may last for days, nocturnal asthma attacks at least 1 time a week, limited exercise tolerance, occasional ER visit, FEV_1 60% to 80% predicted, 20% to 30% variability	Low- or medium-dose inhaled corticosteroids + long-acting bronchodilator, as needed; short-acting beta$_2$ agonist

SEVERE PERSISTENT

Frequent/daily exacerbations, continual symptoms, frequent (more than 4 times a month) nocturnal asthma, exercise intolerance, FEV_1 less than 60%, more than 30% variability, often resulting in hospitalization	High-dose inhaled corticosteroids + long-acting bronchodilator + oral corticosteroid, as needed; short-acting beta$_2$ agonist

FEV_1, Forced expiratory volume in 1 second; ER, emergency room.

inflammatory agents (first tier: corticosteroids; alternatives: leukotriene inhibitors) for the prophylaxis of chronic asthma.[13,35,36] Beta-adrenergic agonists, methylxanthines, and anticholinergic drugs are secondary agents that should be added (i.e., not to be used alone) when anti-inflammatory drugs are inadequate.[29,35] Antileukotrienes are most useful in mild to moderate asthma and in blocking aspirin-induced asthmatic responses.[37]

For persistent asthma, inhaled corticosteroids are recommended over beta-adrenergic agonists because steroids provide better overall control of asthma, less likelihood of a sudden overwhelming attack, and less risk for sudden death.[38,39] Steroids act by reducing the inflammatory response and preventing the formation of cytokines, adhesion molecules, and inflammatory enzymes. Aerosol dosage is two (for mild to moderate disease) to four times daily (severe asthma). Onset of action usually occurs after 2 hours, and peak effects occur 6 hours later. Long-term use of steroid inhalers rarely is associated with systemic adverse effects, provided the maximum recommended dose of 1.5 mg per day of inhaled beclomethasone dipropionate (Vanceril) or equivalent is not exceeded. Use of systemic steroids is reserved for asthma unresponsive to inhaled corticosteroids and bronchodilators, and for use during the recovery phase of a severe acute attack. Corticosteroid-sparing agents (cyclosporine, methotrexate) are used in severe asthma to minimize the adverse effects of high-dose systemic steroids, but they have their own set of adverse effects. Newer agents include molecules that block IgE (monoclonal antibody against human IgE) or the effects of interleukin

(IL)-4 or IL-5.[40,41] To monitor and/or predict response to therapy, noninvasive tests of airway inflammation that measure eosinophilia in sputum or levels of nitric oxide in exhaled breath are being tested but await broad application in clinical practice.[20]

For relief of acute asthma attacks, inhaled beta$_2$-adrenergic agonists are the drugs of choice because of their fast and notable bronchodilatory and smooth muscle relaxation properties (Figure 7-7; see Table 7-1). These agonists produce bronchodilation by activating beta$_2$ receptors on airway smooth muscle cells.[13] Inhalation corticosteroids and cromolyn sodium are used infrequently for this purpose because of slow onset of action. Beta$_2$-adrenergic agonists (administered by a metered-dose inhaler) and cromolyn sodium (Intal) may be used in preventing exercise-induced bronchospasm. They are taken about 30 minutes before exposure to physical activity. Cromolyn sodium decreases airway hyperresponsiveness by stabilizing the membrane of mast cells so mediators are not released when challenged by exercise or cold air.

DENTAL MANAGEMENT
Prevention of Potential Problems

The goal of management for dental patients with asthma must be to prevent an acute asthma attack (Box 7-4). The first step in achieving this goal is to identify patients with asthma by history, learn as much as possible about their problem, and prevent precipitating factors.

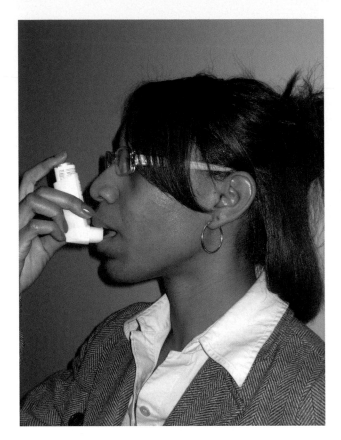

Figure 7-7. Use of an inhaler by a patient.

Through a good history, the dentist should be able to determine the severity and stability of disease. Questions should be asked that ascertain the type of asthma (e.g., allergic, nonallergic), the precipitating substances, the frequency and severity of attacks, the times of day that attacks occur, whether this is a current or past problem, how attacks usually are managed, and whether the patient has received emergency treatment for an acute attack. The clinician must realize that severe disease is associated with frequent exacerbations, exercise intolerance, FEV_1 less than 60%, use of several medications, and a history of visits to an emergency facility for treatment of acute attacks (see Box 7-3).

The stability of the disease can be assessed through clinical and laboratory measures. Features such as shortness of breath, wheezing, increased respiratory rate (more than 50% above normal), FEV_1 that has fallen more than 10% or to below 80% of peak FEV_1, an eosinophil count that is elevated to above 50 per mm,[3] and emergency department visits within the previous 3 months suggest inadequate treatment and poor stability. Also, the use of more than 1.5 canisters of a beta agonist inhaler per month (more than 200 inhalations per month) or doubling of monthly use indicates high risk of a severe asthma attack.[42] For severe and unstable asthma, consultation with the patient's physician is advised. Routine dental treatment should be postponed until better control is achieved.

Modifications during the preoperative and operative phases of dental management of a patient with asthma can

minimize the likelihood of an attack. Patients who have nocturnal asthma should be scheduled for late-morning appointments, when attacks are less likely. Operatory odorants (e.g., methyl methacrylate) should be reduced before the patient is treated. Patients should be instructed to regularly use their medications, bring their inhalers (bronchodilators) to each appointment, and inform the dentist at the earliest sign or symptom of an asthma attack. Prophylactic inhalation of a patient's bronchodilator at the beginning of the appointment is a valuable method of preventing an asthma attack. Alternatively, patients may be advised to bring their spirometer and daily expiratory record to the office. The dentist may request that the patient exhale into the spirometer and record the expired volume. A significant drop in lung function (to below 80% of peak FEV_1 or a greater than 10% drop compared with previous recordings) indicates that prophylactic use of the inhaler or referral to a physician is needed.[43] The use of a pulse oximeter also is valuable for determining the oxygen saturation level of the patient. Healthy patients should remain between 97% and 100%, whereas a drop to 91% or below indicates poor oxygen exchange and the need for intervention.

Because stress is implicated as a precipitating factor in asthma attacks and dental treatment may result in decreased lung function,[44] the dental staff should make every effort to identify patients who are anxious and provide a stress-free environment through establishment of rapport and openness. Preoperative and intraoperative sedation may be desirable. If sedation is required, nitrous oxide/oxygen inhalation is best. Nitrous oxide is not a respiratory depressant, nor is it an irritant to the tracheobronchial tree. Oral premedication may be accomplished with small doses of a short-acting benzodiazepine. Reasonable alternatives with children include the use of hydroxyzine (Vistaril), for its antihistamine/sedative properties, or ketamine, which causes bronchodilation. Barbiturates and narcotics, particularly meperidine, are histamine-releasing drugs that can provoke an attack. Outpatient general anesthesia generally is contraindicated for patients with asthma.

Selection of local anesthetic may require adjustment. In 1987, the US Food and Drug Administration[27] warned that drugs that contained sulfites were a cause of allergic-type reactions in susceptible individuals. Sulfite preservatives are found in local anesthetic solutions that contain epinephrine or levonordefrin, albeit the amount of sulfite in a local anesthetic cartridge is less than the amount commonly found in certain foods. Although rare, at least one case of an acute asthma attack precipitated by exposure to sulfites has been reported.[45] Thus, the use of local anesthetic without epinephrine or levonordefrin may be advisable for patients with moderate to severe disease. Because relevant data remain limited, dentists should discuss with the patient past responses to local anesthetics and allergy to sulfites and should consult with the physician. As an alternative, local anesthetics without a vasoconstrictor may be used in at-risk patients.

BOX 7-4

Dental Management of the Patient With Asthma

1. Identify and assess by history
   - Type of asthma (mild, moderate, or severe)
   - Precipitating factors (and plan for allergen avoidance)
   - Age at onset
   - Level of control (frequency, time of day, and severity of attacks)
     - How usually managed
     - Medications being taken (how often quick-relief medication is used) and taken correctly on the day of the appointment
     - Necessity of emergency care (life-threatening attacks, hospitalizations, emergency department visits)
     - Baseline forced expiratory volume in 1 second (FEV_1) stable (not decreasing)
2. Avoid known precipitating factors
3. Obtain medical consultation for patient with severe persistent asthma
4. Ask patient to bring current medication inhaler to every appointment and to keep it available; (used prophylactically in persons with moderate to severe persistent disease)
5. Drug considerations
   - Avoid aspirin-containing medications (use acetaminophen)
   - Avoid nonsteroidal antiinflammatory drugs (NSAIDs) (see Table 16-3)
   - Avoid barbiturates and narcotics (histamine-releasing drugs)
   - Avoid erythromycin and macrolide antibiotics in patients taking theophylline
   - Discontinue cimetidine 24 hr before intravenous sedation in patients taking theophylline
6. Local anesthetic considerations (may elect to avoid solutions containing epinephrine or levonordefrin because of sulfite preservative)
7. Patients taking chronic corticosteroid medications over the long term may require supplementation (see Chapter 16)
8. Provide stress-free environment through establishment of rapport and openness
9. If sedation is required, nitrous oxide/oxygen inhalation sedation and/or small doses of oral diazepam recommended
10. Recognize signs and symptoms of a severe or worsening asthma attack
    - Inability to finish sentences with one breath
    - Ineffectiveness of bronchodilators to relieve dyspnea
    - Tachypnea equal to or greater than 25 breaths per minute
    - Tachycardia equal to or greater than 110 beats per minute
    - Diaphoresis
    - Accessory muscle usage
    - Paradoxical pulse
11. Administer fast-acting bronchodilator (NOTE: Corticosteroids have delayed onset of action), oxygen, and, if needed, subcutaneous 0.3 to 0.5 ml mL of epinephrine (1:1000)
12. Activate emergency medical system (EMS)
13. Repeat administration of fast-acting bronchodilator every 5 minutes until EMS arrives

Patients with asthma who are medicated over the long term with systemic corticosteroids may require supplementation for major dental procedures (see Chapter 16). However, long-term use of inhaled corticosteroids rarely causes adrenal suppression unless the daily dosage exceeds 1.5 mg beclomethasone dipropionate.[13]

Administration of aspirin-containing medication or other nonsteroidal antiinflammatory drugs to patients with asthma is not advisable because aspirin ingestion is associated with the precipitation of asthma attacks in a small percentage of patients. Likewise, barbiturates and narcotics are best not used because they also may precipitate an asthma attack. Antihistamines have beneficial properties but should be used cautiously because of their drying effects. Patients who are taking theophylline preparations should not be given macrolide antibiotics (i.e., erythromycin and azithromycin) or ciprofloxacin hydrochloride because this may result in a toxic blood level of theophylline. To prevent serious toxicity, the dentist should ask the patient who takes theophylline whether the dosage is being monitored on the basis of serum theophylline levels (recommended to be less than 10 μg/mL).

Approximately 3% of patients who take zileuton experience elevated alanine transaminase levels and liver dysfunction that may affect the metabolism of dentally administered drugs.[46]

Management of Potential Problems: Asthma Attack

An acute asthma attack requires immediate therapy. The signs and symptoms (see Box 7-4) should be recognized quickly and an inhaler provided rapidly. A short-acting beta$_2$-adrenergic agonist inhaler (Ventolin, Proventil) is the most effective and fastest-acting bronchodilator. It should be administered at the first sign of an attack. Long-lasting beta$_2$ agonist drugs like salmeterol (Serevent) and corticosteroids do not act quickly and are not given for an immediate response, but they may provide a delayed response. In cases of a severe asthma attack, use of subcutaneous injections of epinephrine (0.3 to 0.5 mL, 1:1000) or inhalation of epinephrine (Primatene Mist) is the most potent and fastest-acting method for relieving an asthma attack. Supportive treatment includes providing positive-flow oxygenation, repeating bronchodilator doses as necessary, monitoring vital signs (including oxygen saturation, if possible), and activating the emergency medical system, if needed.

Treatment Planning Modifications

No specific treatment planning modifications are required of the patient with asthma.

Oral Complications and Manifestations

Nasal symptoms, allergic rhinitis, and mouth breathing are common with extrinsic asthma. Mouth breathers with asthma may have altered nasorespiratory function that can cause increased upper anterior and total anterior facial height, higher palatal vaults, greater overjets, and a higher prevalence of crossbites.[47]

The medications taken by patients who have asthma may contribute to oral disease. For example, beta$_2$ agonist inhalers decrease salivary flow by 20% to 35%, decrease plaque pH,[48] and are associated with increased prevalence of gingivitis and caries in patients with moderate to severe asthma.[49-51] Gastroesophageal acid reflux is common in patients with asthma and is exacerbated by the use of beta agonists and theophylline.[24] This reflux can contribute to erosion of enamel. Oral candidiasis (acute pseudomembranous type) occurs in approximately 5% of patients who use inhalation steroids for long periods at high dose or frequency.[52] However, this event is rare if a "spacer" or aerosol-holding chamber is attached to the metered-dose inhaler and the mouth is rinsed with water after each use.[53] The condition readily responds to local antifungal therapy, such as nystatin or clotrimazole. Patients should receive instructions on the proper use of their inhaler and the need for oral rinsing. Headache is a frequent adverse effect of antileukotrienes and theophylline. The clinician should be aware of this adverse effect when diagnosing disease in patients with orofacial pain complaints.

REFERENCES

1. Rodarte J. Chronic bronchitis and emphysema. In Goldman L, Ausiello (eds). Cecil Textbook of Medicine, 22nd ed. St. Louis, Elsevier, 2004.
2. World Health Organization. Global initiative for chronic obstructive lung disease. Available at: http://www.goldcopd.com/main.html. Accessed April 7, 2007.
3. American Lung Association. Minority lung disease data—Chronic obstructive pulmonary disease, 2000. Available at: http://www.lungusa.org/pub/minority/copd.html. Accessed April 7, 2007.
4. Centers for Disease Control and Prevention. Mortality patterns—United States, 1989. MMWR 1992;41:121-125.
5. Centers for Disease Control and Prevention. Environmental hazards and health effects: Asthma data and surveillance, 2006. Available at: http://www.cdc.gov/asthma/asthmadata.html. Accessed April 7, 2007.
6. Mannino DM, Gagnon RC, Petty TL, Lydick E. Obstructive lung disease and low lung function in adults in the United States: Data from the National Health and Nutrition Examination Survey, 1988-1994. Arch Intern Med 2000;160:1683-1689.
7. US Department of Health and Human Services. Chronic Obstructive Lung Disease: The Health Consequences of Smoking. A Report of the Surgeon General. USDHHS, Public Health Service, 1984. Publication no. 84-50205.
8. American Lung Association. Chronic obstructive pulmonary disease fact sheet, 2005. Available at: http://www.lungusa.org/site/pp.asp?c=dvLUK9O0E&b=35020. Accessed April 7, 2007.
9. American Thoracic Society. Standards for the diagnosis and care of patients with chronic obstructive pulmonary disease. Am J Respir Crit Care Med 1995;152:S77-S121.
10. Ferguson G. Recommendations for the management of COPD. Chest 2000;117:23S-28S.
11. Abramson MJ, Crockett AJ, Prith PJ, McDonald CF. COPDX: An update of guidelines for the management of chronic obstructive pulmonary disease with a review of recent evidence. Med J Aust 2006;184:342-345.
12. Barnes PJ. Theophylline in chronic obstructive pulmonary disease: New horizons. Proc Am Thorac Soc 2005;2:334-339.
13. Barnes P. Molecular mechanisms of antiasthma therapy. Ann Med 1995;27:531-535.
14. Bellamy D. Progress in the management of COPD. Practitioner 2000;244:24,27-28,30.
15. Crews K, Gordy FM, Penton-Eklund N, et al. Tobacco cessation: A practical dental service. Gen Dent 1999;47:476-483.
16. Vichitvejpaisal H, Joshi GP, Liu J, et al. Effect of severity of pulmonary disease on nitrous oxide washin and washout characteristics. J Med Assoc Thai 1997;80:378-383.
17. Masoli M, Fabian D, Holt S, et al. The global burden of asthma: Executive summary of the GINA Dissemination Committee report. Allergy 2004;59:469-478.
18. Centers for Disease Control and Prevention. Asthma: Basic facts, 2006. Available at: http://www.cdc.gov/asthma/faqs.htm. Accessed April 7, 2007.
19. Centers for Disease Control and Prevention. Surveillance for asthma—United States, 1960-1995. MMWR 1998;47:1-28.
20. Heraghty JL, Henderson AJ. Highlights in asthma 2005. Arch Dis Child 2006;91:422-425.
21. McDaniel M, Paxson C, Waldfogel J. Racial disparities in childhood asthma in the United States: Evidence from the National Health Interview Survey, 1997 to 2003. Pediatrics 2006;117:868-877.
22. McFadden EJ. Asthma. In Kasper DL, et al (eds). Harrison's Principles of Internal Medicine, 16th ed. New York, McGraw-Hill, 2005.
23. Ford-Hutchinson A, Evans J. Leukotriene B$_4$: Biologic properties and regulation of biosynthesis. In Piper P (ed). The Leukotrienes: Their Biological Significance. New York, Raven Press, 1986.
24. Rumbak M, Self T. A diagnostic approach to 'difficult' asthma. Postgrad Med 1992;92:80-90.
25. Mathison D, Stevenson D, Simon R. Precipitating factors in asthma: Aspirin, sulfites, and other drugs and chemicals. Chest 1985;87(suppl 1):50S-54S.

26. Babu K, Salvi S. Aspirin and asthma. Chest 2000;118: 1470-1476.
27. US Department of Health and Human Services. Warning on prescription drugs containing sulfites. FDA Drug Bull 1987;17:2-3.
28. Stevenson D, Simon R. Sulfites and asthma. J Allergy Clin Immunol 1984;74:469-472.
29. National Asthma Education and Prevention Program (National Heart, Lung, and Blood Institute). Second Expert Panel on the Management of Asthma. Expert Panel Report 2: Guidelines for the Diagnosis and Management of Asthma. Bethesda, Md, National Institutes of Health, 1987. Publication no. 97-4051. Available at: http://www.nhlbi.nih.gov/guidelines/asthma/
30. Barrios RJ, Kheradmand F, Batts L, Corry DB. Asthma: Pathology and pathophysiology. Arch Pathol Lab Med 2006;130:447-451.
31. Braman SS. The global burden of asthma. Chest 2006;130(1 suppl):4S-12S.
32. Malamed SF. Medical Emergencies in the Dental Office, 5th ed. St. Louis, Mosby, 2000.
33. Centers for Disease Control and Prevention. Asthma—United States, 1982-1992. MMWR 1995;43:952-953.
34. Lalloo U, Bateman ED, Feldman C, et al. Guideline for the management of chronic asthma in adults—2000 update. S Afr Med J 2000;90:540-541,544-552.
35. National Heart, Lung, and Blood Institute, National Asthma Education and Prevention Program. Guidelines for the diagnosis and management of asthma—Update on selected topics, 2002. J Allergy Clin Immunol 2002;110:S141-S209.
36. Kleerup E, Tashkin D. Outpatient treatment of adult asthma. West J Med 1995;163:49-63.
37. O'Byrne P, Israel E, Drazen J. Antileukotrienes in the treatment of asthma. Ann Intern Med 1997;127:472-480.
38. Ernst P, Spitzer WO, Suissa S, et al. Risk of fatal and near-fatal asthma in relation to inhaled corticosteroid use. JAMA 1992;269:3462-3464.
39. Rees J. Asthma control in adults. BMJ 2006;332:767-771.
40. Milgrom H, Fick RB Jr, Su JQ, et al. Treatment of allergic asthma with monoclonal anti-IgE antibody. N Engl J Med 1999;341:1966-1973.
41. Bergeron C, Boulet LP. Structural changes in airway diseases: Characteristics, mechanisms, consequences, and pharmacologic modulation. Chest 2006;129:1068-1087.
42. Suissa S, Ernst P. Albuterol in mild asthma. N Engl J Med 1997;336:729.
43. Ulrik C, Frederiksen J. Mortality and markers of risk of asthma death among 1,075 outpatients with asthma. Chest 1995;108:10-15.
44. Mathew T, Casamassimo PS, Wilson S, et al. Effect of dental treatment on the lung function of children with asthma. J Am Dent Assoc 1998;129:1120-1128.
45. Schwartz H, Gilbert IA, Lenner KA, et al. Metabisulfite sensitivity and local dental anesthesia. Ann Allergy 1989;62:83-86.
46. Elnabtity MN, Singh RF, Ansong MA, Craig TJ. Leukotriene modifiers in the management of asthma. J Am Osteopath Assoc 1999;7:S1-S6.
47. Bresolin D, Shapiro PA, Shapiro GG, et al. Mouth breathing in allergic children: Its relationship to dentofacial development. Am J Orthod 1983;83:334-340.
48. Kargul B, Tanboga I, Ergeneli S, et al. Inhaler medicament effects on saliva and plaque pH in asthmatic children. J Clin Pediatr Dent 1998;22:137-140.
49. Ryberg M, Moller C, Ericson T. Effect of beta 2-adrenoceptor agonists on saliva proteins and dental caries in asthmatic children. J Dent Res 1987;66:1404-1406.
50. Ryberg M, Moller C, Ericson T. Saliva composition and caries development in asthmatic patients treated with beta 2-adrenoceptor agonists: A 4-year follow-up study. Scand J Dent Res 1991;99:212-218.
51. Reddy DK, Hegde AM, Munshi AK. Dental caries status of children with bronchial asthma. J Clin Pediatr Dent 2003;27:293-295.
52. Barnes P. Efficacy and safety of inhaled corticosteroids: New developments. Am J Respir Crit Care Med 1998;157(suppl):S1-S53.
53. Drugs for ambulatory asthma. Med Lett Drugs Ther 1991;33:9-12.

Smoking and Tobacco Use Cessation

CHAPTER

8

The use of tobacco by smoking (cigarettes, cigars, pipes) or by the use of smokeless products (chewing tobacco, snuff) is an addictive disease that continues to be a major public health problem. Smoking is the leading cause of preventable death and disease in the United States. Smoking causes about 440,000 deaths per year, and more than 8.6 million persons are disabled because of smoking-related diseases.[1,2] Smoking causes more than twice as many deaths as human immunodeficiency virus and acquired immunodeficiency syndrome (AIDS), alcohol abuse, motor vehicle crashes, illicit drug use, and suicide combined.[3] On average, smokers die 10 years earlier than nonsmokers.[4]

The objectives of this chapter are to help the reader to do the following:
- Understand the physical and psychological effects of smoking and tobacco usage;
- Understand the basic principles involved in a smoking cessation program;
- Be familiar with approaches used for smoking cessation and the success rates of each;
- Be familiar with available nicotine replacement products and describe how they are used;
- Be familiar with drugs used in smoking cessation programs and explain how they are used;
- Be able to provide assistance to a patient who wishes to stop smoking.

SYSTEMIC AND ORAL EFFECTS OF SMOKING

Cigarette smoking is a major risk factor for stroke, myocardial infarction, peripheral vascular disease, aortic aneurysm, and sudden death. It is the leading cause of lung disease, including chronic bronchitis, emphysema, pneumonia, and lung cancer. It is also strongly linked to cancers of the esophagus, stomach, pancreas, cervix,

kidney, colon, and bladder. Other effects include premature skin aging and an increased risk for cataracts. Cigar and pipe smokers are subject to similar addictive and general health risks as are cigarette smokers, although pipe and cigar users typically do not inhale. Oral effects of smoking include squamous cell carcinoma (Figure 8-1), leukoplakia (Figure 8-2), nicotine stomatitis (Figure 8-3), smoker's melanosis, hairy tongue (Figure 8-4), and halitosis. It increases the risk of failure of intraosseous implants and the risk of dry socket, and it impairs wound healing. Smokers also have an impaired sense of taste and smell.

The adverse effects of smokeless tobacco primarily consist of addiction and its effects on the oral mucosa, including squamous cell carcinoma, tobacco or snuff dipper's pouch (Figure 8-5), verrucous carcinoma (Figure 8-6), gingival recession (Figure 8-7), periodontitis, and necrotizing ulcerative gingivitis (Figure 8-8). The sense of taste and smell is diminished as well. Evidence suggests that smokeless tobacco use may be associated with adverse pregnancy outcomes and pancreatic cancer.[5,6]

Health care professionals must be vigilant in identifying those patients who use tobacco with goals of encouraging them to stop smoking and assisting them in their efforts. Studies indicate that 70% of smokers want to quit smoking.[7] However, for every smoker who successfully quits, many more do not succeed. Tobacco dependence is a chronic condition that often requires repeated attempts at intervention. On average, smokers fail about eight attempts to quit before they achieve success.[8]

SCOPE OF THE PROBLEM

It is estimated that approximately 20.9% (44.5 million) of adults in the United States are current smokers, and that of these, 81.7% (36.1 million) smoke every day.[9] The overall prevalence of smokers is lower than the 21.6% prevalence reported in 2003 and is significantly lower

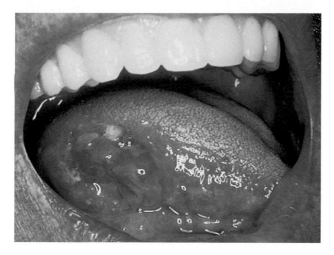

Figure 8-1. Squamous cell carcinoma of the tongue in a heavy cigarette smoker.

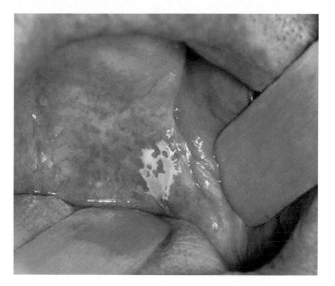

Figure 8-2. Leukoplakia of the palate in a cigarette smoker.

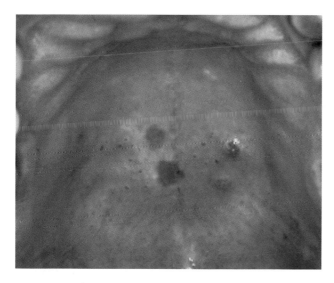

Figure 8-3. Severe nicotine stomatitis in a pipe smoker.

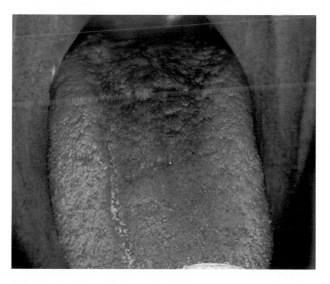

Figure 8-4. Brown hairy tongue in a cigarette smoker.

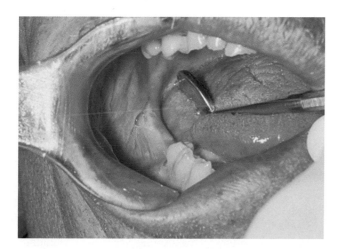

Figure 8-5. Tobacco pouch in the vestibule of a tobacco chewer.

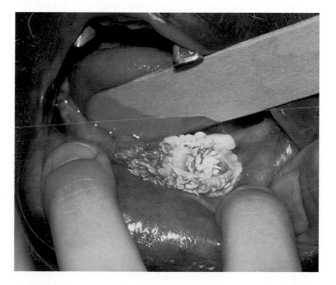

Figure 8-6. Verrucous carcinoma in a snuff user. (Fingers seen in the photo are those of the patient.)

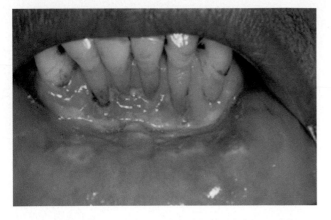

Figure 8-7. Gingival recession and leukoplakia in the area where snuff is held.

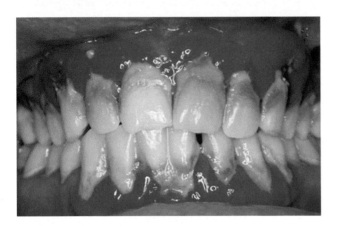

Figure 8-8. Necrotizing ulcerative gingivitis in a cigarette smoker.

TABLE 8-1 Annual Costs of Smoking			
	$3/pack	$4/pack	$5/pack
1 pack/day	$1095	$1460	$1825
2 packs/day	$2190	$2920	$3350
3 packs/day	$3285	$4380	$5475

than the 22.5% prevalence reported in 2002.[10] From 1993 through 2004, the percentage of daily smokers who smoked >25 cigarettes per day (CPD) (i.e., heavy smokers) decreased steadily, from 19.1% to 12.1%. The mean number of CPD among daily smokers was 19.6 in 1993 and 16.8 in 2004. Although this trend is encouraging, the problem continues to be a serious public health issue.

The prevalence of current cigarette smoking varies substantially across population subgroups.[9] Current smoking rates are higher among men (23.4%) than women (18.5%). Among racial/ethnic populations, Asian Americans (11.3%) and Hispanics (15%) have the lowest prevalence of current smoking; Native Americans/Native Alaskans (33.4%) have the highest prevalence, followed by non-Hispanic whites (22.2%) and non-Hispanic blacks (20.2%). By education level, current smoking is most prevalent among adults who have earned a graduate educational development (GED) diploma (39.6%) and among those with a 9th to 11th grade education (34.0%). Smoking prevalence generally decreases with increasing years of education. Persons aged >65 years have the lowest prevalence of current cigarette smoking (8.8%) among all adults. Current smoking prevalence is higher among adults who live below the poverty level (29.1%)

than among those at or above the poverty level (20.6%). Smoking prevalence also varies significantly by state/area, ranging from 10.5% to 27.6%.[11] Current smoking prevalence is highest in Kentucky (27.6%), West Virginia (26.9%), Oklahoma (26.1%), and Tennessee (26.1%). Prevalence is lowest in Utah (10.5%), California (14.8%), and Idaho (17.5%).

The use of smokeless tobacco is primarily seen in men and adolescent boys who are rural residents of southern and western states, whites, Native Americans/Native Alaskans, and persons with lower levels of education.[12] The use of smokeless tobacco became a national public health issue in the early to mid-1980s, when tobacco companies aggressively marketed their products by targeting young people. This practice was halted as a result of Congressional legislation and has since resulted in a gradual decline in prevalence from 6.1% in 1987 to 4.5% in 2000. Of interest is the recommendation by some health care professionals that smokeless tobacco should be promoted to cigarette smokers as a safer alternative for those who are having difficulty quitting smoking (harm reduction).[13,14] This controversial issue will require further research and discussion.

The economics of smoking is staggering. On a national level, the US Public Health Service estimates a total annual cost of $50 billion for the treatment of patients with smoking-related disease, in addition to $47 billion in lost wages and productivity. For the individual smoker, the economic impact of smoking can be substantial, especially given that many smokers have limited financial resources. The cost of a pack of cigarettes varies primarily as a function of excise taxes levied by states, counties, and cities. State-imposed cigarette tax ranges from a high of $2.46/pack (Rhode Island) to a low of $0.07/pack (South Carolina); the national median is $0.80/pack. Additional county and city taxes may add as much as $1.50 more (New York City). States may have additional miscellaneous administrative fees. When all taxes and fees are taken into consideration, the average cost of a pack of cigarettes in the United States is higher than $4.00. Table 8-1 presents calculations of the average annual costs incurred by cigarette smokers, depending on how many packs are smoked per day. In comparison, the average daily costs for smoking cessation products are estimated to be $3.91 for the patch, $5.81 for the gum, $4.98 for the lozenges, and $4.30 for sustained-release bupropion.[15] These costs may vary, depending on the strengths used, and products will be used only for a limited period of time (several weeks or months). These cost comparisons should be kept in mind when patients express concern about the cost of purchasing nicotine replacement products or medications.

BENEFITS OF QUITTING

People who quit smoking live longer than those who continue to smoke because of the risk of dying of smoking-related diseases.[16] The extent to which a smoker's risk is reduced by quitting is dependent on several factors, including number of years as a smoker, number of cigarettes smoked per day, and presence or absence of disease at the time of quitting. Data show that persons who quit smoking before the age of 50 have half the risk of dying in the next 15 years compared with those who continue smoking. Risks of dying of lung cancer are 22 times higher among male smokers and 12 times higher among female smokers than in those who have never smoked. Smokers have twice the risk of dying of coronary heart disease compared with lifetime nonsmokers. Compared with lifetime nonsmokers, smokers have about twice the risk of dying from a stroke. Smoking increases the risk of chronic obstructive pulmonary disease by accelerating the age-related decline in lung function. Box 8-1 lists some short-term and long-term benefits of smoking cessation.

ADDICTION TO NICOTINE

Smoking is a learned or conditioned behavior that is reinforced by nicotine.[17] Cigarettes promote this conditioning in that they allow precise dosing that can be repeated as often as necessary to avoid discomfort and produce maximal desired effects. In addition, smoking behavior is reinforced by and associated with common daily events such as awakening, eating, and socializing. Thus, these associations become almost unavoidable parts of smokers' lives.

Nicotine is a highly addictive drug that has been equated with heroin, cocaine, and amphetamine in terms of addiction potential and its effects on brain neurochemistry.[18] The addictive and behavioral effects of nicotine are complex and are due primarily to its effects on dopaminergic pathways. The physiologic and behavioral effects of nicotine include increased heart rate, increased cardiac output, increased blood pressure, appetite suppression, a strong sense of pleasure and well-being, improved task performance, and reduced anxiety.[15] Tolerance develops with repeated exposure, so that over time, it takes more and more nicotine to produce the same level of effect.

Nicotine is absorbed through the skin and the mucosal lining of the nose and mouth and by inhalation into the lungs. A cigarette is a very efficient delivery system for the inhalation of nicotine. Nicotine is rapidly distributed throughout the body after inhalation, reaching the brain in as little as 10 seconds. Mucosal absorption from smoke-less tobacco is slower, but the effects are more sustained. Nicotine that is swallowed is not absorbed in the stomach because of the acidic environment. The effects of nicotine gradually diminish over 30 to 120 minutes; this produces withdrawal effects that may include agitation, restlessness, anxiety, difficulty concentrating, insomnia, hunger, and a craving for cigarettes. The elimination half-life of nicotine is about 2 hours, which allows it to accumulate with repeated exposure to cigarettes throughout the day, with effects persisting for hours.[17] A typical smoker will take 10 puffs of every cigarette over a period of about 5 minutes that the cigarette is lit. Each cigarette delivers

---

BOX 8-1

Benefits of Quitting Smoking (US Surgeon General)

- 20 minutes after quitting: Your heart rate drops. (US Surgeon General's Report, 1988, pp 39, 202)
- 12 hours after quitting: Carbon monoxide level in your blood drops to normal. (US Surgeon General's Report, 1988, p 202)
- 2 weeks to 3 months after quitting: Your circulation improves and your lung function increases. (US Surgeon General's Report, 1990, pp 193, 194, 196, 285, 323)
- 1 to 9 months after quitting: Coughing and shortness of breath decrease; cilia (tiny hairlike structures that move mucus out of the lungs) regain normal function in the lungs, increasing the ability to handle mucus, clean the lungs, and reduce the risk of infection. (US Surgeon General's Report, 1990, pp 285-287, 304)
- 1 year after quitting: The excess risk of coronary heart disease is half that of a smoker's. (US Surgeon General's Report, 1990, p vi)
- 5 years after quitting: Your stroke risk is reduced to that of a nonsmoker 5 to 15 years after quitting. (US Surgeon General's Report, 1990, p vi)
- 10 years after quitting: The lung cancer death rate is about half that of a continuing smoker. Risks of cancer of the mouth, throat, esophagus, bladder, cervix, and pancreas decrease. (US Surgeon General's Report, 1990, pp vi, 131, 148, 152, 155, 164, 166)
- 15 years after quitting: The risk of coronary heart disease is that of a nonsmoker. (US Surgeon General's Report, 1990, p vi)

Quitting helps to stop the damaging effects of tobacco on your appearance, including the following:
- Premature wrinkling of the skin
- Bad breath
- Stained teeth
- Gum disease
- Bad smelling clothes and hair
- Yellow fingernails
- Food tastes better
- Sense of smell returns to normal
- Ordinary activities no longer leave you out of breath (climbing stairs, light housework, etc.)

about 1 mg of nicotine. Thus, a person who smokes about 1½ packs (30 cigarettes) a day gets 300 hits of nicotine to the brain every day, each one within 10 seconds after a puff.[19] This repeated reinforcement is a strong contributor to the highly addictive nature of nicotine.

INTERVENTIONS FOR SMOKING CESSATION

Numerous ways have been devised to encourage and assist cessation of smoking and tobacco use. Public health measures include raising awareness of the dangers of smoking and tobacco use by airing public service television or radio ads, increasing the price of cigarettes and other tobacco products, and banning smoking in public places. Individual methods of smoking cessation include the use of telephone quit lines and nicotine replacement therapy (NRT), along with individual or group counseling. Overall success rates for smoking cessation efforts are generally low, and quitting is associated with high rates of relapse. The 1-year success rate for stopping "cold turkey" is about 5%. The use of telephone quit lines or brief counseling roughly doubles one's chance of success, as does the use of any of the NRT products.[20] The 1-year success rate with bupropion is about 23%.[21] NRT combined with bupropion improves the success rate to about 36%.[22] One study[23] reported a success rate of 38.5% when a combination of NRT plus bupropion was used, along with intensive counseling. It is interesting to note that one study reported that a program that used only intensive counseling reported a success rate of 68%.[24] In general, the chance for success increases when more than one option is used.

On an individual basis, health care providers should ask their patients about smoking or tobacco use, advise current users to quit, and assist those who express an interest in quitting. In 2000, the US Department of Health and Human Services, Public Health Service, published Clinical Practice Guidelines for Treating Tobacco Use and Dependence, to aid health care professionals in helping their patients to quit smoking.[8] These guidelines are based on the 5 As, which include *asking* patients about their tobacco use, *advising* those who use tobacco to quit, *assessing* the willingness of patients to make a quit attempt, *assisting* in the quit attempt, and *arranging* for follow-up. The effectiveness of the 5 As initiative has been disappointing. Very few dentists or physicians are even aware of the 5 As, much less follow them.[25,26] Reasons most often cited by dentists for not incorporating smoking cessation services into their practices include time involved, lack of training, lack of reimbursement, lack of knowledge of available referral sources, and lack of patient education materials. In view of the poor outcomes of the 5 As, a suggested alternative approach is to ask, advise, and then refer (to an internal resource, an external resource, or a telephone quit line).[15] This approach requires the practitioner to be familiar with available referral sources.

INITIATING SMOKING CESSATION THERAPY

It should be made clear to patients that the dental office is a nonsmoking facility. Signs should be posted that clearly state this. No ash trays should be placed in the office. Dental health professionals should ask every patient about their use of tobacco. This can be easily accomplished by inclusion of tobacco use questions on the medical or dental history, followed by a brief interview. For patients who are current tobacco users, additional questions, including the type of tobacco product used, the frequency of use, and the length of time the product has been used, should be asked. Pipe and cigar users should be asked whether they inhale. During the oral mucosal examination, mucosal changes associated with tobacco use should be noted. Patients who use smokeless tobacco should be asked where they hold the tobacco in their mouth, and special attention should be paid to examination of that area. Any oral changes or systemic diseases that are present that may be related to tobacco use can be discussed and used as motivation to quit smoking. Patients should then be asked whether they have ever considered quitting, and whether they would like to quit. They should be made aware that you support and encourage their quitting and will assist them in their efforts in any way that you can.

If a patient does not wish to quit, the subject should be dropped and the patient not badgered. It is generally counterproductive to pursue the issue; however, patients can be told that, if at any time, they would like to quit, you would be happy to speak with them about it. They can then be asked at subsequent recall appointments whether they have changed their mind about quitting. If a patient indicates that he or she does wish to quit, the practitioner can do the following:

- Help to coordinate a program for the patient, or designate another individual in the office to perform that function
- Prescribe smoking cessation medications for the patient
- Refer the patient to an outside program
- Refer the patient to a counseling source, such as a telephone help line

Depending on how involved the practitioner wishes to become, the following sections describe many options and resources that are available to assist patients in the effort to quit smoking.

Patient Education Literature

It is recommended that practitioners have patient education and motivational materials available for patients to read, to encourage and support tobacco use cessation. Posters can be placed on the walls of the waiting room and treatment areas. Brochures may be kept in the waiting room and in treatment areas to be given to patients who express a desire to quit. Patient education materials are readily available from sources such as the American

BOX 8-2

Resources for Support Material

TELEPHONE HELP/QUIT LINES
- 1-800-QUITNOW (US Department of Health and Human Services national quit line)
- 1-877-44-U-QUIT (National Cancer Institute dedicated quit smoking line)
- 1-877-YES-QUIT (American Cancer Society quit line)
- 1-800-4-CANCER (Cancer Information Service of the National Cancer Institute)

HELPFUL WEB SITES
- www.surgeongeneral.gov/tobacco/
- www.smokefree.gov/
- www.nlm.nih.gov/medlineplus/smokingcessation. html
- www.cancer.gov/cancertopics/pdq/prevention/control-of-tobacco-use/HealthProfessional
- www.cdc.gov/tobacco/
- www.cancer.org/docroot/PED/content/PED_10_13X_Guide_for_Quitting_Smoking.asp

Cancer Society, the National Cancer Institute, and the US Surgeon General; these can be ordered by phone or through their Web sites (Box 8-2). Brochures or handouts may be used to provide telephone quit line numbers or for referral to local smoking cessation programs or support groups. Practitioners also may wish to develop their own patient education materials.

Counseling

Even brief counseling, as occurs when a health care professional routinely asks about smoking and encourages quitting, has been shown to increase quit success rates. Telephone counseling help lines have become widely available and have been shown to double success rates over those reported with quitting "cold turkey." Help lines are available on a national, regional, and state level (see Box 8-2). Help lines can provide support for patients, regardless of whether they are considering quitting, attempting to quit, have successfully quit, or have relapsed. Group counseling can be especially effective by providing the social support and encouragement of the group. Counseling typically consists of both cognitive and behavioral therapies. Cognitive therapy attempts to change the way a patient thinks about smoking, while behavioral therapy attempts to help smokers avoid situations that might trigger the desire to smoke. Evidence has shown that the more intensive the counseling, the better the success rate, and that when counseling is combined with other forms of therapy, such as NRT or pharmacotherapy, it is even more effective. Local, regional, and state health departments may be good sources for smoking cessation counseling and other programs.

Nicotine Replacement Therapy

The rationale for NRT is to replace cigarettes or smokeless tobacco with a source of nicotine that does not have the tars and carbon monoxide of tobacco, and then to gradually reduce the use of that replacement product to the point of abstinence. To prevent withdrawal symptoms, a smoker must maintain a baseline blood level of nicotine of about 15 to 18 ng/mL. A cigarette rapidly increases nicotine blood levels to 35 to 40 ng/mL, producing the "hit" or "rush" that a smoker experiences when smoking; this level then gradually returns to baseline within about 25 to 30 minutes. NRT attempts to provide a blood level that is adequate to prevent withdrawal symptoms without producing the "hit" or "rush" caused by the cigarette. The patient then gradually learns to accept progressively lower and lower blood nicotine levels, and then total abstinence.[19] Five distinct nicotine replacement products are available that differ in cost, route of delivery, and efficiency of delivery of nicotine. These include the transdermal patch, gum, lozenges, the inhaler, and nasal spray (Table 8-2).

All of the NRT products are first-line pharmacotherapeutic agents and have been approved by the US Food and Drug Administration (FDA) for smoking cessation. They all appear to be effective when included as part of a program of smoking cessation, and they generally double the chances of success.[20] Selection of an NRT product is dependent on the number of cigarettes smoked per day, its potential adverse effects, and patient preference. Generally, the more dependent the patient is on nicotine, the higher the beginning doses that will be required, and the greater will be the need to titrate nicotine levels. For very dependent smokers, the combination of a patch with a shorter-acting method such as gum, lozenge, or nasal spray may be indicated. The combination of an NRT with counseling often improves chances for success.

Non-NRT Pharmacotherapy

Another first-line, FDA-approved, non-NRT pharmacotherapeutic cessation agent is bupropion SR, an atypical antidepressant that is thought to affect the dopaminergic and/or noradrenergic pathways involved in nicotine addiction. Bupropion is effective when used alone or in combination with an NRT product and/or counseling. An attractive feature of bupropion is that it may prevent weight gain, which is a common adverse effect of smoking cessation. It is contraindicated in patients with seizure disorders or in those who might be prone to seizures. In addition to bupropion, two second-line agents that have not been approved by the FDA but have been shown to be effective for smoking cessation are nortriptyline and clonidine.[8] Nortriptyline is a tricyclic antidepressant, and clonidine is an $alpha_2$ agonist that is used to treat hypertension. Recently, the FDA approved varenicline, a novel pharmacotherapeutic agent, for smoking cessation. This medication is an $alpha_4beta_2$ nicotinic receptor partial agonist that stimulates dopamine and blocks nicotinic receptors, thus preventing the reward and reinforcement associated with smoking[27] (Table 8-3).

TABLE **8-2**
Nicotine Replacement Products

Product	How Supplied	How Used	Adverse Effects	Advantages/ Disadvantages
NICOTINE TRANSDERMAL PATCHES (OTC)				
Nicoderm CQ, Nicorette, Nicotrol, generic	Nicoderm CQ: 7, 14, 21 mg Nicorette: 5, 10, 15 mg Nicotrol: 5, 10, 15 mg	Start with patches of highest concentration, then use patches of progressively lower concentration over a 6- to 12-week period	Skin irritation, insomnia	Slow onset; takes 6 to 8 hours to reach peak blood level; cannot be readily titrated
NICOTINE GUM (OTC)				
Nicorette, generic	Available in strengths of 2 mg and 4 mg	Not to be chewed as normal gum; should be chewed slightly and then "parked" in the vestibule; repeat chew-park sequence every 30 minutes; nicotine is absorbed through the mucosa; do not eat or drink for 15 minutes before using or while using; start with 8 to 24 pieces/day and gradually reduce over several weeks; maximum, 24/day	Mucosal irritation; indigestion	Quicker delivery than patch but not as quick as lozenge; produces less of a "rush" than is produced by cigarettes or lozenges
NICOTINE LOZENGES (OTC)				
Commit	Available in strengths of 2 mg and 4 mg	Strength required is determined by time to first cigarette in the morning; lozenge "parked" and moistened and allowed to dissolve in the mouth; start with 9 to 20/day and use progressively fewer per day over a 12-week period; do not eat or drink for 15 minutes before using or while using; maximum, 20/day	Gingival and throat irritation; indigestion	Peak blood levels in 20 to 30 minutes; 25% higher blood levels than gum; can be titrated as needed; very efficient; produces less of a rush than is caused by cigarettes but more of a rush than is produced by gum
NICOTINE NASAL SPRAY (PRESCRIPTION)				
Nicotrol NS	Supplied in a pump nasal spray bottle	One dose is a spray into each nostril; maximum of 40 doses per day is progressively decreased over 10 to 12 weeks	Nose and throat irritation	Fastest delivery system; provides the rush of cigarettes
NICOTINE INHALER (PRESCRIPTION)				
Nicotrol Inhaler	Supplied as plastic cartridges; each cartridge provides 4 mg of nicotine (only 2 mg is absorbed)	Each inhaler contains 400 puffs; 80 puffs is equal to 1 cigarette; maximum, 16 cartridges/day; gradually decreased usage over several months	Mouth and throat irritation	Inefficient delivery system; expensive

TABLE **8-3**
Non-NRT Pharmacotherapeutic Agents

Drug	Dosage	Adverse Effects	Precautions/Advantages
Bupropion SR (Zyban)	150 mg daily for 3 days, then 150 mg twice a day for 2 to 3 months; begin 1 to 2 weeks prior to quit date and continue for at least 2 to 3 months	Dry mouth, insomnia	Contraindicated in patients with history of seizures or at risk for seizures; may prevent weight gain
Nortriptyline (Pamelor)	25 to 100 mg/day at bedtime starting 2 to 3 weeks prior to quit date	Dry mouth, sedation	Risk of arrhythmias
Clonidine (Catapres; Catapres TTS)	0.10 to 0.30 mg/day in divided doses or as patch	Dry mouth, sedation, dizziness; skin irritation with patch	Rebound hypertension may occur if drug is discontinued abruptly
Varenicline (Chantix)	Starting 1 week prior to quit date, 0.5 mg daily for 3 days, then 0.5 mg twice a day for 4 days, then 1.0 mg twice daily for 12 weeks	Nausea, insomnia, flatulence, headache	No clinically relevant drug interactions have been identified; may cause taste disturbance

NRT, Nicotine replacement therapy.

Additional treatment strategies with less proven efficacy include monoamine oxidase inhibitors, selective serotonin reuptake inhibitors, opioid receptor antagonists, bromocriptine, antianxiety drugs, nicotinic receptor antagonists, and glucose tablets. Various approaches under investigation include the use of partial nicotine agonists, anticonvulsants, inhibitors of the hepatic P-450 enzyme system, cannaboid-1 receptor antagonists, and nicotine vaccines.[28] Alternative or complementary approaches to smoking cessation have been advocated; however, because of the lack of evidence of effectiveness, their use cannot be supported at this time.[29]

Reimbursement for Smoking Cessation Therapy

One of the reasons often cited for not providing smoking cessation services is the lack of meaningful reimbursement for the time and effort required. This continues to be a problem in many states. Inconsistency has been noted in the coverage provided by managed care organizations and by state Medicaid and Medicare programs. The decision to bill for smoking cessation services depends on the amount of time spent and the degree of involvement of the practitioner. In many instances, assessment, advice, and referral may occur within the context of the normal patient health history and examination; thus, the time specifically devoted to smoking cessation counseling would likely be minimal, and the fee would be included as part of the normal examination fee. If more time is spent in actual counseling and monitoring of a patient's progress, billing for that service would certainly be appropriate. If it is decided to bill for a separate procedure, the International Classification of Diseases (ICD)-9 code 350.1 (Tobacco Use Disorder: Tobacco Dependence) should be used. The Code for Dental Terminology (CDT) D1320 (Tobacco Counseling for the Control and Prevention of Oral Disease) is specifically designated for use by dental practitioners. Practitioners should check with individual programs and carriers to determine whether these services are covered.

REFERENCES

1. Centers for Disease Control and Prevention. Cigarette smoking—attributable mortality—United States, 2000. MMWR 2003;52:842-844.
2. Schroeder S. Tobacco control in the wake of the 1998 Master Settlement Agreement. N Engl J Med 2004; 350:293-301.
3. Centers for Disease Control and Prevention. Comparative Causes of Annual Deaths in the United States. Atlanta, Ga, CDC, 2005.
4. Doll R, Peto R, Boreham J, Sutherland I. Mortality in relation to smoking: 50 years' observations on male British doctors. BMJ 2004;328:1519.
5. Alguacil J, Silverman D. Smokeless and other noncigarette use and pancreatic cancer: A case-control study based on direct interviews. Cancer Epidemiol Biomarkers Prev 2004;13:55-58.
6. England L, Levine R, Mills J, et al. Adverse pregnancy outcomes in snuff users. Am J Obstet Gynecol 2003; 189:939-943.
7. Centers for Disease Control and Prevention. Cigarette smoking among adults—United States, 2000. MMWR 2002;51:642-645.
8. Fiore M, Bailey W, Cohen S, et al. Treating Tobacco Use and Dependence: Clinical Practice Guideline. Bethesda, Md, US Department of Health and Human Services, 2000.
9. Centers for Disease Control and Prevention. Cigarette smoking among adults—United States, 2004. MMWR 2005;54:1121-1124.
10. Centers for Disease Control and Prevention. Cigarette smoking among adults—United States, 2003. MMWR 2005;54:509-513.

11. Centers for Disease Control and Prevention. State-specific prevalence of cigarette smoking and quitting among adults—United States, 2004. MMWR 2005;54:1124-1127.

12. Nelson D, Mowery P, Tomar S, et al. Trends in smokeless tobacco use among adults and adolescents in the United States. Am J Public Health 2006;96:897-905.

13. Kozlowski L. Harm reduction, public health, and human rights: Smokers have a right to be informed of significant harm reduction options. Nicotine Tobacco Res 2002;4(suppl 2):S55-S60.

14. Rodu B. An alternative approach to smoking control. Am J Med Sci 1994;308:32-34.

15. Schroeder SA. What to do with a patient who smokes. JAMA 2005;294:482-487.

16. US Department of Health and Human Services. The Health Benefits of Smoking Cessation: A Report of the Surgeon General. Bethesda, Md, Centers for Disease Control Center for Chronic Disease Prevention and Health Promotion, Office of Smoking and Health, 1990.

17. Dani JA, Harris RA. Nicotine addiction and comorbidity with alcohol abuse and mental illness. Nat Neurosci 2005;8:1465-1470.

18. Tobacco Advisory Group: Royal College of Physicians, Nicotine Addiction in Britain. London: RCP; 2000.

19. Cooper TM, Clayton RR. The Cooper/Clayton Method to Stop Smoking. Lexington, Ky, Institute for Comprehensive Behavioral Smoking Cessation, 2004.

20. Silagy C, Lancaster T, Stead L, et al. Nicotine replacement therapy for smoking cessation. Cochrane Database Syst Rev 2004(3):CD000146.

21. Hurt RD, Sachs DP, Glover ED, et al. A comparison of sustained-release bupropion and placebo for smoking cessation. N Engl J Med 1997;337:1195-1202.

22. Jorenby DE, Leischow SJ, Nides MA, et al. A controlled trial of sustained-release bupropion, a nicotine patch, or both for smoking cessation. N Engl J Med 1999;340:685-691.

23. Chatkin JM, Mariante de Abreu C, Haggstram FM, et al. Abstinence rates and predictors of outcome for smoking cessation: Do Brazilian smokers need special strategies? Addiction 2004;99:778-784.

24. Willemse B, Lesman-Leegte I, Timens W, et al. High cessation rates of cigarette smoking in subjects with and without COPD. Chest 2005;128:3685-3687.

25. Hu S, Pallonen U, McAlister AL, et al. Knowing how to help tobacco users: Dentists' familiarity and compliance with the clinical practice guideline. J Am Dent Assoc 2006;137:170-179.

26. Johnson NW, Lowe JC, Warnakulasuriya KA. Tobacco cessation activities of UK dentists in primary care: Signs of improvement. Br Dent J 2006;200:85-89.

27. Corelli RL, Hudmon KS. Pharmacologic interventions for smoking cessation. Crit Care Nurs Clin North Am 2006;18:39-51, xii.

28. Frishman WH, Mitta W, Kupersmith A, Ky T. Nicotine and non-nicotine smoking cessation pharmacotherapies. Cardiol Rev 2006;14:57-73.

29. Dean AJ. Natural and complementary therapies for substance use disorders. Curr Opin Psychiatry 2005;18:271-276.

Tuberculosis

CHAPTER

9

DEFINITION

Tuberculosis (TB) is a major global health problem that is caused by an infectious and communicable organism, *Mycobacterium tuberculosis*. The disease is spread by inhalation of infected droplets and usually demonstrates a prolonged quiescent period. *M. tuberculosis* replication leads to a host inflammatory and granulomatous response and classic pulmonary and systemic symptoms. Although *M. tuberculosis* is by far the most common causative agent in this human infection, other species of mycobacteria are occasionally encountered, such as *M. avium complex, M. kansasii, M. abscessus, M. xenopi, M. bovis, M. africanum, M. microti,* and *M. canetti*. These mycobacteria may cause systemic diseases (pulmonary lymphadenitis, cutaneous or disseminated) that are referred to as *mycobacteriosis*.

EPIDEMIOLOGY

Incidence and Prevalence

TB has a worldwide incidence of 8 to 10 million; the World Health Organization (WHO) estimates that one third of the world population is infected.[1] This disease kills more adults worldwide each year than does any other single pathogen.[2,3] In contrast, the occurrence of TB in the United States has steadily decreased during the past century and has dropped at a rate of 5% per year over the past 40 years. Peak prevalence in Western countries occurred around the beginning of the 19th century. By the turn of the 20th century, approximately 500 new cases of active TB per 100,000 population were identified annually in the United States. By the mid-1980s, reports to the Centers for Disease Control (CDC) indicated that the rate had decreased to 9.3 per 100,000 population.[4] This figure rose to 10.6, or 26,000 cases,[5,6] in 1993, primarily because of adverse social and economic factors, the acquired immunodeficiency syndrome (AIDS) epidemic, and the immigration of foreign-born persons who

had TB. In 2005, 14,093 cases of TB were reported—a rate of 4.8 per 100,000.[7] This was the lowest rate reported during the past century. Although the figures are encouraging, the disease continues to occur in almost every state of the United States and in 5% to 10% of the population (~15 to 30 million people). Moreover, 54% of new US cases occur in foreign-born persons who migrate or travel to the United States—a rate that has continually increased since 1993.[7]

Although the present rate for the United States as a whole is low, minority residents of inner city ghettos, the elderly, the urban poor, persons living in congregate settings (community dwellings, prisons, and shelters), and those with AIDS have occurrence rates that are several times the national average (Box 9-1). Higher risk for the disease (an 8% chance of developing TB per year) also has been noted in HIV-positive persons and in those who are immunosuppressed from use of medications.[8-12] TB is diagnosed most often in men (1.6 men:1 woman), in Hispanics, African Americans, and Asian Americans (rates 7.3, 8.3, and 19.6 times higher than those of whites, respectively), and in persons between 25 and 64 years of age.[7]

Factors important in reducing the spread of TB in the United States during the past century have included improved sanitation and hygiene measures and the use of effective antituberculous drugs. Unfortunately, failure to complete a course of therapy (which occurs in more than 20% of patients) and improper drug selection have contributed to the persistence of this disease and to the rise that has occurred in the percentage of cases of multidrug-resistant TB—from 0.5% in 1982 to about 1.2% in 2004.[7,13]

Etiology

In most cases of human TB, the causative agent is *M. tuberculosis*, an acid-fast, nonmotile, intracellular rod that is an obligate aerobe. Because *M. tuberculosis* is an aerobe,

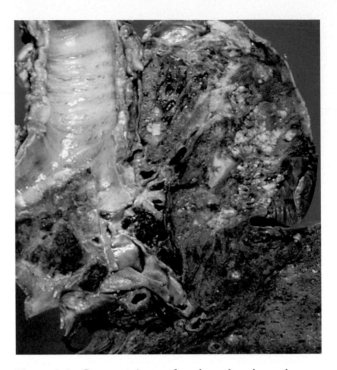

Figure 9-1. Gross specimen of a tuberculous lung, demonstrating caseating granulomas and cavitation. (Courtesy R. Powell, Lexington, Ky.)

it exists best in an atmosphere of high oxygen tension; therefore, it most commonly infects the lung.

M. tuberculosis is typically transmitted by way of infected airborne droplets of mucus or saliva that are forcefully expelled from the lungs, most commonly through coughing but also by sneezing and talking. The quantity and size of expelled droplets influence transmission. Smaller droplets evaporate readily, leaving bacteria and other solid material as floating particles that are easily inhaled. Larger droplets quickly settle to the ground. Transmission by way of fomites rarely occurs.[11,14] Transmission by ingestion (e.g., of contaminated milk) occurs but is rare because of the use of pasteurized milk. A secondary mode of transmission—by ingestion—may occur when a patient coughs up infected sputum, thereby inoculating oral tissues. Oral lesions of TB may be initiated through this mechanism.

The interval from infection to development of active TB is widely variable, ranging from a few weeks to decades. Most cases of TB result from reactivation of a tubercle; only 5% to 10% of cases result at the time of the initial infection. The number of organisms inhaled and the level of immunocompetency largely determine whether the disease is contracted.

Pathophysiology and Complications

TB can affect virtually any organ of the body, although the lung is the most common site of infection. The typical infection of primary pulmonary TB begins with inhalation of infected droplets. These droplets are carried into the alveoli, where bacteria are engulfed by macrophages. Replication occurs within alveolar macrophages, and spread of infection occurs locally to regional (hilar) lymph nodes. Distant dissemination through the bloodstream may occur if the infection is not controlled locally;

however, the vast majority of disseminated bacteria are destroyed by natural host defenses. At approximately 2 to 8 weeks after onset of infection, delayed hypersensitivity to the bacteria develops that is mediated by T (CD4+) helper lymphocytes. This condition manifests as conversion of the tuberculin skin test (purified protein derivative [PPD]) from negative to positive. Subsequently, a chronic granulomatous inflammatory reaction develops that involves activated epithelioid macrophages and formation of granulomas. These natural host defenses usually control and contain the primary pulmonary TB infection, resulting in latent tuberculosis infection. If not contained, the nidus of infection (granuloma) may become a productive tubercle with central necrosis and caseation. Cavitation may occur (Figure 9-1), resulting in the dumping of organisms into the airway for further dissemination into other lung tissue or the exhaled air.

Limitation and local containment of infection may be caused by a variety of factors, including host resistance, host immune capabilities, and virulence of the mycobacterium. Once the infection has been successfully interrupted, the lesion heals spontaneously, then undergoes inspissation, hardening, encapsulation, and calcification. Although the lesion "heals," some bacteria may remain dormant. If infection is not interrupted, dissemination of bacilli may occur through the lung parenchyma, resulting in extensive pulmonary lesions and lymphohematogenous spread. Widespread infection with multiple organ involvement is called *miliary tuberculosis*.

Primary pulmonary TB is seen most often in infants and children; however, cavitation is rare in these age groups. Most children produce no sputum; they usually swallow sputum even if some bacilli are present within the bronchi. Expression of the disease differs somewhat in teenagers and adults in that lymph node involvement and lymphohematogenous spread are not prominent features. However, cavitation commonly occurs. The usual form of disease found in adults is called *secondary* or *reinfection TB*. This occurs with delayed reactivation of persistent dormant viable bacilli and probably represents relapse of a previous infection. This form of the disease usually is confined to the lungs, and cavitation is common. Reasons for relapse include inadequate treatment of the primary infection and the influences of illness, immunosuppressive agents, immunosuppression (AIDS), and age.

Some of the more common sequelae of TB include progressive primary TB, cavitary disease, pleurisy and pleural effusion, meningitis, and disseminated or miliary TB. Isolated organ involvement other than that of the lung may occur and commonly affects the pericardium, peritoneum, kidneys, adrenal glands, and bone (known as Pott's disease when it affects the spine).[15,16] The tongue and other tissues of the oral cavity also are involved infrequently.

Approximately 5% to 10% of persons who develop TB die of the disease.[17] However, the death rate attributable to TB is much greater (54%) in young persons who have AIDS.[17] The advent of effective chemotherapy undoubtedly has been the most significant reason for the lower mortality rate seen in nonimmunosuppressed, TB-infected persons.

CLINICAL PRESENTATION

Signs and Symptoms

Primary infection with *M. tuberculosis* in about 90% of patients results in few manifestations other than a positive tuberculin skin test and radiographic findings. Progression of clinical disease is usually associated with underlying conditions (young and old ages) and diseases that depress the immune response. Once symptoms become apparent, they usually are nonspecific and could be associated with any infectious disease. They include cough, lassitude and malaise, anorexia, unexplained weight loss, night sweats, and fever. Temperature elevation commonly occurs in the evening or during the night and is accompanied by profuse sweating.

Specific local symptoms of the disease are dependent on the organ involved. Persistent cough is the symptom most commonly associated with pulmonary TB, although it may appear late in the course of the disease. Cough is common with cavitary disease. The sputum produced is characteristically scanty and mucoid, but it becomes purulent with progressive disease. Hemoptysis (blood in sputum) is infrequent, occurring in about 20%.[18] Dyspnea is a feature of advanced disease.

Manifestations of extrapulmonary disease occur in about 10% to 20% of cases, more often in human immunodeficiency virus (HIV)-infected persons, and may include localized lymphadenopathy with the development of sinus tracts, back pain over the affected spine, gastrointestinal disturbances (in intestinal TB), dysuria and hematuria (in renal involvement), heart failure, and neurologic deficits.[14] In contrast, in some patients, physical examination may be inconclusive.

Laboratory Findings

The tuberculin (Mantoux) skin test is the most useful and reliable method of determining whether a person has been infected with *M. tuberculosis*. However, the test is only about 95% sensitive and 95% specific. Its limitations are seen in the fact that patients who are initially exposed and are incubating the bacillus during the first 6 to 8 weeks may obtain negative skin test results. Also, 10% to 25% of people with active TB have false-negative skin test results.[19] A positive test result presumptively means that a person has been infected.[20,21] It does not mean that a person has clinically active TB. Some positive skin reactions indicate infection with other mycobacterial species. Physical examination and tests that identify *M. tuberculosis* are required for diagnosis.

Tuberculin is a standardized PPD (PPD-S) of culture extract from *M. tuberculosis*. Specifically, PPD-S is used as the international testing standard. This test is administered by intradermal injection of 0.1 mL of PPD that contains 5 tuberculin units into the volar or dorsal surface of the forearm. The test is read 48 to 72 hours later, and evidence of induration resulting from the delayed hypersensitivity response is noted. An area of induration measuring less than 5 mm is considered a negative result. An area of induration measuring greater than 5 mm is considered positive if the patient has had close contact with an infectious person or an abnormal chest radiograph consistent with TB, or if he or she is suspected or known to be HIV positive or immunosuppressed (Table 9-1). An area of induration that measures 10 mm or greater is considered positive if significant medical risk factors (i.e., diabetes, silicosis, severe kidney disease, cancer) are present, and if the patient is a foreigner or a recent immigrant (<5 years), medically underserved, an alcoholic, an injecting drug abuser, a resident of a congregate setting such as a nursing home, jail, or shelter, or a child (<4 years of age) or adolescent who has been exposed to adults in high-risk categories. Induration of at least 15 mm is considered positive for everyone.[6] A positive test necessitates a physical examination, a radiographic evaluation, and, if necessary, sputum culture to rule out active disease. Without treatment, approximately 5% of skin test converters develop TB within 2 years; another 5% develop it later.[22] Thus, individuals who are at risk for TB—including dentists—should undergo a tuberculin skin test annually.

Although radiographic findings of TB are not pathognomic, chest radiographs are helpful. Patchy or lobular infiltrates in the apical posterior segments of the upper lobes or in the middle or lower lobes, with cavitation and hilar adenopathy, are common findings in active

TABLE 9-1
Categories for Positive PPD Test Results

Induration ≥5 mm	Induration ≥10 mm	Induration ≥15 mm
HIV positive	Children <4 years of age	Persons with no risk factors for TB
Fibrotic changes on chest radiograph consistent with old TB	Injecting drug use	
Recent contacts with TB case	Persons with clinical conditions that place them at high risk*	
Organ transplant or immune suppression	Recent arrivals (<5 yr) from a high-prevalence country	
	Residents of high-risk congregate settings	

HIV, Human immunodeficiency virus; TB, tuberculosis.
*Silicosis, diabetes mellitus, severe kidney disease, leukemia, lymphoma, and head, neck, or lung cancer; weight loss of >10% of ideal body weight; gastrectomy, jejunoileal bypass.

"progressive primary" TB. Healed primary lesions leave a calcified peripheral nodule and a calcified hilar lymph node (Ghon complex).[21]

For preliminary diagnosis, microscopic examination of sputum smear for acid-fast bacilli is advocated because the process is inexpensive and can produce results within 24 hours. Definitive diagnosis of TB is based on culture or direct molecular tests (e.g., nucleic acid amplication) that identify *M. tuberculosis* or other species from body fluids and tissues, usually sputum. Three consecutive morning sputum specimens should be obtained for culturing to ensure positive results.[23] Traditional culture techniques take several weeks to grow mycobacteria on solid medium; however, the use of selective broth (BACTEC-460, Becton-Dickson, Sparks, Md) or similar systems reduces the time to about 1 week.[12,14] Cultures should be accompanied by antimicrobial susceptibility testing for all isolates of *M. tuberculosis* because of the rising incidence of drug resistance. Antibiotic sensitivity testing takes about 7 to 10 days. Molecular tests (nucleic acid amplification and probe kits) are advantageous because they provide results within 24 hours.[24] Some of the previously mentioned tests (skin testing, sputum smears, cultures, and chest films) are less reliable when the patient has HIV infection.

MEDICAL MANAGEMENT

The Advisory Council for the Elimination of Tuberculosis recommends[25] that treatment should begin as soon as TB is diagnosed, and that the case should be reported to the local health department. Within 1 week, an initial treatment plan should be developed that addresses the medical regimen, monitoring for clinical and bacteriologic response and toxicity, patient education, and assessment of the patient's social and behavioral needs and that may affect compliance and completion of therapy, including personal contacts at risk for the disease.

Effective chemotherapy for TB is dependent on (1) patient education and compliance, (2) appropriate selection of drugs, (3) multiple drug use, and (4) drug administration continued for a sufficient time. Selection of a treatment regimen is dictated by the health of the patient and the presence or likelihood of drug-resistant strains (initially based on community infectivity rates, subsequently based on laboratory tests). If a patient is determined to harbor fully susceptible organisms, and the community drug resistance rate is less than 4%, isoniazid, rifampin, and pyrazinamide are given for 8 weeks followed by isoniazid and rifampin (without pyrazinamide) for the next 4 months to complete 6 months of therapy.[26] A larger combination of drugs and increased duration of treatment are recommended when drug-resistant strains are present, the community drug resistance rate is greater than 4%, or the patient is infected with HIV (Box 9-2).[25]

Protection measures also have been introduced to control the spread of disease.[23] For example, hospitalized patients with potentially infectious TB may be placed in isolation rooms with negative pressure during treatment.[3,25,27] In addition, many regional health departments in the United States have implemented "directly observed therapy" to ensure that patients who have TB take the appropriate medicine and dose on schedule.

Following the initiation of chemotherapy, reversal of infectiousness is dependent on proper drug selection and patient compliance. Within 3 to 6 months, approximately 90% of patients become noninfectious, and their sputum cultures convert to negative.[25,28] Patients are allowed to return to normal public contact on the basis of reversal of infectiousness and provided they continue chemotherapy.

Sputum cultures should be tested for drug-resistant bacteria—the most threatening feature of the disease—which occur in approximately 1% of cases in the United States[7] and more than 10% of cases in parts of the Soviet Union and China.[1,13] Ninety percent of drug-resistance cases (defined by the WHO as resistant to the two strongest antituberculous drugs, isoniazid and rifampin) occur in HIV-infected persons.[29] Transmission of drug-

---

BOX 9-2

Common Drug Regimens for the Treatment of Tuberculosis[25,26]

Non–drug-resistant TB
- 3 drugs (isoniazid+rifampin+pyrazinamide) for 2 months
- Followed by 2 drugs (isoniazid and rifampin without pyrazinamide) for 4 months
- 6 months total treatment time

Drug resistance suspected or confirmed to one antituberculous drug, or diagnosis made in a region that has greater than 4% resistance to antituberculousis drug
- 4 drugs (isoniazid+rifampin+pyrazinamide+either ethambutol or streptomycin) for 2 months
- Determination of resistance again; if resistant only to isoniazid: rifampin+pyrazinamide+either ethambutol or streptomycin for 6 months *or* rifampin+ethambutol continued for 12 months
- Immunosuppressed patients to receive treatment for at least 9 months

Confirmed multiple-drug resistance
- 3 to 7 drugs (isoniazid+rifampin+pyrazinamide+ethambutol, an aminoglycoside, or capreomycin, ciprofloxacin, or ofloxacin+either cycloserine, ethionamide, or aminosalicylic acid) to which the organism is susceptible, and continued for 12 to 24 months after the culture becomes negative.
- Rifapentine is available for substitution with rifampin. Dosing is twice weekly.

---

resistant TB has occurred between patients, patients and health care workers, and patients and family members. Multidrug-resistant TB is more common in foreign-born persons,[30] and the outcome is serious. Mortality rates range from 70% to 90%, and the period to death has been 4 to 16 weeks from the time of diagnosis.

The patient who has had a negative skin test result that on retesting has converted to positive is considered infected with *M. tuberculosis*. Once physical examination, radiographs, and sputum culturing have established that the disease is not active (i.e., latent tuberculosis), the patient may be given a course of chemoprophylaxis to prevent the development of clinical disease. Not all patients with positive skin tests are placed on chemoprophylaxis. Those most likely to receive chemoprophylaxis are the young, household contacts of patients with TB, patients who have converted to positive within the past 2 years, and others at high risk for development of the disease (patients who are HIV infected, immunosuppressed, or diabetic, or who have renal failure). Evidence also suggests that the latently infected elderly should be treated.[9] Most commonly, chemoprophylaxis is provided through the oral administration of isoniazid (INH), 300 mg daily for 9 months (10 mg/kg; 9 months for children).[25,31] A higher dose of INH or the addition of ethambutol is recommended for tuberculin-positive persons who have been exposed to patients infected with organisms resistant to INH alone. Even though this usually

prevents the occurrence of active disease, the person retains hypersensitivity to the tuberculin test and will remain positive when skin tested. Major efforts toward development of a TB vaccine are under way.[32,33]

DENTAL MANAGEMENT
Medical Considerations

Many patients with infectious disease, including TB, cannot be clinically or historically identified; therefore, all patients should be treated as though they are potentially infectious, and standard precautions for infection control should be strictly followed. Implementation of infection control measures for patients with TB involves updating each patient's medical history, recognizing the signs and symptoms of TB, and following the guidelines of the CDC for infection control and the prevention of transmission of tuberculosis in health care settings[10,34,35] (see Appendix B). The CDC places most dental facilities in the minimal risk category for potential occupational exposure to TB. On the basis of assignment to this risk category, it recommends that each dental facility have a written TB control protocol that includes instrument reprocessing and operatory cleanup, as well as protocols for identifying, managing, and referring patients with active TB, and educating and training staff.[35] The CDC also recommends that periodic screening of dental care workers with PPD be provided to document any recent exposure, and that protocols should be available that explain how the office assesses, manages, and investigates dental staff with positive PPD tests.

When TB is managed, decisions regarding care are based on the potential infectivity of the patient. The four infectivity categories consist of (1) active TB, (2) a history of TB, (3) a positive tuberculin test, and (4) signs or symptoms suggestive of TB (Box 9-3).

Patients With Clinically Active Sputum-Positive TB. Patients with recently diagnosed, clinically active TB and positive sputum cultures should not be treated on an outpatient basis. Treatment is best rendered in a hospital setting with appropriate isolation, sterilization (mask, gloves, gown), and special engineering control (ventilation) systems and filtration masks.[35] For greater detail, the clinician should refer to the CDC recommendations, which can be found at http://www.cdc.gov/mmwr/PDF/RR/RR4313.pdf. Also, because of the risk of transmission, treatment in the isolation room should be limited to urgent care, and a rubber dam should be used to minimize aerosolization of oropharyngeal microbes. After receiving chemotherapy for at least 2 to 3 weeks and after receiving confirmation from the physician that he or she is noninfectious and lacks any complicating factors, the patient may be treated on an outpatient basis in the same manner as any normally healthy individual (Box 9-4).[36]

A child with active TB who is receiving chemotherapy usually can be treated as an outpatient because bacilli are

---

BOX 9-3

Dental Management of the Patient With a History of Tuberculosis

1. Active sputum-positive tuberculosis
   - Consult with physician before treatment
   - Perform urgent care only; palliate urgent problems with medication if contained facility in a hospital environment is not available
   - Perform urgent care that requires the use of a handpiece (older than 6 years) only in a hospital setting with isolation, sterilization (gloves, mask, gown), and special ventilation
   - Treat those under the age of 6 years as normal patients (noninfectious after consultation with physician to verify status)
   - Treat the patient who produces consistently negative sputum as a normal patient (noninfectious—verify with physician)
2. History of tuberculosis
   - Approach with caution, obtain good history of disease and its treatment duration, make appropriate review of systems mandatory
   - Obtain from patient a history of periodic chest radiographs and physical examination to rule out reactivation or relapse
   - Consult with physician and postpone treatment if there is:
     - Questionable history of adequate treatment time
     - Lack of appropriate medical follow-up since recovery
     - Sign or symptom of relapse
   - Treat as normal patient if present status is free of clinically active disease
3. Recent conversion to positive tuberculin skin test
   - Verify if evaluated by physician to rule out active disease
   - Verify if receiving isoniazid for 6 months to 1 year for prophylaxis
   - Treat as a normal patient
4. Signs or symptoms suggestive of tuberculosis
   - Refer to physician and postpone treatment
   - Treat as in 1 above if treatment is necessary

BOX 9-4

General Guidelines[36] for Determining When During Therapy a Patient With Pulmonary TB Has Become Noninfectious

Patient has:
- Negligible likelihood of multidrug–resistant TB
- Received standard multidrug anti-TB therapy for 2 to 3 weeks
- Demonstrated compliance with treatment
- Demonstrated clinical improvement
- Had three consecutive AFB-negative smear results of sputum specimens
- All close contacts of patient have been identified, evaluated, advised, and, if indicated, started on treatment for latent TB infection

TB, Tuberculosis; AFB, acid-fast bacillus.

rule out the possibility of active disease. If such assurances are not attained, the physician or health department should be contacted to ensure that proper preventive action is taken.

Patients With a Past History of TB. Fortunately, relapse is rare among patients who have received adequate treatment for the initial infection. However, this is not the case in patients who have received inadequate treatment and in those who are immunosuppressed. Regardless of what type of treatment the patient received, any individual with a history of TB initially should be approached with caution. The dentist should obtain a medical history, including diagnosis and dates and type of treatment. Treatment duration of less than 18 months if treatment was provided in past decades, or less than 6 months if treatment was given recently, requires consultation with the physician to determine the patient's status. Patients should provide a history of periodic physical examinations and chest radiographs to check for evidence of reactivation of the disease. Consultation with the physician is advisable to verify current status. The patient who is found free of active disease and immunosuppression may be treated with the use of standard precautions. A good review of systems is important with these patients, and referral to a physician is indicated if questionable signs or symptoms are present.

Patients With a Positive Tuberculin Test. A person with a positive skin test for TB should be viewed as having been infected with mycobacterium. The patient should give a history of being evaluated for active disease by physical examination and chest radiography. In the absence of clinically active disease, these patients have latent tuberculosis and are not considered infectious. A regimen of prophylactic isoniazid may be administered for 6 to 9 months to prevent reactivation and clinical disease. Patients may be treated in a normal manner with the use of standard precautions.

found only rarely in the sputum of young children. The child should be considered noninfectious unless a positive sputum culture has been obtained.[25] Reasons why a child with TB is considered noninfectious include the rarity of cavitary disease in children and their inability to cough up sputum effectively. In this instance, defining exactly what age constitutes a "child" is difficult. As a general rule, children younger than 6 years of age can be confidently treated. Over age 6, some degree of concern may exist. The physician should be consulted before treatment is begun. Of greater concern in this case are the family contacts of the patient because the disease most likely was contracted from an infected adult. All family members who have had contact with the child should provide a history of skin testing and chest radiography to

TABLE **9-2**
Dental Considerations of Antituberculous Drugs

Generic Drug (Trade Drug)	Adverse Effects	Dental Considerations
Isoniazid (INH, Laniazid, Nydrazid, Tubizid)	Hepatotoxicity; elevation in serum aminotransferase activity in 10% to 20% of patients*; rash, fever, peripheral neuropathy	Avoid acetaminophen Increases concentrations of other drugs (e.g., diazepam)
Rifampin (Rifadin, Rimactane)	Hepatotoxicity; gastrointestinal (GI) disturbances, flulike symptoms, thrombocytopenia, rash; turns urine red-orange	Increases incidence of infection, delayed healing, gingival bleeding; decreases metabolism of diazepam, clarithromycin (Biaxin), ketoconazole (Nizoral), itraconazole (Sporanox), fluconazole (Diflucan), and oral contraceptives
Pyrazinamide (generic)	Arthralgias, rash (photoallergy), hyperuricemia, GI disturbance, arthralgias, and hepatitis	—
Ethambutol (Myambutol)	Decreased red-green color discrimination; reduced visual acuity; optic neuritis (rare)	—
Streptomycin (generic)	Ototoxicity, vestibular disturbances, infrequent renal toxicity, perioral numbness	Avoid concurrent use of aspirin
Amikacin (Amikin), kanamycin (Kantrex), capreomycin (Capastat)	Nephrotoxicity and ototoxicity	Avoid concurrent use of aspirin
Ofloxacin (Floxin), ciprofloxacin (Cipro)	GI disturbances; inhibition of bone plate growth	Avoid in children <16 years of age
Aminosalicylic acid (PAS, Teebacin)	GI disturbances	—

*Greater risk of liver damage in persons over 35 years of age; Vitamin B$_6$ is recommended to counteract the adverse effect profile of INH.

Patients With Signs or Symptoms Suggestive of TB. Any time a patient demonstrates unexplained, persistent signs or symptoms that may be suggestive of TB (e.g., dry nonproductive cough, pleuritic chest pain, fatigue, fever, dyspnea, hemoptysis, weight loss) or has a positive skin test and has not been given follow-up medical care, dental care should not be rendered, and the patient should be referred to a physician for evaluation. If a health care provider is exposed to TB, the provider should be evaluated for skin test conversion. Converters should be treated promptly with isoniazid.[37]

Adverse Effects of Drugs

Isoniazid, rifampin, and pyrazinamide therapy may cause hepatotoxicity and elevations in serum aminotransferases (Table 9-2). The prevalence of isoniazid-induced hepatitis is about 1% and increases with advancing age, daily alcohol intake, and previous liver disease.[38] When serum aminotransferases are elevated in patients taking isoniazid, acetaminophen-containing medications should be avoided because of the increased potential for hepatotoxicity. Additional precautions regarding liver dysfunction are discussed in Chapter 11.

Rifampin induces cytochrome P450 enzymes. As a result, the use of rifampin can lower plasma levels of oral contraceptives, diazepam, clarithromycin (Biaxin),

ketoconazole (Nizoral), itraconazole (Sporanox), and fluconazole (Diflucan). In addition, rifampin can cause leukopenia, hemolytic anemia, and thrombocytopenia, resulting in an increased incidence of infection, delayed healing, and gingival bleeding. The use of rifampin combined with pyrazinamide or isoniazid increases the risks for hepatotoxicity and gastrointestinal and neurologic adverse events. Streptomycin should not be administered concurrently with aspirin because of the potential for increased ototoxicity.[39] Nonsteroidal anti-inflammatory drugs should be avoided in patients taking fluoroquinolones (second-line antituberculosis drugs) because of adverse central nervous system effects such as dizziness, insomnia, headache, or psychosis.

Treatment Planning Modifications

Delays in routine treatment must be afforded to patients who are infectious. Treatment may be resumed when patients become noninfectious (see Box 9-4).

Oral Complications and Manifestations

TB manifests infrequently in the oral cavity. Oral lesions can occur at any age but are most frequently seen in men about 30 years of age and in children. The classic mucosal lesion is a painful, deep, irregular ulcer on the dorsum of the tongue. The palate, lips, buccal mucosa, and gingiva

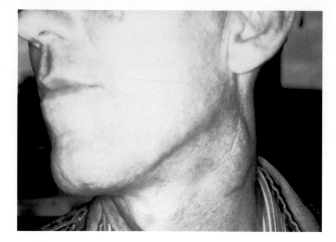

Figure 9-2. Tuberculosis of the cervical lymph nodes.

also may be affected.[40,41] Mucosal lesions have been reported to be granular, nodular, or leukoplakic and sometimes painless.[42] Extension into the jaws can result in osteomyelitis. The cervical and submandibular lymph nodes may become infected with TB; this condition is called *scrofula*. The nodes become enlarged and painful (Figure 9-2), and abscesses may form and drain.[43] Involvement of the salivary glands is rare.[44]

Biopsy in addition to culture can be diagnostic if acid-fast bacilli are found. Resolution of the infectious oral lesion may result from treatment of TB with antituberculous drugs. Pain is managed symptomatically (see Appendix C).

OCCUPATIONAL SAFETY AND HEALTH ASSOCIATION

Dentists should be aware that the Occupational Safety and Health Association (OSHA) issued an enforcement guidance policy in 1993 to protect workers against exposure to *M. tuberculosis*. This policy mandates that employers provide a safe, healthful workplace and permits inspection for occupational exposure to TB in health care settings when complaints are received from public sector employees. Employers who are found to be in violation of the requirements may be fined.

In 1997, OSHA proposed an additional policy based on the CDC guidelines. This newer proposal requires that dentists prepare a written exposure control plan, provide baseline skin test results and medical history, make medical management available after an exposure incident, provide medical removal protection if necessary, provide information and training to employees with exposure potential, and comply with record-keeping requirements. Periodic medical surveillance and respiratory protection would not be required if the dental facility does not admit or treat persons with active TB, has had no confirmed cases of infectious TB within the past year, and is located in a county in which no cases of active TB have been reported within the previous 2 years. By contrast, more strict guidelines (i.e., isolation rooms for patients with suspected or confirmed infectious TB and ventilation equipment) are required when employees may have been exposed to the exhaled air of an individual with suspected or confirmed TB, or were exposed to a high hazard procedure performed on an individual who may have TB that has the potential to generate potentially infectious airborne respiratory secretions. To better familiarize themselves with their legal responsibilities, dentists may visit the OSHA Web site at www.osha. gov/pls/oshaweb/owadisp.show_document?p_table= FEDERAL_REGISTER&p_id=13717 (29 CFR Part 1910).

REFERENCES

1. Aziz MA, Wright A. The World Health Organization/ International Union Against Tuberculosis and Lung Disease Global Project on Surveillance for Anti-Tuberculosis Drug Resistance: A model for other infectious diseases. Clin Infect Dis 2005;41:S258-S262.
2. Sudre P, ten Dam G, Kochi A. Tuberculosis: A global overview of the situation today. Bull World Health Organ 1992;70:149-159.
3. Sbarbaro J. Tuberculosis in the 1990s: Epidemiology and therapeutic challenge. Chest 1995;108:58S-62S.
4. Centers for Disease Control and Prevention. Tuberculosis—United States, 1985. MMWR 1986;35:699-703.
5. Centers for Disease Control and Prevention. Summary of notifiable diseases, United States, 1990. MMWR 1990;39:1-29.
6. Centers for Disease Control and Prevention. Expanded tuberculosis surveillance and tuberculosis morbidity—United States, 1993. MMWR 1994;43:361-366.
7. Centers for Disease Control and Prevention. Trends in Tuberculosis—United States, 2005. MMWR 2006;55:305-308.
8. Calabrese L. The yin and yang of tumor necrosis factor inhibitors. Cleve Clin J Med 2006;73:251-256.
9. Van der Brande P. Revised guidelines for the diagnosis and control of tuberculosis: Impact on management in the elderly. Drugs Aging 2005;8:663-686.
10. Centers for Disease Control and Prevention. Guidelines for preventing the transmission of tuberculosis in healthcare settings, with special focus on HIV-related issues. MMWR 1990;39:1-29.
11. Centers for Disease Control and Prevention. Tuberculosis morbidity in the United States: Final data, 1990. MMWR 1991;40:23-27.
12. Haas D, Des Prez R. Tuberculosis and acquired immunodeficiency syndrome: A historical perspective on recent developments. Am J Med 1994;96:439-450.
13. Bradford W, Daley C. Multiple drug–resistant tuberculosis. Infect Dis Clin North Am 1998;12:157-172.
14. Weir M, Thornton G. Extrapulmonary tuberculosis: Experience of a community hospital and review of the literature. Am J Med 1985;79:467-478.
15. Fowler N. Tuberculous pericarditis. JAMA 1991;266:99-103.
16. Von Lichtenberg F. Infectious disease: Viral, chlamydial, rickettsial, and bacterial diseases. In Cottran RS, Kumar V, Robbins S (eds). Robbins' Pathologic Basis of Disease. Philadelphia, WB Saunders, 1989.

17. Braun M, Cote T, Rabkin C. Trends in death with tuberculosis during the AIDS era. JAMA 1993;269:2865-2868.

18. Lederman MM. Infections of the lower respiratory tract. In Andreolia TE, et al (eds). Cecil Essentials of Medicine, 6th ed. Philadelphia, WB Saunders, 2004.

19. Holden M, Dubin MR, Diamond PH. Frequency of negative intermediate-strength tuberculin sensitivity in patients with active tuberculosis. N Engl J Med 1971;285:1506-1509.

20. American Thoracic Society. The tuberculin skin test. Am Rev Respir Dis 1981;124:356-363.

21. Daniel T. Tuberculosis. In Kasper DL, et al (eds). Harrison's Principles of Internal Medicine, 16th ed. New York, McGraw-Hill, 2005.

22. Centers for Disease Control and Prevention. Epidemiology of tuberculosis. In Self-Study Modules on Tuberculosis. Atlanta, Ga, National Center for Prevention Services, Division of Tuberculosis Elimination, 1995.

23. Diagnostic standards and classification of tuberculosis in adults and children. Am J Respir Crit Care Med 2000;161:1376-1395.

24. Salfinger M, Hale Y, Driscoll J. Diagnostic tools in tuberculosis: Present and future. Respiration 1998;65:163-170.

25. American Thoracic Society. Treatment of tuberculosis and tuberculosis infection in adults and children. Am J Respir Crit Care Med 1994;149:1359-1374.

26. Centers for Disease Control and Prevention. Initial therapy for tuberculosis in the era of multidrug resistance: Recommendations of the Advisory Council for the Elimination of Tuberculosis. MMWR 1993;42(RR-7):1-8.

27. Ravikrishnan K. Tuberculosis: How can we halt its resurgence? Postgrad Med 1992;91:333-338.

28. Centers for Disease Control and Prevention. Bacteriologic conversion of sputum among tuberculosis patients—United States. MMWR 1985;34:747-750.

29. Antonucci G, Girardi E, Raviglione MC, Ippolito G. Risk factors for tuberculosis in HIV-infected persons: A prospective cohort study. JAMA 1995;274:143-148.

30. Centers for Disease Control and Prevention. Recommendations for prevention and control of tuberculosis among foreign-born persons. MMWR 1998;47(RR-16):1-26.

31. Cohn DL. Treatment of latent tuberculosis infection. Semin Respir Infect 2003;18:249-262.

32. Centers for Disease Control and Prevention. Development of new vaccines for tuberculosis. MMWR 1998;47:1-6.

33. Fletcher H, McShane H. Tuberculosis vaccines: Current status and future prospects. Expert Opin Emerg Drugs 2006;11:207-215.

34. Centers for Disease Control and Prevention. Recommended infection-control practices for dentistry, 1993. MMWR 1993;42(RR-8). Available at: http://www.cdc.gov/mmwr/preview/mmwrhtml/00021095.htm. Accessed on March 19, 2007.

35. Centers for Disease Control and Prevention. Guidelines for preventing the transmission of tuberculosis in health-care facilities. MMWR 1994;43(RR-13):1-132. Available at: http://www.cdc.gov/mmwr/PDF/RR/RR4313.pdf. Accessed on March 19, 2007.

36. American Thoracic Society/Centers for Disease Control and Prevention/Infectious Diseases Society of America. Controlling tuberculosis in the United States. Am J Respir Crit Care Med 2005;172:1169-1227.

37. Stead W. Management of health care workers after inadvertent exposure to tuberculosis: A guide for the use of preventive therapy. Ann Intern Med 1995;122:906-912.

38. Forget EJ, Menzies D. Adverse reactions to first-line antituberculosis drugs. Expert Opin Drug Saf 2006;5:231-249.

39. Drug Information for the Health Care Professional. Taunton, Mass. Thomson Micromedex, 2006.

40. Dimitrakopoulos I, Zouloumis L, Lazaridis N, et al. Primary tuberculosis of the oral cavity. Oral Surg 1991;72:712-715.

41. Shafer W, Hine M, Levy B. A Textbook of Oral Pathology, 4th ed. Philadelphia, WB Saunders, 1983.

42. Kolokotronis A, Antoniadis D, Trigonidis D, Papanagiotou P. Oral tuberculosis. Oral Dis 1996;2:242-243.

43. Florio S, Ellis EI, Frost D. Persistent submandibular swelling after tooth extraction. J Oral Maxillofac Surg 1997;55:390-397.

44. Bhargava S, Watmough DJ, Chisti FA, Sathar SA. Case report: Tuberculosis of the parotid gland—Diagnosis by CT. Br J Radiol 1996;69:1181-1183.

CHAPTER
10

SNORING AND OBSTRUCTIVE SLEEP APNEA

Sleep-related breathing disorders constitute a spectrum of clinical entities with variations in sleep structure, respiration, and blood oxygen saturation. The spectrum ranges from mild, intermittent snoring to severe obstructive sleep apnea (OSA) (Figure 10-1). Obesity-hypoventilation syndrome (formerly called pickwickian syndrome) is the term used to describe an extremely severe form of OSA. Snoring, upper airway resistance syndrome (UARS), and OSA are the subjects of this chapter. All of these sleep-related breathing disorders are due to obstructive resistance to airflow during respiration. A related disorder, central sleep apnea, is cessation of breathing that is due to a disorder of the central nervous system ventilatory drive; it is not due to obstruction and thus is not included in this chapter.

Snoring may occur alone or may be a sign of more significant airway impairment. It results from vibration of the soft tissues of the upper airway, primarily during inspiration. Primary snoring (PS) is sometimes referred to as simple snoring or benign snoring; it occurs as an independent entity and is not associated with complaints of sleepiness. It occurs without abnormal ventilation. UARS is a clinical entity midway between PS and OSA that is characterized by snoring, complaints of daytime sleepiness, and fragmentation of sleep with some increased ventilatory effort. OSA is characterized by loud snoring and excessive daytime sleepiness with complete cessation of breathing (apnea) or significantly decreased ventilation (hypopnea) due to airway obstruction during sleep.

GENERAL DESCRIPTION
Epidemiology

Snoring is extremely common in both genders and in all age groups. It is reported to occur in approximately 40% of the adult population, with men having a higher prevalence than women.[1] Estimates of its prevalence vary widely, however, because detection methods rely heavily on subjective reports by bed partners or parents. Reported prevalence of snoring in men varies between 5% and 86% and in women between 2% to 57%. Evidence suggests that in men, the prevalence of snoring increases with age until about age 60, at which time a decrease occurs.[2] In children, snoring is common, with a reported prevalence of between 5% and 15%.[3] Symptoms of sleep-disordered breathing have been reported to increase during pregnancy.[4]

The reported prevalence of OSA varies widely because of differences in assessment methods and in the number of abnormal respiratory events per hour used to define abnormality. On average, it is estimated that about 2% to 5% of the adult population 30 to 60 years of age is affected by OSA.[5] About 0.7% to 3% of children are affected, with the highest prevalence reported between the ages of 2 and 5 years.[6] Variation has been noted between males and females, with males affected more often than females. Variation among racial groups may be due to genetic differences. African Americans, Hispanics, and Asian Americans tend to have a somewhat higher prevalence when compared with whites.

Etiology and Pathophysiology

The primary cause of sleep-related breathing disorders is an anatomically narrowed upper airway combined with pharyngeal dilator muscle collapsibility. The exact pathogenesis, however, is not well understood. Depending on the extent of narrowing, increased resistance to airflow may be clinically expressed as vibration of soft tissues (snoring), hypoventilation (hypopnea), or complete obstruction (apnea).

Anatomic narrowing may occur at any site in the upper airway from the nasal cavity to the larynx. Within the nasal cavity, septal deviation and enlarged turbinates

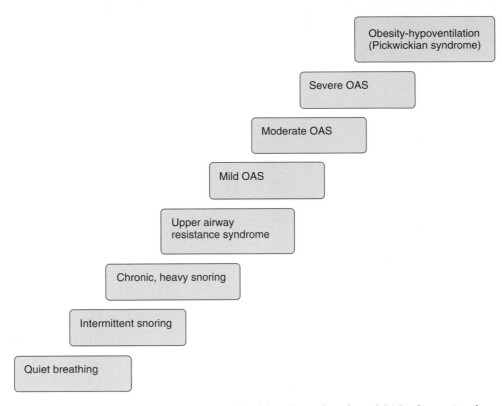

Figure 10-1. Clinical spectrum of sleep-related breathing disorders. OSAS, obstructive sleep apnea syndrome. (Modified from Phillips B, Naughton MT. Fast Facts: Obstructive Sleep Apnea. Oxford, Health Press Limited, 2004.)

may cause narrowing. In the nasopharynx, hypertrophic adenoids, and tonsils, an elongated soft palate and an elongated and edematous uvula may be the cause. In the oropharynx, narrowing may be due to an enlarged tongue, excessive lymphoid tissue, or redundant parapharyngeal folds. The most common sites of airway narrowing or closure during sleep are the retropalatal and retroglossal regions.[7] Most patients with OSA have more than one site of narrowing.[8] A recent study demonstrated that the volume of the upper airway soft tissue structures (i.e., tongue, lateral pharyngeal walls, soft palate, parapharyngeal fat pads) was significantly greater in patients with OSA than in normal controls.[9] Factors that are thought to contribute to enlargement of the upper airway soft tissues in apneic patients include obesity, edema secondary to negative pressures, vibration trauma, male gender, and possibly, genetics.[7]

In addition to anatomic narrowing of the airway, an abnormal degree of collapsibility is observed in the pharyngeal dilator muscles surrounding the airway. Patency of the airway depends on a balance between air pressure within the airway and pressure outside of the airway exerted by the parapharyngeal musculature. Muscles that surround the airway receive phasic activation during inspiration and tend to promote a patent pharyngeal lumen by dilating the airway and stiffening the airway walls.[10] Normally, the intraluminal pressure exceeds the external pressure, and the airway remains patent during inhalation and exhalation. Normal function requires

coordinated timing and activity of agonists and antagonists, and of individual muscles or groups of muscles. The cause of abnormal pharyngeal airway collapse is complex and involves both dynamic and static factors. These factors may include tissue volume, changes in the surface adhesion of mucosal surfaces, changes in neck and jaw posture, decreased tracheal tug, effects of gravity, and decreased intraluminal pressure due to increased upstream resistance in the nasal cavity or pharynx.[7]

Complications and Outcomes

To understand the consequences of sleep-related breathing disorders, it is necessary to review the aspects of normal sleep. Sleep patterns vary with age but are nevertheless similar; thus, for illustrative purposes, the sleep of young adults is discussed here. Normal sleep occurs in two phases: non–rapid eye movement (NREM) sleep and rapid eye movement (REM) sleep (Table 10-1).

The phases of sleep are characterized by distinctive patterns on an electroencephalogram (EEG), as well as by the presence or absence of eye movements. NREM sleep occurs in four stages and is generally characterized by synchronous brain waves, mental inactivity, and physiologic stability (Figure 10-2). Stage 1 NREM is a brief, transitional stage that lasts only a few minutes between wakefulness and sleep and from which a person can be easily aroused. Stage 2 NREM is the initial stage of true sleep from which arousal is more difficult. The appearance of EEG waves called *sleep spindles* or *K-complexes* identifies this stage, which typically lasts 10 to 25 minutes. Stage 3 is characterized by the appearance of EEG high-voltage, slow waves that last for a few minutes and then transition into stage 4, with more frequent and higher-amplitude slow waves. This stage lasts for 20 to 40 minutes. Stages 3 and 4 are often combined, and this combination is referred to as slow wave sleep (SWS).

After a period of NREM sleep, a "lightening" occurs, and REM sleep is entered. REM sleep is very different from NREM sleep and is characterized by asynchronous brain waves, an active brain, and physiologic instability. A key feature is the presence of periodic rapid movement of the eyes with low-voltage EEG waves that resemble wakefulness (Figure 10-3). Variations in blood pressure, heart rate, and respiration occur, along with general muscle atonia and poikilothermia. Dreaming also occurs during REM sleep.

Over the course of a night, sleep cycles between NREM and REM, with each cycle averaging about 90 minutes. Depending on the length of the sleep period, a person typically passes through four to six cycles per night. The length of time in each stage varies, with NREM predominating in the earlier part of the night and REM predominating in the later part of the night (Figure 10-4). It is difficult to define the "normal" length of sleep because of multiple variables, including age, environment, circadian rhythm, and medications; however, most young adults report that they sleep an average of 7.5 hours per weeknight and 8.5 hours on weekend nights.[11]

To gain the restorative benefits of sleep, it is necessary to cycle through the normal stages of sleep. If this does

TABLE 10-1

Percentage of Time Spent in the Various Stages of Sleep in a Normal, Healthy Young Adult

Stage	Percent
RELAXED WAKEFULNESS	<5%
NON-RAPID EYE MOVEMENT SLEEP (NREM)	
Stage 1 (transitional; easy arousal)	2%-5%
Stage 2 (sleep onset; K-complexes, sleep spindles)	45%-55%
Stage 3 (high-voltage slow waves appear)	3%-8%
Stage 4 (increased numbers of high-voltage slow waves)	10%-15%
RAPID EYE MOVEMENT SLEEP (REM) (Desynchronized electroencephalogram [EEG], muscle atonia, bursts of rapid eye movement)	20%-25%

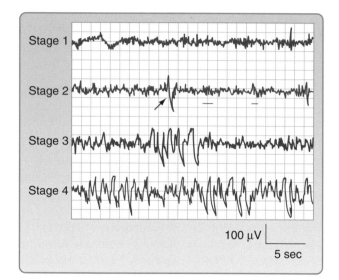

Figure 10-2. Electroencephalographic (EEG) tracings of non–rapid eye movement (NREM) sleep stages. (From Carskadon MA, Dement WC. Normal human sleep: An overview. In Kryger MH, Roth T, Dement WC [eds]. Principles and Practice of Sleep Medicine, 4th ed. Philadelphia, Elsevier, 2005.)

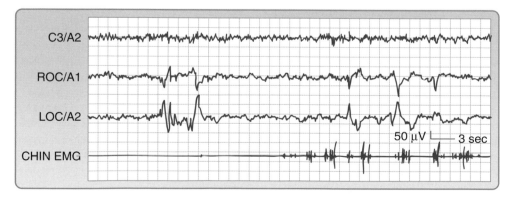

Figure 10-3. Phasic events in human rapid eye movement (REM) sleep. C3/A2 is an electroencephalographic (EEG) lead. ROC/A1 is a lead from the outer canthus of the right eye, and LOC/A2 is a lead from the outer canthus of the left eye. Note the several bursts of activity in the eye leads. (From Carskadon MA, Dement WC. Normal human sleep: An overview. In Kryger MH, Roth T, Dement WC [eds]. Principles and Practice of Sleep Medicine, 4th ed. Philadelphia, Elsevier, 2005.)

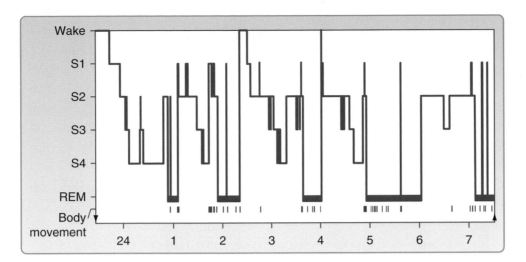

Figure 10-4. Histogram of the progression of sleep stages across a single night in a normal, healthy, young adult. (From Carskadon MA, Dement WC. Normal human sleep: An overview. In Kryger MH, Roth T, Dement WC [eds]. Principles and Practice of Sleep Medicine, 4th ed. Philadelphia, Elsevier, 2005.)

not occur because of sleep deprivation or sleep fragmentation, cognitive and physiologic effects are seen. In the spectrum of sleep-related breathing disorders, different outcomes may be seen. With PS, the degree of airway resistance is such that vibration of the parapharyngeal soft tissues is the only result. No other impairment of airflow or oxygenation is noted. Generally, it is thought that PS has no significant adverse health effects, although evidence suggests that PS may be a risk factor for type 2 diabetes and hypertension.[1]

With OSA, increasing resistance to airflow occurs to the point of obstruction, with partial (hypopnea) or complete (apnea) cessation of breathing, in spite of efforts to continue to breathe. Depending on the degree and duration of the obstruction, hypoxia, anoxia, and hypercarbia may result. This leads to arousal and transition to a lighter stage of sleep (stage 1 or 2), stimulating partial awakening, relief of the obstruction, and resumption of breathing. Depending on the frequency of arousals during the night, sleep can be fragmented (Figure 10-5). Sleep quality is poor and the restorative benefits of sleep are not achieved, leading to a variety of characteristic cognitive and physiologic abnormalities.

Neurocognitive effects of OSA include sleepiness, decreased alertness, irritability, poor concentration, lack of libido, and memory loss. This can lead to poor job performance, marital discord, interpersonal conflicts, and driving impairment. Up to 30% of traffic accidents are attributed to sleepy drivers.[12] Patients with OSA have an eightfold increase in motor vehicle accidents over those without OSA.[13]

In addition to neurocognitive impairment, OSA is associated with numerous cardiovascular effects, including hypertension, stroke, cardiovascular disease, congestive heart failure, pulmonary hypertension, and cardiac arrhythmia. OSA, which is now recognized as one of the treatable causes of hypertension,[14] has also been shown

to significantly increase the risks of stroke and death.[15] Patients with OSA have two- to fourfold greater odds of experiencing complex arrhythmias over those without.[16] It is also thought that treatment of OSA may increase the survival rate of patients with heart failure.[17] In addition, a relationship between OSA, obesity, and metabolic syndrome has been noted.[18] Recent data from the Sleep Heart Health Study provide evidence for an independent relationship between sleep apnea, glucose intolerance, and insulin resistance that may lead to type 2 diabetes.[19]

CLINICAL PRESENTATION
Signs and Symptoms

Major signs and symptoms of sleep-related breathing disorders are those most often described by the bed partner or parent of a patient; they include snoring, snorting, gasping, and breath holding. Snoring is very common, as was previously indicated. Most people who snore do not have OSA, but almost all patients with OSA do snore. In the Wisconsin Sleep Cohort Study of subjects aged 30 to 60 years, 44% of men and 28% of women were habitual snorers, but only 4% of men and 2% of women had OSA.[20] Snoring may be very loud and disruptive to other members of the household. When snoring is the only complaint, it is most often due to PS. If snoring is accompanied by daytime sleepiness and no breathing changes during sleep, UARS must be considered. However, if the snoring is accompanied by snorting, choking, gasping, or a complete cessation of breathing, this is likely a sign of OSA.[21] It should be emphasized that definitive diagnosis of sleep-related breathing disorders cannot be made on the basis of clinical signs and symptoms alone.

Complaints of excessive daytime sleepiness are common in patients with OSA but are not specific and may be due to many factors. A test often used to measure

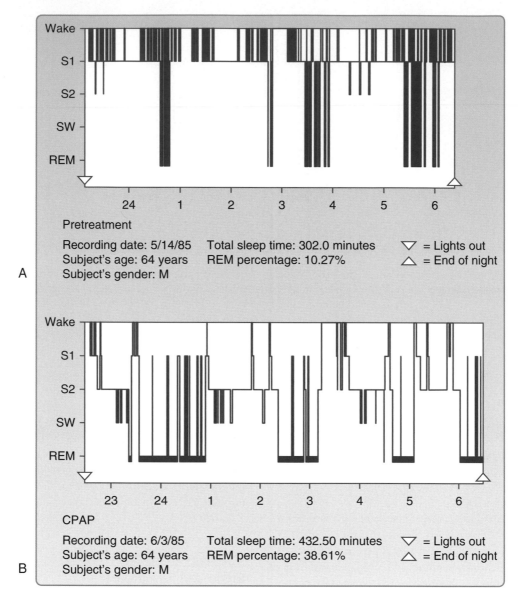

Figure 10-5. A, Histogram of a patient with obstructive sleep apnea. **B,** Histogram of the same patient with the use of continuous positive airway pressure (CPAP). (From Carskadon MA, Dement WC. Normal human sleep: An overview. In Kryger MH, Roth T, Dement WC [eds]. Principles and Practice of Sleep Medicine, 4th ed. Philadelphia, Elsevier, 2005.)

subjective sleepiness is the Epworth Sleepiness Scale (Figure 10-6). It has been validated in clinical studies and correlates with objective measures of sleepiness. It is composed of eight questions or situations in which patients are asked how likely they are to fall asleep. Each question is answered on a scale of 0 to 3, with 3 indicating that they would always fall asleep in a given circumstance. The maximum possible score is 24. A score greater than 10 is associated with significant daytime sleepiness, but it is not specific for sleep-related breathing disorders. Other complaints that may be associated with OSA are nocturia or enuresis, mood changes, memory or learning difficulties, erectile dysfunction, morning headache, and dry mouth upon awakening.

Obesity is a very common finding among patients with OSA. Obesity increases the risk of OSA approximately 10- to 14-fold; the most marked effects are observed during middle age.[22] One measure of obesity is the body mass index (BMI), which is calculated by dividing weight in kilograms by height in meters squared. Adults with a BMI greater than 27 are considered obese. Approximately 40% of individuals with a BMI greater than 40 and 50% of those with a BMI greater than 50 have significantly sleep-disordered breathing.[23] It has been found, however, that neck circumference is more closely related to severity of OSA than is BMI.[24] A neck circumference in men of greater than 17 inches and in women of greater than 16 inches is predictive of OSA.[25] Along with obesity and collar size, other physical features associated with OSA include mandibular retrognathia, long soft palate, large edematous uvula, large tongue, tonsillar and adenoidal hypertrophy, and a high arched palate. In summary, the

THE EPWORTH SLEEPINESS SCALE

Name: _____

Today's date: _____ Your age (years): _____

Your sex (male = M; female = F): _____

How likely are you to doze off or fall asleep in the following situations, in contrast to feeling just tired? This refers to your usual way of life in recent times. Even if you have not done some of these things recently try to work out how they would have affected you. Use the following scale to choose the *most appropriate number* for each situation:

> 0 = would *never* doze
> 1 = *slight* chance of dozing
> 2 = *moderate* chance of dozing
> 3 = *high* chance of dozing

Situation	Chance of dozing
Sitting and reading	_____
Watching TV	_____
Sitting, inactive in a public place (e.g., a theater or a meeting)	_____
As a passenger in a car for an hour without a break	_____
Lying down to rest in the afternoon when circumstances permit	_____
Sitting and talking to someone	_____
Sitting quietly after a lunch without alcohol	_____
In a car, while stopped for a few minutes in the traffic	_____

Thank you for your cooperation

Figure 10-6. Epworth Sleepiness Scale. (From Johns MW. A new method for measuring daytime sleepiness: The Epworth Sleepiness Scale. Sleep 1991;14:540-545.)

most useful predictors of OSA are witnessed apneas, male gender, BMI, and neck circumference.

Laboratory Diagnosis

Definitive diagnosis of a sleep-related breathing disorder is made by polysomnography, which is an overnight sleep study that is performed in a laboratory setting (Figure 10-7). During the performance of a standard laboratory-based polysomnogram (PSG), a technician who is present throughout the night records the activities of the patient during sleep. Multiple physiologic parameters are monitored and recorded on a computer. These include electroencephalogram (EEG) to monitor brain waves, electro-oculogram (EOG) to monitor eye movements, electromyogram (EMG) to monitor jaw muscular activity and leg movements, electrocardiogram (ECG) to monitor heart rate and rhythm, pulse oximetry to monitor blood oxygen saturation, nasal thermistor to monitor nasal airflow and CO_2 levels, and chest and abdominal strain gauges to monitor breathing efforts. After all recording

sensors are attached, the patient is allowed to go to sleep. Most contemporary sleep laboratories have sleeping rooms that are nicely decorated, resembling a normal bedroom. In addition to the sensors attached to the patient, an infrared camera is often used to enable the technician to watch the movements of patients, such as leg movements or sleep walking, or to relate sleeping position to periods of disturbed breathing. A microphone is present in the room to record snoring or other sounds, such as tooth grinding or sleep talking.

A typical PSG encompasses the entire night and is usually sufficient to make a diagnosis, in spite of obvious questions about the "normality" of the night's sleep in such an environment. Often, a diagnosis can be made early in the course of the night, and a trial of therapy with positive airway pressure (PAP) will be attempted. This is called a *split-night study*. If this is not possible, a second sleep study may be necessary to assess the effects of PAP. A computer recording of the entire night is produced; this is then read and interpreted by a qualified physician

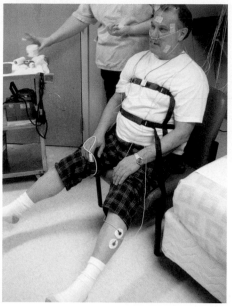

A

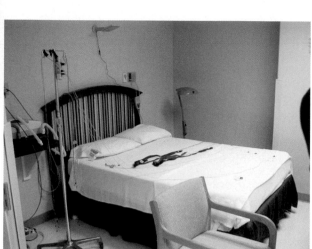

B

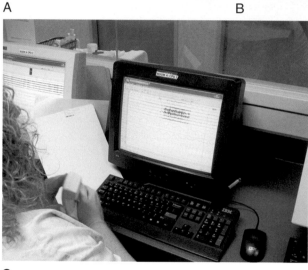

C

Figure 10-7. **A,** Patient being prepared for polysomnogram. Multiple recording leads are in place. **B,** Sleep laboratory/bedroom where the patient spends the night while being recorded. **C,** Sleep technician monitoring the computer printout of the polysomnogram.

trained in sleep medicine, who then makes a diagnosis and recommends treatment (Figure 10-8).

Quantification of the severity of OSA is expressed through the Apnea-Hypopnea Index (AHI) or the Respiratory Disturbance Index (RDI). These two indices are commonly used interchangeably; however, a technical difference between the two has been identified. The AHI is scored by adding all of the apneas that occurred during the night together with all of the hypopneas that occurred over the night, then dividing by the total number of hours slept. The result is expressed as the number of respiratory events per hour. The difference in the RDI is that respiratory effort–related arousals (RERAs) are added to the apneas and hypopneas. It is important to define these terms to understand the diagnosis. According to the American Academy of Sleep Medicine,[26] an apnea is defined as the cessation or near-complete cessation (greater than 70% reduction) of airflow for a minimum of 10 seconds. Hypopnea is a greater than 30% reduction

of amplitude in thoracoabdominal movement or airflow as compared with baseline, with a greater than 4% oxygen desaturation. RERAs are episodes that include a clear drop in respiratory airflow, increased respiratory effort, and a brief change in sleep state (arousal) but do not meet the criteria for apnea or hypopnea.

A diagnosis of OSA is made if the AHI or RDI is greater than 5 per hour and symptoms of excessive daytime sleepiness, witnessed nocturnal apneas, or awakening with choking, breath holding, or gasping are noted. In quantifying the severity of OSA, some disagreement has been expressed; however, a commonly used classification defines an AHI of 0 to 5 per hour as normal, 5 to 15 per hour as mild, 15 to 30 per hour as moderate, and greater than 30 per hour as severe. Along with the AHI, the lowest point (nadir) of oxygen desaturation is reported. UARS is diagnosed in the presence of RERAs, an AHI of less than 5 per hour, and a complaint of excessive daytime sleepiness. PS would yield a completely normal

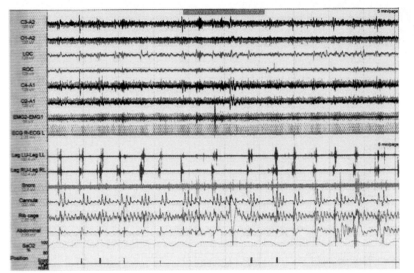

Figure 10-8. A 5-minute epoch of a polysomnogram. C3-A2, O1-A2, C4-A1, and O2-A1 are electroencephalographic leads used to determine sleep stages. LOC and ROC are eyelid leads for recording rapid eye movement. EMG is an electromyogram of the chin used to record jaw movement. ECG is an electrocardiogram that records heart rate and rhythm. Leg LU and RU are leg leads for recording leg movements. Snore is the recording of snoring. Cannula is a measurement of nasal airflow pressure. Rib cage is a recording of rib cage movement. Abdominal is a recording of abdominal movement. SaO_2 is blood oxygen saturation. Position is a recording of body position. (From Phillips B, Naughton M. Fast Facts: Obstructive sleep apnea. Oxford, Heath Press, 2004. Reproduced with permission.)

PSG and no complaint of excessive sleepiness in the presence of snoring.

Other aspects of the PSG that may be reported are total time spent in the various sleep stages, AHI in various sleep stages, and AHI in various sleep positions. In addition, a sleep hypnogram (or histogram), which is a graph of the sleep pattern during the entire night that depicts cycling into and out of the various sleep stages, may be provided. Other tests that may be used include the Multiple Sleep Latency Test (MSLT), which assesses the ability to fall asleep, and the Maintenance of Wakefulness Test (MWT), which assesses the ability to stay awake.

MEDICAL MANAGEMENT

The decision of when and how to treat sleep-related breathing disorders depends on the diagnosis and severity of the disorder. Treatment of PS is elective and is essentially a personal decision that is commonly motivated by the effects of snoring on a spouse or bed partner. It is interesting to note that snoring rarely disturbs the snorer. Parents of children who snore often seek treatment out of concern for the health of the child. Patients who are given a diagnosis of UARS should receive treatment to alleviate the problems associated with snoring, as well as those of sleep fragmentation and resultant sleepiness. UARS is an intermediate condition between PS and OSA that can progress into OSA over time. Patients who are given a diagnosis of OSA require treatment—not only to alleviate snoring and sleepiness, but to prevent or treat the numerous adverse health effects associated with the disease. Even mild sleep apnea is associated with significant morbidity, which increases with severity.[20] An increased mortality rate is associated with an AHI greater than 20 per hour.[27]

General Measures

Several measures may help to decrease or eliminate the signs or symptoms of sleep-related breathing disorders. Weight loss is one of the most effective measures that can

be instituted. It has been shown that even modest weight loss can relieve mild sleep-related breathing disorders and in many cases may be curative.[28] Furthermore, independent of body habitus, regular aerobic exercise has been shown to improve OSA.[29] For patients with obstruction in the nasal cavity, nasal dilator strips may be helpful to physically open the nasal passages, as may the use of nasal decongestants and/or topical corticosteroids.[30] It has been noted that many patients with OSA have positional apnea, with apneas occurring more frequently or more severely in the supine position.[31] For patients with position-dependent apnea, measures to prevent sleeping in a supine position may be helpful and include sewing a tennis ball into a pocket on the back of the pajamas, using a backpack-type device, and using pillows to maintain a side-sleeping posture. Alcohol, sedatives, or muscle relaxants near bedtime should be avoided. Patients who smoke should be encouraged to quit smoking, although the relationship between smoking and OSA remains unclear. Oral or nasal lubricants or sprays, diet supplements, magnets, and hypnosis are some alternative treatment methods purported to relieve snoring; however, credible evidence of effectiveness is lacking.

Positive Airway Pressure

The gold standard for the treatment of OSA is the delivery of positive airway pressure (PAP) to the patient's airway during sleep. This is accomplished with the use of an air compressor that is connected by tubing to a nasal or full face mask attached to the patient's face (Figure 10-9). Room air, under pressure, is delivered to the patient's airway and acts in effect as a pneumatic stent, producing positive intraluminal pressure along the entire pharyngeal airway, thus maintaining patency. It is interesting to note that dilation of the upper airway is greater in the lateral dimension than in the anterior/posterior dimension.[32,33]

An advantage of PAP is that it relieves obstruction at all levels of the airway. Delivery of PAP occurs in one of three ways[34]:

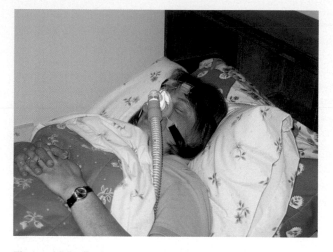

Figure 10-9. Patient using a positive airway pressure device with a nasal mask. (Courtesy June Sorrenson, RRT.)

1. Continuous positive airway pressure (CPAP);
2. Bilevel positive airway pressure (BPAP; BiPAP); or
3. Automatic, self-adjusting positive airway pressure (APAP)

The air may be heated and humidified. CPAP provides air continuously throughout inspiration and exhalation at a single, set pressure, expressed as cm H_2O. BPAP consists of two set pressures, with higher pressure occurring during inhalation and lower pressure noted during exhalation. With APAP, pressures vary continuously according to what is required at a particular moment to maintain airway patency. CPAP, the form most commonly used, is the least expensive. CPAP is most often titrated to an effective level during a PSG in the sleep laboratory, either as part of a split-night study or during a subsequent full-night study. Pressures are typically started at 3 to 5 cm H_2O and are gradually titrated upward, until all measures of OSA are eliminated. With CPAP, typical treatment pressures range between 5 and 15 cm H_2O.[35]

In a recent review of PAP,[36] it was concluded that PAP eliminates respiratory disturbances and reduces AHI when compared with placebo, conservative management, or positional therapy. It also improves stage 3 and 4 sleep and decreases EEG arousals versus placebo. It significantly improves sleep architecture and sleep fragmentation, but these effects are not always consistent. Daytime sleepiness, neurobehavioral performance, psychological functioning, and quality of life may also be improved. The impact on cardiovascular risk is mixed. Compliance with PAP has long been a problem, with the average patient using PAP for only about 4 to 5 hours per night and for only about 5 nights per week.[35,36] Adverse effects with PAP are common and include mask leaks, skin ulceration or irritation under the mask, epistaxis, rhinorrhea, nasal congestion, sinus congestion, dry eyes, conjunctivitis, ear pain, and claustrophobia.

Oral Appliances

Oral appliances (OAs) offer an attractive alternative for many patients with sleep-related breathing disorders who are unable to tolerate the use of PAP, or who refuse to use it. OAs exert their effects by mechanically increasing the volume of the upper airway in the retropalatal and retroglossal areas, as has been confirmed by imaging and physiologic monitoring.[37] These areas of the oropharynx are the most common sites of obstruction in patients with OSA.[38] OAs hypothetically increase airway size more in the retroglossal than in the retropalatal region because they pull the tongue forward.[39,40] However, studies have shown that OAs increase airway size in the retropalatal and retroglossal regions, with increases occurring predominantly in the lateral dimension.[40,41]

Two basic types of oral appliances are available: (1) Mandibular advancement devices (MADs) that engage the mandible and reposition it (and indirectly, the tongue) in an anterior or forward position, and (2) tongue-retaining devices (TRDs) that directly engage the tongue and hold it in a forward position. Currently, more than 50 different designs of OAs are available, but the US Food and Drug Administration (FDA) has approved only 30 of them for use in the treatment of OSA; the remainder have been approved only for snoring (Figure 10-10).

MAD appliances are most commonly used to treat patients with sleep-related breathing disorders. They are typically made of acrylic resin and are composed of two pieces that cover the upper and lower dental arches and are connected in such a way as to hold the mandible forward. The parts may be fused together into a monoblock, nonadjustable appliance, or they may be connected in such a way as to allow some degree of mandibular movement and adjustability. TRDs are generally made of silicone in the shape of a bulb or cavity. The tongue is stuck into the bulb, which is then squeezed and released, producing a suction that holds the tongue forward in the bulb. TRDs have not been approved by the FDA for the treatment of OSA.

Numerous uncontrolled studies have reported varying degrees of success with different types of OAs, ranging from 76% for mild OSA to 40% for more severe OSA.[42-47] Two large prospective studies of patients with a broad range of severity reported an average overall 1-year success rates (AHI <10/hr) of 54%.[47,48] Two randomized, crossover, controlled trials with a total of 97 patients in whom adjustable appliances were used reported complete success (AHI <5/hr) or partial success (AHI reduced by >50% but with an AHI >5/hr) in 63% of subjects.[49,50] A recent comprehensive review of the subject found that the success rate of OAs as defined by the achievement of an AHI of less than 10 per hour was 52%.[37] It should be noted, however, that in some patients, OAs may worsen the symptoms of OSA.[51-54]

Long-term compliance data for OAs are lacking; however, data for 1 year compliance ranges from 48% to 84%.[55,56] Available data suggest that compliance decreases somewhat over time, with compliance at 4 years reported at 62% to 76%.[48,57] A recent report found that 5.7 years after OA treatment was begun, 64% of patients were still using their appliance, 93.7% wore it for longer than 4

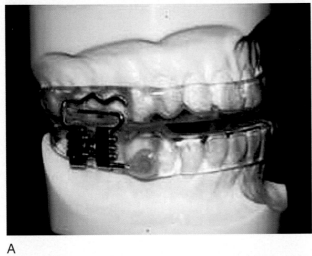

A

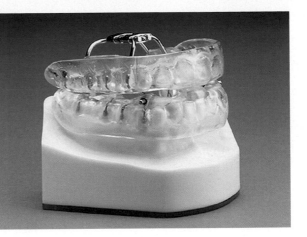

B

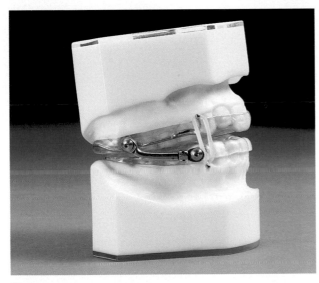

C

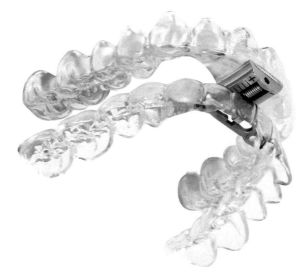

D

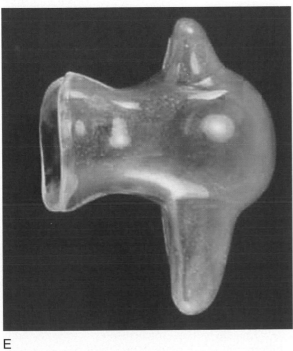

E

Figure 10-10. Examples of oral appliances used for the treatment of obstructive sleep apnea. **A,** Adjustable PM Positioner (Innovative Sleep Products, St. Louis Park, Minn). **B,** Klearway (UBC Sleep Apnea Dental Clinic, Vancouver, BC, Canada). **C,** Herbst (Dentaurum Inc., Newtown, Pa). **D,** TAP-T (Airway Management, Inc., Dallas, Tex). **E,** Tongue-stabilizing device.

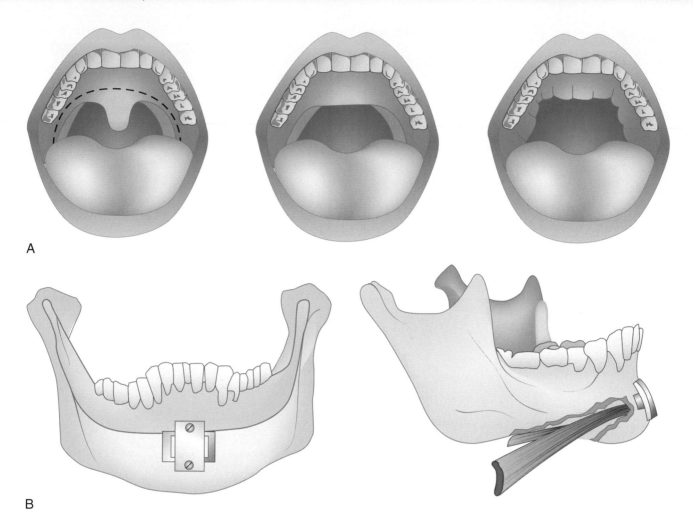

Figure 10-11. Surgical procedures of the upper airway used to treat obstructive sleep apnea.
A, Uvulopalatopharyngoplasty (UPPP). **B,** Genioglossus advancement (GA)

hours a night, and 95% were satisfied with the treatment.[58]

OAs are generally well tolerated, but adverse effects are common.[37] Fortunately, most adverse effects are minor and transient and resolve quickly upon removal of the appliance. Commonly reported adverse effects include temporomandibular (TM) joint pain, muscular pain, tooth pain, hypersalivation, TM joint sounds, dry mouth, gum irritation, and morning-after occlusal changes. On occasion, TM joint pain or dysfunction may become severe enough to prevent continued use of the appliance. Persistent occlusal changes, including retroclination of the maxillary incisors, proclination of the mandibular incisors, and a posterior open bite, have also been reported. Should these occur, and should they be a matter of concern for the patient, orthodontic or restorative treatment may be required for correction.

When compared with CPAP, OAs are not as effective in reducing AHI; however, patients tend to prefer OAs over the use of CPAP.[37] Very few studies have compared OAs with upper airway surgery; however, in two studies in which OAs were compared with uvulopalatopharyngoplasty, OAs were found to be superior.[59,60]

The American Academy of Sleep Medicine has recently published revised guidelines for the use of OAs in the treatment of patients with snoring and OSA.[61]

Oral appliances are recommended for the following:
• Patients with primary snoring;
• Patients with mild to moderate OSA who prefer OAs to CPAP, who do not respond to CPAP, who are not appropriate candidates for CPAP, or who fail treatment attempts with CPAP or behavioral measures; and
• Patients with severe OSA who have failed an initial trial of CPAP

It is further noted that upper airway surgery may supersede the use of OAs in patients for whom these operations are predicted to be highly effective (e.g., tonsillectomy and adenoidectomy, craniofacial operations, tracheostomy).

Upper Airway Surgery

A variety of surgical procedures have been advocated to treat OSA, including tracheostomy, tonsillectomy, adenoidectomy, nasal septoplasty, turbinate reduction, uvulopalatopharyngoplasty (UPPP), laser-assisted uvulo-

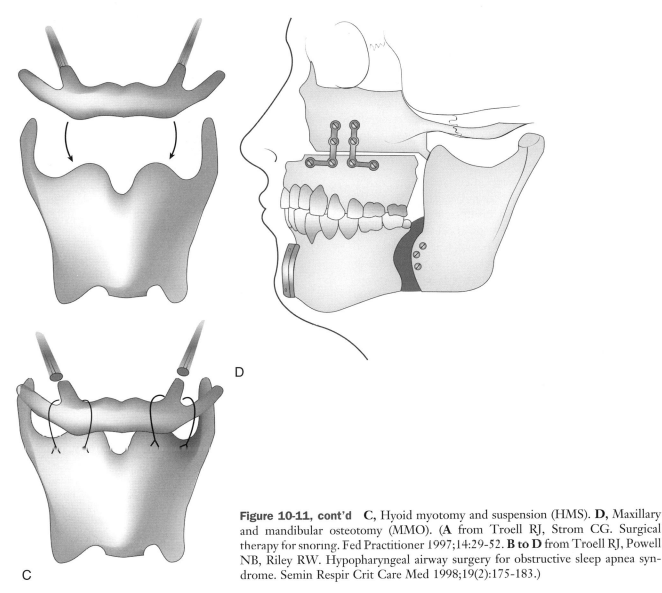

Figure 10-11, cont'd C, Hyoid myotomy and suspension (HMS). **D,** Maxillary and mandibular osteotomy (MMO). (**A** from Troell RJ, Strom CG. Surgical therapy for snoring. Fed Practitioner 1997;14:29-52. **B to D** from Troell RJ, Powell NB, Riley RW. Hypopharyngeal airway surgery for obstructive sleep apnea syndrome. Semin Respir Crit Care Med 1998;19(2):175-183.)

palatoplasty (LAUP), radiofrequency volumetric tissue reduction (RVTR), genioglossus advancement-hyoid myotomy and suspension (GAHMS), tongue base reduction, and maxillary and mandibular advancement osteotomy (MMO) (Figure 10-11). Some of these procedures have relatively modest success rates when performed alone. For example, UPPP, the surgical procedure most commonly performed to correct OSA, has a success rate of less than 50%.[62] Others, however, such as MMO or performance of a combination of procedures, have much higher success rates. The LAUP procedure was found not to be effective and is not recommended for treatment of OSA.[63]

Two forms of surgery are highly effective. Tracheostomy, which bypasses all obstruction in the entire upper airway, is uniformly effective in curing OSA. Its use is limited, however, in that it is unacceptable to most patients but may be used for the occasional patient with very severe OSA who is intolerant of CPAP and who requires urgent treatment.[35] Another predictably successful procedure is the removal of adenoids and tonsils in children. Adenotonsillar hypertrophy is the most common

cause of upper airway obstruction (OSA) in children; adenotonsillectomy is curative in 75% to 100% of cases.[64]

Because upper airway surgery is invasive and irreversible, efforts must be made to identify the site(s) of obstruction to determine which surgical approach should be used and to avoid unnecessary or ineffective surgery.[65] A number of imaging techniques and laboratory modalities, including cephalometrics, computed tomography (CT) scanning, nasopharyngoscopy, and measurements of regional pharyngeal pressure, flow, and resistance, have been used for this purpose. A phased approach to surgery, beginning with less aggressive procedures and advancing to more aggressive interventions when the response to initial treatment is inadequate, is often advocated. The Powell-Riley protocol[66] is a two-phase approach that advocates surgical treatment directed toward specific regions of obstruction during sleep. Phase 1 procedures include nasal reconstruction, UPPP, GAHMS, and possibly, radiofrequency techniques to the soft palate or tongue. Reported success for phase 1 surgical procedures ranges between 23% and 67%.[67] If patients fail to improve after completion of phase 1, they become candidates for phase 2. Phase 2 procedures include MMO and surgical or radiofrequency reduction of the base of the tongue. Reported success with phase 2 procedures ranges between 75% and 100%.[67] Reevaluation of patients after each procedure with the use of PSG is necessary for minimizing further unnecessary surgery. Because of the significant difference in success rates between phase 1 and phase 2 procedures, some surgeons advocate going directly to MMO and bypassing phase 1 interventions.

Complications and adverse effects of upper airway surgery vary with the procedure. For example, UPPP may result in velopharyngeal insufficiency, velopharyngeal stenosis, voice changes, postoperative bleeding, postoperative airway obstruction, and death.[35] MMO and GAHMS may result in lip, cheek, or chin paresthesia or anesthesia, tooth injury, postoperative bleeding, postoperative airway obstruction, and changes in facial appearance.

REFERENCES

1. Hoffstein V. Snoring and upper airway resistance. In Kryger M, Roth T, Dement W (eds). Principles and Practice of Sleep Medicine, 4th ed. Philadelphia, Elsevier, 2005, pp 1001-1012.
2. Lindberg E, Taube A, Janson C, et al. A 10-year follow-up of snoring in men. Chest 1998;114:1048-1055.
3. Anuntaseree W, Kuasirikul S, Suntornlohanakul S. Natural history of snoring and obstructive sleep apnea in Thai school-age children. Pediatr Pulmonol 2005;39:415-420.
4. Pien GW, Fife D, Pack AI, et al. Changes in symptoms of sleep-disordered breathing during pregnancy. Sleep 2005;28:1299-1305.
5. Guilleminault C, Bassiri A. Clinical features and evaluation of obstructive sleep apnea–hypopnea syndrome and upper airway resistance syndrome. In Kryger M, Roth T, Dement W (eds). Principles and Practice of Sleep Medicine, 4th ed. Philadelphia, Elsevier, 2005, pp 1043-1052.
6. Balbani AP, Weber SA, Montovani JC. Update in obstructive sleep apnea syndrome in children. Rev Bras Otorhinolaringol (Engl Ed) 2005;71:74-80.
7. Schwab R, Kuna S, Remmers JE. Anatomy and physiology of upper airway obstruction. In Kryger M, Roth T, Dement W (eds). Principles and Practice of Sleep Medicine. Philadelphia, Elsevier, 2005, pp 983-1000.
8. Morrison DL, Launois SH, Isono S, et al. Pharyngeal narrowing and closing pressures in patients with obstructive sleep apnea. Am Rev Respir Dis 1993;148:606-611.
9. Schwab RJ, Pasirstein M, Pierson R, et al. Identification of upper airway anatomic risk factors for obstructive sleep apnea with volumetric magnetic resonance imaging. Am J Respir Crit Care Med 2003;168:522-530.
10. Series F. Upper airway muscles awake and asleep. Sleep Med Rev 2002;6:229-242.
11. Carskadon M, Dement W. Normal human sleep: An overview. In Kryger M, Roth T, Dement W (eds). Prin-ciples and Practice of Sleep Medicine, 4th ed. Philadelphia, Elsevier, 2005, pp 13-23.
12. George CF. Sleepiness, sleep apnea, and driving: Still miles to go before we safely sleep. Am J Respir Crit Care Med 2004;170:927-928.
13. Dincer HE, O'Neill W. Deleterious effects of sleep-disordered breathing on the heart and vascular system. Respiration 2006;73:124-130.
14. Chobanian AV, Bakris GL, Black HR, et al. Seventh report of the Joint National Committee on Prevention, Detection, Evaluation, and Treatment of High Blood Pressure. Hypertension 2003;42:1206-1252.
15. Yaggi HK, Concato J, Kernan WN, et al. Obstructive sleep apnea as a risk factor for stroke and death. N Engl J Med 2005;353:2034-2041.
16. Mehra R, Benjamin EJ, Shahar E, et al. Association of nocturnal arrhythmias with sleep-disordered breathing: The Sleep Heart Health Study. Am J Respir Crit Care Med 2006;173:910-916.
17. Javaheri S, Wexler L. Prevalence and treatment of breathing disorders during sleep in patients with heart failure. Curr Treat Options Cardiovasc Med 2005;7:295-306.
18. Javaheri S. Sleep and cardiovascular disease: Present and future. In Kryger M, Roth T, Dement W (eds). Principles and Practice of Sleep Medicine, 4th ed. Philadelphia, Elsevier, 2005, pp 1157-1160.
19. Punjabi NM, Shahar E, Redline S, et al. Sleep-disordered breathing, glucose intolerance, and insulin resistance: The Sleep Heart Health Study. Am J Epidemiol 2004;160:521-530.
20. Young T, Peppard PE, Gottlieb DJ. Epidemiology of obstructive sleep apnea: A population health perspective. Am J Respir Crit Care Med 2002;165:1217-1239.
21. Ward Flemons W, McNicholas WT. Clinical prediction of the sleep apnea syndrome. Sleep Med Rev 1997;1:19-32.
22. Redline S. Age-related differences in sleep apnea: Generalizability of findings in older populations. In Kuna S (ed). Sleep and Respiration in Aging Adults. New York, Elsevier, 1991, pp 189-194.
23. Kripke DF, Ancoli-Israel S, Klauber MR, et al. Prevalence of sleep-disordered breathing in ages 40-64 years: A population-based survey. Sleep 1997;20:65-76.
24. Katz I, Stradling J, Slutsky AS, et al. Do patients with obstructive sleep apnea have thick necks? Am Rev Respir Dis 1990;141(5 Pt 1):1228-1231.
25. Davies RJ, Ali NJ, Stradling JR. Neck circumference and other clinical features in the diagnosis of the obstructive sleep apnoea syndrome. Thorax 1992;47:101-105.
26. The International Classification of Sleep Disorders: Diagnostic and Coding Manual, 2nd ed. Westchester, Ill, American Academy of Sleep Medicine, 2005.
27. He J, Kryger MH, Zorick FJ, et al. Mortality and apnea index in obstructive sleep apnea: Experience in 385 male patients. Chest 1988;94:9-14.
28. Peppard PE, Young T, Palta M, et al. Longitudinal study of moderate weight change and sleep-disordered breathing. JAMA 2000;284:3015-3021.
29. Peppard PE, Young T. Exercise and sleep-disordered breathing: An association independent of body habitus. Sleep 2004;27:480-484.

30. Scharf MB, Brannen DE, McDannold M. A subjective evaluation of a nasal dilator on sleep and snoring. Ear Nose Throat J 1994;73:395-401.

31. Oksenberg A, Silverberg DS. The effect of body posture on sleep-related breathing disorders: Facts and therapeutic implications. Sleep Med Rev 1998;2:139-162.

32. Kuna ST, Bedi DG, Ryckman C. Effect of nasal airway positive pressure on upper airway size and configuration. Am Rev Respir Dis 1988;138:969-975.

33. Schwab RJ, Goldberg AN. Upper airway assessment: Radiographic and other imaging techniques. Otolaryngol Clin North Am 1998;31:931-968.

34. Kushida CA, Littner MR, Hirshkowitz M, et al. Practice parameters for the use of continuous and bilevel positive airway pressure devices to treat adult patients with sleep-related breathing disorders. Sleep 2006;29:375-380.

35. Phillips B, Kryger M. Management of obstructive sleep apnea. In Kryger M, Roth T, Dement W (eds). Principles and Practice of Sleep Medicine, 4th ed. Philadelphia, Elsevier, 2005, pp 1109-1121.

36. Gay P, Weaver T, Loube D, Iber C. Evaluation of positive airway pressure treatment for sleep related breathing disorders in adults. Sleep 2006;29:381-401.

37. Ferguson KA, Cartwright R, Rogers R, Schmidt-Nowara W. Oral appliances for snoring and obstructive sleep apnea: A review. Sleep 2006;29:244-262.

38. Rama AN, Tekwani SH, Kushida CA. Sites of obstruction in obstructive sleep apnea. Chest 2002;122:1139-1147.

39. Bennett LS, Davies RJ, Stradling JR. Oral appliances for the management of snoring and obstructive sleep apnoea. Thorax 1998;53(suppl 2):S58-S64.

40. Ryan CF, Love LL, Peat D, et al. Mandibular advancement oral appliance therapy for obstructive sleep apnoea: Effect on awake calibre of the velopharynx. Thorax 1999;54:972-977.

41. Liu Y, Zeng X, Fu M, et al. Effects of a mandibular repositioner on obstructive sleep apnea. Am J Orthod Dentofacial Orthop 2000;118:248-256.

42. Lowe AA, Sjoholm TT, Ryan CF, et al. Treatment, airway and compliance effects of a titratable oral appliance. Sleep 2000;23(suppl 4):S172-S178.

43. Marklund M, Franklin KA, Sahlin C, Lundgren R. The effect of a mandibular advancement device on apneas and sleep in patients with obstructive sleep apnea. Chest 1998;113:707-713.

44. Menn SJ, Loube DI, Morgan TD, et al. The mandibular repositioning device: Role in the treatment of obstructive sleep apnea. Sleep 1996;19:794-800.

45. Pancer J, Al-Faifi S, Al-Faifi M, Hoffstein V. Evaluation of variable mandibular advancement appliance for treatment of snoring and sleep apnea. Chest 1999;116:1511-1518.

46. Pellanda A, Despland PA, Pasche P. The anterior mandibular positioning device for the treatment of obstructive sleep apnoea syndrome: Experience with the Serenox. Clin Otolaryngol Allied Sci 1999;24:134-141.

47. Yoshida K. Effects of a mandibular advancement device for the treatment of sleep apnea syndrome and snoring on respiratory function and sleep quality. Cranio 2000;18:98-105.

48. Marklund M, Stenlund H, Franklin KA. Mandibular advancement devices in 630 men and women with obstructive sleep apnea and snoring: Tolerability and predictors of treatment success. Chest 2004;125:1270-1278.

49. Gotsopoulos H, Chen C, Qian J, Cistulli PA. Oral appliance therapy improves symptoms in obstructive sleep apnea: A randomized, controlled trial. Am J Respir Crit Care Med 2002;166:743-748.

50. Mehta A, Qian J, Petocz P, et al. A randomized, controlled study of a mandibular advancement splint for obstructive sleep apnea. Am J Respir Crit Care Med 2001;163:1457-1461.

51. Ferguson KA, Ono T, Lowe AA, et al. A short-term controlled trial of an adjustable oral appliance for the treatment of mild to moderate obstructive sleep apnoea. Thorax 1997;52:362-368.

52. Hans MG, Nelson S, Luks VG, et al. Comparison of two dental devices for treatment of obstructive sleep apnea syndrome (OSAS). Am J Orthod Dentofacial Orthop 1997;111:562-570.

53. Henke KG, Frantz DE, Kuna ST. An oral elastic mandibular advancement device for obstructive sleep apnea. Am J Respir Crit Care Med 2000;161(2 Pt 1):420-425.

54. Schmidt-Nowara WW, Meade TE, Hays MB. Treatment of snoring and obstructive sleep apnea with a dental orthosis. Chest 1991;99:1378-1385.

55. Clark GT, Sohn JW, Hong CN. Treating obstructive sleep apnea and snoring: Assessment of an anterior mandibular positioning device. J Am Dent Assoc 2000;131:765-771.

56. Fransson AM, Tegelberg A, Leissner L, et al. Effects of a mandibular protruding device on the sleep of patients with obstructive sleep apnea and snoring problems: A 2-year follow-up. Sleep Breath 2003;7:131-141.

57. Ringqvist M, Walker-Engstrom ML, Tegelberg A, Ringqvist I. Dental and skeletal changes after 4 years of obstructive sleep apnea treatment with a mandibular advancement device: A prospective, randomized study. Am J Orthod Dentofacial Orthop 2003;124:53-60.

58. de Almeida FR, Lowe AA, Tsuiki S, et al. Long-term compliance and side effects of oral appliances used for the treatment of snoring and obstructive sleep apnea syndrome. J Clin Sleep Med 2005;1:143-149.

59. Walker-Engstrom ML, Tegelberg A, Wilhelmsson B, Ringqvist I. Four-year follow-up of treatment with dental appliance or uvulopalatopharyngoplasty in patients with obstructive sleep apnea: A randomized study. Chest 2002;121:739-746.

60. Wilhelmsson B, Tegelberg A, Walker-Engstrom ML, et al. A prospective randomized study of a dental appliance compared with uvulopalatopharyngoplasty in the treatment of obstructive sleep apnoea. Acta Otolaryngol 1999;119:503-509.

61. Kushida CA, Morgenthaler TI, Littner MR, et al. Practice parameters for the treatment of snoring and obstructive sleep apnea with oral appliances: An update for 2005. Sleep 2006;29:240-243.

62. Sher AE, Schechtman KB, Piccirillo JF. The efficacy of surgical modifications of the upper airway in adults with obstructive sleep apnea syndrome. Sleep 1996;19:156-177.

63. Littner M, Kushida CA, Hartse K, et al. Practice parameters for the use of laser-assisted uvulopalatoplasty: An update for 2000. Sleep 2001;24:603-619.

64. Schechter MS. Technical report: Diagnosis and management of childhood obstructive sleep apnea syndrome. Pediatrics 2002;109:e69.

65. Practice parameters for the treatment of obstructive sleep apnea in adults: The efficacy of surgical modifications of the upper airway. Report of the American Sleep Disorders Association. Sleep 1996;19:152-155.

66. Powell NB, Riley RW, Guilleminault C. Surgical management of sleep-disordered breathing. In Kryger M, Roth T, Dement W (eds). Principles and Practice of Sleep Medicine, 4th ed. Philadelphia, Elsevier, 2005, pp 1081-1097.

67. Ryan CF. Sleep × 9: An approach to treatment of obstructive sleep apnoea/hypopnoea syndrome including upper airway surgery. Thorax 2005;60:595-604.

PART FOUR

Gastrointestinal Disease

Liver Disease

chapter 11

Liver dysfunction may be attributed to a number of causes, including lifestyle habits and other acquired infections and conditions. The patient with liver disease presents a significant management challenge for the dentist because the liver plays a vital role in metabolic functions, including secretion of bile needed for fat absorption, conversion of sugar to glycogen, and excretion of bilirubin, a waste product of hemoglobin metabolism. Impairment of liver function can lead to abnormalities in the metabolism of amino acids, ammonia, protein, carbohydrates, and lipids (triglycerides and cholesterol). Many biochemical functions performed by the liver, such as synthesis of coagulation factors and drug metabolism, may be adversely affected in the dental patient with acute or chronic liver disease. So, along with impaired drug metabolism, significant bleeding may be a dental problem. Viral hepatitis and alcoholic liver disease are two of the more common liver disorders. In many cases, the liver dysfunction continues to progress over time. Therefore, patients with liver disorders are of significant interest to the dentist, as is their proper management.[1]

HEPATITIS

DEFINITION

Hepatitis is inflammation of the liver that may result from infectious or other causes. Examples of hepatitis with infectious causes are viral hepatitis, infectious mononucleosis, secondary syphilis, and tuberculosis. Noninfectious hepatitis can result from excessive or prolonged use of toxic substances (e.g., drugs [acetaminophen, alcohol, halothane, ketoconazole, methyldopa, methotrexate]; more commonly, alcohol).[1,2]

Etiology

Acute viral hepatitis is the most common form of infectious hepatitis. Five distinct viruses—types A, B, C, D, and E—are associated with this disease (Table 11-1). These viruses each belong to a different family with distinct antigenic properties. They have little in common except for the target organ they infect and some epidemiologic characteristics. Hepatitis A was called *infectious hepatitis*, and hepatitis B was referred to as *serum hepatitis*. Hepatitis D (also known as *delta*) occurs only in association with hepatitis B. Hepatitis C and hepatitis E were known as *non-A non-B hepatitis (NANB)*. They were distinguished by the route of transmission. The parenterally acquired form now is known as *hepatitis C*, and the community-acquired form and enteric subtypes (found in India, Southeast Asia, and Central America) are called *hepatitis E.*

In up to 20% of cases of hepatitis, a standard virus cannot be identified, and the disease is not associated with toxic, metabolic, or genetic conditions. Viruses may be causative. The term *hepatitis non–A-E* is used to describe these conditions. Hepatitis F virus, hepatitis G virus, and transfusion-transmitted virus (TTV) are candidate viruses associated with hepatitis non–A-E. Definitive evidence that these viruses play a pathogenic role in liver disease is lacking.[1,2]

EPIDEMIOLOGY

Incidence and Prevalence

Hepatitis is a worldwide health problem, with more than 5 million new cases occurring annually and more than 300 million persons across the globe carrying the viruses. Regional incidence rates are lowest in the Western hemisphere and northern regions and highest in the Eastern hemisphere and tropical regions. In the United States, viral hepatitis ranks seventh behind chlamydia, gonorrhea, varicella, acquired immunodeficiency virus (AIDS), salmonellosis, and syphilis in reportable infectious diseases. More than 4 million Americans are chronic carriers of hepatitis viruses.[3,4]

TABLE **11-1**
Features of Hepatitis Viruses

	Hepatitis A	Hepatitis B	Hepatitis C	Hepatitis D	Hepatitis E
OLD TERMINOLOGY	Infectious hepatitis	Serum hepatitis	Posttransfusion hepatitis non-A non-B	Delta hepatitis	Hepatitis non-A non-D
FAMILY AND TYPES	Picornavirus 1 serotype, 7 genotypes	Hepadnavirus	Flavivirus 6 major genotypes (40 related subtypes)	Satellite 3 genotypes	Calicivirus 3 genotypes
VIRION STRUCTURE	28-nm RNA nonenveloped virus	42-nm DNA enveloped virus, enveloped Dane particles, spherical and tubular particles	30- to 80-nm ss +RNA enveloped virus	35- to 40-nm defective RNA nonenveloped virus (uses HBsAg for viral envelope)	32- to 34-nm nonenveloped RNA virus
INCUBATION	15-50 days X = 25 days	45-180 days X = 75 days	14-180 days X = 50 days	15-150 days X = 35 days	15-60 days X = 40 days
MAIN ROUTE OF TRANSMISSION	Fecal/oral route	Parenteral, sexual contact*	Parenteral, sexual contact* (low risk)	Parenteral, sexual contact*	Fecal/oral route
DIAGNOSIS[†‡]	Anti-HAV IgG	HBsAg (infectious) Anti-HBsAg (recovery) Anti-HBc (acute, persistently infected, or previously infected nonprotective) HBeAg (infectious) Anti-HBeAg (clearing/cleared infection)	Anti-HCV (previous infection) HCV RNA (infectivity)	Anti-HDV HD-Ag	Anti-HEV
CHRONIC CARRIER STATE	No	Yes, 90% risk of becoming carrier if infected as neonate; 25%-50% risk of becoming carrier if infected as infant; 5%-10% risk of becoming carrier if infected as adult	Yes, risk of becoming carrier is 80%-90%	Yes, carrier state in 20%-70%	No
COMPLICATIONS[§] OF THE LIVER	Rare	Yes, increased risk of liver cirrhosis and hepatocellular carcinoma (HCC) after 25-30 years of infection	Yes, 10-fold increased risk of liver cirrhosis within 20 years; 1%-5% of carriers develop HCC by 20 years; risk of HCC with chronic HCV exceeds risk with chronic HBV	Yes	Rare morbidity and mortality except in pregnant women
ASSOCIATED CLINICAL SYNDROMES		Yes	Yes		

TABLE 11-1
Features of Hepatitis Viruses—cont'd

	Hepatitis A	Hepatitis B	Hepatitis C	Hepatitis D	Hepatitis E
IMMUNIZATION PASSIVE	Immune globulin IG (0.02 mg/kg)	Hepatitis B immune globulin (HBIG) (0.06 mg/kg)	Not available	Not available	Not available
ACTIVE	Harivax, Vaqta, and Twinrix	Recombivax, Engerix,‖ and Twinrix	None (difficult development because of the many genotypes)	Yes; protected with Recombivax, Engerix,‖ and Twinrix	Genentech has applied for vaccine patent

X, Mean; HCC, hepatocellular carcinoma.

*Risk groups include IDUs, HCWs, hemodialysis patients, low socioeconomic level, sexual/household contacts of infected persons, persons with multiple sex partners, and history of transfusion prior to 1991.

†Diagnostic markers of viral hepatitis include elevation of aspartate aminotransferase, alanine aminotransferase, gamma-glutamyl transferase, white blood cell count, and prothrombin time.

‡Preicteric phase: anorexia, nausea, vomiting, fatigue, myalgia, malaise, and fever.

Icterus: Jaundice, discolored stool, dark urine, hepatosplenomegaly, bleeding disorder; serum sickness–like features (arthralgia, rash, angioedema) in 5% to 10%.

§Risk for complications and severe liver disease increases with coinfection of hepatitis B virus and hepatitis C virus and chronic alcohol consumption.

‖Immunization recommended for dental personnel.

During the period from 1980 to 1995, approximately 22,000 to 36,000 cases of hepatitis A were reported annually in the United States, representing an estimated average of 271,000 infections per year when anicteric disease and asymptomatic infections are taken in account.[1] During 1995 and 1996, highly effective hepatitis A vaccines became available in the United States for use among persons older than 2 years of age, providing an opportunity for substantially reduced hepatitis A incidence and potentially eliminating indigenous transmission of hepatitis A virus (HAV).[3]

Hepatitis A occurrence declined for several years; 32,859 cases were reported in 1966 in the United States, whereas 21,532 cases were reported in 1983. Since 1983, a slight increase in reported cases has occurred, with the latest report (in 1998) showing 23,229 cases. Overall, the Centers for Disease Control (CDC) estimates that between 125,000 and 200,000 cases of hepatitis A occur annually. Approximately 47% of acute viral hepatitis cases reported in the United States are caused by HAV.[3]

Between 140,000 and 320,000 new HBV infections occur in the United States annually. This represents approximately 27% of reported cases of acute hepatitis and more than a 50% decrease in the number of cases reported during the past decade. This downward trend likely will continue as a national strategy for eliminating hepatitis B virus (HBV) transmission is implemented. Approximately half of identified patients require hospitalization, and more than 100 infected persons (0.2% to 2%) die annually of fulminant disease. Most infections occur in young adults, and 10% of cases occur in infants and young children. Many transfusion recipients and hemophiliacs who received factor replacement during the 1960s and 1970s were infected with HBV. The current prevalence of volunteer blood donations in the United States that are antibody positive against HBV is 0.2%.

Health professionals estimate that 1.25 million persons in the United States are chronic HBV carriers.[4]

Hepatitis B vaccination is the most effective measure taken to prevent HBV infection and its consequences. Since they were first issued in 1982, recommendations for hepatitis B vaccination have evolved into a comprehensive strategy for eliminating HBV transmission in the United States. A primary focus of this strategy is universal vaccination of infants to prevent early childhood HBV infection and to eventually protect adolescents and adults from infection. Other components include routine screening of all pregnant women for hepatitis B surface antigen (HBsAg) and postexposure immunoprophylaxis of infants born to HBsAg-positive women, vaccination of children and adolescents who were not previously vaccinated, and vaccination of unvaccinated adults who are at increased risk for infection.[5-8]

To date, this immunization strategy has been implemented with considerable success. Recent estimates indicate that more than 95% of pregnant women are tested for HBsAg, and case management has been effective in ensuring high levels of initiation and completion of postexposure immunoprophylaxis among identified infants born to HBsAg-positive women. Hepatitis B vaccine has been successfully integrated into the childhood vaccine schedule, and infant vaccine coverage levels are now equivalent to those of other vaccines in the childhood schedule. During the years from 1990 to 2004, the incidence of acute hepatitis B in the United States declined 75%. The greatest decline (94%) occurred among children and adolescents, coincident with an increase in hepatitis B vaccine coverage. As of 2004, among U.S. children aged 19 to 35 months, more than 92% had been fully vaccinated with three doses of hepatitis B vaccine. This success can be attributed in part to the established infrastructure for vaccine delivery to children and to federal support for perinatal hepatitis B prevention programs.[4-8]

Vaccine coverage among adolescents has also increased substantially. Preliminary data show that 50% to 60% of adolescents aged 13 to 15 years have records that indicate that they received vaccination (with three doses) against hepatitis B (CDC, unpublished data, 2003). As of November 2005, a total of 34 states required vaccination for entry into middle school.[9] Some programs provide hepatitis B vaccine to youth who engage in behaviors that place them at high risk for HBV infection (e.g., injection drug use, having more than one sex partner, male sexual activity with other males), and adolescent hepatitis B vaccination is included as a Health Plan Employer Data Information Set (HEDIS) measure.[4]

Hepatitis C virus (HCV) is a major cause of acute and chronic hepatitis worldwide. Since the time that diagnostic testing was implemented, the rate of new infections declined from an estimated 240,000 in the 1980s to 36,000 reported annually in the United States in the late 1990s. Carrier rates for HCV range from 0.2% to 2.2% in developed countries (0.4% of volunteer blood donations in the United States are antibody positive to HCV). Higher rates (2% to 10%) have been reported in developing nations and inner cities. The prevalence in patients on dialysis ranges from 0.5% to approximately 40%, and rates approach 90% in organ recipients after they have donated an HCV RNA positive organ. Health professionals estimate that 3.5 million to 4 million Americans have chronic HCV infection, making this disease the most common bloodborne infection in the United States. Approximately 10,000 persons die each year in the United States because of HCV-related liver disease. Current estimates predict that mortality rates caused by chronic hepatitis C infection will triple in the United States over the next 10 years, rivaling those of human immunodeficiency virus (HIV).[3]

The incidence of hepatitis D virus (HDV) infection correlates directly with the worldwide rate of chronic HBV infection. Countries with low rates of chronic HBV infection have a low prevalence of HDV infection. In contrast, countries with high endemicity for HBV infection (Southeast Asia and China) have a greater prevalence of HDV infection. HDV accounts for approximately 7500 infections in the United States annually. The prevalence of HDV infection among HBsAg-positive patients is low in the general population (1.4% to 8% in blood donors). The prevalence of HDV infection is highest in persons who are injection drug users (20% to 53%) and those who have hemophilia[4] (48% to 80%). Hepatitis D has a mortality rate of 2% to 20%.[1]

The exact prevalence of hepatitis E virus (HEV) in the United States is not known but is believed to range between 1% and 5%. Reported cases of HEV in the United States have been isolated and have consisted of people who recently traveled to endemic regions (i.e., Asia, India, Southeast Asia, Middle East, Central America, and Mexico). HEV is not a significant factor in the United States, although it has produced a 20% fatality rate in pregnant women during the third trimester of pregnancy. HEV is not considered a problem in developed countries.[1]

Hepatitis A. Hepatitis A virus (HAV) is a 28-nm ribonucleic acid (RNA) virus of the Picornaviridae family that replicates in the liver, is excreted in the bile, and is shed in the stool. HAV has been isolated from feces, grown in culture, and examined by electron microscopy. One serotype and seven genotypes have been identified. Serologic tests for HAV and its antibodies—anti-HAV, immunoglobulin M (IgM), and anti-HAV immunoglobulin G (IgG)—are readily available.

Transmission of HAV occurs almost exclusively through fecal contamination of food or water, usually by traveling in an endemic region, or by direct contact with an infected person.

Common sources include contaminated wells or water supplies, restaurants, and raw shellfish. Because the reservoir for infection is frequently a common food or water source, an occurrence of hepatitis A often becomes an epidemic. Transmission is enhanced by poor personal hygiene, which places school-aged youngsters, food handlers, daycare workers, and travelers in developing countries at greater risk for contracting the disease. Transmission by contaminated blood products is rare, occurring early during the course of the infection when titers in blood can be high and the patient is most infectious.[1,2]

Hepatitis A is a common disease, with serologic evidence of infection noted in approximately 40% of urban populations in the United States. Its incubation period ranges from 15 to 50 days and averages 25 days. Persons of any age may be infected; however, the disease occurs primarily in children and young adults and is often asymptomatic. Hepatitis A tends to be of mild severity and self-limiting; it lasts a couple of weeks and often goes undiagnosed. Hepatitis A may be diagnosed by signs and symptoms such as fatigue, fever, lymphadenopathy, gastrointestinal (GI) upset/nausea, night sweats, and possibly, icteric jaundice. Serologic testing for IgM anti-HAV and IgG anti-HAV may reveal a recent infection. No carrier state is known to exist for it, and recovery usually conveys immunity against reinfection.[1,2]

HAV infection may be effectively prevented by administration of the HAV immune globulin prophylactically or within 2 weeks of exposure. In 1995, two vaccines were developed as a form of immunized protection: Havrix (hepatitis A vaccine, inactivated; GlaxoSmithKline, Research Triangle Park, NC) and Vaqta (hepatitis A vaccine, inactivated; Merck & Co., Whitehouse Station, NJ).[1,2]

Hepatitis B. Hepatitis B virus (HBV) is a deoxyribonucleic (DNA) virus of the Hepadnaviridae family that was first identified in 1965. This virus replicates predominantly in hepatocytes and to a lesser extent in stem cells in the pancreas, bone marrow, and spleen. Electron microscopy has determined several virus-associated particles related to hepatitis B infection. The intact HBV, or Dane particle, is composed of an outer shell and an inner core. The outer shell is the HBsAg. It circulates in the blood as 22-nm spherical and tubular particles for up to 6 months after infection, depending on resolution of the infection. The antibody responsible for clearing the infection is anti-HBs, which signals long-term immunity. The inner core of the particle is the hepatitis B core antigen (HBcAg), with corresponding antibodies IgG anti-HBc and IgM anti-HBc (indicating recent infection). A third particle is the hepatitis B early antigen (HBeAg), an antigenic component derived from cleavage of the core antigen. It is related to hepatitis B infectivity. Its corresponding antibody is anti-HBe. Serologic tests are available for all these antigen/antibody systems, except the HBcAg, which is retained in hepatocytes.[1,2]

Hepatitis B may be transmitted efficiently by percutaneous and permucosal exposure; the most frequent route of transmission in the United States is sexual activity. Exposures that may cause HBV infection include the following:

- Direct percutaneous inoculation, transfusion of infective blood or blood products (serum, plasma, factor concentrates), needle sharing, tattooing, and body piercing
- Indirect percutaneous introduction of infective serum or plasma through minute skin cuts or abrasions
- Absorption of infective serum or plasma through mucosal surfaces of the mouth or eye
- Absorption of infective secretions, such as saliva or semen, through mucosal surfaces, as might occur following heterosexual or homosexual contact
- Transfer of infective serum or plasma via inanimate environmental surfaces or possibly through vectors

Experimental data indicate that fecal transmission of HBV does not occur and airborne spread is not of epidemiologic importance. The incubation period ranges from 45 to 180 days and averages 75 days.[1,2]

The lifetime risk of hepatitis B occurrence among the general population is low; however, some groups have a much higher risk. Included among these are dental personnel and other health care workers, refugees from Indochina and Haiti, residents of mental institutions and prisons, patients on hemodialysis, users of illicit drugs, men who have sex with men, heterosexuals with multiple partners, and recipients of blood transfusions (Box 11-1). The risk of infection is directly related to exposure to blood, resulting in a reported prevalence rate of past infection among general dentists in the 1980s ranging from 13% to 30%. Among oral surgeons, the prevalence rate was as high as 38%. More recent reports cite the prevalence for general dentists at 7.8% to 8.9% and for oral surgeons at 21%. This reduction presumably reflects the effectiveness of vaccination and infection control measures.[5-7]

BOX 11-1

Persons at Substantial Risk for Hepatitis B Who Should Receive Vaccine

- Individuals with occupational risk
- Health care workers
- Public safety workers
- Clients and staff of institutions for the developmentally disabled
- Hemodialysis patients
- Recipients of certain blood products
- Household contacts and sex partners of hepatitis B virus (HBV) carriers
- Adoptees from countries where HBV infection is endemic
- International travelers
- Illicit drug users
- Sexually active homosexual and bisexual men
- Sexually active heterosexual men and women (who have multiple partners)
- Inmates of long-term correctional facilities

From Centers for Disease Control. MMWR 1991;40:14-16.

Although hepatitis B may occur at any age, statistics indicate that the condition is unusual in persons younger than 15 years of age. Of 10,258 cases of type B hepatitis reported to the CDC in 1998, only 282 occurred in patients younger than 15 years of age (2.8%). Compared with hepatitis A, hepatitis B tends to cause greater morbidity and mortality, especially in the very young and in older patients.[7]

Hepatitis C. Hepatitis C virus (HCV) is a 30- to 80-nm-diameter, single-stranded RNA virus of the Flaviviridae family that was identified in 1989. HCV is related to the flaviviruses and the pestiviruses and was previously known as one of the non-A non-B hepatitis viruses (NANB hepatitis). HCV consists of six major genotypes. It causes the most common chronic bloodborne infections in the United States. Serologic tests for the viral antigen and its antibody (anti-HCV) became available in 1991.

HCV is similar to HBV in terms of behavior and characteristics. The incubation period of HCV ranges from 2 weeks to 6 months, with a median of 50 days. Approximately 60% to 90% of HCV cases are transmitted by blood and blood products; approximately 90% of cases of posttransfusion hepatitis were attributed to HCV until routine screening of blood was implemented in 1992. The current risk for posttransfusion hepatitis C in the United States is estimated at 1 in 103,000 patients. Those at greatest risk for this disease are injection drug users and those with large or repeated percutaneous exposures. Injection drug users account for more than 60% of acute HCV infections, and HCV infection is four times more common than HIV in this population. Others at increased risk are patients on hemodialysis, persons who have multiple sexual partners or who have sexual contacts with those who have chronic HCV, health care workers exposed to blood, and recipients of whole blood, blood cellular components, or plasma. The risk of vertical transmission of HCV from infected mother to infant is low, accounting for 5% of cases. Approximately 1% of sexual partners of HCV-infected persons are infected per year. In approximately 30% to 40% of HCV infections, the means of transmission is not known.[1,6,8]

Hepatitis D. Hepatitis D virus (HDV), first described in 1977, is a defective, negative-strand RNA virus that is 35 to 40 nm in diameter. HDV requires HBsAg for its viral envelope and transmissibility, but once inside, a permissive cell replicates without the helper HBV. HDV occurs only in patients with HBV infection, as a coinfection or a superinfection. The hepatitis D antigen (HDAg) and its antibody (anti-HDV) can be detected with serologic testing.

Hepatitis D occurs only as a coinfection with acute hepatitis B or as a superinfection in carriers of hepatitis B. HDV is transmitted parenterally and sexually, similar to HBV. HDV is reported to occur primarily in drug addicts and persons with hemophilia and frequently is associated with more severe fulminant infection than is infection with hepatitis B alone.[1] HDV produces extraordinarily high titers in the blood of infected persons. The incubation period ranges from 15 to 150 days and averages 35 days.[1,6,8]

Hepatitis E. Hepatitis E virus (HEV) is a 32- to 34-nm, nonenveloped RNA-type virus that resembles viruses of the Caliciviridae family. Three genotypes have been detected. This virus is responsible for enterically transmitted (formerly "NANB") hepatitis, a disorder clinically similar to hepatitis A infection. HEV was recognized first in 1983 and was genetically analyzed in 1990. Outbreaks have been documented in developing countries with poor sanitation, such as India, northern Africa, Mexico, and Southeast Asia. Infection by HEV is more common in men than in women. The virus was cloned in 1990, and serologic tests for antigens and antibodies recently became available.[1]

Hepatitis E resembles hepatitis A and is transmitted similarly via fecal/oral contamination. The incubation period ranges from 15 to 60 days, and average incubation lasts 40 days. Viremia occurs during the incubation phase, but the infectious titer has not been determined.

Hepatitis Non–A-E. Cases of acute hepatitis that appear to have a viral origin but that cannot be attributed to any known virus are referred to as *hepatitis non–A-E*. This category includes unknown viruses and emerging viruses associated with hepatitis, such as hepatitis F virus, hepatitis G viruses, and TTV.[1,9]

Occupational Transmission. Little to no risk of transmission of HAV, HEV, and non–A-E hepatitis viruses has been reported to result from occupational exposure of dental health care workers to persons infected with these viruses. In contrast, risk exists for transmission of HBV, and a lesser risk is present for HCV after occupational exposure to infected blood or bodily fluids that contain infected blood. HCV is less infectious and less efficient in transmission when compared with HBV. After percutaneous or other sharp injury of health care workers and exposure to contaminated blood, the risk of contracting HBV is reported to range from 6% to 30%, with potential infectiousness correlating with HBeAg in the serum (i.e., serum with HBeAg and HBsAg may be 10 times more infectious than serum with HBsAg alone). Moreover, HBV can survive for at least 1 week in dried blood on environmental surfaces and on contaminated needles and instruments. In contrast, the seroconversion rate of accidental blood exposure to HCV is between 2% and 8%. For comparison purposes, the risk of contracting HIV after a percutaneous or other sharp injury is 0.3%.[3,10-12]

The role of saliva in HBV transmission, except through percutaneous or permucosal routes, does not appear to be significant. Observations reported to the CDC suggest that transmission of hepatitis B to humans after surface oral contact with HBsAg-positive saliva is unlikely.[7,13] Another study reported that of 19 dental professionals who had cutaneous contact with saliva containing HBsAg and HBeAg, none developed serologic evidence of hepatitis B.[15] Transmission has been reported, however, as a result of a human bite. Permucosal or percutaneous inoculation of infectious saliva is necessary for transmission of hepatitis B. HCV has been detected in saliva. However, HCV is less infectious than HBV and does not appear to be spread through contact with saliva. Spread of HCV rarely has been reported after a human bite and blood splash to the conjunctiva.[9,16,17]

During the past 30 years, HBV transmission has been documented to occur from 9 dental health care workers to dental patients (see Dental Management). Although HCV has not been reported to occur from dental health care worker to patient, it has been reported to be transmitted from two cardiac surgeons to several of their patients. Current data indicate that about 0.7% to 2.0% of general dentists and 2% of oral surgeons are positive for anti-HCV.[12,14,18,19]

Pathophysiology and Complications

Hepatitis viruses replicate in hepatocytes and ultimately damage the host cell. HBV infection produces high serum titers that may reach 10^8 to 10^{11} virions/mL. In contrast, HAV produces a viremia that may reach 10^5 virions/mL in blood but 10^6 to 10^{10} genomes/g in stool.[1]

No single histopathologic lesion is characteristic of viral hepatitis, but the appearances of types A, B, C, D, and E hepatitides are similar and are described together. Commonly, acute viral hepatitis is characterized by ballooning degeneration and necrosis of liver cells (hepatocytes). The entire liver lobule becomes inflamed and consists of lymphocytes and mononuclear phagocytes.[1]

Icterus (jaundice) is associated with hepatitis in approximately 70% of cases of HAV, approximately 30% of cases of HBV infection, and approximately 25% of cases of HCV and HEV. This is caused by an accumulation of bilirubin in the plasma, epithelium, and urine. Bilirubin is a yellowish degradation product of hemoglobin, which is one of the major constituents of bile. Bilirubin normally is transported to the liver by way of the plasma. In the liver, it conjugates with glucuronic acid then is excreted into the intestine, where it aids in the emulsification of fats and stimulates peristalsis. When liver disease is present, bilirubin tends to accumulate in the plasma because of decreased liver metabolism and transport. Jaundice usually becomes clinically apparent when the plasma level of bilirubin approaches 2.5 mg/100 mL (normal is less than 1 mg/100 mL). If plasma bilirubin does not reach this level, the patient is anicteric (without jaundice), thus explaining nonicteric hepatitis.[1]

Most cases of viral hepatitis, especially types A and E, resolve with no complications. HBV, HCV, and HDV may persist and can replicate in the liver when the virus is not completely cleared from the organ. The consequences of hepatitis include recovery, persistent infection (or carrier state), dual infection, chronic active hepatitis, fulminant hepatitis, cirrhosis, hepatocellular carcinoma, and death. Dual infections and chronic consumption of alcohol lead to more severe disease. Approximately 16,000 people die annually because of complications related to hepatitis infection.[1]

Fulminant Hepatitis. A serious complication of acute viral hepatitis is fulminant hepatitis, which is characterized by massive hepatocellular destruction and a mortality rate of approximately 80%. This condition occurs more commonly among the elderly and those with chronic liver disease. Coinfection or superinfection of HBV and HDV or infection by a single hepatitis virus can cause fulminant disease. Mutant strains of these viruses have been proposed to be causative. Each year, more than 100 persons in the United States die of fulminant hepatitis A and E, and approximately 350 persons die of HBV/HDV-associated fulminant disease. HCV rarely causes fulminant hepatitis.[1]

Chronic Infection. Chronic infection (carrier state) is characterized by persistence of low levels of virus in the liver and serum viral antigens (HBsAg, HBeAg, and hepatitis C virus antigen [HCVAg]) for longer than 6 months without signs of liver disease. Individuals with this condition potentially are infectious to others. The rate of carrier establishment varies according to the virus, age, and health of the patient. For example, approximately 50% to 90% of infected infants, 25% of infected children, and 6% to 10% of adults infected with HBV become carriers. In contrast, 70% to 90% of adults infected with HCV develop a persistent carrier state.[20,21] Men and immunosuppressed persons are more com-

monly affected by both viruses. Approximately 0.1% to 0.5% of the general population in the United States (more than 4 million persons) are carriers of HBV and/or HCV, whereas 5% to 15% of the populations of China, Southeast Asia, sub-Saharan Africa, most Pacific Islands, and the Amazon Basin are HBV carriers.[22] This marked difference reflects the endemicity of hepatitis B in these latter countries. The carrier rate of dentists in the United States has decreased, but the risk still is estimated at 3 to 10 times that of the general population. The highest HCV carrier rates are found among injection drug users and persons with hemophilia (20%). Health care workers show approximately 1% to 2% prevalence. The lowest rates of anti-HCV are found among blood donors; about 0.5% to 1.0% are positive. Approximately 2% to 5% of acute coinfections of HBV and HDV progress to chronic infection. Superinfections are more frequent than coinfections, and because of them, more than 70% of persons become chronic carriers.[20,22]

The carrier state may persist for decades or may cause liver disease by progressing to chronic active hepatitis. Chronic active hepatitis is characterized by active virus replication in the liver; HBsAg, HBeAg, or HCVAg in the serum; signs and symptoms of chronic liver disease; persistent hepatic cellular necrosis; and elevated liver enzymes for longer than 6 months. Approximately 3% to 5% of patients infected with HBV, 25% of HBV carriers, and 40% to 50% of those infected with HCV develop chronic active hepatitis.[20,22] HBV- and HCV-related chronic liver destruction and resultant fibrosis lead to cirrhosis in approximately 20% of cases of chronic hepatitis. Approximately 1% to 5% of these patients develop primary hepatocellular carcinoma. An estimated 4000 persons die each year from HBV-related cirrhosis, 10,000 from HCV-related cirrhosis, and more than 800 from HBV- and HCV-related liver cancer. The relationship of liver disease to liver cancer is 30 times to 100 times higher for chronic carriers compared with uninfected persons and is particularly strong in selected Asian populations.[20,22]

CLINICAL PRESENTATION
Signs and Symptoms

After an incubation phase that varies with the infecting virus, approximately 10% of hepatitis A, 60% to 70% of hepatitis C, and 70% to 90% of hepatitis B cases are asymptomatic. When manifestations occur, the clinical features of acute viral hepatitis are similar and are discussed together. Many of the signs and symptoms are common to many viral illnesses and may be described as flulike. This is especially true of the early, or prodromal, phase. Patients classically exhibit three phases of acute illness.[20,22]

The prodromal (preicteric) phase, which usually precedes the onset of jaundice by 1 or 2 weeks, consists of abdominal pain, anorexia, intermittent nausea, vomiting, fatigue, myalgia, malaise, and fever. With hepatitis B, 5%

to 10% of patients demonstrate serum sickness–like manifestations, including arthralgia or arthritis, rash, and angioedema.[20,22]

The icteric phase is heralded by the onset of clinical jaundice, a yellow-brown cast of the eyes, skin, oral mucosa, and urine. Many nonspecific prodromal symptoms may subside, but gastrointestinal symptoms (e.g., anorexia, nausea, vomiting, right upper quadrant pain) may increase, especially early in the phase. Hepatomegaly and splenomegaly frequently are seen. This phase lasts 2 to 8 weeks and is experienced by at least 70% of patients infected with HAV, 30% of those acutely infected with HBV, and 25% to 30% of patients acutely infected with HCV.[20,22]

During the convalescent or recovery (posticteric) phase, symptoms disappear, but hepatomegaly and abnormal liver function values may persist for a variable period. This phase can last for weeks or months, and recovery time for hepatitis B and C is generally longer. The usual sequence includes recovery (clinical and biochemical) within approximately 4 months after the onset of jaundice. HBV infrequently is associated with clinical syndromes, including polyarteritis nodosa, glomerulonephritis, and leukocytoclastic vasculitis. Coagulopathy, encephalopathy, cerebral edema, and fulminant hepatitis are rare.[20,22]

Chronic hepatitis is associated with liver abnormalities but is often asymptomatic for 10 to 30 years. Nonspecific symptoms of chronic hepatitis C (loss of weight, easy fatigue, sleep disorder, difficulty in concentrating, right upper quadrant pain, and liver tenderness) may not appear until hepatic fibrosis, cirrhosis, or hepatocellular carcinoma is present. Hepatic damage is caused by the cytopathic effects of the virus and inflammatory changes related to immune activation. Extrahepatic immunologic disorders associated with chronic HCV infection result from the production of autoantibodies and include immune complex–mediated disease (vasculitis, polyarteritis nodosa), autoimmune disorders (rheumatoid arthritis, glomerulonephritis, thrombocytopenic purpura, thyroiditis, pulmonary fibrosis), and two immunologic disorders: lichen planus and Sjögren's-like syndrome (lymphocytic sialadenitis). If these diseases or signs of advanced liver disease (bleeding esophageal varices, ascites, jaundice, spider angioma, dark urine) are noted, testing for chronic hepatitis is recommended.[2,20,22]

HDV infection often results in severe acute hepatitis or rapidly progressive chronic liver disease. Coinfection usually leads to transient and self-limiting disease, whereas superinfection more often results in severe clinical disease, indicated by sudden exacerbation in a chronic carrier of HBV.

Laboratory Findings

The serum transaminases (aspartate aminotransferase [AST], serum glutamate oxaloacetate transaminase, alanine aminotransferase [ALT], serum glutamate pyruvate transaminase) are sensitive indicators of liver injury and acute viral hepatitis; ALT is a more specific indicator.

Also useful in the diagnosis of hepatitis are elevated levels of serum bilirubin, alkaline phosphatase (heat fraction), gamma-glutamyl transpeptidase, and lactate dehydrogenase, as well as increased white blood cell count and prothrombin time. Antigen/antibody serologic tests are required for identifying the viral agent and for distinguishing acute, resolved, and chronic infections.[23]

Serum transaminase levels become elevated as the result of damage to infected liver cells. Normal levels are lower than 30 to 40 U/L. AST and ALT become elevated usually before serum bilirubin increases. The highest levels, which often correspond to the peak of the icteric phase, gradually subside during the convalescent phase. Jaundice becomes clinically evident as the serum bilirubin level approaches 2.5 mg/100 mL. An elevated bilirubin level may persist after the transaminase level begins to fall. The serum alkaline phosphatase level may be mildly elevated or normal; however, this is a relatively nonspecific test.[23]

An increase in white blood cell count usually occurs, with relative lymphocytosis. Atypical lymphocytes are seen that are identical to those observed in infectious mononucleosis. Monitoring prothrombin time is important because it may become elevated, especially in more extensive disease that results in hepatic cellular destruction. Abnormal hemostasis may occur if the prothrombin time is severely elevated.[23]

Hepatitis A is diagnosed by the presence of elevated IgM anti-HAV for 2 to 4 weeks during the acute phase of the infection, and later by a rise in IgG anti-HAV that indicates the convalescent phase. IgG anti-HAV persists in blood and confers lifelong protection, whereas IgM anti-HAV tends to disappear by the sixth month.[23]

The serologic relationships that occur during hepatitis B virus infection are shown in Figure 11-1 and are summarized as follows:

- The first markers to appear in blood are HBsAg, HBeAg, and HBV DNA, followed by antibodies against the core antigen (IgM anti-HBc and IgG anti-HBc). IgM antibodies are markers of acute infection.
- IgG antibodies contribute to control of disease and indicate immunity.
- The presence of the virus surface antigen (HBsAg) indicates acute or chronic hepatitis B; the patient is infectious.
- The antibody against the surface antigen (anti-HBs) indicates previous exposure to HBV, HBV vaccination, or hepatitis B hyperimmunoglobulin (HBIG) prophylaxis. It connotes recovery and immunity to HBV. If HBsAg is present with antibody response (anti-HBs), the antibody is ineffective and the patient has chronic hepatitis.
- A window occurs between the 24th and 28th weeks when neither HBsAg nor anti-HBs may be present.
- The hepatitis B virus core antigen (HBcAg) is present in liver and is not secreted during acute or chronic disease but elicits an antibody response.

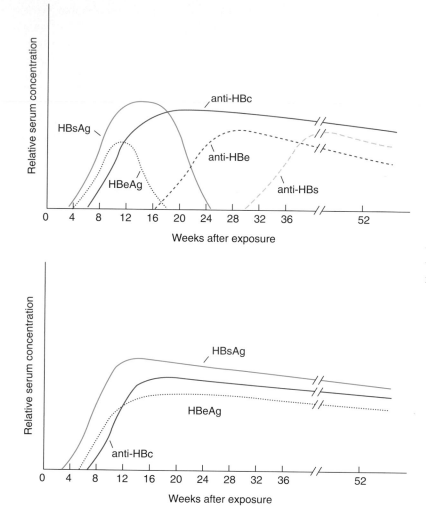

Figure 11-1. Typical sequence of various hepatitis B virus (HBV) markers in **(A)** acute infection with recovery and **(B)** acute infection, resulting in a chronic carrier state.

- HBeAg is a truncated form of HBcAg that is secreted into the blood. The presence of HBeAg correlates with high infectivity. Antibody to HBeAg (anti-HBe) is an indicator of decreased infectivity and recovery.
- The diagnostic markers that most accurately predict acute hepatitis B are HBsAg and IgM anti-HBc.

Screening for HCV is performed by (1) anti-HCV enzyme-linked immunosorbent assay and recombinant immunoblot assay-1, which detect antibodies against recombinant proteins of nonstructural and core regions of the viral genome, and (2) reverse transcriptase polymerase chain reaction (PCR) testing for HCV RNA. Anti-HCV is detected in approximately 90% of patients within 3 months after onset of infection. The presence of anti-HCV is an indication of infectivity; it does not confer recovery or immunity. During chronic HCV infection, ALT levels often are elevated or fluctuate from normal to elevated levels, HCV RNA is detected in blood, and liver disease is evident on tissue biopsy. Screening for HCV infection is recommended for high prevalence groups such as injection drug users, recipients of transfusions, and recipients of solid organ transplants before 1992, recipients of clotting factor concentrate before 1987, persons with persistently elevated ALT levels, and those receiving long-term hemodialysis.[21,24]

Enzyme immunoassays for antibody against HDV (anti-HDV) and anti-HEV tests are available in the United States. The amount of virus in the blood (viral load of HDV RNA and HEV RNA) can be assessed in laboratories with the use of hybridization techniques and PCR.

Biopsy of liver tissue is used to confirm the diagnosis of chronic hepatitis and to rule out other causes of liver damage. The histopathologic report is provided to reveal cause, inflammatory activity and location, and degree of fibrosis.[21,24]

MEDICAL MANAGEMENT

Prevention Through Active Immunization

Risk for viral hepatitis is reduced through active immunization. Currently, two vaccines are available for HAV, two for HBV, one (Twinrix; GlaxoSmithKline, Research Triangle Park, NC) for combination hepatitis A and B, and one (Comvax; Merck, Whitehouse Station, NJ) for combination hepatitis B/*Haemophilus influenzae* type b conjugate for infants. The hepatitis A vaccine was first approved for use in the United States in 1995. Harivax (GlaxoSmithKline, Research Triangle Park, NC) and Vaqta (Merck, Whitehouse Station, NJ) are the formalin-inactivated whole virus vaccines used specifically to prevent HAV infection. Hepatitis A virus vaccines are safe and highly immunogenic and are recommended for persons 2 years of age and older.[25] Hepatitis B vaccines have evolved from the time of first development in 1982. These vaccines originally were derived from pooled donor plasma; however, this form no longer is available. The two vaccines licensed for prevention of HBV infection (Engerix-B [GlaxoSmithKline, Research Triangle Park, NC] and Recombivax HB [Merck, Whitehouse Station, NJ]) are produced by recombinant DNA technology. These vaccines are administered in three doses over a 6-month period and produce an effective antibody response in more than 90% of adults and 95% of infants, children, and adolescents. The conversion rate is based on injections given in the deltoid muscle because injections administered in the buttocks resulted in development of effective antibody titers in only 81% of recipients. Individuals who have received the vaccine in the buttocks should receive serologic confirmation of their antibody titer status. Adverse effects of all three vaccines include soreness at the injection site, fever, chills, flulike symptoms, arthralgia, and rarely, neuropathy. No risk of developing viral infection is associated with these vaccines, including the original plasma-derived vaccine.[25]

The duration of immunity and the need for booster doses remain controversial. Current information based on experience with plasma-derived HBV vaccine and a study by Mahoney[26] indicate that immunity remains effective for longer than 10 years. Current guidelines of the CDC's Advisory Committee on Immunization Practices recommend booster doses only for persons who did not respond to the primary vaccine series.[14,24,26]

During the decade after vaccine licensure, vaccination of target populations who were at high risk for contracting HBV was recommended (see Box 11-1). Health care workers, including dentists, are at the top of the list; it is strongly recommended that they be inoculated with the vaccine. A posttesting strategy is important for identifying those who are nonresponders.[14,24,26]

A strategy for interrupting HBV transmission in all age groups was developed in 1991 and updated in 1995. The current strategy includes the following: (1) prevention of perinatal HBV infection, (2) routine vaccination of all infants, and (3) vaccination of selected adolescents and adults not vaccinated as infants. Implementation of this strategy eventually should lead to control of hepatitis D in parallel with control of hepatitis B.[24,27]

The hepatitis vaccines are not 100% effective in all patients. Recently, it has been noted that rarely occurring variants of the pre-core HBV are not protected under the recombinant HBsAg vaccine. Therefore postvaccination serologic testing is recommended to determine whether the vaccine is effective.[28]

Prevention Through Passive Immunization

Treatment of viral hepatitis can be accomplished through administration of early postexposure immune globulins or postexposure hepatitis B vaccine (see Prevention Through Active Immunization). Immune serum globulin (IG) consists of a pool of antibodies collected from human plasma that is free of HBsAg, HCV, and HIV. This sterile solution contains antibodies against both hepatitis A and hepatitis B. Another type of IG, hepatitis B immune globulin (HBIG), is specially prepared from preselected plasma that is high in titers of anti-HBs. Administration of IG and HBIG is safe, but these globulins interact adversely with live attenuated vaccines (i.e., measles, mumps, rubella [MMR] vaccine) if given within 5 months of each other (Table 11-2).[24]

Treatment

As with many viral diseases, basic therapy is palliative and supportive. Bed rest and fluids may be prescribed, especially during the acute phase. A nutritious, high-calorie diet is advised. Alcohol and drugs metabolized by the liver are not to be ingested. Viral antigen and ALT levels should be monitored for 6 months so that it can be determined whether the hepatitis is resolving.

Chronic hepatitis rarely resolves spontaneously. Standard therapy for patients with chronic hepatitis is interferon (IFN) alfa-2b (3 to 10 million units) administered three times weekly for 6 months to 1 year. Newer modalities have used the pegylated form of IFN with better sustained virologic response.[29] IFN therapy normalizes ALT levels in up to 17% of patients infected with HDV, 30% of those infected with HCV, and 40% of those infected with HBV and reduces the risk for development of hepatocellular carcinoma. Response is better when IFN is initiated early in the course of the disease. Treatment costs, however, are high, and only 10% to 30% of patients achieve long-term remission. Adverse effects (e.g., fatigue, flulike symptoms, bone marrow suppression) are common, and up to 15% of patients experience significant adverse effects that result in discontinuation of treatment. The addition of lamivudine (a nucleoside analog active against HBV) or ribavirin (a guanosine analog active against HCV) results in a virologic response in an additional 15% to 25%.[30] Corticosteroids are usually reserved for fulminant hepatitis. Liver transplantation is a last resort for patients who develop cirrhosis (see Chapter 22).

DENTAL MANAGEMENT
Medical Considerations

Identification of potential or actual carriers of HBV, HCV, and HDV is problematic because in most instances, carriers cannot be identified by history. The inability to identify potentially infectious patients extends to HIV infection and other sexually transmitted diseases. Therefore, all patients with a history of viral hepatitis must be managed as though they are potentially infectious.

TABLE **11-2**

Recommendations Following Accidental Exposure to Blood of a Person Infected With Hepatitis Virus*

Source Person is	Unvaccinated HCW	Vaccinated HCW† Known Responder	Vaccinated HCW Known Nonreceptor	Vaccinated HCW Response Unknown
HBsAg positive	1 dose of hepatitis B immune globulin (HBIG 0.06 mL/kg IM) as soon as possible, preferably within 24 hours + initiate hepatitis B vaccine	No treatment	Administer one dose of HBIG + hepatitis B vaccine, or 2 doses of HBIG with second dose 1 month after the first	Test exposed worker for anti-HBsAg; if inadequate (<10 mU/mL), one dose HBIG + hepatitis B vaccine booster dose
HBsAg negative	Initiate hepatitis B vaccine series	No treatment	No treatment	No treatment
If unknown, not tested	Initiate hepatitis B vaccine series	No treatment	If known high-risk source, consider treating as if source is HBsAg positive	Test exposed worker for anti-HBsAg; if inadequate, initiate revaccination

HCW, Health care worker; HBsAg, hepatitis B surface antigen; IM, intramuscular.

*Adapted from Centers for Disease Control and Prevention. Immunization of health-care workers: Recommendations of the Advisory Committee on Immunization Practices and the Hospital Infection Control Practices Advisory Committee (HICPAC). MMWR 1997;46(RR-18): 1-42.
Following a percutaneous or permucosal exposure, the blood of the source (and exposed) person should be tested for HBsAg, anti–hepatitis C virus (HCV), and human immunodeficiency virus (HIV) antibody. Testing should be done in accordance with state laws and where appropriate pretest and posttest counseling is available. Currently, no treatment is available or recommended for occupational postexposure to HCV, hepatitis E virus (HEV), and non–A-E hepatitis viruses. (Centers for Disease Control. Recommendations for follow-up of health-care workers after occupational exposure to hepatitis C virus. MMWR Morb Mortal Wkly Rep 1997;46[26]:603-606.)
Also, current data suggest that an hepatitis A virus (HAV) percutaneous or permucosal exposure in an occupational setting is unlikely to result in transmission of HAV. Unvaccinated individuals (>2 years of age) recently exposed to HAV are advised to receive a single 0.02-mL/kg intramuscular injection of immune globulin according to the Advisory Committee on Immunization Practices recommendations. (Centers for Disease Control and Prevention: Prevention of hepatitis A through active or passive immunization: Recommendation of the Advisory Committee on Immunization Practice. MMWR Morb Mortal Wkly Rep 1999;48[RR-12]:1-31.)
†Exposed worker vaccinated against hepatitis B virus.

Recommendations for infection control practices in dentistry published by the CDC and the American Dental Association have become the standard of care for preventing cross-infection in dental practice (see Appendix A).[31] These organizations strongly recommend that all dental health care workers who provide patient care should receive vaccination against hepatitis B virus and should implement universal precautions during the care of all dental patients. In addition, standards of the U.S. Occupational Safety and Health Administration require that employers must offer free hepatitis B vaccine to employees who are occupationally exposed to blood or other potentially infectious materials. No recommendations have been provided for immunization against the other hepatitis viruses.[31]

Patients With Active Hepatitis. No dental treatment other than urgent care (absolutely necessary work) should be rendered for a patient with active hepatitis unless the patient is clinically and biochemically recovered. Urgent care should be provided only in an isolated operatory with adherence to strict standard precautions (see Appendix B). Aerosols should be minimized and drugs metabolized in the liver should be avoided as much as possible

(Box 11-2). If surgery is necessary, preoperative prothrombin time and bleeding time should be obtained and abnormal results discussed with the physician. The dentist should refer the patient who has acute hepatitis for medical diagnosis and treatment.[1,2]

Patients With a History of Hepatitis. Most carriers of HBV, HCV, and HDV are unaware that they have had hepatitis. One explanation for this is that many cases of hepatitis B and hepatitis C apparently are mild, subclinical, and nonicteric. These cases may be essentially asymptomatic or may resemble a mild viral disease and therefore remain undetected. Studies of dental school patients who were carriers of hepatitis B found that up to 80% did not report a history of hepatitis infection. Thus, these patients are not identifiable through medical history. Routine laboratory screening of every patient would be required to identify the estimated more than 1 million hepatitis carriers in the United States; this would not be practical. The only practical method of providing protection from these individuals and from other patients with undetected infectious diseases is to adopt a strict program of clinical asepsis for all patients (see Appendix B). Use of the hepatitis B vaccine further decreases the threat of hepatitis B

BOX 11-2

Dental Drugs Metabolized Primarily by the Liver

- Local anesthetics (appear safe for use during liver disease when used in appropriate amounts)
- Lidocaine (Xylocaine)
- Mepivacaine (Carbocaine)
- Prilocaine (Citanest)
- Bupivacaine (Marcaine)
- Analgesics
- Aspirin*
- Acetaminophen (Tylenol, Datril)†
- Codeine†
- Meperidine (Demerol)†
- Ibuprofen (Motrin)*
- Sedatives
- Diazepam (Valium)†
- Barbiturates†
- Antibiotics
- Ampicillin
- Tetracycline
- Metronidazole†
- Vancomycin‡

*Limit dose or avoid if severe liver disease (acute hepatitis and cirrhosis) or hemostatic abnormalities are present.
†Limit dose or avoid if severe liver disease (acute hepatitis and cirrhosis) or encephalopathy is present, or if taken with alcohol.
‡Avoid if severe liver disease (acute hepatitis and cirrhosis) is present.

infection. Inoculation of all dental personnel with hepatitis B vaccine is strongly urged.

For those patients who report a positive history of hepatitis, additional historical information occasionally may be of help to the clinician in determining the type of disease. For instance, an infection that occurred while the person was younger than 15 years of age or that was caused by contaminated food or water would suggest hepatitis A. Disease acquired in a Third World country may indicate hepatitis E. Unfortunately, this approach will not reveal a person who has had infection with both type A and type B or C in whom HBV or HCV infection was subclinical or remained undiagnosed.

An additional consideration in patients with a history of hepatitis of unknown type is the use of the clinical laboratory to screen for the presence of HBsAg or anti-HCV. This may be indicated even in patients who specifically indicate which type of hepatitis they had, because information of this type derived from the patient's history is unreliable 50% of the time.

Patients at High Risk for HBV or HCV Infection.
Several groups are at unusually high risk for HBV and HCV infection (see Box 11-1). Screening for HBsAg and anti-HCV is recommended for individuals who fit into one or more of these categories unless they are already known to be seropositive. Even if a patient is found to be a carrier, no modifications in treatment approach theoretically would be necessary. However, this information still

may be of benefit in certain situations. If a patient is found to be a carrier, the information could be of extreme importance for modification of lifestyle. In addition, the patient might have undetected chronic active hepatitis, which could lead to bleeding complications or drug metabolism problems. Finally, if an accidental needlestick or puncture wound occurs during treatment and the dentist is not vaccinated (or antibody titer status is unknown), knowing whether the patient was HBsAg or HCV positive would be of extreme importance in determining the need for HBIG, vaccination, and follow-up medical care.

Patients Who Are Hepatitis Carriers.
If a patient is found to be a hepatitis B carrier (HBsAg positive) or to have a history of hepatitis C, standard precautions (see Appendix B) are to be followed to prevent transmission of infection. In addition, some hepatitis carriers may have chronic active hepatitis, leading to compromised liver function and interference with hemostasis and drug metabolism. Physician consultation and laboratory screening of liver function are advised for determination of current status and future risks.

Patients With Signs or Symptoms of Hepatitis.
Any patient who has signs or symptoms suggestive of hepatitis should not be given elective dental treatment but instead should be referred immediately to a physician. Necessary emergency dental care should be provided with the use of an isolated operatory and minimal aerosol production.

Dentists Who Are Hepatitis Virus Carriers.
A question also arises concerning dentists who are carriers of HBsAg or HCV. Very few cases of hepatitis B traceable to carrier dentists or oral surgeons have been reported since 1974. No cases of HCV transmission from dentist to patient have been reported. In each instance of HBV transmission, the practitioner was found to be seropositive for HBsAg and (if tested) HBeAg and did not use gloves during dental or surgical procedures. None of the practitioners was aware of chronic infection. As a result of these infections, two patients died. Because of increased awareness of bloodborne pathogens and the implementation of vaccinations and infection control measures in dentistry, no additional outbreaks have been reported since 1987.[32]

After the discovery of a carrier state and the documented transmission of disease, some HBsAg carrier dentists have been forced to quit practice and others have faced lengthy periods of discontinuance until they have undergone seroconversion. The CDC suggests that health care professionals who perform invasive procedures should know their infectivity status; if found positive for a blood-transmissible virus, they should not perform exposure-prone procedures unless they have sought counsel from an expert review panel in their state of practice.[22] If, after discussion with this panel, a carrier dentist elects to continue practice, professional ethics and practice guidelines recommend aggressive efforts to prevent potential transmission through adherence to strict aseptic technique, periodic retesting of HBsAg and HCV RNA, and receipt of informed consent from patients.

CDC Guidelines for Exposure to Blood. To reduce the risk of transmission of hepatitis viruses, the CDC has published postexposure protocols for percutaneous or permucosal exposure to blood. Implementation of these protocols is dependent on the virus present in the source person and the vaccinated state of the exposed person (e.g., a dental health care worker) (see Table 11-2).[22]

Briefly, a vaccinated individual who sustains a needle-stick or puncture wound contaminated with blood from a patient known to be HBsAg positive should be tested for an adequate titer of anti-HBs if those levels are unknown. If levels are inadequate, the individual immediately should receive an injection of HBIG and a vaccine booster dose. The risk that a health care worker will contract HBV from HBV carriers through a sharps injury may approach 30%. If the antibody titer is adequate, nothing further is required. If an unvaccinated individual sustains an inadvertent percutaneous or permucosal exposure to hepatitis B, immediate administration of HBIG and initiation of the vaccine are recommended.[27]

Although no postexposure protocol or vaccine is available at this time for HCV infection, current CDC guidelines recommend that (1) the source person should receive baseline testing for anti-HCV, (2) exposed persons should receive baseline and follow-up testing at 6 months for anti-HCV and liver enzyme activity, (3) anti-HCV enzyme immunoassay positive results should be confirmed by recombinant immunoblot assay (RIBA), (4) postexposure prophylaxis should be avoided with immunoglobulin or antiviral agents, (5) health care workers should be educated regarding the risks and prevention of bloodborne infection.[27]

Exposure Control Plan. With respect to hepatitis viruses, the U.S. Occupational Safety and Health Administration mandates that all employers must maintain an exposure control plan and must protect employees from the hazards of bloodborne pathogens by applying standard precautions and by providing the following as a minimum:
- Hepatitis B vaccinations to employees
- Postexposure evaluation and follow-up
- Recordkeeping of exposures
- Generic bloodborne pathogen training
- Personal protective equipment at no cost to employees

All dentists should be familiar with the agency's compliance directive CPL 2-2.69—Enforcement Procedures for Occupational Exposure to Bloodborne Pathogens; at the time of printing, this information was available at http://www.osha-slc.gov/OshDoc/Directive_data/CPL_2-2.69.html.

Drug Administration

No special drug considerations are required for a patient who has completely recovered from viral hepatitis. However, if a patient has chronic active hepatitis or is a carrier of HBsAg or HCV and has impaired liver function, the dosage of drugs metabolized by the liver should be decreased, or these drugs should be avoided, if possible as advised by the physician. As a guideline, drugs metabolized in the liver should be considered for diminished dosage when one or more of the following are present:
- Aminotransferase levels elevated to greater than 4 times normal values
- Serum bilirubin elevated to above 35 μM/L or 2 mg/dL
- Serum albumin levels lower than 35 mg/L
- Signs of ascites and encephalopathy, and prolonged bleeding time (Table 11-3)

Many drugs commonly used in dentistry are metabolized principally by the liver; they may be used in patients with hepatic disease that is not severe, although in limited amounts (see Box 11-2). A quantity of three cartridges of 2% lidocaine (120 mg) is considered a relatively limited amount of drug.

Treatment Planning Modifications

Treatment planning modifications are not required for the patient who has recovered from hepatitis.

Oral Manifestations and Complications

Abnormal bleeding is associated with hepatitis and significant liver damage. This may result from abnormal synthesis of blood clotting factors, abnormal polymerization of fibrin, inadequate fibrin stabilization, excessive fibrinolysis, or thrombocytopenia associated with splenomegaly that accompanies chronic liver disease. Before any surgery is performed, the platelet count should be obtained, and it should be confirmed that the international normalized ratio (INR) is lower than 3.5 (see Chapter 25). If the INR is 3.5 or greater, the potential for severe postoperative bleeding exists. In this case, extensive surgical procedures should be postponed. If surgery is necessary, an injection of vitamin K usually corrects the problem and should be discussed with the physician. Platelet count and platelet function analysis (see Chapter 25) may indicate whether platelet replacement may be required before surgery and should be discussed with the patient's physician.

Chronic viral hepatitis increases the risk for hepatocellular carcinoma. This malignancy rarely metastasizes to the jaw (fewer than 30 cases in the jaw were reported as of this writing). However, the incidence of hepatocellular carcinoma is on the rise in the United States. Oral metastases primarily present as hemorrhagic expanding masses located in the premolar and ramus regions of the mandible.[1,2]

TABLE **11-3**

Dental Management of the Patient With Alcoholic Liver Disease

1. Detection by such methods as
   - History
   - Clinical examination
   - Alcohol odor on breath
   - Information from family members or friends
2. Referral or consultation with physician to ascertain the following:
   - Verify history
   - Check current status
   - Check medications
   - Check laboratory values
   - Discuss suggestions for management
3. Laboratory screening (if not available from physician) to record the following:
   - Complete blood count (CBC) with differential
   - Aspartate aminotransferase (AST), alanine aminotransferase (ALT)
   - Bleeding time
   - Thrombin time
   - Prothrombin time
4. Assessment of risk of adverse outcomes associated with invasive procedure or infection with prognostic formula (i.e., Modified Child-Pugh Classification found in table below)

KEY POINTS

Parameter	1	2	3
Ascites	None	Moderate	Severe
Encephalopathy	None	Mild (grades 1-2)	Severe (grades 3-4)
Serum bilirubin, mg/dL	<2.0	2.0-3.0	>3.0
Serum albumin, mg/dL	>3.5	2.8-3.5	<2.8
Prothrombin time, seconds increased	1-3	4-6	>6

Patients are scored by adding the numeric value obtained from each row, then are categorized as **class A** (mild disease) = score 5 or 6; **class B** (moderate disease) = score 7 to 9; or **class C** (severe disease) = score 10-15.[36]

5. Minimizing of drugs metabolized by liver (see Box 11-2)
6. If screening tests are abnormal, for surgical procedures, consideration is given to thrombin, gelfoam, antifibrinolytic agents, fresh frozen plasma, vitamin K, platelets—with the help of a physician or PharmD.

ALCOHOLIC LIVER DISEASE

DEFINITION

Alcoholism is a chronic addiction to ethanol in which a person craves and uncontrollably consumes ethanol, becomes tolerant to its intoxicating effects, and has symptoms of alcohol withdrawal when the drinking stops. *The Diagnostic and Statistical Manual of Mental Disorders (DSM-IV)* defines *alcohol dependence* as repeated alcohol-related difficulties in at least three of seven areas of functioning. These include any combination of the following:

- Tolerance
- Withdrawal
- Ingestion of larger amounts of alcohol over longer periods than intended
- Inability to control use
- Giving up important activities to drink
- Spending a great deal of time involved with alcohol use
- Continued use of alcohol despite physical or psychological consequences

Alcohol abuse is the harmful use of alcohol. Individuals who drink alcohol excessively without evidence of dependence have an alcohol abuse disorder. A form of alcohol abuse associated with excessive heavy drinking is "binge drinking." This form of consumption is associated with an increased risk of death due to injury. Alcohol abuse and dependence are not limited to any particular group. All ages and races, both sexes, and all socioeconomic levels are affected. The stereotypical picture of the skid row vagrant applies to only a small percentage of cases.[33]

Alcohol abuse is known to cause or exacerbate many physical conditions. The economic impact of alcohol abuse and dependence in the United States is estimated at $100 billion annually. Because of the widespread use of alcohol, it has been implicated as the leading cause of accidental death and work-related accidents in the United States. Motor vehicle accidents are a major cause of injury-related death, and alcohol is involved in at least half of these. Many behavioral and physical disorders are associated with alcohol abuse; the dentist is required to be knowledgeable about this topic.[33]

EPIDEMIOLOGY

Incidence and Prevalence

Nearly two thirds of Americans older than 14 years of age drink alcoholic beverages; 44% of adults are current drinkers, and 22% are former drinkers. The prevalence of alcohol abuse and dependence in the United States is 7.4% to 9.7%, and the lifetime prevalence is 13.7% to 23.5%. Men are 2 to 5 times more likely than women to develop pervasive alcoholism,[33] although this difference is less pronounced in younger age groups. In all, 14 million Americans satisfy the definition of an alcoholic.[34-36]

Drinking patterns vary by gender and age. For both genders, the prevalence of drinking is highest among persons in the 21- to 34-year age range. Studies have projected that between 7% and 17% of college students have alcohol drinking problems. Overall, 14 million persons in the United States are dependent on alcohol. On the basis of these figures, the average dental practice with 2000 adult patients is predicted to serve 170 to 200 patients who have a problem with alcohol. Whereas problem drinking is seen primarily in adults, its prevalence among teenagers is alarmingly high. One study[32] reported that an estimated 3.3 million persons aged 14 to 17 years could be classified as problem drinkers. Alcoholism among the elderly is also a significant problem, with prevalence estimates ranging between 1% and 10%.[34-36]

Lack of treatment of alcohol abuse leads to significant morbidity and mortality rates. Current figures indicate that 105,000 persons die annually in the United States because of alcohol abuse, and more than 20% of hospital admissions are alcohol related. Cirrhosis is a sequela of alcohol abuse and is the 10th leading cause of death among adults in the United States. Ethanol alone or combined with other drugs such as benzodiazepines is probably responsible for a greater number of toxic overdose deaths than any other agent.[34-37]

Etiology

Alcohol consumption in large or chronic amounts contributes to disease and injury. In contrast, moderate consumption of alcohol (2 to 6 drinks per week) is associated with decreased mortality and cardiovascular disease rates. The quantity and duration of alcohol ingestion required to produce cirrhosis are not clear. However, the typical alcoholic with cirrhosis has a history of at least 10 years of daily consumption of a pint or more of whiskey, several quarts of wine, or an equivalent amount of beer.[34-38]

The relationship between excessive alcohol ingestion and liver dysfunction may lead to cirrhosis. However, the exact effect of alcohol on the liver was not known until researchers demonstrated that alcohol is hepatotoxic and its metabolite, acetylaldehyde, is fibrinogenic. Chemokines also are implicated in the pathogenesis of alcoholic liver disease. Alcohol-induced influx of endotoxin (lipopolysaccharides) from the gut into the portal circulation can activate Kupffer cells, which leads to enhanced chemokine release. Chemokines, in turn, directly and indirectly damage liver hepatocytes. It is curious that only 10% to 15% of heavy alcohol users ever develop cirrhosis—a fact that can probably be explained by hereditary, nutritional, and biochemical differences among individuals.[34-38]

Pathophysiology and Complications

Alcohol has a deleterious effect on neural development, the corticotropin-releasing hormone system, the metabolism of neurotransmitters, and the functions of their receptors. As a result, the acetylcholine and dopaminergic systems are affected, which causes sensory and motor disturbances (e.g., peripheral neuropathies). Prolonged abuse of alcohol contributes to malnutrition (folic acid deficiency), anemia, and decreased immune function. Increased mortality rates have been noted among men who consume more than three drinks daily.[39]

The pathologic effects of alcohol on the liver are expressed by one of three disease entities. These conditions may exist alone but commonly appear in combination. The earliest change seen in alcoholic liver disease is a fatty infiltrate. Hepatocytes become engorged with fatty lobules and distended, and the entire liver is enlarged. Usually, no other structural changes are noted. These changes may be seen after only moderate usage of alcohol for a brief time; however, they are considered completely reversible.[35,36]

A second and more serious form of alcoholic liver disease is alcoholic hepatitis. This is a diffuse inflammatory condition of the liver that is characterized by destructive cellular changes, some of which may be irreversible. The irreversible changes can lead to necrosis. Nutritional factors may play a significant role in the progression of this disease. For the most part, alcoholic hepatitis is considered a reversible condition; however, it can be fatal, if damage is widespread.[35,36]

The third and most serious form of alcoholic liver disease is cirrhosis, which is generally considered an irreversible condition characterized by progressive fibrosis and abnormal regeneration of liver architecture in response to chronic injury or insult (i.e., prolonged and heavy use of ethanol) (Figure 11-2). Cirrhosis results in progressive deterioration of the metabolic and excretory functions of the liver and ultimately leads to hepatic failure. Hepatic failure is manifested by a myriad of health problems. Some of the more important of these are esophagitis, gastritis, and pancreatitis, all of which contribute to generalized malnutrition, weight loss, protein deficiency (including coagulation factors), impairment of urea synthesis and glucose metabolism, endocrine disturbances, encephalopathy, renal failure, portal hypertension, and jaundice. Accompanying portal hypertension is seen as the development of ascites and esophageal varices (Figure 11-3). In some patients with cirrhosis, blood from bleeding ulcers and esophageal varices is incompletely metabolized to ammonia, which travels to the brain and

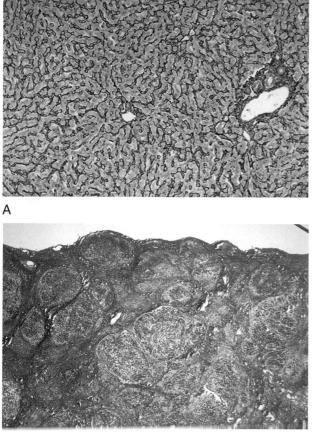

A

B

Figure 11-2. A, Normal liver architecture. **B,** Liver architecture showing alcoholic cirrhosis. (**A,** From Klatt EC. Robbins and Cotran Atlas of Pathology. Philadelphia, Saunders, 2006. **B,** From Kumar V, Cotran RS, Robbins SL. Robbins Basic Pathology, 7th ed. Philadelphia, Saunders, 2003.)

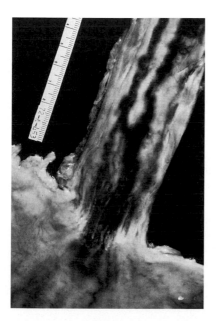

Figure 11-3. Gross section of esophageal varices from an alcoholic patient. (Courtesy A. Golden, Lexington, Ky.)

contributes to encephalopathy. In addition, chronic large consumption of ethanol can result in dementia and psychosis (Wernicke's and Korsakoff's syndromes), cerebellar degeneration, upper alimentary tract cancer and liver cancer, and hematopoietic changes.[40]

Bleeding tendencies are a significant feature in advanced liver disease. The basis for the diathesis is in part a deficiency of coagulation factors, especially the prothrombin group (factors II, VII, IX, and X). These all rely on vitamin K as a precursor for production. Vitamin K is absorbed from the large intestine and stored in the liver, where it is converted into an enzymatic cofactor for the carboxylation of prothrombin complex proteins. Widespread hepatocellular destruction as seen in cirrhosis decreases the capacity of the liver to store and convert vitamin K, leading to deficiencies in prothrombin-dependent coagulation factors. In addition to these deficiencies, thrombocytopenia may be caused by hypersplenism caused by portal hypertension and bone marrow depression. Anemia and leukopenia also may be noted because of the toxic effects of alcohol on the bone marrow and nutritional deficiencies. Accelerated fibrinolysis also may be seen.[40]

The combination of hemorrhagic tendencies and severe portal hypertension sets the stage for episodes of gastrointestinal bleeding, epistaxis, ecchymosis, or ruptured esophageal varix. Most patients with advanced cirrhosis die of hepatic coma, often precipitated by massive hemorrhage from esophageal varices or intercurrent infection.[40]

Ethanol abuse predisposes the individual to infection by several mechanisms. In patients with alcoholism, the resident cell population of the liver is exposed to high concentrations of ethanol. Kupffer cells, which represent more than 80% of tissue macrophages in the body, become impaired because of alcohol bathing of the liver sinusoids. Alcohol-induced impairment of Kupffer cell function and T-cell responses result in increased risk of infection. Although cirrhosis is generally considered to be an end-stage condition, some evidence suggests that at least partial reversibility of the process is possible with complete and permanent removal of the offending agent during the early phase of cirrhosis.[40]

CLINICAL PRESENTATION

Signs and Symptoms

The behavioral and physiologic effects of alcohol vary with the amount of intake, the rate of increase in plasma, the presence of other drugs or medical problems, and the individual's past experience with alcohol. Chronic heavy alcohol intake can result in clinically significant cognitive impairment (even when the person is sober) or distress. The pattern displayed is usually one of intermittent relapse and remission. If the condition is allowed to progress untreated, many individuals develop other psychiatric problems (e.g., anxiety, antisocial behavior, affective disorders), whereas some develop alcohol amnestic

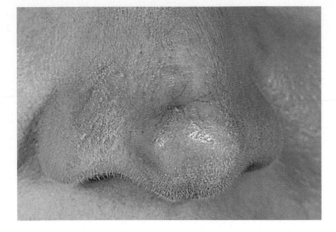

Figure 11-4. Spider angioma. (From Seidel HM, Ball JW, Dain S, Benedict GW. Mosby's Guide to Physical Examination, 6th ed. St. Louis, Mosby, 2006.)

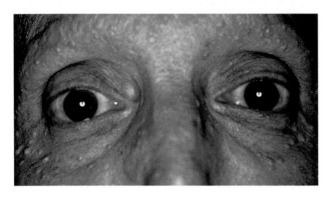

Figure 11-5. Patient with jaundice. Note the yellow sclera. (From Seidel HM, Ball JW, Dain S, Benedict GW. Mosby's Guide to Physical Examination, 6th ed. St. Louis, Mosby, 2006.)

disorder and are unable to learn new material or to recall known material. Alcoholic blackouts may occur. In some individuals, alcohol-induced dementia and severe personality changes are noted.

Clinically, with the possible exception of enlargement, no visible manifestations of fatty liver are present, and the diagnosis usually is made incidentally in conjunction with another illness. The clinical presentation of alcoholic hepatitis often is nonspecific and may include features such as nausea, vomiting, anorexia, malaise, weight loss, and fever. More specific findings include hepatomegaly, splenomegaly, jaundice, ascites, ankle edema, and spider angiomas. With advancing disease, encephalopathy and hepatic coma may ensue, resulting in death.[37]

Alcoholic cirrhosis may remain asymptomatic for many years until sufficient destruction of the liver parenchyma produces clinical evidence of hepatic failure. Ascites, spider angiomas (Figure 11-4), ankle edema, or jaundice (Figure 11-5) may be the earliest signs, but frequently, hemorrhage from esophageal varices is the initial

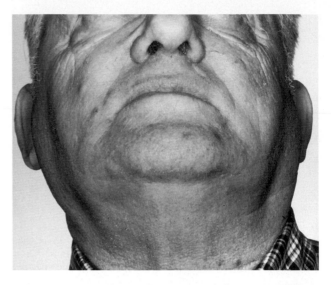

Figure 11-6. Painless enlargement of the parotid glands associated with alcoholism. (Courtesy Valerie Murrah, Chapel Hill, NC.)

sign. The hemorrhagic episode may progress to hepatic encephalopathy, coma, and death. Other less specific signs of alcoholic liver disease include anemia, purpura, ecchymoses, gingival bleeding, palmar erythema, nail changes, and parotid gland enlargement (known as sialadenosis) (Figure 11-6).[40]

Laboratory Findings. Laboratory findings in alcoholic liver disease vary from minimal abnormalities caused by a fatty liver to manifestations of alcoholic hepatitis and cirrhosis. Liver abnormalities cause elevations in bilirubin, alkaline phosphatase, AST, ALT, gamma-glutamyl transpeptidase, amylase, uric acid, triglycerides, and cholesterol. Leukopenia (or leukocytosis) or anemia often is present. For these reasons, a simple screen for alcoholism comes from a sequential multianalyzer-20 and complete blood count (CBC) with differential. Elevated blood levels of gamma-glutamyl transpeptidase and mean corpuscular volume are highly suggestive of alcoholism, whereas an AST/ALT ratio of at least 2 is 90% predictive of alcoholic liver disease. The carbohydrate-deficient transferrin test is also used to screen for and monitor alcohol-dependent patients.[40]

Alcoholic liver disease leads to deficiencies of clotting factors reflected as elevations in prothrombin time and partial thromboplastin time. Thrombocytopenia may be caused by hepatosplenomegaly, resulting in decreased platelet count and increased bleeding time. Increased fibrinolytic activity may be evident in increased bleeding time, prolonged thrombin time, or decreased euglobulin clot lysis time (see Chapter 25).

MEDICAL MANAGEMENT

Treatment of patients with alcoholism consists of three basic steps. The first is identification and intervention. A thorough physical examination is performed to evaluate organ systems that could be impaired. This includes a search for evidence of liver failure, gastrointestinal bleeding, cardiac arrhythmia, and glucose or electrolyte imbalance. Hemorrhage from esophageal varices and hepatic encephalopathy require immediate treatment. Ascites mandates measures to control fluids and electrolytes, alcoholic hepatitis is often treated with glucocorticoids, and infection or sepsis is managed with antimicrobial agents. During this phase, the patient may refuse to accept the diagnosis and may deny that a problem exists.[41]

The second step is withdrawal from alcohol or, in cases of severe dependence, reduction in alcohol consumption. Abrupt alcohol withdrawal results in loss of appetite, tachycardia, anxiety, insomnia, and delirium tremens (DT), characterized by hallucinations, disorientation, impaired attention and memory, and extreme agitation. Physical findings include severe sweating, elevated blood pressure, and tachycardia. The goal of management is to minimize the severity of withdrawal symptoms. Strict dietary modifications, including a high-protein, high-calorie, low-sodium diet and possibly fluid restriction, are required. Patients should receive adequate nutrition and rest, oral multiple B vitamins, including 50 to 100 mg of thiamine daily for at least 1 to 2 weeks, and iron replacement and folic acid supplementation as needed to correct any anemia present.[41]

The third step is to manage central nervous system depression caused by the rapid removal of ethanol. Administration of a benzodiazepine, such as diazepam or chlordiazepoxide, gradually decreases drug levels over a 3- to 5-day period and alleviates alcohol withdrawal symptoms. Beta blockers, clonidine, and carbamazepine have been recently added to the pharmacotherapeutic management options for withdrawal.[37,41]

Once the treatment of withdrawal has been completed, the patient with alcoholism is educated about alcoholism. This involves teaching family members and friends to stop protecting the patient from problems caused by alcohol. Attempts are made to help the patient with alcoholism achieve and maintain a high level of motivation toward abstinence. Steps also are taken to help the patient with alcoholism readjust to life without alcohol and to reestablish a functional lifestyle. The drug disulfiram has been used for some patients during alcohol rehabilitation. Disulfiram inhibits aldehyde dehydrogenase, causing accumulation of acetaldehyde blood levels and thus, sweating, nausea, vomiting, and diarrhea, when taken with ethanol. Naltrexone (an opioid antagonist) and acamprosate (an inhibitor of the γ-aminobutyric acid system) may be used to decrease the amount of alcohol consumed or to shorten the period during which alcohol is used in cases of relapse.[41] Untreated disease that progresses to cirrhosis requires alcohol withdrawal and management of the complications that are present. End-stage cirrhosis cannot be reversed and is remedied only by liver transplantation (see Chapter 22).

DENTAL MANAGEMENT

Medical Considerations

The dentist has an excellent opportunity to assist patients who are at risk for, or who have, alcohol abuse problems. Unfortunately, patients with alcoholism are poorly recognized by health care providers in health care settings unless they have medical complications. Areas of assistance include the following:

- Screening for alcohol risks and abuse
- Providing alcohol prevention information
- Directing patients with abuse problems to health care providers for assessment or treatment
- Supporting dependent patients during the recovery period
- Minimizing relapse in recovering patients

Screening

The patient with chronic alcoholism can be recognized through examination of health problems and behaviors, such as medical signs and symptoms, noncompliance, exacerbated anxieties and fears, failure to fulfill obligations, and emotional fluctuations. During the medical history, the dentist should obtain information from all adolescent and adult patients about the type, quantity, frequency, pattern, and consequences of alcohol use, along with a family history of alcoholism (see Table 11-3). Questioning should be done in a nonjudgmental manner, aided by a standardized questionnaire such as the four-question CAGE questionnaire, the most widely studied and best known instrument, which focuses on impaired control (Cut down), use despite consequences (Annoyed by criticism, experiencing Guilt), and dependence (Eye opener in the morning) (Box 11-3). The CUGE questionnaire replaces the second CAGE question with a question about being Under the influence when driving a car or riding a bike.[35,37,42]

BOX 11-3

CAGE and CUGE Questionnaires for Screening of Alcohol Abuse

C	Have you ever felt the need to **c**ut down on your drinking?
A	Have you ever felt **a**nnoyed by criticism of your drinking?
U	Have you often been **u**nder the influence of alcohol in a situation where it increased your chances of getting hurt, for example, when riding a bicycle or driving a car?
G	Have you ever felt **g**uilty about your drinking?
E	Have you ever taken a drink (**e**ye opener) first thing in the morning?

Data from Mayfield D, McLeod G, Hall P. The CAGE questionnaire: Validation of a new alcoholism screening instrument. Am J Psychiatry 1974;131:1121-1123; and Buntinx BA, et al. The value of the CAGE, CUGE, and AUDIT in screening for alcohol abuse and dependence among college freshmen. Alcoholism Clin Exp Res 2000;24:53-57.

BOX 11-4

Features Suggestive of Advanced Alcoholic Liver Disease

SYSTEMIC COMPLICATIONS
- Traumatic or unexplained injuries (driving under the influence, bruises, cuts, scars, broken teeth)
- Attention and memory deficits
- Slurred speech
- Spider angiomas
- Jaundice (sclerae, mucosa)
- Peripheral edema (edematous puffy face, ankle edema)
- Ascites
- Palmar erythema, white nails, or transverse pale band on nails
- Ecchymoses, petechiae, or prolonged bleeding
- Failure to fulfill role obligations at work, school, home (e.g., missed dental appointments)
- Increased levels of bilirubin, aminotransferases, alkaline phosphates, gamma-glutamyl transpeptidase, and mean corpuscular volume

ORAL COMPLICATIONS
- Poor oral hygiene
- Oral neglect—caries, gingivitis, periodontitis
- Glossitis
- Angular or labial cheilosis
- Candidiasis
- Gingival bleeding
- Oral cancer
- Petechiae
- Ecchymoses
- Jaundiced mucosa
- Parotid gland enlargement
- Alcohol (sweet musty) breath odor
- Impaired healing
- Bruxism
- Dental attrition
- Xerostomia

Family members may be a source of information when interviews are granted in confidence. A high index of suspicion should be followed by clinical examination and a series of laboratory tests for screening purposes, regardless of whether the patient admits to heavy use of alcohol (chronic consumption of more than 14 alcoholic drinks per week for men or more than 4 drinks per occasion, and more than 7 drinks per week for women or more than 3 drinks per occasion). Signs suggestive of alcohol abuse, such as enlargement of the parotid glands (see Figure 11-6) or a distinctive breath odor, may be detectable. Other signs are suggestive of the disease as well (Box 11-4).

Alcoholism transcends age, gender, and socioeconomic spectrum, and many patients are great at hiding their dependence.[42]

Providing Preventive Information. If the dentist suspects that a patient is abusing alcohol, a spouse or significant other can be interviewed to gather additional diagnostic information. If suspicions are confirmed, preventive information should be provided to the patient in a nonthreatening manner. Treatment success depends on motivating the patient to enter treatment and breaking down denial.

Guiding the Patient for Assessment or Treatment and Supportive Care. Facilitating entry of a patient into a treatment program requires that the dentist share concerns aroused by the medical assessment. The dentist can point out destructive patterns of alcohol use and can discuss future problems that may be anticipated if alcohol use continues. Discussions should include talk about the possibilities and successes of treatment. This requires that the dentist be familiar with treatment options within the local community, such as detoxification, inpatient programs, outpatient programs, halfway houses, and continuing care. Active communication and expression of concern from the dentist to the patient and the patient's family during therapy and recovery, along with group meetings, are supportive measures that improve the chances of successful rehabilitation.

Minimizing Relapse. To minimize relapse, the dentist should avoid the use of psychoactive drugs, narcotics, sedatives, and alcohol-containing medications in patients who are recovering from alcoholism (Table 11-4).

If a potentially mood-altering drug is required, the patient's primary care physician (or substance abuse advisor) should be consulted about its use. If approved for use, the drug should be prescribed only in the amount needed without refills. Designating a family member to fill and dispense the drug can minimize the risk of abuse.

Treatment Considerations. In addition to the considerations mentioned earlier, three major dental treatment considerations apply for a patient with alcoholism:
1. Bleeding tendencies
2. Unpredictable metabolism of certain drugs
3. Risk or spread of infection

A CBC with differential, AST and ALT, bleeding time, thrombin time, and prothrombin time are sufficient in screening for potential problems. Abnormal laboratory values, accompanied by abnormal clinical examination or a positive history, provide the basis for referral to a physician for positive diagnosis and treatment. A patient with untreated alcoholic liver disease is not a candidate for elective, outpatient dental care and should be referred to a physician. Once the patient has been managed medically, dental care may be provided after consultation with the physician.[35]

If a patient reveals a history of alcoholic liver disease or alcohol abuse, the physician should be consulted to verify the patient's current status, medications, laboratory values, and contraindications for medications, surgery, or other treatment. In cases where the patient has not been

TABLE 11-4
Alcohol Content of Over-the-Counter Medications

Over-the-counter Medication	Alcohol, %
MOUTHWASH AND GARGLE	
Scope	14.3-15
Signal	14.5
Cepacol	14
Listerine	26.5
Listermint	0
Tom's of Maine	0
ANTIPLAQUE RINSE	
Peridex, Periogard	11.6
Plax	8.7
Peroxyl	6
FLUORIDE RINSE	
ACT	0
SORE THROAT SPRAY AND LIQUID	
Chloraseptic	12.5
TOOTHACHE DROPS AND GEL	
Orajel Maximum Strength Liquid	44.2
Anbesol Maximum Strength	60
DECONGESTANT AND COUGH SUPPRESSANT	
NyQuil	10
Robitussin Alcohol Free	0
Dimetapp Elixir Alcohol Free	0

seen by a physician within the past several months, screening laboratory tests, including CBC with differential, AST and ALT, platelet count, thrombin time, and prothrombin time, should be ordered before invasive procedures are performed (see Table 11-3). Precautionary measures, including an INR test (prothrombin time) that is particularly sensitive to deficiency of factor VII, should be taken to minimize the risk for bleeding (see Chapter 25). Bleeding diatheses should be managed with the assistance of the physician; this may entail the use of local hemostatic agents, fresh frozen plasma, vitamin K, platelets, and antifibrinolytic agents. Hemostatic measures are particularly important when major invasive or traumatic procedures are performed in a patient who has been assigned an American Society of Anesthesiologists (ASA) category of III or greater; who has signs of jaundice, ascites, and clubbing of fingers; or who has been classified as a Child-Pugh class B or C.[43]

A second area of concern in patients with alcoholic liver disease is the unpredictable metabolism of drugs. This concern is twofold. In mild to moderate alcoholic liver disease, significant enzyme induction is likely to have occurred, leading to increased tolerance of local anesthetics, sedative and hypnotic drugs, and general anesthesia. Thus, larger than normal doses of these medications may be required to attain the desired effects.[35]

Also, with advanced liver destruction, drug metabolism may be markedly diminished, which may lead to an increased or unexpected effect. For example, if acetaminophen is given in usual therapeutic doses in chronic alcoholism, or if acetaminophen is taken with alcohol in a fasting state, severe hepatocellular disease with mortality may result. The dentist should use the drugs listed in Box 11-2 with caution when treating patients with chronic alcoholism and should consider adjusting doses (e.g., half the dose if cirrhosis or alcoholic hepatitis is present) or avoiding their use, as advised by the patient's physician. Once again, the occurrence of more than one of the following findings—aminotransferase levels elevated to greater than 4 times normal, serum bilirubin level elevated to above 3.5 μM/L (2 mg/dL), serum albumin level lower than 35 g/L, and signs of ascites, encephalopathy, or malnutrition (see Table 11-3)—suggests that drug metabolism may be impaired.[35]

A third area of concern involves the risk of infection or spread of infection in the patient with alcoholic liver disease. Risk increases with surgical procedures or trauma because oral microorganisms can be introduced into the blood circulation and may not be efficiently eliminated by the reticuloendothelial system. Although patients who have alcoholic liver disease have reduced reticuloendothelial capacity and altered cell-mediated immune function, studies do not indicate that antibiotic prophylaxis should be provided before invasive dental procedures are performed in the absence of an ongoing infection. Despite the lack of evidence, recommendations in the literature call for the use of antibiotic prophylaxis for these patients. Antibiotic prophylaxis is not needed if oral infection is absent. A greater concern is the risk of spread of an ongoing infection because bacterial infections are more serious and are sometimes fatal in patients with liver disease.[2,33] To identify those at risk for responding poorly to invasive procedures and infections, clinicians should consider using one of the assessment formulas for staging liver disease (i.e., Child-Pugh classification scheme; see Table 11-3) and identifying whether a history of bacterial infection (e.g., spontaneous bacterial peritonitis, pneumonia, bacteremia) exists. Consultation with the patient's physician regarding the use of antibiotics should be considered for persons with moderate to severe disease (Child-Pugh class B or C) (i.e., ascites, encephalopathy, elevated bilirubin levels or SBP). Antibiotics should be prescribed when infection develops and is unlikely to resolve without treatment.[43]

Treatment Planning Modifications

Patients with cirrhosis tend to have more plaque, calculus, and gingival inflammation than those without the condition. This seems to be the case in any patient who is a substance abuser and is related to oral neglect rather than to any inherent property of the abused substance. The dentist should not provide extensive care until the patient demonstrates an interest in, and an ability to care for, his or her dentition.

Liver enzyme induction and central nervous system effects of alcohol in patients with alcoholism may require increased amounts of local anesthetic or the use of additional anxiolytic procedures. Appointments with these patients may therefore require more time if this manifestation was not anticipated.

Oral Complications and Manifestations

Poor hygiene and neglect (caries) are prominent oral findings in patients with chronic alcoholism. In addition, a variety of other abnormalities may be found (see Box 11-4). Patients with cirrhosis have been reported to have impaired gustatory function and are malnourished. Nutritional deficiencies can result in glossitis and loss of tongue papillae, along with angular or labial cheilitis, which is complicated by concomitant candidal infection. Vitamin K deficiency, disordered hemostasis, portal hypertension, and splenomegaly (causing thrombocytopenia) can produce spontaneous gingival bleeding, mucosal ecchymoses, and petechiae. In some instances, unexplained gingival bleeding has been the initial complaint of alcoholic patients. A sweet, musty odor to the breath is associated with liver failure, as is jaundiced mucosal tissue.[2,33]

Bilateral, painless hypertrophy of the parotid glands (sialadenosis) is a frequent finding in patients with cirrhosis. The enlarged glands are soft and nontender and are not fixed to the overlying skin. This condition appears to be caused by a demyelinating polyneuropathy that results in abnormal sympathetic signaling, abnormal acinar protein secretion, and acinar cytoplasmic swelling. Because of the origin of this event, the parotid ducts remain patent and produce clear salivary flow.[2,33,44]

Alcohol abuse and tobacco use are strong risk factors for the development of oral squamous cell carcinoma, and the dentist must be aggressive (as with all patients) in the detection of unexplained or suspicious soft tissue lesions (especially leukoplakia, erythroplakia, or ulceration) in chronic alcoholic patients. High-risk sites for oral squamous cell carcinoma include the lateral border of the tongue and the floor of the mouth (see Chapter 26).

REFERENCES

1. Friedman SL. In Keefe FA (ed). Handbook of Liver Disease. New York, NY, Elsevier, 2005, p 496.
2. Golla K, Epstein JB, Cabay RJ. Liver disease: Current perspectives on medical and dental management. Oral Surg Oral Med Oral Pathol Oral Radiol Endod 2004;98:516-521.
3. Fiore AE, Wasley A, Bell BP. Prevention of hepatitis A through active or passive immunization: Recommendations of the Advisory Committee on Immunization Practices (ACIP). MMWR Recomm Rep 2006;55: 1-23.
4. Mast EE, Margolis HS, Fiore AE, et al. A comprehensive immunization strategy to eliminate transmission of hepatitis B virus infection in the United States: Recommendations of the Advisory Committee on Immunization Practices (ACIP). Part 1: Immunization of infants, children, and adolescents. MMWR Recomm Rep 2006;55:1-31.
5. Mosley JW, Edwards VM, Casey G, et al. Hepatitis B virus infection in dentists. N Engl J Med 1975;293: 729-733.
6. Thomas DL, Gruninger SE, Siew C, et al. Occupational risks of hepatitis C infections in North American dentists and oral surgeons. Am J Med 1996;100:41-45.
7. Centers for Disease Control and Prevention. Update: Recommendations to prevent hepatitis B transmission— United States. MMWR Morb Mortal Wkly Rep 1995;44:574-577.
8. Hoofnagle JH. Acute viral hepatitis. In Cecil RL, Goldman L, Bennett JC (eds). Cecil Textbook of Medicine, 21st ed. Philadelphia, Saunders, 2000, p 1433.
9. Chen M, Sonnerborg A, Johansson B, Sallberg M. Detection of hepatitis G virus (GB virus C) RNA in human saliva. J Clin Microbiol 1997;35:973-975.
10. Gerberding JL. Management of occupational exposures to blood-borne viruses. N Engl J Med 1995;332:444-451.
11. Lanphear BP. Management of occupational exposures to blood-borne viruses. Occup Med 12(4):717-730.
12. Cleveland JL, Gooch BF, Shearer BG, Lyerla RA. Risk and prevention of hepatitis C virus infection: Implications for dentistry. J Am Dent Assoc 1999;130: 641-647.
13. Centers for Disease Control. Lack of transmission of hepatitis B to humans after oral exposure to hepatitis B surface antigen–positive saliva. MMWR Morb Mortal Wkly Rep 1978;27:247.
14. Hoofnagle JH, Doo E, Liang TJ, Fleischer R, Lok AS. Management of Hepatitis B: Summary of a clinical research workshop. Hepatology 2007;45(4):1056-1076.
15. SyWassink JM, Lutwick LI. Risk of hepatitis B in dental care providers: A contact study. J Am Dent Assoc 1983;106:182-184.
16. Dusheiko GM, Smith M, Scheuer PJ. Hepatitis C virus transmitted by human bite [letter]. Lancet 1990;336: 503-504.
17. Sartori M, LaTerra G, Aglietta M, et al. Transmission of hepatitis C via blood splash into conjunctiva [letter]. Scand J Infect Dis 1993;25:270-271.
18. Esteban JI, Gomez J, Martell M, et al. Transmission of hepatitis C virus by a cardiac surgeon. N Engl J Med 1996;334:555-560.
19. Klein RS, Freeman K, Taylor PE, Stevens CE. Occupational risk for hepatitis C virus infection among New York City dentists. Lancet 1991;338:1539-1542.
20. Vinayek BE. Acute and chronic hepatitis. In Stein JA (ed). Internal Medicine, 2nd ed. St. Louis, Mosby, 1998, p 876.
21. Alter MJ, Kruszon-Moran D, Nainan OV, et al. The prevalence of hepatitis C virus infection in the United States, 1988 through 1994. N Engl J Med 1999;342: 556-562.
22. Centers for Disease Control. Recommended infection-control practices for dentistry, 1993. MMWR Morb Mortal Wkly Rep 1993;41:1-12.
23. Pratt DS, Kaplan MM. Evaluation of abnormal liver-enzyme results in asymptomatic patients. N Engl J Med 2000;342:1266-1271.

24. Centers for Disease Control. Recommendations for prevention and control of hepatitis C virus (HCV) infection and HCV-related chronic disease. MMWR Morb Mortal Wkly Rep 1998;47:1-38.

25. Thoelen S, Van Damme P, Leentvaar-Kuypers A, et al. The first combined vaccine against hepatitis A and B: An overview. Vaccine 1999;17:1657-1662.

26. Mahoney FJ, Stewart K, Hu H, et al. Progress toward the elimination of hepatitis B virus transmission among health care workers in the United States. Arch Intern Med 1997;157:2601-2609.

27. Centers for Disease Control and Prevention. Immunization of health-care workers: Recommendations of the Advisory Committee on Immunization Practices (ACIP) and the Hospital Infection Control Practices Advisory Committee (HICPAC). MMWR Morb Mortal Wkly Rep 1997;46:1-42.

28. Scully C. Liver disease. In Scully C, Cawson RA (ed). Medical Problems in Dentistry, 5th ed. New York, Elsevier Churchill Livingstone, 2005.

29. Zeuzem S, Feinman SV, Rasenack J, et al. Peginterferon alfa-2a in patients with chronic hepatitis C. N Engl J Med 2000;343:1666-1669.

30. Pianko S, McHutchison JG. Treatment of hepatitis C with interferon and ribavirin. J Gastroenterol Hepatol 2000;15:581-586.

31. ADA Council on Scientific Affairs and ADA Council on Dental Practice. Infection control recommendations for the dental office and the dental laboratory. J Am Dent Assoc 1996;127:672-680.

32. Goodman RA, Solomon SL. Transmission of infectious diseases in outpatient health care settings. JAMA 1991;265:2377-2381.

33. Diamond I. Alcoholism and alcohol abuse. In Goldman L, Bennett JC (eds). Cecil Textbook of Medicine, 21st ed. Philadelphia, WB Saunders, 2000.

34. Beulens JW, Stolk RP, van der Schouw YT, et al. Alcohol consumption and risk of type 2 diabetes among older women. Diabetes Care 2005;28:2933-2938.

35. Friedlander AH, Marder SR, Pisegna YR, Yagiela JA. Alcohol abuse and dependence: Psychopathology, medical management and dental implications. J Am Dent Assoc 2003;134:731-740.

36. McGinnis JM, Foege WH. Mortality and morbidity attributable to use of addictive substances in the United States. Proc Assoc Am Physicians 1999;111:109-118.

37. Diamond I. Alcoholism and alcohol abuse. In Goldman L, Ausiello D (eds). Cecil Textbook of Medicine, 22nd ed. Philadelphia, WB Saunders, 2004.

38. Hanna EZ, Chou SP, Grant BF. The relationship between drinking and heart disease morbidity in the United States: Results from the National Health Interview Survey. Alcohol Clin Exp Res 1997;21:111-118.

39. Watson RR, Borgs P, Witte M, et al. Alcohol, immunomodulation, and disease. Alcohol Alcohol 1994;29:131-139.

40. Podolsky DL. Cirrhosis of the liver. In Harrison TR, Wilson JD (eds). Harrison's Principles of Internal Medicine, 12th ed. New York, McGraw-Hill, 1991, p 1567.

41. O'Connor PG, Schottenfeld RS. Patients with alcohol problem. N Engl J Med 1998;338:592-597.

42. National Institute on Alcohol Abuse and Alcoholism. The Physicians' Guide to Helping Patients With Alcohol Problems. U.S. Department of Health and Human Services, Government Printing Office, 1995.

43. Albers I, Hartmann H, Bircher J, Creutzfeldt W. Superiority of the Child-Pugh classification to quantitative liver function tests for assessing prognosis of liver cirrhosis. Scand J Gastroenterol 1989;24:269-274.

44. Mandel L, Hamele-Bena D. Alcoholic parotid sialadenosis. J Am Dent Assoc 1997;128:411-414.

Gastrointestinal Disease

Gastrointestinal diseases such as peptic ulcer disease, inflammatory bowel disease, and pseudomembranous colitis are common and may affect the delivery of dental care. A patient who has one of these conditions presents several areas of concern to the dental practitioner. The dentist must be cognizant of the patient's condition, must monitor for symptoms indicative of initial disease or relapse, and must be aware of drugs that interact with gastrointestinal medications or that may aggravate these conditions. In addition, oral manifestations of gastrointestinal disease are not rare; thus, the dentist must be familiar with oral patterns of disease.

PEPTIC ULCER DISEASE

DEFINITION

A peptic ulcer is a well-defined break in the gastrointestinal mucosa (greater than 3 mm in diameter, as defined by many industry-sponsored studies) that results from chronic acid/pepsin secretions and the destructive effects of and host response to *Helicobacter pylori*. Peptic ulcers develop principally in regions of the gastrointestinal tract that are proximal to acid/pepsin secretions (Figure 12-1). The first portion of the duodenum is the location of most ulcers in Western populations, whereas gastric ulcers are more frequent in Asia.[1] The upper jejunum rarely is involved. Peptic ulcer disease usually is chronic and focal; only approximately 10% of patients have multiple ulcers.

EPIDEMIOLOGY

Incidence and Prevalence

Peptic ulcer disease is one of the most common human ailments, once affecting up to 15% of the population in industrialized countries. Current estimates suggest that

5% to 10% of the world population is affected, and 350,000 new cases are diagnosed in the United States annually.[2-5] The incidence of peptic ulceration peaked between 1900 and 1950 and progressively decreased thereafter. The decline in Northern Europe and the United States may be the result of decreased cigarette and aspirin consumption, increased use of vegetable cooking oils (a rich source of raw materials for synthesis of prostaglandins, which have cytoprotective properties), and better sanitation.[6] The disease affects 5% to 7% of Northern Europeans and accounts for about 200,000 hospitalizations annually in the United States. Peptic ulcers are rare in Greenlander Eskimos, southwestern Native Americans, Australian aborigines, and Indonesians.[2]

Peak prevalence of peptic ulceration has shifted to the elderly.[4,5] Until the 1980s, the male/female ratio in the United States was 2:1, but current figures approximate this ratio at 1:1.[7] First-degree relatives have a threefold greater risk of developing the disease.[5] Persons who smoke and are heavy drinkers of alcohol are more prone to the disease. An association with blood type O exists. A higher prevalence is seen in patients with hyperparathyroidism and conditions associated with increased gastrin levels (i.e., renal dialysis, Zollinger-Ellison syndrome, mastocytosis). Use of nonsteroidal anti-inflammatory drugs (NSAIDs and aspirin) for longer than 1 month is associated with gastrointestinal bleeding or ulcer complications in 2% to 4% of patients per year who ingest these drugs.[8,9]

The disease is rare in children, with only 1 in 2500 pediatric hospital admissions attributable to peptic ulceration.[10] When a peptic ulcer is diagnosed in a child younger than 10 years of age, the condition most often is associated with an underlying systemic illness, such as severe burn or major trauma.[11] Most deaths that result from peptic ulcer disease occur in patients older than 65 years of age. An average dental practice of 2000 adult

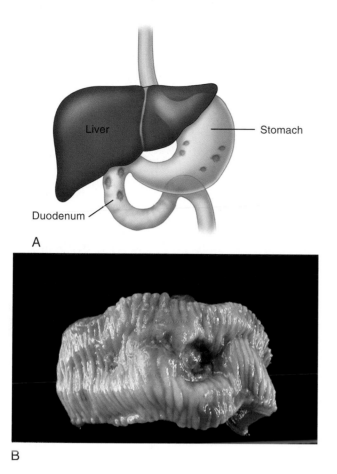

A

B

Figure 12-1. A, Location of peptic ulceration *(shaded areas)*. Darker stipulations are higher-risk sites. **B,** Peptic ulcer of the duodenum. (**B** from Kumar V, Abbas A, Fausto N. Robbins & Cotran Pathologic Basis of Disease, 7th ed. Philadelphia, Saunders, 2005. Courtesy Robin Foss, University of Florida–Gainesville.)

patients is predicted to serve about 100 patients with peptic ulcer disease.

Etiology

Excess acid in the stomach may cause peptic ulcer disease. However, acid hypersecretion is not uniformly found in patients with peptic ulceration.[12] Current evidence supports a complex interaction between aggressive factors that are potentially destructive to the gastrointestinal mucosa and defensive factors that are protective of the mucosa. The primary aggressive factor appears to be *H. pylori* (formerly, *Campylobacter pylori*). This organism is present in 60% to 90% of duodenal ulcers and 50% to 70% of gastric ulcers.[1,13] Use of NSAIDs is the second most common cause of peptic ulcer disease. Other aggressive factors include acid hypersecretion, cigarette smoking, and psychological and physical stress.[14] Cytomegalovirus infection is a rare cause noted in human immunodeficiency virus (HIV)-positive patients.[15]

H. pylori is a microaerophilic, Gram-negative, spiral-shaped bacillus with 4 to 6 flagella.[16] *H. pylori* was first

reported by Marshall and Warren to reside in the antral mucosa.[17,18] The organism is an adherent but noninvasive bacterium that resides at the interface between the surface of the gastric epithelium and the overlying mucous gel. It produces a potent urease that hydrolyzes urea to ammonia and carbon dioxide. This urease may protect bacteria from the immediate acidic environment by increasing local pH while damaging mucosa via the generation of its by-product, ammonia. Chemotaxis of neutrophils and the antibody response are involved in the local tissue damage that subsequently occurs.

Humans are the only known hosts of *H. pylori*. These bacteria display a 0.5% annual infection rate among adults.[19] *H. pylori* is acquired primarily during childhood, possibly as a result of entry from the oral cavity via contaminated food and poor sanitary habits. The organism resides in the oral cavity,[20] from which it probably descends to colonize the gastric mucosa. *H. pylori* can persist in the stomach indefinitely and remains clinically silent in most persons who are infected.[21] The rate of *H. pylori* acquisition is higher in developing than in developed countries.[22] In developing countries, 80% of the population carries the bacterium by the age of 20 years, whereas in the United States, only 20% of 20-year-olds are infected. The prevalence of infection in African Americans and Hispanics is twice that seen in whites in the United States.[23] Infection is correlated with poor socioeconomic status, contaminated drinking water, and familial overcrowding, especially during childhood. Approximately 20% of those infected go on to develop peptic ulcer disease,[14] suggesting that other physiologic and psychological (stress) factors[74] are required for presentation of this disease.

Because of their ability to directly damage mucosa, reduce mucosal prostaglandin production, and inhibit mucous secretion, NSAIDs are associated with 15% to 20% of peptic ulcers.[1,9] Ulcers caused by NSAIDs more often are located in the stomach than in the duodenum. Risk with NSAID use increases with age older than 60 years, high-dosage long-term therapy, use of NSAIDs with long plasma half-lives (e.g., piroxicam) rather than those with short half-lives (i.e., ibuprofen), and concomitant use of alcohol, corticosteroids, anticoagulants, or aspirin. Use of nitrogen-containing bisphosphonate drugs (aledronate, risedronate) for the treatment of osteoporosis and immunosuppressive medications such as mycophenolate is associated with esophageal and gastric ulcers.[1,25]

Pathophysiology and Complications

Ulcer formation is the result of a complex interplay of aggressive and defensive factors (Figure 12-2). Resistance to acidic breakdown is provided normally by mucosal resistance, mucous and prostaglandin production, blood flow, bicarbonate secretion, and ion–carrier exchange. Additional resistance is gained from antibacterial proteins such as lysozyme, lactoferrin, interferon, and defensin/cryptdin.

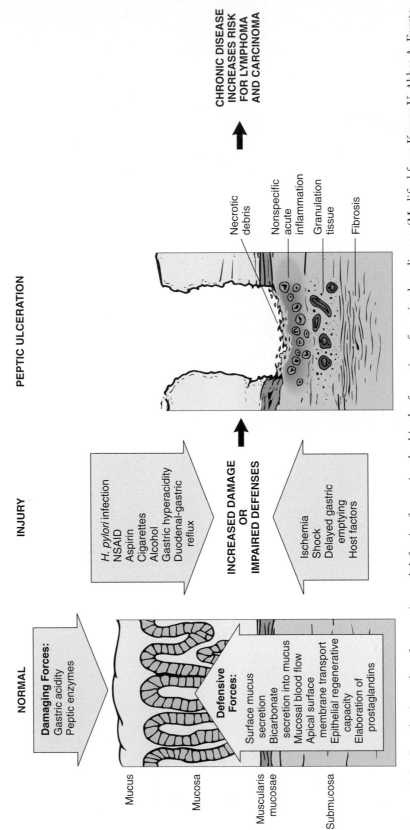
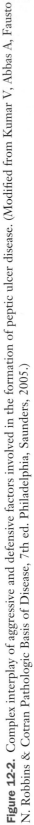

Figure 12-2. Complex interplay of aggressive and defensive factors involved in the formation of peptic ulcer disease. (Modified from Kumar V, Abbas A, Fausto N. Robbins & Cotran Pathologic Basis of Disease, 7th ed. Philadelphia, Saunders, 2005.)

Under normal circumstances, food stimulates gastrin release, gastrin stimulates histamine release by enterochromaffin-like cells in the stomach, and parietal cells secrete hydrogen ions and chloride ions (hydrochloric acid). Vagal nerve stimulation, caffeine, and histamine also are stimulants of parietal cell secretion of hydrochloric acid.[26] Aggressive factors include vagal overactivity and factors that enhance the release of pepsin, gastrin, and histamine. Physical and emotional stress, obsessive-compulsive behavior, parasitic infections, and drugs such as caffeine, high-dose corticosteroids, and phenylbutazone enhance hypersecretion of stomach acid. Alcohol and NSAIDs are directly injurious to gastric mucosa. Alcohol alters cell permeability and can cause cell death. NSAIDs and aspirin disrupt mucosal resistance by impairing prostaglandin production, denaturating mucous glycoproteins, and promoting degranulation of mast cells. Hyperparathyroidism enhances gastrin secretion, and renal dialysis inadequately removes circulating gastrin. Smoking tobacco and family history are risk factors independent of gastric acid secretion for peptic ulcer disease.[7,27] Tobacco smoke, similar to other aggressive factors, can affect gastric mucosa by reducing nitric oxide levels[28]; the latter are important for stimulating mucous secretion and maintaining mucosal blood flow.[29]

H. pylori is strongly associated with peptic ulcer disease; however, the mechanism whereby infection with *H. pylori* results in peptic ulcer disease is not completely understood. *H. pylori* clearly causes inflammation of the gastric mucosa and is responsible for most cases of etiologic gastritis. This bacterium has been implicated in promoting acute gastritis through its ability to disrupt mucosal resistance. The process may involve induction by *H. pylori* of increased gastrin release by G cells,[22,31,32] inflammatory mediators (cytokines), and cells that respond to *H. pylori* antigens, ammonia, and cytotoxin-associated gene (*CagA*) products.[32-35] *H. pylori*–associated antral gastritis is found in 90% to 100% of patients with duodenal ulcers.[36,37] However, no correlation between *H. pylori* and acid hypersecretion exists. In fact, acid secretion in patients with peptic ulcer is similar to that in patients without ulcers,[12] and *H. pylori* alone has been unable to injure stomach mucosa (ex vivo and in vitro).[38] This suggests that the inflammatory response causes mucosal breakdown.[33]

Complications associated with peptic ulcer disease vary with the degree of destruction of the gastrointestinal epithelium and supporting tissues. Superficial ulcers are characterized by necrotic debris and fibrin. Beneath this layer are numerous polymorphonuclear leukocytes, scattered macrophages, and eosinophils. Below is active granulation tissue and fibrosis. A chronic or aggressive ulcer can penetrate through the fibrotic tissue into the muscularis layer (muscularis mucosa). The muscularis layer, weakened by scar tissue, can perforate into the peritoneal cavity (peritonitis) or into the head of the pancreas. Arteries or veins in the muscularis layer may be eroded by ulcers, giving rise to hemorrhage (a bleeding ulcer), anemia, and potential shock. Untreated ulcers often heal by fibrosis, which can lead to pyloric stenosis, gastric outlet obstruction, dehydration, and alkalosis. Complications are more common in the elderly; 5000 people die annually in the United States as a result of these complications.[4]

H. pylori is associated with the development of a low-grade gastric mucosa–associated lymphoid tissue lymphoma.[39] Accordingly, *H. pylori* has been classified by the World Health Organization as a definite (Class I) human carcinogen.[40]

Peptic ulcers rarely undergo carcinomatous transformation. Ulcers of the greater curvature of the stomach have a greater propensity for malignant degeneration than do those of the duodenum. Atrophic gastritis associated with long-term use of proton pump inhibitors (see Medical Management) increases the risk for stomach cancer.[41]

CLINICAL PRESENTATION

Signs and Symptoms

Although many patients with active peptic ulcer have no ulcer symptoms, most develop epigastric pain that is long-standing (several hours) and sharply localized. The pain is described as "burning" or "gnawing" but may be "ill-defined" or "aching." The discomfort of a duodenal ulcer manifests most commonly on an empty stomach, usually 90 minutes to 3 hours after eating, and frequently awakens the patient in the middle of the night. Ingestion of food, milk, or antacids provides rapid relief in most cases. In contrast, patients with gastric ulcers, however, are unpredictable in their response to food and may develop abdominal pain from eating. Symptoms associated with peptic ulceration tend to be episodic and recurrent. Epigastric tenderness often accompanies the condition.

Changes in the character of pain may indicate the development of complications. For example, increased discomfort, loss of antacid relief, or pain radiating to the back may signal deeper penetration or perforation of the ulcer. Protracted vomiting a few hours after a meal is a sign of gastric outlet (pyloric) obstruction. Melena (bloody stools) or black tarry stools indicate blood loss due to gastrointestinal hemorrhage.

Laboratory Findings

A peptic ulcer is diagnosed primarily by fiberoptic endoscopy and laboratory tests for *H. pylori*. Endoscopy affords the opportunity for visualization, access for biopsy, and therapeutic procedures if bleeding is present. Of the many available laboratory tests, urea breath tests (UBTs) are widely used. Serology and/or *H. pylori* stool antigen tests are less commonly used. UBTs are advantageous because they measure indirectly the presence of *H. pylori* before treatment and its eradication after treatment. Serology is useful in determining current or past infection but is limited in documenting the eradication of

H. pylori because antibody titers persist after the organism has been eliminated.

A UBT is a noninvasive test that involves the ingestion of urea labeled with carbon-13 (^{13}C) or carbon-14 (^{14}C). Degradation of urea by the bacillus releases ^{13}C or ^{14}C in expired carbon dioxide. A ^{13}C test can be performed in the office, but ^{14}C tests must be performed in nuclear medicine facilities. Breath tests are advantageous in that they are noninvasive, highly accurate, and highly sensitive.[42] Their accuracy is reduced in patients who take proton pump inhibitors.

A biopsy of the marginal mucosa adjacent to the ulcer is performed during endoscopy to confirm the diagnosis and rule out malignancy. During endoscopy, the rapid urease test can be performed. Microscopic analysis of biopsied tissue with Giemsa, acridine orange, and Warthin-Starry stains is effective in the microscopic detection of *H. pylori* (Figure 12-3). The urease test involves direct inoculation of a portion of the gastric mucosal biopsy into a gel medium that contains urea and phenol red. If the organism is present, the gel is

metabolized to ammonia (raising the pH to greater than or equal to 6.0), which causes the gel to change from yellow to pink. Culture of the organism is reserved for cases in which antimicrobial resistance is suspected because the technique is tedious, difficult, and no more sensitive than routine histologic analysis.

MEDICAL MANAGEMENT

Most patients with peptic ulcer disease suffer for several weeks before going to a doctor for treatment. If the peptic ulcer is confined and uncomplicated and *H. pylori* is not present, antisecretory drugs are administered (Table 12-1). If the patient is infected with *H. pylori*, inhibitors of gastric acid secretion and antimicrobial agents are recommended.[43] Combination therapy is recommended because antisecretory drugs, such as H_2 antagonists and proton pump inhibitors (PPIs), provide rapid relief of pain and accelerate healing, and antibiotics are efficient in eradicating *H. pylori*. As a result, combination treatment accelerates healing and produces an ulcer-free state in 92% to 99% of treated patients.[39,40]

For those with peptic ulcer and *H. pylori* infection, current first-line therapy consists of the administration of at least two antibiotics and one antisecretory drug (Box 12-1). This is known as "triple" therapy. Recommended triple therapy consists of a PPI with clarithromycin and either amoxicillin or metronidazole.[44] Tetracycline and bismuth subsalicylate serve as alternative antibiotic and antisecretory drugs, respectively. Therapy generally is given for 10 days to 2 weeks, and eradication of infection should be confirmed afterward. Quadruple therapy is considered second-line therapy (see Box 12-1).

In the past, more than 50% of patients with peptic ulcer disease experienced recurrences. This occurred because antisecretory drugs alone were the treatment of choice; however, these drugs alone do not eradicate *H. pylori* infection and are noncurative of peptic ulcer disease. Eradication of *H. pylori* with antibiotic treatment reduces

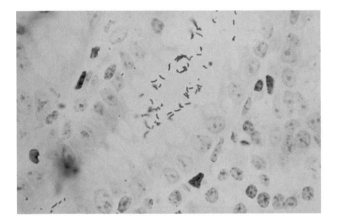

Figure 12-3. *Helicobacter pylori (dark rods)* evident in the lumen of the intestine. (Warthin-Starry stain; courtesy Eun Lee, Lexington, Ky.)

TABLE **12-1**
Antisecretory Drugs

Class	Generic Drug	Trade Name	Dental Management Considerations
H$_2$ histamine antagonist	Cimetidine	Tagamet	Delayed liver metabolism of benzodiazepines; reversible joint symptoms with preexisting arthritis
	Ranitidine	Zantac	—
	Famotidine	Pepcid	Anorexia, dry mouth
	Nizatidine	Axid	Potentially increased serum salicylate levels with concurrent aspirin use
Proton pump inhibitor	Omeprazole	Prilosec	May reduce absorption of ampicillin, ketoconazole, and itraconazole
	Lansoprazole	Prevacid	
	Pantoprazole	Protonix, Protium	
	Esomeprazole	Nexium	
Prostaglandin*	Misoprostol	Cytotec	Diarrhea, cramps

*Not a first-line drug for treating patients with peptic ulcer. Used in the prevention of peptic ulcer and in users of nonsteroidal anti-inflammatory drugs (NSAIDs).

Antimicrobial Regimens for the Treatment of *Helicobacter pylori* Infection in Peptic Ulcer Disease*

FIRST-LINE THERAPY[†]
- Proton pump inhibitor (or ranitidine bismuth citrate) twice daily *plus*
- Clarithromycin (500 mg) twice daily *plus*
- Amoxicillin 1000 mg twice daily or metronidazole 500 mg twice daily

SECOND-LINE THERAPY[†]
- Quadruple therapy subsalicylate proton pump inhibitor twice daily, bismuth subsalicylate/ subcitrate 120 mg 4× daily, plus metronidazole 500 mg twice daily, tetracycline 500 mg four time daily

*Data from Malfertheiner P, et al. Current concepts in the management of *Helicobacter pylori* infection—The Maastricht 2-2000 consensus report. Aliment Pharmacol Ther 2002;16:167-180.[45]
[†]Medications are given over a minimum of 7 days.

the rate of recurrence of peptic ulceration by 85% to 100%.[21,45-48] Reemergence of an ulcer usually is traced to the persistence of *H. pylori* after treatment because of inappropriate drug choice, discontinuance of drug therapy, lack of behavior modification, or bacterial resistance.[1]

In all patients who undergo peptic ulcer therapy, ulcerogenic factors (i.e., continued use of alcohol, aspirin, NSAIDs, and corticosteroids; foods that aggravate symptoms and stimulate gastric acid secretion; stress) should be eliminated to accelerate healing and limit the occurrence of relapse. Patients appear to benefit from smoking cessation, in that perforation rates are higher in smokers, and continued smoking results in a higher rate of relapse after treatment and lower eradication rates of *H. pylori*.[49,50] However, when *H. pylori* is successfully eradicated, cigarette smoking does not appear to increase the risk of recurrence.[51]

Elective surgical intervention (e.g., dissection of the vagus nerves from the gastric fundus) largely has been abandoned in the management of peptic ulcer disease. Today, surgery is reserved primarily for complications of peptic ulcer disease such as significant bleeding (when unresponsive to coagulant endoscopic procedures), perforation, and gastric outlet obstruction. On occasions when peptic ulcer disease is associated with hyperparathyroidism and parathyroid adenoma, surgical removal of the affected gland is the treatment of choice. Resolution of gastrointestinal disease occurs after abnormal endocrine function is terminated. Prototype protein-based vaccines against *H. pylori* continue to be investigated.[52]

DENTAL MANAGEMENT
Medical Considerations

The dentist must identify intestinal symptoms through a careful history that is taken before dental treatment is initiated, because many gastrointestinal diseases, although they are chronic and recurrent, remain undetected for long periods. This history includes a careful review of medications (e.g., aspirin, NSAIDs, oral anticoagulants) and alcohol consumption that may result in gastrointestinal bleeding. If gastrointestinal symptoms are suggestive of active disease, a medical referral is needed. Once the patient returns from the physician and the condition is under control, the dentist should update current medications in the dental record, including the type and dosage, and should follow physician guidelines. Further, periodic physician visits should be encouraged to afford early diagnosis and cancer screenings for at-risk patients.

Of primary importance are the impact and interactions of certain drugs prescribed to patients with peptic ulcer disease (Box 12-2). In general, the dentist should avoid prescribing aspirin, aspirin-containing compounds, and NSAIDs to patients with a history of peptic ulcer disease because of the irritative effects of these drugs on the gastrointestinal epithelium. Acetaminophen and compounded acetaminophen products are recommended instead. If NSAIDs are used, a cyclooxygenase (COX)-2 selective inhibitor (celecoxib [Celebrex]) given in combination with a PPI or misoprostol (Cytotec), 800 μg per day)—a prostaglandin E1 analog—is advised for short-term use to reduce the risk of gastrointestinal bleeding.[1,53] Analgesic selection should be based on patient risk factors (prior gastrointestinal bleeding, age, use of alcohol, anticoagulants or steroids) and should provide the lowest dose for the shortest period to achieve the desired affect. H_2 antagonists and sucralfate are not beneficial selections because they do not appear to protect patients from NSAID-induced complications.[54]

Acid-blocking drugs, such as cimetidine, decrease the metabolism of certain dentally prescribed drugs (i.e., diazepam, lidocaine, tricyclic antidepressants) and enhance the duration of action of these medications (see Table 12-1). Under such circumstances, dosing of anesthetics, benzodiazepines, and antidepressants that are metabolized in the liver may require adjustment. Antacids also impair the absorption of tetracycline, erythromycin, oral iron, and fluoride, and they prevent optimal blood levels of these drugs. To avoid this problem, antibiotics and dietary supplements should be taken 2 hours before or 2 hours after antacids are ingested.

Routine dental treatment may be provided during medical therapy for peptic ulceration; however, the decision should be based on patient comfort and convenience. Should antibiotics become necessary to treat a dental infection during the course of peptic ulcer disease therapy, the choice of antibiotics may be altered by the patient's current medications. For example, tetracycline or metronidazole is not an appropriate choice for most odontogenic infections, and amoxicillin or clarithromycin can be substituted with the approval of the patient's physician.

BOX 12-2

Dental Management Considerations for Patients Who Have or Are Predisposed to Gastrointestinal Disease

1. Evaluate patient, determine health status, and confirm that adequate medical care was received.
2. If patient has recently taken corticosteroids, consider the need for supplemental steroids. Decision should be based on health status and dental procedure (see Box 16-1).
3. Obtain complete blood count if medication profile increases patient risk for anemia, leukopenia, or thrombocytopenia.
4. Provide appropriate treatment for pain and anxiety. Measures include the following:
   a. Patients are advised to obtain proper rest the night before treatment.
   b. Benzodiazepine sedative (e.g., Dalmane) may be prescribed to be taken on the night before treatment.
   c. Appointments are tolerated best when they are scheduled in the morning and are limited in duration.
   d. Patients are advised to reduce business and social obligations on the day of the appointment.
   e. Intraoperative sedation can be provided by an oral, inhalation, or intravenous route.
   f. Analgesic (acetaminophen alone or in combination with opioid) should be provided when postoperative pain is expected. Best to avoid nonselecive and potent nonsteroidal anti-inflammatory drugs

(NSAIDs). If celecoxib is provided, concurrent use of misoprostol (Cytotec [Searle & Co., Chicago, Ill], 800 μg per day) or a proton pump inhibitor (see Table 12-1) is recommended.
4. Lower doses of diazepam, lidocaine, or tricyclic antidepressants may be required if the patient is taking acid-blocking drugs, such as cimetidine, which decreases the metabolism of some dentally prescribed drugs and enhances the duration of action of these medications.
5. Selection of antibiotics for oral infections may be influenced by recent use of antibiotics for peptic ulcer disease.
6. Increased risk for medical complications is associated with the following:
   a. Peptic ulcer disease when age >65 years, previous history of ulcer complications, prolonged use of NSAIDs, and concomitant use of anticoagulants, corticosteroids, or bisphosphonates.
   b. Inflammatory bowel disease when patient has symptomatic disease.
   c. Pseudomembranous colitis when age >65 years, recent hospitalization, broad-spectrum antibiotics (clindamycin, cephalosporins, ampicillin) are used, multiple antibiotics are used, and human immunodeficiency virus (HIV) occurs with immune suppression.

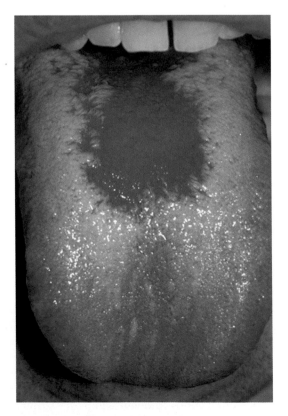

Figure 12-4. Median rhomboid glossitis caused by antibiotic use.

Treatment Planning Modifications

H. pylori is found in dental plaque and may serve as a reservoir of infection and reinfection along the alimentary tract.[20,55] Good oral hygiene measures and periodic scaling and prophylaxis may be useful in reducing the spread of this organism. Rigorous hygiene measures should be discussed with the patient and consideration given to detecting oral organisms in patients who have a history of peptic ulcer disease and are symptomatic or are experiencing recurrences. Routine dental care requires no other modifications in technique for patients with peptic ulcer disease.

Oral Complications and Manifestations

The use of systemic antibiotics for peptic ulcer disease may result in fungal overgrowth (candidiasis) in the oral cavity. The dentist should be alert to identifying oral fungal infections, including median rhomboid glossitis, in this patient population (Figure 12-4). A course of antifungal agents (see Appendix C) should be prescribed to resolve the fungal infection.

Vascular malformations of the lip and erosion of the enamel are two less common oral manifestations of peptic ulcer disease. The former have been reported to range from a small macule (microcherry) to a large venous pool, and they occur in older men with peptic ulcer disease.[56] The latter finding is the result of persistent regurgitation

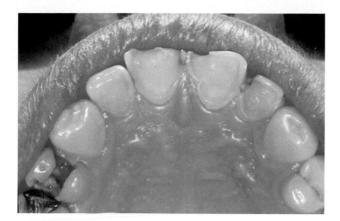

Figure 12-5. Perimylolysis. Destruction of palatal enamel of maxillary incisors in a patient with persistent regurgitation.

of gastric juices into the mouth when pyloric stenosis occurs (Figure 12-5). The finding of enamel erosion combined with a history of reflux indicates that the patient must be evaluated by a physician.

Medications taken by patients for the treatment of peptic ulcer disease can produce oral manifestations. PPIs can alter taste perception. Cimetidine and ranitidine may have a toxic effect on bone marrow; infrequently, they cause anemia, agranulocytosis, or thrombocytopenia. Mucosal ulcerations may be a sign of agranulocytosis, whereas anemia may present as mucosal pallor and thrombocytopenia as gingival bleeding or petechiae. Xerostomia has been associated with the use of famotidine and anticholinergic drugs, such as propantheline (Pro-Banthine). A chronic dry mouth renders the patient susceptible to bacterial infection (caries and periodontal disease) and fungal disease (candidiasis). Erythema multiforme is associated with the use of cimetidine, ranitidine, and lansoprazole.

INFLAMMATORY BOWEL DISEASE

DEFINITION

Inflammatory bowel disease (IBD) describes two idiopathic diseases of the gastrointestinal tract: ulcerative colitis and Crohn's disease. The main criteria that separate the two diseases are the site and extent of tissue involvement; thus, they are discussed together. Ulcerative colitis is a mucosal disease that is limited to the large intestine and rectum. In contrast, Crohn's disease is a transmural process (affects entire wall of the bowel) that may produce "patchy" ulcerations along any point of the alimentary canal from the mouth to the anus but most commonly involves the terminal ileum.

EPIDEMIOLOGY

Incidence and Prevalence

The incidence and prevalence of IBD vary widely by race and geographic location. Occurrence is much higher among Jews and whites than in blacks, and it is considerably higher in the United States and Europe than in Asia and Africa. Approximately 10 to 15 new cases of IBD per 100,000 persons are diagnosed annually in the United States and Europe.[57] Approximately 1 million persons in the United States are affected.[58] Peak age of onset is young adulthood (20 to 40 years of age). However, a second incidence peak of Crohn's disease has been noted in persons older than 60 years of age. Children also have been known to develop IBD. The predilection for ulcerative colitis in men and women is equal, whereas Crohn's disease has a slight predilection for women. A tenfold increased risk of disease in first-degree relatives of patients strongly suggests that genetic factors are involved,[59] although the mode of inheritance is unclear. The environment is a contributory factor, in that Crohn's disease occurs more often in nonsmokers, whereas smoking protects against ulcerative colitis. Breast feeding also appears to reduce the risk of IBD.[60] In the average general dentistry practice with 2000 adult patients, approximately 5 adults are predicted to have IBD.

Etiology

Ulcerative colitis and Crohn's disease are inflammatory diseases of unknown cause that are generally thought to be associated with immune dysfunction in response to environmental factors in genetically susceptible persons. *Nod2/Card15*, a susceptibility gene, has recently been implicated by several research groups in the pathogenesis of Crohn's disease. Mutations in this gene impair the innate immune response, leading to inefficient recognition and clearing of microbes by intestinal epithelium and subsequent inflammation and increased permeability of the intestinal wall.[61-63]

Pathophysiology and Complications

Ulcerative Colitis. Ulcerative colitis is an inflammatory reaction of the large intestine characterized by remissions and exacerbations. The disease starts in the colon/rectum region and may spread proximally to involve the entire large intestine and the ileum. Pathologic findings include edema, vascular congestion, distorted cryptic architecture, and monocellular infiltration. Persistent disease causes epithelial erosions and hemorrhage, pseudopolyp formation, crypt abscesses, and submucosal fibrosis. Chronic deposition of fibrous tissue may lead to fibrotic shortening, thickening, and narrowing of the colon.

Ulcerative colitis usually is lifelong, and progression to its more severe forms predisposes the patient to toxic dilatation (toxic megacolon) and dysplastic changes (carcinoma) of the intestine. Toxic megacolon is the result of disease extension through deep muscular layers. The colon dilates because of weakening of the wall, and intestinal perforation becomes likely. Fever, electrolyte imbalance, and volume depletion are reported. Carcinoma of the colon is 10 times more likely in patients with ulcerative colitis than in the general population.[64] Likelihood of malignant transformation increases with proximal

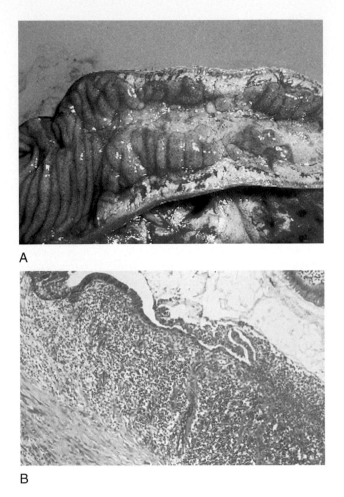

A

B

Figure 12-6. A, Crohn's disease that exhibits ulceration of the intestinal mucosa. **B,** Low-power micrograph showing ulcerated intestinal mucosa of Crohn's disease with dense inflammatory infiltrate. (**A** from Allison MC et al. Inflammatory bowel disease, London, Mosby Ltd., 1998.)

extension of the disease and long-standing disease (greater than 8 to 10 years, at a rate of 0.5% to 2% per year).[65]

Crohn's Disease. Crohn's disease is a chronic, relapsing idiopathic disease that is characterized by segmental distribution of intestinal ulcers (skip lesions) interrupted by normal-appearing mucosa. Although the distal ileum and the proximal colon are affected most frequently, any portion of the bowel may be involved. The rectum is involved in up to 80% of patients—much more often than ulcerative colitis. Macroscopically, the intestine displays sharply delimited regions of thickened bowel wall, irregular glandular openings, mucosal fissuring, ulcerations, erosions, and benign strictures (Figure 12-6). In chronic disease, the intestinal mucosa takes on a nodular or "cobblestoned" appearance as a result of dense inflammatory infiltrates and submucosal thickening. Transmural involvement of the intestinal wall and noncaseating epithelioid granulomas of the intestine and mesenteric lymph nodes are classic features of the disease.

At the microscopic level, ulcerative colitis and Crohn's disease are characterized by infiltrative lesions of the bowel wall that contain activated inflammatory cells (neutrophils and macrophages), immune-based cells (lymphocytes and plasma cells), and noncaseating granulomas. Inflammatory cells appear to be attracted to the region as a result of increased levels of interleukin-1 (IL-1), which stimulates the production of prostaglandins, leukotrienes, and other cytokines (e.g., tumor necrosis factor).[66,67] Crohn's disease is further characterized by defects in mucosal immunity and in the mucosal barrier that result in increased intestinal permeability, increased adherence of bacteria, and decreased expression of defensins.[68] Crohn's disease is characterized clinically by remissions and relapses; relapses are more common in persons who smoke tobacco. Unremitting disease is complicated by small-bowel stenosis and fistulas. Most patients who have Crohn's disease require at least one operation for their condition.[69] Long-standing colonic Crohn's disease increases the risk for the development of colorectal cancer.

CLINICAL PRESENTATION

Signs and Symptoms

Ulcerative Colitis. Patients with ulcerative colitis have three prominent symptoms: (1) attacks of diarrhea, (2) rectal bleeding (or bloody diarrhea), and (3) abdominal cramps. Onset may be sudden or insidious, but the disease continues along a chronic, intermittent course in most patients. Dehydration, fatigue, weight loss, and fever caused by malabsorption of water and electrolytes frequently accompany the condition. Extraintestinal manifestations may include arthritis, erythema nodosum or pyoderma gangrenosum, eye disorders like iritis and uveitis, and growth failure. Although many patients have long periods of remission, less than 5% remain symptom free over a 10-year period; about 50% have a relapse in any given year.[65,70]

Crohn's Disease. Initial manifestations of Crohn's disease consist of recurrent or persistent diarrhea (often without blood) abdominal cramps, anorexia, and weight loss. Unexplained fever, malaise, arthritis, uveitis, and features related to malabsorption often appear next. However, symptoms vary from patient to patient according to the site and extent of involved alimentary tissue. For example, compromised intestinal lumen size may contribute to bowel obstruction and colicky pain that is aggravated by eating. In contrast, the patient may display rectal bleeding, a perirectal abscess or fistula, or dramatic weight loss. Variability in symptoms and the episodic pattern contribute to the average 3-year delay in diagnosis from onset of symptoms.[67] Intestinal complications from chronic inflammatory damage include transmural fibrosis, intestinal fissuring, fistulas, and abscess formation. These complications are common; 70% to 80% of patients require surgery within their lifetime. Malabsorption is an additional complication that can result in striking degrees of weight loss, growth failure, anemia, and clubbing of the fingers. Reduced bone mineral density (i.e., osteoporosis) also results from malabsorption and chronic corticosteroid use. Extraintestinal manifestations (e.g., peripheral arthritis, erythema nodosum, aphthous, episcleritis) occur in about 25% of patients.

Laboratory Findings

The diagnosis of IBD is based primarily on clinical findings, results of colonoscopy and biopsy, and observations on histologic examination of intestinal mucosal. Abdominal radiographs and stool examinations are also supportive. Radiolabeled leukocyte scanning and computed tomography are useful for identifying sites of activity and regions complicated by abscess and fistula formation.[71]

Ulcerative colitis produces friable, granular, erythematous, and eroded mucosa of the colon with regions of edema and chronic inflammation seen upon endoscopic and microscopic inspection. Crohn's disease demonstrates patchy erosions and ulcerations with noncaseating granulomas that can affect any part of the gastrointestinal tract. Blood tests in IBD may show anemia (deficiencies of iron, folate, or vitamin B_{12}) caused by malabsorption, decreased levels of serum total protein and albumin (as a result of malabsorption), inflammatory activity (elevated erythrocyte sedimentation rate and C-reactive protein), and an elevated platelet count, in conjunction with a negative microbial stool sample.

MEDICAL MANAGEMENT

Ulcerative colitis and Crohn's disease can be managed, but not cured, by an array of drugs. Anti-inflammatory medications (e.g., sulfasalazine, 5-aminosalicylic acid, corticosteroids) are generally first-line drugs.[70] Immunosuppressive agents and antibiotics are used as second-line drugs. Third-line approaches for persons with Crohn's disease who are refractory to steroid treatment include monoclonal antibody (infliximab [Remicade]) against tumor necrosis factor[72] and surgical resection to remove the diseased portion of the colon. Supportive therapy that includes bed rest, dietary manipulation, and nutritional supplementation is often required. Dietary intervention with fish oil supplements may be beneficial to those with Crohn's disease.[73]

Sulfasalazine remains a cornerstone of therapy for patients with mild to moderate IBD. It is administered at 4 g/day in divided doses for active disease and at 1 g/day as a maintenance dose during remission.[74,75] Sulfasalazine is made up of 5-aminosalicylic acid (5-ASA) linked to sulfapyridine by an azo bond.[76] After oral administration, the drug is cleaved by colonic bacteria into its two components. The therapeutic properties of sulfasalazine are primarily caused by the local anti-inflammatory effects of 5-ASA within the intestine. Up to a third of patients treated with sulfasalazine report adverse effects (nausea, headache, fever, arthralgia, rash, anemia, agranulocytosis,

cholestatic hepatitis) that are associated with the sulfapyridine component and dose related, and that occur more often after long-term use. The adverse effect profile of sulfasalazine has contributed to its decreased popularity in recent years. Folic acid or iron supplementation is recommended during sulfasalazine therapy to combat associated anemia.

The 5-ASA preparations are just as effective as sulfasalazine and better tolerated, but they are more expensive. Absorption of orally administered 5-ASA occurs in the proximal bowel, thus it can be a problem for the drug to reach the diseased colon. This has led to generic and controlled-release oral formulations of 5-ASA (mesalamine [Asacol {Proctor & Gamble, Pharmaceuticals, Cincinnati, Ohio}, Pentasa {Shire US Inc., Wayne, Pa}], olsalazine, and balsalazide) that dissolve in the distal ileum and colon or are available as rectal suppository or enema.[62] Use of these drugs and of rectally administered 5-ASA drugs is important in the management of ulcerative colitis when the disease is limited to distal segments (sigmoid) of the colon. Renal function is monitored by the physician because 5-ASA drugs are potentially nephrotoxic.

Corticosteroids often are combined with sulfasalazine to induce remission in patients who are moderately to severely ill. Steroids are not recommended for maintenance therapy of disease because adverse effects are associated with long-term use. When severe attacks produce abdominal tenderness, dehydration, fever, vomiting, and severe bloody diarrhea, the patient should be hospitalized, and parenteral corticosteroids administered. After about 2 weeks, or once a satisfactory response is achieved, oral steroids are substituted for parenteral steroids. The dosage is gradually tapered every week so that the total steroid treatment course lasts only 4 to 8 weeks.

Second-line and third-line drugs are used in patients with progressive disease that is unresponsive to sulfasalazine and corticosteroids. Immunosuppressive agents, azathioprine (Imuran), and its metabolite 6-mercaptopurine are used mainly in conjunction with corticosteroids to reduce the amount of steroid needed and to limit dose-dependent adverse effects of steroids. These immunosuppressive agents are limited by their adverse effects (flulike symptoms, leukopenia, pancreatitis, hepatitis, and life-threatening infections). Cyclosporine, an immunosuppressant, also has been used intravenously to heal fistulas caused by ulcerative colitis and Crohn's disease.[65] Bone marrow transplant has been associated with permanent remission.[77]

Methotrexate, an immunomodulator, and infliximab (anti-TNF monoclonal antibody) are used for severe disease (more than one relapse per year) that is refractory to other drugs and for maintenance of remission.[78] Prolonged use of methotrexate is associated with hepatotoxicity and pneumonitis. Infliximab is an expensive drug that is given as a single 2-hour infusion specifically for Crohn's disease.[32] A single infusion induces remission in one third of patients within 4 weeks; however, relapses are likely after 3 months unless infusions are continued at 8- to 12-week intervals.[79]

Antibiotics (metronidazole or ciprofloxacin) have been used for active Crohn's disease and to maintain remission. They also are used after surgery, when toxic colitis develops, and when fever and leukocytosis are present. Although opioids are sometimes used for their anti-diarrheal effect, their use demands caution because these drugs can be addictive and detrimental to the course of therapy. Cromolyn sodium, a mast cell stabilizer, has been used in the rectum to diminish the release of inflammatory substances from mast cells and to alter the course of disease. Supplemental iron is prescribed to some patients to control anemia. A clinical trial of growth hormone has been reported to reduce symptoms in patients with Crohn's disease.[80]

Surgery is recommended for severe cases of IBD when patients do not respond to corticosteroids or when complications (e.g., massive hemorrhage, obstruction, perforation, toxic megacolon, carcinomatous transformation) occur. Total proctocolectomy with ileostomy is the standard but infrequent treatment for intractable ulcerative colitis. Approximately 70% of patients with Crohn's disease require some form of surgery, and 40% have recurrent disease, thus requiring additional resections.

DENTAL MANAGEMENT
Medical Considerations

The use of a steroid drug by a patient with IBD is of concern to the dentist because corticosteroids can suppress adrenal function and reduce the ability of the patient to withstand stress. When a patient is taking corticosteroids, most routine dental care can be provided without the need for additional corticosteroids, as long as adequate control of pain and anxiety is maintained (see Box 12-2). However, an adrenal crisis may be precipitated when a patient has recently discontinued the use of steroids and a particularly stressful or invasive procedure is performed that is associated with severe postoperative pain. In the latter circumstance, the need for administration of supplemental corticosteroids should be determined according to the guidelines delineated in Chapter 16.

Immunosuppressors (azathioprine/6-mercaptopurine) are associated with pancytopenia in approximately 5% of patients. Methotrexate is associated with hypersensitivity pneumonia and hepatic fibrosis, and cyclosporine can induce renal damage. Blood studies (complete blood count with differential, liver and renal function studies) and coagulation studies should be conducted before invasive procedures are performed. For patients who take methotrexate, inquiries should be made as to the patient's breathing capacity. A review of liver enzymes tests (assessed every 3 months) also should be performed. The presence of liver abnormalities dictates that management modifications should be made according to the potential for altered drug metabolism and blood coagulation (see Chapter 11). In addition, a thorough head and neck examination should be performed on patients who take immunosuppressants because of their increased risk for lymphoma and infection (e.g., infectious mononucleosis, recurrent herpes). The development of fever for unknown reasons in this select population mandates prompt referral to the physician.

The criteria for analgesic selection are similar for patients with peptic ulcer disease and those with IBD. Aspirin and other NSAIDs are to be avoided. Acetaminophen may be used alone or in combination with opioids. Alternatively, cotherapy with a COX-2 inhibitor (celecoxib) and a PPI can provide pain relief and simultaneous protection of the gastrointestinal mucosa. A careful drug history should be obtained to avoid prescribing additional opioids to patients who take these medications to manage their intestinal pain.

Treatment Planning Modifications

The severity, clinical course, and ultimate prognosis of patients with IBD are highly variable and can have an impact on routine dental care. Most patients with IBD have intermittent attacks, with asymptomatic remissions between attacks. Patients often require physical rest and emotional support throughout the disease because anxiety and depression may be severe. Only urgent dental care is advised during acute exacerbations of gastrointestinal disease. The clinician can assess the severity of the disease by assessing the patient's temperature and inquiring as to the number of diarrheal bowel movements occurring per day and whether blood is present in the stool.

Elective dental procedures should be scheduled during periods of remission when complications are absent and feelings of well-being have returned. Flexibility in appointment scheduling may be required because of the unpredictability of the disease. When elective surgical procedures are scheduled for patients with IBD who take sulfasalazine, the dentist should review preoperatively the patient's systemic health and obtain a complete blood count with differential and bleeding times. This can be important because, in addition to the immunosuppressive effects of their medications, sulfasalazine is associated with pulmonary, nephrotic, and hematologic abnormalities (i.e., variety of anemias, leukopenia, and thrombocytopenia).

Oral Complications and Manifestations

Several oral complications have been associated with patients who have IBD. Aphthous-like lesions affect up to 20% of patients with ulcerative colitis (Figure 12-7). Oral lesions erupt generally during gastrointestinal flare-ups. The ulcers are mildly painful and may be of the major or minor variety. They affect alveolar, labial, and buccal mucosa, as well as soft palate, uvula, and retromolar trigone, and they may be difficult to distinguish from aphthous. Granularity or irregular margins may be helpful in the diagnosis.

Pyostomatitis vegetans also can affect patients with ulcerative colitis and often aids in the diagnosis. To date,

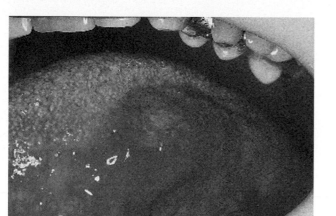

Figure 12-7. Oral ulceration associated with ulcerative colitis. (**A** from Allison MC et al. Inflammatory bowel disease, London, Mosby Ltd., 1998.)

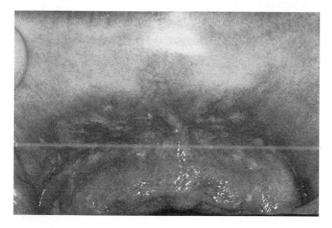

Figure 12-8. Pyostomatitis vegetans. Pustular raised lesions of palate in a patient with ulcerative colitis. **A** from Allison MC et al. Inflammatory bowel disease, London, Mosby Ltd., 1998.

fewer than 50 cases have been reported in the literature.[81,82] This form of stomatitis produces raised papillary, vegetative projections or pustules on an erythematous base of the labial mucosa, gingiva, and palate (Figure 12-8). The tongue rarely is involved. Without treatment, the initial erythematous appearance eventually degenerates into an ulcerative and suppurative mass. Treatment of both the aphthous-like lesions and pyostomatitis vegetans requires medical control of the colitis. Oral lesions that persist after anti-inflammatory drug therapy typically respond to repeated topical steroid applications. The vegetative growths can be eradicated by surgical means.

Unique oral manifestations of Crohn's disease occur in approximately 20% of patients and may precede the diagnosis of gastrointestinal disease by several years. Features include atypical mucosal ulcerations and diffuse swelling of the lips and cheeks (orofacial granulomatosis). Oral ulcers appear as linear mucosal ulcers with hyperplastic margins or papulonodular "cobblestone" proliferations of the mucosa, often in the buccal vestibule and soft palate. Oral lesions are intermittent but chronically present. They become symptomatic when intestinal

disease is exacerbated. Similar to the oral lesions associated with ulcerative colitis, oral ulcerations of Crohn's disease resolve when the gastrointestinal state is medically controlled. Topical steroids are beneficial during symptomatic phases.

Use of sulfasalazine has been associated with toxic effects on bone marrow, resulting in anemia, agranulocytosis, or thrombocytopenia that can present as a bald tongue, an oral infection, or bleeding, respectively. Corticosteroid use can result in osteopenia that may affect the alveolar bone. Methotrexate may cause oral mucositis and increase the frequency of recurrent oral herpes simplex virus infections. A discussion of the oral management of these abnormalities is found elsewhere in the text (see Oral Complications, Peptic Ulcer Disease, and Appendix C).

PSEUDOMEMBRANOUS COLITIS

DEFINITION

Pseudomembranous colitis is a severe and sometimes fatal form of colitis that results from the overgrowth of *Clostridium difficile*. Overgrowth results from the loss of competitive anaerobic gut bacteria, most commonly through the use of broad-spectrum antibiotics, but it can also result from heavy metal intoxication, sepsis, and organ failure. *C. difficile* produces disease via potent enterotoxins that induce colitis and diarrhea. Rarely, other pathogenic microbes may cause pseudomembranous colitis.[83]

EPIDEMIOLOGY

Incidence and Prevalence

Pseudomembranous colitis is the most common nosocomial infection of the gastrointestinal tract. The incidence is about 50 cases per 100,000 persons in the United States, and it is rising.[83] Reported incidence varies with type and frequency of antibiotic exposure. No gender predilection exists; however, the disease is most common in the elderly, patients in hospitals and nursing homes, those who receive tube feeding, and those infected with HIV.[84,85] Infants and young children rarely are affected.

Etiology

C. difficile, the causative agent in 90% to 99% of pseudomembranous colitis cases, is a Gram-positive, spore-forming anaerobic rod that has been found in sand, soil, and feces. Spores may survive on contaminated surfaces for months and are relatively resistant to many disinfectants. *C. difficile* colonizes the gut of 2% to 3% of asymptomatic adults and up to 50% of the elderly.[86] Risk of disease increases in areas where spores are inhaled (e.g., hospitals, farm yards) and when broad-spectrum antibiotics are in prolonged use. The most frequently offending antimicrobial agents are broad-spectrum agents and those that target anaerobic flora of the colon. Highest risk is associated with clindamycin (2% to 20% of usage) or ampicillin or amoxicillin (5% to 9% of usage) and third-generation cephalosporins (less than 2% of usage). Macrolides, penicillins, sulfamethoxazole-trimethoprim (Bactrim, Septra), and tetracycline are involved less frequently, whereas aminoglycosides, antifungal agents, metronidazole, and vancomycin are rarely causative. In general, oral antibiotics are more often causative then parenteral antibiotics.[83,87]

Pathophysiology

As commensal intestinal bacteria are eliminated, *C. difficile* overgrows and produces enzymes that mediate tissue degradation, as well as two toxins (A and B) that bind to intestinal mucosal cells, resulting in cytoskeletal disaggregation and altered vascular permeability, respectively. As cells (enterocytes) die, fluid is lost, and microscopic and macroscopic pseudomembranes form in the distal colon. Mild disease demonstrates anti-inflammatory lesions, whereas severe disease is seen as large, coalescent plaques and extensive denuded areas (Figure 12-9). Histologic findings include epithelial necrosis, distended goblet cells, leukocyte infiltration of the lamina propria,

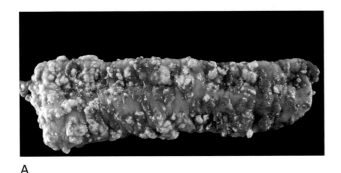

A

B

Figure 12-9. Pseudomembranous colitis from *Clostridium difficile* infection. **A,** Gross photograph showing plaques of yellow fibrin and inflammatory debris adhering to a reddened colonic mucosa. **B,** Low-power micrograph showing superficial erosion of the mucosa and adherent pseudomembrane of fibrin, mucus, and inflammatory debris. (From Kumar V, Abbas A, Fausto N. Robbins & Cotran Pathologic Basis of Disease, 7th ed. Philadelphia, Saunders, 2005.)

and pseudomembranous plaques consisting of inflammatory cells, mucin, fibrin, and sloughed mucosal cells.

CLINICAL PRESENTATION
Signs and Symptoms

Although the course of illness can be variable, diarrhea is the most common symptom. In mild cases, the stool is watery and loose. In severe cases, diarrhea is bloody and is accompanied by abdominal cramps and tenderness and by fever. Diarrhea often occurs within the first 4 to 10 days of antibiotic administration but may develop 1 day to 8 weeks after drug administration. Severe dehydration, metabolic acidosis, hypotension, peritonitis, and toxic megacolon are serious complications of untreated disease.

Laboratory Findings

Pseudomembranous colitis is associated with leukocytosis, leukocyte-laden stools, and a stool sample positive for *C. difficile* or one of its toxins, as determined by tissue culture assay or enzyme immunoassay. Colonic yellow-white pseudomembranes that are 5 to 10 mm in diameter are often visible on sigmoidoscopy.

MEDICAL MANAGEMENT

First-line treatment of pseudomembranous colitis involves discontinuing use of the antimicrobial agent implicated as perturbing the intestinal flora, along with introducing an antibiotic that will eradicate the toxin-producing *C. difficile*. In patients with mild disease, cessation of the offending antibiotic is all that may be needed. In more severe cases, oral metronidazole (Flagyl, 250 mg four times a day for 10 days) is the therapy of first choice. Vancomycin (125 to 500 mg four times a day for 10 days) is recommended for patients who are unresponsive to metronidazole. Both are active against all strains of *C. difficile*. However, *C. difficile* spores can survive treatment, and relapse occurs in about 20% of patients. Hydration and intravenous fluids are provided for electrolyte and fluid imbalances.

DENTAL MANAGEMENT
Medical Considerations

The practitioner should be cognizant that the use of some systemic antibiotics—especially clindamycin, ampicillin, and cephalosporins—is associated with a higher risk of pseudomembranous colitis in elderly, debilitated patients and in those with a previous history of pseudomembranous colitis (see Box 12-2). The decision to use an antibiotic should be based on sound clinical judgment that these drugs are indeed necessary and should not be used in a cavalier manner. The dentist also should be aware that pseudomembranous colitis following short-term use of clindamycin has not been reported after use of the American Heart Association prophylactic regimen.

Treatment Planning Modifications

The dentist should delay elective dental care until after pseudomembranous colitis is resolved.

Oral Complications and Manifestations

The use of systemic antibiotics for the treatment of patients with pseudomembranous colitis can result in fungal overgrowth (candidiasis) in the oral cavity (see Figure 12-4).

REFERENCES

1. Yuan Y, Padol IT, Hunt RH. Peptic ulcer disease today. Nature Clin Pract Gastroenterol Hepatol 2006;3:80-89.
2. Lam S. Aetiological factors of peptic ulcer: Perspectives of epidemiological observations this century. J Gastroenterol Hepatol 1994;9:S93-S98.
3. Lam S. Differences in peptic ulcer between East and West. Baillieres Best Pract Res Clin Gastroenterol 2000;14:41-52.
4. Sandler RS, Everhart JE, Donowitz M, et al. The burden of selected digestive diseases in the United States. Gastroenterology 2002;122:1500-1511.
5. Sonnenberg A, Everhart JE. The prevalence of self-reported peptic ulcer in the United States. Am J Public Health 1996;86:200-205.
6. Hollander D, Tarnawaski A. Dietary essential fatty acids and the decline in peptic ulcer disease—A hypothesis. Gut 1986;27:239-242.
7. Leoci C, Ierardi E, Chiloiro M, et al. Incidence and risk factors of duodenal ulcer: A retrospective cohort study. J Clin Gastroenterol 1995;20:104-109.
8. Derry S, Loke YK. Risk of gastrointestinal haemorrhage with long term use of aspirin: Meta-analysis. BMJ 2000;321:1183-1187.
9. McCarthy D. Nonsteroidal anti-inflammatory drug–related gastrointestinal toxicity: Definitions and epidemiology. Am J Med 1998;105:3S-9S.
10. Drumm B, Rhoads JM, Stringer DA, et al. Peptic ulcer disease in children: Etiology, clinical findings, and clinical course. Pediatrics 1988;82:410-414.
11. Sherman P. Peptic ulcer disease in children: Diagnosis, treatment and implication of *Helicobacter pylori*. Pediatr Gastroenterol 1994;23:707-725.
12. Euler A, Byrne W, Campbell M. Basal and pentagastrin stimulated gastric acid secretory rates in normal children and in those with peptic ulcer disease. J Pediatr 1983;103:766-768.
13. Walsh J, Peterson W. The treatment of *Helicobacter pylori* infection in the management of peptic ulcer disease. N Engl J Med 1995;333:984-991.
14. Borum M. Peptic-ulcer disease in the elderly. Clin Geriatr Med 1999;15:457-471.
15. Varsky CG, Correa MC, Sarmiento N, et al. Prevalence and etiology of gastroduodenal ulcer in HIV-positive patients: A comparative study of 497 symptomatic subjects evaluated by endoscopy. Am J Gastroenterol 1998;93:935-940.
16. Graham D. *Helicobacter pylori* infection in the pathogenesis of duodenal ulcer and gastric cancer: A model. Gastroenterology 1997;113:1983-1991.
17. Marshall B, Warren J. Unidentified curved bacilli in the stomach of patients with gastritis and peptic ulceration. Lancet 1984;1:1311-1315.
18. Warren J, Marshall B. Unidentified curved bacilli on gastric epithelium in active chronic gastritis. Lancet 1983; i:1273-1275.
19. Taylor D, Blaser M. The epidemiology of *Helicobacter pylori* infection. Epidemiol Rev 1991;13:42-59.
20. Shames B, Krajden S, Fuksa M, et al. Evidence for the occurrence of the same strain of *Campylobacter pylori* in the stomach and dental plaque. J Clin Microbiol 1989; 27:2849-2850.
21. Dooley C, Cohen H, Fitzgibbons PL, et al. Prevalence of *Helicobacter pylori* infection and histologic gastritis in asymptomatic persons. N Engl J Med 1989;321:1562-1566.
22. Graham D, Lew GM, Evans DG, et al. Effect of triple therapy (antibiotics plus bismuth) on duodenal ulcer healing: A randomized controlled trial. Ann Intern Med 1991;115:266-269.
23. Malaty H, Evans DG, Evans DJ Jr, Graham DY. *Helicobacter pylori* in Hispanics: Comparison with blacks and whites of similar age and socioeconomic class. Gastroenterology 1992;103:813-816.
24. Levenstein S. Peptic ulcer at the end of the 20th century: Biological and psychological risk factors. Can J Gastroenterol 1999;13:753-759.
25. Lanza FL, Hunt RH, Thomson AB, et al. Endoscopic comparison of esophageal and gastroduodenal effects of risedronate and alendronate in postmenopausal women. Gastroenterology 2000;119:631-638.
26. Scott D, Hersey SJ, Prinz C, Sachs G. Actions of anti-ulcer drugs. Science 1993;262:1453-1454.
27. Kikendall J, Evaul J, Honson L. Effect of cigarette smoking on gastrointestinal physiology and non-neoplastic digestive disease. J Clin Gastroenterol 1984; 6:65-79.
28. Maity P, Biswas K, Roy S, et al. Smoking and the pathogenesis of gastroduodenal ulcer—Recent mechanistic update. Mol Cell Biochem 2003;253:329-338.
29. Chan FKL, Leung WK. Peptic-ulcer disease. Lancet 2002;360:933-941.
30. Moss S, Calam J. Acid secretion and sensitivity to gastrin in patients with duodenal ulcer: Effect of eradication of *Helicobacter pylori*. Gut 1993;34:888-892.
31. Peterson WL, Barnett CC, Evans DJ Jr, et al. Acid secretion and serum gastrin in normal subjects and patients with duodenal ulcer: The role of *Helicobacter pylori*. Am J Gastroenterol 1993;88:2038-2043.
32. Wall G, Heyneman C, Pfanner T. Medical options for treating Crohn's disease in adults: Focus on antitumor necrosis factor—A chimeric monoclonal antibody. Pharmacotherapy 1999;19:1138-1152.
33. Lehman E, Stalder G. Hypotheses on the role of cytokines in peptic ulcer disease. Eur J Clin Invest 1998; 28:511-519.
34. Wallace J, Cucala M, Mugridge K, Parente L. Secretagogue-specific effects of interleukin 1 on gastric acid secretion. Am J Physiol 1991;261:559-564.
35. Tummala S, Keates S, Kelly CP. Update on the immunologic basis of *Helicobacter pylori* gastritis. Curr Opin Gastroenterol 2004;20:592-597.

36. Misiewicz J. *Helicobacter pylori:* Past, present and future. Scand J Gastroenterol 1992;27(suppl 194):25-29.

37. Peterson W. *Helicobacter pylori* and peptic ulcer disease. N Engl J Med 1991;324:1043-1048.

38. Saita H, Murakami M, Teramura S, et al. *Helicobacter pylori* has an ulcerogenic action in the ischemic stomach of rats. J Clin Gastroenterol 1992;141:S122-S126.

39. Zucca E, Bertoni F, Roggero E, et al. Molecular analysis of the progression from *Helicobacter pylori*–associated chronic gastritis to mucosa associated lymphoid tissue lymphoma of the stomach. N Engl J Med 1998;338: 804-810.

40. IARC Working Group on the Evaluation of Carcinogenic Risks to Humans. Schistosomes, liver flukes and *Helicobacter pylori*. IARC Monogr Eval Carcinog Risks Hum 1994;61:1-241.

41. Hansson L. Risk of stomach cancer in patients with peptic ulcer disease. World J Surg 2000;24:315-320.

42. Chiba N, Lahaie R, Fedorak RN, et al. *Helicobacter pylori* and peptic ulcer disease: Current evidence for management strategies. Can Fam Phys 1998;44:1481-1488.

43. National Institutes of Health Consensus Development Panel. Statement: *Helicobacter pylori* in peptic ulcer disease. JAMA 1994;272:65-69.

44. Chiba N, Rao BV, Rademaker JW, Hunt RH. Meta-analysis of the efficacy of antibiotic therapy in eradicating *Helicobacter pylori*. Am J Gastroenterol 1992;87: 1716-1727.

45. Malfertheiner P, Megraud F, O'Morain C, et al. Current concepts in the management of *Helicobacter pylori* infection—The Maastricht 2-2000 consensus report. Aliment Pharmacol Ther 2002;16:167-180.

46. Sonnenberg A, Townsen W. Costs of duodenal ulcer therapy with antibiotics. Arch Intern Med 1995;155: 922-928.

47. Forbes GM, Glaser ME, Cullen DJ, et al. Duodenal ulcer treated with *Helicobacter pylori* eradication: Seven-year follow-up. Lancet 1994;343:258-260.

48. Coghlan JD, Gilligan D, Humphries H, et al. *Campylobacter pylori* and recurrence of duodenal ulcers—A 12-month follow-up study. Lancet 1987;2:1109-1111.

49. Korman MG, Hansky J, Eaves ER, Schmidt GT. Influence of cigarette smoking on healing and relapse in duodenal ulcer disease. Gastroenterology 1983;85:871-874.

50. Svanes C. Trends in perforated peptic ulcer: Incidence, etiology, treatment, and prognosis. World J Surg 2000; 24:277-283.

51. Borody TJ, George LL, Brandl S, et al. Smoking does not contribute to duodenal ulcer relapse after *Helicobacter pylori* eradication. Am J Gastroenterol 1992;87: 1365-1367.

52. Permin H, Andersen LP. Inflammation, immunity, and vaccines for *Helicobacter* infection. Helicobacter 2005; 10(suppl 1):21-25.

53. Wolfe M, Lichtenstein D, Singh G. Gastrointestinal toxicity of nonsteroidal anti-inflammatory drugs. N Engl J Med 1999;340:1888-1899.

54. Ehsanullah R, Page MC, Tildesley G, Wood JR. Prevention of gastroduodenal damage induced by non-steroidal antiinflammtory drugs: Controlled trial with ranitidine. BMJ 1988;297:1017-1021.

55. Nguyen A-M, El-Zaatari F, Graham D. *Helicobacter pylori* in the oral cavity: A critical review of the literature. Oral Surg Oral Med Oral Pathol Oral Radiol Endod 1995;76:705-709.

56. Gius JA, Boyle DE, Castle DD, Congdon RH. Vascular formations of the lip and peptic ulcer. J Am Med Assoc 1963;183:725-729.

57. Jacobsen BA, Fallingborg J, Rasmussen HH, et al. Increase in incidence and prevalence of inflammatory bowel disease in northern Denmark: A population-based study, 1978-2002. Eur J Gastroenterol Hepatol 2006;18: 601-606.

58. Loftus EV Jr. Clinical epidemiology of inflammatory bowel disease: Incidence, prevalence, and environmental influences. Gastroenterology 2004;126:1504-1517.

59. Ogorek C, Fisher R. Differentiation between Crohn's disease and ulcerative colitis. Med Clin N Am 1994; 78:1249-1259.

60. Russel M, Stockbruegger R. Epidemiology of inflammatory bowel disease: An update. Scand J Gastroenterol 1996;31:417-427.

61. Gaya DR, Russell RK, Nimmo ER, Satsangi J. New genes in inflammatory bowel disease: Lessons for complex diseases? Lancet 2006;367:1271-1284.

62. Schreiber S, Rosenstiel P, Albrecht M, et al. Genetics of Crohn disease, an archetypal inflammatory barrier disease. Nat Rev Genet 2005;6:376-388.

63. Schreiber S. Slipping the barrier: How variants in CARD15 could alter permeability of the intestinal wall and population health. Gut 2006;55:308-309.

64. Society for Surgery of the Alimentary Tract, American Gastroenterological Association, American Society for Liver Diseases, American Society for Gastrointestinal Endoscopy, American Hepato-Pancreato-Biliary Association. Ulcerative colitis and colon carcinoma: Epidemiology, surveillance, diagnosis, and treatment. J Gastrointest Surg 1998;2:305-306.

65. Ghosh S, Shand A, Ferguson A. Regular review: Ulcerative colitis. BMJ 2000;320:1119-1123.

66. Cominelli F, Nast CC, Dinarello CA, et al. Regulation of eicosanoid production in rabbit colon by interleukin-1. Gastroenterology 1989;97:1400-1405.

67. Rogler G, Andus T. Cytokines in inflammatory bowel disease. World J Surg 1998;22:382-389.

68. Cobrin GM, Abreu MT. Defects in mucosal immunity leading to Crohn's disease. Immunol Rev 2005;206: 277-295.

69. Becker J. Surgical therapy for ulcerative colitis and Crohn's disease. Gastroenterol Clin N Am 1999;28: 371-390.

70. Carter MJ, Lobo AJ, Travis SP, et al. Guidelines for the management of inflammatory bowel disease in adults. Gut 2004;53(suppl 5):V1-V16.

71. Rampton D. Management of Crohn's disease. BMJ 1999;19:1480-1485.

72. D'Haens G. Infliximab (Remicade), a new biological treatment for Crohn's disease. Ital J Gastroenterol Hepatol 1999;31:519-520.

73. Belluzzi A, Brignola C, Campieri M, et al. Effect of an enteric-coated fish-oil preparation on relapses in Crohn's disease. N Engl J Med 1996;334:1557-1560.

74. Peppercorn M. Advances in drug therapy for inflammatory bowel disease. Ann Intern Med 1990;112:50-60.

75. Ludwig D, Stange E. Treatment of ulcerative colitis. Hepatogastroenterology 2000;47:83-89.

76. Hak S, Dukes G. Therapeutic advances in ulcerative colitis. Pharm Times 1991;Sept:110-120.

77. Kashyap A, Forman S. Autologous bone marrow transplantation for non-Hodgkin's lymphoma resulting in long-term remission of coincidental Crohn's disease. Br J Haematol 1998;103:651-652.

78. Feagan BG, Fedorak RN, Irvine EJ, et al. A comparison of methotrexate with placebo for the maintenance of remission in Crohn's disease. N Engl J Med 2000;342:1627-1632.

79. Rutgeerts P. Review article: Efficacy of infliximab in Crohn's disease—Induction and maintenance of remission. Aliment Pharmacol Ther 1999;13(suppl 4):9-15.

80. Slonim AE, Bulone L, Damore MB, et al. A preliminary study of growth hormone therapy for Crohn's disease. N Engl J Med 2000;342:1633-1637.

81. Soriano ML, Martinez N, Grilli R, et al. Pyodermatitis-pyostomatitis vegetans: Report of a case and review of the literature. Oral Surg Oral Med Oral Pathol Oral Radiol Endod 1999;87:322-326.

82. Ruiz-Roca JA, Berini-Aytes L, Gay-Escoda C. Pyostomatitis vegetans: Report of two cases and review of the literature. Oral Surg Oral Med Oral Pathol Oral Radiol Endod 2005;99:447-454.

83. Surawicz CM. Antibiotic-associated diarrhea and pseudomembranous colitis: Are they less common with poorly absorbed antimicrobials? Chemotherapy 2005;51:81-89.

84. McDonald LC, Owings M, Jernigan DB. *Clostridium difficile* infection in patients discharged from US short-stay hospitals, 1996-2003. Emerg Infect Dis 2006;12:409-415.

85. Bliss DZ, Johnson S, Savik K, et al. Acquisition of *Clostridium difficile* and *Clostridium difficile*–associated diarrhea in hospitalized patient receiving tube feeding. Ann Intern Med 1998;129:1012-1019.

86. Fekety R. Pseudomembranous colitis. In Goldman L, Ausiello D (eds). Cecil Textbook of Medicine, 22nd ed. St. Louis, Elsevier, 2004.

87. Brar H, Surawicz C. Pseudomembranous colitis: An update. Can J Gastroenterol 2000;14:51-56.

PART FIVE

Genitourinary Disease

Chronic Renal Failure and Dialysis

CHAPTER

13

Chronic renal disease and its ultimate result, end-stage renal disease (ESRD), is a worldwide problem that continues to increase.[1] Because patients with ESRD have many serious medical problems, dentists must know how to properly mange them. This chapter reviews the current status of ESRD and presents the principles for dental management.

The kidneys regulate fluid volume and the acid/base balance of plasma; excrete nitrogenous waste; synthesize erythropoietin, 1,25-dihydroxy-cholecalciferol, and renin; and are responsible for drug metabolism. The kidneys also are the target organ for parathormone and aldosterone. Progressive disease of the kidney can result in reduced function and can manifest in several organ systems. The practice of dentistry may be affected by resultant anemia, abnormal bleeding, electrolyte and fluid imbalance, hypertension, drug intolerance, and skeletal abnormalities. In addition, patients who have severe and progressive disease may require artificial filtration of the blood through dialysis or kidney transplantation (see Chapter 22).[2]

DEFINITION

End-stage renal disease (ESRD) refers to bilateral, progressive, chronic deterioration of nephrons, the functional unit of the kidney. The disease results in uremia and can lead to death. ESRD manifests when 50% to 75% of the approximately 2 million nephrons lose function. Under normal physiologic conditions, 25% of circulating blood perfuses the kidney each minute. The blood is filtered through a complex series of tubules and glomerular capillaries. Ultrafiltrate, the precursor of urine, is produced in the nephrons at a rate of about 125 mL/min.[2]

Nephron deterioration leads to ESRD through successive laboratory and clinical stages. The first stage, called *diminished renal reserve*, is usually asymptomatic. This stage is characterized by a mildly elevated creatinine level and a slight decline in glomerular filtration rate (GFR) (10% to 20% change from normal). Progression leads to *renal insufficiency*, a term that is used when the GFR is mildly to moderately diminished (20% to 50% of normal) and nitrogen products begin to accumulate in the blood. In the third stage, called *renal failure*, the ability of the kidney to perform excretory, endocrine, and metabolic functions has deteriorated beyond compensatory mechanisms. This indicates inability of the kidneys to maintain normal homeostasis. The resultant clinical syndrome—caused by renal failure, retention of excretory products, and interference with endocrine and metabolic functions—is called *uremia*. Sequelae involve multiorgan systems, including cardiovascular, hematologic, neuromuscular, endocrine, gastrointestinal, and dermatologic manifestations. The rate of destruction and the severity of disease depend on the underlying causative factors; however, in many cases, the cause remains unknown.[2]

EPIDEMIOLOGY

Incidence and Prevalence

Approximately 8 million people in the United States have some form of kidney disease. Of these, more than 360,000 have irreversible ESRD.[1,3] Each year, approximately 79,000 new cases of ESRD are diagnosed—a rate of 1.3 in 10,000 persons. This disease is increasing by approximately 9% per year, most rapidly in patients over age 65 and in those who have diabetes and hypertension. ESRD occurs more commonly in men; African, Native, and Asian Americans; and those between the ages of 45 and 64 years. More than 90% of patients with ESRD are older than 18 years of age. Approximately 60,000 Americans die annually as a result of ESRD; related cardiovascular disease is the cause of death for most. An average dental practice of 2000 patients can expect to serve 2 patients with ESRD.[1,3]

Etiology

ESRD is caused by any condition that destroys nephrons. The three most common known causes of ESRD are diabetes mellitus (34%), hypertension (25%), and chronic glomerulonephritis (16%). Other common causes include polycystic kidney disease, systemic lupus erythematosus, neoplasm, and acquired immunodeficiency syndrome (AIDS) nephropathy. Hereditary and environmental factors such as amyloidosis, congenital disease, hyperlipidemia, immunoglobulin A nephropathy, and silica exposure also contribute to the disease.[1,2]

Pathophysiology and Complications

Deterioration and destruction of functioning nephrons are the underlying pathologic processes of renal failure. The nephron includes the glomerulus, tubules, and vasculature. Various diseases affect different segments of the nephron at first, but the entire nephron eventually is affected. For example, hypertension affects the vasculature first, whereas glomerulonephritis affects the glomeruli first. Once lost, nephrons are not replaced. However, because of compensatory hypertrophy of the remaining nephrons, normal renal function is maintained for a time. During this period of relative renal insufficiency, homeostasis is preserved. The patient remains asymptomatic and demonstrates minimal laboratory abnormalities such as a diminished GFR. Normal function is maintained until about 50% to 75% of nephrons are destroyed. Subsequently, compensatory mechanisms are overwhelmed, and the signs and symptoms of uremia appear. In terms of morphology, the end-stage kidney is markedly reduced in size, scarred, and nodular (Figure 13-1).[1,2]

A patient with early renal failure may remain asymptomatic, but physiologic changes invariably occur as the disease progresses. These changes occur because of the loss of nephrons. Renal tubular malfunction causes the sodium pump to lose its effectiveness, and sodium excretion occurs. Along with sodium, excessive amounts of dilute urine are excreted, which accounts for the polyuria that is commonly encountered.[1,2]

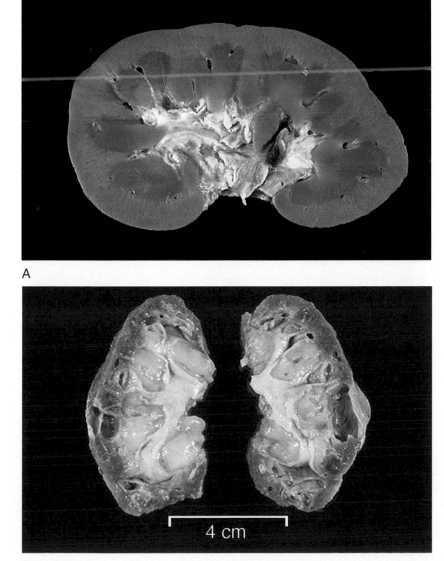

A

B

Figure 13-1. Gross anatomy of (**A**) a normal kidney and (**B**) atrophic kidneys from a patient with "chronic glomerulonephritis." (From Klatt EC. Robbins and Cotran Atlas of Pathology, Philadelphia, Saunders, 2006.)

Patients with advanced renal disease develop uremia, which is uniformly fatal if not treated. Failing kidneys are unable to concentrate and filtrate the intake of sodium, which contributes to the development of fluid overload, hypertension, and risk for cardiac disease. This in part contributes to the fact that approximately 50% of the annual mortality of patients with ESRD is the result of cardiovascular-related events.[1,2]

Loss of glomerular filtration function that results in buildup of nonprotein nitrogen compounds in the blood, mainly urea, is called *azotemia*. Level of azotemia is measured as blood urea nitrogen (BUN). Acids also accumulate because of tubular impairment. The combination of waste products results in metabolic acidosis, the major result of which is ammonia retention. In the later stages of renal failure, acidosis causes nausea, anorexia, and fatigue. Patients may tend to hyperventilate to compensate for the metabolic acidosis. In the patient with ESRD and acidosis, adaptive mechanisms already are taxed beyond normal levels, and any increase in demand can lead to serious consequences. For example, sepsis or a febrile illness can result in profound acidosis and may be fatal.[1,2]

Severe electrolyte disturbances occur in renal failure. Sodium depletion and hyperkalemia develop as azotemia progresses, urine output falls, and acid/base balance continues to deteriorate. Patients with ESRD demonstrate several hematologic abnormalities, including anemia, leukocyte and platelet dysfunction, and coagulopathy. Anemia, caused by decreased erythropoietin production by the kidney, inhibition of red blood cell production and hemolysis, bleeding episodes, and shortened red cell survival, is one of the most familiar manifestations of ESRD. Most of these effects result from unidentified toxic substances in uremic plasma and from other factors.[1,2]

Host defense is compromised by nutritional deficiencies and changes in the production and function of white blood cells. The latter are caused by reduced bioavailability of interleukin-2; downregulation of phagocyte adhesion molecules; increased production of interleukin-1, interleukin-6, and tumor necrosis factor; cell-mediated immune defects; and hypogammaglobulinemia that leads to diminished granulocyte chemotaxis, phagocytosis, and bactericidal activity. Accordingly, individuals with these conditions are more susceptible to infection.[4]

Hemorrhagic diatheses, characterized by tendencies toward abnormal bleeding and bruising, are common in patients with ESRD and are attributed primarily to abnormal platelet aggregation and adhesiveness, decreased platelet factor 3, and impaired prothrombin consumption. Defective platelet production also may play a role. Platelet factor 3 enhances the conversion of prothrombin to thrombin by activated factor X.[4]

The cardiovascular system is affected by a tendency to develop congestive heart failure or pulmonary edema, sometimes both. The most common complication, however, is arterial hypertension, caused by NaCl retention, fluid overload, and inappropriately high renin levels. Hypertrophy of the left ventricle also occurs and may compromise blood supply by way of the coronary vessels. This condition is worsened by anemia. A tendency has been noted for accelerated atherosclerosis to develop in patients with ESRD, and pericarditis is common.[4]

A variety of bone disorders are seen in ESRD; these are collectively referred to as *renal osteodystrophy*. Decreased glomerular filtration occurs with reduced nephron function, which results in decreased 1,25-dihydroxyvitamin D production by the kidney, decreased calcium absorption by the gut, and an increased level of serum phosphate. Because phosphate is the driving force of bone mineralization, excess phosphate tends to cause serum calcium to be deposited in bone (osteoid), leading to a decreased serum calcium level and weak bones. In response to low serum calcium, the parathyroid glands are stimulated to secrete parathormone (PTH), which results in secondary hyperparathyroidism. The functions of PTH are as follows:

- Inhibits the tubular reabsorption of phosphate
- Stimulates renal production of the vitamin D necessary for calcium metabolism
- Enhances vitamin D absorption from the intestine

However, high levels of PTH are sustained because in ESRD, the failing kidney does not synthesize 1,25-dihydroxycholecalciferol, the active metabolite of vitamin D; thus, calcium absorption in the gut is inhibited. PTH, tumor necrosis factor, and interleukin-1 activate bone remodeling, mobilize calcium from the bones, and promote the excretion of phosphate, which can lead to renal and metastatic calcifications. The progression of osseous changes is as follows: osteomalacia (increased unmineralized bone matrix), followed by osteitis fibrosa (bone resorption lytic lesions and marrow fibrosis) (Figure 13-2), and finally, osteosclerosis in varying degrees (enhanced bone density) (Figure 13-3). With renal osteodystrophy, impaired bone growth occurs in children, along with a tendency toward spontaneous fractures with slow healing, myopathy, aseptic necrosis of the hip, and extraosseous calcifications. The incidence of osteomalacia is decreasing because it has been determined that it is most commonly linked to intoxication by aluminum and other heavy metals associated with dialysis treatment of patients with ESRD. Dialysate fluids currently have reduced levels of these intoxicants.[4]

CLINICAL PRESENTATION

Clinical features of renal failure are listed in Box 13-1. Although the type and extent of these clinical manifestations vary with severity and the particular patient, they must be recognized in the context of the patient's overall physical status. Because renal failure can affect multiple systems, attention must be paid to how widespread the effects are on the cardiovascular, nervous, hematologic, gastrointestinal, dermatologic, respiratory, and endocrine systems.[1]

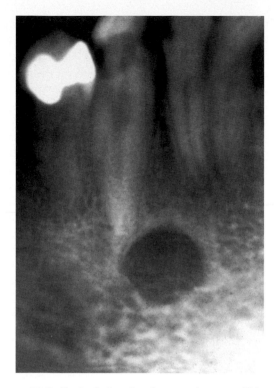

Figure 13-2. Lytic lesion in the anterior mandible of a patient with hyperparathyroidism. (Courtesy L. R. Bean, Lexington, Ky.)

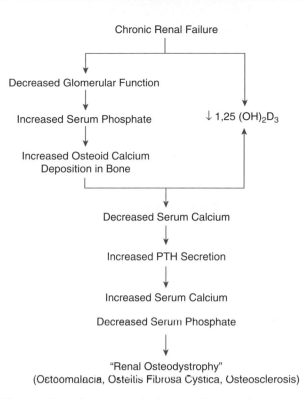

Figure 13-3. Summary of changes that result in renal osteodystrophy.

BOX 13-1

Clinical Features of Chronic Renal Failure

CARDIOVASCULAR
  Hypertension
  Congestive heart failure
  Cardiomyopathy
  Pericarditis
  Accelerated atherosclerosis

GASTROINTESTINAL
  Anorexia
  Nausea and vomiting
  Peptic ulcer and gastrointestinal bleeding
  Hepatitis
  Peritonitis

NEUROMUSCULAR
  Weakness and lassitude
  Drowsiness leading to coma
  Headaches
  Disturbance of vision
  Sensory disturbances—peripheral neuropathy
  Seizures
  Muscle cramps

DERMATOLOGICAL
  Pruritus
  Bruising
  Hyperpigmentation
  Pallor
  Uremic frost

HEMATOLOGICAL
  Bleeding
  Anemia
  Lymphopenia and leukopenia
  Splenomegaly and hypersplenism

IMMUNOLOGICAL
  Prone to infections

METABOLIC
  Nocturia and polyuria
  Thirst
  Glycosuria
  Metabolic acidosis
  Raised serum urea, creatinine, lipids and uric acid
  Electrolyte disturbances
  Secondary hyperparathyroidism

Signs and Symptoms

Patients with renal failure appear ill and anemic and may develop nocturia. Anemia produces pallor of the skin and mucous membranes and contributes to the symptoms of lethargy, listlessness, and dizziness. Widespread effects cause multiorgan system involvement. Hyperpigmentation of the skin is characterized by a brownish-yellow appearance caused by the retention of carotene-like pigments normally excreted by the kidney. These pigments also may cause profound pruritus. An occasional finding is a whitish coating on the skin of the trunk and arms produced by residual urea crystals left when perspiration evaporates ("uremic frost").[1]

Patients with renal failure may demonstrate a variety of gastrointestinal signs such as anorexia, nausea, and vomiting, generalized gastroenteritis, and peptic ulcer disease. Uremic syndrome commonly causes malnutrition and diarrhea. Patients demonstrate mental slowness or depression and become psychotic in later stages. They also may show muscular hyperactivity. Convulsion is a late finding that may be directly correlated with the level of azotemia. Stomatitis manifested by oral ulceration and candidiasis may occur (Figure 13-4). Parotitis may be seen, and a urine-like odor to the breath may be detected.[1]

Because of the bleeding diatheses that accompany ESRD, hemorrhagic episodes are not uncommon, particularly occult gastrointestinal bleeding. However, patients who receive dialysis have improved control of uremia and less severe bleeding. Manifestations include ecchymoses, petechiae, purpura, and gingival or mucous membrane bleeding (epistaxis).

Cardiovascular manifestations of ESRD include hypertension, congestive heart failure (shortness of breath, orthopnea, dyspnea on exertion, peripheral edema), and pericarditis.[1]

Laboratory Findings

Several tests, including urinalysis, BUN, serum creatinine, creatinine clearance, electrolyte measurements, and protein electrophoresis, are used to monitor the progress of ESRD. The most basic test of kidney function is urinalysis, with special emphasis on specific gravity and the presence of protein. Figure 13-5 illustrates laboratory features of the four pathophysiologic stages of chronic renal failure. Table 13-1 lists specific laboratory values indicative of renal function and dysfunction. Of these tests, three are used primarily to assess renal function: creatinine clearance, serum creatinine and GFR. Creatinine is a measure of muscle breakdown and filtration capacity of the nephron. It is proportionate to the glomerular filtration and tubular excretion rates and commonly is used as the index of clearance (creatinine clearance) in a 24-hour urine collection. The BUN is a common indicator of kidney function but is not as specific as creatinine clearance or serum creatinine level.[4]

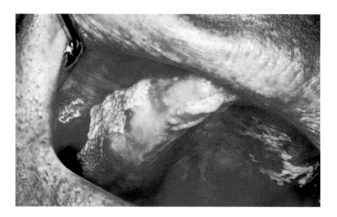

Figure 13-4. Oral candidiasis in a patient with end-stage renal disease.

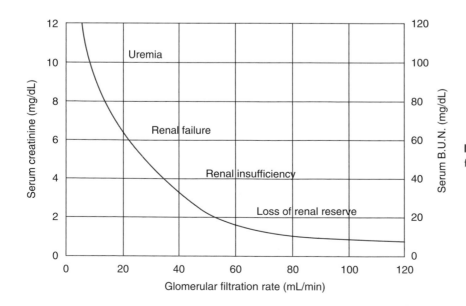

Figure 13-5. Relationship of renal function to serum enzymes.

TABLE **13-1**
Primary Laboratory Values for the Assessment of Renal Function and Failure

Laboratory Test	Reference Value	Indicator of Renal Insufficiency	Indicator of Renal Failure
URINE			
Creatinine clearance	85-125 mL/min (women)	50-90 mL/min	10-50 mL/min (moderate);
	97-140 mL/min (men)		<10 mL/min (severe)
Glomerular filtration rate	100-150 mL/min	50-90 mL/min	10-50 mL/min (moderate);
			<10 mL/min (severe)
SERUM			
Blood urea nitrogen	8 to 18 mg/dL (3 to 6.5 mmol/L)	20-30 mg/dL	30 to 50 mg/dL (moderate);
			>50 mg/dL (severe)
Creatinine	0.6 to 1.20 mg/dL	2 to 3 mg/dL	3 to 6 mg/dL (moderate);
			>6 mg/dL (severe)

Modified in part from Zachee P, Vermylen J, Boogaerts MA. Ann Hematol 1994;69:33-40 and De Rossi SS, Glick M. J Am Dent Assoc 1996;127:211-219.
Secondary indicators of renal function. Normal reference values: calcium, 8.2 to 11.2 mg/dL; chloride, 95 to 103 mmol/L; inorganic phosphorus, 2.7 to 4.5 mg/dL; potassium, 3.8 to 5 mmol/L; sodium, 136 to 142 mmol/L; total carbon dioxide for venous blood, 22 to 26 mmol/L.

As renal failure develops, the patient often remains asymptomatic until the GFR drops to below 20 mL/min, the creatinine clearance drops to below 20 mL/min, and the BUN is above 20 mg/dL. For example, uremic syndrome is rare before the BUN concentration exceeds 60 mg/dL. Other serum tests are used to monitor serum electrolytes involved in acid/base regulation and calcium/phosphate metabolism that are affected by renal disease (see Table 13-1).

Protein and blood in the urine, two predictors of ESRD, have been used to screen large populations. These tests are used to rule out renal disease in the elderly and in persons with diabetes, hypertension, and unexplained fatigue.[4]

MEDICAL MANAGEMENT
Conservative Care

Once the diagnosis of ESRD has been made, the goals of treatment are to retard the progress of disease and to preserve the patient's quality of life. A conservative approach is the first step and may be adequate for prolonged periods. Conservative care, which is designed to slow the progression of renal disease, involves decreasing the retention of nitrogenous waste products and controlling hypertension, fluids, and electrolyte imbalances. This is accomplished by dietary modification—restricting protein and monitoring fluid, sodium, and potassium intake. Any treatable associated condition such as diabetes, hypertension, congestive heart failure, infection, volume depletion, urinary tract obstruction, secondary hyperparathyroidism, and hyperuricemia is corrected or controlled. In particular, secondary hyperparathyroidism is treated with a low-phosphate diet and with the use of nonaluminum phosphate binders (e.g., calcium carbonate), calcitriol, and other vitamin D preparations that

decrease serum parathyroid hormone levels. Conservative care includes the avoidance of nephrotoxic drugs or agents metabolized principally by the kidney.

Anemia that occurs in renal failure usually is treated with the use of recombinant human erythropoietin. In most patients, subcutaneous doses of 50 to 75 IU/kg triweekly normalize hemoglobin levels within 3 months. Adverse effects are infrequent and include seizures, hypertension, and thrombosis. A small percentage of patients develop resistance to recombinant human erythropoietin.[2,4]

Dialysis

Dialysis is a medical procedure that artificially filters blood. Dialysis becomes necessary when the number of nephrons diminishes to the point that azotemia is unpreventable or uncontrollable. The initiation of dialysis is an individual patient decision that becomes important when the serum creatinine is chronically above 3 mg/dL and the creatinine clearance is below 20 mL/min. More than 250,000 individuals receive dialysis in the United States at a cost of more than $7 billion a year. The procedure can be accomplished by peritoneal dialysis or by hemodialysis.[5,6]

Peritoneal dialysis is performed on more than 26,000 Americans. It may be provided as continuous cyclic peritoneal dialysis (CCPD) or chronic ambulatory peritoneal dialysis (CAPD). Both instill a hypertonic solution into the peritoneal cavity via a permanent peritoneal catheter. After a time, the solution and dissolved solutes (e.g., urea) are drawn out. The older method, CCPD, uses a machine at night to perform seven to eight dialysate exchanges while the patient sleeps. During the day, excretory fluids fill the abdomen of the patient until dialysis is repeated that evening.[5,6]

A commonly used method of peritoneal dialysis is CAPD. Dialysis through this method (Figure 13-6) is

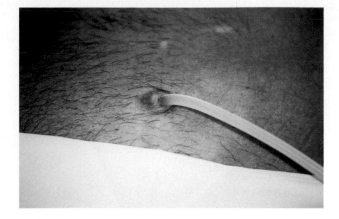

Figure 13-6. Chronic ambulatory peritoneal dialysis catheter site in the abdominal wall. (From Lewis SM, Heitkemper MM, Dirksen SR. Medical Surgical Nursing, 6th ed. St. Louis, Mosby, 2004.)

performed with shorter exchange periods of 30 to 45 minutes, 4 to 5 times per day, usually around breakfast, lunch, and dinner, and before bedtime. Dialysis exchanges are performed manually with 2 to 3 L of dialysate instilled into the peritoneal cavity. The catheter is sealed, and every 4 to 6 hours, the dialysate is allowed to drain into a bag strapped to the patient and new dialysate is instilled. CAPD allows the patient more freedom than CCPD. However, both methods allow patients to perform routine functions between exchanges (e.g., walking, working).

The advantages of peritoneal dialysis are its relatively low cost, ease of performance, reduced likelihood of infectious disease transmission, and lack of anticoagulation. Disadvantages include the need for frequent sessions, risk of peritonitis (approximately 1 per patient every 1.5 years) abdominal hernia, and its significantly lower effectiveness than hemodialysis. Its principal use is for patients in acute renal failure or for those who require only occasional dialysis.[5,6]

Most dialysis patients (90%) receive hemodialysis. Hemodialysis is the method of choice when azotemia occurs and dialysis is needed on a long-term basis. Treatments are performed every 2 or 3 days, depending on need. Usually 3 to 4 hours is required for each session (Figure 13-7). Hemodialysis consumes an enormous amount of the patient's time and is extremely confining. However, daily nocturnal home hemodialysis likely will become available. Between dialysis sessions, patients lead a relatively normal life.[7]

More than 80% of the approximately 240,000 people who receive hemodialysis in the United States do so through a permanent and surgically placed arteriovenous graft or fistula, usually placed in the forearm. Access is achieved by cannulation of the fistula with a large-gauge needle (Figure 13-8). Approximately 18% of patients receive dialysis through a temporary or permanent central catheter while permanent access is healing, or when all other access options have been exhausted. Patients are "plugged in" to the hemodialysis machine at the fistula/graft site, and blood is passed through the machine, fil-

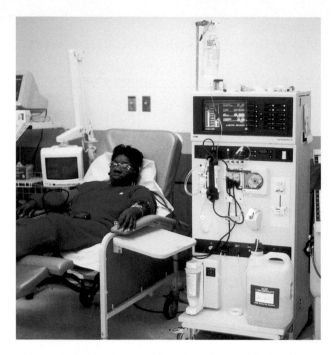

Figure 13-7. Patient undergoing hemodialysis. (From Lewis SM, Heitkemper MM, Dirksen SR. Medical Surgical Nursing, 6th ed. St. Louis, Mosby, 2004.)

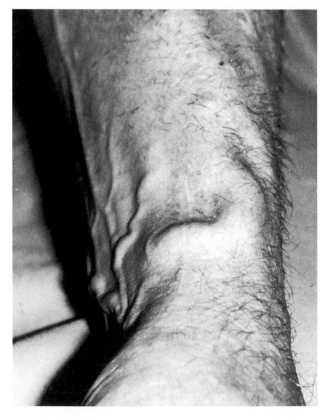

Figure 13-8. Site of a surgically created arteriovenous fistula, with subsequent dilation and hypertrophy of the veins. (Courtesy Dialysis Center, Lexington, Ky.)

tered, and returned to the patient. Heparin is usually administered during the procedure to prevent clotting.[6,7]

Although hemodialysis is a lifesaving technique, dialysis provides only about 15% of normal renal function, and complications develop as a result of the procedure. Serum calcium concentrations require close regulation that is achieved with calcium supplements, calcitriol (active form of vitamin D), or the use of dialysate that contains calcium. Improper blood levels contribute to muscle tetany and oversecretion of parathyroid hormone. Anemia is a common feature of renal failure and dialysis; however, the use of recombinant human erythropoietin has virtually eliminated this problem. In addition, risks of hepatitis B, hepatitis C, and human immunodeficiency virus (HIV) infections are present because dialyzers usually are disinfected—not sterilized—between uses, and patients usually have multiple blood exposures. Risk for transmission of viruses through hemodialysis increases when screening hepatitis tests are not performed, hepatitis B vaccine has not been administered to patients, and separate machines and staff members are not used in the treatment of patients who are carriers of the hepatitis B virus or the hepatitis C virus. A 1997 national survey reported that among chronic hemodialysis patients, the prevalence of hepatitis B surface antigen positivity (carriers of hepatitis B) was 0.9%, of hepatitis C 9.3%, and of HIV 1.3%. Although all three viruses constitute a reservoir of potential infection, only hepatitis B virus and hepatitis C virus have been reported to be transmitted nosocomially in dialysis centers in the United States.[6-8]

Infection of the arteriovenous fistula is an ongoing concern and can result in septicemia, septic emboli, infective endarteritis, and infective endocarditis. *Staphylococcus aureus* is the most common cause of vascular access infection and related bacteremia in these patients. The risk of fistula infection from surgical procedures (e.g., urogenital, oral surgical, dental) is not precisely known but is considered low. A related concern is risk for infection and antibiotic-resistant infection. Long-term hemodialysis patients have a higher rate of tuberculosis and of vancomycin- and methicillin-resistant infections than do members of the general public.[6,7]

As with all patients with ESRD, drugs that are metabolized primarily by the kidney or that are nephrotoxic must be avoided by patients receiving dialysis.

A final problem associated with dialysis is that of abnormal bleeding. As mentioned, patients with ESRD have bleeding tendencies because of altered platelet aggregation and decreased platelet factor III. Hemodialysis is associated with the additional problem of platelet destruction by mechanical trauma of the procedure. Aluminum contamination of the dialysate water may interfere with heme synthesis and contributes to the development of osteomalacia.[6,7] The process of hemodialysis may activate prostaglandin I_2, which can reduce platelet aggregation. However, prostaglandin I_2 has a half-life of 1 to 3 minutes, and its adverse effects may not be demonstrable by routine laboratory tests.[6,7]

The 1-year survival rate of patients on dialysis is 78%. The 5-year survival rate is 28%. An alternative to long-term dialysis is renal transplantation (see Chapter 22). This has obvious advantages but also is associated with a significant number of problems.

DENTAL MANAGEMENT
Patient Under Conservative Care

Medical Considerations. Consultation with the patient's physician is suggested before dental care is provided to patients under care for ESRD. Problems generally do not occur in provision of outpatient dental care if the patient's disease is well controlled and conservative medical care is provided. However, if the patient is in the advanced stages of failure or has another systemic disease common to renal failure (e.g., diabetes mellitus, hypertension, systemic lupus erythematosus), or if electrolyte imbalance is present, dental care may best be provided after physician consultation and in a hospital-like setting. Deferral of treatment may be required until adequate control is attained[1] (Box 13-2).

If the person is to be treated as an outpatient, blood pressure should be closely monitored before and during the procedure (see Chapter 3). Because of the potential for bleeding problems, patients should undergo pretreatment screening for bleeding disorders, including platelet function analyzer-100 (PFA-100) and platelet count (see Chapter 25). Hematocrit level and hemoglobin count also should be obtained for assessment of the status of anemia. Any abnormal values should be discussed with the physician. Few problems are encountered with non-hemorrhagic dental procedures when the hematocrit level is above 25%. If bleeding is anticipated, hematocrit levels can be raised with the use of erythropoietin. A less desirable option is red blood cell transfusion, which carries the risks of sensitization and bloodborne infection. If an orofacial infection occurs, aggressive management with the use of culture and sensitivity tests and appropriate antibiotics is necessary.

When surgical procedures are undertaken, meticulous attention to good surgical technique is necessary to decrease the risks of excessive bleeding and infection. The dentist should consult with the physician to assess the need for antibiotics when invasive procedures are planned. Alterations in drug dosage may be needed according to the amount of kidney function that is present.

If patients with ESRD who are undergoing dialysis or other treatment have been taking large doses of corticosteroids (i.e., 10 mg daily of prednisone or equivalent), it is possible that they may have adrenal hypofunction. To avoid an adrenal crisis, the dental clinician may need to supplement the patient's corticosteroid dose before complex dental procedures are performed (see Chapter 16).[1]

One of the major problems associated with treating a patient with ESRD involves drug therapy. Of concern are drugs that are excreted primarily by the kidney, or that

BOX 13-2

Dental Management of the Patient With End-Stage Renal Disease (Including Emergency Dental Care)

UNDER CONSERVATIVE CARE
- Consult with physician regarding physical status and level of control
- Avoid dental treatment if disease is unstable (poorly controlled or advanced)
- Screen for bleeding disorder before surgery (bleeding time, platelet count, hematocrit, hemoglobin)
- Monitor blood pressure closely
- Pay meticulous attention to good surgical technique
- Avoid nephrotoxic drugs (acetaminophen in high doses, acyclovir, aspirin, nonsteroidal antiinflammatory drugs)
- Adjust dosage of drugs metabolized by the kidney (see Table 13-2)
- Aggressively manage orofacial infections with culture and sensitivity tests and antibiotics
- Consider hospitalization for severe infection or major procedures
- Consider corticosteroid supplementation as indicated

RECEIVING HEMODIALYSIS
- Same as conservative care recommendations
- Beware of concerns of arteriovenous shunt
- Consult with physician about risk for infective endarteritis or endocarditis
- Avoid blood pressure cuff and IV medications in arm with shunt
- Avoid dental care on day of treatment (especially within first 6 hours afterward); best to treat on day after
- Consider antimicrobial prophylaxis (based on guidelines [see Box 13-4])
- Consider corticosteroid supplementation as indicated
- Assess status of liver function and presence of opportunistic infection in these patients because of increased risk for carrier state of hepatitis B and C viruses and human immunodeficiency virus (HIV)

are nephrotoxic. As a general rule, drugs excreted by the kidney are eliminated twofold less efficiently when the GFR drops to 50 mL/min and thus may reach toxic levels at lower GFR. In these circumstances, drug dosage needs to be reduced and timing of administration must be prolonged. Nephrotoxic drugs such as acyclovir, aminoglycosides, aspirin, nonsteroidal anti-inflammatory drugs, and tetracycline require special dosage adjustments. Acetaminophen also is nephrotoxic and may cause renal tubular necrosis at high doses, but it is probably safer than aspirin in these patients because it is metabolized in the liver.

The frequency and dosage of dental drug administration require adjustment during uremia for reasons besides nephrotoxicity and renal metabolism. For example, (1) a low serum albumin value reduces the number of binding sites for circulating drugs, thus enhancing drug effects, (2) uremia can modify hepatic metabolism of drugs

(increasing or decreasing clearance), (3) antacids can affect acid/base or electrolyte balance, further complicating uremic effects on electrolyte balance, and (4) aspirin and nonsteroidal anti-inflammatory drugs potentiate uremic platelet defects; thus, these antiplatelet drugs should be avoided (Table 13-2).

Although nitrous oxygen oxide and diazepam are anti-anxiety drugs that require little modification for use in patients with ESRD, the hematocrit or hemoglobin concentration should be measured before intravenous sedation to ensure adequate oxygenation. Also, drugs that depress the central nervous system (barbiturates, narcotics) are best avoided in the presence of uremia because the blood–brain barrier may not be intact, and excessive sedation may result. When the hemoglobin concentration is below 10 g/100 mL, general anesthesia is not recommended for patients with ESRD.[9]

The risk of bleeding diathesis in patients with uremia dictates that the dentist must have local (topical thrombin, microfibrillar collagen, suture) or systemic (desmopressin 0.3 µg/kg over 30 minutes) hemostatic agents available during surgical procedures. Conjugated estrogens are helpful when longer duration of action is required; however, 1 week of therapy usually is needed to guarantee efficacy. Because of risk of disease transmission, cryoprecipitate (a plasma derivative rich in factor VIII, fibrinogen, and fibronectin) is a less frequently used hemostatic alternative. Platelet transfusions are used infrequently because of the associated risk of immunogenic sensitization.[9]

Treatment Planning Modifications. The goals of dental care for patients receiving conservative treatment for ESRD are to restore the mouth to the healthiest condition possible and to eliminate possible sources of infection. Oral physiotherapy training is important for the maintenance of long-term oral health. Recall appointments may need to be more frequent when salivary flow rates are diminished to reduce the development of oral infections and periodontal disease. Once an acceptable level of oral hygiene has been established, no contraindication exists to routine dental care.

Oral Complications and Manifestations. Several oral changes are seen with chronic renal failure. Box 13-3 lists some of the common oral manifestations of chronic renal failure. One of the most common is pallor of the oral mucosa related to anemia. Red-orange discoloration of the cheeks and mucosa caused by pruritus and deposition of carotene-like pigments occurs when renal filtration is decreased. Salivary flow may be diminished, resulting in xerostomia and parotid infections. Candidiasis is more frequent when salivary flow is diminished. Patients frequently complain of an altered or metallic taste, and the saliva may have a characteristic ammonia-like odor that results from a high urea content.[10]

In severe failure, uremic stomatitis may be present, characterized early by red, burning mucosa covered with

TABLE 13-2
Drug Adjustments in Chronic Renal Disease

Drug	Route of Elimination in Metabolism	Removed by Dialysis	Dosage Adjustment for Renal Failure				Supplement Dose After Hemodialysis
				GFR, mL/min			
			Method	>50	Co-50	<10	
ANALGESIC							
Aspirin	Liver (kidney)	Yes	I	q4h	q6h	Avoid	Yes
Acetaminophen	Liver	Yes (HD); No (PD)	I	q4h	q6h	q8h	No
Ibuprofen (Motrin)	Liver	?	—		No adjustment		No
Propoxyphene* (Darvon)	Liver (kidney)	No	DR	100%	100%	Avoid	No
Codeine	Liver	?	DR	100%	75%	50%	No
Meperidine* (Demerol)	Liver	?	DR	100%	75%	50%	No
ANESTHETIC							
Lidocaine (Xylocaine)	Liver (kidney)	No	—		No adjustment		N/A
ANTIMICROBIAL							
Acyclovir (Zovirax)	Kidney	Yes	I & DR	q8h	q12-24h	50% q24-48h	Yes
Amoxicillin, Penicillin V	Kidney (liver)	No	I	q8h	q8-12h	q24h	Yes
Cephalexin (Keflex)	Kidney	Yes	I	q8h	q12h	q12h	Yes, 50% of usual dose after HD
Clindamycin (Cleocin)	Liver	No	—	100%	100%	100%	No
Erythromycin	Liver	No	DR	100%	100%	50%-75%	No
Ketoconazole (Nizoral)	Liver	No	—	100%	100%	100%	No
Metronidazole (Flagyl)	Liver (kidney)	Yes	DR	100%	100%	50%	Yes (HD); No (PD)
Tetracycline (Doxycycline)	Kidney (liver)	No	I	q8-12h	q12-24th	q24h	No
BENZODIAZEPINE							
Diazepam (Valium); Triazolam (Halcion)	Liver	?	—		No adjustment		No
CORTICOSTEROID							
Dexamethasone	Local site and liver		—		No adjustment		No

Modified from Proctor R et al. Oral and dental aspects of chronic renal failure. J Dent Res 2005;84:199-208, and Singh G. Renal disease. Med Clin North Am 2005;89:240.
DR, Dosage reduction; I, increased interval between doses; GFR, glomerular filtration rate; HD, hemodialysis; PD, peritoneal dialysis.
*Toxic metabolites can build up in severe ESRD.

gray exudates and later by frank ulceration. White patches called *uremic frost* caused by urea crystal deposition are more common on the skin but may be seen on the oral mucosa. These mucosal changes are generally associated with BUN levels greater than 55 mg/dL. Bleeding tendencies are evident as petechiae and ecchymoses on the labial and buccal mucosa, soft palate, and margins of the tongue, as is gingival bleeding (Figure 13-9).[10]

Oral lesions, ulcers, lichen planus (or lichenoid-like) lesions, hairy tongue, and pyogenic granulomas have all been noted in increased frequency in patients with chronic renal failure.[11] These lesions present similarly to other oral lesions and should be treated likewise.

Enamel hypoplasia has been documented in patients with ESRD whose disease began at an early age. In the developing dentition, red-brown discoloration and delayed

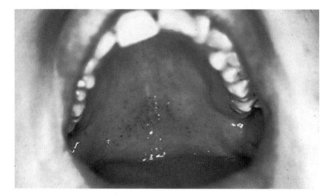

Figure 13-9. Palatal petechiae in a patient with end-stage renal disease.

or altered eruption also have been reported. Tooth erosion from persistent vomiting may be seen. Caries, however, is not a feature because salivary urea inhibits the metabolic end products of bacterial plaque and increases the buffering capacity of saliva, thus preventing a drop in pH sufficient to attain cariogenic levels.[2,9]

Specific osseous changes of the jaws accompany chronic renal failure. The most classically described osseous change is the triad of loss of lamina dura, demineralized bone ("ground glass"), and localized radiolucent jaw lesions (central giant cell granulomas; "brown tumor"). Lytic bone lesions are the result of hyperparathyroidism. Other osseous findings include widened trabeculations, loss of cortication, calcified extraction sites ("socket sclerosis"), and metastatic calcifications within the skull.[2,9]

Patients with chronic renal failure and those with renal transplants who are taking cyclosporine may exhibit gingival enlargement. The clinical presentation is very similar to that caused by phenytoin (Dilantin) or calcium channel blockers. In fact, because of the increased prevalence of hypertension in patients with chronic renal failure, patients may take both cyclosporine and calcium channel blockers. Obviously, the effect on gingival enlargement will not be enhanced. Meticulous oral hygiene and frequent professional prophylaxis will help to reduce the effects of cyclosporine-induced gingival enlargement.

In general, patients with chronic renal failure exhibit increased susceptibility to gingivitis and periodontal disease.

Patient Receiving Dialysis

Medical Considerations. Peritoneal dialysis presents no additional problems in dental management. However, this is not the case with patients who are receiving hemodialysis (see Box 13-1). In hemodialysis patients, a surgically created arteriovenous fistula is created that may be susceptible to infection (endarteritis) and may become a source of bacteremia, resulting in infective endocarditis. Infective endocarditis in patients undergoing hemodialysis occurs even when preexisting cardiac defects are absent. Although the factors that place these patients at risk for infective endocarditis have not been established fully, altered host defenses, altered cardiac output and mechanical stresses, and bacterial seeding and growth on the shunt are important factors.[12-14]

Infective endocarditis occurs in 2% to 9% of patients receiving hemodialysis. This rate is significantly higher than that reported in persons with rheumatic heart disease. Most of these infections are caused by staphylococcal infections that develop at the site of the graft, fistula, or catheter. Approximately 10% to 17% of cases are caused by organisms that can arise from the oral cavity (*Streptococcus viridans;* lactobacillus). Patients with the following devices—dual-lumen cuffed venous catheters and polytetrafluoroethylene grafts, newly placed grafts, and long-term catheters—are at increased risk for bacterial seeding compared with patients with primary arteriovenous fistulas.[12-14] On the basis of an apparently low risk, the American Heart Association (AHA) guidelines (2003)[14] do not include a recommendation for prophylactic antibiotics before invasive dental procedures are performed on patients with intravascular access devices (Box 13-4).

Controversy surrounds the provision of antibiotic prophylaxis for patients on hemodialysis who have known cardiac risk factors as defined by the AHA (see Chapter 2) that place them at increased risk for infective endocarditis when invasive dental procedures are performed. For patients undergoing hemodialysis who do not have known cardiac risk factors, the AHA does not recommend antibiotic prophylaxis; however, the managing physician/nephrologists may be consulted regarding the need for antibiotic prophylaxis. If prophylaxis is selected, the standard regimen of the current AHA guidelines should be used (see Chapter 2).[12-16]

The clinician should be aware of other cardiovascular considerations for patients undergoing hemodialysis. For example, the arm that contains the arteriovenous shunt should be protected from application of the blood pressure cuff, blood drawing, and the introduction of intra-

BOX 13-4

Antibiotic Prophylaxis Recommendations for Use With Placement of Nonvalvular Cardiovascular Devices

PRIMARY PROPHYLAXIS
- Modeled after that used to prevent surgical site infection
- Because of the low incidence of infection with many of the devices, evidence-based data have not been collected that prove efficacy
- Routinely used for placement of electrophysiologic cardiac devices, ventricular assist devices, total artificial hearts, ventriculoatrial shunts, cardiac suture line pledgets, vascular grafts, and arterial patches

SECONDARY PROPHYLAXIS
- Antibiotic prophylaxis is not routinely recommended after device placement for patients who undergo dental, respiratory, gastrointestinal, or genitourinary procedures
- It is recommended for patients with these devices if they undergo incision and drainage of infection at other sites (e.g., abscess) or replacement of an infected device
- It is recommended for patients with residual leak after device placement for attempted closure of the leak associated with patent ductus arteriosus, atrial septal defect, or ventricular septal defect

From Baddour LM, et al. Nonvalvular cardiovascular device-related infections. Circulation 2003;108:2015-2031.

venous medications. An inflated blood pressure cuff or tourniquet may collapse the shunt and render it useless. Likewise, the complication of phlebitis from intravenous medications can produce a clot that may jeopardize the shunt.

Approximately 40% of patients on dialysis have congestive heart failure, and 9% of them die of cardiovascular complications each year. These patients often take several medications to control hypertension, congestive heart failure, or hypercoagulability (i.e., anticoagulation). Dental care must be provided when the patient is medically stable, with an understanding of the medications needed and the dental precautionary measures that are appropriate (see Chapters 3, 4, 6, and 25).[12,13,15,16]

Hemodialysis tends to aggravate bleeding tendencies through physical destruction of platelets and the use of heparin. Therefore, determination of the status of hemostasis is important before oral surgery is performed. A battery of screening tests, including PFA-100, activated partial thromboplastin time (aPTT), and platelet count, should be ordered. Patients at higher risk are those with elevated laboratory values and a history of gastrointestinal bleeding (see Chapter 25). Although increased risk for bleeding is anticipated in these patients, the clinician can perform several management modifications that will reduce the risk. These include the following:

- Providing dental treatment at the optimum time, usually on the day after hemodialysis, because on the day of dialysis, patients are generally fatigued and may have a tendency to bleed. The activity of heparin lasts for 3 to 6 hours after infusion, and delay of treatment is prudent until that medication is eliminated from the bloodstream.
- Obtaining primary closure and, as needed, the use of pressure and hemostatic agents such as thrombin, oxidized cellulose, desmopressin, and tranexamic acid (see Chapter 25).
- Performing major surgical procedures on the day after the end of the week of hemodialysis treatment to provide additional time for clot retention before dialysis is resumed. For example, on a Monday/Wednesday/Friday weekly hemodialysis regimen, surgery performed on Saturday allows an additional day for clot stabilization before hemodialysis is resumed on Monday of the following week.
- Contacting the nephrologist when necessary, and requesting that the heparin dose be reduced or eliminated during the first hemodialysis session after the surgical procedure. Note: Hemodialysis can be performed without heparin when hemostasis and clot retention are important.
- Administering protamine sulfate (usually done by a physician) if immediate care is necessary; doing so will block the anticoagulant effects of heparin.

Patients who are dependent on long-term dialysis, especially those with diabetes, are prone to infection. Such patients also have higher rates of tuberculosis and vancomycin- and methicillin-resistant infections than do members of the general public. Thus, efforts should be made to identify orofacial manifestations of these infections and to eliminate oral sources of infection. Patients with active tuberculosis should not be treated until the disease is rendered inactive (see Chapter 9). Selection of antibiotics for hemodialysis patients with oral infections should be prudent and based on appropriate criteria.

Patients who undergo hemodialysis also can benefit from periodic testing for hepatitis viruses and HIV because vaccination or antiviral agents can be administered to reduce the risk of complications with these diseases. The dentist should be aware that a negative test result in the past is not predictive of a carrier state because patients may have acquired the disease since they were last tested, or they may be carriers of other infectious viruses (e.g., Epstein-Barr virus, cytomegalovirus) that can cause hepatic injury (see Chapter 11) or immune deficiency. Accordingly, all patients should be treated with the use of standard infection control procedures.

Patients who are carriers of hepatitis viruses from infection during hemodialysis may have altered hepatic function. Liver function should be assessed before hemorrhagic procedures are performed (see Chapter 11).

The dentist should be aware that hemodialysis removes some drugs from the circulating blood; this may shorten the duration of effect of prescribed medications. The chance that a given drug will dialyze is governed by four factors: (1) molecular weight and size, (2) degree of protein binding, (3) volume of drug distribution, and (4) endogenous drug clearance. For example, drugs with molecular weights above 500 daltons are poorly dialyzed. Drugs removed during hemodialysis are those with low binding capacity to plasma proteins. However, uremia may greatly alter the normal degree of protein binding. A drug such as phenytoin that normally has high protein binding exhibits lower plasma protein binding during uremia and is available to a greater extent for dialysis removal. Drugs with high lipid affinity have high tissue binding and are not available for dialysis removal. Lastly, efficient liver clearing of a drug greatly reduces the effect of dialysis treatment. Dosage amounts and intervals should be adjusted in accordance with advice from the patient's physician (see Table 13-2).[12,13,15,16]

Oral Complications and Manifestations. Hemodialysis reverses many of the severe oral manifestations associated with ESRD. However, uremic odor, dry mouth, taste change, and tongue and mucosal pain are symptoms that persist in many of these patients. Petechiae, ecchymosis, higher plaque and calculus indices, and lower levels of salivary secretion occur among patients undergoing hemodialysis more frequently than among healthy patients.[12,13,15-17]

Renal Transplant Patient

Patients who have a transplanted kidney may have special management needs, including the need for supplemental corticosteroids or antibiotic prophylaxis and the need for management of oral infection and gingival overgrowth caused by cyclosporine therapy (see Chapter 22).

REFERENCES

1. Proctor R, Kumar N, Stein A, et al. Oral and dental aspects of chronic renal failure. J Dent Res 2005;84: 199-208.
2. Singh G. Renal disease. Med Clin North Am 2005;89: 240.
3. Davidovich E, Davidovits M, Eidelman E, et al. Pathophysiology, therapy, and oral implications of renal failure in children and adolescents: An update. Pediatr Dent 2005;27:98-106.
4. Luke RG. Chronic renal failure. In Goldman L, Bennett JC (eds). Cecil Textbook of Medicine, 9th ed. Philadelphia, WB Saunders, 2000, p 1198.
5. Uribarri J. Past, present and future of end-stage renal disease therapy in the United States. Mt. Sinai J Med 1999;66:14-19.
6. Tokars JI, Miller ER, Alter MJ, et al. National surveillance of dialysis-associated diseases in the United States. Semin Dial 2000;13:75-85.
7. Curtis AS. Treatment of irreversible renal failure. In Goldman L, Bennett JC (eds). Cecil Textbook of Medicine, 9th ed. Philadelphia, Saunders, 2000, pp 579-583.
8. Incidence of end-stage renal disease among persons with diabetes—United States, 1990-2002. MMWR Morb Mortal Wkly Rep 2005;54:1097-1100.
9. Kokko JJ. Chronic renal failure. In Goldman L, Bennett JC (eds). Cecil Textbook of Medicine, 9th ed. Philadelphia, WB Saunders, 2000, pp 546-549.
10. Kho HS, Lee SW, Chung SC, Kim YK. Oral manifestations and salivary flow rate, pH, and buffer capacity in patients with end-stage renal disease undergoing hemodialysis. Oral Surg Oral Med Oral Pathol Oral Radiol Endod 1999;88:316-319.
11. 2006 Report on the Global AIDS Epidemic. Available at: http://www.UNAIDS.org. Accessed May 18, 2006.
12. Goodman JS, Crews HD, Ginn HE, Koenig MG. Bacterial endocarditis as a possible complication of chronic hemodialysis. N Engl J Med 1969;280:876-877.
13. Robinson DL, Fowler VG, Sexton DJ, et al. Bacterial endocarditis in hemodialysis patients. Am J Kidney Dis 1997;30:521-524.
14. Baddour LM, Bettmann MA, Bolger AF, et al. Nonvalvular cardiovascular device–related infections. Circulation 2003;108:2015-2031.
15. DeRossi SS. Dental considerations for the patient with renal disease receiving hemodialysis. J Am Dent Assoc 1996;127:211-219.
16. Tong DC, Rothwell BR. Antibiotic prophylaxis in dentistry: A review and practice recommendations. J Am Dent Assoc 2000;131:366-374.
17. Gavalda C, Bagan J, Scully C, et al. Renal hemodialysis patients: Oral, salivary, dental and periodontal findings in 105 adult cases. Oral Dis 1999;5:299-302.

Sexually Transmitted Diseases

CHAPTER
14

Sexually transmitted diseases (STDs) continue to be a major health problem in the United States and the world, and in many instances, are on the increase. In the United States, some of the highest rates of infection occur in adolescents and young adults. More than 25 STDs have been identified and are listed in Table 14-1. Current estimates predict that more than 65 million Americans are infected with one or more sexually transmitted diseases, and 15 million new infections occur annually.[1] The morbidity and mortality of STDs vary from minor inconvenience or irritation to severe disability and death. The diagnosis of an STD also has psychosocial effects.

STDs have important implications for dentistry. First, STDs are transmitted by intimate interpersonal contact that can result in oral manifestations. The dentist and hygienist must recognize these manifestations so as to refer patients for proper medical treatment. Second, some STDs can be transmitted by direct contact with lesions, blood, or saliva, and because many patients may be asymptomatic, the dentist should approach all patients as though disease transmission were possible and must adhere to standard precautions. Third, a single STD is accompanied by additional STDs in about 10% of cases, and STD-associated genital ulceration increases the risk for human immunodeficiency virus (HIV) infection.[2,3] Fourth, STDs exhibit antimicrobial resistance, and proper treatment is essential.[4] Fifth, some STDs are incurable, but all are preventable. Sixth, dental health care workers can be an important component of STD control by providing diagnosis, education, and information regarding access to treatment.

Although most STDs have the potential for oral infection and transmission, discussion in this chapter is limited to gonorrhea, syphilis, select human herpesvirus, and human papillomavirus infections because these entities are of special interest or importance to dental practice and serve to illustrate basic principles. The reader is referred to Chapters 11 and 19 for information about hepatitis B and AIDS.

GONORRHEA
DEFINITION

Gonorrhea is a worldwide sexually transmitted disease caused by *Neisseria gonorrhoeae*. It produces symptoms in men that usually cause them to seek treatment soon enough to prevent serious sequelae, but maybe not soon enough to prevent transmission to others. Infections in women often do not produce recognizable symptoms until complications have occurred. Because gonococcal infections among women often are asymptomatic, an important component of gonorrhea control in the United States continues to be the screening of women who are at high risk for STDs. Of note, patients infected with *N. gonorrhoeae* are often coinfected with *Chlamydia trachomatis*.

EPIDEMIOLOGY
Incidence and Prevalence

Gonorrhea is the second most commonly reported infectious disease and STD in the United States behind chlamydia. An estimated 700,000 new cases are reported each year in the United States, and about half of these are reported to the Centers for Disease Control and Prevention (CDC).[1,5,6] The reported incidence of gonorrhea in 2004 (i.e., 113.5 cases per 100,000 persons) was the lowest ever reported in the United States and was significantly lower than the incidence in the mid-1970s, when more than 1 million cases were reported.

Humans are the only natural hosts for this disease, and its occurrence is worldwide. Gonorrhea is transmitted almost exclusively via sexual contact, whether genital–genital, oral–genital, or rectal–genital. The primary sites

TABLE 14-1
Sexually Transmitted Diseases

Disease	Organism
Acquired immunodeficiency syndrome (AIDS)	Human immunodeficiency virus (HIV)
Amebiasis	*Entamoeba histolytica*
Bacterial vaginosis	*Bacteroides* spp, *Mobiluncus* spp
Chancroid	*Haemophilus ducreyi*
Condyloma acuminatum (genital warts)	Human papillomavirus infection (HPV-6, HPV-11)
Cytomegalovirus infection	Cytomegalovirus
Enterobiasis	*Enterobius vermicularis*
Epididymitis, mucopurulent cervicitis, lymphogranuloma venereum, nongonococcal urethritis, pelvic inflammatory disease, Reiter's syndrome	*Chlamydia trachomatis*
Epididymitis, gonorrhea, mucopurulent cervicitis, pelvic inflammatory disease	*Neisseria gonorrhoeae*
Genital herpes	Herpes simplex viruses (HSV-1, HSV-2)
Giardiasis	*Giardia lamblia*
Granuloma inguinale (donovanosis)	*Calymmatobacterium granulomatis*
Hepatitis B	Hepatitis B virus (HBV)
Molluscum contagiosum	Poxvirus
Nongonococcal urethritis, nonspecific vaginitis	*Trichomoniasis vaginalis*
Nongonococcal urethritis	*Ureaplasma urealyticum*
Pediculosis	*Pediculus pubis*
Salmonellosis	*Salmonella* spp
Shigellosis	*Shigella* spp
Streptococcal infection	Streptococcal group B spp
Syphilis	*Treponema pallidum*
Vulvovaginal candidiasis	*Candida* spp, *Torulopsis* spp

of infection are the genitalia, the anal canal, and the pharynx.

Gonorrhea can occur at any age, although it is seen most commonly in sexually active teenagers and young adults (4.6 per 1000 in the 15- to 29-year age group) and in the South.[1,5,6] Rates of infection differ by racial background, with African Americans reporting 19 times higher rates of gonorrhea than whites.[1,5,6] Risk factors other than age include first sexual experience at a young age, multiple sexual partners, low level of education, low socioeconomic standing, and living in an urban setting. Through the mid-1990s, cases were reported more commonly in men than in women; however, by the end of the 1990s, CDC data indicated that reportable cases were slightly higher in women.[1,2,5,6] At the current rate of 113.5 per 100,000 population, an average dental practice of 2000 adult patients can expect to provide care for 2 patients with gonorrhea.

Etiology

Gonorrhea is caused by *N. gonorrhoeae*, a gram-negative intracellular diplococcus. *N. gonorrhoeae* is an aerobic microbe that replicates easily in warm, moist areas and preferentially requires high humidity and specific temperature and pH for optimum growth. It is a fragile bacterium that is readily killed by drying, so it is not easily transmitted by fomites. It develops resistance to antibiotics rather easily, and many strains have become resistant

to penicillin and tetracycline, as well as to other antibiotics.

Pathophysiology and Complications

N. gonorrhea displays differential invasiveness based on the type of host epithelium with which it interacts. Columnar epithelium (as found in the mucosal lining of the urethra and cervix) and transitional epithelium (as in the oropharynx and rectum) are highly susceptible to infection, whereas stratified squamous epithelium (skin and mucosal lining of the oral cavity) is generally resistant to infection.[7] This explains the occurrence of rectal, pharyngeal, and tonsillar infections and the relative infrequency of oral infection. Another indication of the resistance of skin to gonococcal infection is the fact that no reported cases of gonorrhea have been reported to occur in the fingers. Figure 14-1 depicts the areas of relative epithelial susceptibility to *N. gonorrhoeae* infection in the oral cavity and oropharynx.

Infection in men usually begins in the anterior urethra. The bacteria invade epithelial tissues and are engulfed within polymorphonuclear leukocytes; this leads to cytokine production and purulent exudates.[7] The infection may remain localized or may extend to the posterior urethra, bladder, epididymis, prostate, or seminal vesicles. It spreads by means of lymphatics and blood vessels. Gonococcemia, although infrequent (1% to 2% of cases), may occur and results in dissemination of the disease to

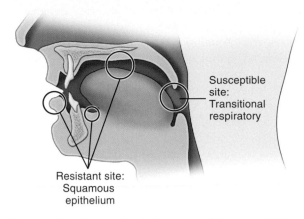

Susceptible
site:
Transitional
respiratory

Resistant site:
Squamous
epithelium

Figure 14-1. Areas of relative epithelial susceptibility to infection by *Neisseria gonorrhoeae* within the oral cavity.

distant body sites. Epididymitis is another complication of infection that can lead to infertility.

Infection in women occurs most commonly in the cervix and the urethra. Invasion of cervical epithelium can lead to the production of a purulent exudate but more often leads to an ascending infection of the endometrium, fallopian tubes, ovaries, and pelvic peritoneum. The ascending infection is a common cause of pelvic inflammatory disease (PID), which affects about one million women each year in the United States.[1] PID can be symptomatic or asymptomatic and may contribute to tubal scarring and infertility or ectopic pregnancy. Disseminated gonorrhea also can occur, with varying frequency. Vertical transmission accounts for a small percentage of cases of gonorrhea in the United States; if untreated, it can cause blindness or joint infection in infants.

In both genders, gonorrhea of the rectum may occur after anal–genital intercourse or through direct anal contamination from genital lesions. Infection of the pharynx and oral cavity is predominantly seen in women and homosexual men after fellatio. It also is occasionally seen after cunnilingus.

Gonococcemia can lead to widespread dissemination and may result in a variety of disorders, including migratory arthritis, skin and mucous membrane lesions, endocarditis, meningitis, PID, and pericarditis.

CLINICAL PRESENTATION
Signs and Symptoms

In men, symptoms usually occur after an incubation period of 2 to 5 days, although they may take as long as 30 days to appear. The most common findings include a mucopurulent (white, yellow, or green) urethral discharge, burning pain on urination, urgency, and frequency. Tenderness and swelling of the meatus may occur.

In women, a significant percentage of cases may be asymptomatic or only minimally symptomatic. Women who have a symptomatic infection may demonstrate vaginal or urethral discharge, dysuria with frequency and urgency, and burning pain when urinating. Backache and abdominal pain also may be present.

Approximately 50% of women and 1% to 3% of men are asymptomatic or only mildly symptomatic. This is unfortunate because patients may not seek medical care for their problem and as a result constitute a large reservoir of infection.

Gonococcal infection of the anal canal is commonly less intense than genital infection, but similar symptoms, including a copious purulent discharge, soreness, and pain, may be noted.

Within the oral cavity, the pharynx is most commonly affected.[8] Pharyngeal infection is detected in 3% to 7% of heterosexual men, 10% to 20% of heterosexual women, and 10% to 25% of homosexual men.[9] It usually is seen as an asymptomatic infection with diffuse, nonspecific inflammation or as a mild sore throat. The likelihood of transmission of pharyngeal gonorrhea to the genitalia seems much less than that of genital–genital transmission.[10,11] Of significance, however, is the fact that *N. gonorrhoeae* has been cultured from the expectorated saliva of two thirds of patients with oropharyngeal gonorrhea.[10]

Gonococcal stomatitis or oral gonorrhea appears to be uncommon; case reports in the literature are limited.[9,12-15] In many reported instances, oral gonorrhea lacked definitive laboratory identification of *N. gonorrhoeae*, and diagnosis was based on presumptive evidence. Chue[16] has presented a review of the varied and nonspecific manifestations of oral gonorrhea. These include acute ulceration, diffuse erythema, necrosis of the interdental papillae, lingual edema, edematous tissues that bleed easily, vesiculations, and a pseudomembrane that is nonadherent and leaves a bleeding surface on removal. Lesions may be solitary or widely disseminated. Symptoms include a burning or itching sensation, dryness, increased salivation, bad taste, fetid breath, fever, and submandibular lymphadenopathy. The lesions of oral gonorrhea may closely resemble the lesions of erythema multiforme, bullous or erosive lichen planus, or herpetic gingivostomatitis.

In a case report, Chue[17] describes acute temporomandibular joint arthritis caused by disseminated gonococcal infection from a genital site.

Laboratory Findings

Laboratory diagnosis of a genital *N. gonorrhoeae* infection can be made presumptively on the basis of a finding of Gram-negative diplococci within polymorphonuclear leukocytes in a smear of urine or of purulent discharge (Figure 14-2). However, culture is the gold standard for the diagnosis of *N. gonorrhoeae*. Nucleic acid amplification testing (NAAT) is highly sensitive and specific for the organism[18] and can be used to simultaneously test for *C. trachomatis*. In suspected cases of oropharyngeal gonorrhea, because other species of *Neisseria* are normal inhabitants of the oral cavity, a smear and Gram stain are not as helpful. Therefore, culturing with selective media or use of NAAT is necessary.

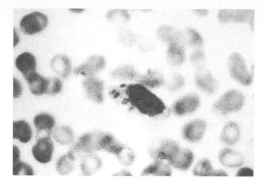

Figure 14-2. Smear demonstrates Gram-negative diplococci within a leukocyte. (Courtesy H. D. Wilson, MD, Lexington, Ky.)

MEDICAL MANAGEMENT

The CDC recommendations[19-21] offer several choices for the treatment of uncomplicated gonococcal infection of the cervix, urethra, and rectum. All are single-dose regimens. They include oral cefixime 400 mg in a single dose, or injectable ceftriaxone 125 mg (intramuscularly [IM]) in a single dose), or a single oral dose of a quinolone (ciprofloxacin [Cipro] 500 mg, or ofloxacin [Floxin] 400 mg or levofloxacin [Levaquin] 250 mg) plus coverage against the common coinfecting organism *Chlamydia trachomatis* with azithromycin 1 g given orally in a single dose, or doxycycline 100 mg orally two times a day for 7 days. For patients who cannot take ceftriaxone, spectinomycin (2 g IM) is a recommended alternative.[19,21] A very low (0.9%) treatment failure rate has been reported with ceftriaxone-doxycycline in the United States, and follow-up cultures are not considered essential unless symptoms persist. After antibiotic therapy is begun, infectiousness is diminished rapidly (within a matter of hours).[11,19] Infections detected after treatment are generally the result of reinfection by a sexual partner—not treatment failure. Quinolone-resistant strains (QRNs) are increasing and are more common in the Far East, Hawaii, and California.[21] Thus, the treatment of patients with gonorrhea with quinolones is becoming inadvisable in many areas.

The clinician should be aware that gonococcal pharyngitis is more difficult to eradicate than infections at urogenital and anorectal sites. Few antigonococcal regimens can reliably cure such infections more than 90% of the time, and IM cefixime is recommended.[21] Also, as with all STDs, all sex partners of patients who have *N. gonorrhoeae* infection should be assessed and treated.

SYPHILIS

DEFINITION

Syphilis is an acute and chronic STD caused by *Treponema pallidum* that produces skin and mucous membrane lesions in the acute phase, and bone, visceral, cardiovascular, and neurologic disease in the chronic phase. The variety of systemic manifestations associated with the later stages of syphilis resulted in historical designation of it as the "great imitator" disease. As with gonorrhea, humans are the only known natural hosts for syphilis. The primary site of syphilitic infection is the genitalia, although primary lesions also occur extragenitally.[7] In the United States, persons who live in the South are more frequently infected.[22] Syphilis remains an important infection in contemporary medicine because of the morbidity it causes, and because it enhances the transmission of human immunodeficiency virus (HIV).[23]

EPIDEMIOLOGY

Incidence and Prevalence

Syphilis is the fifth most frequently reported STD in the United States today, surpassed only by chlamydia, gonorrhea, salmonellosis, and acquired immunodeficiency syndrome (AIDS). In 1990, the incidence of primary and secondary syphilis reached 50,223 cases.[10] The number of cases of primary and secondary syphilis dropped to 20,627 in 1994 and fluctuated between 6800 and 8000 between 1999 and 2004.[21,22] This represents a rate of decline of 86%—from 20.3 cases/100,000 population to 2.7/100,000 during the past decade.[1,21] A disproportionately high number of cases continue to occur in the South and among Hispanic and non-Hispanic African American men and women. Syphilis occurs more commonly in persons aged 25 to 39 years. Its incidence in males is greater than that in females, with a ratio of more than 5:1.[1,5,21]

Congenital syphilis occurs when the fetus is infected in utero by an infected mother. In 2004, a total of 353 cases of congenital syphilis were reported to the CDC. This represents a rate of 8.6 per 100,000 live births—a dramatic decline from a peak of 107.3 cases per 100,000 live births in 1991.[1,5,21]

Etiology

The etiologic agent of syphilis is *Treponema pallidum*, which is a slender, fragile anaerobic spirochete. It is transmitted predominantly sexually, including by oral–genital and rectal–genital contact with contaminated sores. However, transmission also can occur via nonsexual means such as kissing, blood transfusion, or accidental inoculation with a contaminated needle. Indirect transmission by fomites is possible but uncommon because the organism survives for only a short time outside the body.[7,22] *T. pallidum* is easily killed by heating, drying, disinfecting, and using soap and water. The organism is difficult to stain, except through certain silver impregnation methods. Demonstration is best done with dark-field microscopy with a fresh specimen.

Pathophysiology

It is believed that *T. pallidum* does not invade completely intact skin; however, it can invade intact mucosal epithelium and gain entry via minute abrasions or hair follicles. Within a few hours after invasion, bacterial spread to the

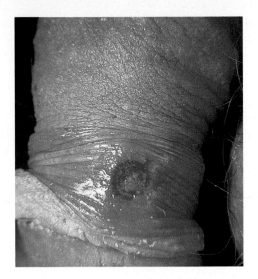

Figure 14-3. Primary syphilis: Chancre of the penis. (From Habif TP, Campbell JI Jr, Chapman MS, et al. Skin Disease: Diagnosis and Treatment, 2nd ed. St. Louis, Mosby, 2005.)

lymphatics and the bloodstream occurs, resulting in early widespread dissemination of the disease. The early response to bacterial invasion consists of endarteritis and periarteritis.[7,22] The risk of transmission occurs during the primary, secondary, and early latent stages of disease, but not in late syphilis.[74] Overall, patients are most infectious during the first 2 years of the disease.

CLINICAL PRESENTATION

Signs and Symptoms

Manifestations and descriptions of syphilis are classically divided according to stages of occurrence, with each stage having its own peculiar signs and symptoms that are related to time and antigen-antibody responses. These stages are primary, secondary, latent, tertiary, and congenital. It is important to note that many infected persons do not develop symptoms for years, yet they remain at risk for late complications if not treated.

Primary Syphilis. The classic manifestation of primary syphilis is the chancre, a solitary firm, round, granulomatous lesion that develops at the site of contact with the infectious organism. The chancre usually occurs within 2 to 3 weeks (range, 10 to 90 days) after exposure (Figure 14-3). Patients are infectious, however, before it appears. The lesion begins as a small papule and enlarges to form a surface erosion or ulceration that commonly is covered by a yellowish hemorrhagic crust and teems with *T. pallidum*. It is commonly painless. Associated with the chancre are enlarged, painless, hard regional lymph nodes. The chancre usually subsides in 3 to 6 weeks without treatment, leaving variable scarring in the form of a healed papule.[7,22,25] The genitalia, oral cavity (lips, tongue), fingers, nipples, and anus are common sites for chancres. Figure 14-4 presents examples of extragenital syphilitic chancres (lip and perioral). If adequate treat-

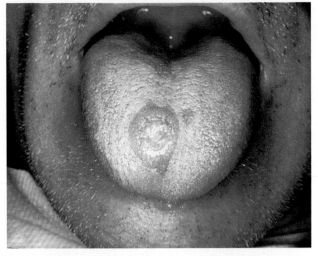

A

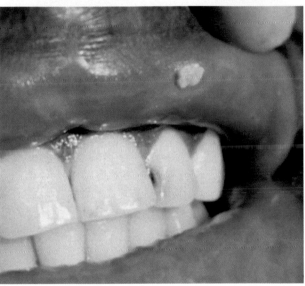

B

Figure 14-4. Primary syphilis. **A,** Chancre on tongue seen in primary syphilis. **B,** Extragenital chancre of the lip. (**A** from Ibsen DAC, Phelan JA. Oral pathology for the hygienist, 4th ed, St. Louis, Saunders, 2003.)

ment is not provided, the infection progresses to secondary syphilis.

Secondary Syphilis. The manifestations of secondary syphilis appear 6 to 8 weeks after initial exposure. The chancre may or may not have completely resolved by this time. The symptoms and signs of secondary syphilis include fever, arthralgia and malaise, generalized lymphadenopathy, and patchy hair loss and develop in 80% of patients. Generalized eruptions of the skin and mucous membranes (Figure 14-5, *A*). The papules of the rash are well demarcated and reddish brown and have a predilection for the palms and soles; they are typically not itchy. Oral manifestations of secondary syphilis include pharyngitis, papular lesions, erythematous or grayish white erosions (mucous patches) (see Figure 14-5, *B*), irregular linear erosions, and, rarely, parotid gland enlargement.

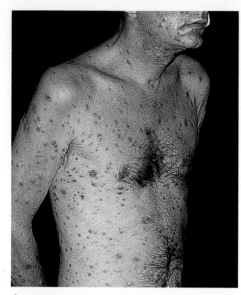

A

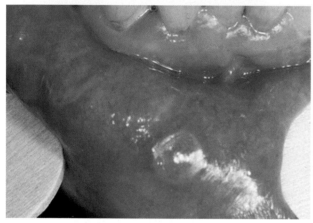

B

Figure 14-5. Lesions of secondary syphilis. **A,** Profuse papular rash. **B,** Mucous patch of the lower lip (**A** from Habif TP, Campbell JI Jr, Chapman MS, et al. Skin Disease: Diagnosis and Treatment, 2nd ed. St. Louis, Mosby, 2005.)

The lesions of skin and mucous membranes are highly infectious.[7,22,25] Without treatment, secondary syphilis ultimately resolves; however, infection progresses to latent or late stages.

Latent Syphilis. Latent syphilis is defined as the third stage of the untreated infection. Patients are seroreactive but are asymptomatic and show no clinical evidence of disease. Latent syphilis is divided into early latent syphilis (acquired the disease within the preceding year) and late latent syphilis (longer than 1 year). During the first 4 years of latent syphilis, patients may have mucocutaneous relapses and are considered infectious. After 4 years, relapses do not occur, and patients are considered noninfectious (except for blood transfusions and pregnant women).[7,22] The latent stage may last for many years or, in fact, for the remainder of the person's life. In some untreated patients, however, progression to tertiary syphilis occurs.

Tertiary (Late) Syphilis. The tertiary (late) stage occurs in 10% to 40% of untreated persons, generally several years after disease onset.[26] It is the destructive stage of the disease. Patients are noninfectious. Any organ of the body (mucocutaneous, osseous, visceral, or neural) may become involved. Signs and symptoms of this stage do not occur until years after the initial infection.

The gumma, which is the classic localized lesion of tertiary syphilis, may involve the skin, mucous membranes, bone, nervous tissue, and/or viscera. It is believed to be the end result of a hypersensitivity reaction and is basically an inflammatory granulomatous lesion with a central zone of necrosis. It is not infectious.

All other manifestations of tertiary syphilis are essentially vascular in nature and result from an obliterative endarteritis. Cardiovascular syphilis is most commonly seen as an aneurysm of the ascending aorta. Neurosyphilis can result in a meningitis-like syndrome, Argyll Robertson pupils (which react to accommodation but not to light), altered tendon reflexes, general paresis, tabes dorsalis (degeneration of dorsal columns of the spinal cord and sensory nerve trunks), difficulty in coordinating muscle movements, or insanity.

The oral lesions of tertiary syphilis consist of diffuse interstitial glossitis and the gumma. Interstitial glossitis should be considered a premalignant condition. The tongue may appear lobulated and fissured with atrophic papillae, resulting in a bald and wrinkled surface. Leukoplakia frequently is present. The oral gumma is a rare lesion that most commonly involves the tongue and palate. It appears as a firm tissue mass with central necrosis. Palatal gummas may perforate into the nasal cavity or maxillary sinus.

Congenital Syphilis. Syphilis or its sequelae occur in the newborn if the mother is infected while carrying the child. The disease is transmitted to the fetus in utero, usually after the 16th week, because before this time, the placenta prevents transmission of bacteria. The disease persists worldwide because a substantial number of women do not receive syphilis serologic testing during pregnancy, or they receive the testing too late in pregnancy and often do not receive prenatal care.[27] Physical manifestations vary according to the time of infection. The sequelae of early infection include osteochondritis, periostitis (frontal bossing of Parrot), rhinitis, rash, and ectodermal changes. Syphilis contracted during late pregnancy may involve bones, teeth (see Oral Manifestations), eyes, cranial nerves, viscera, skin, and mucous membranes. A classic triad of congenital syphilis known as Hutchinson's triad includes interstitial keratitis of the cornea, eighth nerve deafness, and dental abnormalities (i.e., Hutchinson's incisors [Figure 14-6] and mulberry molars).

Laboratory Findings

T. pallidum has never been cultured successfully on any type of medium; therefore, the definitive diagnosis of

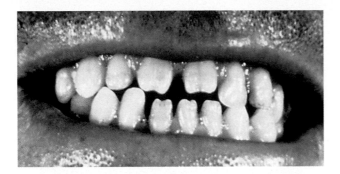

Figure 14-6. Congenital syphilis: Hutchinson's teeth.

syphilis is made from a positive dark-field microscopic examination or on the basis of direct immunofluorescent antibody tests on fresh lesion exudates. Dark-field examination is consistently positive only during primary and early secondary stages. Definitive diagnosis of oral lesions by this method is difficult because other *Treponema* species are indigenous to the oral cavity.

Syphilis is typically diagnosed by a two-step process involving a nonspecific (screening) antibody test followed by a treponeme-specific test. Screening antibody tests of blood are also known as serologic tests for syphilis (STS). These tests are of two basic types (indirect and direct) and are differentiated by the types of antibodies they investigate.

Screening Serologic Tests for Syphilis: Nontreponemal Tests (VDRL and RPR). Standard screening tests for syphilis consist of the Venereal Disease Research Laboratory (VDRL) slide test, the rapid plasma reagin (RPR) test, and the automated reagin test (ART). These indirect, nontreponemal serologic tests are designed to detect the presence of an antibody-like substance called *reagin* that is produced when *T. pallidum* reacts with various body tissues. They are equally valid. A disadvantage of reaginic tests is the occasional biologic false-positive result that can occur.

Nontreponemal tests produce titers (reported quantitatively as serologic dilutions [e.g., 1:2, 1:4, 1:8]) that usually correlate with disease activity. They are consistently positive and yield the highest titers between 3 and 8 weeks after the appearance of the primary chancre. In primary syphilis, nontreponemal tests usually revert to negative within 12 months after successful treatment. In secondary syphilis, up to 24 months may be required for the patient to become seronegative. Occasionally, a patient will remain seropositive for the rest of his or her life, or will test positive with an associated infection or condition (false positive). With tertiary syphilis, many patients remain seropositive for life.[2]

Confirmatory Serologic Tests for Syphilis: Treponemal Tests (FTA-ABS and MHA-TP). Treponemal tests are designed to detect the specific antibody produced against treponemes that cause syphilis, yaws, and pinta.[7,22] They are more specific than reaginic tests but

less sensitive. Thus, they typically are performed after a positive VDRL or RPR. The fluorescent treponemal antibody (FTA) test, fluorescent treponemal antibody absorption (FTA-ABS) test, and *T. pallidum* particle agglutination test (TP-PA) are examples.[2,21] Treponemal antibody titers wane over time but remain positive in about 80% of patients, regardless of treatment. Thus, they should not be used to assess response to treatment.

Polymerase chain reaction (PCR) for specific treponemal DNA sequences may be helpful in confirming the diagnosis when other studies are not helpful.[28]

MEDICAL MANAGEMENT

Parenteral injection of long-acting benzathine penicillins (e.g., penicillin G, 2.4 million U IM in a single dose) remains the recommended treatment for primary, secondary, or early latent syphilis. Additional doses for 3 weeks are recommended for someone who has had syphilis for longer than a year (late latent). Alternative drugs for patients allergic to penicillin include oral doxycycline (100 mg orally two times a day for 2 weeks for the primary stage) and erythromycin (500 mg orally four times a day for 2 weeks for the primary stage) or ceftriaxone sodium IM injection.[21] Testing for HIV status and treatment of sexual partners also are recommended. After completing treatment, patients should be retested at 6 and 12 months to monitor for seroconversion status. A low failure rate has been reported in the treatment of syphilis. An important aspect to note in the management of syphilis is that, as with gonorrhea, infectiousness is reversed rapidly, probably within a matter of hours, on initiation of medical treatment.[20,22]

The Jarisch-Herxheimer reaction is an acute febrile reaction that is frequently accompanied by chills, myalgias, and headache that occur within 24 hours after initiation of therapy for syphilis. It occurs most often (i.e., in 50% patients) after treatment for early syphilis.

Congenital syphilis is best managed through implementation of preventive measures. This requires that all pregnant women be tested for syphilis by serology at the first prenatal visit. If positive, the expectant mother should be treated with penicillin and retested at the 28th week and again at delivery. Infants born to seroreactive mothers should be assessed by means of clinical, radiographic, and laboratory tests of blood and cerebrospinal fluid (CSF) for VDRL. If results prove the disease or suggest that syphilis is highly probable, then infants should be treated with IV penicillin G for at least 10 days. The treatment response for congenital and tertiary stages of syphilis is limited by the extent of damage already incurred.

GENITAL HERPES

DEFINITION

Genital herpes is a recurrent, incurable viral disease of the genitalia that is caused by one of two closely related types of herpes simplex virus (HSV)—type 1 and type 2. Most genital herpes infections are caused by HSV-2. The disease consists of acute and recurrent phases and is associated with high rates of subclinical infection and asymptomatic viral shedding. The prevalence of genital herpes has increased by 30% since the late 1970s.[29,30]

EPIDEMIOLOGY

Incidence and Prevalence

Genital herpes is an important STD in the United States and in the world. Its exact incidence is unknown because it is not a reportable disease, and most persons have not been diagnosed because their disease is mild or asymptomatic. It is estimated that 50 million persons, or more than 25% of persons 12 years and older, in the United States are infected.[21,29] An estimated 1.6 million new cases of HSV-2 occur annually in the United States.[31,32] The prevalence in developing countries is between 40% and 60%.[32] Many cases of genital herpes are acquired from persons who are asymptomatic at the time of sexual contact, or who do not know that they have genital herpes. About 70% to 95% of first-episode cases of genital herpes are caused by HSV-2, whereas up to 30% are caused by HSV-1.[21] Prevalence in women (25%) and in African Americans (46%) is reportedly higher than in men (20%) and in whites (18%).[29]

Etiology

HSV belongs to a family of eight human herpesviruses that includes cytomegalovirus, Epstein-Barr virus, varicella-zoster virus, human herpesvirus type 6 (HHV-6), human herpesvirus type 7 (HHV-7), and Kaposi's sarcoma–associated herpesvirus (HHV-8). HSV-1 is the causative agent of most herpetic infections that occur above the waist, especially on the mucosa of the mouth (herpetic gingivostomatitis, herpes labialis), nose, eyes, brain, and skin. Infection with HSV-1 is extremely common; most adults demonstrate antibodies to this virus. It is thought that many primary infections with HSV-1 are subclinical and thus are never known to the infected person. Transmission usually occurs through close contact, such as touching or kissing, and transfer of infective saliva. HSV-1 also is transmitted via sexual contact. Airborne droplet infection has not been well demonstrated, although it is possible.[33] Autoinoculation via face, fingers, eyes, and genitalia is a persistent clinical problem.

HSV-2 is the causative agent of most herpes infections that occur below the waist, such as in or around the genitalia (genital herpes). HSV-2 is transmitted predominantly by sexual contact but may also be passed nonsexually. Its primary mode of transmission is through an asymptomatic viral shedder. HSV-2 can be transmitted to a newborn from an infected mother.

Although the primary site of occurrence of HSV-1 is above the waist and of HSV-2 below the waist, each infection may occur at either site and in fact can be inoculated

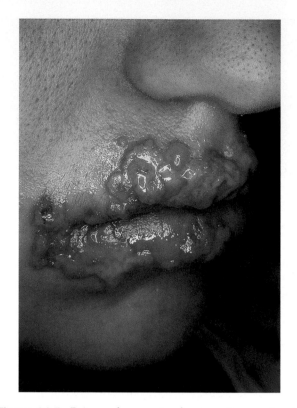

Figure 14-7. Primary herpes simplex type 2 occurring in the oral cavity documented by laboratory testing. (From Sapp JP et al. Contemporary oral and maxillofacial pathology, ed 2, St. Lous, Mosby, 2004.)

from one site to the other (Figure 14-7). Furthermore, the two types cannot be differentiated clinically.

Pathophysiology and Complications

The pathologic processes of herpesvirus infections HSV-1 and HSV-2 are essentially identical; thus, the lesions of skin and mucous membranes are identical. Infection arises from intimate contact with a lesion or infective fluid (e.g., saliva). Epithelial cells are invaded, and viral replication occurs. Characteristic cellular changes include ballooning degeneration, intranuclear inclusion bodies, and the formation of multinucleated giant cells. With cellular destruction come inflammation and increasing edema, which result in formation of a papule that progresses to a fluid-filled vesicle. These vesicles rupture, leaving an ulcerated or crusted surface.

Lymphadenopathy and viremia are prominent features. In normal individuals, the infection is contained by usual host defenses and runs its course within 10 to 20 days. However, spread to other epidermal sites (e.g., herpetic whitlow [infection of the fingers], keratoconjunctivitis [eyes]) and in neonates during childbirth has been documented. In rare cases, infants and immunosuppressed persons can develop systemic (meningitis) and widespread infection that may result in significant morbidity and death.

During the epithelial infection, progeny enter the ends of local peripheral neurons and migrate up the axon to the regional ganglion (HSV-1 primarily in the trigeminal, and HSV-2 primarily in the sacral), where they reside. After stimulation such as trauma, sunlight, menses, or intercourse, the virus reactivates, migrates down the axon, and produces recurrent infection with lesions similar to the primary, but less severe in nature and more localized. Of the two HSV serotypes that can infect the sacral ganglia, HSV-2 is more efficient in reactivating and producing recurrent genital lesions, whereas HSV-1 may pose a greater risk of neonatal herpes.[34] Also, immune suppression increases the risk for more frequent and severe recurrences.

CLINICAL PRESENTATION

Signs and Symptoms

Most (about 60%) new cases of HSV-2 infection are asymptomatic[32]; newly acquired cases are asymptomatic more frequently in men than in women. After an incubation period of 2 to 7 days, lesions (i.e., papules, vesicles, ulcers, crusts, and fissures) of primary genital herpes may appear. In women, both internal and external genitalia may be involved, as well as the perineal region and the skin of the thighs and buttocks. In men, the external genitalia may be involved, as may the skin of the inguinal area. Lesions in moist areas tend to ulcerate early, are painful, and may cause dysuria. Lesions on exposed dry areas tend to remain pustular or vesicular and then crust over. Painful regional lymphadenopathy accompanies infection, along with headache, malaise, myalgia, and symptoms of fever. These subside in about 2 weeks, and healing occurs in 3 to 5 weeks.

Outbreaks of recurrent genital herpes typically occur 2 to 6 times per year and are generally less severe than the primary infection. Recurrences are frequently precipitated by menses, intercourse, or immune suppression. A *prodrome* of localized itching, tingling, paresthesia, pain, and burning may be noted and is variably followed by a vesicular eruption (Figure 14-8). Healing occurs in 10 to 14 days. Constitutional symptoms are generally absent. Between recurrences, infected persons shed virus intermittently through the genital tract.

HSV-1 and HSV-2 lesions are highly infectious and therefore can be transmitted to other individuals or to other sites on the patient. Orogenital contact may result in spread from the source to the oral cavity or genitals of the sexual partner. The infectious period of herpetic lesions is of uncertain length, but positive viral cultures are detected most often from stages prior to crusting. Therefore, one should assume that all herpetic lesions (i.e., papular, vesicular, pustular, and ulcerative) prior to completion of crusting are infectious.

Laboratory Findings

Cytologic examination of a smear taken from the base of a herpetic lesion reveals typical features, including ballooning degeneration of cells, intranuclear inclusion bodies, and multinucleated (fused) giant cells. However,

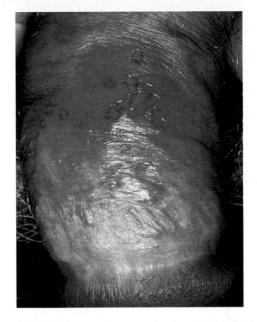

Figure 14-8. Recurrent herpes simplex virus infection of the foreskin. (From Habif TP, Campbell JI Jr, Chapman MS, et al. Skin Disease: Diagnosis and Treatment, 2nd ed. St. Louis, Mosby, 2005.)

cytology is nonspecific and less sensitive than viral culture. Diagnosis is best established by swabbing an infected secretion or ulcer and isolating the virus by cell culture. The virus is identified by staining the infected cells for HSV antigen with the use of immunofluorescence or immunoperoxidase. Alternatively, NAAT may be used[21,30] and is particularly useful when neurologic symptoms develop and cerebrospinal fluid is sampled. Serologic detection of antibodies to HSV-1 glycoprotein G1 or HSV-2 glycoprotein G2 aids in diagnosis and management (e.g., counseling the patient about the potential for recurrence).

MEDICAL MANAGEMENT

Management of patients with a first clinical episode of genital herpes includes antiviral therapy and counseling regarding the natural history of genital herpes, sexual and perinatal transmission, and ways to reduce transmission. Current CDC recommendations[21] call for the use of acyclovir (Zovirax), famciclovir (Famvir), or valacyclovir (Valtrex). All three are nucleoside analog drugs that act as DNA chain terminators during virus replication in infected cells. Some of these agents are available in oral, topical, and intravenous formulations. Topical acyclovir therapy is substantially less effective than systemic drug administration, and its use is not recommended for genital herpes. Use of systemic antiviral drugs can shorten the duration, frequency, and symptoms of outbreaks and can reduce the frequency of asymptomatic shedding and the risk of transmission.[35] However, antiviral agents do not eliminate the virus from the latent state, nor do they affect subsequent risk, frequency, or severity of recur-

BOX 14-1

Regimens Recommended by the Centers for Disease Control and Prevention for the Treatment of Genital Herpes

PRIMARY EPISODE OF GENITAL HERPES*
- Acyclovir 400 mg orally three times a day for 7-10 days, or
- Acyclovir 200 mg orally five times a day for 7-10 days, or
- Famciclovir 250 mg orally three times a day for 7-10 days, or
- Valacyclovir 1 g orally twice a day for 7-10 days

RECURRENT INFECTION
- Acyclovir 400 mg orally three times a day for 5 days, or
- Acyclovir 200 mg orally five times a day for 5 days, or
- Acyclovir 800 mg orally twice a day for 5 days, or
- Famciclovir 125 mg orally twice a day for 5 days, or
- Valacyclovir 500 mg orally twice a day for 3 to 5 days, or
- Valacyclovir 1000 mg orally once a day for 5 days.

DAILY SUPPRESSIVE THERAPY
- Acyclovir 400 mg twice daily, or
- Famciclovir 250 mg orally twice a day, or
- Valacyclovir 500 mg orally once a day, or
- Valacyclovir 1000† mg orally once a day

*Note: Treatment may be extended if healing is incomplete after 10 days of therapy. Higher dosages of acyclovir (e.g., 400 mg orally five times a day) were used in treatment studies of first-episode herpes proctitis and first-episode oral infection. However, comparative studies with respect to genital herpes have not been performed. Valacyclovir and famciclovir probably are also effective for acute HSV proctitis or oral infection, but clinical experience is lacking.[20]

†Higher doses may be required for patients who have more than 10 recurrences per year.

rence after drug use is discontinued. Antiviral drugs are most effective when given preventatively at least 1 day within the appearance of symptoms, whether for primary or recurrent disease. Current treatment recommendations[21] (Box 14-1) are directed toward primary, recurrent, and suppressive genital herpes therapy. These protocols may also be used for oral infection. Intravenous antiviral agents (cidofovir [Vistide; Gilead Sciences Inc., Foster City, Calif] and foscarnet [Foscavir]) are reserved for severe or complicated infections and may be required for immune suppressed patients.

Daily suppressive antiviral therapy can be implemented for patients with frequent recurrences (more than five recurrences per year). Suppressive therapy reduces the frequency of recurrence by 70% to 80% among persons who have six or more recurrences per year and reduces asymptomatic viral shedding between outbreaks.[19,21] Safety and efficacy have been documented among patients given daily therapy with acyclovir for as long as 6 years, and among those given valacyclovir and

famciclovir for 1 year. Suppressive therapy has not been associated with emergence of clinically significant acyclovir resistance among immunocompetent patients. Because the frequency of recurrence tends to diminish over time in many patients, current recommendations include discussing periodically the possibility of discontinuing suppressive therapy to reassess the need for continued therapy.

Acyclovir, famciclovir, and valacyclovir have been assigned pregnancy category C, B, and B, respectively, by the US Food and Drug Administration (FDA). Accordingly, famciclovir and valacyclovir are considered relatively safe to administer to pregnant women.[36]

INFECTIOUS MONONUCLEOSIS

DEFINITION

Although not classically defined as an STD, infectious mononucleosis is discussed in this chapter because transmission occurs through intimate personal contact. Infectious mononucleosis is an infection that is caused, in at least 90% of cases, by the Epstein-Barr virus (EBV), a lymphotropic herpesvirus. Other viruses may also produce features of acute infectious mononucleosis. Infectious mononucleosis produces the classic clinical triad of fever, pharyngitis, and lymphadenopathy. Transmission of the virus occurs primarily by way of the oropharyngeal route during close personal contact (i.e., intimate kissing). Children, adolescents, and young adults are most commonly affected. About 40% of asymptomatic herpesvirus-seropositive adults carry EBV in their saliva on any given day.[37]

EPIDEMIOLOGY

Incidence, Prevalence, and Etiology

More than 90% of adults worldwide have been infected with EBV.[37] In the United States, about 50% of 5-year-old children and 70% of college freshmen have evidence of prior EBV infection.[38,39] The peak age of acquisition in the United States is reportedly between 15 and 19 years of age. The annual incidence in this adolescent age group is 3.4 to 6.7 cases per 1000 persons.[38] Incidence has been reported as 30 times higher in whites than in blacks in the United States.[38] No gender predilection has been noted. Having numerous sexual partners increases the risk for acquisition of EBV.

Pathophysiology

EBV is a lymphotropic herpesvirus that is transmitted primarily through exposure to oropharyngeal secretions. Infrequently, it is transmitted through shared infected drinks, eating utensils, or infected blood products. Incubation time is 30 to 50 days. A prodromal period of 3 to 5 days precedes the clinical phase, which lasts 7 to 20 days. During the prodromal phase, the virus infects oropharyngeal epithelial cells and spreads to B lymphocytes in the tonsillar crypts. Infected B lymphocytes circulate through the reticuloendothelial system, triggering a marked lymphocytic response. In normal blood smears, large reactive lymphocytes represent about 1% to 2% of cells. In infectious mononucleosis, they constitute 10% to 40% of circulating white blood cells. Reactive lymphocytes are not EBV-infected B lymphocytes but are T lymphocytes that react to the infection (Figure 14-9).[39] The combination of reactive lymphocytes, the cytokines they produce, and the B-cell–produced (heterophile) antibodies directed against EBV antigens contributes to the clinical manifestation of the acute infection. Hepatosplenomegaly develops in about 40% to 50% of patients, splenic rupture occurs in 0.1% to 0.2% of all cases, and death is a rare outcome.[37,39] After the acute infection, the virus remains latent in B lymphocytes for the life of the host. As effective transforming agents, EBV-associated lymphomas and carcinomas are common.

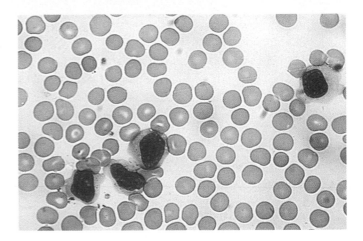

Figure 14-9. Atypical lymphocytes in infectious mononucleosis. (From Kumar V, Abbas A, Fausto N. Robbins & Cotran's Pathologic Basis of Disease, 7th ed. Philadelphia, Saunders, 2005.)

CLINICAL PRESENTATION

Signs and Symptoms

Infectious mononucleosis usually is asymptomatic when found in children; however, when young adults are affected, about 50% are mildly symptomatic. Fever, sore throat, tonsillar enlargement, and lymphadenopathy occur in 70% to 90% of patients.[37,39,40] Additional features include malaise, fatigue, an absolute lymphocytosis (>10% reactive lymphocytes), and a positive heterophil antibody test.[36] About a third of patients develop palatal petechiae during the first week of the illness, and about 30% of patients experience an exudative pharyngitis.[39-41] Generalized skin rash and petechiae of the lips are seen in about 10% of cases. Also, the liver and spleen can enlarge and become tender. Symptoms tend to dissipate within 3 weeks of onset.

Laboratory Findings

The diagnosis of infectious mononucleosis is made on the basis of symptoms and a laboratory profile characterized by peripheral lymphocytosis (e.g., 50% lymphocytes [primarily T lymphocytes]) and at least 10% atypical lymphocytes (see Figure 14-9), along with a positive heterophile antibody test.[37] Heterophile antibodies are immunoglobulin (Ig)M antibodies that bind (agglutinate) to erythrocytes from nonhuman species such as sheep and horses.[42] This process forms the basis for the Monospot (Ortho-Clinical Diagnostics, Rochester, NY, USA) rapid latex agglutination test. Symptomatic patients who have a negative heterophile antibody test should be retested in 7 to 10 days because this test can be insensitive during the first week. If the second test is negative, tests for viral capsid antigen (VCA)-IgG and VCA-IgM antibody and EBV nuclear antigen (EBNA) should be performed.[38-40] These tests are more specific for EBV infection. If test results are positive, the patient has heterophile-negative infectious mononucleosis. A few patients with the classic disease description may be heterophile antibody negative and EBV-IgM negative. For these patients, tests for cytomegalovirus (CMV), *Toxoplasma gondii*, HHV-6, human immunodeficiency virus (HIV), and adenovirus should be performed.[38,39] Once EBV-associated mononucleosis has been diagnosed, EBV copy numbers in the blood can be used to monitor the severity and progression of the infection.[43]

MEDICAL MANAGEMENT

Although a number of antiviral drugs can inhibit EBV replication in culture, no drug is licensed for use in the clinical treatment of EBV infection. The lack of efficacy of antivirals results from the fact that mononucleosis is largely due to the immune response. As such, treatment of patients with infectious mononucleosis remains symptomatic and consists of bed rest, fluids, acetaminophen or nonsteroidal anti-inflammatory agents for pain control, and gargling and irrigation with saline solution or lidocaine to relieve symptoms of pharyngitis and stomatitis. Vigorous activity is to be avoided to reduce the risk of splenic rupture. In some patients with severe toxic exudative pharyngotonsillitis, pharyngeal edema and upper airway obstruction, or seizures, a short course of prednisone may be given. About 20% of patients with symptomatic infectious mononucleosis have concurrent beta-hemolytic streptococcal pharyngotonsillitis and should be treated with penicillin V, if they are not allergic to penicillin. Ampicillin should be avoided because at least 90% of patients develop a hypersensitivity skin rash when treated with this drug.[22] Most persons feel better and return to normal activities within a month.

HUMAN PAPILLOMAVIRUS INFECTION

DEFINITION

Human papillomaviruses (HPVs) are small, double-stranded, nonenveloped DNA viruses that infect and replicate in epithelial cells. More than 100 genotypes of

TABLE **14-2**
Human Papillomavirus–Associated Oral
Mucosal Lesions

Lesion	Most Common HPV Type
Condyloma acuminatum	6, 11
Epithelial dysplasia, carcinoma in situ, squamous cell carcinoma	2, 16, 18
Focal epithelial hyperplasia (Heck's disease)	13, 32
Lichen planus	11, 16
Oral bowenoid papulosis	6, 11, 16
Squamous papilloma	6, 11
Verruca plana	3, 10
Verruca vulgaris	2, 4, 6, 11, 16
Verrucous carcinoma	2, 6, 11, 16, 18

HPV have been identified, and more than 30 types are known to be sexually transmitted and to affect the ano-genital epithelium.[21] Each HPV subtype exhibits preferential anatomic sites of infection and a propensity for altering epithelial growth and replication. The spectrum of disease that is induced is dependent on the type of HPV infection, location, and immune response. Subtypes of HPV have been classified as "high-risk" or "low-risk" types. Low-risk HPVs (HPV-6, -11) produce benign proliferative lesions of mucocutaneous structures. High-risk HPV types (HPV-16, -18, -31, -33, -35, -45) are strongly associated with dysplasia and carcinoma of the uterine and anal tract and other mucosal sites.[44,45] Table 14-2 lists HPV-associated lesions.

EPIDEMIOLOGY

Incidence and Prevalence

HPV infections are one of the three most common STDs in the United States. An estimated 20 million people in the United States have genital HPV infections[1] that can be transmitted through sexual contact.[45] Although the exact incidence of HPV infection remains unknown, because it is not a reportable STD and most cases are asymptomatic or subclinical, it is estimated that more than 6 million new infections occur every year in the United States,[1] and up to 40% of sexually active individuals are infected with the virus.[46] By age 50, more than 80% of women will have acquired genital HPV infection. The infection is more common among African American women than white women. The highest rates of infection occur between the ages of 19 and 26 years.[1] Approximately 1% of sexually active adults in the United States have visible genital warts.[47] The lifetime number of sexual partners is the most important risk factor that has been identified for the development of genital warts.[48,49]

Etiology

Genital HPV can be transmitted by direct contact during sexual intercourse or passage of a fetus through an infected birth canal, or by autoinoculation. Genital lesions usually appear after an incubation period of HPV in epithelium for 3 weeks to 8 months. The most common manifestation of HPV replication is the venereal wart (or condyloma acuminatum). HPV types 6 and 11 are the subtypes most frequently associated with condyloma acuminatum. HPV types 2 and 6 also have been identified in condylomata but are not considered the primary etiologic agents.

Pathophysiology

HPV is transmitted through intimate or sexual contact. The virus replicates in the nuclei of epithelial cells and increases the turnover of infected cells, or it remains episomally in a latent state. Benign types such as HPV-6 and -11 have a strong tendency to induce epithelial hyperplasia such as condylomata and a spreading infection. HPV-16 and -18 have a propensity to induce dysplasia and malignant transformation. HPV types 31, 33, 35, 39, 45, 51, 52, 54, 56, and 58 convey intermediate to high risk for inducing carcinoma. Cofactors such as smoking contribute to the progression to cancer.

CLINICAL PRESENTATION

Signs and Symptoms

Most individuals infected with HPV are asymptomatic, and the infection clears on its own. Visible genital warts caused by HPV-6 or -11 are typically diagnosed as condyloma acuminatum. These growths are seen in sexually active individuals in warm, moist, intertriginous areas such as the anogenital skin and mouth, where friction and microabrasion allow entrance of the pathogen. Condylomata appear as small, soft, exophytic papillomatous growths (Figure 14-10, A). The surface is cauliflower-like or broccoli-like; the base is sessile. The borders are raised and rounded. The color varies from pink to dusky gray. Lesions often are multiple and recurrent and can coalesce to form large, pebbly warts. Most condylomata are asymptomatic; however, patients may report itching, irritation, pain, or bleeding as a result of manipulation or trauma. During pregnancy, condylomata may enlarge as the result of increased vascularity. Condylomata can occur on the vagina, anus, mouth (see Figure 14-10, B), pharynx, or larynx, and may appear weeks or months after the onset of infection.

HPV types 16, 18, 31, 33, and 35 have an infrequent association with genital warts and a more common association with dysplasia and carcinoma of the cervix. These high-risk HPV types also contribute to the development of squamous intraepithelial neoplasia (Bowen's disease) of the genitalia.

Laboratory Findings

HPV does not grow in cell culture, and serologic tests are not routinely performed, in part because 90% of infected persons become serologically HPV negative

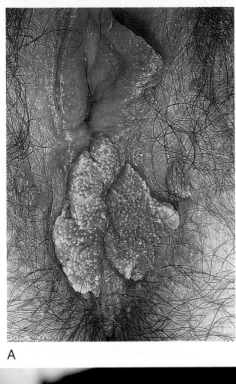

A

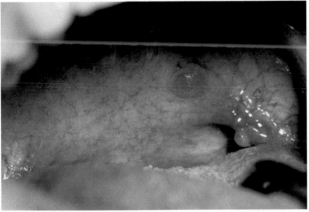

B

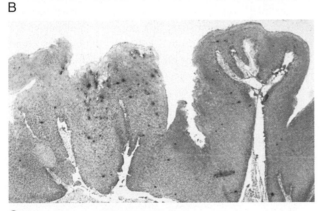

C

Figure 14-10. Human papillomavirus (HPV) infections. **A,** Large, cauliflower-like wart of the vagina. **B,** Dome-shaped HPV-induced lesions of the soft palate and retromolar trigone. **C,** In situ hybridization showing HPV DNA as indicated by dark purple stains in the epithelium of a condyloma acuminatum. (**A** from Habif TP, Campbell JI Jr, Chapman MS, et al. Skin Disease: Diagnosis and Treatment, 2nd ed. St. Louis, Mosby, 2005.)

within 2 years. Therefore, lesions of condyloma acuminatum should be biopsied and examined microscopically, if the clinical diagnosis is uncertain. Its microscopic appearance consists of a sessile base, with raised epithelial borders, a thick spinous spinosum layer (acanthosis), and hyperkeratosis. Identification of HPV within the lesion confirms the diagnosis. This is generally achieved with the use of commercial in situ hybridization kits that use RNA probes to detect viral DNA specific to HPV genotypes (see Figure 14-10, *C*). Viral subtyping may be important for determining risk of carcinogenesis when cervical tissue and an abnormal Papanicolaou smear are involved (see Chapter 26, Cervical Cancer section).

MEDICAL MANAGEMENT

A major advance occurred in 2006 with the introduction of the HPV vaccine (Gardasil).[49] This vaccine is 95% to 100% effective in preventing infection with HPV types 6, 11, 16, and 18. It has been approved for use in girls and women aged 9 to 26 years and is administered in a 3-shot regimen over a 6-month period. Additional vaccines are under investigation and are likely to enter the market soon. These vaccines prevent infection by four HPV types, and thus the major risk for cervical cancer. However, they have not been shown to eliminate or cure HPV and do not work against all HPV types.

At present, most persons in the United States have not been vaccinated and, if sexually active, are at risk for HPV infection. HPV-induced genital warts can be completely removed with chemicals, antiviral drugs, or surgery. The best response is attained with small warts that have been present for less than 1 year. The CDC[21] recommends podofilox 0.5% (Condylox) be the medication of first choice. It causes necrosis by arresting cells in mitosis. This patient-applied medication should be used twice a day for 3 days, with no treatment given for the next 4 days and the cycle repeated up to 4 times. Alternatively, the patient may apply imiquimod (Aldara) 5% cream at bedtime, 3 times per week for up to 16 weeks. Imiquimod is an immune response modifier drug. Most warts dissipate within 8 weeks. Other available therapies include surgery (excision, cryotherapy, laser), weekly topical therapy with podophyllum 10% to 25% in tincture of benzoin, and trichloroacetic acid 80% to 90% or bichloroacetic acid. Topical and intralesional therapy with 5-fluorouracil, an antimetabolite, has resulted in a greater than 60% response rate,[51] and cidofovir is an antiviral that yields an effective response. Intralesional interferon is an option, but it is rarely recommended because of cost and adverse effects. Recurrences are common despite the use of first-line therapies (in about 10% to 25% of cases, generally within 3 months), even when the entire lesion, including the base, is removed. As with all STDs, treatment should include the patient's sexual partner to avoid reinfection. Without treatment, lesions may enlarge and spread. Spontaneous regression occurs in about 20% of patients.[51]

DENTAL MANAGEMENT
Medical Considerations

The dental management of patients with an STD begins with identification. Because they are potentially infectious, the obvious goal is to identify all individuals who have active disease. Unfortunately, this is not possible in every case because some persons will not provide a history or may not demonstrate significant signs or symptoms suggestive of their disease. The inability of clinicians to identify potentially infectious patients applies to other diseases as well, such as HIV infection and viral hepatitis. Therefore, it is necessary for all patients to be managed as though they were infectious. The U.S. Public Health Service, through the CDC, has published recommendations for standard precautions to be followed in controlling infection in dentistry that have become the standard for preventing cross-infection[53] (see Appendix B). Strict adherence to these recommendations will, for all practical purposes, eliminate the danger of disease transmission between dentist and patient.

Even though these procedures are followed, several significant facts regarding STDs should be remembered. See Box 14-2 for these facts.

Gonorrhea. The patient with (nonoral) gonorrhea poses little threat of disease transmission to the dentist. This is because of specific requirements for transmission of the disease and because of early reversal of infectiousness

once antibiotics have been administered. Patients in this category can receive dental care within days of beginning antibiotic treatment.

Syphilis. Lesions of untreated primary and secondary syphilis are infectious, as are the patient's blood and saliva. Even after treatment has begun, its absolute effectiveness cannot be determined except through conversion of the positive serologic test to negative; however, early reversal of infectiousness is to be expected after antibiotic treatment has been initiated. The time required for this conversion varies from a few months to longer than a year. Therefore, patients who are currently under treatment or who have a positive STS test after receiving treatment should be viewed as potentially infectious. Still, any necessary dental care may be provided with adherence to standard precautions, unless oral lesions are present. Dental treatment can commence once oral lesions have been successfully treated.

Genital Herpes. Localized uncomplicated genital herpes infection poses no problem for the dentist. In the absence of oral lesions, any necessary dental work may be provided. If oral lesions are present, elective treatment should be delayed until lesions scab over, to avoid inadvertent inoculation of adjacent sites. Antiviral agents may be required to prevent recurrence after dental treatment has been provided.

Infectious Mononucleosis. Patients with infectious mononucleosis may come to the dentist because of oral signs and symptoms. Patients with clinical findings of fever, sore throat, petechiae, and cervical lymphadenopathy must be assessed so that a diagnosis of their condition can be established. Screening clinical laboratory tests can be ordered by the dentist (complete blood count [CBC], heterophil [Monospot] antibody test, and EBV antigen testing), or the patient may be referred to a physician for evaluation and treatment. Routine dental treatment should be delayed for about 4 weeks until the patient has recovered, the patient's liver is capable of normal metabolism of drugs, and the blood count, spleen and immune system have returned to normal.

Human Papillomavirus Infection. Although genital condylomata acuminatum do not affect dental management, oral warts are infectious, and standard precautions apply during oral treatment of patients. The presence of oral lesions necessitates referral to a physician to rule out genital lesions of the patient or his or her sexual partner. Excisional biopsy is recommended for HPV oral lesions.

Patients With a History of STD

Patients who have had an STD should be assessed carefully. They are at higher risk for additional STDs and recurrent infection. The clinician should ensure that adequate treatment was provided for any previous infec-

---

> ### BOX 14-2
>
> **Dental Management of the Patient With a Sexually Transmitted Disease***
>
> - **Gonorrhea**—Little threat of transmission to dentist; oral lesions are possible
> - **Syphilis**—Untreated primary and secondary lesions infectious; blood also is potentially infectious
> - **Genital herpes**—Little threat of transmission to dentist; oral lesions (possible from autoinoculation) are infectious
> - **HPV infection**—Little threat of transmission to dentist; oral lesions are possible
>
> Persons with sexually transmitted disease (STD) are at risk for human immunodeficiency virus (HIV) infection.
>
> New cases of syphilis, gonorrhea, and acquired immunodeficiency syndrome (AIDS) should be reported to the local/state health department.

*Because many patients with an active STD (as well as with other infectious diseases such as AIDS and hepatitis B) cannot be identified by the dentist, all patients should be considered potentially infectious and should be managed with the use of standard precautions. Preventive measures should be implemented that include patient education, as well as evaluation, treatment, and counseling of sexual partners.

tion and that new infections have not developed. Special attention should be given to unexplained lesions of the oral, pharyngeal, or perioral tissues. Also, a review of systems may reveal urogenital symptoms. Patients with a history of gonorrhea or syphilis should report a history of antibiotic therapy. Patients treated for syphilis should receive a periodic STS test for 1 year to monitor conversions from positive to negative. Adequate medical follow-up care should have been provided; if it was not, consultation and referral to a physician should be considered.

Patients With Signs, Symptoms, or Oral Lesions Suggestive of an STD

Patients who have signs or symptoms that suggest an STD, or who have unexplained oral or pharyngeal lesions, should be treated with caution. The index of suspicion should be higher if the patient is between 15 and 29 years of age and has risk factors such as being an urban dweller, being single, and belonging to a lower socioeconomic group. Any patient who has unexplained lesions should be questioned about possible relationships of the lesions to past sexual activity and should be advised to seek medical care. Herpetic lesions in or around the oral cavity should be recognizable. Patients with oral herpes lesions should not receive routine dental care but should be given palliative treatment only. For a severe primary oral infection or for infectious mononucleosis, the patient may require specific therapy and referral to a physician.

Treatment Planning Modifications

No modifications in the technical treatment plan are required for a patient with an STD. No adverse interactions have been reported between the usual antibiotics or drugs used to treat STDs and drugs commonly used in dentistry. No drugs are contraindicated. Patients with Hutchinson's incisors due to congenital syphilis may request aesthetic repair of their anterior teeth.

Reporting to State Health Officials

Dentists should be aware of local statutory requirements regarding reporting STDs to state health officials. Syphilis, gonorrhea, and AIDS are diseases that must be reported in every state. Local health departments and state STD programs are sources of information regarding this matter.

Oral Manifestations

Gonorrhea. The presentation of oral gonorrhea is infrequent, nonspecific, and varied, that is, it may range from slight erythema of the oropharynx to severe ulceration with a pseudomembranous coating. Lesions usually develop within 1 week of contact with an infected person; often, a history of fellatio is reported.[8] In terms of the oropharynx, patients describe that they have a sore throat and the mucosa becomes fiery red, with tiny pustules and an itching and burning sensation (Figure 14-11). When

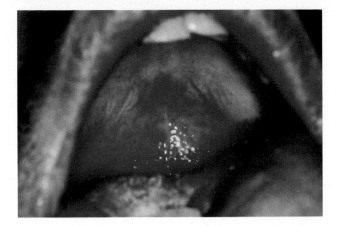

Figure 14-11. Gonococcal infection of the oral pharynx.

the tonsils become involved, they are invariably enlarged and inflamed with or without a yellowish exudate. The patient may be asymptomatic or incapacitated, with limited oral function (eating, drinking, talking), depending on the degree of inflammation. Diagnosis of oral lesions should be attempted with a smear and Gram stain followed by confirmatory tests.

The initial step in treatment is to ensure that the patient is under the care of a physician and is receiving proper antimicrobial therapy. After this, treatment of oral lesions is symptomatic (see Appendix C). The patient should be assured that oral infection will resolve with the use of appropriate antibiotics.

Syphilis. Syphilitic chancres and mucous patches are usually painless, unless they become secondarily infected. Both lesions are highly infectious. The chancre begins as a round papule that erodes into a painless ulcer with a smooth grayish surface (see Figure 14-4). Size can vary from a few millimeters to 2 to 3 cm. A key feature is lymphadenopathy that may be unilateral. The intraoral mucous patch often appears as a slightly raised, asymptomatic papule(s) with an ulcerated or glistening surface. The lips, tongue, and buccal or labial mucosa may be affected. Both the chancre and the mucous patch (see Figure 14-5) regress spontaneously with or without antibiotic therapy, although chemotherapy is required to eradicate the systemic infection. The gumma is a painless lesion that may become secondarily infected. It is noninfectious and frequently occurs on and destroys the hard palate. Interstitial glossitis, the result of contracture of the tongue musculature after healing of a gumma, is viewed as a premalignant lesion. Oral manifestations of congenital syphilis include peg-shaped permanent central incisors with notching of the incisal edge (Hutchinson's incisors) (see Figure 14-6), defective molars with multiple supernumerary cusps (mulberry molars), atrophic glossitis, a high narrow palate, and perioral rhagades (skin fissures).

Genital Herpes. HSV-1–induced ulcers are more common in the oral cavity than are those caused by HSV-

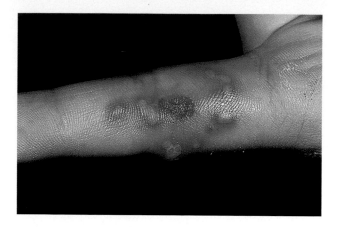

Figure 14-12. Herpetic whitlow. (From Habif TP, Campbell JI Jr, Chapman MS, et al. Skin Disease: Diagnosis and Treatment, 2nd ed. St. Louis, Mosby, 2005.)

2; however, these lesions cannot be differentiated clinically, and both should be treated similarly with antiviral agents (see Box 14-1 and Appendix C). Oral and perioral herpetic lesions are infectious during the papular, vesicular, and ulcerative stages, and elective dental treatment should be delayed until the herpetic lesion has completely healed. Dental manipulation during these infectious stages poses risks of (1) inoculation to a new site on the patient, (2) infection to the dental care worker, and (3) aerosol or droplet inoculation of the conjunctivae of the patient or of dental personnel. Once the lesion has crusted, it can be considered as relatively noninfectious.

A problem of particular concern to dentists is herpetic infection of the fingers or nail beds contracted by dermal contact with a herpetic lesion of the lip or oral cavity of a patient. The infection is called a herpetic whitlow, or a herpetic paronychia (Figure 14-12). It is serious, debilitating, and recurrent. Herpetic whitlow can be triggered to recur as a result of trauma or vibration from operating dental handpieces. Also, asymptomatic HSV shedding at oral or nonoral sites can trigger erythema multiforme, a mucocutaneous eruption characterized by "target" papules and ulcers that result from an immune response to the virus.

Infectious Mononucleosis. Head, neck, and oral manifestations of infectious mononucleosis include fever, severe sore throat, palatal petechiae, and cervical lymphadenopathy. Lymph nodes in the anterior and posterior cervical chain often are enlarged and tender to palpation. Postrecovery, EBV is associated with oral hairy leukoplakia, a benign entity, as well as with Hodgkin's and non-Hodgkin's lymphomas.

Human Papillomavirus Infection. Condylomata acuminatum commonly occur on the ventral tongue, gingiva, labial mucosa, and palate (see Figure 14-10, *B*). Transmission occurs by direct contact with infected anal, genital, or oral sites, or by self-inoculation. Lesions can be surgically excised, chemically removed with podophyllin, or

laser ablated. Caustic chemicals such as podophyllin are to be used with great caution to avoid damage to adjacent uninfected tissue and should be rinsed several hours after application. In addition, high-speed evacuation should be used during laser therapy to avoid inhalation of the virion-laden plume. Transmission of human papillomavirus (HPV) via inhalation of the plume has been documented to cause laryngeal condylomata.[53]

The dentist also should be cognizant that a condyloma identified in children raises the suspicion of sexual child abuse when autoinoculation by hand-to-genital contact, nonsexual contact, or maternal fetal transmission has been ruled out. Failure to report signs of an STD to state health officials is a legal offense in some states.

REFERENCES

1. Centers for Disease Control. STD surveillance, 2004. Available at: http://www.cdc.gov/std/stats/. Accessed April 5, 2007.
2. Centers for Disease Control. Sexually transmitted disease treatment guidelines, 1993. MMWR 1993; 42(RR-14):1-93.
3. Gwanzura L, McFarland W, Alexander D, et al. Association between human immunodeficiency virus and herpes simplex virus type 2 seropositivity among male factory workers in Zimbabwe. J Infect Dis 1998;177:481-484.
4. Fox K, Knapp J. Antimicrobial resistance in *Neisseria gonorrhoeae*. Curr Opin Urol 1999;9:65-70.
5. Centers for Disease Control. Summary of notifiable diseases, United States, 1998. MMWR 1999;47:1-93.
6. Miller WC, Zenilman JM. Epidemiology of chlamydial infection, gonorrhea, and trichomoniasis in the United States—2005. Infect Dis Clin North Am 2005;19: 281-296.
7. McAdam AJ, Sharpe AH. Infectious diseases. In Kumar V, Abbas AK, Fausto N (eds). Robbins and Cotran's Pathologic Basis of Disease, 7th ed. Philadelphia, WB Saunders, 2005.
8. Balmelli C, Gunthard HF. Gonococcal tonsillar infection—A case report and literature review. Infection 2003;31:362-365.
9. Escobar V, Farman A, Arm R. Oral gonococcal infection. Int J Oral Surg 1984;13:549-554.
10. Centers for Disease Control. Summary of notifiable diseases, United States, 1990. MMWR 1990;39:1-65.
11. Giunta J, Fiuamara N. Facts about gonorrhea and dentistry. Oral Surg 1986;62:529-531.
12. Jamsky R, Christen A. Oral gonococcal infections: Report of two cases. Oral Surg 1982;53:358-362.
13. Kohn S, Shaffer J, Chomenko A. Primary gonococcal stomatitis. JAMA 1972;219:86.
14. Merchant H, Schuster G. Oral gonococcal infection. J Am Dent Assoc 1977;95:807-809.
15. Schmidt H, Hjørting-Hanssen E, Philipsen H. Gonococcal stomatitis. Acta Derm Venereol 1961;41: 324-327.
16. Chue P. Gonorrhea—Its natural history, oral manifestations, diagnosis, treatment, and prevention. J Am Dent Assoc 1975;90:1297-1301.
17. Chue P. Gonococcal arthritis of the temporomandibular joint. Oral Surg 1975;39:572-577.

18. Van Dyck E, Ieven M, Pattyn S, et al. Detection of *Chlamydia trachomatis* and *Neisseria gonorrhoeae* by enzyme immunoassay, culture, and three nucleic acid amplification tests. J Clin Microbiol 2001;39:1751-1756.

19. Centers for Disease Control. 1998 guidelines for treatment of sexually transmitted diseases. MMWR 1998;47:1-118.

20. Little JW. Gonorrhea: An update. Oral Surg Oral Med Oral Pathol Oral Radiol Endod 2006;101:137-148.

21. Centers for Disease Control. Sexually transmitted diseases treatment guidelines—2002. MMWR 2002;51:1-80.

22. Centers for Disease Control. Summary of notifiable diseases, United States, 1994. MMWR 1995;43:1-80.

23. Grosskurth H, Mosha F, Todd J, et al. Impact of improved treatment of sexually transmitted diseases on HIV infection in rural Tanzania: Randomised controlled trial. Lancet 1995;346:530-536.

24. Lowhagen G. Syphilis: Test procedures and therapeutic strategies. Semin Dermatol 1990;9:152-159.

25. Little JW. Syphilis: An update. Oral Surg Oral Pathol Oral Med Oral Radiol Endod 2005;100:3-9.

26. Hook WE 3rd. Acquired syphilis in adults. N Engl J Med 1992;326:1060-1069.

27. Southwick K, Guidry H, Weldon M, et al. An epidemic of congenital syphilis in Jefferson County, Texas, 1994-1995: Inadequate prenatal syphilis testing after an outbreak in adults. Am J Public Health 1999;89:557-560.

28. Zoechling N, Schluepen E, Soyer H, et al. Molecular detection of *Treponema pallidum* in secondary and tertiary syphilis. Br J Dermatol 1997;136:683-686.

29. Fleming D, McQuillan G, Johnson R, et al. Herpes simplex virus type 2 in the United States, 1976 to 1994. N Engl J Med 1997;337:1105-1111.

30. Miller KE, Ruiz DE, Graves JC. Update on the prevention and treatment of sexually transmitted diseases. Am Fam Physician 2003;67:1915-1922.

31. Armstrong G, Schillinger J, Markowitz L, et al. Incidence of herpes simplex virus type 2 infection in the United States. Am J Epidemiol 2001;153:912-920.

32. Langenberg A, Corey L, Ashley R, et al. A prospective study of new infections with herpes simplex virus type 1 and type 2. N Engl J Med 1999;341:1432-1438.

33. Nahmias AJ, Roizman B. Infection with herpes simplex viruses 1 and 2. N Engl J Med 1973;289:781-789.

34. Brown ZA, Wald A, Morrow RA, et al. Effect of serologic status and cesarean delivery on transmission rates of herpes simplex virus from mother to infant. JAMA 2003;289:203-209.

35. Corey L, Wald A, Patel R, et al. Once-daily valacyclovir to reduce the risk of transmission of genital herpes. N Engl J Med 2004;350:11-20.

36. Drug Information for the Health Care Professional, 29th ed, vol IA, IB. Rockville, Md, United States Pharmacopeial Convention, 2006.

37. Miller CS, Avdiushko SA, Kryscio RJ, et al. Effect of prophylactic valacyclovir on the presence of human herpesvirus DNA in saliva of healthy individuals after dental treatment. J Clin Microbiol 2005;43:2173-2180.

38. Ebell MH. Epstein-Barr virus infectious mononucleosis. Am Fam Physician 2004;70:1279-1287.

39. Godshall S, Kirchner J. Infectious mononucleosis: Complexities of a common syndrome. Postgrad Med 2000;107:175-186.

40. Auwaerter P. Infectious mononucleosis in middle age. JAMA 1999;281:454-459.

41. Bailey R. Diagnosis and treatment of infectious mononucleosis. Am Fam Physician 1994;49:879-888.

42. Linderholm M, Boman J, Juto P, et al. Comparative evaluation of nine kits for rapid diagnosis of infectious mononucleosis and Epstein-Barr virus–specific serology. J Clin Microbiol 1994;32:259-261.

43. Balfour HH Jr, Holman CJ, Hokanson KM, et al. A prospective clinical study of Epstein-Barr virus and host interactions during acute infectious mononucleosis. J Infect Dis 2005;192:1505-1512.

44. Brown T, Yen-Moore A, Tyring S. An overview of sexually transmitted disease, Part II. J Am Acad Dermatol 1999;41:661-677.

45. Frisch M, Glimelius B, van den Brule A, et al. Sexually transmitted infection as a cause of anal cancer. N Engl J Med 1997;337:1350-1358.

46. Koutsky L, Gallowy D, Holmes K. Epidemiology of genital human papillomavirus infection. Epidemiol Rev 1988;10:122-163.

47. Borg A, Medley G, Garland S. Polymerase chain reaction: A sensitive indicator of the prevalence of human papillomavirus DNA in a population with sexually transmitted disease. Acta Cytol 1995;39:654-658.

48. Cates W Jr. Estimates of the incidence and prevalence of sexually transmitted diseases in the United States, American Social Health Association Panel. Sex Transm Dis 1999;26:S2-S7.

49. Munk C, Svare E, Poll P, et al. History of genital warts in 10,838 women 20 to 29 years of age from the general population: Risk factors and association with Papanicolaou smear history. Sex Transm Dis 1997;24:567-572.

50. FDA licenses new vaccine for prevention of cervical cancer and other diseases in females caused by human papilloma virus. http://www.fda.gov/bbs/topics/NEWS/2006/NEW01385.html. Accessed April 5, 2007.

51. Swinehart J, Skinner R, McCarty J, et al. Development of intralesional therapy with fluorouracil/adrenaline injectable gel for management of condyloma acuminata: Two phase II clinical studies. Genitourin Med 1997;73:481-487.

52. Carson D. Common sexually transmitted diseases. Am Druggist 1994;October:43-49.

53. Centers for Disease Control and Prevention. Recommended infection-control practices for dentistry, 1993. MMWR 1993;41(RR-8):1-12.

54. Hallmo P, Naess O. Laryngeal papillomatosis with human papillomavirus DNA contracted by a laser surgeon. Eur Arch Otorhinolaryngol 1992;248:425-427.

PART SIX

Endocrine and Metabolic Disease

Diabetes Mellitus

CHAPTER

15

Diabetes mellitus is the third most common cause of death in the United States, and it is increasing significantly.[1,2] In 2006, the Centers for Disease Control and Prevention (CDC) Data and Trends: National Diabetes Surveillance Program reported a 6% increase in the incidence of diabetes mellitus in the United States in only 1 year (Figure 15-1).[3] The major reason for this dramatic increase in cases of diabetes is obesity. Nearly 20 million Americans, or 6.5% of the entire population, have diabetes. Of these, approximately 6 million cases have not been diagnosed.[4]

Diabetes mellitus is a disease complex with metabolic and vascular components. This chronic disease is characterized by hyperglycemia and complications that include microvascular disease of the kidney and eye and a variety of clinical neuropathies.[1,2]

Diabetes is associated with chronic, premature macrovascular disease and serious microvascular disease. The metabolic component involves the elevation of blood glucose associated with alterations in lipid protein metabolism, resulting from a relative or absolute lack of insulin. Maintenance of good glycemic control can prevent or retard the development of microvascular complications of diabetes. The vascular component includes an accelerated onset of nonspecific atherosclerosis and a more specific microangiopathy that particularly affects the eyes and kidneys. Retinopathy and nephropathy are eventual complications, given sufficient duration, in nearly every individual with diabetes. These complications result in serious morbidity and are so characteristic of diabetes that the classification of diabetic type is dependent on their presence.[1,5]

The American Diabetes Association (ADA) classification of diabetes is summarized in Box 15-1.[6] Diabetes mellitus is of great importance to dentists because they are in a position as members of a health care team to detect new cases of diabetes. They also must be able to render dental care to patients who are already being treated for diabetes without endangering their well-being. A crucial aspect of identification of the dental patient with diabetes is the ability of the dentist to recognize the level of severity and of glycemic control, as well as the presence of complications from diabetes, so that he or she can treat the patient appropriately. Essential to this determination is knowledge of the patient's blood glucose level at the time that dental treatment is provided.

DEFINITION

Incidence and Prevalence

More than 240 million persons worldwide have diabetes mellitus, and health officials estimate that this figure will double or triple within the next 10 years. Of the nearly 20 million Americans, or 6.5% of the entire population, who have diabetes, approximately 6 million cases have not been diagnosed. The prevalence of diabetes mellitus has increased more than sixfold in the United States over the past 40 years.[3,6]

From 1980 through 2003, the number of hospital discharges with diabetes as any listed diagnosis more than doubled (from 2.2 million to 5.1 million discharges). During this period, the number of discharges with diabetes as any listed diagnosis increased the most among persons with diabetes who were aged 75 years and older (from 0.5 million to 1.6 million discharges).[3,6]

The same studies estimate that more than 20% of Americans are classified as obese, which represents a 57% increase over the past 10 years. This problem is increasing, and the prevalence of diabetes will also increase. Although the problem extends across all age groups, the largest group of individuals in this category are 30 to 39 years old.[3,6]

Approximately 1 million new cases of diabetes emerge in the United States each year, and about half of these individuals are unaware of their condition. An estimated

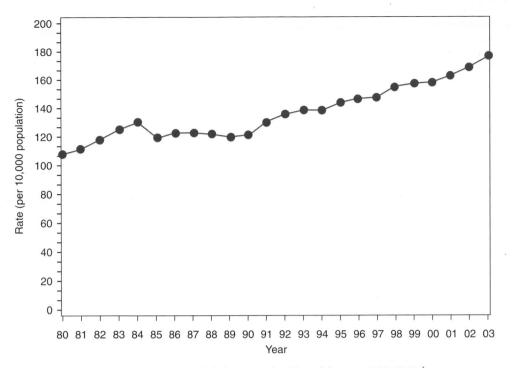

Figure 15-1. Increasing incidence of diabetes in the United States, 1980-2003.[3]

BOX 15-1	
Current Classification of Diabetes (American Diabetes Association, 1997)	
Type 1	Beta-cell destruction or defect in beta-cell function, usually leading to absolute insulin deficiency
Immune mediated	Presence of islet cell or insulin antibodies that identify the autoimmune process leading to beta-cell destruction
Idiopathic	No evidence of autoimmunity
Type 2	Insulin resistance with relative insulin deficiency
Other specific types	Genetic defects of beta-cell function or insulin action, pancreatic diseases, endocrinopathies, malnutrition, or drug- or chemical-induced diabetes
	Impaired fasting glucose (impaired glucose tolerance)
	Abnormalities of fasting glucose (abnormal glucose tolerance)
Gestational	Any degree of abnormal glucose tolerance during pregnancy diabetes

The incidence of type 1 diabetes has increased several-fold in children and teenagers over the past 30 years. About 210,000 people younger than 20 years of age have diabetes. This represents 0.26% of all people in this age group. Approximately 1 in every 400 to 500 children and adolescents has type 1 diabetes.[3,6]

Mortality and Morbidity: Relative to Glycemic Control. Diabetes mellitus accounts for about 40,000 deaths per year.[7-11] Rates of associated morbidity are extremely high. The relative risk that individuals with diabetes will acquire end-stage renal disease is 25 times that of individuals without diabetes.[12] Additionally, 25% of all new cases of end-stage renal disease result from diabetes mellitus.[13,14] The relative risk that patients with diabetes will require the amputation of an extremity because of diabetic complications is more than 40 times that of normal persons; more than 20,000 amputations are performed per year on patients with diabetes mellitus, which represents nearly 50% of all nontraumatic amputations.[1,15-17] Retinopathy occurs in all forms of diabetes.[1,15-17] As with other complications of diabetes, the development of retinopathy (and blindness) varies with duration and control of the disease.[17] The relative risk that an individual with diabetes will become blind is 20 times greater than that of other individuals. Susceptibility to myocardial infarction and stroke in patients with diabetes is 2 to 5 times greater than in those without the disease. The severity of these (and other) complications of diabetes is largely dependent on the degree and level of control of hyperglycemia.[12]

12% of the general population in the United States has impaired glucose tolerance.[7] Of patients with diabetes in the United States, 90% to 95% have type 2 disease. Thus, the prevalence of type 2 diabetes is approximately 10 times that of type 1. The vast majority of undiagnosed cases of diabetes are of the type 2 variety.

Nathan and colleagues[1] reported in a longitudinal retrospective study that lasted longer than 17 years, that diabetic patients with good glycemic control (hemoglobin [HbA]1c levels <7%) had 42% fewer systemic complications and 57% fewer deaths than those with diabetes with poorly controlled hyperglycemia (>8%).

The most significant risk factors for type 2 diabetes are family history and obesity. About 60% to 70% of patients with type 2 diabetes are obese at the time of diagnosis.[1]

The number of cases of diabetes in the United States will continue to rise for the following reasons[3,6]:

- The population is increasing
- Life expectancy is increasing
- The number of people with obesity is increasing
- Persons with diabetes are living longer because of better medical management, and they are having children who will pass on the disease.

The glycosylated hemoglobin value (HbA1c) is the primary target for glycemic control. The American Diabetes Association recommends that the blood test—which measures average levels of glycemia over the preceding 2 to 3 months—should be performed at least twice a year in patients whose treatment goals are being met (and who have stable glycemic control), and quarterly in patients whose treatment has changed or whose goals are not being met. The goal for patients in general is an HbA1c value of less than 7%, and the goal for each individual patient is as close to normal (less than 6%) as is possible without the occurrence of clinically significant hypoglycemia (see Figure 15-2). Unfortunately, these goals are often unmet. In 1999 and 2000, only 37% of adults 20 years of age or older with diagnosed diabetes nationwide were estimated to have values below 7%. Moreover, many people with diabetes do not know their HbA1c values, because they have not been tested, or because they have not been informed about their results or do not recall them.[7]

Etiology

Diabetes mellitus may be the result of any of the following:

- A genetic disorder
- Primary destruction of islet cells through inflammation, cancer, or surgery
- An endocrine condition such as hyperpituitarism or hyperthyroidism
- An iatrogenic disease that occurs after steroids have been administered.

In this chapter, discussion is limited to the genetic type of diabetes, the most common type, which also has been called primary, hereditary, or essential diabetes (see Box 15-1).[6]

The two types of genetic diabetes are type 1 and type 2 diabetes. A genetic component is involved in the origin of both; however, the role of genetics in type 2 diabetes is much greater than in type 1 diabetes. In addition to the weak genetic role that has been noted in type 1 diabetes, environmental factors such as viral infection and autoimmune reaction appear to be causative. Studies of identical twins have shown that if one twin develops type 1 diabetes, the other twin has about a 50% chance of getting the disease. Additionally, if one identical twin develops type 2 diabetes, the other has a 100% chance of also developing it. Obesity plays an important part in the development of type 2 diabetes, but how this occurs is not well understood.[1,6]

Gestational diabetes mellitus (GDM) occurs as the onset of impaired glucose tolerance (IGT) or clinical diabetes during pregnancy. The condition of patients usually returns to normal after the birth of the child, but they have an increased risk of developing diabetes within 5 to 10 years. GDM enhances risk for loss of the fetus and is associated with increased size of surviving fetuses. Several groups of patients fit into the classification of previous abnormality of glucose tolerance (pre-AGT), including patients who have had gestational diabetes, formerly obese individuals who have lost weight, patients with hyperglycemia that occurs after myocardial infarction, and those with posttraumatic hyperglycemia.[18]

Patients who have never had an abnormal glucose tolerance test result but who are by genetic background at increased risk of developing diabetes mellitus fit into the potential abnormalities of glucose tolerance (post-AGT) classification. Figure 15-2 illustrates the various types of glycemic abnormalities and their classification, along with requirements for insulin.[12]

Patients with clinical signs and symptoms of diabetes mellitus may have type 1, type 2, or another type of diabetes. These individuals exhibit an elevation in fasting blood glucose, abnormal glucose tolerance test results, and microangiopathy.[1]

In type 1 diabetes, sudden onset of clinical symptoms usually occurs; this condition often is diagnosed in individuals younger than 40 years of age; it may, however, occur at any age. Type 2 diabetes generally occurs after age 40 in obese individuals. The incidence of type 2 diabetes increases with age, and insulin secretion may be low, normal, or high. Although most persons with type 2 diabetes are able to secrete insulin for some time, they have decreased numbers of insulin receptors within target cells, and their postreceptor activity is reduced.[4]

Although little progress has been made in understanding the pathogenesis of type 2 diabetes, researchers know of a strong genetic influence in its origin (Table 15-1). Defects in insulin secretion, rather than insulin sensitivity, are most likely the major genetic predisposing factor to the development of type 2 diabetes. Obesity plays a major role in onset of the disease; between 60% and 70% of individuals with type 2 diabetes are obese.[6,19-22]

Pathophysiology and Complications

Glucose is the most important stimulus for insulin secretion. Insulin remains in circulation for only several minutes (half-life [$t_{1/2}$], 4 to 8 minutes); it then interacts with target tissues and binds with cell surface insulin receptors. Secondary intracellular messengers are activated and interact with cellular effector systems,

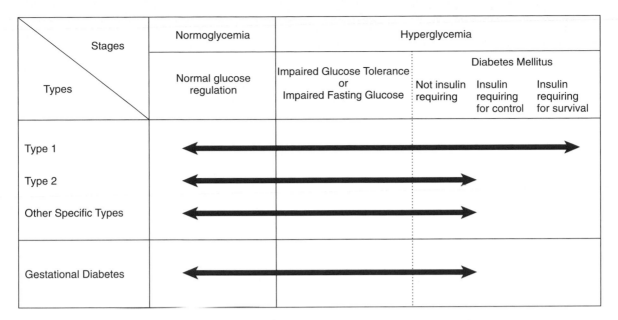

Figure 15-2. Disorders of glycemia: Classification and requirements for insulin.

TABLE **15-1**
Hereditary Probability of Developing Type 2
Diabetes Among Members of Families

Family Member A	Family Member B	Chance of Developing Diabetes Mellitus, %
Parent	Parent	85
Parent	Grandparent, aunt, uncle	60
Parent	First cousin	40
One parent		20
One grandparent		14
One first cousin		2

From Saadoun AP. Hereditary probability of developing Type 2 diabetes among members of families. Periodont Abstr 1980;28: 116-137.

including enzymes and glucose transport proteins. Lack of insulin or insulin action allows glucose to accumulate in the tissue fluids and blood.[19,23,24]

The mechanisms by which hyperglycemia may lead to microvascular complications include increased accumulation of polyols through the aldose reductase pathway and of advanced glycosylation end products.

The patient with uncontrolled diabetes is deprived of insulin or its action but will continue to use carbohydrates at the usual rates in the brain and nervous system because these tissues do not require insulin. However, other tissues in the body are unable to take glucose into the cells or to use it at a normal rate. Increased production of glucose from glycogen, fat, and protein may occur; thus, the rise in blood glucose in diabetic persons results from a combination of underutilization and overproduction attained through glycogenolysis and fat metabolism.

Hyperglycemia leads to glucose excretion in the urine, which results in increased urinary volume. The increase in fluid lost through urine may lead to dehydration and loss of electrolytes. With type 2 diabetes, prolonged hyperglycemia can lead to significant losses of fluid in the urine. When this type of severe dehydration occurs, urinary output drops, and a hyperosmolar nonketotic coma may result. This condition is seen most often in elderly patients with type 2 diabetes.[12,23,25,26]

Lack of glucose utilization by many cells of the body leads to cellular starvation. The patient often increases intake of food but in many cases still loses weight. If these events continue to progress, the person with type 1 diabetes develops metabolic acidosis. For a time, the body may be able to maintain the pH at nearly normal levels; but as the buffer system and respiratory and renal regulators fail to compensate, body fluids become more acidic (i.e., pH falls). Severe acidosis will lead to coma and death if it is not identified and treated. The primary manifestations of diabetes—hyperglycemia, ketoacidosis, and vascular wall disease—contribute to the inability of patients with uncontrolled diabetes to fight infection and prevent their wounds from healing.

The end results of these effects, as well as others yet to be identified, are that the patient with uncontrolled diabetes is rendered much more susceptible to infection, the patient's ability to deal with an infection once it has been established is reduced, and healing of traumatic and surgical wounds is delayed.[12,23,25-27]

Patients with type 1 diabetes demonstrate significant effects of the disease on long-term survival. Few deaths occur among these patients before the age of 30 years. By age 55, only 48% of women and 34% of men are still alive. When compared with the general population, women with diabetes live 22 fewer years than women without the disease, and men with diabetes live 24 fewer

TABLE 15-2

Expected Years of Additional Life in Individuals With and Without Diabetes Compared With Given-Age Cohorts

Attained Age of Individual With Diabetes, y	Expected Years Additional Life of Individual Without Diabetes	Expected Years Additional Life of Individual With Diabetes	Years Lost Because of Diabetes
10	61.5	44.3	17.2
20	51.9	36.1	13.8
30	42.5	30.1	12.4
40	33.3	23.7	9.6

TABLE 15-3

Prevalence of Complications in Patients With Insulin-Dependent Diabetes Mellitus (IDDM)

Complication	Cumulative Prevalence
Visual impairment	14%
Blindness	16%
Renal failure	22%
Stroke	10%
Amputation	12%
Myocardial infarction	21%
Median years of survival after diagnosis of type 1 diabetes	39
Median age at death, y	49

BOX 15-2

Complications of Diabetes Mellitus

- Ketoacidosis (type 2 diabetes)
- Hyperosmolar nonketotic coma (type 2 diabetes)
- Diabetic retinopathy/blindness
- Cataracts
- Diabetic nephropathy/renal failure
- Accelerated atherosclerosis (coronary heart disease[1])
- Ulceration and gangrene of feet
- Diabetic neuropathy (dysphagia, gastric distention, diarrhea, impotence, muscle weakness/cramps, numbness, tingling, deep burning pain)
- Early death

years than those without the disease. Diabetes mellitus diagnosed at the age of 10 years is estimated to cause a loss of 17.2 years of life expectancy (Table 15-2). In addition to decreasing life expectancy, the complications of diabetes mellitus lead to significant signs and symptoms that affect the quality of life. Data on the prevalence of diabetic complications are presented in Table 15-3.[12,28,29]

Complications of diabetes are related to the level of hyperglycemia and pathologic changes that occur within the vascular system and the peripheral nervous system (Box 15-2). Vascular complications result from microangiopathy and atherosclerosis.

Therefore, the case is strong for appropriate glycemic control to prevent or reduce progression of complications. In any case, vessel changes include thickening of the intima, endothelial proliferation, lipid deposition, and accumulation of para-aminosalicylic acid–positive material. These changes can be seen throughout the body but have particular clinical importance when they occur within the retina and the small vessels of the kidney.[12,13,28,29]

Diabetic retinopathy consists of nonproliferative changes (microaneurysms, retinal hemorrhages, retinal edema, retinal exudates) and proliferative changes (neovascularization, glial proliferation, vitreoretinal traction) and is the leading cause of blindness in the United States. The incidence of blindness in all persons with diabetes is 0.2% per year; it is 0.6% per year for diabetic individuals with retinopathy. Proliferative retinopathy is most common among patients with type 1 diabetes; a much lower incidence is seen in type 2 diabetes. Cataracts occur at an earlier age and with greater frequency in those with type 1 diabetes. The typical cataract, senile cataract, is identified in 59% of individuals with diabetes aged 35 to 55 years but in only 12% of those without the disease. Young persons with diabetes are prone to the development of metabolic cataracts.[12,17]

Diabetic nephropathy leads to end-stage renal disease in 30% to 40% of individuals with type 1 diabetes (Figure 15-3). Renal failure occurs in only 5% of individuals with type 2 diabetes. However, because type 2 diabetes is much more common than type 1, the number of persons with renal failure is equal for the two types of diabetes. Renal failure is the leading cause of death in patients with type 1 diabetes. Of all patients who undergo dialysis, 25% have diabetes. Microangiopathy in the kidney usually involves the capillaries of the glomerulus.[12,13,30]

Macrovascular disease (atherosclerosis) occurs earlier and is more widespread and more severe in persons with diabetes. In patients with type 1 diabetes, atherosclerosis seems to develop independent of microvascular disease (microangiopathy). Hyperglycemia plays a role in the evolution of atherosclerotic plaques. Individuals with uncontrolled diabetes have increased levels of low-density lipoprotein (LDL) cholesterol and reduced levels of high-density lipoprotein (HDL) cholesterol. Attainment of normal glycemia often improves the LDL/HDL ratio.[12,13,28,30]

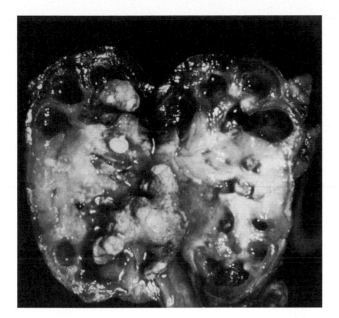

Figure 15-3. Diabetic nephropathy (cross section of kidney). (Courtesy Richard Estensen, Minneapolis, Minn.)

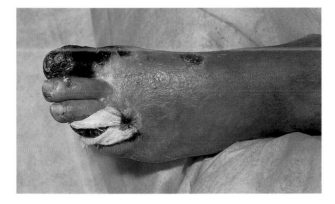

Figure 15-4. Diabetic gangrene of the feet. (From Swartz MH. Textbook of Physical Diagnosis: History and Examination, 5th ed. Philadelphia, Saunders, 2006.)

A major determinant of the morbidity associated with poor glycemic control in diabetes is accelerated atherosclerosis. Atherosclerosis increases the risks of ulceration and gangrene of the feet (Figure 15-4), hypertension, renal failure, coronary insufficiency, myocardial infarction, and stroke. The most common cause of death in patients with type 2 diabetes is myocardial infarction. By age 55, a third of all individuals with diabetes die of complications from coronary heart disease (CHD). Death rate from CHD in the general population up to age 55 is approximately 8% for men and 4% for women. Women with diabetes treated with insulin have greater risks for CHD than do non–insulin-treated women. This is not true for insulin-treated men. A person with diabetes also has less chance of surviving a myocardial infarction than does a nondiabetic person.[1,23,28]

In the extremities, diabetic neuropathy may lead to muscle weakness, muscle cramps, a deep burning pain,

tingling sensations, and numbness. In addition, tendon reflexes, two-point discrimination, and position sense may be lost. Some cases of oral paresthesia and burning tongue are caused by this complication.[12,15,31]

Diabetic neuropathy also may involve the autonomic nervous system. Esophageal dysfunction may cause dysphagia, stomach involvement may cause a loss of motility with massive gastric distention, and involvement of the small intestine may result in nocturnal diabetic diarrhea. Sexual impotence and bladder dysfunction also may occur. Diabetic neuropathy is common with type 1 and type 2 diabetes and may occur in more than 50% of patients. Neuropathy progresses over time in type 2 diabetes, and this increase may be greater in patients with hypoinsulinemia.[12,15,31]

Other complications include decubitus ulcerations, gangrenous extremities, cataracts, skin rashes, and deposits of fat in the skin (xanthoma diabeticorum). In individuals who were diagnosed early and are now well controlled, these complications may not develop as quickly or to as great an extent as in those in whom the disease was detected late or was poorly managed.[12,15,31]

CLINICAL PRESENTATION

Signs and Symptoms

In patients with type 1 diabetes, the onset of symptoms is sudden and more acute. Symptoms include polydipsia, polyuria, polyphagia, loss of weight, loss of strength, marked irritability, recurrence of bed wetting, drowsiness, and malaise. Patients with severe ketoacidosis may experience vomiting, abdominal pain, nausea, tachypnea, paralysis, and loss of consciousness. The onset of symptoms in type 2 diabetes usually is insidious, and the cardinal signs (polydipsia, polyuria, polyphagia, weight loss, and loss of strength) are less commonly seen.[2,6] The signs and symptoms of type 1 and type 2 diabetes are summarized in Table 15-4 and Box 15-3.

Other signs and symptoms related to the complications of diabetes include skin lesions, cataracts, blindness, hypertension, chest pain, and anemia. The rapid onset of myopia in an adult is highly suggestive of diabetes mellitus.

Laboratory Findings

Two groups of patients should be screened for diabetes mellitus: (1) those individuals with signs and symptoms of diabetes or its complications, and (2) high-risk ethnic groups (i.e., African Americans, Hispanics, Native Americans, Asian Americans, and Pacific Islanders). Persons with HDL cholesterol levels lower than 35 mg/100 mL or triglyceride levels greater than 250 mg/100 mL, those who have relatives with diabetes, persons who are obese or older than 45 years of age, those who have had GDM, and individuals who have delivered large babies (>9 lb) or who have had spontaneous abortions or stillbirths should be screened at periodic intervals. For individuals older

TABLE **15-4**
Clinical Pictures of Type 1 and Type 2 Diabetes

	Type 1	Type 2
Frequency, % of person with diabetes	5-10	90-95
Age at onset, y	15	40 and over
Body build	Normal or thin	Obese
Severity	Extreme	Mild
Insulin	Almost all	25% to 30%
Plasma glucagons	High, suppressible	High, resistant
Oral hypoglycemic agents	Few respond	50% respond
Ketoacidosis	Common	Uncommon
Complications	90% in 20 years	Less common
Rate of clinical onset	Rapid	Slow
Stability	Unstable	Stable
Genetic locus	Chromosome 6	Chromosome 11(?)
HLA and abnormal autoimmune reactions	Present	Not present
Insulin receptor defects	Usually not found	Often found

HLA, Human lymphotrophic antigen.

BOX 15-3

Symptoms of Diabetes

TYPE 1
- Cardinal symptoms (common): Polydipsia, polyuria, polyphagia, weight loss, loss of strength
- Other symptoms: Recurrence of bed wetting, repeated skin infections, marked irritability, headache, drowsiness, malaise, dry mouth

TYPE 2
- Cardinal symptoms (much less common): Polydipsia, polyuria, polyphagia, weight loss, loss of strength
- Usual symptoms: Slight weight loss or gain, gastrointestinal upset, nausea, urination at night, vulvar pruritus, blurred vision, decreased vision, paresthesias, dry flushed skin, loss of sensation, impotence, postural hypotension

---

than age 45, the screening should occur routinely at 3-year intervals. Most of the screening for diabetes involves those individuals with undiagnosed type 2 diabetes. Obese individuals, high-risk ethnic groups, and those with low HDL cholesterol levels or high triglyceride levels should be screened earlier and more frequently.[2,6,32-34]

The diagnosis of diabetes is established by the presence of a symptom complex that consists of the following:
- Cardinal symptoms of polydipsia, polyphagia, polyuria, loss of strength, and unexplained weight loss
- Microangiopathy involving the retina
- Abnormal glucose metabolism seen on clinical laboratory test results that show glucose and acetone in the urine
- Fasting blood glucose (no caloric intake for at least 8 hr) level at or above 126 mg/100 mL
- 2-Hour postprandial (after a 75-g glucose load) blood glucose level at or above 200 mg/100 mL
- Lowered oral glucose tolerance level

The use of laboratory tests for the diagnosis of diabetes mellitus has changed since 1997. Before then, the glucose tolerance test was considered the diagnostic laboratory test. Since then, fasting glucose level has become the standard laboratory test.

Additionally, levels of glycohemoglobin (HbA1c), also known as *glycosylated hemoglobin*, in red blood cells are used for the general assessment of the long-term level (and control) of hyperglycemia in diabetic patients. The use and interpretation of various clinical laboratory tests for the evaluation and diagnosis of diabetes are described here in general terms.[2,4,32]

Blood Glucose Determination. When interpreting blood glucose level, the dentist should keep in mind that the source of blood, the age of the patient, the nature of the diet, and the physical activity level of the patient often affect the results. Also of great importance is the method used to measure the amount of sugar present in the blood sample.

If the diet has been poor in carbohydrate for several days, and the person is given 75 or 100 mg of glucose just before the blood glucose level is measured, a condition called *starvation hyperglycemia* possibly may be produced, which could be misdiagnosed as diabetes mellitus. To prevent this from occurring, the diet should contain at least 250 to 300 g of carbohydrate on each of the 3 days before testing.

Physical activity tends to lower blood glucose level. Patients whose blood glucose level is going to be assessed should not participate in excessive physical activity.

The most accurate technique for determining blood glucose levels is one that measures only glucose. The Folin and Wu method yields higher results because it also measures other blood sugars (e.g., fructose and lactose). Methods that use glucose oxides produce the lowest blood sugar value because they are specific for glucose. Most autoanalyzers use a ferricyanide method, which results in values a little higher than those attained with methods that use glucose oxides.

TABLE 15-5
Criteria for the Diagnosis of Diabetes Mellitus*

Objective Criteria	Definition
1. Symptoms of diabetes plus casual plasma glucose level of 200 mg/dL or greater	Casual is defined as any time of day without regard to time since last meal Classic symptoms of diabetes include polyuria, polydipsia, and unexplained weight loss
OR	
2. Fasting plasma glucose of 126 mg/dL or greater	Fasting is defined as no caloric intake for 8 hours or longer
OR	
3. 2-hour plasma glucose level of 200 mg/dL or greater during an oral glucose tolerance test	The test should be performed using a glucose load containing the equivalent of 75 g of anhydrous glucose dissolved in water; this test is not recommended for routine clinical use
In the absence of unequivocal hyperglycemia with acute metabolic decompensation, these criteria should be confirmed by repeated testing on a different day.	

From Report of the expert committee on the diagnosis and classification of diabetes mellitus. Diabetes Care 26(Suppl 1):S5-S20, 2003.
*If the first test performed is the 2-hr postprandial test and the value is 200 mg/dl or greater, the physician should order a fasting blood glucose test. Fasting requires no caloric intake for 8 hours. The postprandial test is the ingestion of the equivalent of 75 g of glucose 2 hours before determination of blood glucose.

Fasting venous blood glucose. The 1997 ADA criteria for the diagnosis of diabetes mellitus state that diabetes is present if the fasting blood glucose level is 126 mg/100 mL or greater on two or more occasions.

Two-hour postprandial glucose. For the 2-hour postprandial glucose test, the patient is given a 75- or 100-g glucose load after a night of fasting. Blood glucose levels taken at 2 hours that are 200 mg/100 mL or higher on two or more occasions are diagnostic of diabetes mellitus (Table 15-5).[2,4-6]

Oral Glucose Tolerance Test. The glucose tolerance test reflects the rate of absorption, uptake by tissues, and excretion in the urine of glucose. The glucose load can be given as Glucola, which contains 75 g of glucose in each 7–fl oz bottle. Some laboratories use a 75-g glucose load; others use a 100-g glucose load after a night of fasting. Venous blood samples are drawn from the arm just before and 1, 2, and 3 hours after ingestion of glucose. Urine samples also are collected at each interval.

The most characteristic alterations seen in diabetes are an increased fasting blood glucose (126 mg/100 mL or higher), an increased peak value (200 mg/100 mL or higher), and a delayed return to normal in the 2- and 3-hour samples. Hypoglycemia may occur in those with early, mild diabetes 3 to 5 hours after ingestion of glucose. For this reason, some physicians extend the glucose tolerance test to 5 hours for some patients. Urine samples should not contain glucose at any point during the test.

As was previously mentioned, the glucose tolerance test is no longer the standard for diagnosing diabetes mellitus. This test is used to identify patients with impaired glucose absorption and gestational diabetes. Special tests may be performed to measure the release of insulin at various intravenous (IV) glucose infusion levels. However, these are basically used to detect special problems and are not part of the routine testing undertaken to diagnose diabetes mellitus.[4-6]

Glycohemoglobin. The extent of glycosylation of hemoglobin A (a nonenzymatic addition of glucose) that results in formation of HbA1c in red blood cells is used for general assessment of the long-term level (and control) of hyperglycemia in patients with diabetes.[4-6] Measurement of HbA1c levels is of value in the detection and evaluation of patients (Table 15-6). HbA1c is an electrophoretically fast-moving hemoglobin component found in normal persons; it increases in the presence of hyperglycemia and may reflect glucose levels in the blood over the 6 to 12 weeks preceding administration of the test. Normally, patients should have 6% to 8% HbA1c. In well-controlled diabetes cases, the level should stay below 7%. The level of hyperglycemia as indicated by the HbA1c may reach as high as 20% in some uncontrolled cases. Patients do not have to fast before they undergo testing, which can be useful in monitoring the progress of the disease. Normal values must be established for each laboratory. It is now standard practice to measure HbA1c levels at least quarterly in patients who are taking insulin for diabetes mellitus. Complications from diabetes are accelerated in individuals with elevated HbA1c. Therefore, this monitoring is particularly important for those patients who are not monitoring their blood glucose at home on a regular basis.[4-6]

Urinary Glucose and Acetone. Determination of urinary glucose and acetone is of limited value in detecting overt diabetes.

MEDICAL MANAGEMENT

Diabetes mellitus is not a curable disease. Current evidence supports no precise relationship between hyperglycemia and the vascular complications of diabetes.

TABLE 15-6
American Diabetes Association and American College of Endocrinology: Targets for Glycemia Management

Parameter	Normal	ADA*	ACE
Premeal plasma glucose (mg/dL)	<100 (mean ~90)	90-130	<110
Postprandial plasma glucose* (mg/dL)	<140	<180	<140
A1c	4%-6%	<7%	<6.5%

The ADA further recommends: (1) goals should be individualized; (2) certain populations (children, pregnant women, and elderly) require special considerations; (3) less-intensive goals may be indicated in patients with severe or frequent hypoglycemia; (4) based on epidemiologic analysis, more stringent glycemic goals (i.e., a normal A1C, <6%) may further reduce complications at the cost of increased risk of hypoglycemia; and (5) postprandial glucose may be targeted if A1c goals are not met despite reaching preprandial glucose goals.

Modified from American Diabetes Association: Standards of medical care in diabetes. Diabetes Care 27:S15-S35, 2004; and American College of Endocrinologists: American College of Endocrinology consensus statement on guidelines for glycemic control. Endocr Pract 8(Suppl 1):5-11, 2002.
*Postprandial glucose measurements should be made 1-2 hours after the beginning of the meal, generally peak levels in patients with diabetes.

However, the bulk of evidence weighs in favor of such a relationship; hence, good control of glucose levels is a must. It is projected that the risk of serious cardiovascular disease in type 1 diabetic patients is more than 10 times that in nondiabetic patients.[1]

In a recent report from the Diabetes Control and Complications Trial (DCCT),[1] during 17 years of follow-up, intensive glycemic control in patients with diabetes resulted in a reduction of 57% of adverse cardiovascular events. A key observation supporting the concept that good hyperglycemic control prevents complications in individuals with diabetes is to note what happens in transplanted kidneys. When a kidney is transplanted from a healthy person to one with the disease, it develops nephropathy within 3 to 5 years. However, if pancreatic transplantation also is performed, no nephropathy appears to develop. Another example of how proper hyperglycemic control can prevent diabetic complications from occurring is found in the eye. The rate of developing proliferative retinopathy is reduced with good diabetic control.[12] (Box 15-4 and Table 15-7).

Therapy must be a highly individualized process and usually must continue for the rest of the patient's life. This need for lifelong compliance is a problem for many patients. Results of treatment and of testing must be reevaluated on a continual basis, and patient education regarding the disease, its complications, and its management is an ongoing process. Therapeutic goals for most patients include the following: (1) to maintain blood glucose levels as close to normal as possible without repeated episodes of hypoglycemia, (2) to strive to maintain normal body weight, (3) to control hypertension and hyperlipidemia, and (4) to develop a flexible treatment plan that does not dominate the patient's life any more than is necessary.[12,35,36]

The patient with diabetes may be treated through control of diet and physical activity, along with administration of oral hypoglycemic agents and insulin (see Box 15-4). In many cases of type 2 diabetes, the disease can be controlled by weight loss, diet, and physical activity.

BOX 15-4

Treatment of Patients With Diabetes Mellitus

TYPE 1 DIABETES
• Diet and physical activity
• Insulin
  • Conventional
  • Multiple injections
  • Continuous infusion
  • Pancreatic transplantation (see Chapter 22)

TYPE 2 DIABETES
• Diet and physical activity
• Oral hypoglycemic agents
• Insulin plus oral hypoglycemic agents
• Insulin

Total calories must be balanced with physical activity and body weight, and a balanced diet is indicated (with rigid control of the total caloric content). Some physicians will start a patient with diabetes on a diet that has a certain balance of carbohydrate, protein, and fat; others will allow the patient more freedom and will control only the total caloric content.[12,35,36]

DCCT[1] showed that the most effective strategies for the prevention and treatment of complications from diabetes involved intensive treatment of the patient with hyperglycemia. Aldose reductase inhibitors and aminoguanidine may be effective therapeutic agents. Antihypertensive drugs (angiotensin-converting enzyme [ACE] inhibitors such as captopril [Capoten; Bristol-Myers Squibb, Princeton, NJ, USA]) may be effective in treating nephropathy. Dietary protein restriction also may be effective. Control of hyperglycemia is beneficial in reducing diabetic neuropathy[12,16,35-38] (see Table 15-7).

If control of the patient's diet and physical activity fails to affect blood glucose level, hypoglycemic agents are used. Many patients with type 2 diabetes may be treated with oral hypoglycemic agents. Four classes of oral hypoglycemic agents are known (Table 15-8). The largest class

TABLE 15-7
Effective Strategies for the Prevention and
Treatment of Complications of Diabetes

Effect of Reduction of Complications

Complication/Strategy	Prevention	Therapy
RETINOPATHY		
Intensive therapy of hyperglycemia	Yes	Yes
Photocoagulation	Yes	—
Vitrectomy	Yes	—
Aldose reductase inhibitors	Experimental	—
Aminoguanidine	Experimental	—
Antiplatelet therapy	Experimental	—
NEPHROPATHY		
Intensive therapy of hyperglycemia	Yes	Yes
Antihypertensive drugs	Yes	Yes
Dietary protein restriction	Possible	Possible
Aldose reductase inhibitors	Experimental	—
Aminoguanidine	Experimental	—
NEUROPATHIC SYNDROMES		
Intensive therapy of hyperglycemia	Yes	Yes
Aldose reductase inhibitors	Experimental	—
PERIPHERAL NEUROPATHY		
Amitriptyline	Yes	—
Antidepressant drugs	Yes	—
Capsaicin	Yes	—
Phenytoin	Possible	—
Carbamazepine	Possible	—
GASTROPARESIS		
Erythromycin	Yes	—
Metoclopramide	Yes	—
Cisapride	Yes	—
Domperidone	Possible	—
Aminoguanidine	Experimental	—

TABLE 15-8
Oral Antidiabetic (Hypoglycemic) Drugs

Class Drug	Daily Dose	Doses/Day
SULFONYLUREAS (ENHANCE INSULIN SECRETION)		
First generation		
Chlorpropamide	100-500 mg	1
Acetohexamide	1500 mg	1
Tolazamide	100-1000 mg	1-2
Tolabutamide	500-3000 mg	2-3
Second generation		
Glipizide	5-40 mg	1-2
Glyburide	1.25-20 mg	1-2
Glimepiride	1-8 mg	1
BIGUANIDES (REDUCE HEPATIC GLUCOSE PRODUCTION)		
Metformin	1500-2500 mg	1-2
Glucovance	?	
GAMMA-GLUCOSIDASE INHIBITORS (DELAY CARBOHYDRATE DIGESTION)		
Acarbose	75-300 mg	3
THIAZOLIDINEDIONES (ENHANCE INSULIN SENSITIVITY)		
Troglitazone*	400-600 mg	1
Rosiglitazone	4-16 mg	2
Pioglitazone†	15-45 mg	1

*Recent reports of severe drug-related hepatotoxicity. This drug has been removed from the market.
†Recent approval as treatment for type 2 diabetes.

- Monthly visits and monitoring; patient self-monitoring of blood glucose levels 4 times per day
- Multiple daily insulin injections or use of an insulin infusion device
- Frequent adjustment of the insulin dosage relative to the patient's blood glucose level, diet, and exercise regimen

Predefined goals to be attained in the DCCT were fasting blood glucose level 70 to 120 mg/100 ml; postprandial blood glucose level 180 mg/100 ml; and Hb A1c two standard deviations above the mean value in normal subjects. The results of the DCCT indicated significant improvement in diabetic status and reduction of diabetic complications across the board. Once complications have started, they progress without intensive therapy for controlling the hyperglycemia. The DCCT supported early intensive therapy, which had a significant effect on limiting the complications of diabetes.

ACE inhibitors can delay the onset and progression of diabetic nephropathy. In one study, patients with type 1 diabetes who were treated with captopril experienced a 50% decrease in renal complications. Another study showed the positive effects of blood pressure control on the progression of complications from type 1 diabetes. This study concluded that control of blood pressure with the use of ramipril (an ACE inhibitor) improved diabetic nephropathy with respect to slowing the decline of overall renal function, slowing the rate of progression to end-

is sulfonylurea drugs (Table 15-9), followed by the biguanides. The third largest class of drugs consists of the gamma-glucosidase inhibitors. The last group of drugs is the recently approved thiazolidinediones.

Certain oral hypoglycemic agents, specifically, tolbutamide and related sulfonylurea drugs, were indicted in a report from the University Group Diabetes Program as ineffective and tending to increase the risk of cardiovascular disease. Since the time of that report, no additional studies seemed to support these conclusions. Intensive treatment for hyperglycemia in DCCT consisted of the following[1,12,35,36]:

- Hospitalization to initiate therapy
- Intensive patient education about diet and diabetes

TABLE 15-9

Metabolism, Potency, and Activity of Oral Hypoglycemic Agents (Sulfonylurea drugs) Used for Type 2 Diabetes

Agent	Maximum Daily Dose, mg/day	Rate of Metabolism	Duration of Known Activity, hr
Tolazamide	1000	Rapid	24
Acetohexamide	1500	Intermediate	12-18
Glyburide	2220	Intermediate	24
Glipizide	2245	Intermediate	24

stage renal disease, slowing the clinical course of protein-uria, and improving morbidity and mortality from diabetes. Antihypertensive therapy also is beneficial in slowing the progression of diabetic complications, especially diabetic nephropathy.[39,40]

Thiazide diuretics are not recommended for use in patients with diabetes because they cause hyperglycemia, hypokalemia, and hypercholesterolemia. Their use has been associated with increased mortality due to cardio-vascular disease.

The ideal treatment, an artificial pancreas, is still on the drawing board but significant progress is being made toward that goal.[37] Patients with Type 1 diabetes are treated with some form of insulin. The insulin in most cases is injected subcutaneously. In 2006 an insulin inhaler became available for patients needing large amounts of insulin (60 units or more) each day.[38] Many patients wear an external insulin pump used to deliver insulin via sub-cutaneous injection; a very few have a pump implanted into the abdominal subcutaneous tissue that can supply insulin on a programmed basis into the peritoneal cavity.[5,8]

Diabetics with kidney failure are candidates for com-bined pancreas and kidney transplantation that is very successful. The transplantation of only the pancreas has not been nearly as successful. The transplantation of islet cells from the pancreas to the recipient's liver has shown great promise, but long-term success rate is low.[39]

Pharmacologic Treatment of Type 1 Diabetes

Patients with Type 1 diabetes are treated with insulin.[5,9] Insulin therapies were introduced in 1922 and for the first 60 years consisted of animal insulins obtained from bovine or porcine pancreatic extracts. Porcine insulin differs from human insulin by one amino acid and bovine insulin by three amino acids. The use of animal insulins was complicated by incomplete purification and tendency to induce the formation of anti-insulin antibodies. In the 1980s recombinant human insulin was introduced, which resolved these issues. During the last few years insulin analogues were developed that provide advantageous pharmacokinetics. Recombinant human insulin and the newer analogues are now the main preparations used to treat Type 1 diabetes. Highly purified animal insulins are also now available.[5]

The parameters for the selection of the type of insulin to be used are the speed of onset, peak affect, and dura-tion of action. Available human insulins and analogues include rapid-acting, short-acting, intermediate-acting, and long-acting preparations. Rapid-acting and short-acting preparations are used as meal (or bolus) insulins and intermediate-acting and long-acting insulins serve as basal insulins.[5]

Regular human insulin is a short-acting preparation that has a delayed onset of action compared to endoge-nous insulin due to the formation of hexamers that slow the rate of absorption. The more rapid-acting insulin analogues are now being used more often as the primary meal or bolus insulin.

Intermediate-acting human insulins were developed to mimic the basal insulin secretion seen in non-diabetic individuals. Neutral Protamine Hagedorn (NPH) insulin was first introduced in 1946. It consists of a suspension of insulin complexed with protamine and zinc. Another intermediate-acting insulin is lente, a crystalline suspen-sion of insulin with zinc and acetate (Table 15-10). NPH and lente show a substantial variation in subcutaneous absorption and can result in variable glycemic control.[5]

Ultralente is a long-acting human insulin that consists of a zinc suspension of insulin. Its effects are similar to those of intermediate-acting insulin with a possible greater variation in absorption (see Table 15-10). With the avail-ability of intermediate-acting preparations and new long-acting analogues it now has limited clinical use.[5]

Two rapid-acting insulin analogues are now available: lispro and aspart. These products more closely match the actions of endogenous insulin at meal times. Lispro is identical to human insulin except for the reversal of the 28th and 29th amino acid residues (proline and lispro) of the normal insulin B chain. This change produces a steric hindrance involved in dimerization that reduces dimer formation. Thus, clinically, lispro acts similarly to mono-meric human insulin and mimics the normal prandial insulin surge in response to carbohydrate ingestion. Insulin aspart consists of the replacement of the proline residue at position 28 of the B chain with aspartic acid. The negative charge of the aspartic acid residue causes repulsion from other negatively charged amino acids that results in decreased self-association of insulin aspart monomers. Insulin aspart has a similar pharmacokinetic profile to that of lispro (see Table 15-10).[5]

Two long-acting insulin analogues have been devel-oped. The first commercially available long-acting ana-logue, insulin glargine, was introduced in 2001.[5,40] It

TABLE **15-10**
Insulin Preparations Classified According to Their Pharmacodynamic Profiles

	Onset of Action (h)	Peak Action (h)	Duration of Action (h)
RAPID-ACTING			
Insulin lispro*	0.25-0.5	0.5-2.5	≤5
Insulin aspart*	<0.25	1-3	3-5
SHORT-ACTING			
Regular (soluble)	0.5-1	2-4	5-8
INTERMEDIATE-ACTING			
NPH (Isophane)	1-2	2-8	14-24
Lente (insulin zinc suspension)	1-2	3-10	20-24
LONG-ACTING			
Ultralente	0.5-3	4-20	20-36
Insulin glargine*	2-4	Peak less	20-24
PREMIXED COMBINATIONS			
50% NPH, 50% regular	0.5-1	Dual	14-24
70% NPH, 30% regular	0.5-1	Dual	14-24
70% NPA, 30% aspart*	<0.25	Dual	14-24
75% NPL, 25% lispro*	<0.25	Dual	14-24

From Wolfsdorf JI, Weinstein DA: Management of Diabetes in Children. In DeGroot LJ, Jameson JL: Endocrinology, ed 5, Saunders, 2006.

*Insulin analogue developed by modifying the amino acid sequence of the human insulin molecule. Data are from the manufacturers. These data are for human insulins and are approximations from studies in adult test subjects. Time-action profiles are reasonable estimates only. The times of onset, peak, and duration of action vary within and between patients and are affected by numerous factors, including size of dose, site and depth of injection, dilution, exercise, temperature, and other factors.

NPA, Neutral protamine aspart; NPL, neutral protamine lispro. Both NPA and NPL are stable premixed combinations of intermediate- and short-acting insulins.

Pharmacodynamic effects of insulin lispro and insulin aspart appear to be equivalent. Most of the human insulins and insulin analogues are available in insulin cartridges and/or disposable insulin pens.

consists of two modifications to human insulin; two arginines added to the carboxy terminus of the B chain and replacement of asparagines by glycine at position A21.[5] These changes make the analogue soluble in the acidic injection solution but much less soluble at the neutral physiologic pH of subcutaneous tissue. This allows a much slower absorption rate from the injection site (see Table 15-10). Insulin detemir is the second long-acting analogue to be developed. Detemir is not yet commercially available. In detemir the B30 amino acid of human insulin has been removed and a 14-carbon aliphatic fatty acid has been acylated to the B29 amino acid.[5] This allows for reversible binding between albumin and the added fatty acid. After injection, equilibrium develops between free and bound detemir with about 98% of the analogue being bound to albumin. Only the free analogue binds to the insulin receptor, thus the duration of action is prolonged based on the sustained release of the analogue bound to circulating albumin.[5]

Some patients are able to use premixed human insulin or premixed insulin analogues.[41,42] Premixed human insulin (70/30) consisting of 70% of a regular insulin and 30% of a long-acting insulin has been used but resulted in too many variations in peak glucose levels, duration of action, and time of onset. Two premixed insulin analogues are now being used that have overcome these problems. The first is insulin lispro (75/25), consisting of 75% insulin lispro protamine suspension and 25% insulin lispro. The second is biphasic insulin aspart (70/30), consisting of 70% insulin aspart protamine suspension and 30% insulin aspart (see Table 15-10).[42]

A new drug, pramlintide, has been approved for the treatment of patients with Type 1 and Type 2 diabetes who have failed to achieve targets for glucose control despite optimal insulin therapy.[43] Pramlintide is an amylinomimetic, a synthetic analog of human amylin. Amylin is co-secreted from beta cells of the pancreas with insulin and modulates gastric emptying. It prevents postprandial rise in serum glucagon and decreases satiety and caloric intake. It is administered by a separate injection (cannot mix it with insulin) just before meals, starting with a 15-µg dose and increasing in increments of 15 µg as needed (wait 3 to 7 days before increasing dosage; if nausea occurs dosage must be reduced). The insulin dosage must be adjusted based on blood glucose monitoring.[43]

Intensive Insulin Therapy. Intensive insulin therapy is recommended for all patients with Type 1 diabetes.[5] Two regimens are available: multiple daily injection (MDI) of insulin and continuous subcutaneous infusion of insulin (CSII). Both regimens attempt to mimic physiologic insulin secretion through appropriate meal and basal insulin replacement. The choice is generally determined by patient directed factors, such as lifestyle, finances, and personal preference.[5]

A multiple daily injection regimen involves at least four injections of insulin per day. It consists of boluses of meal insulin before each meal and at least one injection of basal insulin, usually at bedtime. If needed, a second injection of basal insulin can be added at breakfast or before lunch.[5] The choice of meal insulin is a rapid-acting analogue, lispro or aspart. Basal insulin replacement in the past has consisted of NPH, lente, or Ultralente. Now more patients are being given insulin glargine.[44] However, large-scale studies evaluating the efficacy of multiple daily injection regimens using rapid-acting analogues for meal insulin and long-acting analogues for basal coverage are still pending. It is anticipated that this combination will be shown to provide the most physiologic insulin replacement available.[5]

In the late 1970s the first external insulin infusion pump was developed. This provided the basis for modern continuous subcutaneous insulin infusion (CSII).[5] In CSII, an external infusion pump delivers a continuous infusion of rapid-acting or short-acting insulin through a catheter inserted into the subcutaneous tissue of the abdominal wall.[5,45,46] The pump is programmed to deliver insulin continuously at a specified rate to meet the patient's basal insulin needs. For meal coverage the patient uses the pump to deliver a specified bolus of insulin before eating. The rapid-acting insulin analogues are the insulins of choice in CSII. The major limitation with CSII is the cost of pump and necessary supplies (tubing) that must be changed every 48 to 72 hours. There is also a small risk of infection it the insertion site of the catheter. Lastly, pump malfunction or catheter disruption can lead rapidly to hyperglycemia or ketoacidosis.[5]

Insulin delivery. MDI and CSII both have insulin delivered into subcutaneous fat tissue. In CSII, insulin is delivered through a needle or Siastic infuser placed subcutaneously. The needle and its injection site are changed every 48 to 72 hours to reduce the risk of infection. In MDI therapy, insulin is injected subcutaneously using either syringes or pen-and-cartridge devices. The MDI method uses disposable plastic syringes to draw insulin from multiple-use vials for injection into the subcutaneous tissue. Meal and basal insulins that are being taken at the same time can be drawn into the same syringe with the exception of glargine, which can't be mixed with other insulins.[5]

In MDI therapy using pen-and-cartridge devices to deliver insulin, replaceable cartridges containing insulin are placed into a pen-shaped delivery device (insulin pen) and then the insulin is injected subcutaneously. Insulin

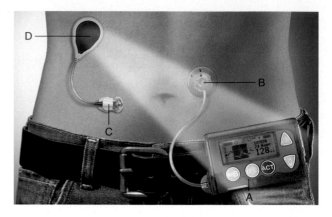

Figure 15-5. The MiniMed Paradigm 522 Insulin Pump. The insulin pump (**A**) is small and can be worn under clothing or on a belt. It delivers insulin through a tube or cannula (**B**) that is inserted into the subcutaneous tissue. The pump can be disconnected for bathing, swimming, or changing clothes. A small sensor for glucose (**C**) is inserted into the subcutaneous tissue using an automatic insertion device. Sensor data is sent to a transmitter (**D**) that is attached to the skin with a waterproof adhesive patch. The transmitter sends data to the insulin pump using wireless technology. The sensor and tube (new tubing) from the pump must be relocated every 3 days to minimize the risk of infection obstruction of the tube. (Courtesy Medtronics, Minneapolis.)

pens offer the advantage of more accurate dosing and easier administration. However, basal and meal insulins that are being taken at the same time can't be mixed and require separate injections. The insulin pen mode of delivery has become the choice for most diabetics using MDI therapy.[5]

External insulin pumps are now available. They are worn around the waist and the patient controls the amount of insulin that is injected into subcutaneous tissue. Medtronic has developed an external pump system (Figure 15-5) that allows for real-time continuous glucose monitoring (MiniMed Paradigm REAL-Time System [models 522 and 722]).[47]

FDA approval for the use of the MiniMed Paradigm systems was granted on April 13, 2006.[48]

Alterative routes for insulin delivery. Even with the best efforts, a full imitation of normal physiologic insulin secretion generally can't be achieved with the subcutaneous delivery of current insulin preparations. Thus the search for alternative routes of delivery of insulin continues to be of great interest. Options that are being considered include nasal, pulmonary, oral, transdermal, and peritoneal delivery of insulin. These options have had only limited success to date. The intrapulmonary and intraperitoneal options appear to offer the best promise for the future.[5]

The FDA just approved the first inhaled version of insulin, called Exubera, from Pfizer Inc. (Figure 15-6) and it became available in September 2006.[38,49,50] It is

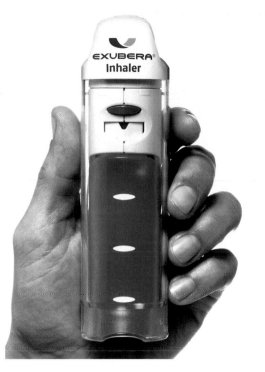

Figure 15-6. Exubera inhaled insulin system, EXUBERA® (insulin human [rDNA origin]) shown in the closed position. Inhalation powder is the first diabetes treatment that can be inhaled. It can be used to treat patients with Type 1 diabetes and patients with Type 2 diabetes requiring insulin. Patients with Type 1 diabetes still require a long-acting injected insulin in addition to Exubera. It may be part of a treatment plan that includes hypoglycemic medications for patients with Type 2 diabetes. (Courtesy Pfizer Inc., New York.)

approved for those over 18 years of age with Type 1 or Type 2 diabetes.[51,52]

Intraperitoneal insulin delivery may soon be commercially available in the United States by using an implantable insulin pump. These implanted pumps (Medtronic Inc.) are now being used in Europe, with over 181 being placed since 1995.[53] The insulin pump is implanted directly into the abdominal subcutaneous tissues, with a catheter inserted directly into the peritoneal cavity. Insulin secretion is regulated by the patient from a handset, which signals the pump via the catheter to deliver insulin on demand. The pump reservoir holds a 2- to 3-month supply of insulin.

Treatment of Type 2 Diabetes

The management of Type 2 diabetes involves lifestyle interventions, drug therapy, and control of risk factors for cardiovascular disease.[1,2] This includes control of blood glucose levels, blood pressure, lipid levels, and antiplatelet therapy as indicated.[2] Recent evidence shows that tight control of blood glucose levels reduces the risk for microvascular (renal and retinal) and neuropathic complications of Type 2 diabetes. It has also been shown to slow the onset of macrovascular (coronary artery disease, myocardial infarction, and stroke) complications.[1,2,54]

The monitoring of blood glucose levels and hemoglobin A1c is an important part of the management of patients with Type 1 and Type 2 diabetes and is covered in other media, as is the approach to intensive insulin therapy.[32]

Drug Treatment of Type 2 Diabetes. Since 1995 a number of new classes of drugs have become available for the treatment of Type 2 diabetes. These oral agents can be divided by mechanism of action into the following: insulin sensitizers with primary action in the liver, insulin sensitizers with primary action in peripheral tissues, insulin secretagogues, and drugs that slow the absorption of carbohydrates. Injectable drugs used to treat Type 2 diabetes include two new agents, exenatide and pramlintide, and insulin (Table 15-11).[2,55,56] Exubera, inhaled insulin, became available in 2006 and can serve as the source for meal insulin, with basal insulin still being provided by injection.[57,58] Potential drug interactions with agents used in dentistry are shown in Table 15-12.

Oral agents

Insulin sensitizers acting in liver—biguanides. Metformin (Glucophage) is the only biguanide available in the United States. Its major action is to reduce hepatic insulin resistance, gluconeogenesis, and glucose release.[2] Metformin does not increase insulin levels and thus is not associated with significant risk of hypoglycemia. A rare complication, lactic acidosis, is of concern in patients who are at risk for this complication independent of metformin treatment. Weight gain is not a significant problem with metformin use. It is contraindicated in patients with symptomatic congestive heart failure, renal insufficiency, or hepatic insufficiency.[2] Metformin extended release (Glucophage XR) was recently approved and provides effective and well-tolerated glycemic control with once-daily dosing.[59]

Insulin sensitizers acting in peripheral tissues—thiazolidinediones. This class of drugs is also referred to as TZDs or glitazones. Troglitazone, approved in 1997, was withdrawn from the United States market in 2000 due to rare reports of fulminant hepatic necrosis.[2] Two drugs, pioglitazone (Actos) and rosiglitazone (Avandia), from this class are on the market for use in the United States. Glitazones decrease insulin resistance by making muscle and adipose cells more sensitive to insulin and by decreasing hepatic glucose production. These drugs appear to work by binding to and modulating the activity of a family of nuclear transcription factors termed peroxisome-proliferator-activated receptors (PPARs). They cause a slow improvement in glycemic control over time (weeks to months) along with improvement in insulin sensitivity and reduction of free fatty acid levels. They are well tolerated, with the only significant adverse effects being weight gain and fluid retention. These drugs should not be used in patients with active liver disease or elevated alanine aminotransferase levels greater than 2.5 times the upper limit of normal. They are also contraindicated in patients with symptomatic heart failure.

TABLE **15-11**
Comparison of Therapies for Type 2 Diabetes Mellitus

Treatment	Delivery	Target Tissue	Stimulates Insulin Secretion	Improves Insulin Sensitivity	Severe Hypoglycemia	Weight Gain	Rare Problems
LIFESTYLE	Self directed	Muscle Fat	No	Yes	No	No	Injury
INSULIN Human Analogs Lispro, Aspart Glargine Detemir*	Injected	Beta cell support	No	No	Yes	Yes	Skin lesions
Exubera	Inhaled						
SECRETAGOGUES Glipizide Glyburide Glimepiride	Oral	Beta cell	Yes	No	Yes	Yes	Sulfa allergy
BIGUANIDES Metformin	Oral	Liver	No	Modest	No	No	Lactic acidosis
ALPHA GLUCOSIDASE INHIBITORS Acarbose Miglitol	Oral	Gut	No	No	No	No	Liver disease
GLITAZONES Pioglitazibe Rosiglitazone	Oral	Fat Muscle	No	Yes	No	Yes	Congestive heart failure
MEGLITINIDES Repaglinide Nateglinide	Oral	Beta cell	Yes	No	Yes	Yes	
INCRETIN MIMETICS Exenatide Liraglutide*	Injected	Beta cell	Yes	No	No	Yes	Nausea, vomiting, diarrhea
AMYLINOMIMETICS Pramlintide	Injected	Beta cell	Yes	No	Possible	Slight	Nausea
DIPEPTIDYL PEPTIDASE 4 INHIBITORS Vildagliptin* Sitagliptin* Saxagliptin*	Oral	Beta cell	Yes	No	No	No	?

Based on Buse JB: Management of Type 2 Diabetes Mellitus. In DeGroot LJ, Jameson JL: Endocrinology, ed 5, Saunders, 2006, p 493.
*Drugs still in clinical testing.

Another concern with these agents is weight gain.[2] Rosiglitazone in combination with metformin has been shown to significantly improve the control of fasting plasma glucose/A1c in patients in whom metformin therapy alone failed.[60]

Insulin secretagogues. These agents all bind to the sulfonylurea receptor on the plasma membrane of pancreatic beta cells. The major clinical differences between these agents is the duration of action and subtle variations in their hypoglycemic potential.[2]

Sulfonylureas have been available since the 1950s. They are the most cost-effective glucose-lowering agents on the market. They have a slow onset of action and variable duration of action. First generation sulfonylureas include chlorpropamide (Diabinese), tolazamide, acetohexaminde (Dymerlor), and tolbutamide. The second-generation sulfonylureas include glipizide (Glucotrol, Glucotrol XL), glyburide (Micronase, Glynase, DiaBeta), and glimepiride (Amaryl) (see Table 15-9). The second-generation agents are more potent and have fewer adverse

TABLE **15-12**
Drug Interactions With Agents Used in Dentistry*

Diabetic Drug	Drug Interactions

Insulin
Human
Analogs
  Lispro, Aspart
  Glargine
  Exubera
	Salicylates, NSAIDs (large doses and chronic use) and alcohol increase the hypoglycemic effect
	Corticosteroids and epinephrine increase glucose levels

Secretagogues Glipizide Glyburide Glimepiride	Salicylates and ketoconazole increase the hypoglycemic effect Corticosteroids decrease the action
Biguanides Metformin	None reported concerning dentistry
Alpha Glucosidase Inhibitors Acarbose Miglitol	None reported concerning dentistry
Glitazones Pioglitazibe Rosiglitazone	None reported concerning dentistry
Meglitinides Repaglinide Nateglinide	Risk of increased hypoglycemia with salicylates, non-selective beta-blockers and NSAIDs Metabolism may be inhibited by ketoconazole, miconazole, and erythromycin
Incretin Mimetics Exenatide Liraglutide	Exenatide is a new drug and does not appear to have any interactions with agents used in dentistry Liraglutide is not on the market yet
Amylinomimetics Pramlintide	New drug that has the potential to delay absorption of drugs taken orally, such as analgesics; these drugs should be taken at least 1 hour before or 2 hours after the injection of pramlintide
Dipeptidyl Peptidase 4 Inhibitors Vildagliptin Sitagliptin Saxagliptin	Drugs not on the market yet

Based on Mosby's 2007 Dental Drug Consult; Including Therapeutic Classification, Elsevier, St. Louis, 2007.

effects and drug interactions than the first-generation drugs. The extended-release glipizide and glimepiride are preferred drugs as they can be dosed once daily and have a relatively low risk of hypoglycemia and weight gain.[2] Side effects include weight gain and, much less commonly, nausea, vomiting, rashes, purpura, and pruritis. Rare adverse effects are leukopenia, thrombocytopenia, hemolytic anemia, and cholestasis.[2]

Meglitinides. Meglitinides increase the secretion of insulin in the presence of glucose. Repaglinide (Prandin) is a meglitinide and is distinct from the sulfonylureas. It is dosed with each meal and provides good postprandial control of glucose. It is associated with less hypoglycemia and weight gain than the second-generation sulfonylureas.[2]

Nateglinide (Starlix) is a derivative of phenylalanine and has a quicker onset and shorter duration of action than Repaglinide. It is best used when fasting glucose levels are modestly elevated, as in early diabetes, or in combination with insulin sensitizers or long-acting evening insulin.[62] Nateglinide plus metformin in one study was found to be equally effective in terms of HbA1c control and more effective in postprandial glucose control than metformin plus gliclazide.[61]

Alpha-glucosidase inhibitors (AGIs). AGIs inhibit the terminal step of carbohydrate digestion at the brush border of the intestinal epithelium. Administered with the first bite of a carbohydrate-containing meal, they cause a delay in carbohydrate absorption, which allows the sluggish insulin-secretory dynamics typical of Type 2 diabetes to catch up with carbohydrate absorption.[2] Two AGI drugs are now marketed in the United States, acarbose (Precose) and miglitol (Glyset). Their use has been limited by frequent gastrointestinal complaints, the need to administer the drugs at the beginning of each meal, only modest reduction in A1c, and limited effect on fasting glucose levels. However, factors supporting their use include the ability to lower glucose in most patients without hypoglycemia or weight gain. The major adverse effects are flatulence, abdominal distress or distension, and diarrhea.[2]

Fixed combination pills. Several combinations of oral hypoglycemic agents are available. Two combinations of a sulfonylurea and a biguanide on the market are Glucovance (Glyburide plus Metformin) and Metaglip (Glipizide plus Metformin). A combination of a thiazolidinedione and a biguanide, Avandamet (Rosiglitazone plus Metformin)[2], is also available.

Dipeptidyl peptidase-4 inhibitors. New oral agents are being developed for the treatment of Type 2 diabetes. The incretin effect is described below under injectable agents. Natural glucagon-like peptide (GLP-1) accounts for much of the incretin effect and when injected is quickly degraded by the enzyme dipeptidyl peptidase-4 (DPP-4).[62] Agents that can inhibit DPP-4 are now under study as drugs for the treatment of Type 2 diabetes. The following drugs are in phase 1 to phase III study: vildagliptin (Galvus), sitagliptin (Januvia), and saxagliptin (BMS-477118). These agents are being tested in monotherapy and in combination with other drugs used to treat diabetes. Sitagliptin, for example, has been shown to provide good glycemic control in monotherapy or combined with metformin. It is well tolerated and does not cause weight gain or hypoglycemia.[62-64]

Injectable agents

Insulin. Patients with Type 2 diabetes with failing beta cell function will require insulin therapy. In addition, to gain tighter glycemic control, which reduces the risks of microvascular and neuropathic complications, many other patients with Type 2 diabetes are now being treated by insulin. Available human insulins and analogues include rapid-acting, short-acting, intermediate-acting, and long-acting preparations. Rapid-acting and short-acting preparations are used as meal (or bolus) insulins and intermediate-acting and long-acting insulins serve as basal insulins[5] (see the section on insulin therapy).

Incretin mimetics. New drugs are being developed that approach the treatment of Type 2 diabetes in novel ways. One approach is to stimulate the incretin effect.[65,66] Orally ingested glucose leads to a much higher insulin response than intravenous glucose. Two gastrointestinal (GI) hormones that promote the incretin effect (increased insulin response) are glucagon-like peptide-1 (GLP-1) and gastric inhibitory polypeptide (GIP). These GI hormones account for up to 60% of the postprandial insulin secretion and this response is diminished in Type 2 diabetes.[65,66] Thus Type 2 diabetes is characterized by an incretin defect.

GIP does not appear to stimulate insulin secretion directly, and GLP-1 will stimulate insulin secretion only under hyperglycemic conditions and will not produce hypoglycemia.[62] Other actions of GLP-1 include inhibition of glucagon secretion and delaying of gastric emptying. Native GLP-1 is degraded rapidly when injected by subcutaneous or IV administration and is not effective for treatment. Incretin mimetics have been developed that are long-acting GLP-1 analogs that are resistant to degradation. Liraglutide is in phase III testing. Exendin-4 (exenatide, Byetta) has just been approved for the treatment of Type 2 diabetes.[62]

Exenatide, derived from a compound found in the saliva of the Gila monster, is an incretin mimetic agent that enhances glucose-dependent insulin secretion and has several other antihyperglycemic actions.[67] Exenatide is subcutaneously injected and has recently been approved

for clinical use. It is indicated as adjunctive therapy in patients with Type 2 diabetes failing to gain glycemic control with metformin, a sulfonylurea, or both.[67] Weight gain, nausea, vomiting, diarrhea, jitteriness, dizziness, and headache are adverse effects associated with the use of exenatide.[67]

Liraglutide is a GLP-1 long-acting analogue that has yet to be approved for clinical use.[68] Studies to date indicate that it is effective and well tolerated. It appears to have the potential to increase beta-cell replication. Adverse effects include headache, vomiting, and nausea. Liraglutide in combination with metformin has been shown to be effective in the treatment of Type 2 diabetes.[69]

Amylinomimetics. Another approach that has been developed is to use an analog of human amylin. Amylin is co-secreted from beta cells of the pancreas with insulin and modulates gastric emptying. It prevents postprandial rise in serum glucagon and decreases satiety and caloric intake. Pramlintide has just been approved for the treatment of patients with Type 2 diabetes who have failed to achieve targets for glucose control despite optimal insulin therapy.[70] Pramlintide is administered by a separate injection (cannot mix it with insulin) just before meals, starting with a 15-μg dose and increasing in increments of 15 μg as needed (wait 3 to 7 days before increasing dosage, if nausea occurs dosage must be reduced). The insulin dosage must be adjusted based on blood glucose monitoring.[70]

Insulin Shock

Patients who are treated with insulin must closely adhere to their diet. If they fail to eat in a normal manner but continue to take their regular insulin injections, they may experience a hypoglycemic reaction caused by an excess of insulin (insulin shock). A hypoglycemic reaction also may be due to an overdose of insulin or an oral hypoglycemic agent. Reaction or shock caused by excessive insulin usually occurs in three well-defined stages, each more severe and dangerous than the one preceding it (Box 15-5).

Mild Stage. The mild stage, which is the most common, is characterized by hunger, weakness, trembling, tachycardia, pallor, and sweating; paresthesias may be noted on occasion. It occurs before meals, during exercise, and when food has been omitted or delayed (see Box 15-5).

Moderate Stage. In the moderate stage, because blood glucose substantially drops, the patient becomes incoherent, uncooperative, and sometimes belligerent or resistive; judgment and orientation are defective. The chief danger during this stage is that patients may injure themselves or someone else (e.g., if the patient is driving) (see Box 15-5).

Severe Stage. Complete unconsciousness with or without tonic or clonic muscular movements occurs during the severe stage. Most of these reactions take place

BOX 15-5

Signs and Symptoms of Insulin Reaction

MILD STAGE
- Hunger
- Weakness
- Tachycardia
- Pallor
- Sweating
- Paresthesias

MODERATE STAGE
- Incoherence
- Uncooperativeness
- Belligerence
- Lack of judgment
- Poor orientation

SEVERE STAGE
- Unconsciousness
- Tonic or clonic movements
- Hypotension
- Hypothermia
- Rapid thready pulse

during sleep, after the first two stages have gone unrecognized. This stage also may occur after exercise or after the ingestion of alcohol, if earlier signs have been ignored. Sweating, pallor, rapid and thready pulse, hypotension, and hypothermia may be present (see Box 15-5).

The reaction to excessive insulin can be corrected by giving the patient sweetened fruit juice or anything with sugar in it. Patients in the severe stage (unconsciousness) are best treated with an IV glucose solution; glucagon or epinephrine may be used for transient relief.

DENTAL MANAGEMENT
Medical Considerations

Any dental patient whose condition remains undiagnosed but who has the cardinal symptoms of diabetes (i.e., polydipsia, polyuria, polyphagia, weight loss, and weakness) should be referred to a physician for diagnosis and treatment. Patients with findings that may suggest diabetes (headache, dry mouth, marked irritability, repeated skin infection, blurred vision, paresthesias, progressive periodontal disease, multiple periodontal abscesses, loss of sensation) should be referred to a clinical laboratory or a physician for screening tests.

Today, patients may be able to readily monitor their blood glucose level with the use of a personal blood glucose monitoring device (e.g., Glucometer, Glucowatch). Patients with an estimated fasting blood glucose level of 126 mg/100 mL or higher should be referred to a physician for medical evaluation and treatment, if indicated. Those with a 2-hour postprandial blood glucose level of 200 mg/100 mL or higher also should be referred.[2,71]

In a study of patients with diabetes who entered a dental clinic, fasting blood glucose was determined as part of the initial dental examination in a total of 97 patients (mean age, 57.7 years); 28 patients (28.9%) were found to be hyperglycemic (greater than 130 mg/100 mL) (mean, 174.8 ± 40.8 mg/100 mL), and 2 were noted to be hypoglycemic (less than 70 mg/100 mL). This fact illustrates for dental practitioners that patients with diabetes commonly are not under good glycemic control.[32]

Patients who are obese, who are older than 45 years of age, or who have close relatives with diabetes should be screened once a year for any indication of hyperglycemia that may reveal the onset of diabetes. Women who have given birth to large babies (greater than 10 lb) or who have had multiple spontaneous abortions or stillbirths also should be screened once a year for diabetes. The use of oral contraceptive agents is not contraindicated in patients with diabetes; however, adverse effects of oral contraceptive agents on the progression of complications from diabetes have been reported. Patients described here are best screened by their physician.[2,71]

All patients with diagnosed diabetes must be identified by history, and the type of medical treatment they are receiving must be established. The type of diabetes (type 1, type 2, or other types of diabetes) should be determined, and the presence of complications noted. Patients who are being treated with insulin should be asked how much insulin they use and how often they inject themselves each day. They should also be asked whether they monitor their own blood glucose, by which method, how often, and the value of the most recent level. The frequency of insulin reactions and when the last one occurred should be determined. The frequency of visits to the physician should be established, as should the timing and results of the last HbA1c test. Whether the patient checks his or her blood for glucose should be determined. Those in whom diabetes has been diagnosed should be monitoring their blood glucose with a glucose monitoring system. This provides the dentist with information regarding the severity of diabetes and the level of control that has been attained[2,71] (Box 15-6).

Vital signs also serve as a guide to the control and management of disease in the diabetic patient. Patients with abnormal pulse rate and rhythm and/or elevated blood pressure should be approached with caution. Functional capacity is important for determination of the severity and level of control of diabetes and should be part of the patient's evaluation prior to dental treatment. Overall poor physical status (i.e., <4 metabolic equivalent levels [METs]) increases the risk of complications during and after dental treatment. The risk for serious cardiovascular events increases substantially in patients with <4 METs (see Chapter 1).[2,71] Daily activities that equate to approximately 4 METs and can be used to assess the patient's status include comfortably doing light yard work (i.e., raking leaves, mowing the lawn, weeding, etc.), walking about 5 km/hour (20 minutes/mile); or doing light carpentry. In addition to these examples, other

BOX 15-6

Detection of the Patient With Diabetes

KNOWN DIABETIC PERSON
1. Detection by history:
   a. Are you diabetic?
   b. What medications are you taking?
   c. Are you being treated by a physician?
2. Establishment of severity of disease and degree of "control"
   a. When were you first diagnosed as diabetic?
   b. What was the level of the last measurement of your blood glucose?
   c. What is the usual level of blood glucose for you?
   d. How are you being treated for your diabetes?
   e. How often do you have insulin reactions?
   f. How much insulin do you take with each injection, and how often do you receive injections?
   g. Do you test your urine for glucose?
   h. When did you last visit your physician?
   i. Do you have any symptoms of diabetes at the present time?

UNDIAGNOSED DIABETIC PERSON
1. History of signs or symptoms of diabetes or its complications
2. High risk for developing diabetes
   a. Parents who are diabetic
   b. Gave birth to one or more large babies
   c. History of spontaneous abortions or stillbirths
   d. Obese
   e. Over 40 years of age
3. Referral or screening test for diabetes

BOX 15-7

Dental Management of the Patient With Diabetes*

1. Non–insulin-dependent patient:
   If diabetes is well-controlled,[†] all dental procedures can be performed without special precautions.
2. Insulin-controlled patient:
   - If diabetes is well-controlled,[†] all dental procedures can be performed without special precautions.
   - Morning appointments are usually best.
   - Patient advised to take usual insulin dosage and normal meals on day of dental appointment; information confirmed when patient comes for appointment.
   - Advise patient to inform dentist or staff if symptoms of insulin reaction occur during dental visit.
   - Glucose source (orange juice, soda, Glucola) should be available and given to the patient if symptoms of insulin reaction occur.
3. If extensive surgery is needed:
   - Consult with patient's physician concerning dietary needs during postoperative period.
   - Antibiotic prophylaxis can be considered for patients with brittle diabetes and those taking high doses of insulin who also have chronic states of oral infection.

If not well-controlled (i.e., does not meet ANY of above criteria: fasting blood glucose <70 mg/dL or >200 mg/dL and ANY complications [post MI, renal disease, congestive heart failure, symptomatic angina, old age, cardiac dysrrhythmia, cerebrovascular accident], and blood pressure ≥180/110 mm Hg, or functional capacity <4 metabolic equivalents):
   - Provide appropriate emergency care only.
   - Request referral for medical evaluation, management, and risk factor modification
     - If symptomatic, seek IMMEDIATE referral
     - If asymptomatic, request routine referral

*Special precautions may be needed for patients with complications of diabetes, renal disease, heart disease, etc.
†Well-controlled: fasting blood glucose between 70 mg/dL and 200 mg/dL and no complications (i.e., post MI, renal disease, congestive heart failure, symptomatic angina, old age, cardiac dysrrhythmia, cerebrovascular accident), blood pressure <180/110 mm Hg and functional capacity >4 metabolic equivalents.

equivalent physical activities may be substituted and evaluated. Dental patients in the poor functional capacity category (<4 METs) should be approached with caution.[2,71]

Patients with type 2 diabetes who have no evidence of complications and whose disease is under good medical control, as determined by consultation with the patient's physician, require little or no special attention when receiving dental treatment, unless they develop a significant dental or oral infection that is possibly accompanied by swelling or fever. By contrast, patients with complications such as renal disease or cardiovascular disease may need to be managed in special ways. Those who are treated with insulin or who are not under good medical management also require special attention (Box 15-7). This typically involves consultation with the patient's physician.

Patients who have not seen their physician for a long time, who have had frequent episodes of insulin shock, or who report signs and symptoms of diabetes may have disease that is unstable. These patients should be referred to their physician for evaluation, or the physician should be consulted to establish the patient's current status.

Some patients with type 1 diabetes who are being treated with large doses of insulin have periods of extreme hyperglycemia and hypoglycemia (brittle diabetes), even when given the best of medical management. For these patients, close consultation with the physician is required before any dental treatment is started.[2,71]

A major goal in the dental management of patients with diabetes who are being treated with insulin is to prevent insulin shock during the dental appointment. Patients should be told to take their usual insulin dosage and to eat normal meals before their dental appointment, which is usually best scheduled in the morning. When such a patient comes for the appointment, the dentist should confirm that the patient has taken insulin and has eaten breakfast. In addition, patients should be instructed to tell the dentist whether at any time during the appointment, they feel symptoms of an insulin reaction. A source of sugar such as orange juice, cake icing, soda, or Glucola must be available in the dental office to be given to the patient if symptoms of an insulin reaction occur (see Box 15-7) (see Appendix A).

Any patient with diabetes who is going to undergo extensive periodontal or oral surgery procedures other than single simple extractions should be given special dietary instructions after surgery. It is important that the total caloric content and the protein/carbohydrate/fat ratio of the diet remain the same so that control of the disease and proper blood glucose balance are maintained. The patient's physician should be consulted about dietary recommendations for the postoperative period. One suggestion is to have the patient use a blender to prepare his or her usual diet so that it can be ingested with minimum discomfort; alternatively, special food supplements in a liquid form may be used. The physician also may alter the patient's insulin regimen according to his or her ability to eat properly, and according to the extent of the surgery to be performed.

Patients who have brittle diabetes (very difficult to control) or who require a high dosage of insulin (type 1 diabetes) may be at increased risk for postoperative infection. However, prophylactic antibiotics usually are not indicated. If the patient develops an infection, appropriate systemic antibiotics may be given. A protocol for IV sedation often involves fasting before the appointment (i.e., nothing by mouth after midnight); using only half the usual insulin dose; and then supplementing with IV glucose during the procedure. Patients with well-controlled diabetes may be given general anesthesia, if necessary; however, in a dental office, management with local anesthetics is preferable.[2,71]

Any patient with diabetes and an acute dental or oral infection presents a significant management problem (Box 15-8). This problem will be even more difficult for patients who take a high insulin dosage and for those who have type 1 diabetes. Infection often leads to loss of control over the diabetic condition; as a result, infection is not handled by the body's defenses as well as it would be in the normal patient. Patients with brittle diabetes (i.e., difficult to control, requires a high dosage of insulin) may require hospitalization during management of an infection. The patient's physician should be consulted and should become a partner during this period.[2,71]

The risk for infection in patients with diabetes is directly related to fasting blood glucose levels. If fasting blood glucose level is below 206 mg/100 mL, no increased risk is present; however, if fasting blood glucose level is between 207 and 229 mg/100 mL, the risk is increased by 20%. Additionally, if fasting blood glucose level rises to above 230 mg/100 mL, an 80% increase has occurred in the risk of infection. Therefore, dentists must be aware of the level of glycemic control in patients undergoing complex oral surgical procedures because of their

---

BOX 15-8

Dental Management of the Patient With Diabetes and Acute Oral Infection

1. Non–insulin-controlled patients may require insulin; consultation with physician required
2. Insulin-controlled patients usually require increased dosage of insulin; consultation with physician required
3. Patient with brittle diabetes or receiving high insulin dosage should have culture(s) taken from the infected area for antibiotic sensitivity testing
   a. Culture sent for testing
   b. Antibiotic therapy initiated
   c. In cases of poor clinical responses to the first antibiotic, a more effective antibiotic is selected according to sensitivity test results
4. Infection should be treated with the use of standard methods
   a. Warm intraoral rinses
   b. Incision and drainage
   c. Pulpotomy, pulpectomy, extractions, etc.
   d. Antibiotics

---

increased risk of infection. Judicious monitoring and appropriate use of antibiotics must be considered in the management of these patients.[2]

The basic aim of treatment is to simultaneously cure the oral infection and respond to the need to regain control of the diabetic condition. Patients who are receiving insulin usually require additional insulin, which should be prescribed by their physician; non–insulin-controlled patients may need more aggressive medical management of their diabetes, which may include insulin, during this period. The dentist must treat the infection very aggressively by incision and drainage, extraction, pulpotomy, warm rinses, and antibiotics. Antibiotic sensitivity testing is recommended for patients with brittle diabetes and for those who require a high insulin dosage for control. For these patients, penicillin therapy can be initiated; then, if the clinical response is poor, a more effective antibiotic can be selected on the basis of results of antibiotic sensitivity testing. Attention also must be paid to the patient's electrolyte balance and to fluid and dietary needs.[2]

Local Anesthetics and Epinephrine

For most patients with diabetes, routine use of local anesthetic with 1:100,000 epinephrine should be tolerated well. However, epinephrine has a pharmacologic effect that is opposite that of insulin, so blood glucose could rise with the use of epinephrine. In diabetic patients with hypertension, post myocardial infarction, cardiac arrhythmia caution may be indicated with epinephrine. Guidelines for these patients are similar to those for patients with cardiovascular conditions and may be even more strict for those with diabetes and cardiovascular conditions, as along with determination of functional capacity

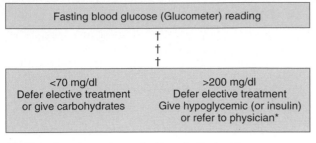

*Oral hypoglycemic agent prescribed by patient's physician.

Figure 15-7. Decision-making diagram for the dental treatment of patients with diabetes according to blood glucose (Glucometer) reading.

via METs. Diabetic patients with more than 4 METs are usually more stable, and when other indicators of physical status are also present (e.g., glycemic control), they are able to tolerate most dental procedures (see Chapter 1). Conversely, patients with METs values lower than 4 may be more likely to encounter complications and should be approached with caution. Obviously, diabetic patients may fluctuate between these states from time to time and from appointment to appointment (see Box 15-7).[2,72]

Treatment Planning Modifications

The patient with diabetes who is receiving good medical management and is under good glycemic control without serious complications such as renal disease, hypertension, or coronary atherosclerotic heart disease can undergo any indicated dental treatment. If diabetes is under good control, even cardiac transplantation can be safely performed.[2]

However, in patients with diabetes who have serious medical complications, the plan of dental treatment may need to be altered (see Chapters 3, 4, 5, 6, and 13). Studies have indicated that many dental patients with diabetes are not under good glycemic control. Elevated fasting blood glucose levels render the dental patient more susceptible to complications. Another concern is that the patient experiences too much glycemic control (hypoglycemia), resulting in low glucose levels (<70 mg/dl). This situation must also be recognized and managed appropriately (Figure 15-7). Therefore, careful and continuous monitoring of the patient's physical status is mandatory.[32]

Oral Complications and Manifestations

Oral complications of poorly controlled diabetes mellitus may include xerostomia; bacterial, viral, and fungal infections (including candidiasis); poor wound healing; increased incidence and severity of caries; gingivitis and periodontal disease; periapical abscesses; and burning mouth symptoms. Oral findings in patients with uncontrolled diabetes most likely relate to excessive loss of fluids through urination, altered response to infection, microvascular changes, and possibly, increased glucose concentrations in saliva.[73-77]

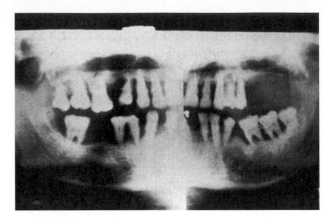

Figure 15-8. Panoramic radiograph of a young adult with severe, progressive periodontitis. After positive screening for diabetes, the patient was referred to a physician, and the diagnosis of diabetes mellitus was established. The patient required insulin treatment.

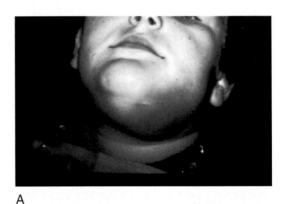

A

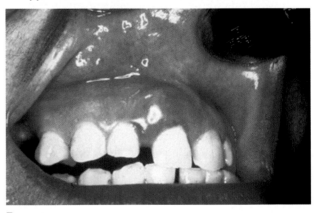

B

Figure 15-9. A, Patient with cellulitis resulting from a mandibular tooth abscess. **B,** Periodontal abscess in a patient with multiple abscesses. After evaluation by a physician, the diagnosis of diabetes was established.

The effects of hyperglycemia lead to increased amounts of urine, which deplete the extracellular fluids and reduce the secretion of saliva, thus resulting in dry mouth. A high percentage of patients with diabetes present with xerostomia.[73-77] The parotid saliva of persons with uncontrolled diabetes has been reported to contain a slightly increased amount of glucose. Several studies

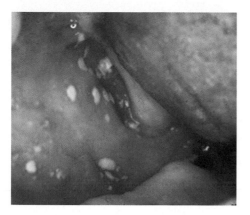

Figure 15-10. Oral moniliasis in a patient with diabetes. Note the multiple small white lesions on the buccal mucosa. The lesions could be scraped off. Cytologic study and cultures confirmed the clinical impression of infection by *Candida albicans.*

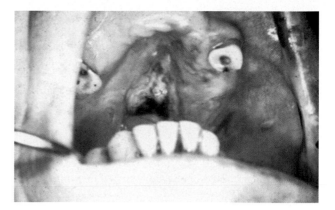

Figure 15-11. Lesion involving the palate in a patient with diabetes. Cultures established the diagnosis of mucormycosis, a serious fungal infection that may occur in patients with systemic diseases such as diabetes or cancer. Treatment usually includes control of diabetes, surgical excisions of the lesion, and administration of antibiotics and fungicides.

have reported increased incidence and severity of gingival inflammation, periodontal abscess, and chronic periodontal disease in diabetic patients (Figures 15-8 and 15-9).[73-77]

Small blood vessel changes may occur in the gingival tissues of patients with diabetes. Also, adults with uncontrolled diabetes who are prone to periodontal disease have more severe manifestations of periodontal disease than do individuals without diabetes who are prone to periodontal disease. This relationship remains unclear in the patient with controlled diabetes. As a group, patients with diabetes appear to have more severe periodontal disease than those without it, but the differences are not great. Investigators have concluded that glucose tolerance test results are not a reliable predictor of a patient's periodontal status. The time relationship between the occurrence of the diabetic state and the onset of periodontal disease has yet to be established. Periodontal disease is clearly a complication of type 1 diabetes. The increase in periodontal disease that is found in patients with type 1 diabetes cannot be explained solely by increased supragingival plaque accumulations. The periodontal disease found in these young adults (older than 30 years of age) usually is asymptomatic and remains undetected. The increased risk of periodontal disease is particularly significant when hyperglycemia is poorly controlled.[73-77]

In 1999, the American Academy of Periodontology pointed out in the context of refined standards for the classification of diabetes that uncontrolled or poorly controlled diabetes is indeed associated with increased risk for periodontitis. On the basis of results reported by multiple studies, the academy determined that periodontal disease is more severe and frequent in patients with poorly controlled diabetes.

Caries may be more significant in patients with diabetes who have poor glycemic control.[33] Oral fungal infections, including candidiasis and the more rare mucormycosis (Figures 15-10 and 15-11), may be noted in the patient with uncontrolled diabetes (see Appendix

C). Generally, it is agreed that healing is delayed in individuals with uncontrolled diabetes, and that they are more prone to various oral infections after undergoing surgical procedures.[78]

Oral lesions are more common in patients with diabetes. A significantly higher percentage of oral lesions, especially candidiasis, traumatic ulcers, lichen planus, and delayed healing, has been noted in individuals with type 1 diabetes, as compared with a control population. It is possible that alterations in the immune system may be responsible for the appearance of lichen planus in diabetes.[2,75-79]

Diabetic neuropathy may lead to oral symptoms of paresthesias and tingling, numbness, burning, or pain caused by pathologic changes involving nerves in the oral region. Diabetes has been associated with oral burning symptoms. Early diagnosis and treatment of diabetes may allow for regression of these symptoms, but in long-standing cases, the changes may be irreversible.[80,81]

REFERENCES

1. Nathan DM, Cleary PA, Backlund JY, et al. Intensive diabetes treatment and cardiovascular disease in patients with type 1 diabetes. N Engl J Med 2005;353:2643-2653.
2. Miley DD, Terezhalmy GT. The patient with diabetes mellitus: Etiology, epidemiology, principles of medical management, oral disease burden, and principles of dental management. Quintessence Int 2005;36:779-795.
3. Geiss LS, Pan L, Cadwell B, et al. Changes in incidence of diabetes in U.S. adults, 1997-2003. Am J Prev Med 2006;30:371-377.
4. Mensing C. Standards of medical care in diabetes—2006. Diabetes Care 2006;29(suppl 1):S4-S42.
5. Retnakaran R, Zinman B. Treatment of Type 1 Diabetes Mellitus in Adults. In: De Groot LJ, Jameson JL, editors. Endocrinology. Philadelphia: Saunders (Elsevier); 2006. p. 1167-1185.
6. Mensing C. Diagnosis and classification of diabetes mellitus. Diabetes Care 2006;29(suppl 1):S43-S48.

7. Steinhauer T, Bsoul SA, Terezhalmy GT. Risk stratification and dental management of the patient with cardiovascular diseases. Part II: Oral disease burden and principles of dental management. Quintessence Int 2005;36:209-227.

8. Norris AW, Svoren BM. Complications and comorbidities of type 2 diabetes. Pediatr Ann 2005;34:710-718.

9. Mauer M, Fioretto P. Preventing microalbuminuria in type 2 diabetes. N Engl J Med 2005;352:833-834; author reply 833-834.

10. Booth GL, Kapral MK, Fung K, Tu JV. Recent trends in cardiovascular complications among men and women with and without diabetes. Diabetes Care 2006;29: 32-37.

11. Juutilainen A, Lehto S, Ronnemaa T, et al. Type 2 diabetes as a "coronary heart disease equivalent": An 18-year prospective population-based study in Finnish subjects. Diabetes Care 2005;28:2901-2907.

12. Nathan DM. Complications of diabetes. In Kahn HS (ed). Joslin's Diabetes Mellitus, 14th ed. Philadelphia, Pa, Lippincott, Williams and Wilkins, 2005, p 1808.

13. Mlynarski WM, Placha GP, Wolkow PP, et al. Risk of diabetic nephropathy in type 1 diabetes is associated with functional polymorphisms in RANTES receptor gene (CCR5): A sex-specific effect. Diabetes 2005;54: 3331-3335.

14. Jaber BL, Madias NE. Atorvastatin in patients with type 2 diabetes mellitus undergoing dialysis. N Engl J Med 2005;353:1858-1860; author reply 1858-1860.

15. Bloomgarden ZT. Clinical diabetic neuropathy. Diabetes Care 2005;28:2968-2974.

16. Incidence of end-stage renal disease among persons with diabetes—United States, 1990-2002. MMWR Morb Mortal Wkly Rep 2005;54:1097-1100.

17. Aiello LP. Angiogenic pathways in diabetic retinopathy. N Engl J Med 2005;353:839-841.

18. Greene MF, Solomon CG. Gestational diabetes mellitus—Time to treat. N Engl J Med 2005;352:2544-2546.

19. Asai M, Yoshida M, Miura Y. Immunologic tolerance to intravenously injected insulin. N Engl J Med 2006;354: 307-309.

20. Mensing C. Technical reviews. Diabetes Care 2006; 29(suppl 1):S70-S72.

21. Parving HH, Hovind P, Rossing P. Telmisartan vs. enalapril in type 2 diabetes. N Engl J Med 2005;352:835-836; author reply 835-836.

22. Lu HK, Yang PC. Cross-sectional analysis of different variables of patients with non–insulin dependent diabetes and their periodontal status. Int J Periodontics Restorative Dent 2004;24:71-79.

23. Bloomgarden ZT. Developments in diabetes and insulin resistance. Diabetes Care 2006;29:161-167.

24. Lernmark A. Type 1 diabetes—Does suppressing T cells increase insulin? N Engl J Med 2005;352:2642-2644.

25. Perkins BA, Krolewski AS. Early nephropathy in type 1 diabetes: A new perspective on who will and who will not progress. Curr Diab Rep 2005;5:455-463.

26. Zammitt NN, Frier BM. Hypoglycemia in type 2 diabetes: Pathophysiology, frequency, and effects of different treatment modalities. Diabetes Care 2005;28: 2948-2961.

27. Selvin E, Wattanakit K, Steffes MW, et al. HbA1c and peripheral arterial disease in diabetes: The atherosclerosis risk in communities study. Diabetes Care 2006;29:877-882.

28. Perkins BA, Bril V. Early vascular risk factor modification in type 1 diabetes. N Engl J Med 2005;352: 408-409.

29. Kahn HS. The lipid accumulation product is better than BMI for identifying diabetes: A population-based comparison. Diabetes Care 2006;29:151-153.

30. Deghaye N, Pawinski RA, Desmond C. Financial and economic costs of scaling up the provision of HAART to HIV-infected health care workers in KwaZulu-Natal. S Afr Med J 2006;96:140-143.

31. Tesfaye S, Chaturvedi N, Eaton SE, et al. Vascular risk factors and diabetic neuropathy. N Engl J Med 2005; 352:341-350.

32. Rhodus NL, Vibeto BM, Hamamoto DT. Glycemic control in patients with diabetes mellitus upon admission to a dental clinic: Considerations for dental management. Quintessence Int 2005;36:474-482.

33. Nield-Gehrig JS, Daniels AH. Improving awareness and dental care of diabetic patients. Pract Proced Aesthet Dent 2004;16:85-87.

34. Ramseier CA. Potential impact of subject-based risk factor control on periodontitis. J Clin Periodontol 2005;32(suppl 6):283-290.

35. Cefalu WT. Glycemic control and cardiovascular disease—Should we reassess clinical goals? N Engl J Med 2005;353:2707-2709.

36. Campbell A. Tackling "diabesity" head-on: Joslin Diabetes Center's new nutrition guideline. Diabetes Self Manag 2005;22:40,42-44.

37. Asgari AA, Sarvghadi F, Zahed N. Telmisartan vs. enalapril in type 2 diabetes. N Engl J Med 2005;352:835-836; author reply 835-836.

38. Silva AI, de Matos AN, Brons IG, Mateus M. An overview on the development of a bio-artificial pancreas as a treatment of insulin-dependent diabetes mellitus. Med Res Rev 2006;26(2):181-222.

39. Dunn C, Curran MP. Spotlight on inhaled human insulin (Exubera®) in diabetes mellitus. Treat Endocrinol 2006;5(5):329-331.

40. Weir GC, Gaglia JL. Pancreatic and islet transplantation. In De Groot LJ, Jameson JL, editors. Endocrinology. Philadelphia: Saunders (Elsevier); 2006. p. 1271-1292.

41. Chen JW, Lauritzen T, Bojesen A, Christiansen JS. Multiple mealtime administration of biphasic insulin aspart 30 versus traditional basal-bolus human insulin treatment in patients with type 1 diabetes. Diabetes Obes Metab 2006;8(6):682-689.

42. Garber AJ. Premixed insulin analogues for the treatment of diabetes mellitus. Drugs 2006;66(1):31-49.

43. Ferri FF, Kabongo ML, Fox CR, Bodenner D, Plodkowski R. Diabetes mellitus type 1 in adults. Philadelphia: Elsevier; 2006.

44. Varanauskiene E, Varanauskaite I, Ceponis J. [An update on multiple insulin injection therapy in type 1 and 2 diabetes]. Medicina (Kaunas) 2006;42(9):770-779.

45. Heptulla RA, Allen HF, Gross TM, Reiter EO. Continuous glucose monitoring in children with type 1 diabetes: before and after insulin pump therapy. Pediatr Diabetes 2004;5(1):10-15.

46. Liberatore R, Jr., Perlman K, Buccino J, Artiles-Sisk A, Daneman D. Continuous subcutaneous insulin infusion pump treatment in children with type 1 diabetes mellitus. J Pediatr Endocrinol Metab 2004;17(2):223-226.

47. Medtronic. MiniMed Paradigm REAL-Time System (models 522 or 722): Medtronic; 2006.

48. Warren J, Sabicer S. Medtronic Receives FDA Approval for World's First Insulin Pump with Real-Time Continuous Glucose Monitoring: Medtronic Media Contacts; 2006. Available at http://www.medtronic.com/Newsroom.

49. Freemantle N, Strack TR. Will availability of inhaled human insulin (Exubera®) improve management of type 2 diabetes? The design of the Real World trial. Trials 2006;7:25.

50. Inhaled insulin (Exubera). Med Lett Drugs Ther 2006;48(1239):57-58.

51. Iltz JL, Baker DE, Setter SM, Keith Campbell R. Exenatide: an incretin mimetic for the treatment of type 2 diabetes mellitus. Clin Ther 2006;28(5):652-665.

52. Simsek S, de Galan BE, Tack CJ, Heine RJ. [Treatment of patients with diabetes mellitus by means of inhaled insulin]. Ned Tijdschr Geneeskd 2006;150(15):829-832.

53. Tucker ME. Implanted insulin pump continues to work for patients with type 1 diabetes: Elsevier; 2006.

54. Courtney CH, Olefsky JM. Type 2 Diabetes Mellitus: Etiology, Pathogenesis and Natural History. In De Groot LJ, Jameson JL, editors. Endocrinology. Philadelphia: Saunders (Elsevier); 2006. p. 1093-1119.

55. Bray GM. Exenatide. Am J Health Syst Pharm 2006;63(5):411-418.

56. Hoogwerf RJ. Exenatide and pramlintide: new glucose-lowering agents for treating diabetes mellitus. Cleve Clin J Med 2006;73(5):477-484.

57. Inhaled insulin (Exubera). Med Lett Drugs Ther 2006;48(1239):57-58.

58. Dunn C, Curran MP. Spotlight on inhaled human insulin (Exubera®) in diabetes mellitus. Treat Endocrinol 2006;5(5):329-331.

59. Schwartz SL, Wu JF, Berner B. Metformin extended release for the treatment of type 2 diabetes mellitus. Expert Opin Pharmacother 2006;7(6):803-809.

60. Beale S, Bagust A, Shearer AT, Martin A, Hulme L. Cost-effectiveness of rosiglitazone combination therapy for the treatment of type 2 diabetes mellitus in the UK. Pharmacoeconomics 2006;24 Suppl 1:21-34.

61. Ristic S, Collober-Maugeais C, Pecher E, Cressier F. Comparison of nateglinide and gliclazide in combination with metformin, for treatment of patients with Type 2 diabetes mellitus inadequately controlled on maximum doses of metformin alone. Diabet Med 2006;23(7):757-762.

62. Gallwitz B. Therapies for the treatment of type 2 diabetes mellitus based on incretin action. Minerva Endocrinol 2006;31(2):133-147.

63. Barnett A. DPP-4 inhibitors and their potential role in the management of type 2 diabetes. Int J Clin Pract 2006;60(11):1454-1470.

64. Bergman AJ, Stevens C, Zhou Y, Yi B, Laethem M, De Smet M, et al. Pharmacokinetic and pharmacodynamic properties of multiple oral doses of sitagliptin, a dipep-tidyl peptidase-IV inhibitor: a double-blind, randomized, placebo-controlled study in healthy male volunteers. Clin Ther 2006;28(1):55-72.

65. Ahren B. [New strategy in type 2 diabetes tested in clinical trials. Glucagon-like peptide 1 (GLP-1) affects basic caused of the disease]. Lakartidningen 2005;102(8):545-549.

66. Drucker DJ, Nauck MA. The incretin system: glucagon-like peptide-1 receptor agonists and dipeptidyl peptidase-4 inhibitors in type 2 diabetes. Lancet 2006;368(9548):1696-1705.

67. Yoo BK, Triller DM, Yoo DJ. Exenatide: a new option for the treatment of type 2 diabetes. Ann Pharmacother 2006;40(10):1777-1784.

68. Feinglos MN, Saad MF, Pi-Sunyer FX, An B, Santiago O. Effects of liraglutide (NN2211), a long-acting GLP-1 analogue, on glycaemic control and body-weight in subjects with Type 2 diabetes. Diabet Med 2005;22(8):1016-1023.

69. Nauck MA, Hompesch M, Filipczak R, Le TD, Zdravkovic M, Gumprecht J. Five weeks of treatment with the GLP-1 analogue liraglutide improves glycaemic control and lowers body weight in subjects with type 2 diabetes. Exp Clin Endocrinol Diabetes 2006;114(8):417-423.

70. Nogid A, Pham DQ. Adjunctive therapy with pramlintide in patients with type 1 or type 2 diabetes mellitus. Pharmacotherapy 2006;26(11):1626-1640.

71. Fiske J. Diabetes mellitus and oral care. Dent Update 2004;31:190-196,198.

72. Brown RS, Rhodus NL. Epinephrine and local anesthesia revisited. Oral Surg Oral Med Oral Pathol Oral Radiol Endod 2005;100:401-408.

73. Aren G, Sepet E, Ozdemir D, et al. Periodontal health, salivary status, and metabolic control in children with type 1 diabetes mellitus. J Periodontol 2003;74:1789-1795.

74. Campus G, Salem A, Uzzau S, et al. Diabetes and periodontal disease: A case-control study. J Periodontol 2005;76:418-425.

75. Lalla E, Park DB, Papapanou PN, Lamster IB. Oral disease burden in Northern Manhattan patients with diabetes mellitus. Am J Public Health 2004;94:755-758.

76. Negishi J, Kawanami M, Terada Y, et al. Effect of lifestyle on periodontal disease status in diabetic patients. J Int Acad Periodontol 2004;6:120-124.

77. Promsudthi A, Pimapansri S, Deerochanawong C, Kanchanavasita W. The effect of periodontal therapy on uncontrolled type 2 diabetes mellitus in older subjects. Oral Dis 2005;11:293-298.

78. Belazi M, Velegraki A, Fleva A, et al. Candidal overgrowth in diabetic patients: Potential predisposing factors. Mycoses 2005;48:192-196.

79. Rhodus NL, Myers S, Kaimal S. Diagnosis and management of oral lichen planus. Northwest Dent 2003;82:17-19,22-25.

80. Rhodus NL, Carlson CR, Miller CS. Burning mouth (syndrome) disorder. Quintessence Int 2003;34:587-593.

81. Rhodus NL, Myers S, Bowles W, et al. Burning mouth syndrome: Diagnosis and treatment. Northwest Dent 2000;79:21-28.

Adrenal Insufficiency

CHAPTER 16

BACKGROUND

The adrenal glands are small (6 to 8 g) endocrine glands that are located bilaterally at the superior pole of each kidney. Each gland contains an outer cortex and an inner medulla. The adrenal medulla functions as a sympathetic ganglion and secretes catecholamines, primarily epinephrine, whereas the adrenal cortex secretes several steroid hormones with multiple actions (Figure 16-1). This chapter focuses on primary disorders caused by adrenal cortical function and hypofunction (i.e., insufficiency).

The adrenal cortex makes up about 90% of the gland and consists of three zones. The outer zone is the zona glomerulosa. The middle zone is the zona fasciculata, and the innermost zone is the zona reticularis. The cortex manufactures three classes of adrenal steroids: glucocorticoids, mineralocorticoids, and androgens. All are derived from cholesterol and share a common molecular nucleus. The predominant hormone of the zona glomerulosa is aldosterone, a mineralocorticoid. Aldosterone regulates physiologic levels of sodium and potassium and is relatively independent of pituitary gland feedback. The zona fasciculata secretes glucocorticoids, and the zona reticularis secretes androgens, or sex hormones.

Cortisol, the primary glucocorticoid, is responsible for a wide variety of functions and effects. Some of the more important ones include regulation of carbohydrate, fat, and protein metabolism, maintenance of vascular reactivity, inhibition of inflammation, and maintenance of homeostasis during periods of physical or emotional stress.[1] Cortisol acts as an insulin antagonist (Figure 16-2), increasing blood levels and peripheral use of glucose; increasing liver glucose output; and initiating lipolysis, proteolysis, and gluconeogenic mechanisms. The anti-inflammatory action of cortisol is modulated by its inhibitory action on (1) lysosome release, (2) prostaglandin production, (3) eicosanoid and cytokine release, (4) endothelial cell expression of intracellular and extracellular adhesion molecules (ICAMs and ECAMs, respectively) that attract neutrophils, and (5) the function of leukocytes.

Regulation of cortisol secretion occurs via the hypothalamic-pituitary-adrenal (HPA) axis (Figure 16-3). Central nervous system afferents mediating circadian rhythm and responses to stress stimulate the hypothalamus to release corticotropin-releasing hormone (CRH), which stimulates the production and secretion of adrenocorticotropic hormone (ACTH) by the anterior pituitary. ACTH, then stimulates the adrenal cortex to produce and secrete cortisol. Plasma cortisol levels are increased within a few minutes after stimulation. Circulating levels of cortisol inhibit the production of CRH and ACTH, thus completing a negative feedback loop.[2]

Cortisol secretion normally follows a diurnal pattern. Peak levels of plasma cortisol occur about the time of awakening in the morning and are lowest in the afternoon and evening[3] (Figure 16-4). This pattern is reversed in an individual who habitually works nights and sleeps during the day. The normal secretion rate of cortisol over a 24-hour period is approximately 20 mg.[2,3] During periods of stress, the HPA axis is stimulated, resulting in increased secretion of cortisol. Anticipation of surgery or an athletic event usually is accompanied by only minimal increases in cortisol secretion. However, surgery itself is one of the most potent activators of the HPA axis.[4-7] Various stressors such as trauma, illness, burns, fever, hypoglycemia, and emotional upset can trigger this effect. The greatest response is noted in the immediate postoperative period. However, this can be reduced by morphine-like analgesics, benzodiazepines, or local anesthesia, suggesting that the pain response mechanism increases the requirement for cortisol.[8-10]

Synthetic glucocorticoids (cortisol-like drugs) are used in the treatment of many diseases (e.g., rheumatoid arthritis, systemic lupus erythematosus, asthma, hepatitis, inflammatory bowel disease, dermatoses, mucositis) and can affect adrenal function. Glucocorticoids are used on

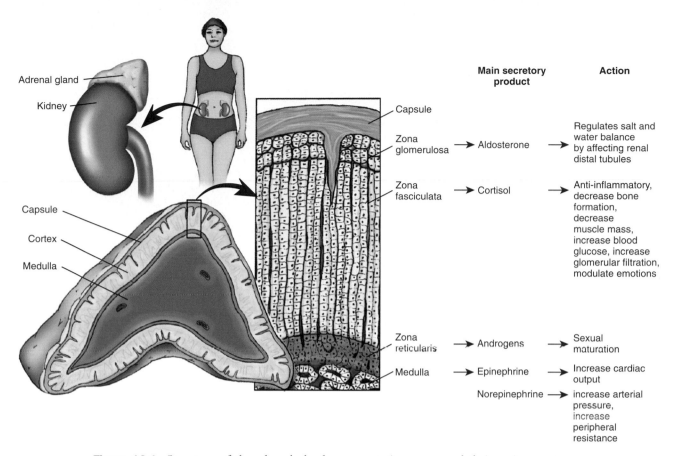

Figure 16-1. Structure of the adrenal gland, representative zones, and their main secretory products and physiologic actions. (Modified from Thibodeau GA, Patton KT. Anatomy & Physiology, 6th ed. St. Louis, Mosby, 2006.)

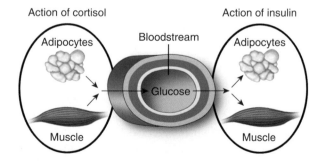

Figure 16-2. Effects of cortisol and insulin on glucose in the bloodstream.

a long-term basis in patients during immunosuppressive therapy for organ transplantation and joint replacement. In dentistry, corticosteroids are used during perioperative periods for reduction of pain, edema, and trismus after oral surgical and endodontic procedures.[11,12] Many synthetic glucocorticoids are available, and they differ in potency relative to cortisol and in their duration of action (Table 16-1).

Mineralocorticoids

Aldosterone is the primary mineralocorticoid secreted by the adrenal cortex. It is essential to sodium and potassium balance and to the maintenance of extracellular fluid (i.e., intravascular volume). Its actions occur primarily on the distal tubule and the collecting duct of the kidney, where it promotes sodium retention, potassium excretion, and fluid retention. Aldosterone secretion is regulated by the renin-angiotensin system, ACTH, and plasma sodium and potassium levels. It is stimulated by a fall in renal blood pressure, which results from decreased intravascular volume or a sodium imbalance,[3] and causes release of renin, which activates angiotensin. Angiotensin causes aldosterone to be secreted. When blood pressure rises, renin-angiotensin release diminishes, serving as a negative feedback loop that inhibits additional production of aldosterone (Figure 16-5).

Adrenal Androgens

Dehydroepiandrosterone is the principal androgen secreted by the adrenal cortex. The effects of adrenal androgens are the same as those of testicular androgens (i.e., masculinization and the promotion of protein anabolism and growth). The activity of the adrenal androgens, however, is only about 20% that of the testicular androgens and is of relatively minor importance.[3] Estrogen precursors are secreted from the zona reticularis of the adrenal cortex.

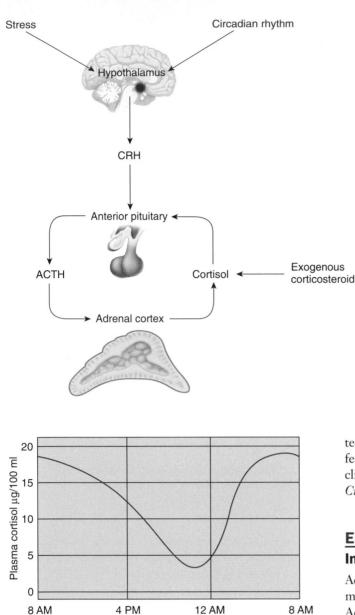

Stress

Circadian rhythm

Hypothalamus

CRH

Anterior pituitary

ACTH

Cortisol ← Exogenous corticosteroid

Adrenal cortex

Figure 16-3. Hypothalamic-pituitary-adrenal axis and the regulation of cortisol secretion.

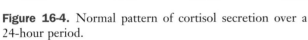

Figure 16-4. Normal pattern of cortisol secretion over a 24-hour period.

DEFINITION

Disorders that affect the adrenal glands result in overproduction or underproduction of adrenal products. Excess production of the adrenal glands results in the overproduction of cortisol, mineralocorticoids, androgens, or estrogen, in isolation or combination. The most common type of overproduction is due to glucocorticoid excess and, when caused by pathophysiologic processes, is known as *Cushing's disease.*

Insufficient adrenocortical function may occur primarily or secondarily. Primary adrenocortical insufficiency is uncommon and is known as Addison's disease. The more common form, secondary adrenocortical insufficiency, results from hypothalamic or pituitary disease or from the administration of exogenous corticosteroids. Both downregulate adrenal production of cortisol. Long-

term excessive use of glucocorticoids can result in clinical features mimicking Cushing's disease. This collection of clinical features of glucocorticoid excess is known as *Cushing's syndrome.*

EPIDEMIOLOGY

Incidence and Prevalence

Adrenal insufficiency occurs in 40 to 60 persons per 1 million adults. Primary adrenocortical insufficiency, or Addison's disease, occurs at a rate of approximately 8 cases per 1 million people per year. Secondary adrenocortical insufficiency is about 5 times more common than primary adrenal insufficiency. Approximately 5% of adults in the United States chronically use corticosteroids and thus are at risk for secondary adrenocortical insufficiency. A dental practice serving 2000 adults can expect to encounter 50 patients who use steroids or who have potential adrenal abnormalities.

Pathophysiology and Complications

Primary adrenocortical insufficiency is caused by progressive destruction of the adrenal cortex, usually of an idiopathic nature (most commonly, autoimmune) but also resulting from hemorrhage, sepsis, infectious disease (tuberculosis, human immunodeficiency virus [HIV], cytomegalovirus, and fungal infection), malignancy, adrenalectomy, or drugs.[13] Signs and symptoms of the disease are the result of deficiencies of adrenocortical hormones. Clinical evidence of deficiency generally arises only after 90% of the adrenal cortices have been destroyed.

TABLE **16-1**

Glucocorticoids and Their Relative Potency

Compound	Antiinflammatory Potency	Mineralocorticoid Potency	Approximate Equivalent Dose, mg
SHORT-ACTING (<12 hr)			
Cortisol	1	2	20
Cortisone	0.8	2	25
INTERMEDIATE-ACTING (12-36 hr)			
Prednisone	4	1	5
Prednisolone	4	1	5
Methylprednisolone	5	0	4
Triamcinolone	5	0	4
LONG-ACTING (>36 hr)			
Paramethasone	10	0	2
Betamethasone	25	0	0.75
Dexamethasone	25	0	0.75

Modified from Schimmer BP, Parker KL. In Brunton LL, et al (eds). Goodman and Gilman's The Pharmacological Basis of Therapeutics, 11th ed. New York, McGraw-Hill, 2006.[1]

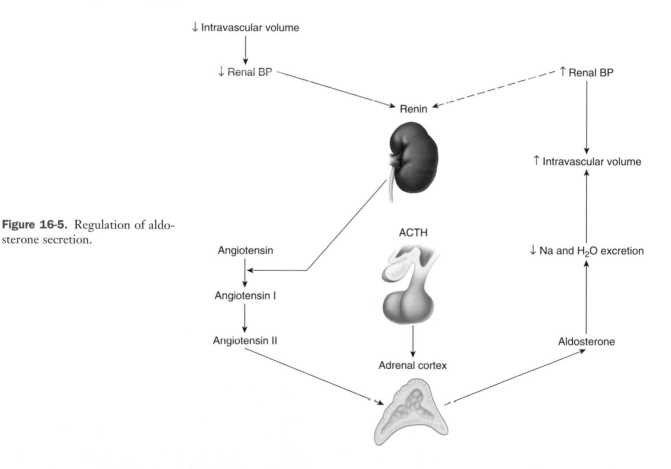

Figure 16-5. Regulation of aldosterone secretion.

The major hormones of the adrenal cortex are cortisol and aldosterone. Addison's disease is caused by the lack of these compounds. Lack of cortisol results in impaired metabolism of glucose, fat, and protein, as well as hypotension, increased ACTH secretion, impaired fluid excretion, excessive pigmentation, and an inability to tolerate stress. The relationship between corticosteroids and response to stress is not well understood but probably involves the maintenance of vascular reactivity to vasoactive agents and the maintenance of normal blood pressure and cardiac output. Aldosterone deficiency results in an inability to conserve sodium and eliminate potassium and hydrogen ions, leading to hypovolemia, hyperkalemia, and acidosis.[4]

Secondary adrenocortical insufficiency is a far more common problem and results from hypothalamic or pituitary disease, administration of exogenous corticosteroids, or, less commonly, administration of specific drugs (e.g., desferrioxamine in the treatment of thalassemia).[14] The secretion of cortisol is directly dependent on the level of circulating ACTH. As plasma cortisol level increases, the production of ACTH decreases by virtue of negative feedback to the pituitary and the hypothalamus. With the administration of corticosteroids, the feedback system senses the elevated plasma steroid levels and inhibits ACTH production, which, in turn, suppresses adrenal production of cortisol (see Figure 16-3). The result is partial adrenal insufficiency. The production of aldosterone, because it is ACTH independent, is not appreciably affected.

Determination of the degree of adrenocortical hypofunction (i.e., suppression) resulting from corticosteroid use for a given patient is controversial and generally has been thought to depend on the dose, as well as the timing and duration of administration. In the past, suppression was thought to be more likely with supraphysiologic doses taken daily over an extended period. However, the prediction of suppression that is based on the history of dosage or length of administration has been unreliable.[15] Assessment of suppression is best accomplished through laboratory evaluation with the use of stimulation tests for functional cortisol production.

A common treatment modification of steroid therapy that attempts to minimize adrenal suppression is the alternate-day regimen. This consists of giving steroids in the morning every other day instead of daily, but at a higher dose to maintain an elevated serum level. Because the cortisol level normally is higher in the morning, a single, large dose given at that time has less suppressant effect on ACTH, and the HPA axis is allowed to function normally and produce endogenous steroids on the off day. The result is less adrenal suppression than is seen with twice-a-day therapy. Unfortunately, this approach often is not adequate to control symptoms, and many patients must return to daily therapy.

Topically applied and inhaled corticosteroids are rare inducers of adrenal suppression by absorption through the skin, mucous membranes, or pulmonary alveoli. Although the amount of topical steroid required to treat small, noninflamed areas probably does not cause significant suppression, prolonged treatment of large inflamed areas may be a cause for concern, especially if occlusive dressings are used.[16-18] Similar comments may be made regarding the use of inhaled corticosteroids, if they are given in frequent and high doses.[19,20] Doses of 1000 to 1500 mg/day (in four divided doses) of beclomethasone dipropionate or budesonide in adults (depending on body mass) generally are considered to represent the cutoff point, indicating that adrenal suppression is probable.[21]

Once corticosteroid administration has ceased, the HPA axis regains its responsiveness, and normal ACTH and cortisol secretion resumes eventually. The time required to regain normal adrenal responsiveness is thought to vary from days to months. However, studies from a large review[22] demonstrated a return to stress stimulation of HPA function within 14 days, in spite of the fact that supraphysiologic doses were given for a month or longer.

CLINICAL PRESENTATION
Signs and Symptoms

Hypoadrenalism. Primary adrenal insufficiency (Addison's disease) produces signs and symptoms that relate to a deficiency of aldosterone and cortisol. The most common complaints are weakness, fatigue, and abnormal pigmentation of the skin and mucous membranes (Figure 16-6). Hypotension, anorexia, and weight loss are additional common findings. If a patient with Addison's disease is challenged by stress (e.g., illness, infection, surgery), an adrenal crisis may be precipitated. This medical emergency manifests as severe exacerbation of the patient's condition, including sunken eyes, profuse sweating, hypotension, weak pulse, cyanosis, nausea, vomiting, weakness, headache, dehydration, fever, dyspnea, myalgias, arthralgia, hyponatremia, and eosinophilia. If not treated rapidly, the patient may develop hypothermia, severe hypotension, hypoglycemia, and circulatory collapse that can result in death.[23]

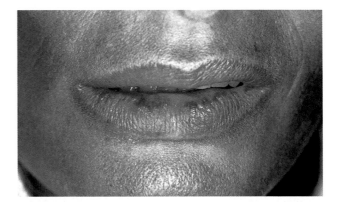

A

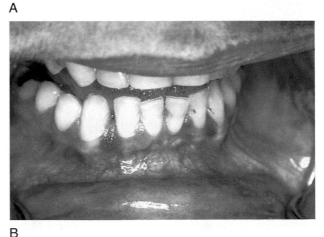

B

Figure 16-6. Patient with Addison's disease. Note the bronzing of the skin with pigmentation of **(A)** the lip and **(B)** the oral mucosa.

Secondary adrenal insufficiency caused by long-term corticosteroid administration may cause a partial insufficiency that is limited to glucocorticoids. The condition usually does not produce any symptoms unless the patient is significantly stressed and does not have adequate circulating cortisol during times surrounding stress. In this event, an adrenal crisis is possible. However, an adrenal crisis in a patient with secondary adrenal suppression is rare and tends not to be as severe as that seen with primary adrenal insufficiency because aldosterone secretion is normal. Thus, hypotension, dehydration, and shock seldom are encountered.[4]

Hyperadrenalism. Adrenal hyperfunction can produce four syndromes that are dependent on the adrenal product that is in excess—androgen, estrogen, mineralocorticoid, and cortisol. Androgen-related disorders are rare and primarily affect the reproductive organs. Mineralocorticoid excess (primary aldosteronism) is associated with hypertension, hypokalemia, and dependent edema (see Chapter 3). The most common form of hyperadrenalism is due to glucocorticoid excess (endogenous or exogenous), and it leads to a syndrome known as Cushing's syndrome. This syndrome classically produces weight gain, round or moon-shaped facies (Figure 16-7), a "buffalo hump" on the upper back, abdominal striae, hypertension, hirsutism, and acne. Other findings may include glucose intolerance (e.g., diabetes mellitus), heart failure, osteoporosis and bone fractures, impaired healing, and psychiatric disorders (mental depression, mania, anxiety disorders, cognitive dysfunction, and psychosis).[23] Long-term steroid use may also increase risks for insomnia, peptic ulceration, cataract formation, glaucoma, growth suppression, and delayed wound healing.

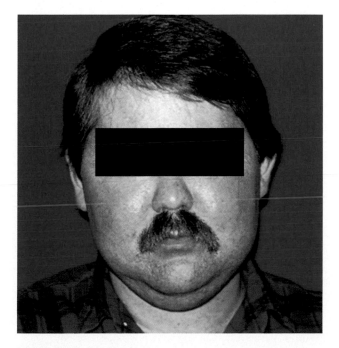

Figure 16-7. Moon-shaped face: A clinical manifestation of Cushing's disease.

Laboratory Findings

Because cortisol deficiency is the primary concern from a dental management perspective, remarks in this chapter are limited to tests for the determination of adrenal function associated with cortisol secretion. Cortisol levels can be measured in urine, plasma, and saliva. Of the three bodily fluids, saliva appears to be the most sensitive. However, the clinician must provide screening with the knowledge that cortisol values may be altered by a variety of factors, including circadian rhythm, diet, and stress. For example, normal plasma cortisol concentrations in the early morning range from 10 to 20 µg/dL, whereas late afternoon values typically range from 3 to 10 µg/dL. To minimize the effects of circadian rhythm, late-night salivary cortisol testing is recommended.[24]

A positive screening cortisol screening test should be followed by provocative (stimulation) tests of the HPA axis. These tests include the synthetic ACTH (cosyntropin) stimulation test, the CRH test, and the dexamethasone suppression test. The ACTH stimulation test, the most reliable screening test for adrenal hypofunction, directly evaluates the level of adrenal reserve. A positive response (i.e., an increase in plasma cortisol level after ACTH administration) is indicative of adrenal function. However, a subnormal test response, although suggestive of adrenal insufficiency, has limited correlation with the patient's clinical ability to respond to stress.[25] The CRH test differentiates ACTH-dependent from ACTH-independent disorders; the dexamethasone suppression test can be used to screen for adrenal hyperfunction but has specificity issues associated with false-positive and false-negative results.

MEDICAL MANAGEMENT
Primary Adrenal Insufficiency

The primary medical needs of the addisonian patient are (1) management of the adrenal disease (e.g., elimination of the infectious agent or malignant disease), and (2) hormonal replacement therapy. Glucocorticoid replacement is accomplished at levels that correspond to normal physiologic output of the adrenal cortex, usually about 20 to 30 mg of hydrocortisone or cortisone acetate per day, with a range of 12.5 to 50 mg daily. Cortisone 30 mg daily or prednisone 7.5 mg daily provides adequate substitution therapy. Current practice recommends that two thirds of the dose should be given in the morning and one third in the later afternoon to reflect the normal diurnal cycle. Mineralocorticoid replacement is accomplished by daily administration of fludrocortisone (0.05 to 0.1 mg). Patients are also encouraged to ingest adequate sodium.[23] Although patients with Addison's disease can lead essentially normal lives with appropriate treatment, the need for supplemental glucocorticoids during periods of illness, trauma, or "stress" continues indefinitely.

Secondary Adrenal Insufficiency

Secondary adrenal insufficiency may result from destructive hypothalamic-pituitary disorders or long-term steroid use. In the former case, treatment involves correcting the ACTH-dependent disorder and replacing the missing glucocorticoid. In the latter situation, the clinician may be challenged by trying to balance the beneficial effects of steroids with their unwanted adverse effects. Steroids are prescribed in the management of nonendocrine disorders for their anti-inflammatory and immunosuppressive properties. Selection is based on potency, route of administration, duration of action, and anticipated adverse effects. The goal is to achieve resolution of disease symptoms while minimizing adverse effects. Depending on the condition, dosages are generally targeted to be equal to or less than the daily replacement dose of the preparation used. For example, hydrocortisone is usually dispensed at about 20 mg/day, prednisone or prednisolone at 5 mg/day, and dexamethasone at 0.5 mg/day (see Table 16-1). Such regimens given as a morning dose are less suppressive. Higher and divided daily doses are more suppressive and usually take at least 3 weeks to result in clinical manifestation of glucocorticoid deficiency. A method for minimizing the adverse effects of long-term systemic steroid therapy is the alternate-day regimen. This method allows the adrenal gland to function normally during the off day and thus does not tend to cause axis suppression. A tapered dosage schedule is often implemented for discontinuation of steroid usage, but this may not be necessary in many cases.[26]

Patients who are provided steroids for low adrenal reserve and to prevent adrenal crisis during and after surgery have been of concern ever since Fraser et al[27] reported in 1952 that a patient experienced refractory hypotension at the end of a routine surgical procedure and died 3 hours later. A similar case was reported a year later.[28] The general consensus has been that these "at-risk" patients should be provided supplemental steroids during periods of stress, trauma, or illness.[13,23,29] However, this philosophy has been examined over the past decade, and a new approach has emerged. The basis for this change comes from knowledge of adrenal cortical response to physical stressors that has been refined over the past 20 years,[5] and from evidence that few well-documented cases of adrenal crisis have been reported in the literature.[6,30]

The newer recommendations, as described by Salem and colleagues[30] and others,[31] base the need for glucocorticoid replacement on three factors: (1) the duration and severity of surgery and level of pain control, (2) the amount of cortisol produced during the physiologic response to surgical stress, and (3) the overall health of the patient who takes daily steroids.

Surgery is known to cause increased plasma corticosteroid levels during and after operations. Plasma cortisol levels peak at twofold to tenfold above baseline between 4 and 10 hours after the operation.[32,33] The level of response is based on the magnitude of the surgery and whether general anesthesia is used. Postoperative pain is also contributory, and urine levels of cortisol metabolites have been shown to remain increased for 3 to 6 days after the surgery.[33] Kehlet[6] estimates that adults secrete 75 to 150 mg a day in response to major surgery and 50 mg a day during minor procedures. Cortisol secretion in the first 24 hours after surgery rarely exceeds 200 mg.[7,30]

Under conditions of general anesthesia, corticosteroid-treated patients have a significantly lower plasma cortisol response to surgery than do patients who have not received corticosteroid drugs.[34,35] This may be an effect of steroid-induced adrenal insufficiency or the use of barbiturate anesthetic drugs that can reduce cortisol production.[36,37] Likewise, midazolam administration reduces stress associated with oral surgery, as determined by salivary cortisol levels.[8]

For minor surgery, the risk of adrenal crisis appears to be low. Several studies have shown that the vast majority of patients who take daily equivalent or lower doses of steroid (e.g., mean dose 5 to 10 mg prednisone daily) on a long-term basis for conditions such as renal transplant or rheumatoid arthritis maintain adrenal function and do not require supplementation for minor surgical procedures.[26,34,38,39] In addition, a significant proportion of patients who took 5 to 50 mg prednisone daily for between 6 days and 10 years and stopped therapy before surgery produced plasma cortisol levels similar to those of normal subjects for up to 7 days after minor or major surgery; they also followed a normal postoperative course.[31,38,40]

If doubt exists as to the adrenal cortical status of a patient scheduled for surgery, a stimulation test of the HPA axis (e.g., ACTH stimulation test) is recommended as a preoperative screening evaluation of adrenal function. If biochemical evaluation demonstrates inadequate HPA axis function or insufficient adrenal reserve, or if preoperative testing is not performed, perioperative glucocorticoid coverage should be provided according to the recommendations below.

The current recommendations for general surgery, which have been put forth by Salem et al,[30] are as follows:

- For minor surgical stress, the glucocorticoid target is about 25 mg of hydrocortisone equivalent on the day of surgery. For example, an asthmatic patient who takes 5 mg of prednisone every other day should receive 5 mg of prednisone on the day of surgery, preoperatively.
- For moderate surgical stress, the glucocorticoid target is about 50 to 75 per day of hydrocortisone equivalent for up to 1 to 2 days. For example, a patient with systemic lupus erythematosus who takes 10 mg prednisone daily should receive 10 mg of prednisone (or parenteral equivalent) preoperatively and 50 mg of hydrocortisone intravenously intraoperatively. On the first postoperative day, 20 mg of hydrocortisone is administered intravenously every 8 hours (i.e., 60 mg per day).

The patient is returned to the preoperative glucocorticoid dose on postoperative day 2.

- For major surgical stress, the glucocorticoid target is about 100 to 150 mg per day of hydrocortisone equivalent given for 2 to 3 days. For example, a patient with Crohn's disease who takes 40 mg prednisone daily for several years should receive 40 mg prednisone (or the parenteral equivalent) preoperatively and 50 mg hydrocortisone intravenously every 8 hours after the initial dose for the first 48 to 72 hours after surgery. In comparison, a patient who takes 5 mg prednisone daily who is undergoing similar major surgery is recommended to receive 5 mg prednisone (or the parenteral equivalent) as a preoperative dose, with 25 mg of hydrocortisone given intraoperatively and 25 mg administered every 8 hours after surgery for the subsequent 48-hour period.

The above protocol recommends that the steroid should be taken within 2 hours of the surgical procedure, and the surgeon, anesthetist, and nurses should be advised of possible complications. If the postoperative course is uneventful, the patient is returned to the usual glucocorticoid dosage upon completion of the regimen.

Factors that may complicate the postoperative course and exacerbate adrenal insufficiency include liver dysfunction, febrile illness, sepsis, nausea and vomiting, and some drugs.[41] Drugs that can lower plasma cortisol levels include aminoglutethimide (an adrenolytic), etomidate (an anesthetic agent), ketoconazole, and inducers of hepatic cytochrome P450 oxygenases (e.g., phenytoin, barbiturates, rifampin) that accelerate degradation of cortisol. It is also important to note that the action of oral anticoagulants can be potentiated (resulting in increased risk of bleeding) by the intravenous (IV) administration of high-dose methylprednisolone.[42]

Adrenal Crisis

A rare and potentially life-threatening outcome in spite of steroid supplementation is acute adrenal insufficiency (adrenal crisis). This condition requires immediate treatment, including IV injection of a glucocorticoid—usually a 100-mg hydrocortisone bolus and fluid and electrolyte replacement. Intramuscular (IM) injection results in slow absorption and is not preferred for emergency treatment. Over the first 24 hours, 100 mg is administered IV slowly every 6 to 8 hours; if needed, blood pressure is supported with fluid replacement and vasopressors, along with correction of hypoglycemia. Resolution of the event or condition that precipitated the crisis is required.

DENTAL MANAGEMENT

In developing recommendations for dental patients with adrenal disease, the dentist must consider the type and degree of adrenal dysfunction and the dental procedure planned. Patients with hyperadrenalism have an increased likelihood of hypertension and osteoporosis and increased risk for peptic ulcer disease. To minimize the risk of an adverse outcome, blood pressure should be taken at baseline and monitored during dental appointments. Osteoporosis has a relationship with periodontal bone loss, implant placement, and bone fracture. Treatment planning should address the risk for periodontal bone loss, and measures should be instituted that promote bone mineralization and avoid extensive neck manipulation if osteoporosis is severe. Because of the risk of peptic ulceration, postoperative analgesics selection should not include aspirin and nonsteroidal anti-inflammatory drugs for long-term steroid users.

Evidence indicates that the vast majority of patients with adrenal insufficiency may undergo routine dental treatment without the need for supplemental glucocorticoids.[6,31,38,39,43] Individuals at risk for adrenal crisis are those who undergo stressful surgical procedures and have no or extremely low adrenal function because of primary or secondary adrenal insufficiency.

To determine who is at risk for adrenal insufficiency or crisis, a thorough medical history must be taken. Past or present history of tuberculosis, histoplasmosis, or HIV increases the risk for adrenal disease (insufficiency) in that opportunistic infectious agents may attack the adrenal glands. In addition, adrenal crisis is possible when adrenally insufficient patients discontinue treatment or simply do not take their glucocorticoid before a stressful surgical procedure.

Other than major surgical procedures (e.g., extraction of bony impaction, osteotomy, bone resection, cancer surgery), few dental procedures appear to warrant the use of supplemental steroids before, during, or after the operative period. Patients who are currently taking corticosteroids generally have enough exogenous and endogenous cortisol to handle routine dental procedures, if their usual steroid dose is taken within 2 hours of the surgery. Furthermore, routine dental procedures do not stimulate cortisol production at levels comparable with those that occur at the time of surgery.[31,43]

Studies[4,32,40,44] investigating the stress response to minor general and oral surgical procedures have concluded that significant cortisol increases are not generally seen before or during the operation but are increased in the postoperative period approximately 1 to 5 hours after the procedure is begun. The postoperative increase in plasma cortisol levels is likely a response to pain because postoperative cortisol increases correlate with loss of local anesthesia[43] and are blunted by the use of analgesics and midazolam.[8,32] Consistent with this, Ziccardi and colleagues[45-47] reported that supplementation is not required for patients who take corticosteroids when uncomplicated minor surgical procedures of the orofacial complex are performed with local anesthesia with or without conscious sedation.

To identify who needs supplementation for moderate to severe surgical procedures, the ACTH stimulation test may be performed. A low biochemical test result demonstrating inadequate adrenal cortical function indicates that supplemental steroids should be provided at a level sufficient for the stress response. However, even if a patient has adrenal cortical suppression as diagnosed by an abnormal stimulation test, this does not necessarily reflect how he or she will react clinically or whether an adverse reaction will even occur.[5,21,22] Patients who had their glucocorticoid medications discontinued within a week before surgery have withstood general surgical procedures without the development of adrenal crisis.[5,7,38,40]

On the basis of these studies and the limited number of purported adrenal crisis cases associated with dental procedures,[46,48-50] four clinical factors appear to contribute to the risk of adrenal crisis during the perioperative period of oral surgery. These include severity of surgery, drugs administered, overall health of the patient, and extent of pain control. Additional factors (e.g., amount of blood loss, fasting state) may contribute to hypotension and hypoglycemia that can be confused with adrenal crisis but do not require glucocorticoids for resolution.

At present, for minor oral and periodontal surgery, adrenal insufficiency is prevented when circulating levels of glucocorticoids are about 25 mg of hydrocortisone equivalent per day. This is equivalent to a dose of about 6 mg of prednisone. If the patient is to gain the benefit of the corticosteroid, the drug should be taken within 2 hours of the surgical procedure. Preferably, surgery is scheduled in the morning and stress reduction measures are implemented.

For major oral surgical stress involving the use of general anesthesia, procedures of longer than 1 hour duration, or significant blood loss, the glucocorticoid target is about 50 to 100 mg per day of hydrocortisone equivalent on the day of surgery and for at least 1 postoperative day. Patients should take their normal dose and should be given supplemental hydrocortisone intraoperatively to achieve 100 mg. Hospitalization should be considered for these patients because blood pressure can be more closely monitored postoperatively in this setting.[51] Hydrocortisone 25 mg is usually prescribed every 8 hours subsequent to surgery for 24 to 48 hours, depending on the procedure and the anticipated level of postoperative pain. Box 16-1 shows recommendations for supplementa-

---

BOX 16-1

Dental Management of the Patient With Possible Adrenal Insufficiency

1. Patient past history of systemic corticosteroid use
   a. Evaluate the patient.
   b. Determine whether systemic corticosteroid was taken within the past 2 weeks and the reason for discontinuing usage.
   c. Determine type, dose, and duration of systemic corticosteroid used.
   d. Identify signs and symptoms of possible adrenal insufficiency.
   e. If major invasive oral procedure is planned and corticosteroid was taken within the past 2 weeks, consult with the physician regarding status and stability (adrenocorticotropic hormone [ACTH] or perform corticotropin-releasing hormone [CRH] test performed). If adrenal insufficient, implement steroid supplementation protocol.* Note that risk of medical complications increases when major surgical procedures are performed on persons who have low adrenal reserve.
2. Patient currently taking systemic corticosteroids
   a. Evaluate the patient.
   b. Determine dose and duration of systemic corticosteroid used.

   c. Identify signs and symptoms of possible adrenal insufficiency.
   d. For diagnostic and minimally invasive procedures, have patient take the usual daily dose, and perform oral procedure in the morning, shortly after the corticosteroid is taken. Stress reduction measures should be implemented, blood pressure recorded during the procedure.
   e. For major invasive oral procedures, consult with the physician regarding status and stability (ACTH or CRH test performed). Implement the steroid supplementation protocol.*
3. Patient not taking systemic corticosteroids, but may have adrenal insufficiency
   a. Evaluate the patient for historical findings associated with risk for adrenal insufficiency.
   b. Identify signs and symptoms of adrenal insufficiency.
   c. Refer to the physician for ACTH testing.
   d. If the patient is found to be adrenally insufficient, defer dental treatment until stabilized with corticosteroid treatment. Then, follow the steroid supplementation protocol* as defined in 2d and 2e.

*Steroid supplementation protocol for major surgical procedure:
- Discontinue drugs that decrease cortisol levels (e.g., ketoconazole) at least 24 hours before surgery with the consent of the patient's physician.
- Have patient take usual morning dose (or the parenteral equivalent as a preoperative dose), and provide supplemental hydrocortisone preoperatively and intraoperatively to achieve 100 mg within first hour of surgery. Give hydrocortisone 25 mg every 8 hours subsequent to surgery for 24 to 48 hours. Perform in hospital environment.
- Provide adequate operative and postoperative analgesia.
- Use barbiturates with caution and knowledge of the potential for adverse effects on plasma cortisol levels.
- Monitor blood pressure (BP) and blood loss throughout the procedure. If BP drops to below 100/60 mm Hg and the patient is unresponsive to fluid replacement and vasopressive measures, administer supplemental steroids.
- Communicate with the patient at the end of the appointment and within 4 hours postoperatively to determine whether features of weak pulse, hypotension, dyspnea, myalgias, arthralgia, ileus, and fever are present. Signs and symptoms of adrenal crisis dictate transport to a hospital for emergency care.

tion when oral maxillofacial surgical procedures are planned.

Additional measures are recommended to minimize the risk of adrenal crisis associated with surgical stress. Surgery should be scheduled in the morning when cortisol levels are highest. Proper stress reduction should be provided because anxiety increases cortisol demand. Nitrous oxide–oxygen inhalation and benzodiazepine sedation[8,52] are helpful in minimizing stress and reducing cortisol demand.[33] In contrast, reversal of and recovery from general anesthesia and extubation, and not the trauma of surgery itself, are major determinants of secretion of ACTH, cortisol, and epinephrine.[52,53] Thus, general anesthesia increases glucocorticoid demand for these patients. Barbiturates also should be used cautiously because these drugs enhance the metabolism of cortisol and reduce blood levels of cortisol.[29,37,54] In addition, inhibitors of corticosteroid production (e.g., ketoconazole metyrapone, aminoglutethimide) should be discontinued at least 24 hours before surgery with the consent of the patient's physician.

Surgeries that last longer than 1 hour are more stressful than shorter surgeries and should be performed with consideration of the need for steroid supplementation. Blood and fluid volume loss exacerbate hypotension and increase the risk of adrenal insufficiency–like symptoms. Thus, methods of reducing blood loss should be used. Patients who take anticoagulants are at increased risk for postsurgical bleeding and hypotension. In addition, inadequate pain control during the postoperative period increases the risk of adrenal crisis. Clinicians should provide good postoperative pain control by providing long-acting local anesthetics (e.g., bupivacaine) at the end of the procedure.

Monitoring of blood pressure throughout the procedure is critical for recognition of the development of an adrenal crisis. During surgery, blood pressure should be evaluated at 5-minute intervals and before the patient leaves the office. A systolic blood pressure below 100 mm Hg or a diastolic pressure at or below 60 mm Hg represents hypotension. The diagnosis of hypotension dictates that the clinician must take corrective action. This would include proper patient positioning (i.e., head lower than feet), fluid replacement, administration of vasopressors, and evaluation for signs of adrenal dysfunction versus hypoglycemia. Immediate treatment during an adrenal crisis consists of the administration of 100 mg of hydrocortisone or 4 mg dexamethasone IV and immediate transportation to a medical facility.

Treatment Planning Modifications

Dental treatment of a patient with undiagnosed and untreated adrenal insufficiency should be delayed until the patient has been medically stabilized. Otherwise, treatment modifications are not required for patients with medically stable adrenal disorders.

Oral Complications and Manifestations

In primary adrenal insufficiency, diffuse or focal brown macular pigmentation of the oral mucous membranes is a common finding (see Figure 16-6). Pigmentation of sun-exposed skin often follows the appearance of oral pigmentation. Patients with secondary adrenal insufficiency may be prone to delayed healing and may have increased susceptibility to infection.

REFERENCES

1. Schimmer BP, Parker KL. Adrenocorticotropic hormone; adrenocortical steroids and their synthetic analogs: Inhibitors of the synthesis and actions of adrenocortical hormones. In Brunton LL, et al (eds). Goodman and Gilman's The Pharmacologic Basis of Therapeutics, 11th ed. New York, McGraw-Hill, 2006.
2. Guyton AC, Hall JE. Textbook of Medical Physiology, 10th ed. Philadelphia, WB Saunders, 2000.
3. Genuth SM. The adrenal glands. In Physiology, 5th ed. Philadelphia, Elsevier, 2004.
4. Stewart PM. The adrenal cortex. In Larsen PR, Kronenberg HM, Melmed S, Polonsky KS (eds). Williams Textbook of Endocrinology, 10th ed. Philadelphia, WB Saunders, 2003.
5. Chernow B, Alexander HR, Smallridge IIC, et al. Hormonal responses to graded surgical stress. Arch Intern Med 1987;147:1273-1278.
6. Kehlet H. Clinical course and hypothalamic-pituitary-adrenocortical function in glucocorticoid-treated surgical patients. Copenhagen, 1976, FADL's Forlag.
7. Kehlet H, Binder C. Adrenocortical function and clinical course during and after surgery in unsupplemented glucocorticoid-treated patients. Br J Anaesth 1973;45:1043-1048.
8. Jerjes W, Jerjes WK, Swinson B, et al. Midazolam in the reduction of surgical stress: A randomized clinical trial. Oral Surg Oral Med Oral Pathol 2005;100:564-570.
9. George JM, Reier CE, Lanese RR, Rower M. Morphine anesthesia blocks cortisol and growth hormone response to surgical stress in humans. J Clin Endocrinol Metab 1974;38:736-741.
10. Raff H, Norton AJ, Flemma RJ, Findling JW. Inhibition of the adrenocorticotropin response to surgery in humans: Interactions between dexamethasone and fentanyl. J Clin Endocrinol Metab 1987;65:295-298.
11. Gersema L, Baker K. Use of corticosteroids in oral surgery. J Oral Maxillofac Surg 1992;50:270-277.
12. Kaufman E, Heling I, Rotstein I, et al. Intraligamentary injection of slow-release methylprednisolone for the prevention of pain after endodontic treatment. Oral Surg Oral Med Oral Pathol 1994;77:651-654.
13. Loriaux DL, McDonald WJ. Adrenal insufficiency. In Degroot LJ (ed). Endocrinology, 3rd ed, vol 2. Philadelphia, WB Saunders, 1995.
14. Al-Elq AH, Al-Saeed HH. Endocrinopathies in patients with thalassemias. Saudi Med J 2004;25:1347-1351.
15. Schlaghecke R, Kornely E, Santen RT, Ridderskamp P. The effect of long-term glucocorticoid therapy on pituitary-adrenal responses to exogenous corticotropin-releasing hormone. N Engl J Med 1992;326:226-230.

16. Coskey RJ. Adverse effects of corticosteroids. I. Topical and intralesional. Clin Dermatol 1986;4:155-160.

17. Patel L, Clayton PE, Addison GM, et al. Adrenal function following topical steroid treatment in children with atopic dermatitis. Br J Dermatol 1995;132:950-955.

18. Plemons JM, Rees TD, Zachariah NY. Absorption of a topical steroid and evaluation of adrenal suppression in patients with erosive lichen planus. Oral Surg 1990; 69:688-693.

19. Hanania NA, Chapman KR, Kesten S. Adverse effects of inhaled corticosteroids. Am J Med 1995;98:196-208.

20. Maxwell DL. Adverse effects of inhaled corticosteroids. Biomed Pharmacother 1990;44:421-427.

21. Toogood JH, Jennings B, Baskerville J, Lefcoe NM. Personal observations on the use of inhaled corticosteroid drugs for chronic asthma. Eur J Respir Dis 1984; 65:321-338.

22. Glick M. Glucocorticosteroid replacement therapy: A literature review and suggested replacement therapy. Oral Surg 1989;67:614-620.

23. Williams GH, Dluky RG. Diseases of the adrenal cortex. In Kasper DL, et al (eds). Harrison's Principles of Internal Medicine, 16th ed. New York, McGraw-Hill, 2005.

24. Findling JW, Raff H. Screening and diagnosis of Cushing's syndrome. Endocrinol Metab Clin North Am 2005;34:385-402.

25. Bethune JE. The diagnosis and treatment of adrenal insufficiency. In Degroot LJ, et al (eds). Endocrinology, 2nd ed, vol 2. Philadelphia, WB Saunders, 1989.

26. Shapiro R, Carroll PB, Tzakis AG, et al. Adrenal reserve in renal transplant recipients with cyclosporine, azathioprine, and prednisone immunosuppression. Transplantation 1990;49:1011-1013.

27. Fraser CG, Preuss FS, Bigford WD. Adrenal atrophy and irreversible shock associated with cortisone therapy. JAMA 1952;149:1542-1543.

28. Lewis L, Robinson RF, Yee J, et al. Fatal adrenal cortical insufficiency precipitated by surgery during prolonged continuous cortisone treatment. Ann Intern Med 1953; 39:116-126.

29. Parnell AG. Adrenal crisis and the dental surgeon. Br Dent J 1964;116:294-298.

30. Salem M, Tainsh RE Jr, Bromberg J, et al. Perioperative glucocorticoid coverage: A reassessment 42 years after emergence of a problem. Ann Surg 1994;4:416-425.

31. Miller CS, Dembo JB, Falace DA, Kaplan AL. Salivary cortisol response to dental treatment of varying stress. Oral Surg Oral Med Oral Pathol Oral Radiol Endod 1995;79:436-441.

32. Banks P. The adreno-cortical response to oral surgery. Br J Oral Surg 1970;8:32-44.

33. Thomasson B. Studies on the Content of 17-Hydroxy-corticosteroid and Its Diurnal Rhythm in the Plasma of Surgical Patients. Turku, Finland, Mercators Tryckeri Helsingfors, 1959.

34. Jasani MK, Freeman PA, Boyle JA, et al. Cardiovascular and plasma cortisol responses to surgery in corticosteroid-treated RA patients. Acta Rheumatol Scand 1968;14: 65-70.

35. Jasani MK, Freeman P, Boyle J, et al. Studies of the rise in plasma 11-hydroxycorticosteroids (11-OHCS) in

36. Lehtinen A-M, Hovorka J, Widholm O. Modification of aspects of the endocrine response to tracheal intubation by lignocaine, halothane and thiopentone. Br J Anaesth 1984;56:239-245.

37. Oyama T, Takiguchi M, Aoki N, Kudo T. Adrenocortical function related to thiopental-nitrous oxide-oxygen anesthesia and surgery in man. Anesth Analges Curr Res 1971;50:727-731.

38. Bromberg JS, Baliga P, Cofer JB, et al. Stress steroids are not required for patients receiving a renal allograft and undergoing operation. J Am Coll Surg 1995;180: 532-536.

39. Friedman RJ, Schiff CF, Bromberg JS. Use of supplemental steroids in patients having orthopaedic operations. J Bone Joint Surg Am 1995;77:1801-1806.

40. Plumpton FS, Besser GM, Cole PV. Corticosteroid treatment and surgery. 2. The management of steroid cover. Anesthesia 1969;24:12-18.

41. Singh N, Gayowski T, Marino IR, Schlichtig R. Acute adrenal insufficiency in critically ill liver transplant recipients. Transplantation 1995;59:1744-1745.

42. Costedoat-Chalumeau N, Amoura Z, Aymard G, et al. Potentiation of vitamin K antagonists by high-dose intravenous methylprednisolone. Ann Intern Med 2000; 132:631-635.

43. Miller CS, Little JW, Falace DA. Supplemental corticosteroids for dental patients with adrenal insufficiency: Reconsideration of the problem. J Am Dent Assoc 2001;132:1570-1579.

44. Shannon IL, Isbell G, Prigmore J, Hester JW. Stress in dental patients. II. The serum free 17-hydroxycortico-steroid response in routinely appointed patients undergoing simple exodontias. Oral Surg Oral Med Oral Pathol 1970;15:1142-1146.

45. Ziccardi VB, Abubaker AO, Sotereanos GC, Patterson GT. Maxillofacial considerations in orthotopic liver transplantation. Oral Surg Oral Med Oral Pathol 1991;71:21-26.

46. Ziccardi VB, Abubaker AO, Sotereanos GC, Patterson GT. Precipitation of an Addisonian crisis during dental surgery: Recognition and management. Compendium 1992;13:518,520,522-524.

47. Ziccardi VB. Personal communication, 2000.

48. Broutsas MG, Seldin R. Adrenal crisis after tooth extractions in an adrenalectomized patient: Report of case. J Oral Surg 1972;30:301-302.

49. Cawson RA, James J. Adrenal crisis in a dental patient having systemic corticosteroids. Br J Oral Surg 1973; 10:305-309.

50. Schietler LE, Tucker WM, Christian DG. Adrenal insufficiency: Report of a case. Spec Care Dent 1984;4: 22-24.

51. Glowniak JV, Loriaux DL. A double-blind study of perioperative steroid requirements in secondary adrenal insufficiency. Surgery 1997;121:123-129.

52. Hempenstall PD, Campbell JP, Bajurnow AT, et al. Cardiovascular, biochemical, and hormonal responses to intravenous sedation with local analgesia versus general

anesthesia in patients undergoing oral surgery. J Oral Maxillofac Surg 1986;44:441-446.

53. Udelsman R, Norton JA, Jelenich SE, et al. Responses of the hypothalamic-pituitary-adrenal and renin-angiotensin axes and the sympathetic system during controlled surgical and anesthetic stress. J Clin Endocrinol Metab 1987;64:986-994.

54. Siker SE, Lipschitz E, Klein R. The effect of preanesthetic medications on the blood level of 17-hydroxycorticosteroids. Ann Surg 1956;143:88.

Thyroid Diseases (Hyperthyroidism, Hypothyroidism, Thyroiditis, and Neoplastic Disease)

CHAPTER 17

The patient with thyroid disease is of concern to the dentist from several aspects. The dentist may detect early signs and symptoms of thyroid disease and may refer the patient for medical evaluation and treatment. In some cases, this may be lifesaving, whereas in others, quality of life can be improved and complications of certain thyroid disorders avoided.

In this chapter, emphasis is placed on disorders involving hyperfunction of the gland (hyperthyroidism or thyrotoxicosis), hypofunction of the gland (hypothyroidism or myxedema or cretinism), thyroiditis, and the detection of lesions that may be cancerous (Table 17-1). The standard abbreviations used for thyroid gland function and terminologies are defined in Box 17-1. In an average dental practice, an estimated 20 to 150 patients will have a thyroid disorder.

THYROID GLAND

LOCATION

The thyroid gland, which is located in the anterior portion of the neck just below and bilateral to the thyroid cartilage, develops from the thyroglossal duct and portions of the ultimobranchial body (Figure 17-1).[1,2] It consists of two lateral lobes connected by an isthmus. The right lobe is normally larger than the left,[3] and in some individuals, a superior portion of glandular tissue, or a pyramidal lobe, can be identified. Thyroid tissue may be found anywhere along the path of the thyroglossal duct, from its origin (midline posterior portion of the tongue) to its termination (thyroid gland, in the neck).[1] In rare cases, the entire thyroid is found in the anterior mediastinal compartment; however, in most individuals, remnants of the duct atrophy and disappear.[1,2] The thyroglossal duct passes through the region of the developing hyoid bone, and remnants of the duct may become enclosed or surrounded by bone.[1,3] Ectopic thyroid tissue may secrete thyroid hormones or may become cystic (Figure 17-2) or neoplastic.[4] In a few individuals, the only functional thyroid tissue is found in these ectopic locations.[2]

The parathyroid glands develop from the third and fourth pharyngeal pouches and become embedded within the thyroid gland.[1] Neural crest cells from the ultimobranchial branchial body give rise to thyroid medullary C cells that produce calcitonin, a calcium-lowering hormone.[1,2] These C cells are found throughout the thyroid gland.[1,2]

ENLARGEMENT AND NODULES OF THE THYROID GLAND

Generalized enlargement of the thyroid gland, referred to as a *goiter*, may be diffuse (Figure 17-3), nodular (Figure 17-4), functional, or nonfunctional.[1,2] On a functional basis, thyroid enlargement can be divided into three types: primary goiter (simple goiter and thyroid cancer), thyrostimulatory secondary goiters (Graves' disease, Hashimoto's thyroiditis, and congenital hereditary goiter), and thyroinvasive secondary goiters (Hashimoto's thyroiditis, subacute painful thyroiditis, Riedel's thyroiditis, and metastatic tumors to the thyroid). Simple goiter accounts for about 75% of all thyroid swellings.[1] Most of these goiters are nonfunctional and thus do not cause hyperthyroidism. The goiter of Graves' disease is associated with hyperthyroidism.[1,5] Hashimoto's thyroiditis leads to hypothyroidism and thyroid enlargement.[1] In contrast, patients with enlargement due to subacute thyroiditis develop a transient period of hyperthyroidism.[1] Nodules found in the thyroid may be hyperplastic nodules, adenomas, or carcinomas. Hyperplastic nodules and adenomas can be functional (Figure 17-5) or nonfunctional. Most carcinomas are nonfunctional.[1,6,7] Thyroid cancer most often presents as a single nodule but can present as multiple lesions or in rare cases can occur within a benign goiter.[1,6,7]

TABLE **17-1**
Thyroid Disorders

Thyroid Condition	Causes
Hyperthyroidism	Primary thyroid hyperfunction
	Graves' disease
	Toxic multinodular goiter
	Toxic adenoma
	Secondary thyroid hyperfunction
	Pituitary adenoma—TSH secretion
	Inappropriate TSH secretion (pituitary)
	Trophoblastic hCG secretion
	Without thyroid hyperfunction
	Hormonal leakage—Subacute thyroiditis
	Thyroid hormone use (factitia)
	Bovine thyroid in ground beef
	Metastatic thyroid cancer
	Iatrogenic (overdosage of thyroid hormone)
Hypothyroidism (cretinism, myxedema)	Primary atrophic hypothyroidism
	Insufficient amount of thyroid tissue
	Destruction of tissue by autoimmune process
	Hashimoto's thyroiditis (atrophic and goitrous)
	Graves' disease—End stage
	Destruction of tissue by iatrogenic procedures
	^{131}I therapy
	Surgical thyroidectomy
	External radiation to thyroid gland
	Destruction of tissue by infiltrative process
	Amyloidosis, lymphoma, scleroderma
	Defects of thyroid hormone biosynthesis
	Congenital enzyme defects
	Congenital mutations in TSH receptor
	Iodine deficiency of excess
	Drug induced: Thionamides, lithium, others
	Agenesis or dysplasia
	Secondary hypothyroidism
	Pituitary
	Panhypopituitarism (neoplasm, radiation, surgery)
	Isolated TSH deficiency
	Hypothalamic
	Congenital
	Infection
	Infiltration (sarcoidosis, granulomas)
	Transient hypothyroidism
	Silent and subacute thyroiditis
	Thyroxine withdrawal
	Generalized resistance to thyroid hormone
Thyroiditis	Acute suppurative
	Subacute painful
	Subacute painless
	Hashimoto's
	Chronic fibrosing (Riedel's)
Thyroid neoplasms	Adenomas
	Carcinomas
	Others

TSH, Thyroid-stimulating hormone; hCG, human chorionic gonadotropin.

BOX 17-1

Standard Abbreviations Used for Thyroid Gland Function and Terminology	
T_4	Thyroxine
T_3	Triiodothyronine
rT_3	Reverse triiodothyronine
TSH	Thyroid-stimulating hormone
TRH	Thyrotropin-releasing hormone
TT_4	Total thyroxine
TT_3	Total triiodothyronine
FT_3	Free triiodothyronine
FT_4	Free thyroxine
T_3U	Triiodothyronine uptake
FT_4I	Free thyroxine index
FT_3I	Free triiodothyronine index
TTG	Thyroid globulin
TBG	Thyroid-binding globulin
TTR	Transthyretin
TBA	Thyroid-binding albumin

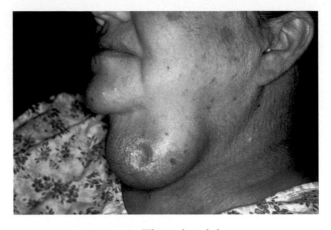

Figure 17-2. Thyroglossal duct cyst.

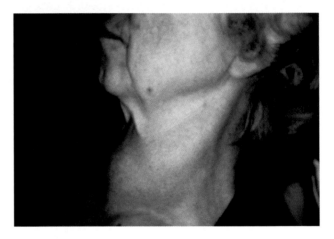

Figure 17-3. Diffuse enlargement of the thyroid gland due to Graves' disease (goiter).

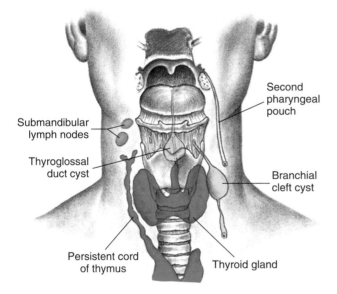

Figure 17-1. Thyroglossal duct cyst and branchial cleft cyst development. (From Seidel HM, Ball JW, Dains JE, Benedict GW. Mosby's Guide to Physical Examination, 6th ed. St. Louis, Mosby, 2006.)

FUNCTION OF THE THYROID GLAND

The thyroid gland secretes three hormones: thyroxine (T_4), triiodothyronine (T_3), and calcitonin.[2] Thyroid hormone influences the growth and maturation of tissues, cell respiration, and total energy expenditure. This hormone is involved in the turnover of essentially all substances, vitamins, and hormones.[2] Some thyroid hormone actions take place at the level of the mitochondria to influence oxidative metabolism, or at the level of the plasma membrane and endoplasmic reticulum to influence the activity of Ca^{2+}-ATPase (calcium/adenosine triphosphatase), as well as the transcellular flux of substrates and cations.[1,2]

Calcitonin is involved, along with parathyroid hormone and vitamin D, in regulating serum calcium and phosphorous levels and skeletal remodeling. (This hormone and its actions are considered further in Chapter 13.) T_4 and T_3 are hormones that affect metabolic processes throughout the body and are involved with oxygen use.[1,2]

Epidemiology

Incidence and Prevalence. Low iodine intake is associated with an increased prevalence of thyrotoxicosis (hyperthyroidism) in general. However, high iodine intake is associated with an increased prevalence of Graves' disease. In all, 60% to 80% of all cases of thyrotoxicosis are caused by Graves' disease. Populations with a lower percentage of cases caused by Graves' disease have a lower iodine intake, and those with a high iodine intake have a higher prevalence of Graves' disease. Graves' disease occurs in up to 2% of women, in whom it is only one-tenth as frequent as in men. Graves' disease is rare before adolescence; it usually occurs when the individual is between 20 and 50 years of age, and it does occur in the elderly.[1,8,9]

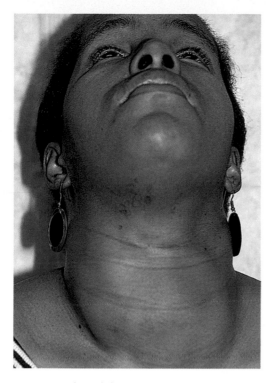

Figure 17-4. Multinodular goiter. (From Swartz MH. Textbook of Physical Diagnosis: History and Examination, 5th ed. Philadelphia, Saunders, 2006.)

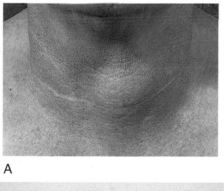

A

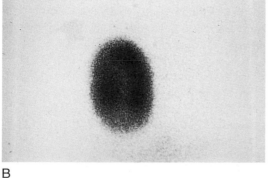

B

Figure 17-5. Toxic adenoma of the thyroid gland causing hyperthyroidism **(A).** Toxic adenoma in the right thyroid demonstrated with the use of Tc-pertechnetate scanning **(B).** (From Forbes CD, Jackson WF. Color Atlas and Text of Clinical Medicine, 3rd ed. Edinburgh, Mosby Ltd., 2003.)

Congenital hypothyroidism occurs in about 1 in 4000 newborns. A few cases may be transient, but the vast majority are permanent. Most cases (80% to 85%) are due to thyroid gland dysgenesis, and developmental abnormalities are twice as common in girls. The annual incidence rate of autoimmune hypothyroidism is 4 per 1000 women and 1 per 1000 men. It is more common in certain populations such as the Japanese because of genetic factors and long-term exposure to a high-iodine diet. Prevalence increases with age, and mean age at diagnosis is 60 years. Subclinical hypothyroidism is diagnosed in 6% to 8% of women (10% in women over 60 years of age) and 3% of men.[1,8,10]

Acute suppurative thyroiditis, which is rare, is due to suppurative (usually bacterial) infection of the thyroid. Subacute painful thyroiditis (most likely of viral origin) has a peak incidence at 30 to 50 years, and women are affected three times more often than men. It accounts for 5% of all medical consultations for thyroid disease. Subacute painless thyroiditis is not rare and occurs in patients with underlying autoimmune thyroid disease. It is reported in up to 5% of women 3 to 6 months after pregnancy and is then called *postpartum thyroiditis*. In all, 80% of cases of the sporadic type affect women between the ages of 30 and 40 years. Focal chronic thyroiditis (Hashimoto's thyroiditis) is present in 20% to 40% of euthyroid autopsy cases. Chronic thyroiditis (Hashimoto's thyroiditis) results in serologic evidence of autoimmunity with the presence of thyroid peroxidase (TPO) antibodies. These antibodies are 4 to 10 times more common in "healthy" women than in men. Hashimoto's thyroiditis is the most prevalent form of thyroid autoimmune disease, affecting 3% to 4% of the population in the United States. It is 3 times more common in women and is most frequently diagnosed between the third and fifth decades of life. Riedel's thyroiditis is a rare form of chronic thyroiditis that typically occurs in middle-aged women.[1,8]

Thyroid nodules can be found in about 5% of the adult population in the United States.[1,7,11] The frequency of cancer in solitary thyroid nodules has been reported to be about 1% to 5%.[1,7,11] Thyroid cancer is identified in 8% to 20% of surgically removed thyroid nodules. Among autopsy studies of thyroid nodules, about 3% are cancerous.[6,12] The estimated number of cases of thyroid cancer in the United States in the year 2000 was 18,400, with 75% of cases occurring in women.[13] In 2001, 19,500 cases of thyroid cancer were reported, and about 1200 deaths were due to thyroid cancer.[14] In 2002, 10 cases of thyroid cancer were reported per 100,000 population.[11] Over the past 10 years, the incidence of thyroid cancer has increased at a rate of 5% per year.[11] The overall incidence of thyroid cancer is increasing worldwide.[15] More papillary carcinomas have been reported, along with fewer follicular and anaplastic carcinomas.[15]

Differentiated cancers can occur at any age, but the median age at diagnosis is 45 to 50 years.[15] Anaplastic cancers are usually diagnosed in individuals 60 years of

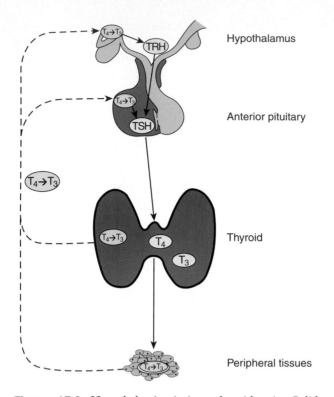

Figure 17-6. Hypothalamic-pituitary-thyroid axis. Solid lines correspond to stimulatory effects, and dotted lines depict inhibitory effects. Conversion of T4 to T3 in the pituitary and the hypothalamus is mediated via 5′-deiodinase type II. This event is also important throughout the central nervous system, thyroid, and muscle. 5′-deiodinase type I (propylthiouracil-sensitive) plays a major role in liver, kidney, and thyroid. TRH, thyrotropin-releasing hormone; TSH, thyroid-stimulating hormone. (Redrawn from DeGroot LJ, Jameson JL. Endocrinology, 5th ed, vol 2. Philadelphia, Saunders, 2006.)

age or older.[15] Differentiated cancers are 3 times more common in women than in men.[15] However, beyond the age of 50, the incidence is the same for men and for women.[15] Thyroid cancer, which is uncommon in children, accounts for only about 3% of pediatric malignancies.[16]

Thyroid cancer is more common in areas with endemic goiter.[15] The greatest incidence of thyroid cancer is found in Hawaii and the Polynesian Islands.[15] Poland has one of the lowest incidences of thyroid cancer worldwide.[15]

Pathophysiology and Etiology

Blood levels of T_4 and T_3 are controlled through a servofeedback mechanism mediated by the hypothalamic-pituitary-thyroid axis (Figure 17-6). Increased or decreased metabolic demand appears to be the main modifier of the system. Drugs, illness, thyroid disease, and pituitary disorders may affect control of this balance.[1,2,17,18] Studies also show that age has some effect on the system.

Under normal conditions, thyrotropin-releasing hormone (TRH) is released by the hypothalamus in response to external stimuli (e.g., stress, illness, metabolic

demand, low levels of T_3 and, to a lesser degree, T_4). TRH stimulates the pituitary to release thyroid-stimulating hormone (TSH), which causes the thyroid gland to secrete T_4 and T_3.[1,2] T_4 and T_3 also have a direct influence on the pituitary. High levels turn off the release of TSH, and low levels turn it on. In the blood, T_4 and T_3 are almost entirely bound to plasma proteins.

Binding plasma proteins consist of thyroxine-binding globulin (TBG), transthyretin, and thyroid-binding albumin (TBA). Small amounts of T_3 and T_4 are bound to high-density lipoproteins.[2] The most important thyroid hormone–binding serum protein is TBG, which binds about 70% of T_4 and 75% to 80% of T_3.[2] Only 0.02% to 0.03% of free thyroxine (FT$_4$) and about 0.3% of free triidothyroxine (FT$_3$) is found in plasma.[1,2]

Low T_4 and T_3 plasma levels often are found in ill and medicated older persons. Protein abnormalities can affect total T_4 and T_3 levels. Illness can reduce the conversion of T_4 to T_3 and can increase reverse T_3 (rT_3). Drugs and illness also can affect free levels of T_4 and T_3. The main age-related change seen in much older individuals is a fall in T_3 due to the reduced peripheral conversion of T_4 to T_3.[19]

Antibodies to various structures within the thyroid are associated with autoimmune diseases of the thyroid. Graves' disease and Hashimoto's thyroiditis have such an association. Three autoantibodies are most often involved in autoimmune thyroid disease: TSH receptor antibodies (TSHRAb), thyroid peroxidase antibodies (TPOAb), and thyroglobulin antibodies (TgAb).[20] TSHRAb are not found in the general population but are found in 80% to 95% of patients with Graves' disease and in 10% to 20% of those with autoimmune thyroiditis. Most TSHRAb in Graves' disease are stimulating antibodies, which stimulate the release of thyroid hormone. However, blocking antibodies to the TSH receptor (TSHR-blocking Ab) also are found, which block the release of thyroid hormone. The ratio of these TSH receptor antibodies determines the clinical status of the patient with regard to function of the thyroid gland.[8,9,20]

TgAb are found in about 10% to 20% of the general population. These antibodies are found in 50% to 70% of patients with Graves' disease and in 80% to 90% of those with autoimmune thyroiditis.[8,9,20,21] TPOAb are found in 8% to 27% of the general population. About 50% to 80% of patients with Graves' disease have these antibodies. TPOAb are found in 90% to 100% of patients with autoimmune thyroiditis.[8,9,20,21]

Laboratory Tests

Direct tests of thyroid function involve the administration of radioactive iodine. Measurement of thyroid radioactive iodine uptake (RAIU) is the most common of these tests. [131]I has been used for this test, but ^{123}I is preferred because it exposes the patient to a lower radiation dose. RAIU, which is measured 24 hours after administration of the isotope, varies inversely with plasma iodide concentration and directly with the functional state of the thyroid. In the United States, normal 24-hour RAIU is 10% to 30%. RAIU discriminates poorly between normal and hypothyroid states. Values above the normal range usually indicate thyroid hyperfunction.[22,23]

Several tests are available that measure thyroid hormone concentration and binding in blood. Highly specific and sensitive radioimmunoassays are used to measure serum T_4 and T_3 concentrations and rarely to measure rT_3 concentration. The normal range for T_4 is 64-154 nmol/L (5-12 mg/dL). The normal range for T_3 is 1.2-2.9 nmol/L (80-190 mg/dL).[23] Elevated levels usually indicate hyperthyroidism, and lower levels usually indicate hypothyroidism. Free hormone levels usually correlate better with the metabolic state than do total hormone levels. Indirect assays are used to estimate the free T_4 level.[22,23]

Measurement of basal serum TSH concentration is useful in the diagnosis of hyperthyroidism and hypothyroidism. Very sensitive methods, such as immunoradiometric or chemiluminescent techniques, are now available to measure serum TSH. The normal range for TSH is 0.5-4.5 mμ/L. In cases of hyperthyroidism, the TSH level is almost always low or nondetectable. Higher levels indicate hypothyroidism, and lower levels signify hyperthyroidism.[22,23]

Other tests used in selected cases include the TSH stimulation test, the T_3 suppression test, and radioassay techniques for measuring TSHRAb, TSHR-blocking Ab, TPOAb, and TgAb.[22,23] A thyroid scan is commonly used to localize thyroid nodules and to locate functional ectopic thyroid tissue. ^{123}I or ^{99}Tc (technetium) is injected, and a scanner localizes areas of radioactive concentration. This technique allows for the identification of nodules 1 cm or larger. When a pinhole thyroid scan is used, 2- to 3-mm lesions may be detected.[21,24]

Ultrasonography may be used to detect thyroid lesions. Nodules 1 to 2 mm in size can be identified. This technique also is used to distinguish solid from cystic lesions, to measure the gland, and to guide needles for aspiration of cysts or for biopsy of thyroid masses. Computed tomography (CT) and magnetic resonance imaging (MRI) are expensive procedures that are helpful mainly in the postoperative management of patients with thyroid cancer. They are used for the preoperative evaluation of larger lesions of the thyroid (greater than 3 cm) that extend beyond the gland into adjacent tissues.[21,24]

THYROTOXICOSIS (HYPERTHYROIDISM)
Etiology, Pathophysiology, and Complications

The term *thyrotoxicosis* refers to an excess of T_4 and T_3 in the bloodstream. This excess may be caused by ectopic thyroid tissue, Graves' disease, multinodular goiter, thyroid adenoma, subacute thyroiditis (painful and painless), ingestion of thyroid hormone (thyrotoxicosis factitia), food-containing thyroid hormone, or pituitary disease involving the anterior portion of the gland (Table 17-2). In this section, the signs and symptoms, laboratory tests, treatment, and dental considerations for the patient with Graves' disease are considered in detail and serve as a model for other conditions that can result in similar clinical manifestations. It should be emphasized that multinodular goiter, ectopic thyroid tissue, and neoplastic causes of hyperthyroidism are rare compared with toxic goiter.[8,9,22]

The basic cause of Graves' disease is not understood, but an immunoglobulin or a family of immunoglobulins directed against the TSH receptor mediate thyroid stimulation. These include TSHRAb and TSHR-blocking Ab, which inhibit the binding of TSH to its receptors. Graves' disease is now considered to be an autoimmune disease.[8,9,22] The chief risk factor for Graves' disease is female gender, in part because of modulation of the autoimmune response by estrogen. This disorder is much more common in women (10:1) and may manifest during puberty, pregnancy, or menopause (see Figure 17-3). Emotional stress such as severe fright or separation from loved ones has been reported to be associated with its onset. The disease may occur in a cyclic pattern and may then "burn itself out" or continue in an active state.[8,9,21]

Clinical Presentation

Signs and Symptoms. Direct and indirect effects of excessive thyroid hormones contribute to the clinical picture in Graves' disease. The most common symptoms are nervousness, fatigue, rapid heartbeat or palpitations, heat intolerance, and weight loss (see Table 17-2). These symptoms are reported in more than 50% of all patients in whom the disease is diagnosed. With increasing age, weight loss and decreased appetite become more common, and irritability and heat intolerance are less common. Atrial fibrillation is rare in patients younger than 50 years old but occurs in approximately 20% of older patients. The patient's skin is warm and moist and the complexion rosy; the patient may blush readily. Palmar erythema may be present, profuse sweating is common, and excessive melanin pigmentation of the skin occurs in many patients; however, pigmentation of the oral mucosa has not been reported. In addition, the patient's hair becomes fine and friable, and the nails soften.[8,9,21,25]

Graves' ophthalmopathy, which is identified in approximately 50% of patients, is characterized by edema and inflammation of the extraocular muscles, as well as an increase in orbital connective tissue and fat. Ophthalmopathy is an organ-specific autoimmune process that is strongly linked to Graves' hyperthyroidism. Although hyperthyroidism may be successfully treated, ophthalmopathy often produces the greatest long-term disability for patients with this disease. Figures 17-7 and 17-8 demonstrate the signs associated with ophthalmopathy (eyelid retraction, proptosis, periorbital edema, chemosis, and bilateral exophthalmos). This disease may progress to visual loss through exposure keratopathy or compressive optic neuropathy.[25,26]

Most thyrotoxic patients show eye signs not related to the ophthalmopathy of Graves' disease. These signs (i.e., stare with widened palpebral fissures, infrequent

TABLE 17-2
Clinical Findings and Treatment of Thyroid Disorders

Condition	Signs and Symptoms	Laboratory Test	Treatment
Hyperthyroidism	**Skeletal**—Osteoporosis **Cardiovascular**—Palpitations, tachycardia, arrhythmias, cardiomegaly, congestive heart failure, angina, myocardial infarction **Gastrointestinal**—Weight loss, increased appetite, pernicious anemia **Central nervous system**—Anxiety, restlessness, sleep disturbances, emotional lability, impaired concentration, weakness, tremors (hands, fingers, tongue) **Skin**—Erythema, thin fine hair, areas of alopecia, soft nails **Eyes**—Retraction of upper lid, exophthalmos, corneal ulceration, ocular muscle weakness **Other**—Increased risk for diabetes, decreased serum cholesterol level, increased risk for thrombocytopenia, sweating	T_4—Elevated T_3—Elevated **TSH**—None or greatly decreased **TBG**—Elevated Normal range: T_4 5-12 mg/dL or 64-154 nmol/L T_3 80-190 mg/dL or 1.2-2.9 nmol/L TSH 0.5-4.5 mμ/L TBG 1-25 mg/mL	Antithyroid agents: Propylthiouracil Carbimazole Methimazole Radioactive iodine Subtotal thyroidectomy Propranolol—Rx for the adrenergic component in thyrotoxicosis (sweating, tremor, and tachycardia)
Hypothyroidism	**Musculoskeletal**—Arthritis, muscle cramps **Cardiovascular**—Shortness of breath, hypertension, slow pulse **Gastrointestinal**—Constipation, anorexia, nausea or vomiting **Central nervous system**—Mental and physical slowness, sleepiness, headache **General**—Dry, thick skin/dry hair, fatigue, edema (puffy hand, face, eyes), cold intolerance, hoarseness, weight gain	T_4—Decreased T_3—Decreased **TSH**—Elevated **TBG**—Decreased	Sodium levothyroxine (Synthroid, LT_4) or sodium liothyronine (Leotrix, LT_3)
Thyroiditis	**Hashimoto's**—Rubbery, firm goiter, hypothyroidism develops later	Later in disease, T_4, T_3, and TBG are decreased, TSH becomes elevated	Thyroid hormone, surgery in rare cases (compression of vital tissues)
	Subacute painful—Enlarged, firm, tender gland, with pain that may radiate to ear or jaw	Hyperthyroid returning to euthyroid status	Aspirin, prednisone, propranolol for symptoms of thyrotoxicosis
	Acute suppurative—Pain, tenderness in gland, fever, malaise	Euthyroid	Incision and drainage, appropriate antibiotics
	Chronic fibrosing—Hard, fixed, enlarged gland	Usually remains euthyroid; hypothyroid status may occur	Usually none, surgery if vital tissues compressed, thyroid hormone
	Subacute painless—Firm, nontender, enlarged gland	Hyperthyroid for 5 to 6 months returning to euthyroid status	Propranolol for symptoms of thyrotoxicosis

T_4, Thyroxine; T_3, triiodothyronine; TSH, thyroid-stimulating hormone; TBG, thyroxine-binding globulin.

blinking, lid lag, jerky movements of the lids, and failure to wrinkle the brow on upward gaze) result from sympathetic overstimulation and usually clear when thyrotoxicosis is corrected.[25,26]

Another complication, which is found in about 1% to 2% of patients with Graves' disease, is dermopathy (Figure 17-9). In focal areas of the skin, hyaluronic acid and chondroitin sulfate concentrations in the dermis are increased. This may occur as the result of lymphokine activation of fibroblasts. Accumulation causes compression of the dermal lymphatics and nonpitting edema. Early lesions contain a lymphocytic infiltrate. Nodular and plaque formation may occur in chronic lesions. These lesions are most common over the anterolateral aspects of the shin. Patients with dermopathy almost always develop severe ophthalmopathy.[8,9,25]

Increased metabolic activity caused by excessive hormone secretion increases circulatory demand; increased stroke volume and heart rate often develop in addition to widened pulse pressure, resulting in palpitations. Supraventricular cardiac dysrhythmias develop in many patients. Congestive heart failure may occur and often is somewhat resistant to the effects of digitalis. Patients with untreated or incompletely treated thyro-

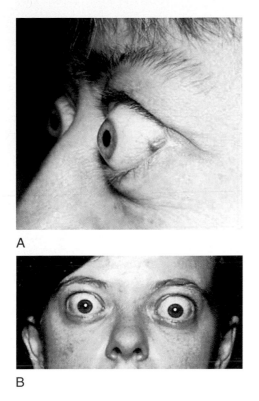

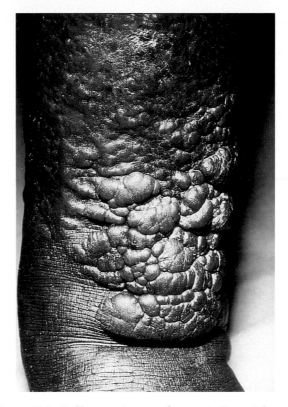

Figure 17-7. A, Lid retraction is a common eye sign in Graves' disease. It is recognized when the sclera is visible between the lower margin of the upper lid and the cornea. **B,** Proptosis in Graves' disease results from enlargement of muscles and fat within the orbit as a result of mucopolysaccharide infiltration. (**A,** From Goldman L, Ausiello D. Cecil Textbook of Medicine, 22nd ed. Philadelphia, Saunders, 2004. **B,** From Seidel H. Mosby's Guide to Physical Examination, 4th ed. St. Louis, Mosby, 1999.)

Figure 17-9. Infiltrative dermopathy seen in Graves' disease. Hyperpigmented, nonpitting induration of the skin of the legs is usually found in the pretibial area (pretibial myxedema). Lesions are firm, and clear edges can be seen. (From Larsen PR, et al. Williams Textbook of Endocrinology, 10th ed. Philadelphia, Saunders, 2003.)

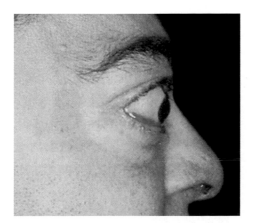

Figure 17-8. Exophthalmos of Graves' disease can be unilateral or bilateral and causes protrusion of the globe forward; it results from an increase in volume of the orbital contents. (From Seidel HM, Ball JW, Dains JE, Benedict GW. Mosby's Guide to Physical Examination, 6th ed. St. Louis, Mosby, 2006.)

toxicosis are highly sensitive to the actions of epinephrine or other pressor amines, and these agents must not be administered to them; however, once the patient has been well managed from a medical standpoint, administration of these agents can be resumed.[8,9,25]

Dyspnea not related to the effects of congestive heart failure may occur in some patients. The respiratory effect is caused by reduction in vital capacity related to weakness of the respiratory muscles. Weight loss, even with an increased appetite, is a common finding in younger patients. Stools are poorly formed, and the frequency of bowel movements is increased. Anorexia, nausea, and vomiting are rare but, when they occur, may be forerunners of thyroid storm. Gastric ulcers are rare in patients with thyrotoxicosis. Many of these patients have achlorhydria, and about 3% develop pernicious anemia.[8,9,25]

Thyrotoxic patients tend to be nervous and often show a great deal of emotional lability, losing their tempers easily and crying often; severe psychiatric reactions may occur. Patients cannot sit still and are always moving. A tremor of the hands and tongue, along with lightly closed eyelids, is often present; in addition, generalized muscle weakness may lead to easy fatigability (see Table 17-2).[8,9,25]

The effect of excessive thyroid hormone production on mineral metabolism is complex and not well understood. The role of calcitonin only complicates the problem. However, thyrotoxic patients have increased excretion of calcium and phosphorus into their urine and stools, and radiographs show increased bone loss. Hypercalcemia occurs sometimes, but serum levels of alkaline phosphatase usually are normal. The bone age of young individuals is advanced (see Chapter 13).[8,9,25] Glucose intolerance and, rarely, diabetes mellitus may accompany hyperthyroidism. Those with diabetes who are treated with insulin require an increased dose of insulin if they develop Graves' disease.[25]

Individual red blood cells (RBCs) in patients with thyrotoxicosis are usually normal; however, the RBC mass is enlarged to carry the additional oxygen needed for increased metabolic activities. In addition to the increased total numbers of circulating RBCs, the bone marrow reveals erythroid hyperplasia, and requirements for vitamin B_{12} and folic acid are increased. White blood cell (WBC) count may be decreased because of a reduction in the number of neutrophils, whereas the absolute number of eosinophils may be increased. Enlargement of the spleen and lymph nodes occurs in some patients. The platelets and the clotting mechanism usually are normal, but thrombocytopenia has been reported.[8,9,25] Increased metabolic activity associated with thyrotoxicosis leads to increased secretion and breakdown of cortisol; however, serum levels remain within normal limits.

Laboratory Findings. T_4, T_3, TBG, and TSH tests can be used to screen for hyperthyroidism. However, current practice is to screen patients suspected of being hyperthyroid with use of the TSH serum level and to measure or estimate the free T_4 concentration. A low TSH level and a high free T_4 concentration are classically combined in hyperthyroidism (see Table 17-2). Some patients are hyperthyroid with a low TSH level and a normal free T_4 concentration, but they have an elevated free T_3 level. A few patients have normal or elevated TSH and high free T_4. These patients have a TSH-secreting pituitary adenoma or thyroid hormone resistance syndrome.[8,9,25]

Medical Management

Treatment of patients with thyrotoxicosis may involve antithyroid agents that block hormone synthesis, iodides, radioactive iodine, or subtotal thyroidectomy (Box 17-2). The antithyroid agents most often used in the United States are propylthiouracil and methimazole, both of which inhibit thyroid peroxidase and thus the synthesis of thyroid hormone. Propylthiouracil also blocks extrathyroidal deiodination of T_4 to T_3. Carbimazole is the drug of choice in the United Kingdom, and propylthiouracil is the drug of choice in North America. The usual length of treatment ranges up to 18 months. When the "block-replace" regimen is used, no added benefit occurs after 6 months of treatment with an antithyroid agent that is given along with T_4. Antithyroid agents may cause a mild leukopenia, but drug therapy is not stopped unless the WBC count is more severely depressed. In rare cases, agranulocytosis may occur (Box 17-3). If sore throat, fever, and/or mouth ulcers develop, most physicians advise the patient to stop the antithyroid medication and have a WBC count performed.[8,9,25]

Radioactive iodine is the preferred initial treatment for patients with Graves' disease in North America. It is

---

BOX 17-2

Treatment of Thyrotoxicosis[8,9]

SEVERE THYROTOXICOSIS
- Propylthiouracil (PTU)—100 to 150 mg q 8 hr; in some cases, PTU 200 to 300 mg q 6 hr.
- With improvement of symptoms, PTU dosage can be lowered. As improvement continues, can switch to once-a-day methimazole (MMI) 2.5 to 5.0 mg once per day for 12 to 24 months.

MODERATE THYROTOXICOSIS
- Start with methimazole (MMI), which is 10 times more potent than propylthiouracil (PTU). MMI also has longer intrathyroid residence time but does not inhibit conversion of T_4 to T_3 as PTU does. Start with 20 to 30 mg once per day. Within 4 to 6 weeks, the patient will be euthyroid. Reduce dosage to 2.5 to 5 mg per day for 12 to 24 months.
- No surgical complications or radiation hazards. Frequent relapses occur, and drug adverse effects may complicate treatment.

^{131}I THERAPY
- This is the most common form of treatment in the United States. Antithyroid drugs are given to make the patient euthyroid. The antithyroid medicine is stopped for 3 to 5 days, and then 6000 to 8000 rad dosage of ^{131}I is given. More than 80% of patients are cured with a single dose of ^{131}I.
- Delayed control of thyrotoxicosis, lower efficacy in large goiters, easy to perform, no surgical risk, questionable radiation hazard, and transient worsening of preexisting eye disease. Rare, mild, and transient adverse effects.

SURGERY
- Patient must be euthyroid before surgery is performed. This is usually done with one of the antithyroid drugs (PTU or MMI). Subtotal thyroidectomy is the treatment of choice.
- Hypoparathyroidism occurs in 0.9% to 2.0% of cases, and recurrent laryngeal nerve damage is found in 0.1% to 2.0% of cases. Bleeding, infection, and anesthetic complications may occur. Results in fast correction of thyrotoxicosis but at a high cost.

---

contraindicated in pregnant women and in those who are breast feeding. Radioactive iodine can induce or worsen ophthalmopathy, particularly in smokers. Weetman[25] recommends antithyroid drug treatment for patients younger than 50 years of age at their first episode of Graves' disease; radioactive iodine is recommended for those older than 50 years of age. The main adverse effect associated with radioactive iodine treatment is hypothyroidism. The incidence of cancer is unchanged or slightly reduced in patients treated with radioactive iodine, but the risk of death from thyroid cancer and possibly other cancers is slightly increased. Patients with severe hyperthyroidism should be treated with an antithyroid drug for 4 to 8 weeks before radioactive iodine therapy is initiated.

BOX 17-3

Adverse Effects of Antithyroid Drugs (propylthiouracil and methimazole)

SEVERE
- Agranulocytosis (0.2%-0.5%)
- Only rare cases reported
  - Hepatitis (can result in hepatic failure)
  - Cholestatic jaundice
  - Thrombocytopenia
  - Hypoprothrombinemia
  - Aplastic anemia
  - Lupus-like syndrome with vasculitis
  - Hypoglycemia (insulin antibodies)

LESS SEVERE
Most frequent (1% to 5%)
- Rash
- Urticaria
- Arthralgia
- Decreased leukocyte level (drop in white blood cell count by 2-3 × 10³)
- Fever
Less frequent
- Arthritis
- Diarrhea
- Decreased sense of taste

From Dillmann WH. The thyroid. In Goldman L, Ausiello D (eds). Cecil Textbook of Medicine, 22nd ed. Philadelphia, Saunders, 2004.

This approach reduces the slight risk of thyrotoxic crisis if radioactive iodine was given initially.[25]

Subtotal thyroidectomy is preferred by some patients with a large goiter and is indicated in those with a coexistent thyroid nodule whose nature is unclear. The patient is first treated with an antithyroid drug until euthyroidism is achieved. Then, inorganic iodide is administered for 7 days before surgery. In major centers, hyperthyroidism is cured in more than 98% of cases, and low rates of operative complications are reported. Postoperative hypothyroidism is a complication of more frequent surgical treatment as near-total thyroidectomy is approached.[25]

If exophthalmos is present, it follows a course independent of the therapeutic metabolic response to antithyroid treatment modalities and usually is irreversible. The adrenergic component in thyrotoxicosis can be managed with beta-adrenergic antagonists such as propranolol. Propranolol alleviates adrenergic manifestations such as sweating, tremor, and tachycardia.[8,9,25]

A delay in recovery of the hypothalamus-pituitary-thyroid axis occurs in most patients with Graves' disease who are treated with ^{131}I and manifests as a transient central hypothyroid phase.[8,9,25] The clinical presentations of thyroid disorders often are subtle in older adults and may be confused with "normal" aging. To avoid delay in diagnosis, some authors recommend routine TSH screening in the primary care practice of all patients age 60 and older. When hyperthyroidism is caused by Graves'

disease, symptomatic therapy with a beta blocker or antithyroid drugs is initiated and is followed by definitive thyroid ablation with radioiodine.[8,27]

Management of Thyrotoxic Crisis. Patients with thyrotoxicosis who are untreated or incompletely treated may develop thyrotoxic crisis, a serious but fortunately rare complication of abrupt onset that may occur at any age. Thyrotoxic crisis occurs in less than 1% of patients hospitalized for thyrotoxicosis.[8,9] Most patients who develop thyrotoxic crisis have a goiter, wide pulse pressure, eye signs, and a long history of thyrotoxicosis. Precipitating factors include infection, trauma, surgical emergencies, and operations. Early symptoms of extreme restlessness, nausea, vomiting, and abdominal pain have been reported; fever, profuse sweating, marked tachycardia, cardiac arrhythmias, pulmonary edema, and congestive heart failure soon develop. The patient appears to be in a stupor, and coma may follow. Severe hypotension develops, and death may occur. These reactions appear to be associated, at least in part, with adrenal cortical insufficiency.[8,9,28] Immediate treatment for the patient in thyrotoxic crisis consists of large doses of antithyroid drugs (200 mg of propylthiouracil), potassium iodide, propranolol (to antagonize the adrenergic component), hydrocortisone (100 to 300 mg), dexamethasone (2 mg orally every 6 hours, to inhibit release of hormone from the gland and peripheral conversion of T_4 to T_3), intravenous (IV) glucose solution, vitamin B complex, wet packs, fans, and ice packs. Cardiopulmonary resuscitation is sometimes needed.[8,9]

Thyrotoxicosis Factitia. Thyrotoxicosis that results from the ingestion, usually chronic, of excessive quantities of thyroid hormone is referred to as *thyrotoxicosis factitia*. This condition usually occurs in patients with underlying psychiatric disease, or in individuals such as nurses and physicians who have access to the medication. In other cases, patients may not be aware that they are taking the hormone or some other thyroid active agent (iodocasein) as part of a weight reduction program.[1,8]

Other Causes of Thyrotoxicosis. Thyrotoxicosis has been reported to occur in patients who ate ground beef containing large quantities of bovine thyroid. Functional ectopic thyroid tissue can cause thyrotoxicosis. Thyroid tissue may be found in ovarian teratomas (struma ovarii). In rare cases, hyperfunctioning metastases of follicular carcinoma may cause thyrotoxicosis.[1,8]

THYROIDITIS

DEFINITION

Thyroiditis is inflammation of the thyroid gland that may occur for a variety of reasons. Five types of thyroiditis have been identified: Hashimoto's, subacute painful, subacute painless, acute suppurative, and Riedel's (Table 17-3).[1,29] Radiation therapy and drugs such as lithium,

TABLE 17-3
Thyroiditis

Type	Cause	Clinical Findings	Thyroid Function	Treatment
Hashimoto's thyroiditis	Autoimmune related	Goiter—Moderate in size, rubbery, firm	Euthyroid early Few with transient hyperfunction Most develop hypothyroidism	Thyroid hormone In rare cases, compression of vital tissues; surgery is indicated
Subacute painful thyroiditis	Viral infection	Enlarged, firm, tender gland with pain that may radiate to ear, jaw, or occipital region	Hyperthyroidism with return to euthyroid state	Aspirin Prednisone Propranolol for symptoms of thyrotoxicosis
Acute suppurative thyroiditis	Bacterial infection	Pain and tenderness in gland, fever, malaise, skin over the gland warm and red	Euthyroid	Incision and drainage, appropriate antibiotics
Chronic fibrosing thyroiditis (Riedel's)	Unknown	Enlarged gland that is stony, hard, and fixed to surrounding tissues	Usually remain euthyroid, but in some cases, hypothyroidism may occur	Usually none; if vital structures are compressed, surgery is indicated; thyroid hormone
Subacute painless thyroiditis	Not established but related to autoimmune thyroid disease	Enlarged gland that is firm and nontender; may occur in women 5 to 6 months after pregnancy	Hyperthyroidism for 5 to 6 months, then return to euthyroid state	Propranolol for symptoms of thyrotoxicosis

interlukin-2, interferons, and amiodarone also may cause thyroiditis iatrogenically.[1,8] In some cases (subacute painful thyroiditis), inflammation may result from transient hyperthyroidism due to follicle damage and release of preformed thyroid hormone.[29] In contrast, Hashimoto's thyroiditis (chronic autoimmune thyroiditis) results in progressive hypothyroidism.[1,29]

Hashimoto's thyroiditis is the most common cause of primary hypothyroidism in the United States.[29] It is an autoimmune disorder that presents most often as an asymptomatic diffuse goiter. High titers of circulating thyroid autoantibodies and thyroid antigen–specific T cells are observed. It usually affects young and middle-aged women. However, it can occur in men (3 to 4 times more common in women) and persons at any age.[29] By the time the diagnosis has been established, most patients are hypothyroid. A family history of Hashimoto's thyroiditis or other autoimmune thyroid disorders is often reported.[1,29] It may be associated with other autoimmune diseases such as pernicious anemia and type 1 diabetes mellitus. Early in the disease course, the thyroid becomes enlarged and firm and may have a nodular consistency. Late in the disease, the gland may become atrophied and no longer palpable.[1,29]

Subacute painful thyroiditis is uncommon and often follows upper respiratory tract viral infection.[29] Patients often present with an enlarged, painful, tender gland with signs and symptoms of hyperthyroidism.[1,29] A marked increase in erythrocyte sedimentation rate (ESR) occurs,

along with a low radioactive iodine uptake. A brief phase of hypothyroidism may be noted. Recovery of normal thyroid function can be expected. Subacute painful thyroiditis has a peak incidence in the third through fifth decades. It is about 4 times more common in women than in men.[1,29]

Subacute painless thyroiditis is another autoimmune disorder.[29] Patients usually present with signs and symptoms of hyperthyroidism without thyroid pain or tenderness or fever. ESR is normal, and radioactive iodine uptake is abnormally low. Transient hypothyroidism may occur before normal thyroid function returns. This condition occurs in up to 5% of postpartum women and is more common among women than men.[1,8]

Acute suppurative thyroiditis is caused by microbial infection of the thyroid.[29] Patients present with severe neck pain, fever, focal thyroid tenderness, and erythema of the overlying skin. This acute infection may require fine-needle aspiration and culture for determination of the appropriate antibiotic therapy.[1,29] It may also require surgical incision and drainage if an abscess is present. This condition is rare and, when found, is seen in immunocompromised individuals and those with penetrating neck wounds.[29]

Riedel's thyroiditis is fibrous infiltration of the thyroid gland of unknown origin.[29] This condition, which may represent a variant of Hashimoto's thyroiditis, presents as a slowly enlarging stony neck mass, which may extend beyond the thyroid gland. As it gets larger, it may cause compressive symptoms such as dyspnea, dysphagia, hoarseness, and a sensation of choking.[1,8] The clinical course is unpredictable, and patients may require surgery. It occurs predominantly in women and may eventually lead to clinically significant hypothyroidism.[29]

Because Hashimoto's thyroiditis is the most common type of thyroiditis, it is discussed in greater detail in the following section.

CLINICAL PRESENTATION—HASHIMOTO'S THYROIDITIS

Signs and Symptoms

Goiter is the hallmark of Hashimoto's thyroiditis (Figure 17-10). The goiter is usually moderate in size and rubbery firm in consistency, and it moves freely with swallowing. In cases of sudden onset, the clinical picture suggests subacute thyroiditis with pain. Patients may be euthyroid during early phases of the disease. Over time, most patients develop hypothyroidism as lymphocytes replace functioning tissue. In a few cases, the patient develops transient hyperthyroidism, to be followed later by hypothyroidism.[1,8,30]

Laboratory Findings

Early in the course of Hashimoto's disease, the patient is euthyroid, but TSH level is often slightly increased and RAIU is increased. Increasing titers of autoantibodies are found early in the disease; anti-TPOAb and anti-TgAb are the most important from a clinical standpoint. Fine-needle biopsy of the thyroid gland at this stage helps to confirm the diagnosis. Later in the disease, serum levels

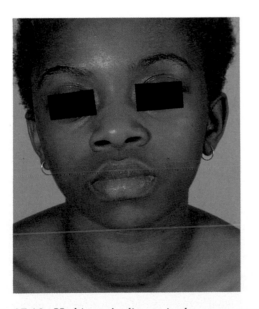

Figure 17-10. Hashimoto's disease is the most common cause of goitrous hypothyroidism. The initial lesion consists of a diffuse goiter, and the patient may be euthyroid. Later, the patient becomes hypothyroid, and very late in the disease, the gland atrophies. (From Forbes CD, Jackson WF. Color Atlas and Text of Clinical Medicine, 3rd ed. Edinburgh, Mosby Ltd., 2003.)

of T_4 and T_3 start to fall, and the level of TSH continues to increase. At this stage the patient is hypothyroid and requires treatment with hormone replacement.[1,8,30]

MEDICAL MANAGEMENT

Early in the course of the disease, patients with Hashimoto's disease have small goiters, are asymptomatic, and do not require treatment. Patients with larger goiters and/or mild hypothyroidism are treated with thyroid hormone replacement. More recent goiters usually respond by decreasing in size. Long-standing goiters often do not respond to hormone treatment. In these cases, unsightly goiters or those compressing adjacent structures may be treated by surgery after an attempt has been made to decrease their size with the use of hormone therapy. Patients with full-blown hypothyroidism require hormone replacement treatment.[1,8,30]

HYPOTHYROIDISM

DEFINITION

The causes of hypothyroidism can be divided into four main categories (see Table 17-1):
1. Primary atrophic
2. Secondary
3. Transient
4. Generalized resistance to thyroid hormone

Ninety-five percent of cases of hypothyroidism are caused by primary and goitrous hypothyroidism. Acquired impairment of thyroid function affects about 2% of adult women and about 0.1% to 0.2% of adult men in North America.[1,8,10] Hypothyroidism may be congenital or acquired. Permanent hypothyroidism occurs about once in every 4000 live births in the United States. Transient hypothyroidism occurs in 1% to 2% of newborns. Most infants with permanent congenital hypothyroidism have thyroid dysgenesis, that is, ectopic, hypoplastic, or thyroid agenesis. The acquired form may follow thyroid gland or pituitary gland failure. Radiation of the thyroid gland (radioactive iodine), surgical removal, and excessive anti-thyroid drug therapy are responsible for most of these cases of hypothyroidism; however, some occur with no identifiable cause.[1,8,10]

Subclinical hypothyroidism is a prevalent condition that is characterized by elevated serum TSH concentration and normal serum FT_4 and T_3.[10] It occurs in about 75 of 1000 women and in 28 of 1000 men. It is most common in women and older adults and is caused by chronic autoimmune thyroiditis, postpartum thyroiditis, ^{131}I therapy, thyroidectomy, and antithyroid drugs. Subclinical hypothyroidism caused by chronic autoimmune thyroiditis has a predictable clinical course.[10] Spontaneous return to normal TSH values occurs in 5% to 6% of cases. Progression to overt hypothyroidism occurs at a rate of about 5% per year. Some patients report fatigue, weight gain, poor memory, poor ability to concentrate, and depressed feelings.[10]

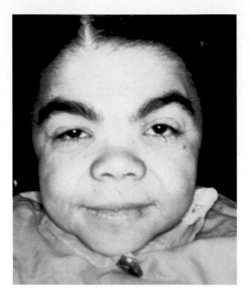

Figure 17-11. Cretinism.

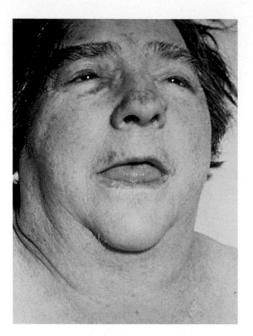

Figure 17-12. Clinical hypothyroidism showing characteristic nonpitting edematous changes in the skin of the face. Note the dry, puffy facial appearance and coarse hair. (Courtesy Paul W. Ladenson, MD, The Johns Hopkins University and Hospital, Baltimore, Md. In Seidel HM, Ball JW, Dains JE, Benedict GW. Mosby's Guide to Physical Examination, 6th ed. St. Louis, Mosby, 2006.)

CLINICAL PRESENTATION
Signs and Symptoms

Neonatal cretinism is characterized by dwarfism; being overweight; a broad, flat nose; wide-set eyes; thick lips; a large, protruding tongue; poor muscle tone; pale skin; stubby hands; retarded bone age; delayed eruption of teeth; malocclusions; a hoarse cry; an umbilical hernia; and mental retardation. All of these characteristics can be prevented by early detection and treatment (Figure 17-11).

The onset of hypothyroidism in older children and adults (Figure 17-12) is characterized by a dull expression; puffy eyelids; alopecia of the outer third of the eyebrows; palmar yellowing; dry, rough skin; dry, brittle, and coarse hair; increased size of the tongue; slowing of physical and mental activity; slurred, hoarse speech; anemia; constipation; increased sensitivity to cold; increased capillary fragility; weight gain; muscle weakness; and deafness (see Table 17-2).

Accumulation of subcutaneous fluid (intracellularly and extracellularly) is usually not as pronounced in patients with pituitary myxedema as it is in those with primary (thyroid) myxedema. Serum cholesterol levels are elevated in thyroid myxedema and are closer to normal values in patients with pituitary myxedema. Untreated patients with severe myxedema may develop hypothermic coma that usually is fatal. T_4, T_3, TBG, and TSH tests are used to screen for hypothyroidism.[1,8,10] Results that indicate hypothyroidism are shown in Table 17-2.

MEDICAL MANAGEMENT

Patients with hypothyroidism are treated with synthetic preparations that contain sodium levothyroxine (T_4) (Box 17-4) or sodium liothyronine (T_3).[5] The usual prescription for patients of ideal body weight for sodium levothyroxine is 75 µg to 100 µg per day. Hypothyroid patients receiving warfarin or other related oral anticoagulants when treated with T_4 may have further prolongation of prothrombin time and could be at risk for hemorrhage. In addition, hypothyroid patients with diabetes with a decreased need for insulin or sulfonylureas may become hyperglycemic when treated with T_4.[1,8,10]

Congestive heart failure may occur in severe cases of myxedema. Levothyroxine therapy can correct this condition (Figure 17-13). The treatment of hypothyroid children with levothyroxine can result in a dramatic reversal of the signs and symptoms (Figure 17-14).

Patients with untreated hypothyroidism are sensitive to the actions of narcotics, barbiturates, and tranquilizers, so these drugs must be used with caution. Smoking can worsen the disease. Stressful situations such as cold, operations, infections, or trauma may precipitate a hypothyroid (myxedema) coma in untreated hypothyroid patients. External manifestations of severe myxedema, bradycardia, and severe hypotension are just about always present. Myxedematous coma occurs most often in severely hypothyroid elderly patients. It is more common during the winter months and has a high mortality rate. Hypothyroid coma is treated by parenteral levothyroxine (T_4) and steroids; the patient is covered to conserve heat and artificial respiration. Hypertonic saline and glucose may be required to alleviate dilutional hyponatremia and occasional hypoglycemia.[1,8,10]

THYROID CANCER

DEFINITION

Three main histologic types of thyroid cancer have been identified: differentiated, medullary, and anaplastic. Differentiated cancers are subdivided into papillary, follicular, mixed, and Hürthle cell carcinomas (Table 17-4).[1,15,31,32] In addition, primary lymphomas may occur in the thyroid gland, and other cancers may metastasize to the thyroid. An important neoplastic syndrome, multiple endocrine neoplasia type 2 (MEN2), involves the thyroid gland. MEN2 consists of medullary thyroid carcinoma (MTC), pheochromocytoma in 50% of cases, and parathyroid hyperplasia/adenoma in 10% to 35% of cases.[15] In rare cases, cancer from other locations may metastasize to the thyroid gland.[33] The kidney is the most common site of origin for metastasis to the thyroid gland; other sites include cancer of the breast and lung, and melanoma.[15,33]

Etiology and Clinical Findings

External radiation to the cervical region is believed to be one cause of thyroid cancer.[15] Children who underwent thymic irradiation are at increased risk. Teenagers with acne that was treated by irradiation also are at greater risk for thyroid cancer. Patients with other types of neck cancer treated with irradiation have increased risk for thyroid cancer.[15] Children exposed to radioactive fallout from Chernobyl have been found to have an increase in thyroid cancer.[15] External medical diagnostic radiation can add to the risk for thyroid cancer; however, dental radiographs do not appear to add to this burden.[15] Radiation to the thyroid from internal sources and diagnostic

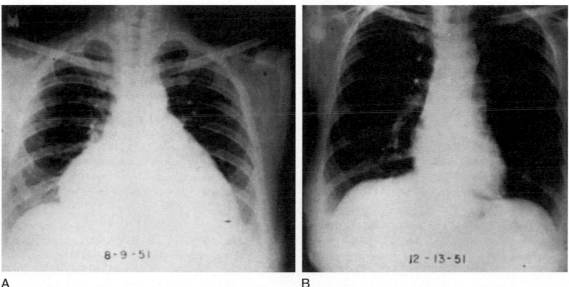

A   B

Figure 17-13. Radiography showing enlargement of the heart in a patient with heart failure due to myxedema **(A).** Same patient after treatment with thyroid hormone; radiography shows a return to normal heart size **(B).** (From Larsen PR, Kronenberg HM, Melmed S, Polonsky KS. Williams Textbook of Endocrinology, 10th ed. Philadelphia, Saunders, 2003.)

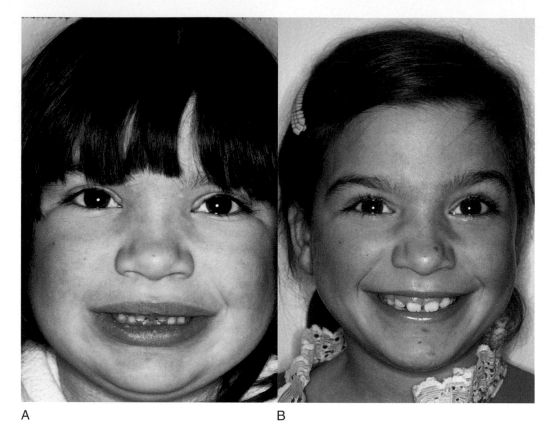

A   B

Figure 17-14. A, A 9-year-old girl with severe hypothyroidism. **B,** The same girl 1 year after treatment with thyroid hormone replacement. Note the return to normal facial appearance. (From Neville B, Damm DD, Allen CM, et al. Oral and Maxillofacial Pathology, 2nd ed. Philadelphia, Saunders, 2002.)

TABLE 17-4
Classification of Thyroid Cancer[14,31,32]

Type	Frequency, %	10-Year Survival, %
Differentiated—Papillary	75-80	>90
Differentiated—Follicular	8-10	80
Differentiated—Hürthle cell	1	70
Anaplastic	1-5	<2
Medullary	5-8	40
Lymphoma	1-5	45
Metastases to the thyroid	<1	Determined by primary

or therapeutic doses of ^{131}I have not been associated with an increased risk for thyroid cancer.[15] Environmental factors such as high dietary iodine intake (papillary cancer) or a very low iodine intake (follicular cancer) appear to increase the risk for thyroid cancer.[15] A genetic factor is suggested by an increased risk for thyroid cancer when a family member has had thyroid cancer or MEN2.[1,15,31,32] In some cases, no risk factor can be identified.

On physical examination, manifestations of thyroid malignancy, including firm consistency of the nodule, irregular shape, fixation to underlying or overlying tissue, and suspicious regional lymphadenopathy, should be sought.[1,15,31,32] Signs and symptoms that may be associated with thyroid cancer include a lump in the region of the gland, a dominant nodule(s) in multinodular goiter, a hard painless mass, fixation to adjacent structures, enlarged cervical lymph nodes, a rapidly growing mass, hemoptysis, dysphagia, stridor, and hoarseness.[15]

DIAGNOSIS

The cornerstone for the diagnosis of thyroid nodules is ultrasonography and fine-needle aspiration biopsy (FNAB).[1,15,31,32] Clinically detected nodules should be evaluated through ultrasonography. Hypoechoic nodules should be submitted for FNAB (Figure 17-15). Ultrasound also can be used in cases of nonpalpable nodules, to guide FNAB. Overall rates of sensitivity and specificity for FNAB of thyroid nodules exceed 90% in iodine-sufficient areas.[1,15,31,32] FNAB is easy to perform and safe; very few complications have been reported.[15] The key to accuracy of the technique is to obtain an adequate specimen. This usually involves obtaining three to six aspirations that will contain at least five or six groups of 10 to 15 well-preserved cells.[15] Nodules found in patients living in iodine-deficient areas may require surgical removal before a diagnosis can be established.[15]

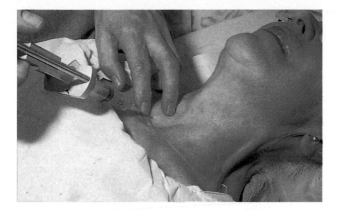

Figure 17-15. Fine-needle aspiration of a thyroid nodule is the investigation of choice in a patient with a solitary nodule of the thyroid. (From Forbes CD, Jackson WF. Color Atlas and Text of Clinical Medicine, 3rd ed. Edinburgh, Mosby Ltd., 2003.)

TREATMENT

For most papillary carcinomas, surgery is the indicated treatment.[1,15,31,32] Options include lobectomy and total thyroidectomy. The recurrence rate is higher for lobectomy, but complications are fewer.[15] Radioiodine ablation of residual thyroid tissue does not improve survival but does allow for interpretation of thyroglobulin levels.[15] Radioiodine ablation is useful in metastatic disease and locally invasive disease, and in cases where cervical lymph nodes cannot be resected.[15] Suppression of levothyroxine can be used to limit thyrotropin stimulation of tumor growth, but adverse effects may be difficult for the patient to deal with.[15]

Treatment of follicular carcinomas involves surgery, followed by radioiodine ablation and lifelong thyrotropin suppression through levothyroxine replacement therapy.[1,15,31,32] Initial surgery may consist of thyroid lobectomy or total thyroidectomy.[15] Other available options for minimally invasive disease include lobectomy and levothyroxine suppression of thyrotropin secretion alone; if cancer recurs, the rest of the thyroid is surgically removed, and radioiodine scanning for recurrence or radioiodine ablation of remaining thyroid tissue is performed.[15]

Hürthle cell cancers and medullary carcinomas are treated by total thyroidectomy with cervical lymph node dissection.[1,15,31,32] Patients with medullary carcinoma should undergo regular monitoring of serum calcitonin for evidence of recurrence.[15] The main objective of treatment for patients with anaplastic carcinomas is to control symptoms and relieve airway obstruction.[15] Any combination of surgery, external beam radiotherapy, and chemotherapy may be used. However, at best, these treatments occasionally may add several months to the life span.[15] External beam radiotherapy is used to manage bony pain caused by metastases.[15]

Complications associated with total or subtotal thyroidectomy are hypoparathyroidism, recurrent laryngeal nerve damage, hemorrhage, and general risks associated with surgery.[1,15,31,32] Complications of external beam radiotherapy include damage to the spinal cord, skin damage, and mucosal ulceration.[15] Complications associated with chemotherapy include nausea and vomiting, mucosal damage, hair loss, infection, and bleeding (see Chapter 26).[15]

PROGNOSIS

The best prognosis for differentiated cancers is based on age of the patient, metastases, and extent and size of the lesion. The best outlook is projected for young people with localized cancers that are smaller than 2 cm.[15] Overall 10-year survival rates for papillary carcinoma are 80% to 90%, follicular carcinoma 65% to 75%, and medullary carcinoma 60% to 70%.[15] Involvement of cervical nodes predicts recurrence in older patients (older than 45 years) but does not predict overall survival. Patients with distant metastases of a differentiated carcinoma have a long-term survival of 43%. The prognosis for anaplastic carcinoma is very poor, and 5-year survival is rare (see Table 17-4).[15]

DENTAL MANAGEMENT
Clinical Examination

Examination of the thyroid gland should be included as part of a head and neck examination performed by the dentist.[34,35] The anterior neck region may be scanned for indications of old surgical scars, the posterior dorsal region of the tongue should be examined for a nodule that could represent lingual thyroid tissue, and the area just superior and lateral to the thyroid cartilage should be palpated for the presence of a pyramidal lobe. Although difficult to detect, the normal thyroid gland can be palpated in many patients.[34] It may feel rubbery and may be more easily identified by having the patient swallow during the examination. As the patient swallows, the thyroid rises; lumps in the neck that may be associated with it also rise (move superiorly). Nodules in the midline area of the thyroglossal duct move upward with protrusion of the patient's tongue.[34]

An enlarged thyroid gland caused by hyperplasia (goiter) feels softer than the normal gland. Adenomas and carcinomas involving the gland are firmer on palpation and are usually seen as isolated swellings. Patients with Hashimoto's disease or Riedel's thyroiditis have a gland that on palpation is much firmer than the normal gland (see Table 17-4).[31]

If a diffuse enlargement of the thyroid is detected, auscultation should be used to examine for a systolic or continuous bruit that can be heard over the hyperactive gland of thyrotoxicosis or Graves' disease as a result of engorgement of the gland's vascular system.

MEDICAL CONSIDERATIONS
Thyrotoxicosis

The dentist should be aware of the clinical manifestations of thyrotoxicosis, so that undiagnosed or poorly treated

TABLE 17-5
Dental Management of the Patient With Thyroid Disease

Clinical Setting	Hyperthyroid	Hypothyroid
Detection of undiagnosed disease	Symptoms Signs Refer for medical Dx and Rx	Symptoms Signs Refer for medical Dx and Rx
Diagnosed disease	Determine original diagnosis and Rx Past treatment Current treatment Lack of signs and symptoms Presence of any complications	Original diagnosis and Rx Past treatment Current treatment Lack of signs and symptoms Presence of any complications
Untreated or poorly controlled	Avoid surgical procedures Treat any acute infection Avoid use of epinephrine or pressor amines	Avoid surgical procedures Treat oral infection Avoid central nervous system (CNS) depressants such as narcotics, barbiturates, etc.
Well controlled	Treat acute infection (avoid if possible) Treat chronic infection Implement normal procedures and management	Avoid oral infections Implement normal procedures and management
Medical crisis (rare)	Recognition and initial management of **thyrotoxic crisis** Seek medical aid Wet packs, ice packs Hydrocortisone (100-300 mg) Cardiopulmonary resuscitation Propylthiouracil Intravenous (IV) glucose solution	Recognition and initial management of **myxedema coma** Seek medical aid Cover to conserve heat Hydrocortisone (100-300 mg) Cardiopulmonary resuscitation Parental levothyroxine IV saline and glucose

disease can be detected and the patient referred for medical evaluation and treatment (Table 17-5; see also Table 17-2). By doing this, dentists may be able to help reduce the morbidity and mortality rates associated with thyrotoxicosis.[34,35]

Patients with untreated or poorly treated thyrotoxicosis are susceptible to developing an acute medical emergency called *thyrotoxic crisis*, which is another important reason for detection and referral. Symptoms include restlessness, fever, tachycardia, pulmonary edema, tremor, sweating, stupor, and finally, coma and death, if treatment is not provided. If a surgical procedure is performed on these patients, a crisis may then be precipitated. In addition, an acute oral infection could precipitate a crisis. If a crisis occurs, the dentist should be able to recognize what is happening, begin emergency treatment, and seek immediate medical assistance (see Table 17-5). The patient can be cooled with cold towels, given an injection of hydrocortisone (100 to 300 mg), and started on an IV infusion of hypertonic glucose (if equipment is available). Vital signs must be monitored, and cardiopulmonary resuscitation initiated, if necessary. Immediate medical assistance should be sought, and, when available, other measures such as antithyroid drugs and potassium iodide may be started.[8,9,34]

Although the role of chronic infection and thyrotoxicosis is unclear, these conditions should be treated, as in any other patient. Once the patient has been identified and referred for medical management, oral foci of infec-

tion can be treated. Patients with extensive dental caries or periodontal disease, or both, can be treated after medical management of the thyroid problem has been effected.

The use of epinephrine or other pressor amines (in local anesthetics or gingival retraction cords, or to control bleeding) must be avoided in the untreated or poorly treated thyrotoxic patient. However, the well-managed or euthyroid thyrotoxic patient presents no problem in this regard and may be given normal concentrations of these vasoconstrictors.[34] Care must be taken with patients who are being controlled with nonselective beta blockers. When epinephrine is given to these patients, it is possible that blood pressure can be increased through inhibition of the vasodilatory action of epinephrine attained through blocking of beta$_2$ receptors.[35] Clinical experience has shown that small amounts of epinephrine can be used safely in these patients. More concentrated preparations of epinephrine (retraction cords and those used to control bleeding) should be avoided (see Chapter 3).

Adverse reactions to propylthiouracil include agranulocytosis and leukopenia (Box 17-5). If these should occur, the patient is at risk for serious infection. The physician should monitor the patient for these adverse reactions. The dentist can consult with the patient's physician, or he or she can order a complete blood count to rule out the presence of these complications prior to undertaking surgical procedures. It has been reported that propylthiouracil can induce sialolith formation. This

---

BOX 17-5

Medical Problems of Concern to the Dentist in Treating a Patient With Undiagnosed or Poorly Controlled Thyroid Disease

HYPERTHYROIDISM
- Adverse interaction with epinephrine
- Life-threatening cardiac arrhythmias
- Congestive heart failure
- Complications of underlying cardiovascular pathologic conditions
- Thyrotoxic crisis can be precipitated by the following:
  - Infection
  - Surgical procedures

HYPOTHYROIDISM
- Exaggerated response to central nervous system (CNS) depressants
- Sedatives
- Narcotic analgesics
- Myxedematous coma can be precipitated by the following:
  - CNS depressants
  - Infection
  - Surgical procedures

---

drug also can increase the anticoagulant effects of warfarin. Aspirin and nonsteroidal anti-inflammatory drugs can increase the amount of circulating T_4 and make control of thyroid disease more difficult.[35]

Once the thyrotoxic patient is under good medical management, the dental treatment plan can proceed without alteration (see Table 17-5). If acute oral infection occurs, however, consultation with the patient's physician is recommended as part of the management program.[34] Box 17-5 lists the medical concerns the dentist should be aware of regarding the hyperthyroid patient.

Hypothyroidism

In general, the patient with mild symptoms (see Table 17-2) of untreated hypothyroidism is not in danger when receiving dental therapy. Central nervous system (CNS) depressants, sedatives, or narcotic analgesics may cause an exaggerated response in patients with mild to severe hypothyroidism (see Table 17-5). These drugs must be avoided in all patients with severe hypothyroidism and must be used with care (reduced dosage) in patients with mild hypothyroidism; however, a few patients with untreated severe symptoms of hypothyroidism may be in danger if dental treatment is rendered (see Box 17-5). This is particularly true of elderly patients with myxedema. A myxedematous coma can be precipitated by CNS depressants, surgical procedures, and infections; thus, once again, the major goal of the dentist is to detect these patients and refer them for medical management before any dental treatment is rendered (see Tables 17-2 and 17-5).[8,10,36] If myxedema coma should occur, the

dentist should call for medical aid; while waiting for this assistance, the dentist can inject 100 to 300 mg of hydrocortisone, cover the patient to conserve heat, and apply cardiopulmonary resuscitation (CPR) as indicated. Once medical aid becomes available, parental levothyroxine is administered, and IV hypertonic saline and glucose are given as needed.

Patients with less severe forms of hypothyroidism should be identified when possible, because the quality of their life can be greatly improved with medical treatment. In young individuals, permanent mental retardation can be avoided with early medical management. In addition, oral complications of delayed eruption of teeth, malocclusion, enlargement of the tongue, and skeletal retardation can be prevented through early detection and medical treatment.

Once the hypothyroid patient is under good medical care, no special problems in terms of dental management remain, except for the need to address malocclusion and enlarged tongue, if they are present.

Thyroid Cancer

Palpation and inspection of the thyroid gland should be included as part of the routine head and neck examination performed by the dentist. If thyroid enlargement is noted, even though the patient may appear euthyroid (normal thyroid function), a referral should be made for evaluation before dental treatment is rendered. A diffuse enlargement may be a simple goiter, subacute thyroiditis, or chronic thyroiditis. The patient may be hyperthyroid, hypothyroid, or euthyroid. Isolated nodules may turn out to be an adenoma or carcinoma. Growing nodules in diffusely enlarged glands or in glands with multinodular involvement may be the manifestation of thyroid carcinoma and must be evaluated by a physician.[37]

ORAL COMPLICATIONS AND MANIFESTATIONS

Thyrotoxicosis

Osteoporosis involving the alveolar bone may occur, and dental caries and periodontal disease appear rapidly in these patients. The teeth and jaws develop rapidly, and premature loss of deciduous teeth with early eruption of permanent teeth is common. Euthyroid infants of hyperthyroid mothers have been reported to have erupted teeth at birth. A few patients with thyrotoxicosis have been found to have a lingual "thyroid," consisting of thyroid tissue below the area of the foramen cecum.[34,35]

If the dentist detects a lingual tumor in a euthyroid patient, a physician should examine the patient before the mass is surgically removed (Figure 17-16). This usually is done with radioactive iodine scanning.[34,38]

Hypothyroidism

Infants with cretinism may present with thick lips, enlarged tongue, delayed eruption of teeth, and resulting malocclusion. The only specific oral change manifested

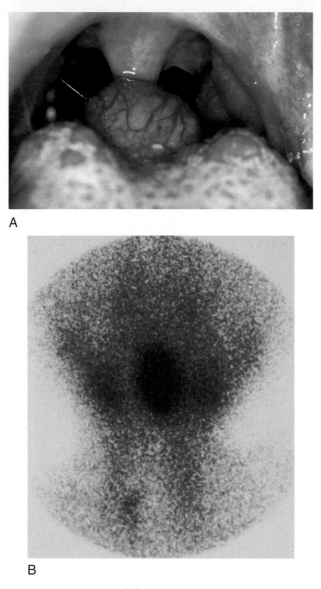

Figure 17-16. Lingual thyroid nodule in a 4-year-old girl **(A).** Thyroid scan of the lingual nodule **(B).** (From Neville BW, Damm DD, Allen CM, et al. Oral and Maxillofacial Pathology, 2nd ed. Philadelphia, Saunders, 2002.)

by adults with acquired hypothyroidism is an enlarged tongue.[36,38]

Thyroiditis

The pain associated with subacute painful thyroiditis may radiate to the ear, jaw, or occipital region. Hoarseness and dysphagia may occur. Patients may report palpitations, nervousness, and lassitude. On palpation, the thyroid is enlarged, firm, often nodular, and usually very tender.[36,39]

REFERENCES

1. Jameson JL, Weetman AP. Diseases of the thyroid gland. In Kasper DL, Braunwald E, Fauci AS, et al (eds). Harrison's Online Principles of Medicine, 16th ed. New York, McGraw-Hill, 2005, pp 2104-2127.

2. Larsen PR, Davies TF, Schlumberger M-J. Thyroid physiology and diagnostic evaluation of patients with thyroid disorders. In Larsen PR, Kronenberg HM, Melmed D, Polonsky KS (eds). Williams Textbook of Endocrinology, 10th ed. Philadelphia, Saunders, 2003, pp 331-365.

3. Mazzaferri EL. The thyroid. In Mazzaferri EL (ed). Endocrinology, 3rd ed. New York, Medical Examination Publishing, 1986.

4. Marinovic D, Garel C, Czernichow P, Leger J. Ultrasonographic assessment of the ectopic thyroid tissue in children with congenital hypothyroidism. Pediatr Radiol 2004;34:109-113.

5. Larsen PW, Davies TF. Hypothyroidism and thyroiditis. In Larsen PR, Kronenberg HM, Melmed D, Polonsky KS (eds). Williams Textbook of Endocrinology, 10th ed. Philadelphia, Saunders, 2003, pp 415-465.

6. Emerson CH. Thyroid nodules and goiter. In Greene H, Fincher RE, Johnson WP, et al (eds). Clinical Medicine, 2nd ed. St. Louis, Mosby, 1996, pp 259-262.

7. Kabongo ML, Jones RC, Scherger JE, et al. Thyroid Nodule. Philadelphia, Elsevier, 2004.

8. Dillmann WH. The thyroid. In Goldman L, Ausiello D (eds). Cecil Textbook of Medicine. Philadelphia, Saunders, 2004, pp 1391-1412.

9. Marino M, Chiovato L, Pinchera A. Graves' disease. In DeGroot LJ, Jameson JL (eds). Endocrinology, 5th ed. Philadelphia, Saunders (Elsevier), 2006, pp 1995-2029.

10. Wiersinga WM. Hypothyroidism and myxedema coma. In DeGroot LJ, Jameson JL (eds). Endocrinology, 5th ed. Philadelphia, Saunders (Elsevier), 2006, pp 2081-2101.

11. Pacini F, DeGroot LJ. Thyroid neoplasia, Thyroid Manager, updated Feb., 2006, accessed Jan. 22, 2007. Available at http://www.thyroidmanager.org.

12. Cooper DS. Solitary thyroid nodule. In Bardin CW (ed). Current Therapy in Endocrinology and Metabolism, 5th ed. St. Louis, Mosby, 1994, pp 102-104.

13. Greenlee R, Murray T, Bolden S, Wingo PA. Cancer statistics: 2000. CA Cancer J Clin 2000;50:7-33.

14. Schlurnberger M-J, Filetti S, Hay ID. Benign and malignant nodular thyroid disease. In Larsen PR, Kronenberg HM, Melmed D, Polonsky KS (eds). Williams Textbook of Endocrinology, 10th ed. Philadelphia, Saunders, 2003, pp 465-491.

15. Saver DF, Scherger JE, Pearson RL, et al. Thyroid Carcinoma. Philadelphia, Elsevier, 2004.

16. Skinner MA. Cancer of the thyroid gland in infants and children. Semin Pediatr Surg 2001;10:119-126.

17. Nickolai TF. The thyroid gland. In Rose LF, Kaye D (eds). Internal Medicine for Dentistry, 2nd ed. St. Louis, Mosby-Year Book, 1990, pp 997-1019.

18. Green MF. The endocrine system. In Pathy MSJ (ed). Principles and Practice of Geriatric Medicine, 2nd ed. New York, John Wiley & Sons, 1991, pp 1061-1122.

19. Germain DLS. Thyroid hormone metabolism. In DeGroot LJ, Jameson JL (eds). Endocrinology, 5th ed. Philadelphia, Saunders (Elsevier), 2006, pp 1861-1873.

20. Weetman AP. Autoimmune thyroid disease. In DeGroot LJ, Jameson JL (eds). Endocrinology, 5th ed. Philadelphia, Saunders (Elsevier), 2006, pp 1979-1995.

21. Reed Larson P, Davies TF, Hay ID. The thyroid gland. In Wilson JD, Foster DW, Kronenberg HM, Reed

Larson P (eds). Williams Textbook of Endocrinology, 9th ed. Philadelphia, WB Saunders, 1998, pp 389-515.

22. Wartofsky L. Diseases of the thyroid. In Fauci AS, Braunwald E, Isselbacher KJ, et al (eds). Harrison's Principles of Internal Medicine, 14th ed. New York, McGraw-Hill, 1998, pp 2012-2035.

23. Weiss RE, Wu SY, Refetoff S. Diagnostic tests of the thyroid. In DeGroot LJ, Jameson JL (eds). Endocrinology, 5th ed. Philadelphia, Saunders (Elsevier), 2006, pp 1899-1963.

24. Blum M. Thyroid imaging. In DeGroot LJ, Jameson JL (eds). Endocrinology, 5th ed. Philadelphia, Saunders (Elsevier), 2006, pp 1963-1979.

25. Weetman AP. Graves' disease. N Engl J Med 2000;343: 1236-1248.

26. Burch HB, Bahn RS. Graves' ophthalmopathy. In DeGroot LJ, Jameson JL (eds). Endocrinology, 5th ed. Philadelphia, Saunders (Elsevier), 2006, pp 2029-2043.

27. Hollenberg AN, Jameson JL. Mechanisms of thyroid hormone action. In DeGroot LJ, Jameson JL (eds). Endocrinology, 5th ed. Philadelphia, Saunders (Elsevier), 2006, pp 1873-1899.

28. Mazzaferri EL. Recognizing thyrotoxicosis. Hosp Pract (Off Ed) 1999;34:43-46,49-51,55-56 passim.

29. Saver DF, Pollak FF, McCartney C, et al. Thyroiditis. Philadelphia, Elsevier, 2004.

30. Amino M, Hidaka Y. Chronic (Hashimoto's) thyroiditis. In DeGroot LJ, Jameson JL (eds). Endocrinology, 5th ed. Philadelphia, Saunders (Elsevier), 2006, pp 2055-2069.

31. McHenry CR. Thyroid cancer. In Rakel RE, Bope ET, editors. Conn's Current Therapy, 58th ed, Philadelphia, Saunders, 2006. Available at http://home.mdconsult. com/thyroidcancer. Accessed Oct. 10, 2006.

32. Weigel RJ, Macdonald JS, Haller D. Cancer of the endocrine system. In Abeloff MD, Armitage JO, Niederhuber JE, et al (eds). Clinical Oncology, 3rd ed. London, Churchill Livingstone, 2004, pp 1612-1621.

33. Wood K, Vini L, Harmer C. Metastases to the thyroid gland: The Royal Marsden experience. Eur J Surg Oncol 2004;30:583-588.

34. Little JW. Thyroid disorders: Part I, Hyperthyroidism. Oral Surg Oral Med Oral Pathol Oral Radiol Endod 2006;101:276-284.

35. Pinto A, Glick M. Management of patients with thyroid disease: Oral health considerations. J Am Dent Assoc 2002;133:849-858.

36. Little JW. Thyroid disorders: Part II, Hypothyroidism and thyroiditis. Oral Surg Oral Med Oral Pathol Oral Radiol Endod 2006;102:148-153.

37. Little JW. Thyroid disorders: Part III, Neoplastic thyroid disease. Oral Surg Oral Med Oral Pathol Oral Radiol Endod 2006;102:275-280.

38. Neville BW, Damm DD, Allen CA, Bouquot JE. Oral & Maxillofacial Pathology, 2nd ed. Philadelphia, Saunders, 2002.

39. Guimaraes VC. Subacute and Riedel's thyroiditis. In DeGroot LJ, Jameson JL (eds). Endocrinology, 5th ed. Philadelphia, Saunders (Elsevier), 2006, pp 2069-2081.

Pregnancy and Breast Feeding

CHAPTER

18

A pregnant patient, although not considered medically compromised, poses a unique set of management considerations for the dentist. Dental care must be rendered to the mother without adversely affecting the developing fetus, and although routine dental care of pregnant patients is generally safe to perform, the delivery of dental care involves some potentially harmful elements, including ionizing radiation and drug administration. In contrast, the provision of select dental care can be beneficial to the developing infant. Thus, the prudent practitioner must balance the beneficial aspects of dentistry while minimizing or avoiding exposure of the patient to potentially harmful procedures.

Additional considerations arise during the postpartum period if the mother elects to breast-feed her infant. Although most drugs are only minimally transmitted from maternal serum to breast milk, and the infant's exposure is not significant, the dentist should avoid using any drug that is known to be harmful to the infant.

DEFINITION
Physiology and Complications

To define rational management guidelines, a review of the normal processes of pregnancy and fetal development is provided. Endocrine changes are the most significant basic alterations that occur with pregnancy. They result from the increased production of maternal and placental hormones and from modified activity of target end organs.

Fatigue is a common physiologic finding during the first trimester that may have a psychological impact. A tendency toward syncope and postural hypotension has also been noted. During the second trimester, patients typically have a sense of well-being and relatively few symptoms. During the third trimester, increasing fatigue and discomfort and mild depression may be reported.

Several cardiovascular changes occur as well. Blood volume increases by 40%, cardiac output by 30% to 40%, and red blood cell volume by only about 15% to 20%.[1] In spite of the increase in cardiac output, blood pressure falls (usually to 100/70 mm Hg or lower) during the second trimester, and a modest increase is noted in the last month of pregnancy. This increase in blood volume is associated with high-flow/low-resistance circulation, tachycardia, and heart murmurs, and it may unmask glomerulopathies, peripartum cardiomyopathy, arterial aneurysms, or arteriovenous malformations. A benign systolic murmur is one of the more common complications; it develops in 90% of pregnant women but disappears shortly after delivery.[2] A murmur of this type is considered physiologic or functional. However, a murmur that preceded pregnancy or persisted after delivery would require further evaluation for determination of its significance.

During late pregnancy, a phenomenon known as *supine hypotensive syndrome* may occur that manifests as an abrupt fall in blood pressure, bradycardia, sweating, nausea, weakness, and air hunger when the patient is in a supine position.[1,3] Symptoms are caused by impaired venous return to the heart that results from compression of the inferior vena cava by the gravid uterus. This leads to decreased blood pressure, reduced cardiac output, and impairment or loss of consciousness. The remedy for the problem is to roll the patient over onto her left side, which lifts the uterus off the vena cava. Blood pressure should rapidly return to normal.

Blood changes in pregnancy include anemia and a decreased hematocrit value.[1] Anemia occurs because blood volume increases more rapidly than red blood cell mass. As a result, a fall in hemoglobin and a marked need for additional folate and iron occur. Approximately 20% of pregnant women have iron deficiency—a problem that is exaggerated by significant blood loss. Although changes in platelets are usually insignificant, several blood clotting factors (especially fibrinogen; von Willebrand factor; factors VII, VIII, IX, and X; and fibrin-split products) are increased. This hypercoagulation state increases the risk of thrombosis 7- to 10-fold.[1,4,5]

Several WBC changes occur. WBC count increases because of neutrophilia, and this increased level of neutrophils may complicate interpretation of the complete blood count during infection. Also, during pregnancy, the immune system shifts from helper T-cell 1 (TH1) dominance to TH2 dominance.[2] This leads to immune suppression. During the postpartum period, rebound and heightened inflammatory activity occurs.

Changes in respiratory function during pregnancy include reduced expiratory reserve volume caused by enlargement of the uterus in the cephalad direction and increased demand on the lungs for oxygen. These ventilatory changes produce an increased rate of respiration (tachypnea) and dyspnea that is aggravated by the supine position.

Pregnancy predisposes the expectant mother to an increased appetite and often a craving for unusual foods. As a result, the diet may be unbalanced, high in sugars, or nonnutritious. This can adversely affect the mother's dentition and contribute to significant weight gain. Taste alterations and an increased gag response are also common; the latter may make up to 90% of pregnant women vulnerable to nausea and vomiting ("morning sickness"). Symptoms of nausea and vomiting are linked to an increase in human chorionic gonadotropin and estrogen[2] and are worse during the first trimester.

The general pattern of fetal development should be understood when dental management plans are being formulated. Normal pregnancy lasts approximately 40 weeks. During the first trimester, organs and systems are formed. Thus, the fetus is most susceptible to malformation during this period. After the first trimester, the majority of formation is complete, and the remainder of fetal development is devoted primarily to growth and maturation. Thus, the chances of malformation are markedly diminished after the first trimester. A notable exception to this is the fetal dentition, which is susceptible to malformation from toxins or radiation, and to tooth discoloration caused by administration of tetracycline.

Complications of pregnancy are infrequent when prenatal care is provided and the mother is healthy. Unfortunately, complications occur more often in expectant mothers who harbor pathogens (oral and extraoral) and smoke, and in nonwhites over whites in the United States.[6] Common complications include infection, inflammatory response, glucose abnormalities, and hypertension.[4] Each increases the risks for preterm delivery, perinatal mortality, and congenital anomalies. Insulin resistance is a contributing factor to the development of gestational diabetes mellitus (GDM), which occurs in 2% to 6% of pregnant women. GDM increases the risks for infection and large birth weight babies. Hypertension is of particular interest because it can lead to end organ damage or preeclampsia, a clinical condition of preg-

nancy that manifests as hypertension, proteinuria, edema, and blurred vision. Preeclampsia progresses to eclampsia if seizures or coma develop. The cause of eclampsia is unknown but appears to involve sympathetic overactivity associated with insulin resistance, the renin-angiotensin system, lipid peroxidation, and inflammatory mediators.[7] Complications of pregnancy that are unresponsive to diet modification and palliative care ultimately require drugs or hospitalization for adequate control.

Another consideration related to fetal growth is spontaneous abortion (miscarriage). Spontaneous abortion, the natural termination of pregnancy before the 20th week of gestation, occurs in more than 15% of all pregnancies; most cases are caused by intrinsic fetal abnormalities.[8] Therefore, it is most unlikely that any dental procedure would be implicated in spontaneous abortion, provided fetal hypoxia and exposure of the fetus to teratogens are avoided. Febrile illness and sepsis also can precipitate a miscarriage; therefore, prompt treatment of odontogenic infection and periodontitis is advised.

Because of immature liver and enzyme systems, the fetus has a limited ability to metabolize drugs. Pharmacologic challenge of the fetus is to be avoided when possible.

During the postpartum period, the mother may suffer from lack of sleep and postpartum depression. Also during the postpartum period, risks for autoimmune disease, particularly rheumatoid arthritis, multiple sclerosis, and thyroiditis, are increased.

DENTAL MANAGEMENT
Medical Considerations

Management recommendations during pregnancy should be viewed as general guidelines—not as immutable rules. The dentist should assess the general health of the patient through a thorough medical history. Inquiries should be made regarding current physician, medications taken, use of tobacco, alcohol, or illicit drugs, history of gestational diabetes, miscarriage, hypertension, and morning sickness. If possible, contacting the patient's obstetrician or physician to discuss her medical status, dental needs, and proposed dental treatment is helpful. This is beneficial from the standpoint of planning treatment and also demonstrates to the patient a caring concern about her and her baby. In a 1992 survey of obstetricians,[9] 91% of respondents indicated that they preferred not to be contacted in regard to "routine" dental care. However, 88% wanted to be consulted before the dentist prescribed antibiotics, and 54% wanted to participate in a consultation before the dentist prescribed analgesics (Box 18-1).

Pregnancy is a special event in a woman's life; hence, it is an emotionally charged experience. Establishing a good patient/dentist relationship that encourages openness, honesty, and trust is an integral part of successful management. This kind of relationship greatly reduces stress and anxiety for both patient and dentist.

BOX 18-1

Dental Management Considerations for Patients Who Are Pregnant

1. Evaluate patient; determine trimester and health status.
2. Confirm that medical prenatal care was provided, or facilitate entry into medical care.
3. Provide periodontal therapy and oral hygiene instructions.
4. Educate the patient: Discuss the importance and benefits of good plaque control and fluoride.
5. Minimize radiographic exposure.
6. Minimize drug use. Drug selection should be based on safety profile, risk to mother and fetus, and potential for interactions and adverse effects.
7. Avoid prolonged appointment time in the dental chair (i.e., risk of supine hypothesion).
8. The safest time for provision of dental treatment is the second trimester.

As with all patients, monitoring of vital signs is important for identifying undiagnosed abnormalities and the need for corrective action. At a minimum, blood pressure, pulse, and respirations should be measured. Systolic pressure values at or above 140 mm Hg and diastolic pressure at or above 90 mm Hg are signs of hypertension (see Chapter 3). Also diagnostic of hypertension is an increase of 30 mm or more in systolic blood pressure or an increase of 15 mm Hg in diastolic blood pressure compared with prepregnancy values.[10] Confirmed hypertensive values dictate that the patient should be referred to a physician to ensure that preeclampsia and other cardiovascular disorders are properly diagnosed and managed.

Preventive Program. An important objective in planning dental treatment for a pregnant patient is to establish a healthy oral environment and an optimum level of oral hygiene. This essentially consists of a plaque control program that minimizes the exaggerated inflammatory response of gingival tissues to local irritants that commonly accompany the hormonal changes of pregnancy.[11] This is important because maternal periodontal disease increases the infant's risk for preterm birth and low birth weight.[12,13] This is speculated to be caused by bacteria or bacterial products transported through the systemic circulation that elicit inflammatory responses within the placental membranes.[14] In addition, maternal plaque control has implications for caries risk for the infant. Studies conducted over the past 25 years have shown that reduced oral streptococcal levels in the pregnant mother reduce the risk that the infant will become infected and develop caries.[15-17]

Because of these apparent risks to the infant, acceptable oral hygiene techniques should be taught, reinforced, and monitored. Diet counseling, with emphasis on limiting the intake of refined carbohydrates and carbonated soft drinks, should be provided. Coronal scaling and polishing or root curettage may be performed whenever necessary. Preventive plaque control measures, including daily rinses with 0.12% chlorhexidine, should be provided and emphasized throughout pregnancy, including the first trimester, for benefit to the pregnant mother and the developing baby.[14]

The benefits of prenatal fluoride are also apparent. Studies by Glenn[18] and Glenn and associates[19] have shown that a daily 2.2-mg tablet of sodium fluoride administered to mothers during the second and third trimesters in combination with fluoridated water resulted in 97% of the offspring being caries free for up to 10 years. Not only were medical or dental defects, including fluorosis, absent in these children, but an association with decreased premature delivery and increased birth weight was seen in the fluoride treatment group. The conclusion was that fluoride tablet supplementation from the third through ninth months of pregnancy was safe and effective. In another study sponsored by the National Institute of Dental Research, more than 1200 women and their offspring were studied. Half of the women received prenatal fluoride and the other half were given placebo.[20] After 5 years, offspring from the prenatal fluoride group had 45% fewer caries than did placebo group offspring, and 96% were free of caries. Similarly, in a study of 65 pregnant women, salivary streptococcal levels were significantly reduced in mothers and their offspring following a regimen that included diet counseling, prophylaxis, systemic fluoride, daily fluoride, and chlorhexidine mouth rinsing.[17] These findings indicate that prenatal fluoride and oral hygiene measures provide benefit to the mother and the newborn without risk and should be discussed with the patient and the obstetrician.

Treatment Timing

Other than as part of a good plaque control program, elective dental care is best avoided during the first trimester because of potential vulnerability of the fetus (Table 18-1). The second trimester is the safest period during which to provide routine dental care. Emphasis should be placed on controlling active disease and eliminating potential problems that could occur later in pregnancy or during the immediate postpartum period, because providing dental care during these periods is often difficult. Extensive reconstruction or significant surgical procedures are best postponed until after delivery.

The early part of the third trimester is still a good time to provide routine dental care. However, after the middle of the third trimester, elective dental care is best postponed. This is because of the increasing feeling of discomfort that many expectant mothers may experience. Prolonged time in the dental chair should be avoided to prevent the complication of supine hypotension. If supine hypotension develops, rolling the patient onto her left side affords return of circulation to the heart. Scheduling short appointments, allowing the patient to assume a semireclined position, and encouraging frequent changes of position can minimize problems.

TABLE 18-1
Treatment Timing During Pregnancy

First Trimester	Second Trimester	Third Trimester
Plaque control	Plaque control	Plaque control
Oral hygiene instruction	Oral hygiene instruction	Oral hygiene instruction
Scaling, polishing, curettage	Scaling, polishing, curettage	Scaling, polishing, curettage
Avoid elective treatment; urgent care only	Routine dental care	Routine dental care

Dental Radiographs

Dental radiography is one of the more controversial areas in the management of a pregnant patient. Irradiation should be avoided during pregnancy, especially during the first trimester, because the developing fetus is particularly susceptible to radiation damage.[21] However, should dental treatment become necessary, radiographs may be required to accurately diagnose and treat the patient. Therefore, the dentist must be aware of how to proceed safely in this situation.

The safety of dental radiography has been well established, provided features such as fast exposure techniques (e.g., high-speed film, digital imaging), filtration, collimation, and lead aprons are used. Of all aids, the most important for the pregnant patient is the protective lead apron. Studies have shown that when an apron is used during contemporary dental radiography, gonadal and fetal radiation is less than 0.01 microSieverts (μSv).[22-24]

The dentist must keep in perspective the facts of radiation biology. Animal and human data[25-30] clearly support the conclusion that no increase in gross congenital anomalies or intrauterine growth retardation occurs as a result of exposures during pregnancy totaling less than 5 to 10 centiGray (cGy).[31]* For comparison, the following may be considered[28,29] (Table 18-2):
- A medical chest radiograph results in an estimated fetal or embryonic dose of 0.008 cGy
- A skull radiograph results in 0.004 cGy
- Natural background radiation is approximately 0.0004 cGy daily
- A full mouth series of dental radiographs with a lead apron results in 0.00001 cGy

When risks of dental radiography are further assessed during pregnancy, three reports should be kept in mind. The first states that the maximum risk attributable to 1 cGy (which is more than 1000 full mouth series with E-speed film and rectangular collimation or 10% to 20% of the threshold dose) of in utero radiation exposure is estimated[26] to be approximately 0.1%. This is a quantity thousands of times less than the normal anticipated risks of spontaneous abortion, malformation, or genetic disease. The second report calculates the risk of a first-generation fetal defect from a dental radiographic examination to be 9 in 1 billion.[32] The third report found that

TABLE 18-2
Comparative Radiation Exposures to Fetal or Embryonic Tissues

Source of Radiation	Absorbed Exposure, cGy
Upper gastrointestinal series	0.330
Chest radiograph	0.008
Skull radiograph	0.004
Daily (cosmic) background radiation	0.0004
Full mouth dental series (18 intraoral radiographs, D film, lead apron)	0.00001

Modified from National Council on Radiation Protection and Measurements. Medical radiation exposure of pregnant and potentially pregnant women. NCRP Report No. 54, Washington, DC, NCRP Publications, 1977[28]; and DiSaia PJ. In Scott JR, et al (eds). Danforth's Obstetrics and Gynecology, 6th ed. Philadelphia, JB Lippincott, 1990.[29]

the gonadal dose to women, after full mouth radiography, is less than 0.01 μSv, which is at least 1000-fold below the threshold shown to cause congenital damage to newborns.[24] These figures indicate that with use of the lead apron, rectangular collimation, and E-speed film or faster techniques, one or two intraoral films are truly of minute significance in terms of radiation effects on the developing fetus. In terms that can be explained to a patient, one should consider the following: The gonadal/fetal dose of 2 periapical dental films (when a lead apron is used) is 700 times less than 1 day of average exposure to natural background radiation in the United States.[33,34]

Despite the negligible risks of dental radiography, the dentist should not be cavalier regarding its use during pregnancy (or at any other time, for that matter). Radiographs should be used selectively and only when necessary and appropriate to aid in diagnosis and treatment. Bitewing, panoramic, or selected periapical films are recommended for minimizing patient dose. To further reduce the radiation dose, the following measures should be employed: rectangular collimation, E-speed film or faster techniques (digital imaging reduces radiographic exposure by at least 50% compared with E-speed exposures), lead shielding (abdominal and thyroid collar), high kilovoltage (kV) or constant beams, and an ongoing quality assurance program.

An additional consideration is the pregnant dental auxiliary or dentist. The maximum permissible radiation

---

*1 cGy (0.01 Gy) = 1 rad (roentgen, R) (e.g., IR = 0.01 Gy = 0.01 Sievert [Sv] = 10 mSv). For diagnostic radiology, 1 Sv = 1 Gy.

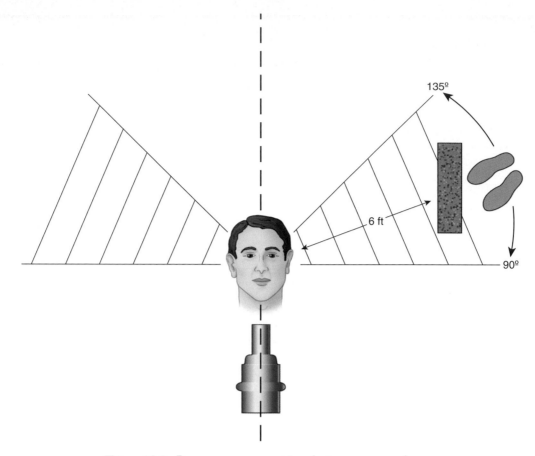

Figure 18-1. Proper operator position during exposure of x-rays.

dose for whole body exposure of the pregnant dental care worker is 0.005 Gy or 5 mSv per year. This is equivalent to the maximum permissible radiation dose of the nonoccupationally exposed public and ten-fold less than the level of occupationally exposed nonpregnant workers (50 mSv).[31] The National Commission of Radiation Protection and Measurements reports that production of congenital defects is negligible from fetal exposures of 50 mSv.[31,35] To further ensure safety, the pregnant operator should wear a film badge, stand more than 6 feet from the tube head, and position herself at between 90 and 130 degrees of the beam, preferably behind a protective wall (Figure 18-1). When these guidelines are followed, no contraindication to pregnant women operating the x-ray machine occurs. However, dentists should familiarize themselves with federal (Code of Federal Regulations, Code 10, Part 20, Section 20.201) and state regulations that would supersede these guidelines.

Drug Administration

During Pregnancy. Another controversial area in treatment of the pregnant dental patient is drug administration. The principal concern is that a drug may cross the placenta and be toxic or teratogenic to the fetus. Additionally, any drug that is a respiratory depressant may cause maternal hypoxia, resulting in fetal hypoxia, injury, or death.

Ideally, no drug should be administered during pregnancy, especially during the first trimester. However, adhering to this rule is sometimes impossible. Most of the commonly used drugs in dental practice can be given during pregnancy with relative safety, although a few exceptions are notable. Table 18-3 presents a suggested approach to drug usage for pregnant patients.

Before prescribing or administering a drug to a pregnant patient, the dentist should be familiar with the U.S. Food and Drug Administration[36] categorization of prescription drugs for pregnancy based on their potential risk of fetal injury. These pregnancy risk classification categories, although not without limitations,[37] are meant to aid clinicians and patients in making decisions about drug therapy. Counseling should be provided to ensure that women who are pregnant clearly understand the nature and magnitude of the risk associated with a drug.

The current pregnancy labeling categories are as follows:

A Controlled studies in humans have failed to demonstrate a risk to the fetus, and the possibility of fetal harm appears remote.

B Animal studies have not indicated fetal risk, and human studies have not been conducted; *or* animal studies have shown a risk, but controlled human studies have not.

TABLE **18-3**
Drug Administration During Pregnancy and Breast Feeding

Drug	FDA Pregnancy Risk Category	Use During Pregnancy	Risk	Use During Breast Feeding
LOCAL ANESTHETICS				
Articaine	C	Use with caution; consult physician		Unknown
Bupivacaine	C	Use with caution; consult physician	Fetal bradycardia	Yes
Etidocaine	B	Yes		Yes
Lidocaine	B	Yes		Yes
Mepivacaine	C	Use with caution; consult physician	Fetal bradycardia	Yes
Prilocaine	B	Yes		Yes
ANALGESICS (NONNARCOTIC)				
Acetaminophen	B	Yes		Yes
Aspirin	C/D[3]	Caution; avoid in third trimester	Postpartum hemorrhage Constriction ductus arteriosus	Avoid
Cyclooxygenase (COX)-2 inhibitor	C	Avoid in third trimester	May lead to constriction, ductus arteriosus	Yes
Diflunisal, etodolac, mefenamic acid	C/D[3]	Use with caution; avoid in third trimester; consult physician	Delayed labor	No
Ibuprofen, flurbiprofen	B/D[3]	Caution; avoid in third trimester	Delayed labor	Yes
Naproxen	B/D[3]	Caution; avoid in third trimester	Delayed labor	Yes
ANALGESICS (NARCOTIC)				
Codeine	C/D*	Use with caution (low dose, short duration); consult physician	Neonatal respiratory depression	Yes
Hydrocodone	C/D[3]	Use with caution (low dose, short duration); consult physician	Neonatal respiratory depression	—
Oxycodone	C/D[3]	Use with caution (low dose, short duration); consult physician	Neonatal respiratory depression	Yes
Pentazocine	C	Use with caution (low dose, short duration); consult physician	Neonatal respiratory depression	Yes
Propoxyphene	C	Use with caution (low dose, short duration); consult physician	Neonatal respiratory depression	Yes
ANTIBIOTICS				
Cephalosporins	B	Yes		Yes
Clindamycin	B	Yes		Yes
Fluoroquinolones (norfloxacin, ciprofloxacin, ofloxacin, and enoxacin)	C	Use with caution; consult physician	Arthropathy	Caution
Macrolides				
Erythromycin	B	Yes; avoid estolate form		Yes
Azithromycin	B	Yes		Yes
Clarithromycin	C	Use with caution; consult physician		Yes
Metronidazole	B	Yes		Yes
Penicillins	B	Yes		Yes
Tetracycline	D	Avoid	Tooth discoloration, inhibits bone formation	Avoid
Tetracycline (periodontal dosages)	C	Avoid	Tooth discoloration, inhibits bone formation	Avoid

TABLE 18-3
Drug Administration During Pregnancy and Breast Feeding—cont'd

Drug	FDA Pregnancy Risk Category	Use During Pregnancy	Risk	Use During Breast Feeding
ANTIVIRALS				
Acyclovir	C	Yes		Yes
Famciclovir	B	Yes		Yes
Valacyclovir	B	Yes		Yes
ANTIFUNGALS				
Fluconazole	C	Yes		Yes
Nystatin	B/C	Yes		Yes
CORTICOSTEROIDS				
Prednisone	B	Yes		Yes
SEDATIVE/HYPNOTICS				
Barbiturates	D	Avoid	Neonatal respiratory depression	Avoid
Benzodiazepines (diazepam, lorazepam)	D	Avoid	Possible risk for oral clefts with prolonged exposure	Avoid
Triazolam	X			
Nitrous oxide	Not assigned		Best used in second and third trimesters and for <30 minutes; consult physician	Yes
SIALOGOGUES				
Cevimeline	C	No information		No information
Pilocarpine	C	Yes		Avoid

Modified from Moore PA. Selecting drugs for the pregnant dental patient. J Am Dent Assoc 1998;129:1281-1286[39]; Drug Information for the Health Care Professional, 2nd ed. Rockville, Md, United States Pharmacopeial Convention, 2000[40]; and Briggs GG, Freeman RK, Yaffe SJ. Drugs in Pregnancy and Lactation: A Reference Guide to Fetal and Neonatal Risk, 5th ed. Baltimore, Williams & Wilkins, 1998.[41]
D*, = Risk category D if used for prolonged period or high dose; D[3], Risk category D if administered during the third trimester.

C Animal studies have shown a risk, but controlled human studies have not been conducted, or studies are not available in humans or animals.

D Positive evidence of human fetal risk exists, but in certain situations, the drug may be used despite its risk.

X Evidence of fetal abnormalities and fetal risk exists based on human experience, and the risk outweighs any possible benefit of use during pregnancy.

Obviously, drugs in category A or B are preferable for prescribing during pregnancy. However, many drugs that fall into category C are administered during pregnancy; therefore, these drugs present the greatest difficulty for the dentist and the physician in terms of therapeutic and medicolegal decisions.

Physicians may advise against the use of some of the approved drugs or conversely may suggest the use of a questionable drug. The listed guidelines are general ones. An example of the occasional use of a questionable drug would be a narcotic for a pregnant patient who is in severe pain.

Anesthetics. Local anesthetics administered with epinephrine are considered relatively safe for use during pregnancy and are assigned to pregnancy risk classification categories B and C. Although both the local anesthetic and the vasoconstrictor cross the placenta, subtoxic threshold doses have not been shown to cause fetal abnormalities. Because of adverse effects associated with high levels of these drugs, it is advisable to limit the dose to the amount required. Concerns include risk for methemoglobinemia with high-dose prilocaine and articaine, as well as embryocidal effects associated with toxic doses of bupivacaine.[38]

Analgesics. The analgesic of choice during pregnancy is acetaminophen (category B). Aspirin and nonsteroidal anti-inflammatory drugs convey risks for constriction of the ductus arteriosus, as well as for postpartum hemorrhage and delayed labor (see Table 18-3).[39,40] The risk of these adverse events increases when agents are administered during the third trimester. Risk also is more closely associated with prolonged administration, high dosage, and selectively potent anti-inflammatory drugs, such as indomethacin.

Prolonged or high doses of opioids are associated with congenital abnormalities and respiratory depression.[41,42] For this reason, opioid-containing drugs should generally be avoided.

Antibiotics. Penicillins, erythromycin (except in estolate form), and cephalosporins (first and second generation) are considered safe for the expectant mother and the developing child. However, these antibiotics have lower maternal blood levels compared with controls because of a shorter half-life and increased volume of distribution. For example, in one study, 2 of 10 pregnant mothers failed to have detectable drug blood levels of erythromycin up to 4 hours after antibiotic administration.[43] An increased dose or more frequent administration may be required if an infection is not readily brought under control with antibiotic use. The use of tetracycline is contraindicated during pregnancy. Tetracyclines bind to hydroxyapatite, causing brown discoloration of teeth, hypoplastic enamel, inhibition of bone growth, and other skeletal abnormalities.[44]

The dental community's concern for potential interactions between antibiotics and oral contraceptives requires mention in this chapter.[45] This concern arises from the ability of select antibiotics such as rifampin, an antituberculosis drug, to reduce plasma levels of circulating oral contraceptives. However, studies to date regarding other antibiotics have been less convincing. To address this concern, the American Dental Association Council on Scientific Affairs issued the following recommendations: "The dentist should (1) advise the patient of the potential risk of the antibiotic's reducing the effectiveness of the oral contraceptive, (2) recommend that the patient discuss with her physician the use of an additional nonhormonal means of contraception, [and] (3) advise the patient to maintain compliance with oral contraceptives when concurrently using antibiotics." The application of these recommendations appears prudent until the findings of larger studies become available.

Anxiolytics. Few anxiolytics are considered safe during pregnancy. However, a single exposure to nitrous oxide–oxygen (N_2O–O_2) for less than 35 minutes has not been associated with any human fetal anomalies, including low birth rate.[46] In contrast, chronic N_2O-O_2 inhalation analgesia may cause inactivation of methionine synthetase and vitamin B_{12} and altered DNA metabolism that can lead to cellular abnormalities in animals and birth defects. Accordingly, the following guidelines are recommended if N_2O-O_2 is used during pregnancy:

- Use of N_2O—O_2 inhalation should be minimized to 30 minutes.
- At least 50% oxygen should be delivered to ensure adequate oxygenation at all times.

- Appropriate oxygenation should be provided to avoid diffusion hypoxia at the termination of administration.
- Repeated and prolonged exposures to nitrous oxide are to be prevented.
- The second and third trimester are safer periods for treatment because organogenesis occurs during the first trimester.[1]

An additional consideration involves the female dentist or dental auxiliary who is pregnant. These practitioners should not be exposed to persistent trace levels of nitrous oxide in the operatory. Female dental health care workers who are chronically exposed to nitrous oxide for more than 3 hours per week, when scavenging equipment is not used, have decreased fertility and increased rates of spontaneous abortion.[47] Implementation of National Institute for Occupational Safety and Health recommendations can reduce occupational exposure to nitrous oxide (Box 18-2).[48,49]

During Breast Feeding. A potential problem arises when a nursing mother requires the administration of a drug in the course of dental treatment. The concern is that the administered drug may enter the breast milk and be transferred to the nursing infant, in whom exposure may result in adverse effects.

Data on which to draw definitive conclusions about drug dosages and effects via breast milk are limited.

BOX 18-2

Control of Nitrous Oxide in the Dental Office During Pregnancy

1. Inspect nitrous oxide equipment, and replace defective tubing and parts.
2. Check pressure connections for leaks, and fix leaks.
3. Ensure that mask fits well and is secure. Check that the reservoir bag is not overinflated or underinflated.
4. Provide operatory ventilation of 10 or more room air exchanges per hour.
5. Use a scavenging system and appropriate mask sizes. Vacuum should provide up to 45 L/min.
6. Connect and turn on the vacuum pump of the scavenging system before providing nitrous oxide.
7. Regularly conduct air sampling. Maintain low exposure limits (e.g., 25 ppm*) when pregnant dental health care workers are involved.

Modified from McGlothlin JD, Crouch KG, Mickelsen RL. Control of Nitrous Oxide in Dental Operatories. Cincinnati, Ohio, U.S. Department of Health and Human Services, Public Health Service, Centers for Disease Control and Prevention, National Institute for Occupational Safety and Health, Division of Physical Sciences and Engineering, Engineering Control Technology Branch, 1994. DHHS publication no. (NIOSH) 94-129. ETTB report no. 166-04.[48]
*This limit is an NIOSH recommendation. In contrast, Yagiela suggests a time-weighted average (TWA) lower limit of 100 ppm for an 8-hour workday. (Yagiela JA. Health hazards and nitrous oxide: A time for reappraisal. Anesth Prog 1991;38:1-11.[50])

However, retrospective clinical studies and empiric observations, coupled with known pharmacologic pathways, allow recommendations to be made. A significant fact is that the amount of drug excreted in the breast milk usually is not more than 1% to 2% of the maternal dose. Therefore, most drugs are of little pharmacologic significance to the infant.[41,51]

Agreement exists that a few drugs, or categories of drugs, are definitely contraindicated for nursing mothers. These include lithium, anticancer drugs, radioactive pharmaceuticals, and phenindione.[41,52,53] Table 18-3 contains recommendations adapted from the American Academy of Pediatrics regarding the administration of commonly used dental drugs during breast feeding.[54] As with drug use during pregnancy, individual physicians may wish to modify these recommendations, which should be viewed only as general guidelines for treatment.

In addition to careful drug selection, authorities suggest that nursing mothers take the drug just after breast feeding and avoid nursing for 4 hours or longer if possible. This should result in reduced drug concentrations in the breast milk.[53,54]

Treatment Planning Modifications

No technical modifications are required for the pregnant patient. However, full mouth radiographs, reconstruction, crown and bridge procedures, and significant surgery are best delayed until after pregnancy. A prominent gag reflex also may dictate a delay in certain dental procedures. Although dental amalgam has not been shown to be hazardous to pregnant women or the developing fetus,[55,56] several European countries and Canada have national recommendations advising dentists to limit or avoid the placement and replacement of amalgams during pregnancy.[57,58]

Oral Complications and Manifestations

The most common oral complication of pregnancy is pregnancy gingivitis (Figure 18-2). This condition results from an exaggerated inflammatory response to local irritants and less than meticulous oral hygiene during periods of increased secretion of estrogen and progesterone and altered fibrinolysis.[11] Pregnancy gingivitis begins at the marginal and interdental gingiva, usually in the second month of pregnancy. Progression of this condition leads to fiery red and edematous interproximal papillae that are tender to palpation. In approximately 1% of gravid women, the hyperplastic response may exacerbate in a localized area, resulting in a pyogenic granuloma or "pregnancy tumor" (Figure 18-3). The most common location for a pyogenic granuloma is the labial aspect of the interdental papilla. The lesion is generally asymptomatic; however, toothbrushing may traumatize the lesion and cause bleeding. Hyperplastic gingival changes become apparent around the second month and continue until after parturition, at which time the gingival tissues usually regress and return to normal, provided proper oral hygiene measures are implemented and any calculus

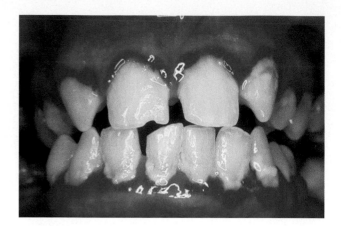

Figure 18-2. Generalized gingivitis—"pregnancy gingivitis"—in a woman in the sixth month of pregnancy.

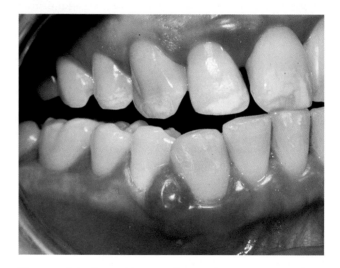

Figure 18-3. Pyogenic granuloma—"pregnancy tumor"—occurring during pregnancy.

present is removed.[11] Surgical or laser excision is occasionally required if symptoms, bleeding, or interference with mastication dictates. Pregnancy does not cause periodontal disease but may modify and worsen what is already present. Gestational diabetes mellitus, however, is associated with increased risk for periodontal disease.[59] Because periodontal disease in a pregnant women increases the risk of a low-birthweight baby,[14] oral hygiene measures and plaque control programs should be offered to mothers during pregnancy.

A relationship between dental caries and the physiologic processes of pregnancy has not been demonstrated. Caries activity is attributed to the presence of cariogenic bacteria in the mouth, a diet containing fermentable carbohydrates, and poor oral hygiene. Control of the carious process through fluoride and chlorhexidine is important because maternal saliva is the primary vehicle for transfer of cariogenic streptococci to the infant.[60,61]

Many women are convinced that pregnancy causes tooth loss (i.e., "a tooth for every pregnancy"), or that calcium is withdrawn from the maternal dentition to supply fetal requirements (i.e., "soft teeth"). Calcium is present in the teeth in a stable crystalline form and hence is not available to the systemic circulation to supply a calcium demand. However, calcium is readily mobilized from bone to supply these demands. Therefore, although calcium supplementation for the purpose of preventing tooth loss or soft teeth is unwarranted, the physician may prescribe calcium to fulfill the general nutritional requirements of mother and infant.

Tooth mobility, localized or generalized, is an uncommon finding during pregnancy. Mobility is a sign of gingival disease, disturbance of the attachment apparatus, and mineral changes in the lamina dura. Because vitamin deficiencies may contribute to this and other congenital problems (e.g., folate deficiency, spina bifida), the dentist, when discussing oral hygiene, should take this opportunity to educate the patient about the benefits of the use of multivitamins. Daily removal of local irritants, adequate levels of vitamin C, and delivery of the newborn should result in reversal of tooth mobility.

Pregnant women often have a hypersensitive gag reflex. This, in combination with morning sickness, may contribute to episodes of regurgitation and lead to halitosis and enamel erosion. The dentist should advise the patient to rinse after regurgitation with a solution that neutralizes the acid (e.g., baking soda, water).

REFERENCES

1. Suresh L, Radfar L. Pregnancy and lactation. Oral Surg Oral Med Oral Pathol Oral Radiol Endod 2004;97: 672-682.
2. Cunningham FG, Bloom SL, Hauth JC, et al. Williams Obstetrics, 22nd ed. New York, NY, McGraw-Hill, 2005.
3. Turner M, Aziz SR. Management of the pregnant oral and maxillofacial surgery patient. J Oral Maxillofac Surg 2002;60:1479-1488.
4. Kaaja RJ, Greer IA. Manifestations of chronic disease during pregnancy. JAMA 2005;294:2751-2757.
5. Merck Manual, 18th ed. Whitehouse Station, NJ, Merck Research Laboratories, 2006.
6. Ventura SJ, Martin JA, Curtin SC, et al. Births: Final data for 1998. Natl Vital Stat Rep 2000;48:1-100.
7. Rudra CB, Qiu C, David RM, et al. A prospective study of early-pregnancy plasma malondialdehyde concentration and risk of preeclampsia. Clin Biochem 2006;39: 722-726.
8. Branch WE, Scott JR. Early pregnancy loss. In Scott JR, et al (eds). Danforth's Obstetrics and Gynecology, 9th ed. Philadelphia, Lippincott Williams & Wilkins, 2003.
9. Shrout MK, Comer RW, Powell BJ, McCoy Bp. Treating the pregnant dental patient: Four basic rules addressed. J Am Dent Assoc 1992;123:75-80.
10. Solomon CG, Seely EW. Hypertension in pregnancy— A manifestation of insulin resistance syndrome? Hypertension 2001;37:232-239.
11. Löe H. Periodontal changes in pregnancy. J Periodontol 1965;36:209-217.
12. Offenbacher S, Boggess KA, Murtha AP, et al. Progressive periodontal disease and risk of very preterm delivery. Obstet Gynecol 2006;107:29-36.
13. Khader YS, Ta'ani Q. Periodontal diseases and the risk of preterm birth and low birth weight: A meta-analysis. J Periodontol 2005;76:161-165.
14. Lopez NJ, Da Silva I, Ipinza J, Gutierrez J. Periodontal therapy reduces the rate of preterm low birth weight in women with pregnancy-associated gingivitis. J Periodontol 2005;76:2144-2153.
15. Kohler B, Bratthall D, Krasse B. Preventive measures in mothers influence the establishment of the bacterium Streptococcus mutans in their infants. Arch Oral Biol 1983;28:225-231.
16. Kohler B, Andréen I. Influence of caries—Preventive measures in mothers on cariogenic bacteria and caries experience in their children. Arch Oral Biol 1994;39: 907-911.
17. Brambilla E, Felloni A, Gagliani M, et al. Caries prevention during pregnancy: Results of a 30-month study. J Am Dent Assoc 1998;129:871-877.
18. Glenn FB. Immunity conveyed by a fluoride supplement during pregnancy. J Dent Child 1977;44:391-395.
19. Glenn FB, Glenn WD III, Duncan RC. Fluoride tablet supplementation during pregnancy for caries immunity: A study of the offspring produced. Am J Obstet Gynecol 1982;143:560-564.
20. Leverett DII. Clinical Trial of the Effect of Prenatal Fluoride Supplements In Preventing Dental Caries. Bethesda, Md, National Institute of Dental Research, April 1992. Final Report (7/83-6/91), pp 1-54.
21. Serman NJ, Singer S. Exposure of the pregnant patient to ionizing radiation. Ann Dent 1994;53:13-15.
22. Bean LR Jr, Devore WD. The effects of protective aprons in dental roentgenography. Oral Surg 1969;28: 505-508.
23. Laws PW. The X-Ray Information Book: A Consumer's Guide to Avoiding Unnecessary Medical and Dental X-Rays. New York, Farrar, Straus, and Giroux, 1983.
24. White SC. 1992 assessment of radiation risk from dental radiography. Dentomaxillofac Radiol 1992;21:118-126.
25. Brent RL. Environmental factors: Radiation. In Brent RL, Harris MI (eds). Prevention of Embryonic, Fetal and Perinatal Disease. Fogarty International Center Series on Preventive Medicine, vol 3. Washington, DC, U.S. Department of Health, Education, and Welfare, 1976. Publication no. 76-853, pp 1799-1807.
26. Brent RL. The effects of embryonic and fetal exposure to x-ray, microwaves, and ultrasound. Clin Obstet Gynecol 1983;26:484-510.
27. Brent RL. Ionizing radiation. Contemp Obstet Gynecol 1987;30:20-29.
28. National Council on Radiation Protection and Measurements. Medical Radiation Exposure of Pregnant and Potentially Pregnant Women. Washington, DC, NCRP Publications, 1977. NCRP report no. 54.
29. DiSaia PJ. Radiation therapy in gynecology. In Scott JR, et al (eds). Danforth's Obstetrics and Gynecology, 8th ed. Philadelphia, JB Lippincott, 1999.
30. Mole RH. Radiation effects on pre-natal development and their radiological significance. Br J Radiol 1979;52: 89-101.

31. National Council on Radiation Protection and Measurements. Recommendations on Limits for Exposure to Ionizing Radiation. Bethesda, Md, NCRP, 1987. NCRP report no. 91.

32. Danforth RA, Gibbs SJ. Diagnostic dental radiation: What's the risk? J Calif Dent Assoc 1980;28:28-35.

33. Gonad Doses and Genetically Significant Dose from Diagnostic Radiology: United States, 1964 and 1970. Washington, DC, Department of Health Education and Welfare (DHEW), 1976. FDA Publication no. 76-8034.

34. Freeman JP, Brand JW. Radiation doses of commonly used dental radiographic surveys. Oral Surg Oral Med Oral Pathol 1994;77:285-289.

35. National Council on Radiation Protection and Measurements. Ionizing radiation exposure of the population of the United States. Bethesda, Md, NCRP, 1987. NCRP report no. 93.

36. Pregnancy categories for prescription drugs. FDA Drug Bull 1982;12:24-25.

37. U.S. Food and Drug Administration. Content and format of labeling for human prescription drugs: Pregnancy labeling, public hearing—FDA. Notice of public hearing; request for comments. Fed Regist 1997;62:41061-41063.

38. Denson DD, Coyie DE, Thompson GA. Bupivacaine protein binding in the term parturient: Effect of lactic acidosis. Clin Pharmacol Ther 1984;35:702.

39. Moore PA. Selecting drugs for the pregnant dental patient. J Am Dent Assoc 1998;129:1281-1286.

40. Drug Information for the Health Care Professional. Taunton, Mass, Thomson Micromedex, 2006.

41. Briggs GG, Freeman RK, Yaffe SJ. Drugs in Pregnancy and Lactation: A Reference Guide to Fetal and Neonatal Risk, 5th ed. Baltimore, Williams and Wilkins, 1998.

42. Heinonen OP, Slone D, Shapiro S. Birth Defects and Drugs in Pregnancy. Littleton, Mass, Publishing Sciences Group, 1977.

43. Larsen B, Glover DD. Serum erythromycin levels in pregnancy. Clin Ther 1998;20:971-977.

44. Cohlan SW, Bevelander G, Tiamsic T. Growth inhibition of prematures receiving tetracycline. Am J Dis Child 1963;105:453-461.

45. American Dental Association Health Foundation Research Institute. Antibiotic interference with oral contraceptives. JADA 1991;122:79.

46. Crawford JS, Lewis M. Nitrous oxide in early human pregnancy. Anaesthesia 1986;41:900-905.

47. Rowland AS, Baird DD, Shore DL, et al. Nitrous oxide and spontaneous abortion in female dental assistants. Am J Epidemiol 1995;141:531-538.

48. McGlothlin JD, Jensen PA, Fischbach TJ, et al. Control of anesthetic gases in dental operatories. Scand J Work Environ Health 1991;18(suppl 2):103-105.

49. NIOSH ALERT: 1994 DHHS (NIOSH) Publication No. 94-100. Request for assistance in controlling exposures to nitrous oxide during anesthetic administration. Available at: http://www.cdc.gov/niosh/noxidalr.html. Accessed April 5, 2007.

50. Yagiela JA. Health hazards and nitrous oxide: A time for reappraisal. Anesth Prog 1991;38:1-11.

51. Ito S, Lee A. Drug excretion into breast milk—Overview. Adv Drug Deliv Rev 2003;55:617-627.

52. American Academy of Pediatrics Committee on Drugs. The transfer of drugs and other chemicals into human milk. Pediatrics 1994;93:137-150.

53. Yankowitz J. Drugs in pregnancy and lactation. In Scott JR, et al (eds). Danforth's Obstetrics and Gynecology, 9th ed. Philadelphia, Lippincott Williams & Wilkins, 2003.

54. Berlin CM. Pharmacologic considerations of drug use in the lactating mother. Obstet Gynecol 1981;58(suppl 5):17S-23S.

55. Larrson K. Teratological aspects of dental amalgam. Adv Dent Res 1992;6:114-119.

56. Hujoel PP, Lydon-Rochelle M, Bollen AM, et al. Mercury exposure from dental filling placement during pregnancy and low birth weight risk. Am J Epidemiol 2005;161:734-740.

57. Anderson BA, et al. Dental amalgam—A report with reference to the medical devices directive 93/42/EEC from an Ad Hoc Working Group mandated by DGIII of the European Commission. Angelholm, Sweden, Nordiska Dental AB, 1998.

58. Minister of Supply and Services, Canada. Health Canada: The Safety of Dental Amalgam. Montréal, The Minister, 1996.

59. Novak KF, Taylor GW, Dawson DR, et al. Periodontitis and gestational diabetes mellitus: Exploring the link in NHANES III. J Public Health Dent 2006;66:163-168.

60. Caufield PW. The fidelity of initial acquisition of mutans streptococci by infants from their mothers. J Dent Res 1995;74:681-685.

61. Berkowitz RJ, Hones P. Mouth to mouth transmission of the bacterium Streptococcus mutans between mother and child. Arch Oral Biol 1985;4:377-379.

PART SEVEN

Immunologic Disease

AIDS, HIV Infection, and Related Conditions

CHAPTER 19

On June 5, 1981, when the Centers for Disease Control (CDC) reported five cases of *Pneumocystis carinii* pneumonia in young homosexual men in Los Angeles, few suspected that it heralded a pandemic of acquired immunodeficiency syndrome (AIDS). In 1983, a retrovirus (later named the human immunodeficiency virus, or HIV) was isolated from a patient with AIDS. In the 25 years since the first report, more than 67 million persons have been infected with HIV, and more than 25 million have died of AIDS. The total number of deaths has exceeded those caused by the Black Death of 14th century Europe and the influenza pandemic of 1918 and 1919. Worldwide, more than 40% percent of new infections among adults occur in young people 15 to 24 years of age.[1,2]

AIDS is an infectious disease that is transmitted predominantly through intimate sexual contact and parenteral means by HIV. Given the nature of this bloodborne pathogen, HIV and AIDS have important implications for dental practitioners. Although HIV has rarely been transmitted from patients to health care workers, this may occur, and of course, the patient with HIV or AIDS is certainly medically compromised and needs special dental management considerations.

DEFINITION

The definition of AIDS provided by the CDC includes a cluster of differentiation 4 (CD4) lymphocyte count of less than 200 in a patient who is infected with HIV. This definition also includes individuals who are HIV infected with pulmonary tuberculosis, recurrent episodes of pneumonia, or invasive cervical carcinoma. Previously, Kaposi's sarcoma or lymphoma, *P carinii* pneumonia or other life-threatening opportunistic infection, the wasting syndrome, and/or central nervous system (CNS) syndromes with dementia and associated immunosuppression would fulfill the definition, regardless of the CD4 count. With continuing improvements in the pharmacologic management of patients with AIDS, most opportunistic infections do not occur, even with extremely low CD4 counts.[3,4]

Incidence and Prevalence

At the end of 2003, an estimated 1,039,000 to 1,185,000 persons in the United States were living with HIV/AIDS; in 24% to 27%, the condition remained undiagnosed, and patients were unaware of their HIV infection. In 2004, more than 4.9 million people were infected by HIV, and about 3.1 million individuals died (Table 19-1).[4]

In 2006, the CDC estimated that more than 1.8 million Americans were infected with HIV, and that more than 950,000 cases of AIDS had been diagnosed, primarily in adults; about 10,000 cases occurred in children younger than 13 years of age. More than 530,000 related deaths have been reported in the United States, again primarily in adults; only 5000 deaths were reported in children younger than age 13, and approximately 25% were unaware of the diagnosis. Worldwide, more than 25 million persons have died of AIDS (see Table 19-1).[2,3]

The estimated number of diagnoses of AIDS in the United States per year is approximately 42,000. Most are adult and adolescent AIDS cases, which account for about 99% of all cases. In 2004, AIDS cases totaled 42,466; 31,024 cases occurred in males and 11,442 cases in females. In all, 48 cases of AIDS were estimated in children younger than age 13.[3,4] The AIDS epidemic continues to progress in the United States, although the rate has slowed somewhat over the past few years, according to the CDC. Still, the CDC reports approximately 3500 new cases per month.

No vaccine or definitive treatment exists for this nationwide epidemic. Currently approved groups of antiretroviral drugs (highly active antiretroviral therapy [HAART]) may help slow the progression of infection, but no cure is yet known. The best treatment approach

TABLE **19-1**

Acquired Immunodeficiency Syndrome (AIDS) Cases, According to Year of Diagnosis and Selected Characteristics of Persons: United States, 1999-2003*

Gender, Race and Hispanic Origin, Age at Diagnosis, and Region of Residence	All Years[1]	Year of Diagnosis				
		1999	2000	2001	2002	2003
		Estimated Number of Cases[2]				
All persons[3]	929,985	41,356	41,267	40,833	41,289	43,171
GENDER						
Male, 13 years and over	749,887	31,159	30,387	30,074	30,517	31,614
Female, 13 years and over	170,679	10,010	10,763	10,639	10,666	11,498
Children, under 13 years	9,419	187	117	119	105	59
Not Hispanic or Latino						
White	376,834	12,626	12,047	11,620	11,960	12,222
Black or African American	368,169	19,960	20,312	20,291	20,476	21,304
American Indian or Alaska Native	3,026	162	186	179	196	196
Asian or Pacific Islander	7,166	369	373	409	452	497
Hispanic or Latino[4]	172,993	8,141	8,233	8,204	8,021	8,757
AGE AT DIAGNOSIS						
Under 13 years	9,419	187	117	119	105	59
13-14 years	891	57	56	76	68	59
15-24 years	37,599	1,541	1,642	1,625	1,810	1,991
25-34 years	311,137	11,349	10,385	9,947	9,504	9,605
35-44 years	365,432	17,165	17,295	16,890	17,008	17,633
45-54 years	148,347	8,099	8,566	8,929	9,310	10,051
55-64 years	43,451	2,218	2,422	2,468	2,724	2,888
65 years and over	13,711	739	783	779	759	886
REGION OF RESIDENCE						
Northeast	285,040	11,885	12,516	11,350	10,551	11,461
Midwest	91,926	4,069	4,139	4,094	4,337	4,198
South	337,409	17,224	16,757	17,693	18,482	19,609
West	186,100	6,892	6,661	6,468	6,843	6,667
U.S. dependencies, possessions, and associated nations	29,511	1,286	1,194	1,228	1,075	935
		Percent Distribution[5]				
All persons[3]	100.0	100.0	100.0	100.0	100.0	100.0
GENDER						
Male, 13 years and over	80.6	75.3	73.6	73.7	73.9	73.2
Female, 13 years and over	18.4	24.2	26.1	26.1	25.8	26.6
Children, under 13 years	1.0	0.5	0.3	0.3	0.3	0.1
Not Hispanic or Latino						
White	40.5	30.5	29.2	28.5	29.0	28.3
Black or African American	39.6	48.3	49.2	49.7	49.6	49.3
American Indian or Alaska Native	0.3	0.4	0.5	0.4	0.5	0.5
Asian or Pacific Islander	0.8	0.9	0.9	1.0	1.1	1.2
Hispanic or Latino[4]	18.6	19.7	20.0	20.1	19.4	20.3
AGE AT DIAGNOSIS						
Under 13 years	1.0	0.5	0.3	0.3	0.3	0.1
13-14 years	0.1	0.1	0.1	0.2	0.2	0.1
15-24 years	4.0	3.7	4.0	4.0	4.4	4.6
25-34 years	33.5	27.4	25.2	24.4	23.0	22.2
35-44 years	39.3	41.5	41.9	41.4	41.2	40.8
45-54 years	16.0	19.6	20.8	21.9	22.5	23.3
55-64 years	4.7	5.4	5.9	6.0	6.6	6.7
65 years and over	1.5	1.8	1.9	1.9	1.8	2.1

TABLE 19-1

Acquired Immunodeficiency Syndrome (AIDS) Cases, According to Year of Diagnosis and Selected Characteristics of Persons: United States, 1999-2003—cont'd

Gender, Race and Hispanic Origin, Age at Diagnosis, and Region of Residence	All Years[1]	Year of Diagnosis				
		1999	2000	2001	2002	2003
		Percent Distribution[5]				
REGION OF RESIDENCE						
Northeast	30.6	28.7	30.3	27.8	25.6	26.5
Midwest	9.9	9.8	10.0	10.0	10.5	10.4
South	36.3	41.6	40.6	43.3	44.8	45.4
West	20.0	16.7	16.1	15.8	16.6	15.4
U.S. dependencies, possessions, and associated nations	3.2	3.1	2.9	3.0	2.6	2.2

*Data based on reporting by state health departments.

[1]Based on cases reported to the Centers for Disease Control and Prevention from the beginning of the epidemic through 2003.

[2]Numbers are point estimates that result from adjustments for reporting delays to AIDS case counts. The estimates do not include adjustments for incomplete reporting. Data are provisional. See Appendix I, AIDS Surveillance.

[3]Total for all years includes 1,796 persons of unknown race or multiple races and one person of unknown sex. All persons totals were calculated independent of values for subpopulations. Consequently sums of subpopulations may not equal total for all persons.

[4]Persons of Hispanic origin may be of any race.

[5]Percents may not sum to 100 percent due to rounding and because 0.2 percent unknown race and Hispanic origin are included in totals.

NOTES: See Appendix II, AIDS, for discussion of AIDS case reporting definitions and other issues affecting interpretation of trends. This table presents adjusted data (point estimates) by year of diagnosis and replaces surveillance data by year of report in previous editions of Health, United States.

SOURCES: Centers for Disease Control and Prevention, National Center for HIV, STD, and TB Prevention, Division of HIV/AIDS Prevention–Surveillance and Epidemiology, AIDS Surveillance; HIV/AIDS Surveillance Report, 2003 (vol. 15) table 3. Atlanta: US Department of Health and Human Services, Centers for Disease Control and Prevention. 2004. Also available at www.cdc.gov/hiv/stats/hasrlink.htm. From Health, United States, 2005.

for AIDS, as for other infectious diseases, continues to be public health measures such as preventive education, early detection, and counseling for infected patients and their contacts (family, lover, friends, coworkers) and the use of drugs to slow the progress of the disease. Recent changes in the epidemiology of AIDS have been a positive testimony to this approach.[5]

From the time of diagnosis, 30% of patients with AIDS can be expected to live approximately 2 to 3 years, with most others living 10 years or longer. Death usually results from an opportunistic infection and, in some cases, from complications associated with the various malignancies seen with AIDS. The onset of these complications generally is associated with a low CD4 count. All individuals infected with HIV-1 eventually develop AIDS. This will remain true until effective antiviral treatment agents become available. Presently, however, most individuals with AIDS are living longer, including some with CD4 counts that are extremely low (i.e., 10 to 40).[5]

Several cases of HIV-2 infection have been reported by the CDC and others from various countries, including Canada, the United States, South America, and Europe. HIV-2 has been shown to provide some natural immunity to HIV-1 and develops much less rapidly. Immunosuppression is not as severe. However, ultimate mortality from HIV-2 remains unknown.[5]

In the United States, AIDS is the leading cause of death in men 25 to 44 years of age; more than 30 million adults and 1 million children throughout the world are infected. Over the past 5 years, a steady increase in heterosexual transmission of AIDS has occurred in the United States, and the number of cases of AIDS associated with blood and blood products has declined (Figure 19-1 and Table 19-2). However, over that same period, a 31% decrease was reported in the incidence of HIV infection in males who have had sex with men. The overall prevalence in that group (over 13 years of age) is 15.9 per 100,000.[6]

Recently, much progress has been made in the treatment of AIDS. Although no cure is known, HAART has made a significant difference in survival and reduction of systemic complications, as well as in the quality of life of individuals infected with HIV.[7]

The impact and importance of AIDS in dentistry have been significant. The CDC has made specific recommendations for dentists who treat HIV-infected patients. The American Dental Association has established national guidelines and standards for infection control, identification of potential patients with AIDS, and treatment of these patients in the dental setting. The Occupational Safety and Health Administration has mandated certain standards of practice designed to reduce the likelihood of transmission of bloodborne pathogens to employees in the dental office.

Among other changes that recently occurred in the epidemiology of AIDS is an increase in the ratio of

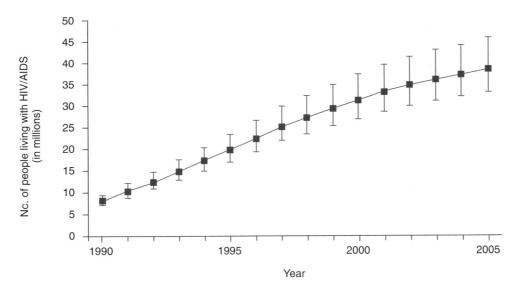

Figure 19-1. Number of people in the world living with HIV/AIDS. (Modified from Merson MH. The HIV-AIDS pandemic at 25—The global response. N Engl J Med 2006;354: 2414-2417.)

TABLE **19-2**

AIDS Cases by Exposure Category*

Exposure Category	Estimated # of AIDS Cases in 2003		
	Male	Female	Total
Male-to-male sexual contact	17,969	—	17,969
Injection drug use	6,353	3,096	9,449
Male-to-male sexual contact and injection drug use	1,877	—	1,877
Heterosexual contact	5,133	8,127	13,260
Other[†]	281	276	557

Exposure Category	Estimated # of AIDS Cases through 2003		
	Male	Female	Total
Male-to-male sexual contact	440,887	—	440,887
Injection drug use	175,988	70,558	246,546
Male-to-male sexual contact and injection drug use	62,418	—	62,418
Heterosexual contact	56,403	93,586	149,989
Other[†]	14,191	6,535	20,726

From the CDC HIV/AIDS Surveillance Report: HIV Infection and AIDS in the United States, 2004.
*Data includes the distribution of the **estimated number** of diagnoses of AIDS among adults and adolescents by exposure category. A breakdown by sex is provided where appropriate.
[†]Includes hemophilia, blood transfusion, perinatal, and risk not reported or not identified.

infected women to men, particularly in the 30- to 40-year age group in black women (see Tables 19-1 and 19-2). A reduction in the number of AIDS cases reported in the transfusion and hemophiliac groups has occurred because of the testing (started in 1985) of donor blood for HIV antibodies and the heating of factor VIII replacement preparations. Table 19-2 describes the distribution of AIDS cases in terms of exposure through 2003.[6]

Risk of Transmission From Health Care Personnel

In 1990, an HIV-infected Florida dentist transmitted, in some undetermined way, HIV infection to six of his patients. All of these patients are now deceased.[8] To date, this is the only documented case of HIV transmission from an infected health care professional to patients. The risk of HIV transmission from infected patients to health care workers is very low, reportedly about 3 out of every 1000 cases (0.3%) in which a needlestick or other sharp instrument transmitted blood from infected patients to health care workers.[9,10] This rate of transmission can be reduced by postexposure prophylaxis with zidovudine (AZT) and other agents.[10] The risk of transmission in the dental setting is minimized by the application of standard infection control procedures.[11] The only other report of HIV transmission involving dentistry came from Bucaramanga, Colombia, in 1997,[12] where 14 cases of HIV infection occurred among hemodialysis patients at a university hospital. Transmission of the virus appeared to occur through contaminated dental instruments.[12]

Etiology

In 1984, the etiologic agent for AIDS was identified independently by three laboratories. A French team from the Pasteur Institute identified a retrovirus called the *lymphadenopathy-associated virus* and reported it as the causative agent for AIDS. In the United States, a team from the National Institutes of Health isolated a retrovirus identified as the human T lymphotropic virus III (HTLV-III) and labeled it as the etiologic agent for AIDS. A team in San Francisco also isolated a retrovirus, AIDS-related virus (ARV), and designated it as the causative agent for

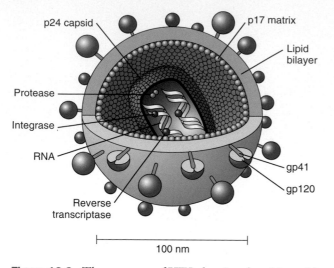

Figure 19-2. The structure of HIV, showing the p24 capsid protein surrounding two strands of viral RNA. (From Copstead LC, Banasik JL. Pathophysiology, 3rd ed. St. Louis, Saunders, 2005.)

AIDS. All three viruses were similar retroviruses, but minor differences were observed in their amino acid sequences. Variation in disease patterns may be accounted for by the slight differences among AIDS viruses, which also makes difficult the production of a vaccine. The three groups essentially were describing the same retrovirus, which can change its antigenicity. Until 1986, most workers in the field referred to the virus as HTLV-III and considered it to be the causative agent for AIDS. In 1986, the World Health Organization recommended that the AIDS virus be called the *human immunodeficiency virus* (Figure 19-2).[5,13]

What first appeared to be a single virus is now actually known as a complex family of lentiviruses composed of two subtypes (HIV-1 and HIV-2) with many different strains. HIV can infect most human cells; however, the cells most commonly infected are those with CD4 receptors, including T-helper lymphocytes (CD4 cells) and macrophages; hence, these cells are most deeply involved in HIV infection. Research has suggested that other receptors are active in allowing HIV to infect human cells. Evidence has surfaced that HIV/antibody complexes interact with Fc or a complement receptor, which facilitates entry of the virus into the cell. Other cell surface receptors include galactosylcerebroside glycolipids, LFA-1 adhesion receptor, and certain proteases.[5,13]

A small portion of the carboxyterminal half of the viral envelope (gp120), which represents less than 5% of the total genome, is associated with the most virulent features of HIV infection (see Fig. 19-2). This segment of gp120, which has been referred to as the V_3 loop, may represent the best site for vaccine development. Long-term survivors of HIV infection have been found to have less virulent HIV strains, without the enhancing antibodies to HIV and with strong CD8m T-cell antiviral activity.[5,13]

HIV-1 gene expression is divided into two temporal phases: an early regulatory phase and a later structural phase. In the early phase, a set of small messenger ribonucleic acids (mRNAs) are produced that encode the regulatory proteins tat, rev, and nef. These are powerful viral regulators and activators that are necessary for viral replication. Efforts toward the development of a vaccine have revolved around these regulatory proteins. When the viral regions responsible for neutralization enhancement are defined, the development of nef proteins to block HIV replication may be possible.[5,13] (For an indepth discussion of the function of these viral genes and their products, the reader is referred to Chapter 17 by Fauci AS, Lane HC. HIV disease: AIDS and related disorders. In Kasper DL, et al [eds]. Harrison's Online Principles of Medicine, 16th ed. New York, McGraw-Hill, 2005.)

Current attempts to develop a vaccine are directed toward (1) preventing HIV infection, and (2) interfering with viral replication, to render the HIV infection less severe. Major efforts to develop a vaccine thus far have centered around the most virulent portion of HIV, with goals of identifying and producing the antiviral agent produced by CD8+ cells, or developing nef (or other) proteins to block HIV replication.[14]

Pathophysiology and Complications

In addition to its transfer by sexual means and the parenteral transfer of infected blood, AIDS may be transmitted vertically, probably at birth, or transplacentally to infants born of infected mothers. The most common method of sexual transmission in the United States is homosexual anal intercourse; however, heterosexual transmission has been documented from infected males to noninfected females. Transmission from infected females to noninfected males also has been reported. Heterosexual transmission of HIV can occur through sexual contact of carriers who are heterosexual intravenous (IV) drug users, bisexual males, or blood recipients of either gender. HIV has been found in saliva, but transmission via saliva has not been demonstrated. HIV has also been isolated from tears, breast milk, cerebrospinal fluid, amniotic fluid, and urine. However, blood, semen, breast milk, and vaginal secretions are the only fluids that have been shown to be associated with transmission of the virus. Casual contact has not been demonstrated as a means of transmission.[14]

By the year 2006, more than 1.9 million Americans were estimated to have been exposed to the AIDS virus. Current data suggest that most if not all of these individuals will develop AIDS as defined by the CDC. Antibody positivity to HIV means that the person has been infected with the virus and can be viremic. Individuals who appear to be most susceptible to developing AIDS are those with repeated exposure to the virus who also have an immune system that has been challenged by repeated exposure to various antigens (semen, hepatitis B, or blood products).[6,12]

Individuals infected with the virus develop antibodies, usually within 6 to 12 weeks. Most infected individuals

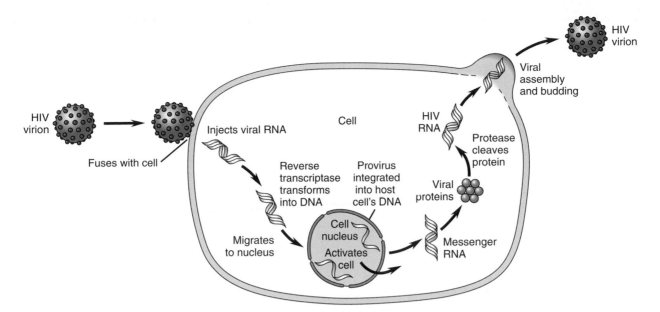

Figure 19-3. The HIV life cycle. (From Copstead LC, Banasik JL. Pathophysiology, 3rd ed. St. Louis, Saunders, 2005.)

develop a viremia within 2 to 6 weeks. A few may take up to 6 months to achieve seroconversion. In rare cases, as long as 35 months may be required for seroconversion to occur. The incubation period for AIDS appears to be lengthy for most individuals (mean, 10 to 12 years). Only about 30% of individuals with AIDS are dead within 3 years of diagnosis, whereas approximately 50% live beyond 10 years.[6,12]

Once it has gained access to the bloodstream, HIV selectively seeks out T lymphocytes (specifically T4 or T-helper lymphocytes) (Figure 19-3). The virus binds to the CD4 lymphocyte cell surface specifically through the highly glycosylated outer surface envelope (gp120) proteins. Upon infection, reverse transcriptase catalyzes the synthesis of a haploid, double-stranded DNA provirus, which becomes incorporated into the chromosomal DNA of the host cell. Thus integrated, the provirus genetic material may remain latent in an unexpressed form until events occur that activate it, at which time DNA transcription rapidly occurs and new virions are produced. The virus is lymphotropic; hence, the cells it selects for replication are soon destroyed. Once the virus has taken hold, it soon causes a reduction in the total number of T-helper cells, and a marked shift in the ratio of T4 to T8 lymphocytes occurs. The normal ratio of T-helper to T-suppressor lymphocytes is about 2:1 (60% T-helper, 30% T-suppressor). In AIDS, the T4/T8 ratio is reversed. This marked reduction in T-helper lymphocytes, to a great degree, explains the lack of immune response seen in patients with AIDS and most likely is related to the increase in malignant disease that has been found to be associated with AIDS, including Kaposi's sarcoma, lymphoma, carcinoma of the cervix, and carcinoma of the rectum.[6,12]

Table 19-3 presents the clinical stages of HIV infection through frank AIDS. Most (more than 50%) indi-

viduals exposed to the virus at first develop an acute, brief viremia (seroconversion sickness) within 2 to 6 weeks of HIV exposure. A concomitant, temporary fall occurs in CD4 cells (lymphopenia, along with high titers of plasma HIV), but patients do not develop evidence of immune suppression. Various flulike symptoms occur in this acute seroconversion sickness that usually last about 2 to 4 weeks. Only an estimated 20% of these individuals seek medical attention. These individuals respond by producing antibodies to HIV (i.e., anti-gp120 and anti-p24), and cytotoxic T lymphocyte levels increase. Immune abnormalities in HIV disease consist of progressive depletion of CD4+ T lymphocytes with ultimate pancytopenia, impaired lymphocyte proliferation, and cytokine responses to mitogens and antigens; impaired cytotoxic lymphocyte function and natural killer cell activity; anergy to skin testing; and diminished antibody responses to new antigens.[6,12]

The virus also may infect neurons or macrophages in the CNS, allowing its presence within the body in latent form. Individuals may demonstrate a viremia on occasion and hence are considered carriers of the virus who have the potential to infect others. Of special concern is the fact that circulating antibodies fail to neutralize the virus because it has the capacity to alter its antigenicity (see Fig. 19-3). An alarming characteristic of these patients, in addition to their potential to be infectious and to develop AIDS, is that approximately 50% develop signs of dementia that can be rapidly progressive. In most cases, after a long asymptomatic period, the CD4 count continues to drop and HIV continues to proliferate; in addition, the infected individual may develop signs and symptoms such as lymphadenopathy, fever, weight loss, diarrhea, night sweats, pharyngitis, rashes, myalgia and arthralgia, headache, neuropathy and malaise, and eventually, AIDS (Figure 19-4).[6,12]

TABLE 19-3
Clinical Stages of HIV Infection

Status	Signs/Symptoms	Laboratory Findings	Comments
Recent infection	No signs or symptoms.	HIV nucleic acid: positive p24 antigen, positive DNA PCR, positive ELISA and Western blot	Patient is unaware of his or her HIV infection. Can transmit the infection by blood or sexual activity.
Acute seroconversion syndrome	Symptoms occur within about 1 to 3 wk after infection in about 70% of infected patients: Fever, diarrhea, nausea, vomiting Skin rashes (roseola-like or urticarial) Weight loss Pharyngitis Myalgia, headache Lymphadenopathy Symptoms clear in about 1 to 2 wk.	HIV antibody negative at start of syndrome. Seroconversion occurs near end of the syndrome. CD4+ and CD8+ lymphocytes reduced in numbers. After acute symptoms, they tend to return toward normal levels. ELISA and Western blot +.	The severity of the acute syndrome varies among infected individuals. The period for seroconversion of the 30% of patients without acute symptoms varies and can be 1-6 months or longer.
Latent period (asymptomatic stage)	Median time from initial infection to onset of clinical symptoms is 8 to 10 years. About 50% to 70% of patients develop persistent generalized lymphadenopathy (PGL).	ELISA and Western blot +. A slow but usually steady increase in viral load. Usually, a steady decline in CD4+ cell count.	Viral replication is ongoing and progressive. A steady decline in CD4+ cell counts occurs, except in the less than 1% who are nonprogressors (also have low viral load).
Early symptomatic HIV infection (B symptoms, AIDS-related complex)	Without treatment, lasts for 1 to 3 years. Any of the following: PGL Fungal infections Vaginal yeast and trichomonal infections Oral hairy leukoplakia Herpes zoster Herpes simplex HIV retinopathy Constitutional symptoms Fever, night sweats, fatigue diarrhea, weight loss	ELISA and Western blot +. HIV antigen, RNA, and DNA tests are positive. Signs and symptoms increase as the CD4+ cell count declines and approaches 200/mm^3. Viral load continues to increase. Platelet count may decrease in about 10% of patients.	The spectrum of disease changes as CD4 + cell count declines.
AIDS	Signs and symptoms of any of the following: Opportunistic infection(s) *Pneumocystis carinii* pneumonia Cryptococcosis Tuberculosis Toxoplasmosis Histoplasmosis Others Malignancies Kaposi's sarcoma Burkitt's lymphoma Non-Hodgkin's lymphoma Primary CNS lymphoma Invasive cervical cancer Slim (wasting) disease	High viral load. CD4+ cell count below 200/mm^3 indicates AIDS. CD4+ cell count below 50/mm^3 at high risk for lymphoma and death. Platelet count may be low. Neutrophil count may be low. ELISA and Western blot +. HIV antigen, RNA, and DNA tests are positive.	Death usually occurs because of wasting, opportunistic infection, or malignancies. The use of combination antiretroviral agents has slowed the death rate, but long-term outlook must depend on vaccines for prevention and treatment because the virus promotes resistance to these agents.

HIV, Human immunodeficiency virus; ELISA, enzyme-linked immunosorbent assay; AIDS, acquired immunodeficiency syndrome; CNS, central nervous system.

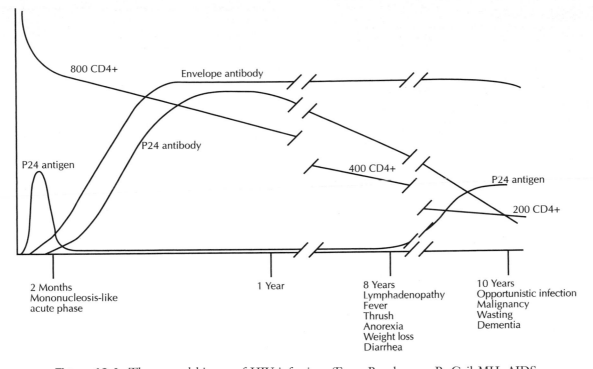

Figure 19-4. The natural history of HIV infection. (From Brookmeyer R, Gail MH. AIDS Epidemiology: A Quantitative Approach. New York, Oxford University Press, 1994, pp 1-18.)

Generally, when the CD4 count drops to below 200, the patient is susceptible to several opportunistic infections, including *P carinii* pneumonia, toxoplasmosis, influenza, histoplasmosis, cytomegalovirus (CMV) infection, and mucocutaneous diseases such as candidiasis. The neoplasms previously discussed also may appear during AIDS.[6,12]

Cases of tuberculosis (TB) in HIV-infected patients have risen dramatically during the past 5 years. The CDC reports that coincident cases of HIV/AIDS and TB increased from 8% to 17% during that time. The number of cases of TB in the United States during that period increased from approximately 21,000 to 26,000 per year. Most of these cases have occurred among HIV-infected populations as have the increasing number of multidrug resistant strains of TB (see Chapter 9).

CLINICAL PRESENTATION

Signs and Symptoms

During the first 2 to 6 weeks after initial infection with HIV, more than 50% of patients develop an acute flulike viremia that may last 10 to 14 days. Others may not manifest this symptom complex. Patients have HIV but are antibody negative. They usually experience seroconversion within 6 weeks to 6 months and then demonstrate antibodies. The severity of the initial acute infection with HIV is predictive of the course the infection will follow. In one study, 78% of individuals with a long-lasting acute illness developed AIDS within 3 years; by contrast, only 10% of those individuals with no acute illness at serocon-

---

BOX 19-1

Categorization of HIV Exposures

GROUP 1
HIV antibody positive—asymptomatic

GROUP 2
CD4 <400
Constitutional symptoms (i.e., fever, malaise, lymphadenopathy, diarrhea); opportunistic infections

GROUP 3
AIDS; CD4 <200
Kaposi's sarcoma, lymphoma, pneumonia, cervical carcinoma, etc.

HIV, Human immunodeficiency virus; AIDS, acquired immunodeficiency syndrome.

---

version developed AIDS within 3 years. Once exposure to HIV and seroconversion have occurred, three groups of patients may be identified (Boxes 19-1 and 19-2; see Figure 19-4).[6,12]

Group 1. Immediate post-HIV exposure. After a brief postseroconversion sickness syndrome, these individuals are antibody positive to HIV but are asymptomatic and show no other laboratory abnormalities.

Group 2. Progressive immunosuppression, HIV-symptomatic stage. Individuals who demonstrate various laboratory changes (i.e., lymphopenia: T-helper/T-

Signs and Symptoms of HIV Infection

**INITIAL EXPOSURE OR INFECTION
(SEROCONVERSION SYNDROME)**
- Flulike symptoms—fever, weakness, 10 to 14 days
- Asymptomatic stage
- Serologic evidence of infection
- No signs or symptoms

SYMPTOMATIC STAGE
- Serologic evidence of infection
- T4/T8 ratio reduced to about 1
- Persistent lymphadenopathy
- Oral candidiasis
- Constitutional symptoms—night sweats, diarrhea, weight loss, fever, malaise, weakness

ADVANCED SYMPTOMATIC STAGE
- Serologic evidence of infection
- T4/T8 ratio suppressed to less than 0.5
- HIV encephalopathy
- HIV wasting syndrome
- Major opportunistic infections
- Neoplasms—Kaposi's sarcoma, lymphoma, carcinoma of rectum

HIV, Human immunodeficiency syndrome.

TABLE **19-4**

Common Immunosuppression-Related Diseases Based on T-Helper Cell Level*

T-Helper Cell Count	Disease
>400	Most patients have no signs of immunosuppression-associated disease
301 to 400	Bacterial skin infections = staphylococcal
201 to 300	Herpes zoster
	Candidiasis
	Tinea pedis
	Oral hairy leukoplakia
101 to 200	Tuberculosis
	Pneumocystis carinii pneumonia
	Histoplasmosis
	Coccidioidomycosis
	Cryptococcal meningitis
	Toxoplasmosis
	Herpes simplex
	Cryptosporidiosis
	Kaposi's sarcoma
0 to 100	Wasting syndrome
	Cytomegalovirus
	Lymphoma
	Mycobacterium avium complex

*The T-helper cell range is the common range for onset of the disease. The disease could first appear at a higher or lower T-cell level.[53]

suppressor ratio usually less than 1) in addition to HIV antibody positivity also may show some clinical signs or symptoms, such as enlarged lymph nodes, night sweats, weight loss, oral candidiasis, fever, malaise, and diarrhea.

Group 3. Individuals who have AIDS, including Kaposi's sarcoma, wasting syndrome, lymphoma, cervical or rectal carcinoma, CNS symptoms with dementia, a life-threatening opportunistic infection (i.e., tuberculosis, pneumonia), a CD4 count of less than 200, and an altered T-helper/T-suppressor ratio of 0.5 or less. They are HIV antibody positive and can demonstrate generalized lymphadenopathy with severe weight loss, fatigue, chronic diarrhea, chronic fever, and night sweats (Table 19-4). HIV may infect the CNS and often leads to a progressive form of dementia.

Patients may become confused and disoriented or may experience short-term memory deficits. Others develop severe depression or paranoia and show suicidal tendencies. Table 19-3 describes the clinical stages of HIV infection through frank AIDS.

Laboratory Findings

HIV can be isolated from the blood, semen, breast milk, tears, and saliva of many patients with AIDS. Most patients exposed to the virus, with or without clinical evidence of disease, show antibodies to the virus. Patients with advanced HIV infection or AIDS have an altered ratio of T4/T8 lymphocytes, a decrease in total number of lymphocytes, thrombocytopenia, anemia, a slight alteration in the humoral antibody system, and a decreased ability to show delayed allergic reactions to skin testing (cutaneous anergy).[14]

In 1985, several screening tests became available for identification of antibodies to HIV. The enzyme-linked immunosorbent assay (ELISA) is sensitive but has a high rate of false-positive results. Current practice is to screen first with ELISA. If the first results are positive, a second ELISA is performed. All positive results are then rescreened with a second test, the Western blot analysis. This combination of screening tests is accurate more than 99% of the time. Positive ELISA and Western blot test results indicate only that the individual has been exposed to the AIDS virus. If results of the Western blot are indeterminate, HIV infection is rarely, if ever, positive. These tests, however, do not indicate the status of the HIV infection or whether AIDS is present. Neither do they show if the patient is viremic because a special test, the DNA polymerase chain reaction (PCR) for direct detection of the virus, would need to be performed. This test is considerably more expensive. However, patients with positive results from the ELISA and Western blot tests are considered potentially infectious. An ELISA test developed by Wellcome is 98% sensitive in detecting antibodies to HIV in saliva. A test to detect salivary secretory immunoglobulin A antibodies of nonmaternal origin in newborns of women at risk for HIV infection has been found accurate in detecting infected infants.[5,12,15,16]

Since 1989, HIV DNA sequences may be readily detected by the DNA PCR assay, which was found to be an equivalent method of culturing the virus itself. Direct detection of HIV by PCR is superior to testing for HIV antigen in serum.[17]

Viral load (degree of viremia in blood plasma) is determined with the use of a PCR-based test such as that available through Roche Molecular Systems Inc. Detection ranges from 50 copies per milliliter to more than 750,000 copies per milliliter. The greatest viral load is found during the first 3 months after initial infection and during late stages of the disease.

MEDICAL MANAGEMENT

No effective treatment or cure for AIDS is known. Antiviral agents have been unsuccessful in killing the HIV virus. However, zidovudine (AZT or Retrovir) has been shown to exert significant inhibitory effects on in vitro replication and the cytopathogenicity of HIV. AZT has been found to prolong life in both asymptomatic and symptomatic HIV-infected individuals, although no evidence suggests that AZT is effective in preventing infection once exposure to the virus has occurred (Table 19-5).[18]

Medical management of the HIV-infected patient must include counseling regarding safe sexual practices, how to avoid the spread of HIV, and how to minimize exposure to high-risk pathogens. The physician provides baseline and ongoing assessments of the patient, as well as antiretroviral therapy and preventive treatment in the form of vaccine and prophylaxis against opportunistic infection. One goal is to achieve maximum reduction of the viral load and to maintain this reduction for as long as possible to slow disease progression. Another goal is to restore the CD4 count back to a normal range. The physician should use HAART in a manner that will achieve viral suppression and immune reconstitution while at the same time preventing emergence of resistance and limiting drug toxicity. Long-term goals are to delay disease progression, prolong life, and improve quality of life.

Antiretroviral Therapy

Table 19-5 lists the antiretroviral agents that are currently available for the management of HIV/AIDS. The first antiretroviral agent used in the AIDS epidemic was zidovudine (AZT); however, viral resistance emerged often during the initial 6 to 12 months of therapy.[19] Therapy now consists of a combination of regimens, including at least one potent agent that will minimize viral replication, thus reducing mutation rates that can lead to resistance.[19] The development of more potent antiretroviral agents in the mid-1990s and the recognition that combination therapy was more effective than monotherapy have led to improved clinical benefits.[19] These regimens have represented a major advance in the treatment of HIV-infected patients who have access to

medical care and are capable of taking these drugs and willing to do so.[19] Taking these drugs, given their toxicities, costs, and inconvenience, presents a major challenge for patients.[19]

The antiretroviral agents are used to restore immune dysfunction by inhibiting viral replication. Four different types of agents that are now available—protease inhibitors (PIs), nucleoside reverse transcriptase inhibitors (NRTIs), non-nucleoside reverse transcriptase inhibitors (NNRTIs), and nucleotides and the fusion inhibitors (enfuvirtide is the first member of this class to become available)—have just received approval from the U.S. Food and Drug Administration (FDA) for clinical use (see Table 19-5).[4] These agents are usually used in combinations known as HAART. Patients who are on these medications must be closely monitored for effectiveness and drug toxicity.[4]

The drug regimen that is initiated should be potent enough to suppress the viral load to below the level of assay detection for a prolonged period.[19] This requires at least two drugs, including at least one that is a PI, an NNRTI, or abacavir.[19] Usually, two NRTIs are used.[19] Currently, regimens consisting of efavirenz or nevirapine or lopinavir-ritonavir plus lamivudine plus either zidovudine or tenofovir are popular.[19] The first drug that allows AIDS to be treated with one pill a day has just recently won federal approval—a development that government officials said would both simplify and improve treatment of the disease. The drug, called *Atripla*, is a combination of three once-a-day drugs that are already on the market—Sustiva (Bristol-Myers Squibb), and Viread and Emtriva (Gilead Sciences). Only a decade ago, when cocktails of AIDS drugs began to be used, patients sometimes had to take two dozen or more pills a day.

All patients with acute antiretroviral syndrome and patients within 6 months of seroconversion should be offered antiretroviral treatment.[4,20] Also, all patients with symptoms ascribed to HIV infection and symptomatic patients with CD4+ T-cell count less than 350/mm^3 are offered treatment.[4,20] Another group of patients who should be offered treatment with antiretroviral agents are those with plasma HIV RNA levels greater than 55,000 copies/mL.[4,20] Treatment is generally initiated for asymptomatic patients who have a rapid drop in CD4+ T-cell count or high viral loads (730 to 55,000 copies/mL). Asymptomatic patients with stable CD4+ T-cell counts and low viral loads are generally followed without treatment.[4,20] Antiretroviral therapy is strongly recommended for patients with CD4+ T-cell counts of fewer than 200/mm^3 and for those with AIDS.[4,20]

Vaccination. Immunization with killed microbial products or recombinant products is considered safe in HIV-infected adults. The HIV-infected adult should receive the following products before his/her CD4+ T-cell count drops to below 200/mm^3: 23-valent polysaccharide pneumococcal vaccination, hepatitis A vaccine (all patients negative for HAV antibody), hepatitis B vaccine (all

TABLE 19-5
Antiretroviral Drugs Used to Treat HIV Infection

Class	Drugs	Toxicity	Interactions	Comments
PROTEASE INHIBITORS (PIs)	Amprenavir Indinavir Lopinavir Nelfinavir Ritonavir Saquinavir	Nausea, vomiting Diarrhea Abdominal discomfort Paresthesias Fatigue Anemia, leukopenia Thrombocytopenia Altered taste Hypercholesterolemia Hypertriglyceridemia Xerostomia	Amiodarone Quinidine Rifampin Ergotamine St. John's wort Midazolam Triazolam	PIs act at the end of the virus replication cycle, blocking the catalytic center of the protease enzyme, resulting in viral particles that are ineffective and immature.
NUCLEOSIDE REVERSE TRANSCRIPTASE INHIBITORS (NRTIs)	Abacavir Emtricitabine Didanosine Lamivudine Stavudine Zalcitabine Zidovudine	Headache Insomnia Fatigue Anemia, neutropenia Nausea Diarrhea Neuropathy Pancreatitis Myopathy Xerostomia	Avoid mixing zidovudine and stavudine, ribavirin, or doxorubicin. Ganciclovir and interferon-α must be avoided.	Drug adverse effects are often dose related and can be minimized with lower doses of the agents. Use of zalcitabine is restricted because of the small therapeutic window. Stavudine is the most frequently used drug in the group.
NON-NUCLEOSIDE REVERSE TRANSCRIPTASE INHIBITORS (NNRTIs)	Delavirdine Efavirenz Nevirapine	Dizziness, insomnia Confusion, agitation Hallucinations Depression, mania Skin rashes Nausea, vomiting Diarrhea Stevens-Johnson syndrome Xerostomia, taste alteration	Midazolam Triazolam Clarithromycin (rash, <drug concentration) Sertraline (<drug concentration) Warfarin (>drug effect) Ketoconazole (<drug concentration)	The most important negative adverse effects are neuropsychiatric events, skin reactions, GI alterations, and liver alterations.
NUCLEOTIDES	Adefovir Tenofovir	Dizziness Nausea, diarrhea Weakness Depression, anxiety Skin rash—allergy Neuropathy Liver, kidney failure Lactic acidosis (rapid breathing, drowsiness, muscle aches)	NSAIDs, acyclovir, and ganciclovir affect the metabolism of tenofovir. Vancomycin, NSAIDs, and cyclosporine increase risk for kidney disease.	Adefovir is not used often because of GI and renal toxicity. Tenofovir is used in patients on multiple drug therapy who are not responding. Tenofovir is usually well tolerated.
FUSION INHIBITORS (FIs)	Enfuvirtide	Bacterial pneumonia Rash, fever Nausea, vomiting Glomerulonephritis Guillain-Barré syndrome Taste disturbance Hyperglycemia Myalgia Xerostomia Anorexia	No significant drug interactions	Inhibits fusion of HIV-1 and CD4+ T cells. Only one fusion inhibitor has been approved (enfuvirtide), and it has to be injected. Two other fusion inhibitors are at early stages of clinical testing.

TABLE **19-5**
Antiretroviral Drugs Used to Treat HIV Infection—cont'd

Initial treatment of established HIV infection should consist of one choice from each of sets A1 and B1:
- **Set A1:** efavirenz, indinavir, nelfinavir, ritonavir plus indinavir, ritonavir plus lopinavir, ritonavir plus saquinavir
- **Set B1:** stavudine plus didanosine, stavudine plus lamivudine, zidovudine plus didanosine, zidovudine plus lamivudine

An alternative, although less strongly recommended, option provides one from each of sets A2, B2, and C2:
- **Set A2:** abacavir, amprenavir, lopinavir, delavirdine, nelfinavir plus saquinavir (soft gel capsule), nevirapine, ritonavir, saquinavir (soft gel capsule)
- **Set B2:** tenofovir, an NRTI. It is the oral prodrug of PMPA, an acyclic nucleotide phosphonate analog related to adefovir, which is active against simian immunodeficiency virus (SIV), HIV-1, and HIV-2
- **Set C2:** didanosine plus lamivudine, zidovudine plus zalcitabine

Response to treatment is measured by the plasma HIV RNA level. A change in therapy should be considered if any of the following occurs:
- Viral load reduction is <0.5-0.75-$\log_{10}$ at 4 weeks or is <1-$\log_{10}$ at 8 weeks
- Viral load has not been suppressed to undetectable levels at 4-6 months
- Virus is repeatedly detected after initial suppression to undetectable levels, suggesting the development of viral drug resistance
- A significant increase (threefold or greater) in viral load not attributable to infection, vaccination, or test methodology
- Persistently declining CD4+ T-cell count
- Clinical deterioration
- Undetectable viral load in a patient on double nucleoside therapy

Treatment failure is defined by U.S. Department of Health and Human Services (DHHS) guidelines as virologic, immunologic, or clinical according to the following criteria:
- Virologic failure:
  - VL >400 c/mL at 24 wk
  - VL >50 c/mL at 48 wk
  - VL rebound to >400 c/mL after viral suppression
- Immunologic failure:
  - Failure of CD4 count to increase by >25-50 (increase averages 50/mm^3 at 4 months with successful highly active antiretroviral therapy [HAART]) (JID 2002;185:471)
- Clinical failure:
  - Occurrence or recurrence of an HIV-related event >3 months after therapy (this does not include the immune reconstitution syndrome)

Failure of therapy may be ascribed to the following:
- Nonadherence to drug regimen
- Inadequate potency of drugs or suboptimal levels of antiretroviral agents
- Viral resistance to certain drugs
- Poor oral absorption or drug interactions
- Other reasons that are poorly understood

GI, Gastrointestinal; NSAIDs, nonsteroidal antiinflammatory drugs; HIV, human immunodeficiency virus; VL, viral load.
Also see www.ATDN.org (AIDS Treatment Data Network).

patients negative for previous exposure), tetanus booster, and yearly influenza vaccine; patients who are seronegative for varicella-zoster or who have no history of chickenpox or shingles who are exposed to chickenpox or shingles should receive varicella-zoster immune globulin within 48 hours.[4]

Over the course of the AIDS epidemic, a small group of HIV-infected individuals have been identified in whom infection could be controlled for 20 years or longer without antiretroviral drug therapy.[21] It appears that this group of individuals developed persistent immune control against HIV. An understanding of how this occurred provides information on the clinical sequelae of infection and improves prospects for the development of vaccine against HIV.[21]

Effective vaccination offers the best hope for containing the HIV epidemic.[22] HAART is effective now in containing infection in individuals who are able to receive the drugs and willing to accept the difficulty involved in taking them and the toxicity associated with the drugs. However, the long-term effectiveness of HAART is in doubt because of developing resistance. With the epidemic still spreading and the fact that HAART is not available for most infected individuals, the development of effective vaccines is essential from a therapeutic and a preventive standpoint.[22]

The optimal type of immune response for an HIV vaccine has yet to be determined. Thus, a variety of approaches are being explored. Some are at various stages of preclinical development, others have entered or completed phase 1 and 2 trials in humans, and two vaccine candidates (recombinant gp120 proteins) have completed phase 3 efficacy trials.[22]

The following approaches are under consideration for the development of an HIV-1 vaccine (Table 19-6): whole virus vaccines, envelope protein vaccines, synthetic peptide vaccines, internal core protein vaccines, live vector vaccines, nucleic acid vaccines, and live-attenuated virus vaccines.[22]

DENTAL MANAGEMENT

Health history, head and neck examination, intraoral soft tissue examination, and complete periodontal and dental examinations should be performed on all new patients. History and clinical findings may indicate that the patient has HIV/AIDS. Patients with HIV/AIDS and those at high risk for it realize their lack of true privacy on questionnaires; in addition, an AIDS phobia or homophobia may exist among members of the dental staff. Thus, answers to certain questions may be less than honest. As a result, a patient's history should be obtained whenever possible via caring, understanding, verbal communication, with sharing of knowledge and facts through honesty, avoidance of direct personal questions, and openness with the patient. Because of the sensitive social and legal issues associated with AIDS, direct questions are not recommended for inclusion in the health history questionnaire, but certain questions suggestive of a high risk for AIDS or related conditions may be included on the health questionnaire, and verbal follow-up is required.

Patients who, on the basis of history or clinical findings, are found to be at high risk for AIDS or related conditions should be referred for HIV testing, medical evaluation, other appropriate diagnostic procedures, and psychosocial intervention. The dentist should not undertake diagnostic laboratory screening but rather should refer the patient to an appropriate medical facility. This

---

TABLE 19-6
Approaches for HIV Vaccine Development

Approaches for Vaccine Development	Comments and Status
Whole virus	Whole virus vaccines have received relatively little emphasis, primarily because of safety considerations. The chief concern is related to the potential hazard of retained genetic material in such a vaccine, which has the potential for transmission of the virus.
Envelope protein	Envelope protein vaccines composed of HIV-1 envelope proteins have undergone the most extensive study in humans. Envelope HIV-1 vaccines studied in humans have been generated through recombinant DNA expression systems, which provide an efficient means by which to prepare large quantities of purified proteins and bypass concerns about possible contamination with other HIV-1 components.
Synthetic peptides	Synthetic peptides offer another approach to the development of envelope vaccines. Synthetic peptides are generated that include only epitopes of immunologic interest. This affords the opportunity for inclusion of only those epitopes that are most important for a protective response in the vaccine and for exclusion of minor or even potentially deleterious epitopes. An example of this approach is a vaccine candidate that consists of synthetically produced peptides from the V3 loops of multiple strains of HIV-1, linked to an oligolysine backbone.
Internal core proteins	Internal core proteins composed of HIV-1 internal proteins, either entirely or in part, have received relatively less attention than the envelope protein vaccines. An example of a vaccine candidate based on internal proteins is a 30 amino acid peptide of p17 of HIV-1 (HGP-30).
Live vectors	Considerable interest exists in the development of live vector vaccines for HIV-1. Such vaccines have the potential to present HIV-1 antigens in the context of a replicating microbial system; in addition, in the case of an obligate intracellular organism such as a virus, host cells express the antigens. The most extensively studied live vectors for HIV-1 vaccine development are the poxvirus vectors vaccinia and canarypox.
Nucleic acid	Nucleic acid vaccines are based on the observation that segments of nucleic acid genomes or plasmids ("naked DNA") administered intramuscularly undergo transcription and express proteins; this observation has led to the use of this technique as a means by which to deliver antigens for immunization. DNA vaccination is being studied for a variety of potential viral vaccines, including phase 1 studies with HIV-1 vaccines.
Live-attenuated virus	Live-attenuated virus vaccines have been highly successful in the control of several important viral diseases, including measles, rubella, and polio. These vaccines present in a manner that most closely resembles naturally occurring infection, and that stimulates a broad array of humoral and cell-mediated immune responses. The major concern in the development of live-attenuated HIV-1 vaccine candidates is safety. As a result, the development of live-attenuated HIV-1 vaccine is proceeding cautiously.

HIV, Human immunodeficiency virus.

should follow a discussion concerning the clinical findings and the possibility that AIDS or a related condition is present. At this time, sexual preference, IV drug use, and so forth may be discussed and often are mentioned by the patient. The patient should be strongly encouraged to seek diagnostic and supportive medical services.

Patients at high risk for AIDS and those in whom AIDS or HIV has been diagnosed should be treated identically to any other patient, that is, with standard precautions. Several guidelines have emerged regarding the rights of dentists and patients with AIDS, including the following:

- Dental treatment may not be withheld because the patient refuses to undergo testing for HIV exposure. The dentist should assume that this type of patient is a potential carrier of HIV and should treat the person using standard precautions, just as the dentist would for any other patient.
- A patient with AIDS who needs emergency dental treatment may not be refused care because the dentist does not want to treat patients with AIDS.
- No medical or scientific reason exists to justify why patients with AIDS who seek routine dental care may be declined treatment by the dentist, regardless of the dentist's reason. However, if the dentist and the patient agree, the dentist may refer this patient to someone who would be more willing to provide treatment.
- A patient who has been under the care of a dentist and then develops AIDS or a related condition must be treated by that dentist or by a referral that is satisfactory for and agreed to by the patient. The CDC and the American Dental Association recommend that infected dentists should inform the patient of his or her HIV status and should receive consent or refrain from performing invasive procedures.

Treatment Planning Considerations

A major consideration in dental treatment of the patient with HIV/AIDS involves determining the current CD4+ lymphocyte count and level of immunosuppression of the patient. Other points of emphasis in dental treatment planning include the level of viral load, which may be related to susceptibility to opportunistic infections and rate of progression of AIDS. The dentist should be knowledgeable about the presence and status of opportunistic infections and the medications that the patient may be taking for therapy or prophylaxis for these opportunistic infections.[9,23] Patients who have been exposed to the AIDS virus and are HIV seropositive but asymptomatic may receive all indicated dental treatment. Generally, this is true for patients with a CD4+ cell count of more than 400. Patients who are symptomatic for the early stages of AIDS (i.e., CD4+ cell count lower than 200) have increased susceptibility to opportunistic infection and may be effectively medicated with prophylactic drugs.[9,23]

The patient with AIDS can receive almost any dental care needed and desired once the possibility of significant immunosuppression, neutropenia, or thrombocytopenia has been ruled out. Complex treatment plans should not be undertaken before an honest and open discussion about the long-term prognosis of the patient's medical condition has occurred.

Dental treatment of the HIV-infected patient without symptoms is no different from that provided for any other patient in the practice. Standard precautions must be used for *all* patients. Any oral lesions found should be diagnosed, then managed by appropriate local and systemic treatment or referred for diagnosis and treatment. Patients with lesions suggestive of HIV infection must be evaluated for possible HIV.

Patients may be medicated with drugs that are prophylactic for *P carinii* pneumonia, candidiasis, herpes simplex virus (HSV) or CMV, or other opportunistic disease, and these medications must be carefully considered in dental treatment planning. Care in prescribing other medications must be exercised with these, or any, medications after which the patient may experience adverse drug effects, including allergic reactions, toxic drug reactions, hepatotoxicity, immunosuppression, anemia, serious drug interactions, and other potential problems. Most often, consultation with the patient's physician is mandatory.[9,23]

Patients with severe thrombocytopenia may require special measures (platelet replacement) before any surgical procedures (including scaling and curettage) are performed. Patients with advanced immunosuppression and neutropenia may require prophylaxis for invasive procedures (CD4 cell count below 200/mm³ and/or neutrophil count lower than 500/mm³).[9,23] Acetaminophen should be used with caution in patients treated with zidovudine (Retrovir) because studies have suggested that granulocytopenia and anemia, associated with zidovudine, may be intensified; also, aspirin should not be given to patients with thrombocytopenia. Antacids, phenytoin, cimetidine, and rifampin should not be given to patients who are being treated with ketoconazole because of the possibility of altered absorption and metabolism.[9,23]

Medical consultation is necessary for symptomatic HIV-infected patients before surgical procedures are performed. Current platelet count and white blood cell count should be available. Patients with abnormal test results may require special management. All these matters must be discussed in detail with the patient's physician.[9,23] Any source of oral or dental infection should be eliminated in HIV-infected patients, who often require more frequent recall appointments for maintenance of periodontal health. Daily use of chlorhexidine mouth rinse may be helpful.[9,23]

In patients with periodontal disease whose general health status is not clear, periodontal scaling for several teeth can be provided to allow assessment of tissue response and bleeding. If no problems are noted, the rest of the mouth can be treated. Root canal therapy may carry a slightly increased risk for postoperative infection in patients with advanced HIV disease. Infection can be treated through local and systemic measures.[9,23]

Individuals with severe symptoms of AIDS may be best managed by treatment of their more urgent dental needs to prevent pain and infection, with deferment of extensive restorative procedures. The main objectives of care are to prevent infection and to keep the patient free of dental or oral pain. When one is planning invasive dental procedures, attention must be paid to the prevention of infection and excessive bleeding in patients with severe immunosuppression, neutropenia, and thrombocytopenia.[9,23] This may involve the use of prophylactic antibiotics in patients with neutrophil count lower than 500 cells/mm[3]. White blood cell and differential counts, as well as a platelet count, should be ordered before any surgical procedure is undertaken. If significant thrombocytopenia occurs, platelet replacement may be needed. If severe neutropenia is present, antibiotic prophylaxis may be necessary. Medical consultation should precede any dental treatment.

Occupational Exposure to HIV

Postexposure antiretroviral prophylaxis is recommended in cases of high-risk exposure to HIV-infected blood.[4] High-risk exposure includes the following: high level of viremia in the source patient, exposure to large volume of infected fluid, deep penetrating injury with sharp device covered with visible blood from the infected patient, and needlestick injury during injection of the infected patient.[4] Postexposure prophylaxis should consist of two NRTIs with or without a potent PI to minimize toxicity and afford high tolerability.[4] If drug resistance in the source patient is identified, an alternative regimen should be considered. Prophylaxis should be initiated within a few hours of exposure, if possible. This should be continued for 4 weeks. The exposed dental health care worker should be followed with antibody testing for HIV infection at baseline, 6 weeks, 12 weeks, and 6 months.[4] If the exposed dental health care worker is pregnant, unknown but possible risks of postexposure prophylaxis to the fetus versus the risk of infection should be discussed.[4]

Oral Complications and Manifestations

Clinical findings that may suggest a high risk for AIDS or related conditions include candidiasis of the oral mucosa (Figures 19-5 to 19-8), bluish purple or red lesion or lesions that upon biopsy are identified as Kaposi's sarcoma (Figures 19-9 to 19-12), hairy leukoplakia of the lateral borders of the tongue (Figure 19-13), and other oral lesions associated with HIV infection, such as HSV, herpes zoster, recurrent aphthous ulcerations, linear gingival erythema (Figure 19-14), necrotizing ulcerative periodontitis (Figure 19-15), and necrotizing stomatitis (Table 19-7).[24] Other oral conditions noted to occur in association with HIV infection are oral warts (Figure 19-16), facial palsy, trigeminal neuropathy, salivary gland

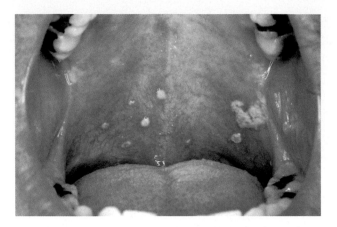

Figure 19-5. White lesion on the palate in a patient with AIDS. The lesion could be removed with a tongue blade. The underlying mucosa was erythematous. Clinical and cytologic findings supported the diagnosis of pseudomembranous candidiasis. (From Silverman S Jr. Color Atlas of Oral Manifestations of AIDS, 2nd ed. St. Louis, Mosby, 1996.)

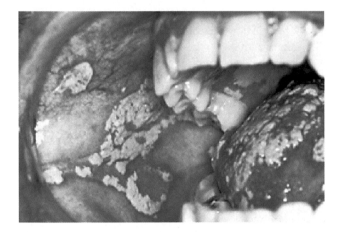

Figure 19-6. Note the white lesions on the oral mucosa. The diagnosis of pseudomembranous candidiasis was established. (Courtesy Eric Haus, Chicago.)

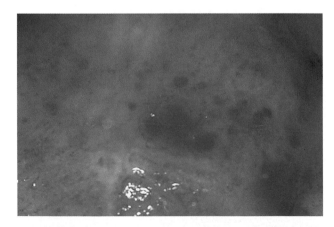

Figure 19-7. Erythematous palatal lesion in an HIV antibody–positive patient. Smears taken from the lesion showed hyphae and spores consistent with *Candida*. The lesion healed after a 2-week course of antifungal medications. A diagnosis of erythematous candidiasis was made on the basis of clinical laboratory findings. (Courtesy Eric Haus, Chicago.)

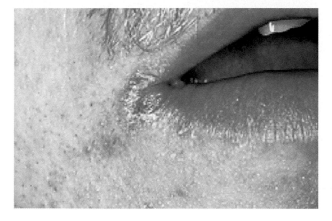

Figure 19-8. Patients with AIDS with angular cheilitis. The lesion responded to antifungal medication. (Courtesy Eric Haus, Chicago.)

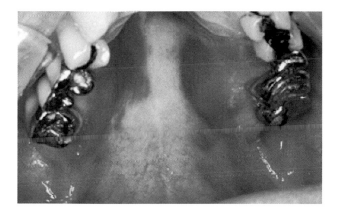

Figure 19-10. Multiple large, flat, erythematous lesions involve the palatal mucosa. Biopsy revealed the lesions to be Kaposi's sarcoma, and the patient was eventually given a diagnosis of AIDS. (Courtesy Sol Silverman, San Francisco, Calif.)

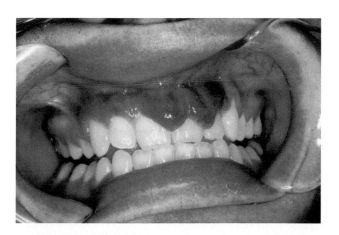

Figure 19-12. Kaposi's sarcoma of the gingiva. (From Silverman S Jr. Color Atlas of Oral Manifestations of AIDS, 2nd ed. St. Louis, Mosby, 1996.)

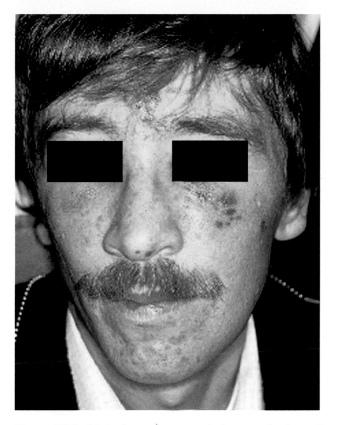

Figure 19-9. Multiple erythematous lesions on the face of a patient with AIDS. With the use of biopsy, lesions were established as Kaposi's sarcoma. (Courtesy Sol Silverman, San Francisco, Calif.)

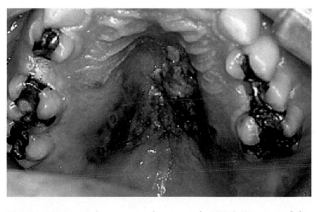

Figure 19-11. A homosexual man with AIDS. Biopsy of the palatal lesion revealed Kaposi's sarcoma. (Courtesy Sol Silverman, San Francisco, Calif.)

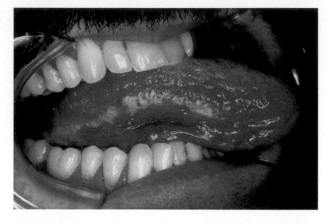

Figure 19-13. Diffuse white lesion involving the tongue. Biopsy supported the diagnosis of hairy leukoplakia. (From Silverman S Jr. Color Atlas of Oral Manifestations of AIDS, 2nd ed. St. Louis, Mosby, 1996.)

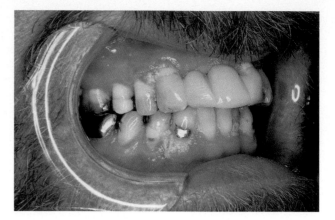

Figure 19-16. Multiple areas of condyloma acuminata on the gingivae of an HIV-positive patient. (From Silverman S Jr. Color Atlas of Oral Manifestations of AIDS, 2nd ed. St. Louis, Mosby, 1996.)

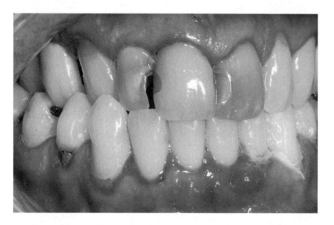

Figure 19-14. Band of linear gingival erythema involving the free gingival margin of an HIV-infected patient. (From Neville BW, Damm DD, Allen CM, Bouguot JE. Oral and Maxillofacial Pathology, 2nd ed. Philadelphia, Saunders, 2002.)

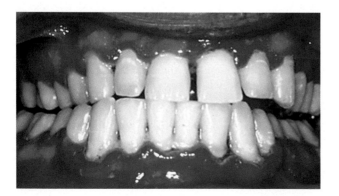

Figure 19-15. Necrotizing ulcerative periodontitis in an HIV-infected patient. The diagnosis was established after the patient was referred for medical evaluation. (Courtesy Sol Silverman, San Francisco, Calif.)

enlargement, xerostomia, and melanotic pigmentation (Table 19-8).[9,23,25] Candidiasis, hairy leukoplakia, specific forms of periodontal disease (i.e., linear gingival erythema and necrotizing ulcerative periodontitis), Kaposi's sarcoma, and non-Hodgkin's lymphoma are believed to be strongly associated with HIV infection.[9,23,25] The stages at which oral lesions appear have been described by several investigators and are summarized in Table 19-9. Management of the oral manifestations of HIV infection is discussed in Tables 19-10 and 19-11.

Worldwide, candidiasis is the most common oral manifestation of HIV infection. Oral candidiasis diagnosed in HIV-infected patients with persistent generalized lymphadenopathy may be of predictive value for the subsequent development of AIDS. The appearance of pseudomembranous candidiasis in HIV-infected individuals has been shown to be a strong indicator for the progression of infection to AIDS. The erythematous form of candidiasis also indicates progression toward AIDS.[24] The percentage of patients with HIV/AIDS and candidiasis has been described by several investigators and is summarized in Table 19-12. This information might be helpful to dental clinicians in evaluating patients for the initial diagnosis of HIV/AIDS or in determining stage of infection and level of immunosuppression. However, the oral manifestations of candidiasis that occurred more recently may be masked by earlier use of prophylactic antifungal agents.[24]

The variant of Kaposi's sarcoma that is associated with AIDS has been called *epidemic*. Epidemic Kaposi's sarcoma most often is disseminated throughout the body and runs a fulminant clinical course, with a lower than 20% survival rate at 2 years if associated with opportunistic infection.[9,23,25]

The literature suggests that Epstein-Barr virus (EBV) is not associated with any other oral white lesions that must be differentiated from hairy leukoplakia. Thus, hairy leukoplakia may be caused by reactivation of EBV

TABLE **19-7**
Oral Lesions Commonly Associated With HIV Infection and AIDS

Oral Condition	Comment
Persistent generalized lymphadenopathy	An early sign of HIV infection, found in about 70% of infected patients during the latent stage of infection.
	Must be present longer than 3 months and in two or more extrainguinal locations.
	Anterior and posterior cervical, submandibular, occipital, and axillary nodes are most frequently involved.
Oral candidiasis	Most common intraoral manifestation of HIV infection. First found during the early symptomatic stage of infection. Once found, this indicates that AIDS will develop within 2 years in untreated patients.
Pseudomembranous	
Erythematous	
Hyperplastic	About 90% of patients with AIDS will develop oral candidiasis at some timen during their disease course.
Angular cheilitis	
HIV-associated periodontal disease	Linear gingival erythema does not respond to improved plaque control procedures (may represent an unusual pattern of candidiasis).
Linear gingival erythema	
Necrotizing ulcerative gingivitis (NUG)	NUG relates to ulceration and necrosis of one or more interdental papillae with no loss of periodontal attachment.
Necrotizing ulcerative periodontitis (NUP)	
	NUP consists of gingival ulceration and necrosis with attachment loss and does not respond to conventional periodontal therapy.
Necrotizing stomatitis	May be seen as an extension of NUP or may involve oral mucosa separate from the gingiva.
Herpes simplex virus (HSV)	Immunocompetent individuals and HIV-infected patients experience about the same rate of recurrent HSV infection (10%-15%), but in HIV-infected individuals, the lesions are more widespread, occur in an atypical pattern, and may persist for months.
Varicella-zoster virus (VZV)	Recurrent VZV infection is common in HIV-infected patients, but the course is more severe. Intraoral lesions are often severe and can lead to bone involvement with loss of teeth.
Oral hairy leukoplakia (OHL)	White lesion most often found on the lateral border of the tongue. OHL on rare occasions has been found on the buccal mucosa, soft palate, and pharynx. Associated with Epstein-Barr virus infection.
	When found in a nontreated patient with early HIV symptomatic infection, the finding of OHL indicates that AIDS will develop in the near future.
Kaposi's sarcoma (KS)	Human herpes virus type 8 (HHV-8) appears to be involved in KS development. About 50% of patients with KS have oral lesions, and the oral cavity is the initial site of involvement in 20% to 25% of cases. The most common sites are the hard palate, gingival, and tongue. KS found in an HIV-infected individual is diagnostic of AIDS.

HIV, Human immunodeficiency virus; AIDS, acquired immunodeficiency syndrome.

in the oral mucosa in association with HIV-induced immune deficiency. The diagnosis of hairy leukoplakia is based on the clinical appearance of the lesion, its lack of response to antifungal therapy, and histologic findings. The finding of hairy leukoplakia also has predictive value for the subsequent development of AIDS.[9,23,25]

Lymphadenopathy at cervical and submandibular locations often is an early finding in patients infected with HIV. This condition is persistent and may be found in the absence of any current infection or medications known to cause lymph node enlargement. The nodes tend to be larger than 1 cm in diameter, and multiple sites of enlargement may be found.[9,23,25]

The overall general dental management of the patient with AIDS is depicted in Box 19-3. The dentist should perform head and neck and intraoral soft tissue examinations on all patients. White lesions in the mouth must be found and the patient managed in such a way that a diagnosis is established. This may involve cell study, culture, and biopsy by the dentist or referral to an oral surgeon. If red or purple lesions are found that cannot be explained by history (e.g., trauma, burn, chemical, physical) or proved by clinical observation (healing within 7 to 10 days), biopsy must be performed. Persistent lymphadenopathy must be investigated by referral for medical evaluation, diagnosis, and treatment.

TABLE 19-8
Less Common Oral Conditions Associated With HIV Infection

Oral Condition	Comment

Aphthous ulcerations
  Minor
  Major
  Herpetiform
	About 66% of lesions are of the more uncommon forms—major and herpetiform. With more severe reduction of CD4+ cell count, major lesions become more prevalent. Lesions that are chronic or atypical, or that do not respond to treatment should be biopsied.

Human papillomavirus (HPV)
  Verruca vulgaris (wart)
  Oral squamous papilloma
	The usual HPV types are found in oral lesions, but some uncommon variants such as HPV-7 and HPV-32 also are found. Lesions are usually multiple and may be found on any oral mucosal site.

Histoplasmosis	Histoplasmosis is the most common endemic respiratory fungal infection in the United States and is usually subclinical and self-limiting. Dissemination of infection occurs in about 5% of patients with AIDS who live in areas in the United States where the fungus is endemic.
Molluscum contagiosum	Molluscum contagiosum is caused by a poxvirus. The lesions are small papules with a central depressed crater. In immunocompetent individuals, the lesions are self-limiting and are found on the genitals and trunk. In patients with AIDS, multiple lesions (hundreds) are found that do not regress (5% to 10% of patients with lesions have lesions of the facial skin).
Thrombocytopenia	Thrombocytopenia is found in about 10% of HIV-infected individuals. It may occur during any stage of the disease. Skin manifestations are most common, but petechiae, ecchymosis, and spontaneous gingival bleeding can occur in the oral cavity.
HIV-associated salivary gland disease	Found in 5% of HIV-infected patients and can occur any time during the infection. Swelling of the parotid is most common. Bilateral involvement is common. In some patients, CD8 lymphocytes infiltrate the gland and are associated with lymphadenopathy. Xerostomia may occur. Patients are at increased risk for B-cell lymphoma.
Hyperpigmentation	Melanin pigmentation has been reported to occur in HIV-infected patients. Several of the medications (ketoconazole, clofazimine, and zidovudine) used to treat these patients may cause melanin pigmentation. Addison's-like pigmentation also may occur because of destruction of the adrenal gland. HIV infection itself may cause melanin pigmentation.
Lymphoma	Found in about 3% of patients with AIDS. Most are found in extranodal locations. Most lesions are non-Hodgkin's B-cell lymphoma and are related to the EBV. The CNS is the most common site, but oral lesions occur in the palate and gingiva and in other locations.
Oral squamous cell carcinoma	Squamous cell carcinoma can be found in the oral cavity, pharynx, and larynx in HIV-infected individuals. The same risk factors apply as for the general population, but the cancer occurs at a younger age (it appears that HIV infection accelerates onset of carcinoma).

HIV, Human immunodeficiency virus; AIDS, acquired immunodeficiency virus; EBV, Epstein-Barr virus; CNS, central nervous system.

TABLE 19-9
Specific Oral Lesions Related to Stage of HIV Infection: Percentage of Patients With Lesions

Lesion	Seronegative High Risk (%)	Seropositive, But Data Not Separated into Clinical Stages (%)	Asymptomatic & PGL (%)	ARC (%)	AIDS (%)
Hairy leukoplakia	0.3-3	19	8-21	9-44	4-23
Candidiasis	0.8-10	11-31	5-17	11-85	29-87
Kaposi's sarcoma	0	0.3-3	1-2	0	35-38
Herpes simplex	0-0.5	0-1	0-5	11-29	0-9
Aphthous ulcerations	0-2	0-1	2-8	11-14	2-7
Venereal warts	0-0.7	0-1	0-1	0	0-1
ANUG	0-0.2	1-5	0-1	0	51
HIV periodontitis	0	0	0-2	0-21	19

Based on Barone R, et al. Oral Surg 1990;69:169-173; Barr C, et al. IADR 1990;1443:289; Feigal DW, et al. IADR 1989;65:190; Little JW, Melnick SL, Rhame FS. Gen Dent 1994;42:446-450; Melnick SL, et al. Oral Surg 1989;68:37-43; Roberts MW, Brahim JS, Rinne NF. J Am Dent Assoc 1988;116:863-866; Silverman S Jr, et al. J Am Dent Assoc 1986;112:187-192.
ANUG, Acute necrotizing ulcerative gingivitis; AIDS, acquired immunodeficiency syndrome; ARC, AIDS-related complex; HIV, human immunodeficiency virus; PGL, persistent generalized lymphadenopathy.

TABLE 19-10
Treatment of Oral Lesions Commonly Associated With HIV Infection and AIDS

Oral Condition	Treatment and Management
Persistent generalized lymphadenopathy	Usually not treated directly, may need biopsy to rule out lymphoma or other conditions

Oral candidiasis
  Pseudomembranous
  Erythematous
  Hyperplastic
  Angular cheilitis
	Nystatin is often ineffective. Topical clotrimazole is effective but has high rate of recurrence. Systemic fluconazole, ketoconazole, and itraconazole are effective but have a number of drug interactions and may result in drug-resistant candidiasis. If azoles fail, then intravenous amphotericin B can be administered.

HIV-associated periodontal disease
  Linear gingival erythema (LGE)
  Necrotizing ulcerative gingivitis (NUG)
  Necrotizing ulcerative periodontitis (NUP)
  Necrotizing stomatitis (NS)
	LGE usually responds to plaque removal, improved oral hygiene, and chlorhexidine rinses. Cases that fail to respond usually respond to systemic antifungal medications. Therapy for NUG, NUP, and NS involves debridement (removal of necrotic tissue and povidone-iodine irrigation), chlorhexidine rinses, metronidazole, follow-up care, and long-term maintenance.

Herpes simplex virus (HSV)	Acyclovir suspension used as a rinse and swallow during the first 3 days can be effective. An elixir or syrup of diphenhydramine (Benadryl) of 12.5 mg/5 mL can be used for pain control. In patients with severe immunosuppression, acyclovir capsules, 200 mg, 50 capsules, taken 5 times per day for 10 days (risk for viral resistance). Acyclovir ointment or penciclovir cream can be used for topical treatment of herpes labialis.
Varicella-zoster virus (VZV)	Intravenous acyclovir is recommended for severe herpes zoster in patients with immunosuppression.
Oral hairy leukoplakia (OHL)	Treatment often is not needed. Acyclovir or desciclovir can result in rapid resolution, but recurrence is likely. Retinoids or podophyllum resin therapy can lead to temporary remission. HIV therapy with zidovudine can result in significant regression.
Kaposi's sarcoma (KS)	Treatment objectives are usually palliative and involve radiation or systemic chemotherapy. Intraoral lesions causing severe pain or bleeding or interfering with function can be injected with vinblastine or a sclerosing agent (sodium tetradecyl sulfate) or removed by surgical excision. Other options for dealing with these types of lesions are cryotherapy, laser ablation, and electrosurgery, but care must be taken to protect operating personal from aerosolization of viral particles when the laser or electrosurgery is used.

HIV, Human immunodeficiency virus; AIDS, acquired immunodeficiency syndrome.

BOX 19-3

Dental Management of the Patient With AIDS or a Related Condition: General Procedures

KEY POINTS
- Consult whenever possible with the patient's physician to establish current status; if severe thrombocytopenia is present (<50,000), platelet replacement may be needed before surgical procedures are performed.
- Determine whether prophylactic antibiotics are needed to protect patients with severe immune neutropenia (<500 cells/mm^3) from postoperative infection.

- Render only more immediately needed treatment for patients with advanced AIDS.
- In most cases, provide dental procedures in accordance with the patient's wants and needs.
- Inform all personnel working with patients with AIDS of the relative risks involved and how they can be minimized.

AIDS, Acquired immunodeficiency syndrome.

TABLE **19-11**

Treatment of Less Common Oral Conditions Associated With HIV Infection

Oral Condition	Treatment and Management

Aphthous ulcerations
  Minor
  Major
  Herpetiform
	Treatment of major lesions that persist involves potent topical or intralesional corticosteroids. Systemic steroids are generally avoided to prevent further immune suppression. Thalidomide treatment has yielded good response but should be used only for a short time because the drug can enhance HIV replication. Granulocyte colony-stimulating factor has produced significant results in a limited number of patients.

Human papillomavirus (HPV)
  Verruca vulgaris (wart)
  Oral squamous papilloma
	Treatment of choice is surgical removal of the lesion(s). Other treatment modalities include topical podophyllin, interferon, and cryosurgery. Laser ablation and electrocoagulation have been used, but care must be taken because the plume may contain infectious HPV.

Histoplasmosis	The treatment of choice for disseminated histoplasmosis is intravenous amphotericin B. Oral itraconazole has also been found to be effective and has fewer adverse effects and better compliance.
Molluscum contagiosum	Curettage, cryosurgery, and cautery have been used to treat these lesions, but they are painful and recurrences are common. Resolution of multiple lesions has been reported with HAART.
Thrombocytopenia	Platelet counts below 50,000/mm^3 may result in significant bleeding with minor surgical procedures. Platelet replacement may be indicated for these patients.
HIV-associated salivary gland disease	Risk is increased for cysts of the parotid and lymphoma. Treatment may involve prednisone or antiretroviral therapy. Associated xerostomia can be managed with sialogogues and saliva substitutes.
Hyperpigmentation	Usually, no treatment is indicated. Single lesions may have to be biopsied so that melanoma can be ruled out. Patients with Addison's disease may require corticosteroids.
Lymphoma	Treatment usually involves a combination of chemotherapy and radiation and is used for local control of disease. Prognosis is very poor with death occurring within months of the diagnosis. HAART has reduced the prevalence of opportunistic infections and Kaposi's sarcoma in HIV-infected patients but has not affected the prevalence of lymphoma.
Oral squamous cell carcinoma	Treatment of oral squamous cell carcinoma is the same as for non–HIV-infected patients: surgery, radiation, chemotherapy, or combination therapy.

HIV, Human immunodeficiency virus; HAART, highly activated antiretroviral therapy.

TABLE **19-12**

Summary of Statistics Related to Oral Candidiasis in HIV-Infected Individuals Taken From 17 Published Reports in the United States

Disease State	Papers	Range*	Prevalence Frequencies Weighted Mean, %	Mean
Oral candidiasis	17	11-96	30.0	45.2
Erythematous	7	10-96	40.5	33.0
Pseudomembranous	6	6-69	22.2	25.6
Hyperplastic	6	2-20	3.8	3.8
Angular cheilitis	4	1-23	12.5	16.0

From Samaranayake LP, Holmstrup P. J Oral Pathol Med 1989;18:554-564.

HIV, Human immunodeficiency virus.

*Weighted by overall number of patients with oral candidiasis in each study.

REFERENCES

1. Merson MH. The HIV-AIDS pandemic at 25: The global response. N Engl J Med 2006;354:2414-2418.
2. Joint United Nations Programme on HIV/AIDS. 2006 report on the global AIDS epidemic. Available at: http://www.UNAIDS.org. Accessed May 18, 2006.
3. The HIV/AIDS epidemic: The first 10 years. MMWR Morb Mortal Wkly Rep 1991;40:357-363.
4. Baustian GH, et al. AIDS, 2006. Available at: http:/www.firstconsult.com/home. Accessed May 25, 2006.
5. Fauci AS. HIV disease: AIDS and related disorders. In Harrison's Online Principles of Medicine. New York, NY, McGraw-Hill, 2006.
6. Racial/ethnic disparities in diagnoses of HIV/AIDS—33 states, 2001-2004. MMWR Morb Mortal Wkly Rep 2006;55:121-125.
7. Bravo IM, Correnti M, Escalona L, et al. Prevalence of oral lesions in HIV patients related to CD4 cell count and viral load in a Venezuelan population. Med Oral Patol Oral Cir Bucal 2006;11:E33-E39.
8. Centers for Disease Control. Update: Transmission of HIV infection during an invasive dental procedure in

Florida. MMWR Morb Mortal Wkly Rep 1991;40: 21-27.

9. Little JW, et al. AIDS and related conditions. In Dental Management of the Medically Compromised Patient. St. Louis, Mosby, 2002, pp 221-248.

10. Scheld WM. Introduction to HIV and associated disorders. In Goldman L, Ausiello D (eds). Cecil Textbook of Medicine. Philadelphia, WB Saunders, 2004, pp 2135-2137.

11. Centers for Disease Control. Guidelines for infection control in dental health-care settings. MMWR Morb Mortal Wkly Rep 2003;52:1-5.

12. Bautista LE, Orostegui M. Dental care associated with an outbreak of HIV infection among dialysis patients. Rev Panam Salud Publica 1997;2:194-202.

13. Public Health Service Workshop on Human-T-Lymphotropic Virus Type III—United States. MMWR Morb Mortal Wkly Rep 1985;34:477-479.

14. Fox RI. Clinical features, pathogenesis, and treatment of Sjögren's syndrome. Curr Opin Rheumatol 1996;8: 438-445.

15. Rolinski B, Wintergerst U, Matuschke A, et al. Evaluation of saliva as a specimen for monitoring zidovudine therapy in HIV-infected patients. AIDS 1991;5:885-888.

16. Deeks SG. Antiretroviral therapy. In Treatment of HIV Infection, 3rd ed. San Francisco, Calif, University of San Francisco Press, 1999.

17. Cheng B, Rhodus NL, Williams B, et al. Detection of apoptotic cells in whole saliva of patients with oral premalignant and malignant lesions: A preliminary study.

Oral Surg Oral Med Oral Pathol Oral Radiol Endod 2004;97:465-470.

18. Carpenter CC, Fischl MA, Hammer SM. Antiretroviral therapy for HIV infection in 1998: Updated recommendations of the International AIDS Society—USA panel. JAMA 1998;280:75-79.

19. Masur H. Treatment of HIV infection and AIDS. In Goldman L, Ausiello D (eds). Cecil Textbook of Medicine. Philadelphia, Saunders, 2004, pp 2183-2191.

20. Fauci AS, Lane HC. HIV disease: AIDS and related disorders. In Kasper DL (ed). Harrison's Online Principles of Medicine. New York, McGraw-Hill, 2005.

21. Sax PE, Walker BD. Immunology related to AIDS. In Goldman L, Ausiello D (eds). Cecil Textbook of Medicine. Philadelphia, Saunders, 2004, pp 2137-2138.

22. Barouch DH, Baden LR, Dolin R. Human immunodeficiency virus vaccines. In Mandell GL, Bennett JE, Dolin R (eds). Principles and Practices of Infectious Diseases. St. Louis, Elsevier (Churchill Livingstone), 2005, pp 1707-1717.

23. Scully C, Cawson RA. Medical Problems in Dentistry—Immunodeficiencies and HIV Disease, 5th ed. Edinburgh, Elsevier, 2005, p 683.

24. Challacombe SJ, Coogan MM, Williams DM. Overview of the Fourth International Workshop on the Oral Manifestations of HIV Infection. Oral Dis 2002;8(suppl 2):9-14.

25. Regezi JA, Sciubba JJ, Jordan RCK. Oral Pathology: Clinical Pathologic Correlations, 4th ed. St. Louis, Elsevier (Saunders), 2003, p 544.

Allergy

20

Allergic diseases are increasing in prevalence and are contributing significantly to health care costs. For example, the number of children with allergies has recently doubled.[1]

One of the most common medical emergencies that can occur in the dental office is that of an acute allergic reaction. The following four reasons signify why the dentist must know about allergy:

1. To identify patients with a true allergic history, so acute medical emergencies that might occur in the dental office because of an allergic reaction can be prevented
2. To recognize oral soft tissue changes that might be caused by an allergic reaction
3. To identify and plan appropriate dental care for patients who have severe alterations of their immune system because of radiation, drug therapy, or immune deficiency disorders
4. To recognize signs and symptoms of acute allergic reactions and manage these problems appropriately

To accomplish these goals, the dentist first must acquire a basic understanding of allergy.

DEFINITION

Epidemiology: Incidence and Prevalence

It is estimated that 15% to 25% of all Americans are allergic to some substance, including about 4.5% who have asthma, 4% who are allergic to insect stings, and 5% who are allergic to one or more drugs. Allergic reactions account for about 6% to 10% of all adverse drug reactions. Of these, 46% consist of erythema and rash, 23% urticaria, 10% fixed drug reactions, 5% erythema multiforme, and 1% anaphylaxis. About a 1% to 3% risk for an allergic reaction is possible when a drug is used. Fatal drug reactions occur in about 0.01% of surgical inpatients and 0.1% of medical inpatients.[1-3]

Drugs are the most common cause of urticarial reaction in adults, and food and infection are the most common causes of these lesions in children. Urticaria occurs in 15% to 20% of young adults. In approximately 70% of patients with chronic urticaria, no etiologic agent can be identified.[1-4]

Use of iodinated organic compounds as radiographic contrast media results in about 1 death for every 1,400 to 60,000 diagnostic procedures. Animal insulin used to treat patients with type 1 diabetes causes an allergic reaction in about 10% to 56% of these individuals, and reports have stated that some 25% of patients with diabetes who are allergic to insulin react to penicillin.[1-3]

About 5% to 10% of individuals who are given penicillin develop an allergic reaction, and 0.04% to 0.2% of these experience an anaphylactic reaction to the drug. Death occurs in about 10% of those individuals who experience an anaphylactic reaction. Usually, in anaphylactic reactions to penicillin, death occurs within 15 minutes after administration of the drug; 50% of the time, the allergic reaction starts immediately after drug administration. About 70% of individuals report that they have taken penicillin previously (Box 20-1). The most common causes of anaphylactic death are penicillin, bee stings, and wasp stings; individuals with an atopic history are more susceptible to anaphylactic death than are patients with no history of allergy. Causes of anaphylaxis of significance to the dentist are listed in Box 20-2.[1-3]

In rare cases, antihistamines have been reported to cause urticaria through an allergic response to the colored coating material of the capsule. In addition, azo and nonazo dyes used in toothpaste have been reported to cause anaphylactic-like reactions. Aniline dyes used to coat certain steroid tablets have caused serious allergic reactions as well.[1-3]

Parabens (used as preservatives in local anesthetics) have caused anaphylactoid reactions. Sulfites (sodium

Summary of 151 Cases of Penicillin-Related Anaphylactic Deaths

- 21 (14%) of cases had a history of allergies
- 106 (70%) of cases had received penicillin before; 25% had experienced a sudden allergic reaction
- 128 (85%) of cases died within 15 minutes of administration
- 75 (50%) of cases experienced symptoms right after first administration of the drug
- 3 (2%) of cases were related to oral penicillin

Data from Idsoe O, et al. Bull WHO 1968;38:159-188.

Causes of Human Anaphylactic Reactions of Importance to the Dentist

CAUSATIVE AGENTS
Antibiotics
- Penicillins
- Sulfonamides
- Vancomycin
- Amphotericin B
- Cephalosporins
- Nitrofurantoin
- Ciprofloxacin
- Tetracyclines
- Streptomycin
- Chloramphenicol

MISCELLANEOUS DRUGS/THERAPEUTIC AGENTS
- Acetylsalicylic acid
- Succinylcholine
- d-Tubocurarine
- Antitoxins
- Progesterone
- Thiopental
- Vaccines
- Protamine sulfate
- Nonsteroidal anti-inflammatory drugs (NSAIDs)
- Opiates
- Mechlorethamine

DIAGNOSTIC AGENTS
- Sodium dehydrocholate
- Radiographic contrast media
- Sulfobromophthalein
- Benzylpenicilloyl polylysine (Pre-Pen)

HORMONES
- Insulin
- Parathormone
- Corticotropin
- Synthetic adrenocorticotropic hormone (ACTH)

ENZYMES
- Streptokinase
- Penicillinase
- Chymotrypsin
- Asparaginase
- Trypsin
- Chymopapain

BLOOD PRODUCTS
- Whole blood
- Plasma
- Gamma globulin
- Cryoprecipitate
- Immunoglobulin A (IgA)

LATEX

Modified from Patterson R. In Patterson R (ed). Allergies, 5th ed. Philadelphia, JB Lippincott, 1997, pp 593-596.

metabisulfite or acetone sodium bisulfite) used in local anesthetic solutions to prevent oxidation of the vasoconstrictors can cause serious allergic reactions. The group most susceptible to allergic reactions caused by sulfites includes the 9 to 11 million persons in the United States in whom asthma has been diagnosed.[1-3]

Etiology

Allergic diseases result from an immunologic reaction to a noninfectious foreign substance (antigen). They comprise a series of repeat reactions to a foreign substance. These reactions involve different types of immunologic hypersensitivity (Box 20-3) and elements of the nonspecific and specific branches of the immune system (Box 20-4). The three branches of the immune system are the humoral, cellular, and nonspecific branches. Functions of the humoral and cellular branches of the immune system are shown in Table 20-1.[1-4]

Foreign substances that trigger hypersensitivity reactions are called *allergens* or *antigens*. Box 20-5 shows some of the characteristics of antigens. Two types of lymphocytes play central roles in the two branches of the specific immune system: B lymphocytes in the humoral branch, and T lymphocytes in the cellular branch. The three branches of the immune system do not operate independently. T lymphocytes play an important role in the regulation of B lymphocytes. The initial function of the humoral and cellular branches of the immune system involves the recognition of antigens; however, cells and chemicals from the nonspecific branch of the immune system are needed to eradicate antigens.[1-4]

Under some circumstances, repeated contact with or exposure to an antigen may cause an inappropriate response (hypersensitivity) that can be harmful or destructive to host tissues; thus, hypersensitivity reactions can involve cellular or humoral components of the immune system.[1-4] Reactions that involve the humoral system most often occur soon after contact has been made with the antigen; three types of hypersensitivity reaction (types I, II, and III) involve elements of the humoral immune system. Type IV hypersensitivity reactions involve the cellular immune system. Allergic reactions that involve the cellular immune system often have delayed onset.

Examples include contact dermatitis, graft rejection, graft-versus-host disease, some drug reactions, and some types of autoimmune disease.[1-4]

Pathophysiology and Complications

Humoral Immune System. B lymphocytes recognize specific foreign chemical configurations via receptors on their cell membranes. For the antigen to be recognized by specific B lymphocytes, it must first be processed by T lymphocytes and macrophages. Each clone (family) of B lymphocytes recognizes its own specific chemical structure. Once recognition has taken place, the B lymphocytes differentiate and multiply, forming plasma cells and memory B lymphocytes. Memory B lymphocytes remain inactive until contact is made with the same type of antigen. This contact transforms the memory cell into a plasma cell that produces immunoglobulins (antibodies) specific for the antigen involved. Box 20-6 lists the functions of the five classes of immunoglobulins. Note that immunoglobulin E (IgE) is the key antibody involved in the pathogenesis of type I hypersensitivity reactions.

BOX 20-3

Coombs and Gell Classification of Immunologic Hypersensitivity Reactions

- Type I = Anaphylactic or IgE mediated
- Type II = Cytotoxic
- Type III = Immune complex mediated
- Type IV = Cell mediated or delayed

IgE, Immunoglobulin E.

BOX 20-4

The Immune System

1. Nonspecific
   a. Mechanical reflexes
      (1) Coughing, sneezing
      (2) Action of cilia
      (3) Sphincter control of bladder
   b. Secretion of bactericidal substances
      (1) Stomach acid
      (2) Earwax (cerumen)
      (3) Enzymes in tears or saliva
   c. Phagocytic cells
      (1) Neutrophils
      (2) Monocytes
      (3) Macrophages
   d. Circulating chemicals
      (1) Complement
      (2) Interferon
2. Specific
   a. Humoral immunity
      (1) Protection against bacterial infection
      (2) Clones of B lymphocytes
      (3) Recognition of chemical configuration
      (4) Production of antibodies by plasma cells
      (5) Eradication of antigen
   b. Cellular immunity
      (1) Protection against viral infection, tuberculosis, leprosy
      (2) Transplant rejection
      (3) Production of cytokines by T lymphocytes
      (4) Eradication of antigen

Modified from Thomson NC, Kirkwood EM, Lever RS. In Thomson NC, et al (eds). Handbook of Clinical Allergy. Oxford, Blackwell Scientific, 1990, pp 1-36.

TABLE 20-1
Functions of the Immune System

Function	Humoral	Cellular
Processing of antigen	T-helper cells and macrophages	Macrophages plus antigens of major histocompatibility complex (MHC)
Cellular recognition of antigen	Receptors on B lymphocytes are sensitive to specific chemical configurations	T lymphocytes with receptors to specific subsets of MHC antigens
Cellular response to presentation of antigen	Specific clones of B lymphocytes multiply and produce plasma cells and memory cells	Specific clones of T lymphocytes multiply and produce effector T cells and memory T cells
Cellular action against antigen	Plasma cells produce specific immunoglobulins (antibodies); memory cells become plasma cells, with later antigen contact	Effector T cells produce cytokines; Memory T cells become effector T cells, with later antigen contact
Eradication of antigen	Reaction with specific antibody is facilitated by nonspecific branch of the immune system; antigen is removed by cells of a nonspecific branch	Destruction of antigen by cytokines and elements of a nonspecific branch of the immune system

Modified from Thomson NC, Kirkwood EM, Lever RS. In Thomson NC, et al (eds). Handbook of Clinical Allergy. Oxford, Blackwell Scientific, 1990, pp 1-36.

BOX 20-5

Antigens

- Materials considered foreign by the body
- Large molecular size
- Certain degree of molecular complexity
- Cell-mediated immune response rarely induced by polysaccharides (T-independent antigens)
- Multiple antigenic determinants or antibody-binding sites (epitopes)
- Various reactions in humans

Modified from Thomson NC, Kirkwood EM, Lever RS. In Thomson NC, et al (eds). Handbook of Clinical Allergy. Oxford, Blackwell Scientific, 1990, pp 1-36.

BOX 20-6

Functions of Immunoglobulins

1. Immunoglobulin (Ig)G
   a. Most abundant immunoglobulin
   b. Small size allows diffusion into tissue spaces
   c. Can cross the placenta
   d. Opsonizing antibody—facilitates phagocytosis of microorganisms by neutrophils
   e. Four subclasses: IgG1, IgG2, IgG3, IgG4 (IgG can bind to mast cells)
2. IgA
   a. Two types
      (1) Secretory (dimer, secretory components)— found in saliva, tears, and nasal mucus; secretory component protects from proteolysis
      (2) Serum (monomer)
   b. Does not cross the placenta
   c. Last immunoglobulin to appear in childhood
3. IgM
   a. Large molecule
   b. Confined to intravascular space
   c. First immunoglobulin produced
   d. Activates complement
   e. Good agglutinating antibody
4. IgE
   a. Very low concentration in serum (0.004%)
   b. Increased in parasitic and atopic diseases
   c. Binds to mast cells and basophils
   d. Key antibody in pathogenesis of type I hypersensitivity reactions
5. IgD
   a. Low concentration in serum
   b. Little importance

Modified from Thomson NC, Kirkwood EM, Lever RS. In Thomson NC, et al (eds). Handbook of Clinical Allergy. Oxford, Blackwell Scientific, 1990, pp 1-36.

BOX 20-7

Functions of the Humoral Immune System

1. First encounter with antigen (primary response)
   a. Latent period
      (1) Antigen is processed
      (2) B lymphocyte clone is selected
      (3) Differentiation and proliferation
      (4) Plasma cells produce specific immunoglobulins
   b. Specific immunoglobulin (Ig)M level increases first in serum followed by IgG
   c. IgM levels later fall to zero
   d. IgG levels fall; however, some stay the same
2. Second encounter with antigen (secondary response)
   a. Latent period is shorter
      (1) Antigen is processed
      (2) Memory cells are selected; become plasma cells
      (3) Plasma cells produce specific immunoglobulins
   b. IgM levels increase first
   c. IgG levels increase to 50 times the level found in the primary response
   d. IgM levels fall later
   e. IgG levels fall later, but a significant serum level is usually maintained

Modified from Thomson NC, Kirkwood EM, Lever RS. In Thomson NC, et al (eds). Handbook of Clinical Allergy. Oxford, Blackwell Scientific, 1990, pp 1-36.

BOX 20-8

Type I Hypersensitivity[4]

1. Immunoglobulin (Ig)E antibody mediated
2. Immediate response
3. Usual allergens (antigens)
   a. Dust
   b. Mites
   c. Pollens
   d. Animal danders
   e. Food
   f. Drugs (haptens)
4. Symptoms
   a. Anaphylaxis
   b. Hay fever
   c. Asthma
   d. Urticaria, angioedema
   e. Symptoms on occasion
5. Frequency: Affects about 10% of the population
6. Inherited tendency

Modified from Thomson NC, Kirkwood EM, Lever RS. In Thomson NC, et al (eds). Handbook of Clinical Allergy. Oxford, Blackwell Scientific, 1990, pp 1-36.

Normal functions of the humoral immune system are shown in Box 20-7.[1-4]

Type I, type II, and type III hypersensitivities involve elements of the humoral immune system. Type I hypersensitivity is summarized in Box 20-8. These are IgE- mediated reactions that lead to the release of chemical mediators from mast cells and basophils in various target tissues. The role of IgE is clear in these reactions, but that of the other sensitizing antibody, IgG4, is not well understood.[1-4]

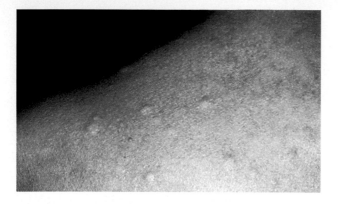

Figure 20-1. This patient had taken penicillin a number of times without any problem. However, he developed a generalized urticarial reaction after injection of penicillin for treatment of an acute oral infection.

Type I hypersensitivity reactions. Type I hypersensitivity reactions, which are related to the humoral immune system, usually occur soon after second contact has been made with an antigen; however, many individuals have repeated contacts with a drug or material before they finally become allergic to it (Figure 20-1). *Anaphylaxis* is an acute reaction involving the smooth muscle of the bronchi in which the antigen/antibody complex that is formed causes histamine release from mast cells. The smooth muscle contracts, and this may lead to acute respiratory distress or failure. *Atopy* is a hypersensitivity state that is influenced by hereditary factors. Hay fever, asthma, urticaria, and angioneurotic edema are examples of atopic reactions. Lesions most commonly associated with atopic reactions include urticaria, which is a superficial lesion of the skin, and angioneurotic edema, which is a lesion that occurs in the deeper layer of the skin or in other tissues such as the larynx or tongue. In true allergic reactions, these lesions result from the effects of antigens and their antibodies (IgE) on mast cells in various locations in the body. The antigen/antibody complex causes the release of mediators (histamine) from mast cells; these mediators then produce an increase in the permeability of adjacent vascular structures, resulting in loss of intravascular fluid into surrounding tissue spaces. This reaction accounts for the edematous lesions of urticaria, angioneurotic edema, and secretions associated with hay fever.[1-4]

Agents that commonly cause acute urticaria include shellfish, nuts, eggs, milk, antibiotic drugs, and insect bites (bee stings). Humoral antibodies involved in anaphylaxis and atopy are IgE antibodies that are fixed to and sensitize mast cells, so that when they encounter the antigen, they release histamine.[1-4]

Type II hypersensitivity reactions. The key elements involved in type II hypersensitivity are shown in Box 20-9. These reactions are IgG or IgM mediated. The classic example of type II (cytotoxic) hypersensitivity is transfusion reaction caused by mismatched blood.[1-4]

BOX 20-9

Type II Hypersensitivity

1. Antibody mediated
2. Cytotoxic hypersensitivity
   a. Antibodies combine with host cells recognized as foreign
   b. Foreign antigens bind to host cell membranes during induced hemolytic anemia or thrombocytopenia
3. Common examples
   a. Transfusion reactions from mismatched bloods
   b. Rhesus incompatibility
   c. Goodpasture's syndrome

Modified from Thomson NC, Kirkwood EM, Lever RS. In Thomson NC, et al (eds). Handbook of Clinical Allergy. Oxford, Blackwell Scientific, 1990, pp 1-36.

BOX 20-10

Type III Hypersensitivity

1. Antibody mediated via immune complex formation
2. Also known as immune complex–mediated hypersensitivity
3. Local form is Arthus reaction
4. Immune complex formation
   a. Hypersensitivity state: Complexes persist and lodge in blood vessel walls, initiating inflammatory reaction
   b. Large complexes
   c. Removed by neutrophils and macrophages
   d. Soluble complexes (more antigen than antibody)
      (1) Most harmful
      (2) Penetrate vessel wall
      (3) Lodge in the basement membrane
   e. Complement is activated
      (1) Vascular permeability increased
      (2) Neutrophils attracted
      (3) Neutrophils release enzymes
      (4) Vasculitis results
5. Sensitive sites
   a. Renal glomeruli
   b. Synovial membranes
6. Examples
   a. Systemic lupus erythematosus
   b. Poststreptococcal glomerulonephritis

Modified from Thomson NC, Kirkwood EM, Lever RS. In Thomson NC, et al (eds). Handbook of Clinical Allergy. Oxford, Blackwell Scientific, 1990, pp 1-36.

Type III hypersensitivity reactions. Type III hypersensitivity is summarized in Box 20-10. These reactions take place in blood vessels and involve soluble immune complexes. They constitute what is referred to as *immune complex–mediated hypersensitivity*. Their key feature is vasculitis. Clinical examples include systemic lupus erythematosus and streptococcal glomerulonephritis.[1-4]

Type IV Hypersensitivity

SIGNS AND SYMPTOMS SUGGESTIVE OF AN ALLERGIC REACTION
1. Mediated by T lymphocytes
2. Does not involve antibodies
3. Also called delayed-type hypersensitivity (response not seen until about 2 days after antigenic exposure)
4. Examples include the following:
   a. Contact dermatitis
   b. Graft rejection
   c. Graft-versus-host reaction
   d. Some type of drug hypersensitivity
   e. Some types of autoimmune disease

Modified from Thomson NC, Kirkwood EM, Lever RS. In Thomson NC, et al (eds): Handbook of Clinical Allergy. Oxford, Blackwell Scientific, 1990, pp 1-36.

Cellular Immune System. In the cellular or delayed immune system, T lymphocytes play the central role. The primary function of this system is to recognize and eradicate antigens that are fixed in tissues or within cells. This system is involved in protection against viruses, tuberculosis, and leprosy. Antibodies are not operative in the cell-mediated immune system. Effector T lymphocytes produce various cytokines that serve as active agents of this system.[1-4]

Type IV hypersensitivity reactions. Type IV hypersensitivity reactions, which involve the cellular immune system, include infectious contact dermatitis, transplant rejection, and graft-versus-host disease (Box 20-11). Events in type IV hypersensitivity (contact dermatitis), which may involve dendritic cells and Langerhans cells, present the antigen to undifferentiated T lymphocytes. Some of the more common antigens that cause contact dermatitis include metal jewelry, perfumes, rubber products, chemicals such as formaldehyde, and medicines such as topical anesthetics. Type IV hypersensitivity reactions usually are delayed and appear about 48 to 72 hours after contact has been made with the antigen.[1-4]

Infectious-type allergic reactions are exemplified by the tuberculin skin test, in which a person who has previously been exposed to *Mycobacterium tuberculosis* develops, along with a second exposure in the form of an intradermal injection of altered bacteria, a delayed response—usually within 48 to 72 hours. This response is characterized by induration, erythema, swelling, and sometimes ulceration at the site of injection.

Contact allergy occurs when a substance of low molecular weight that is not antigenic by itself comes in contact with a tissue component (primarily a protein) and forms an antigenic complex. This small molecule is called a *hapten* (or one half of an antigen), and the resulting complex causes sensitization of T lymphocytes. Poison ivy is an example of a contact allergy wherein the reaction

is delayed (with response occurring 48 to 72 hours after contact is made with the allergen).

Graft rejection occurs when organs or tissues from one body are transplanted into another body. Cellular rejection of transplanted tissue occurs, unless the donor and recipient are genetically identical or the host's immune response has been suppressed.

Graft-versus-host reaction is an unusual phenomenon that occurs in bone marrow transplant recipients whose cellular immune system has been rendered deficient by whole body irradiation. Lymphocytes transferred to the host attempt to destroy host tissues.[1-4]

Nonallergic Reactions. Other agents may cause mast cells to release their mediators without inciting a true allergic reaction; this occurs in cases of chronic urticaria caused by certain drugs, temperature changes, and emotional states and in some reactions to drugs. Most so-called anaphylactic reactions to local anesthetics do not involve an antigen/antibody reaction but result from damage to the mast cells caused by other mechanisms. These reactions are referred to as anaphylactoid or *anaphylaxis-like.*[1-4]

From the clinical standpoint, approaches to management of anaphylactic and anaphylactic-like reactions are similar; therefore, these types of drug reactions are viewed as true allergic reactions. Some cases of urticaria and angioneurotic edema have a similar pathogenesis and are not considered true allergic reactions.

Nonallergic cases of urticaria, angioneurotic edema, and anaphylactic-like reactions are caused by the nonspecific release of vasoactive amines from mast cells or by the activation of some other form of nonspecific immunologic effector mechanism. The reader is referred to a text on allergic diseases for an in-depth discussion of the origin of these reactions.[1-4]

MEDICAL MANAGEMENT

Patients with atopy may be given injections to gradually desensitize them so that they are no longer allergic to the antigen. Some individuals with severe asthma may be forced to move to an area of the country that does not contain the antigen (e.g., in the case of allergy to pollen). Patients with asthma (see Chapter 7), immune complex injury, or cytotoxic immune reactions may be treated with systemic steroids, whereas those with hay fever or urticaria are treated with antihistamines.

Newer antihistamines are highly effective and produce fewer adverse effects (e.g., drowsiness) (Table 20-2). All of these are good. They differ in a number of ways, such as size of the tablets, length of time for which they act, how effective they are, extent to which they may have a slight tendency to cause sleepiness (although all are superior to old antihistamines in terms of this), adverse effects, and drug interactions, as well as price.

Patients who have received an organ transplant often take steroids and immunosuppressive drugs. A variety of

TABLE 20-2
Examples of Newer and Safer Antihistamines

Official Name	Trade Names	OTC?*
Acrivastine	Semprex, Benadryl Allergy Relief capsules	No
Cetirizine	Zirtec, Zyrtec	Yes
Desloratadine	Neoclarityn	No
Fexofenadine	Telfast 120, Telfast 180, Allegra	No
Loratadine	Clarityn, Clarityne, Boots Antihistamine Tablets, Claritin	Yes
Mizolastine	Mizollen, Mistamine (superseded by fexofenadine)	No
Terfenadine	Triludan, Seldane, Aller-Eze, Histafen	Yes

*OTC means some or all medicines in this row can be purchased "over the counter" in the United States without a doctor's prescription.

treatments, including topical steroids, have been used for patients with contact dermatitis. From a dental standpoint, the patient who is being treated for allergies has an increased chance of being allergic to another substance; in addition, if this individual is taking steroids, his or her reaction to stress may be impaired (see Chapter 16). Further, if the patient should receive an organ transplant, he or she may be susceptible to infection (see Chapter 22).

DENTAL MANAGEMENT
Medical Considerations

The dentist is often confronted with problems related to allergy. One of the most common concerns is the patient who reports an allergy to a local anesthetic, antibiotic, or analgesic. The history then must be expanded, with specific efforts made to determine exactly what the offending substance was and exactly how the patient reacted to it. If the adverse reaction was of an allergic nature, one or more of the classic signs or symptoms of allergy should have been present (Box 20-12). If these signs or symptoms were not reported, the patient probably did not experience a true allergic reaction. Common examples of mislabeled allergy include syncope after injection of a local anesthetic and nausea or vomiting after ingestion of codeine. Adverse drug reactions are listed in Box 20-13.

Local Anesthetics. The reaction most often associated with local anesthetics is a toxic reaction, which usually results from inadvertent intravenous injection of the anesthetic solution (Box 20-14). Excessive amounts of an anesthetic also can cause a toxic reaction or a reaction to the vasoconstrictor. Signs and symptoms associated with toxic reactions to a local anesthetic are shown in Box 20-15. Signs and symptoms of a vasoconstrictor reaction include tachycardia, apprehension, sweating, and hyperactivity. Another common reaction to local anesthetics

---

BOX 20-12

Signs and Symptoms Suggestive of an Allergic Reaction[3]

- Urticaria
- Swelling
- Skin rash
- Chest tightness
- Dyspnea, shortness of breath
- Rhinorrhea
- Conjunctivitis

BOX 20-13

Adverse Drug Reactions[4]

SIGNS AND SYMPTOMS OF A TOXIC REACTION TO LOCAL ANESTHETIC
Predictable
- Dose related
- No immunologic basis
- Account for about 80% of all adverse reactions to drugs
- Direct toxicity
- Overdose
- Drug interaction
- Adverse effects of drugs

Unpredictable
- Not dose related
- Unrelated to expected pharmacologic effects
- Allergy
- Pseudoallergy (anaphylactoid reactions)
- Idiosyncrasy
- Intolerance
- Paradoxical reactions (cause histamine release but not IgE mediated)
- Underlying genetic defect often present

BOX 20-14

Adverse Reactions to Local Anesthetics[5]

- Toxicity
- Central nervous system stimulation
- Central nervous system depression
- Vasoconstrictor effects
- Anxiety
- Allergic reaction

---

involves the anxious patient who, because of concern about receiving a "shot," experiences tachycardia, sweating, paleness, and syncope (Box 20-16). True allergic reactions to the local anesthetics (amides) most often used in dentistry are rare.[5]

If the patient's history supports a toxic or vasoconstrictor reaction, the dentist should explain the nature of the

BOX 20-15

Signs and Symptoms of a Toxic Reaction to Local Anesthetic[5]

- Talkativeness
- Slurred speech
- Dizziness
- Nausea
- Depression
- Euphoria
- Excitement
- Convulsions

BOX 20-16

Signs and Symptoms of a Psychomotor Response to Injection of a Local Anesthetic[15]

- Hyperventilation
- Vasovagal syncope (bradycardia, pallor, sweating)
- Sympathetic stimulation (anxiety, tremor, tachycardia, hypertension)

BOX 20-17

Referral to an Allergist of a Patient With a History of Anesthetic Allergy

1. History shows reaction consistent with allergic response
   a. Allergic to anesthetic that is identified
   b. Allergic to anesthetic that cannot be identified
   c. Allergic to several anesthetics involving both amides and esters
2. Skin testing not indicated because of variable results
3. Provocative dose testing (PDT)
4. Selection and recommendation of alternative local anesthetic based on results of PDT

previous reaction (see Box 20-15) and avoid injecting the local anesthetic solution intravenously by aspirating before the injection and limiting the amount of solution to the recommended dose. If the patient's history supports an interpretation of fainting and not a toxic or allergic reaction, the dentist's primary task will be to work with the patient to reduce anxiety during dental visits. If the history supports a true allergic reaction to a local anesthetic, the dentist should try to identify the type of local anesthetic that was used. Once this has been done, a new anesthetic with a different basic chemical structure can be used. The two main groups of local anesthetics in dentistry consist of the following:

1. Para-aminobenzoic acid (PABA) esters (procaine [Novocain] and tetracaine [Pontocaine])
2. Amides (lidocaine [Xylocaine], mepivacaine [Carbocaine], and prilocaine [Citanest])

Benzoic acid ester anesthetics may cross-react with each other, whereas amide anesthetics usually do not cross-react. Cross reaction does not occur between ester and amide local anesthetics.[5,6]

Procaine is the local anesthetic associated with the highest incidence of allergic reactions. Its antigenic component appears to be PABA, one of the metabolic breakdown products of procaine. Cross-reactivity has been reported between lidocaine and procaine; however, this could be traced to the presence of a germicide, methylparaben, which has been used in small amounts as a preservative and is chemically similar to PABA. Thus, a patient who is allergic to procaine may react to lidocaine solution if it contains methylparaben. Lidocaine that does not contain methylparaben can now be readily obtained and should be used for patients with an allergic history to procaine.[5,6]

Patients who have been allergic to local anesthetics but who cannot identify the specific agent to which they reacted present more of a problem. The nature of the reaction must be established, and if it is consistent with an allergic reaction, the next step should be to attempt to identify the anesthetic used. When the patient is unable to provide this information, the dentist can attempt to contact the previous dentist involved. If this fails, the following two options are available:

1. An antihistamine (diphenhydramine [Benadryl]) can be used as the local anesthetic
2. The patient may be referred to an allergist for provocative dose testing (PDT) (Box 20-17)

The use of diphenhydramine is often the more practical option. A 1% solution of diphenhydramine that contains 1:100,000 epinephrine can be easily compounded by a pharmacist, but it must be confirmed that methylparaben is not used as a preservative. This solution induces anesthesia of about 30 minutes average duration and can be used for infiltration or block injection. When it is used for a mandibular block, 1 to 4 mL of solution is needed. Some patients have reported a burning sensation, swelling, or erythema after a mandibular block with 1% diphenhydramine, but these effects were not serious and cleared within 1 or 2 days. No more than 50 mg of diphenhydramine should be given during a single appointment. Diphenhydramine also can be used in the patient who states that he or she is allergic to both ester and amide local anesthetics.[5,6]

The dentist may elect to refer the patient to an allergist for evaluation and testing, which usually includes both skin testing and PDT. Most investigators agree that skin testing alone for allergy to local anesthetics is of little benefit because false-positive results are common; therefore, the allergist also should perform PDT. Sending samples for specific testing of one's usual anesthetic agents without vasoconstrictors is of great help.

On the basis of patient history, the allergist selects a local anesthetic for testing that is least likely to cause an allergic reaction; this is usually an anesthetic from the amide group because they generally do not cross-react with each other. At 15-minute intervals, 0.1 mL of test solution is injected subcutaneously, with concentrations increasing from 1:10,000 to 1:1000 to 1:100 to 1:10, followed by undiluted solution; next, 0.5 mL of undiluted test solution is tried; and finally, 1 mL of undiluted solution is given. During PDT, the allergist should be prepared to deal with any adverse reaction that might occur and should report to the dentist on the drug selected, the final dose given, and the absence of any adverse reaction. Under these conditions, a local anesthetic that causes no reaction can be used in the tested patient, and the risk of an allergic reaction is no greater than in the general population. Malamed has reported that he has not dealt with a single patient for whom a safe local anesthetic could not be found through the PDT procedure.[5]

When administering an alternative anesthetic to a patient with a history of a local anesthetic allergy, the dentist should follow these steps:

1. Inject slowly, aspirating first to make sure that a vessel is not being injected.
2. Place 1 drop of the solution into the tissues.
3. Withdraw the needle, and wait 5 minutes to see what reaction, if any, occurs. If no allergic reaction occurs, as much anesthetic as is needed for the procedure should be deposited. Be sure to aspirate before giving the second injection (Box 20-18).

BOX 20-18

Dental Management of a Local Anesthetic Allergy[4]

1. Establish history of previous reaction after use of local anesthetic
2. Establish history of previous reaction and type of anesthetic used
   a. Syncopal
   b. Allergic
      (1) Soft tissue swelling
      (2) Skin rash
      (3) Rhinitis
      (4) Difficulty breathing
3. If reaction was consistent with allergic reaction, the following should be done:
   a. Select anesthetic from a different chemical group
      (1) Para-aminobenzoic acid (procaine)
      (2) Amide (lidocaine, mepivacaine)
   b. Aspirate, inject 1 drop of alternate anesthetic, and wait 5 minutes; if no reaction occurs, inject after the rest of the anesthetic needed is aspirated (be prepared to deal with an allergic reaction, should one occur)
   c. In cases of allergic reaction to several local anesthetic agents, or when a previously used anesthetic cannot be identified, consider using diphenhydramine
4. If history of multiple allergies is present, or if type of local anesthetic used previously cannot be identified, refer the patient to an allergist for provocative dose testing (PDT).

Penicillin. The use of penicillin has been increasing tremendously throughout the world during the past 30 years, particularly in the United States. Approximately 2.5 million persons in the United States are allergic to penicillin, and allergic reactions occur in 5% to 10% of patients who receive penicillin and related drugs. About 0.04% to 0.2% of patients treated with penicillin develop an anaphylactic reaction, and about 10% of these individuals die, accounting for some 400 to 800 deaths per year. Box 20-19 shows the risk assessment of penicillin reactions.[1,3,4,7]

The possibility of sensitizing a patient to penicillin increases according to the route of administration as follows[2,4,6]: Oral administration results in sensitization of only about 0.1% of patients, intramuscular (IM) injection in about 1% to 2%, and topical application in about 5% to 12%. On the basis of these data, the use of penicillin in a topical ointment is contraindicated. Additionally, if the dentist has a choice, the oral route is preferable for administration whenever possible. Parenteral administration of penicillin will evoke a more serious reaction than will oral administration. Some investigators have suggested that the risk is equally great for a serious allergic reaction with both routes. Antibodies produced against penicillin cross-react with the semisynthetic penicillins and may cause severe reactions in patients who are allergic to penicillin. Nevertheless, the synthetic penicillins seem to cause fewer new sensitizations in patients who are not allergic to penicillin at the time of administration. Patients with a history of penicillin allergy should be given erythromycin or clindamycin for the treatment of oral infection or clindamycin for prophylaxis against infective endocarditis.[1,3,4,6]

BOX 20-19

Penicillin Reactions[4]

ANAPHYLAXIS
- In 0.04% to 0.2% of patients
- Fatal reaction in 1 per 100,000 treated individuals
- Atopic predisposition not a risk factor for anaphylaxis, but is a risk factor for fatal reaction
- Risk of reaction is dependent on
  - History of prior reaction
  - Time interval since prior reaction
  - Persistence of specific immunoglobulin (Ig)E antibodies
  - History of multiple drug sensitivities
- Most useful parameter to assess risk in patients with a history of penicillin reaction is skin testing with major and minor determinants
  - Negative result—Very little risk
  - Positive result—High risk for serious reaction to penicillin; risk for cross reaction with cephalosporin

Skin testing for allergy to penicillin is much more reliable than is skin testing for allergy to a local anesthetic; however, some risk is involved, and the allergist must be prepared for adverse reactions. Several points should be considered in the use of skin testing for penicillin sensitivity. To be cost-effective, the test should be conducted only on patients with a history of penicillin reaction who need penicillin for a serious infection. An important fact to remember is that penicillin reactivity declines with time; hence, a patient may have reacted to the drug years ago but is now no longer sensitive (negative skin test). The length of time for retaining sensitivity is variable and is dependent on IgE levels. Most anaphylactic reactions to penicillin occur in patients who have been treated in the past with penicillin but reported no adverse reactions.[1,3,4,6]

When skin testing for penicillin sensitivity is performed, both metabolic breakdown products of penicillin (the major derivative, penicilloyl polylysine, and the minor derivative mixture) must be tested; 95% of penicillin is metabolized to the major determinant and 5% to the minor determinants. If skin tests are negative to both breakdown products, the patient is considered not allergic to penicillin; however, if positive tests are obtained for one or both of the breakdown products, the patient is considered to be allergic to penicillin, and the drug should not be used. When penicillin must be used, the patient with a positive skin test can be desensitized to it. Patients with a positive skin test to minor derivative mixture have a higher incidence of anaphylactic reactions than do patients with a positive test to the major derivative.[1,3,4,6]

In dentistry, wherein alternative antibiotics can be selected, reactions to penicillin are preventable by mere avoidance of the use of penicillin in patients who have a history of penicillin allergy. Additionally, drugs that may cross-react, including ampicillin, carbenicillin, and methicillin, should be avoided in these patients.[4,6]

Cephalosporins cross-react in 5% to 10% of penicillin-sensitive patients. The risk is greatest with first- and second-generation drugs. Cephalosporins are metabolized to their major determinant, cephaloyl, which may cross-react with the major determinant of penicillin. Cephalosporins usually can be used in patients with a history of distant, nonserious reaction to penicillin. However, skin testing is recommended by some authors for these patients. If the patient's skin test to penicillin is negative, then penicillin or a cephalosporin may be used. If the penicillin skin test is positive, a skin test for the specific cephalosporin selected should be performed. If this skin test is negative, the cephalosporin that was tested can be used. Box 20-20 summarizes the use of cephalosporins in patients with a history of penicillin hypersensitivity.[4-6]

Patients with a negative history of allergy to penicillin can be treated with the drug when indicated, and it should be given by the oral route. The patient is observed for 30 minutes after the first dose, if possible, and is advised to

---

BOX 20-20

Use of Cephalosporins in Patients With a History of Penicillin Hypersensitivity

1. Cephalosporins metabolized to major determinant, cephaloyl
2. Cephaloyl can cross-react with major determinant of penicillin (penicilloyl polylysine)
3. Risk of adverse reaction to cephalosporin is controversial
   a. Greatest with first- or second-generation drugs
      (1) Cephaloridine, 16.5%
      (2) Cephalothin, 5%
      (3) Cephalexin, 5.4%
   b. Anaphylaxis
      (1) Positive history of penicillin reaction, 0.1%
      (2) Negative history of penicillin reaction, 0.4%
   c. Urticaria
      (1) Positive history of penicillin reaction, 1.3%
      (2) Negative history of penicillin reaction, 0.4%
4. Patient with history of penicillin reaction, first skin test for penicillin sensitivity
   a. Negative—Use penicillin or a cephalosporin
   b. Positive
      (1) Avoid penicillin
      (2) Skin test is specific for cephalosporin; use if result is negative

From Lichtenstein LM, Busse WW, Geha RS. Current Therapy in Allergy, Immunology and Rheumatology, 6th ed. London, Mosby Ltd, 2003.

---

seek immediate care if any of the signs or symptoms of an allergic reaction occur after he or she has left the dental office (Box 20-21).

Analgesics. Aspirin may cause gastrointestinal upset, but this can be avoided if it is taken with food or a glass of milk. The discomfort may include "heartburn," nausea, vomiting, or gastrointestinal bleeding. Aspirin should not be used by patients with an ulcer, gastritis, or a hiatal hernia and should be used with care by patients whose condition predisposes them to nausea, vomiting, dyspepsia, or gastric ulceration. Aspirin also is known to prolong prothrombin time and to inhibit platelet function, which is usually of little clinical importance, except in patients with a hemorrhagic disease or a peptic ulcer. In these patients, aspirin must be avoided. Many individuals ($\approx$2 per 1000) are allergic to salicylates. Allergic reactions to aspirin can be serious, and deaths have been reported.[1,3,4]

Aspirin provokes a severe reaction in some patients with asthma. They may react in the same way to other nonsteroidal anti-inflammatory drugs (NSAIDs) that inhibit cyclooxygenase, which is the key enzyme involved in the generation of prostaglandin from arachidonic acid. The typical reaction consists of acute bronchospasm, rhinorrhea, and urticaria. Most individuals with asthma who react to NSAIDs also have nasal polyps and lack IgE-mediated allergy to airborne allergens. The mechanism

BOX 20-21

Procedures for Prevention of a
Penicillin Reaction

1. Have emergency kit for treatment.
2. Take medical history on all patients, including the following:
   a. Previous contact with penicillin
   b. Reactions to penicillin
   c. Allergic reactions to other agents
3. Do not use penicillin in patient with a history of reactions to drugs.
4. Tell patient when you are going to give penicillin.
5. Do not use penicillin in topical preparations.
6. Do not use penicillinase-resistant penicillins unless infection is caused by penicillinase-producing staphylococci.
7. Use oral penicillin whenever possible.
8. Use disposable syringes for injection of penicillin.
9. Have patient wait in office for 30 minutes after first dose of penicillin is given.
10. Inform patient about signs and symptoms of allergic reaction to penicillin, and if these occur, to seek immediate medical assistance.

for this reaction does not appear to be allergic but remains undefined.[8]

The dentist should be aware of the many multiple-entity analgesic preparations that include aspirin or other salicylates. These agents must not be given to the patient who may be endangered by an adverse reaction associated with aspirin or other salicylates.[1,4]

Many NSAIDs are now available, and most can cause some degree of gastrointestinal irritation. NSAIDs also are inhibitors of prostaglandin formation, platelet aggregation, and prothrombin synthesis. Most have the potential for cross-sensitivity in patients who exhibit an asthma-like reaction to aspirin. NSAIDs should not be given to certain patients with asthma, patients with an ulcer or hemorrhagic disease, and those who are pregnant or nursing. The new cyclooxygenase (COX)-2 inhibitors that are now available and effective cause much less gastrointestinal disturbance.[8] However, selective COX-2 inhibitors may cause renal dysfunction and elevated blood pressure, which, in turn, may precipitate heart failure in vulnerable individuals. Although NSAID-related cardiotoxicity is relatively rare and is most commonly seen in elderly individuals with concomitant disease, the widespread long-term use of these drugs in high-risk groups is potentially hazardous. Pending comprehensive safety analyses, the use of NSAIDs in high-risk patients should be discouraged.

Codeine is a narcotic analgesic that is commonly used in dentistry. Emesis, nausea, and constipation may occur with analgesic doses of codeine. Miosis and adverse renal, hepatic, cardiovascular, and bronchial effects are not likely to occur with therapeutic doses, however. Most of the reported reactions to codeine consist of nonallergic

gastrointestinal manifestations; nevertheless, these may be severe enough to preclude the use of codeine in certain patients. Alternate drug selections may be made after a current pharmacology text, such as *Physicians' Desk Reference* or *Accepted Dental Therapeutics*, is consulted.[5]

Rubber Products. A number of reports have demonstrated that certain health care workers and patients are at risk for hypersensitivity reactions to latex or agents used in the production of rubber gloves or related materials (e.g., rubber dam, blood pressure cuff, catheters). Latex from surgical gloves has been know to cause cardiovascular collapse in surgical patients, anaphylaxis in an obstetrics and gynecology physician, hypersensitivity reactions in other health care workers, and anaphylaxis in other patients. About 3% of hospital physicians and nurses have been affected by hypersensitivity reactions to latex. However, most of these cases were type IV reactions, which were caused by agents used in the production of rubber products. Type I allergic reactions to latex are rare. On the basis of these findings, it can be concluded that serious type I hypersensitivity reactions may occur in physicians, dentists, other health care workers, and patients as the result of contact with latex products such as gloves, rubber dam, balloons, or catheters.[9]

Dentists should be aware that latex allergy can present as anaphylaxis during dental work when the patient or the dentist has been sensitized to latex. Anaphylaxis may occur in the sensitized individual after contact has been made with rubber gloves, rubber dam material, blood pressure cuffs, or any other product containing latex. Studies have shown that latex-allergic individuals have IgE antibodies for specific latex proteins. Latex skin tests are a satisfactory means of identifying individuals who may be sensitized to latex.[9,10]

Dental Materials and Products. Type I, type III, and type IV hypersensitivity reactions have been reported to result from various dental materials and products. Topical anesthetic agents have been reported to cause type I reactions consisting of urticarial swelling. Mouth rinses and toothpastes containing phenolic compounds, antiseptics, astringents, or flavoring agents have been known to cause type I, type III, and type IV hypersensitivity reactions involving the oral mucosa or lips. Hand soaps used by dental care workers also have been reported as a cause of type IV reactions. Some of the dental agents that can lead to type IV hypersensitivity (contact stomatitis) include dental amalgam, acrylic, composite resin, nickel, eugenol, rubber products, talcum powder, mouthwashes, and toothpastes.[10,11]

Other Conditions. Allergic patients who are being treated with steroids should be managed as described in Chapter 16. Patients who have received an organ transplant should be managed as described in Chapter 22. The dental management of patients with asthma is primarily concerned with preventing severe asthma attacks from

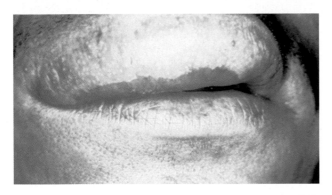

Figure 20-2. Angioneurotic edema of the upper lip that occurred soon after injection of a local anesthetic.

occurring in the dental office and dealing with an attack if one happens. In addition, certain important drug considerations must be applied to these patients (see Chapter 7).[8]

Treatment Planning Modifications

The dentist should obtain from each patient a history of any allergic reactions. If a patient has a history of allergy to drugs or materials that may be used in dentistry, a clear entry should be made in the dental record, and any further contact with or use of the antigen(s) should be avoided in that patient. Most allergic patients can receive any indicated dental treatment as long as the antigen is avoided and special preparations are made for those patients receiving steroids.

Oral Complications and Manifestations

Hypersensitivity.

Type I hypersensitivity. Oral lesions can be produced by type I hypersensitivity reactions. An atopic reaction to various foods, drugs, or anesthetic agents may occur within or around the oral cavity and is usually characterized by urticarial swelling or angioneurotic edema (Figure 20-2). This reaction is generally rapid, with the lesion developing within a short time after coming into contact with the antigen. This painless, soft tissue swelling produced by transudate from the surrounding vessels may cause itching and burning. The lesion is usually present for 1 to 3 days and then begins to resolve spontaneously. Oral antihistamines should be given; oral diphenhydramine, 50 mg every 4 hours, is the recommended regimen. Treatment is provided for 1 to 3 days. Further contact with the antigen must be avoided (Box 20-22).[5,12]

Type III hypersensitivity. Foods, drugs, or agents that are placed within the oral cavity can cause white, erythematous, or ulcerative lesions as determined by the presence of type III hypersensitivity or immune complex reactions. These lesions develop rather quickly, usually within a 24-hour period, after contact is made with the offending antigen. Some cases of aphthous stomatitis (Figure 20-3) may be caused by type III hypersensitivity, but most are related to lymphocyte dysfunction. Figure

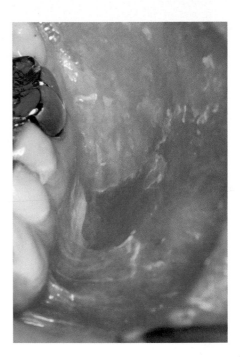

Figure 20-3. Stomatitis that occurred in a patient who was found to be allergic to the toothpaste he was using. (From Neville BW, Damm DD, Allen CM, Bouguot JE. Oral and Maxillofacial Pathology, 2nd ed. Philadelphia, Saunders, 2002.)

BOX 20-22

Oral or Paraoral Type I Hypersensitivity Reactions

1. Urticarial swelling (or angioneurotic edema)
   a. Reaction occurs soon after contact with antigen
   b. Reaction consists of painless swelling
   c. Itching and burning may occur
   d. Lesion may remain for 1 to 3 days
2. Treatment
   a. Reaction not involving tongue, pharynx, or larynx and with no respiratory distress noted requires 50 mg of diphenhydramine 4 times a day until swelling diminishes
   b. Reaction involving tongue, pharynx, or larynx with respiratory distress noted requires the following:
      (1) 0.5 mL of 1:1000 epinephrine, IM or SC
      (2) Oxygen
      (3) Once immediate danger is over, 50 mg of diphenhydramine should be given 4 times a day until swelling diminishes

IM, Intramuscular; SC, subcutaneous.

20-4 shows an allergic dermatitis that occurred after orthodontic brackets and archwires (containing nickel) were placed. Erythema multiforme represents an immune complex reaction.[13]

About half of patients in whom erythema multiforme is diagnosed (Figure 20-5) are found to have a predisposing factor such as a drug allergy or a herpes simplex infection that is involved in the onset of their disease.

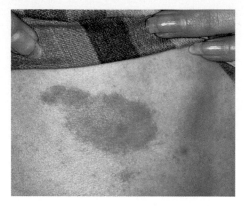

Figure 20-4. Allergic rash on the abdomen of a patient in whom orthodontic brackets and archwires were just placed. The patient was tested and was found to be allergic to the nickel in the wires.

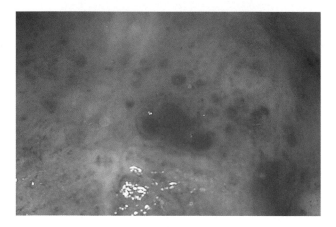

Figure 20-5. Erythema multiforme that developed after oral administration of a drug used to treat an oral infection. Ulceration of the palatal mucosa.

Sulfa antibiotics are most commonly associated with the onset of erythema multiforme; sulfonyl urea hypoglycemic agents (e.g., tolbutamide, tolazamide, glyburide, glipizide), which are used to treat some individuals with diabetes, have been found to be associated with the onset of erythema multiforme as well. Many patients with erythema multiforme can be treated with symptomatic therapy, including a bland mouth rinse, syrup of diphenhydramine, and triamcinolone acetonide (Kenalog) in Orabase. A few patients with more severe involvement may require systemic steroids. (See Appendix B for treatment regimens.) If a drug appears to be associated with onset of the disease, any further contact with it should be avoided. Box 20-23 summarizes oral type III hypersensitivity reactions.[4,9,11]

Type IV hypersensitivity. Contact stomatitis is a delayed allergic reaction that is associated with the cellular immune response in most cases. Because of the delayed nature of the reaction after contact is made with the allergen in cases of contact stomatitis, the dentist

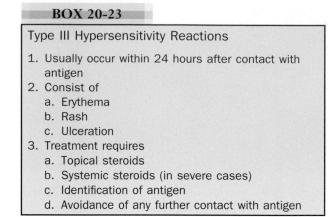

BOX 20-23

Type III Hypersensitivity Reactions

1. Usually occur within 24 hours after contact with antigen
2. Consist of
   a. Erythema
   b. Rash
   c. Ulceration
3. Treatment requires
   a. Topical steroids
   b. Systemic steroids (in severe cases)
   c. Identification of antigen
   d. Avoidance of any further contact with antigen

must inquire about contacts with materials that may have occurred 2 to 3 days before the lesions appeared. The antigen may be found in dental materials, toothpaste, mouth rinses, lipsticks, face powders, and so forth. In many cases, no further treatment is necessary once the source of the antigen has been identified and removed from further contact with the patient; however, if the tissue reaction is severe or persistent, topical corticosteroids should be used. A good preparation for topical use is triamcinolone acetonide in Orabase (see Appendix C for treatment regimens).[4,9,11]

Various dental materials have been reported as the cause of allergic reactions in patients. Impression materials containing an aromatic sulfonate catalyst have been reported to cause a delayed allergic reaction in postmenopausal women. The reaction consisted of tissue ulceration and necrosis that became progressively worse with each exposure.[9,11]

Some authors have reported that oral lesions may be found in close association with amalgam restorations. These (mucosal) lesions have been described as whitish, reddish, ulcerative, or lichenoid and were thought to be caused by toxic irritation or a hypersensitivity reaction to the silver amalgam restoration. When these restorations were removed, the lesions most often cleared. In some studies, skin testing for mercury sensitivity was performed. All reports suggested that some of the oral lesions resulted from toxic injury to the mucosa, and others were a result of type IV hypersensitivity reaction to mercury in the amalgam.[14]

No thorough studies relate nonspecific symptoms such as depression, fatigue, and headache to the effects of mercury in amalgam restorations. The practice of avoiding the use of amalgam restorations in patients with nonspecific symptoms has, at present, no scientific basis. However, removal of any amalgam restorations in contact with oral mucosa that shows lesions consistent with a toxic or hypersensitivity reaction to mercury is rational.[14]

On rare occasions, dental composite materials have been reported to cause allergic reactions. The acrylic monomer used in denture construction has caused an

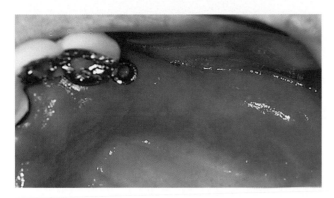

Figure 20-6. Allergic reaction to removable partial denture framework. Note the erythematous demarcation.

allergic reaction; however, the vast majority of tissue changes under dentures result from trauma and secondary infection with bacteria or fungi. Gold, nickel, and mercury have been reported to cause allergic reactions that result in tissue erythema and ulceration (Figure 20-6).[11-13]

The dentist may wish to test agents that are thought to be possible antigens that cause oral lesions. Oral epimucous testing for contact stomatitis consists of placing the suspected antigen in contact with the oral mucosa and observing for any reaction over a period of several days (e.g., erythema, sloughing, ulceration) that might indicate an allergy to the test material. In most cases, a reaction is not expected to develop for at least 48 to 72 hours. Various techniques have been used to conduct epimucous testing for suspected allergens. One of these involves placing the suspected allergen in a rubber suction cup, placing the cup on the buccal mucosa, and observing at intervals for erythema or ulceration under the cup. Another technique is to place a sample of the suspected antigen in a depression on the palatal aspect of an overlay denture. The denture is inserted and holds the allergen in contact with the palatal mucosa.

Another technique consists of incorporating the allergen into Orabase, applying Orabase in the mucobuccal fold, and periodically observing for a reaction. Alternately, the antigen can be incorporated into an oral adhesive spray. Skin testing and oral epimucous testing for potential antigens are not foolproof, by any means; in certain patients, they yield unreliable tissue responses. The response in some cases may be caused by trauma; in others, in which no tissue reaction occurs, the patient may still be allergic to the substance.

Basic management of contact stomatitis requires removal of common sources of antigens known to cause hypersensitivity reactions to discover whether the lesions clear. Skin or mucosal testing for sensitivity also can be performed. Once the offending agent or antigen has been identified, the patient should be told to avoid any future contact with the antigen. Again, if the lesions persist, topical steroids can be applied (see Appendix C).

Lichenoid Drug Eruptions. Some patients with skin and/or oral lesions identical to those of lichen planus will be found to have taken certain drugs before the onset of their lesions. If these drugs are withdrawn, the lesions clear within several days (in most patients) or within a few weeks. The agents most commonly associated with the onset of lichenoid lesions are levamisole (Levantine) and the quinidine drugs. Other agents found to be associated are the thiazide drugs, methyldopa, and photographic dyes (e.g., paraphenylenediamine). Biopsy of a lichenoid lesion shows the same microscopic picture as is seen in lichen planus, with the additional finding of eosinophils in the subepithelial infiltrate. These lesions are related to the cellular immune system and therefore could be placed under the heading of contact stomatitis; however, the true nature of the reactions is not clear.[14]

MANAGEMENT OF SEVERE TYPE I HYPERSENSITIVITY REACTIONS

Even when the dentist has taken appropriate precautions, an allergic reaction may occur. Most of these are mild and of a nonemergency nature; however, some may be severe and life threatening (anaphylactic). The dentist must be ready to deal with either type. In handling the anaphylactic reaction, the dentist should remember that it has an allergic origin. In other words, the reaction should occur soon after (i.e., minutes) the injection, ingestion, or application of a topical anesthetic, medication, drug, local anesthetic, or dental product. The dentist must take the following actions immediately (see Appendix A):

- Place the patient in a head-down or supine position.
- Make certain that the airway is patent.
- Administer oxygen.
- Be prepared to send for help and to support respiration and circulation. The rate and depth of respiration should be noted, as should the patient's other vital signs. Most reactions in dental patients consist of simple fainting, which can be well managed by the preceding actions. In addition, the dentist may administer aromatic spirits of ammonia through inhalation, which encourages breathing through reflex stimulation.
- If these initial steps have not solved the emergency problem, and the problem is of an allergic cause, the dentist is faced with an edematous-type or an anaphylactic reaction.

Angioneurotic Edema. If an immediate type I hypersensitivity reaction has resulted in edema of the tongue, pharyngeal tissues, or larynx, the dentist must take additional emergency steps to prevent death from respiratory failure. At this point, if the patient has not responded to the initial procedures and is in acute respiratory distress, the dentist should do the following:

BOX 20-24

Signs and Symptoms of Anaphylaxis

- Itching of soft palate
- Nausea, vomiting
- Substernal pressure
- Shortness of breath
- Hypotension
- Pruritus
- Urticaria
- Laryngeal edema
- Bronchospasm
- Cardiac arrhythmias

BOX 20-25

Anaphylaxis

BASIS

1. First contact with antigen results in formation of antibodies by plasma cells.
2. Antibodies circulate in bloodstream (immunoglobulin [Ig]E antibodies).
3. Antibodies attach to target tissues (mast cells near smooth muscle of bronchi).
4. Next contact with antigen may result in combination of antigen with antibody.
5. Antigen/antibody complex causes degranulation of mast cell(s) with release of histamine.
6. Smooth muscle contracts and vessels lose fluid, etc.
7. Acute respiratory distress and cardiovascular collapse may occur within minutes.

MANAGEMENT

1. Call for medical help.
2. Place patient in the supine position.
3. Check for open airway.
4. Administer oxygen.
5. Check pulse, blood pressure, and respiration.
   a. If depressed or absent, inject 0.3 to 0.5 mL 1:1000 epinephrine IM into the tongue.
   b. Provide cardiopulmonary resuscitation if needed.
   c. Repeat injection of 0.5 mL 1:1000 epinephrine if no response.

IM, Intramuscular.

- Inject 0.3 to 0.5 mL of 1:1000 epinephrine through an IM (into the tongue) or subcutaneous (SC) route.
- Support respiration, if indicated, by mouth-to-mouth breathing or bag and mask; the dentist should make sure the chest moves when either of these methods is used.
- Check the carotid or femoral pulse; if a pulse cannot be detected, closed chest cardiac massage should be

initiated. By this time, someone in the office should have called a nearby physician or hospital.

Anaphylaxis. An anaphylactic reaction usually takes place within minutes. The signs and symptoms associated with anaphylactic reactions are listed in Box 20-24. In contrast to a severe edematous reaction, in which respiratory distress occurs first, both respiratory and circulatory depression occur early in the anaphylactic reaction. Anaphylaxis often is fatal unless vigorous, immediate action is taken. Because it occurs within minutes after contact with the antigen, the dentist should take the following steps (Box 20-25):

- Have someone in the office call for medical aid from a nearby physician or hospital.
- Place the patient in a supine position.
- Make certain the airway is patent.
- Administer oxygen.
- Check the carotid or femoral pulse and respiration; determine whether no pulse is present and the respiration is depressed.
- Inject 0.3 to 0.5 mL of 1:1000 epinephrine through an IM (into the tongue) or SC route. Support circulation through closed chest cardiac massage. Support respiration by mouth-to-mouth breathing. Repeat the injection of epinephrine if no response occurs.

REFERENCES

1. Kay AB. Allergies and allergic diseases: First of two parts. N Engl J Med 2001;344:30-37.
2. Hagner RR. Disorders of the immune system. In Kasper DL, Harrison TR (eds). Harrison's Principles of Internal Medicine, 16th ed. New York, McGraw-Hill, 2003.
3. Patterson R. Anaphylaxis. In Grammer LC, Greenberger PA (eds). Allergic Diseases: Diagnosis and Management, 5th ed. Philadelphia, JB Lippincott, 1997.
4. Lichtenstein LM, Busse WW, Geha RS (eds). Current Therapy in Allergy, Immunology, and Rheumatology, 6th ed. Philadelphia, Mosby, 2004.
5. Malamed SF. Allergy and toxic reactions to local anesthetics. Dent Today 2003;22:114-116, 118-121.
6. Council on American Dental Associations. Accepted Dental Therapeutics. Chicago, The American Dental Association, 2005.
7. Wang L, Lopes LG, Oliveira GC, et al. Antibiotic prophylaxis in a patient with penicillin allergy and recurrent bacterial endocarditis: A case report. Spec Care Dent 2005;24:283-286.
8. Coke JM. The asthma patient and dental management. Gen Dent 2003;51:504-507.
9. Cullinan P, Field A, Hourihane J, et al. Latex allergy: Position paper of the British Society of Clinical Immunology. Clin Exp Allergy 2003;33:1489-1493.
10. Hamann CP, DePaola LG, Rodgers PA. Occupation-related allergies in dentistry. J Am Dent Assoc 2005;136:500-510.

11. Pretorius E. Allergic reactions caused by dental restorative products. SADJ 2002;57:372-375.

12. Maeda S, Miyawaki T, Nomura S, et al. Management of oral surgery in patients with hereditary or acquired angioedemas: review and case reports. Oral Surg Oral Med Oral Pathol Oral Radiol Endod 2003;96:540-543.

13. Kalimo K, Mattila L, Kautiainen H. Nickel allergy and orthodontic treatment. J Eur Acad Dermatol Venereol 2004;18:543-545.

14. Kato Y, Hayakawa R, Shiraki R, Ozeki K. A case of lichen planus caused by mercury allergy. Br J Dermatol 2003;148:1268-1269.

Rheumatologic and Connective Tissue Disorders

CHAPTER

21

Arthritis is a nonspecific term that means "inflammation of the joints." Arthritic disease encompasses a group of disorders of the rheumatic diseases that affect bones, joints, and muscles. Laypersons often use the term *arthritis* interchangeably with *rheumatism*, to denote aches, pains, and stiffness in the joints and muscles. More than 100 arthritic (or rheumatic) diseases affect various parts of the body. Some of the more common types include rheumatoid arthritis, osteoarthritis, systemic lupus erythematosus, juvenile arthritis, scleroderma, Sjögren's syndrome, gout, ankylosing spondylitis, Lyme disease, fibromyalgia, and psoriatic arthritis.[1]

Arthritic diseases have significant personal and economic impact. According to the Arthritis Foundation, more than 40 million Americans suffer from various forms of arthritis, and more than 8 million of these are disabled. In terms of its overall economic impact, arthritis costs the American economy more than $18 billion annually, and more than 27 million workdays are lost per year.[1]

Although arthritis comprises a group of more than 60 important diseases, this chapter is limited to a discussion of rheumatoid arthritis, osteoarthritis, systemic lupus erythematosus (SLE), Lyme disease, and Sjögren's syndrome, which are among the most common forms encountered and can serve as models for the other forms. Several important items regarding the dental management of patients with rheumatologic and connective tissue disorders, including effects on the temporomandibular joint (TMJ), salivary glands, and oral mucosal tissues, organ and system involvement, and drug therapy, are discussed here.

RHEUMATOID ARTHRITIS

DEFINITION

Incidence and Prevalence

Rheumatoid arthritis (RA) is an autoimmune disease of unknown origin that is characterized by symmetric inflammation of joints, especially of the hands, feet, and knees. Severity of the disease varies widely from patient to patient and from time to time within the same patient. Determination of prevalence is somewhat difficult to determine because of lack of well-defined markers of the disease; however, estimates of prevalence range from 1% to 2% of the population. Disease onset usually occurs between ages 35 and 50 years and is more prevalent in women than men by a 3 : 1 ratio. This gender differentiation implies involvement of sex hormones in the susceptibility and sensitivity of the disease. Other factors, such as socioeconomic status, education, and psychosocial stress, have been suggested to play predisposing roles.[2]

Etiology

The cause of RA is unknown; however, evidence seems to implicate an interrelationship of infectious agents, genetics, and autoimmunity. One theory suggests that a viral agent alters the immune system in a genetically predisposed individual, leading to destruction of synovial tissues. Although researchers sometimes discover a particular gene that is related to the disease, it usually is the occurrence of disease within families that suggests a genetic component. For most autoimmune diseases, however, aggregation in families is rather modest; in most cases, a person with RA or SLE does not have a close relative with the same illness. Therefore, investigators

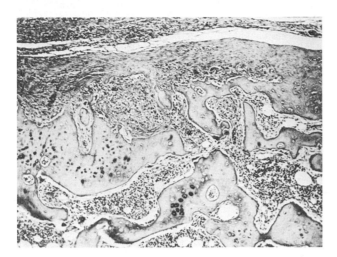

Figure 21-1. The joint surface *(top)* has lost its cartilage and consists of granulation tissue with scar tissue. Subchondral bone shows degenerative changes and areas of necrosis. (Courtesy A. Golden, Lexington, Ky.)

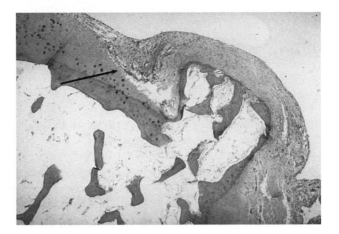

Figure 21-2. A micrograph of a pannus resulting from severe synovitis in rheumatoid arthritis. The pannus is eroding articular cartilage and bone *(arrow)*. (Courtesy Richard Estensen, Minneapolis, Minn.)

must study carefully the prevalence of disease among populations of individuals with different degrees of genetic relatedness. The most useful types of populations for these comparisons consist of genetically identical individuals (monozygotic twins), individuals who share approximately 50% of their genes (dizygotic twins and siblings), and unrelated individuals within the population. Many persons who develop RA have a genetic predisposition that occurs in the form of a tissue marker called HLA-DR4; however, not everyone with this tissue type develops the disease. Some questions have been raised as to whether vitamins or foods are implicated in RA. Currently, circumstantial evidence suggests that food may play a role in the origin and treatment of RA; however, studies to date are of limited value, and further research is warranted.[2,3]

Pathophysiology and Complications

With RA, the fundamental abnormality involves microvascular endothelial cell activation and injury.[2] Primary changes occur within the synovium, which is the inner lining of the joint capsule. Edema of the synovium occurs, followed by thickening and folding. This excessive tissue, composed of proliferative and invasive granulation tissue, is referred to as *pannus* (Figure 21-1). In addition, marked infiltration of lymphocytes and plasma cells into the capsule occurs. Eventually, granulation tissue covers the articular surfaces and destroys the cartilage and subchondral bone through enzymatic activity (Figure 21-2). This process also extends to the capsule and ligaments, causing distention and rupture. New bone or fibrous tissue then is deposited, resulting in fusion or loss of mobility.[2]

A likely sequence of events begins with a synovitis that stimulates immunoglobulin G (IgG) antibodies. These antibodies form antigenic aggregates in the joint space, leading to the production of rheumatoid factor (autoantibodies). Rheumatoid factor then complexes with IgG

complement, a process that produces an inflammatory reaction that injures the joint space.[1,2]

An associated finding in 20% of patients with RA is the presence of subcutaneous nodules, which are commonly found around the elbow and finger joints. These nodules are thought to arise from the same antigen/antibody complex that is found in the joint. Vasculitis confined to small and medium-sized vessels also may occur and is probably caused by the same complexing.[1,2]

RA is a pleomorphic disease with variable expression. The most progressive period of the disease occurs during the earlier years; thereafter, it slows. Gradual onset occurs in more than 50% of patients, and as many as 20% follow a monocyclic course that abates within 2 years. Another 10% experience relentless crippling that leads to nearly complete disability. The remainder follow a polycyclic or progressive course.[2] The long-term prognosis for people with abrupt onset of disease is similar to that for people with gradual disease onset. The course and severity of RA are unpredictable, but the disorder is characterized by remissions and exacerbations. For most patients, however, the disease is a sustained, lifelong problem that can be controlled or modified to allow a normal or nearly normal life.[1,2]

The life expectancy of persons with severe RA is shortened by 10 to 15 years. This increased mortality rate usually is attributed to infection, pulmonary and renal disease, and gastrointestinal bleeding.[1,2]

Many complications may accompany RA. Included among these are digital gangrene, skin ulcers, muscle atrophy, keratoconjunctivitis sicca (Sjögren's syndrome), TMJ involvement, pulmonary interstitial fibrosis, pericarditis, amyloidosis, anemia, thrombocytopenia, neutropenia, and splenomegaly (Felty's syndrome).[1-3]

CLINICAL PRESENTATION

Signs and Symptoms

The usual onset of RA is gradual and subtle (Table 21-1), and the disorder is commonly preceded by a prodromal

TABLE **21-1**
Comparison of Rheumatoid Arthritis and Osteoarthritis

Rheumatoid Arthritis	Osteoarthritis
Multiple symmetric joint involvement	Usually one or two joints (or groups) involved
Significant joint inflammation	Joint pain usually without inflammation
Morning joint stiffness for longer than 1 hour	Morning joint stiffness lasting less than 15 minutes
Symmetric, spindle-shaped swelling of proximal interphalangeal joints joints and volar subluxation of metacarpophalangeal joints and Bouchard's nodes of proximal interphalangeal joints	Heberden's nodes of distal interphalangeal joints
Systemic manifestations (fatigue, weakness, malaise)	No systemic involvement

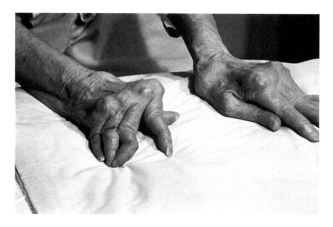

Figure 21-3. Hands of a patient with advanced rheumatoid arthritis. (From Damjanov I. Pathology for the Health Professions, 3rd ed. St. Louis, Saunders, 2006.)

BOX 21-1

Criteria for the Diagnosis of Rheumatoid Arthritis*

- Morning stiffness
- Arthritis of three or more joint areas
- Arthritis of hand joints
- Symmetric arthritis
- Rheumatoid nodules
- Serum rheumatoid factor
- Radiographic changes

Modified from Arnett FC, Edworthy SM, Bloch DA, et al. Arthritis Rheum 1988;31:315-324.

*At least four must be present for a diagnosis of rheumatic arthritis.

phase of general fatigue and weakness with joint and muscle aches. Characteristically, these symptoms come and go over varying periods. Then, painful joint swelling, especially of the hands and feet, occurs in several joints and progresses to other joints in a symmetric fashion. Joint involvement persists and gradually progresses to immobility, contractures, subluxation, deviation, and other deformities. Characteristic features include pain in the affected joints aggravated by movement, generalized joint stiffness after inactivity, and morning stiffness that lasts longer than 1 hour. The joints most commonly affected are fingers, wrists, feet, ankles, knees, and elbows. Multiple joint changes noted in the hands include a symmetric spindle-shaped swelling of the proximal interphalangeal (PIP) joints, with dorsal swelling and characteristic volar subluxation of the metacarpophalangeal (MCP) joint (Figure 21-3). The TMJ is reported to be involved in up to 75% of patients.[3]

Extra-articular manifestations include rheumatoid nodules, vasculitis, skin ulcers, Sjögren's syndrome, interstitial lung disease, pericarditis, C-spine instability, entrapment neuropathies, and ischemic neuropathies. The American Rheumatism Association has developed revised criteria for the diagnosis and classification of RA to be used in clinical trials and epidemiologic studies (Box 21-1). These criteria have high specificity (89%) and sensitivity (91% to 94%) compared with controls when used

to classify patients with RA. For the diagnosis of RA to be made, four of seven criteria must be met.[1]

Laboratory Findings

No laboratory tests are pathognomonic or diagnostic of RA, although they are used in conjunction with clinical findings to confirm the diagnosis. Laboratory findings most commonly seen in RA include an increased erythrocyte sedimentation rate, the presence of C-reactive protein, a positive rheumatoid factor in 85% of affected patients, and a hypochromic/microcytic anemia. In patients with Felty's syndrome (RA with splenomegaly), a marked neutropenia may be present.[3]

Diagnosis

The American College of Rheumatology has established criteria for the diagnosis of RA, the classification of severity by radiography, functional classes, and the definition of remission. Although they were not designed for managing individual patients, these criteria are useful as a frame of reference and for describing clinical phenomena.[1]

By definition, the diagnosis of RA cannot be made until the disease has been present for at least several weeks. Many extra-articular features of RA, the characteristic symmetry of inflammation, and the typical serologic findings may not be evident during the first month or two after disease onset. Therefore, the diagnosis of RA usually is presumptive early in its course.[1]

Although extra-articular manifestations may dominate in some patients, documentation of an inflammatory synovitis is essential for a diagnosis. Inflammatory synovitis can be documented by demonstration of synovial fluid leukocytosis, defined as white blood cell (WBC) counts greater than 2000/mm^3, histologic evidence of synovitis, or radiographic evidence of characteristic erosions.[1]

MEDICAL MANAGEMENT

Over the past several years, major advances in the treatment of RA were due to three trends:

1. Recognition that drug therapies, especially when used early in the disease, can alter outcomes and reduce severity, disability, and mortality
2. Improved understanding of the pathogenetic mechanisms involved in immunologic and inflammatory processes
3. Development of therapies that target specifically the pathophysiologic processes and mediators involved in the pathogenesis of RA

As a consequence, rheumatologists and other practitioners are more willing than they were before to prescribe medications that may ameliorate symptoms, slow or even halt disease progression, and modify the disease course, thereby preventing damage to the joints and resultant functional limitations. An accurate diagnosis provides the foundation for proper management of RA. Appropriate and timely therapeutic intervention can alleviate symptoms and improve overall prognosis.[1]

The treatment approach to RA is, by necessity, palliative because no cure as yet exists for the disease. Treatment goals are to reduce joint inflammation and swelling, relieve pain and stiffness, and facilitate and encourage normal function. These goals are accomplished through a basic treatment program that consists of patient education, rest, exercise, physical therapy, and aspirin or other nonsteroidal anti-inflammatory drugs (NSAIDs).[1]

When an understanding of the determinants of disease outcome is acquired, a treatment strategy that will be useful and acceptable to the individual patient can be devised. These determinants include presence of rheumatoid factor, early onset of severe synovitis with functional limitation, joint erosions, persistent elevation of erythrocyte sedimentation rate or C-reactive protein, presence of extra-articular manifestations, and a family history of severe RA.

The major goals of therapy are to relieve pain, swelling, and fatigue; improve joint function; stop joint damage; and prevent disability and disease-related morbidity. These goals are constant throughout the disease course, although emphasis may shift to address specific patient needs. For example, some patients with advanced joint damage experience minimal swelling or constitutional symptoms and benefit most from physical therapy, joint reconstruction, and pain control. Most patients, however, require continued efforts to control the inflammatory process through disease-modifying therapy.[1]

Drugs for the management of RA have been traditionally, but imperfectly, divided into two groups: those used primarily for the control of joint pain and swelling, and those intended to limit joint damage and improve long-term outcome. Symptoms of pain and swelling in RA are mediated, at least in part, by intense cytokine activity. NSAIDs inhibit proinflammatory prostaglandins and are effective treatments for pain, swelling, and stiffness, but they have no effect on the disease course or on risk of joint damage. On the other hand, anti-inflammatory properties have been noted for several disease-modifying antirheumatic drugs (DMARDs), which are used principally to control disease and to limit joint damage. These include methotrexate and biologic response modifiers with actions targeted against specific cytokines, such as tumor necrosis factor-α (TNF-α). Corticosteroids are powerful, nonspecific inhibitors of cytokines and, in some studies that compared them with placebo, are reported to effectively delay joint erosion.[4]

NSAIDs, especially aspirin, constitute the cornerstone of treatment. Aspirin may be prescribed in large doses on an individual basis. A common approach is to start a patient on three 5-grain tablets 4 times a day, then to adjust the dosage on the basis of patient response. The most common sign of aspirin toxicity is tinnitus. Should this occur, dosage is decreased. In addition to aspirin, many NSAIDs are available for use. Some of the more common of these include the new cyclooxygenase (COX)-2 inhibitors, namely, rofecoxib (Vioxx) and celecoxib (Celebrex), ibuprofen (Motrin, Advil, Rufen, Nuprin), naproxen (Naprosyn, Aleve), sulindac (Clinoril), tolmetin (Tolectin), fenoprofen (Nalfon), piroxicam (Feldene), diclofenac (Voltaren), flurbiprofen (Ansaid), diflunisal (Dolobid), etodolac (Lodine), and nabumetone (Relafen). All NSAIDs can cause a qualitative platelet defect that may result in prolonged bleeding, especially when given in high doses. The effects of aspirin are irreversible for the life of the platelet (10 to 12 days); thus, this effect continues until new platelets have replaced the old. The effect of the other NSAIDs on platelets is reversible and lasts only as long as the drug is present in the plasma (see Chapter 25).[5-7]

In addition to NSAIDs, a variety of other drugs are used to treat patients with RA (Table 21-2). Many of these drugs cause blood dyscrasias that may lead to more frequent infection, delayed healing, and prolonged bleeding.[5-7]

DMARDs, which are commonly employed in the treatment of patients with RA, are classified in various groups, each of which consists of multiple drugs (e.g., antimalarials, penicillamine, gold compounds) (see Table 21-2).[5-7]

Gold compounds may be effective in decreasing inflammation and retarding the progress of the disease, but the incidence of associated toxicity is high, and dermatitis with mucosal ulceration, proteinuria,

TABLE 21-2
Drugs Used in the Management of Rheumatoid Arthritis and Systemic Lupus Erythematosus

Generic Name (Trade Name)	Dental and Oral Considerations
SALICYLATES	
Aspirin, Ascriptin, Bufferin, Anacin, Ecotrin, Empirin	Prolonged bleeding but not usually clinically significant
NONSTEROIDAL ANTI-INFLAMMATORY DRUGS	
Ibuprofen, Fenoprofen, Indomethacin, Naproxen, Meclofenamate, Piroxicam, Sulindac, Tolmetin, Diclofenac, Flurbiprofen, Diflunisal, Etodolac, Nabumetone, Motrin, Nalfon, Indocin, Feldene, Naprosyn, Meclomen, Clinoril, Tolectin, Voltaren, Ansaid, Dolobid, Lodine, Relafen, Oxaprozin, Ketorolac	Prolonged bleeding but not usually clinically significant; oral ulceration, stomatitis
CYCLOOXYGENASE (COX)-2 INHIBITORS	
Celecoxib	None
Rofecoxib	
TUMOR NECROSIS FACTOR-α INHIBITORS	
Etanercept	None
Infliximab	
INJECTABLE GLUCOCORTICOIDS	
Triamcinolone hexacetonide	Adrenal suppression, masking of oral infection, impaired healing
Triamcinolone acetonide	
Prednisolone tebutate	
Methylprednisolone acetate	
Dexamethasone acetate	
Hydrocortisone acetate	
Triamcinolone diacetate	
Betamethasone sodium phosphate and acetate	
Dexamethasone sodium phosphate	
Prednisolone sodium phosphate	
SYSTEMIC GLUCOCORTICOIDS	
Hydrocortisone, Cortisone, Prednisone, Prednisolone, Dexamethasone, Methylprednisolone (Deltasone, Meticorten, Orasone, Articulose-50, Delta-Cortef, Medrol)	Adrenal suppression, masking of oral infection, impaired healing
DISEASE-MODIFYING ANTIRHEUMATIC DRUGS	
Antimalarial agents	
Hydroxychloroquine, Quinine, Chloroquine (Plaquenil)	
Penicillamine	
(Cuprimine, Depen)	
Gold compounds	
Gold sodium thiomalate (Auranofin, Aurothioglucose, Myochrysine Ridaura, Solganal)	Increased infections, delayed healing, prolonged bleeding, oral ulcerations
Aralen	Increased infections, delayed healing, prolonged bleeding, glossitis, stomatitis
Sulfasalazine	
Azulfidine	Increased infections, delayed healing, prolonged bleeding, intraoral pigmentation
Immunosuppressives	
Azathioprine, Cyclophosphamide	Increased infections, delayed healing, prolonged bleeding
Methotrexate, Cyclosporine, Chlorambucil (Imuran, Cytoxan, Rheumatrex)	Increased infections, delayed healing, prolonged bleeding, stomatitis

neutropenia, and thrombocytopenia may result. Antimalarial drugs (e.g., chloroquine, hydroxychloroquine) are also used to treat patients with RA; they are usually given in combination with aspirin or corticosteroids. Adverse effects include severe eye damage and blue-black intraoral pigmentation. Penicillamine also is used in the treatment of patients with RA. Both the antimalarials and penicillamine, however, are associated with significant toxicity—a fact that limits their use. Corticosteroids (e.g., prednisone, prednisolone) frequently are useful in controlling acute symptoms; however, because of multiple adverse effects, long-term usage is avoided if possible. One of the more potentially significant associated adverse effects is adrenal suppression (see Chapter 16).[5-7]

In cases of refractory disease, immunosuppressive therapy has been used successfully and may include methotrexate, cyclophosphamide, or azathioprine. These drugs may produce significant adverse effects, including severe oral ulceration. Methotrexate also may cause hepatic toxicity. COX-2 inhibitors and TNF-α inhibitors have recently proved effective in relieving the symptoms of RA (see Table 21-2). Although COX-2 inhibitors (e.g., celecoxib [Celebrex], rofecoxib [Vioxx]) have shown considerable efficacy in relieving inflammatory pain associated with RA, problems have been reported with these agents, and myocardial infarction has occurred in patients who have used these treatments over the long term. In fact, Vioxx was taken off the market by the U.S. Food and Drug Administration (FDA). Celebrex remains on the market, but warnings regarding potential heart problems are provided to long-term users. Standard NSAIDs inhibit both cyclooxygenases (COX-1 and COX-2)—the enzymes involved in production of prostaglandins. Whereas COX-2 is active on demand, COX-1 is critical for normal cellular function. A complication that may result from the use of NSAIDs for arthritis (and other conditions) is the adverse effect of gastrointestinal distress. Because COX-2 inhibitors are selective for this enzyme, they produce fewer gastrointestinal adverse effects.[5-7]

As treatment options for RA become more effective and more complex, greater attention will be paid to the costs of drug treatments and associated adverse effects with respect to disease control and remission. Drugs that improve the long-term outcomes of disease will be prescribed more frequently, and efforts will be made to limit the use of NSAIDs in persons who are coping with joint pain and swelling.

In two studies reported in the *New England Journal of Medicine,*[5-7] the biological agents etanercept and infliximab, both TNF-α inhibitors, were shown to be highly effective in the treatment of patients with early rheumatoid arthritis when compared with the gold standard, methotrexate. Although costly and difficult to administer (intravenous route), etanercept (e.g., Enbrel, Immunex) was shown to significantly reduce symptoms of RA and to more effectively slow joint damage when compared with methotrexate. Infliximab (costly and somewhat difficult to administer by subcutaneous injection) likewise when used with methotrexate significantly reduced RA symptoms and slowed joint damage to a greater extent when compared with methotrexate therapy alone. Although these biologic agents are novel and show great promise, they have had limited widespread use in RA therapy.[5-7]

Combination Therapies

In people with moderate to severe disease activity, methotrexate often is used in combination with other agents. In patients who have acute and severe disease, initial therapy often consists of a combination of DMARDs, corticosteroids, and NSAIDs. Combinations of DMARDs also are used to improve disease control; approximately 50% of people with RA who are treated by rheumatologists are prescribed combination therapies with two or three DMARDs. The combination of methotrexate, hydroxychloroquine, and sulfasalazine is among the most popular regimens, although study results are not readily duplicated among prescribing physicians. Other successful combination therapies include methotrexate used with such agents as cyclosporine, TNF-α antagonists, leflunomide, and azathioprine.

Surgical management of severely deformed or dysfunctional joints often is necessary and may involve a variety of procedures, including arthroplasty, reconstruction, synovectomy, and total joint replacement.

Much research that is currently under way regarding certain genetic factors may provide useful information on the likely disease course and may help to guide treatment. Poor socioeconomic status and low levels of educational achievement are important predictors of poor disease outcome. Health-related beliefs, goals, and desires of patients are important predictors of compliance with treatment and outcome. Willingness on the part of health care providers to understand and work with these beliefs, and to educate patients about the disease, is as fundamental to the successful treatment of RA as is any medication that can be prescribed. Access to rheumatologists and other health care professionals skilled in the treatment of RA is fundamental to lessening the burden of disease.[3] This is important for correct diagnosis and initiation of patient-specific treatment early in the disease course; both are critical factors in the successful management of RA. Although joint destruction progresses at variable rates and with variable intensity, many patients experience joint damage early in the disease, as evidenced by radiography, emphasizing the need for timely and aggressive use of disease-modifying agents to prevent long-term disability. Still, the median time between onset of symptoms of RA and its diagnosis is 36 weeks.[1-3]

Clinical tools for monitoring a patient's well-being and the efficacy of therapy include patient assessments of the duration of morning stiffness and severity of fatigue, as well as functional, social, emotional, and pain status, as measured by a health assessment questionnaire. A patient-derived global assessment based on a visual analog scale is a simple and effective means of recording patient well-being. The number of tender and swollen joints is a useful measure of disease activity, as is the presence of anemia, thrombocytosis, and elevated sedimentation rate or C-reactive protein. Serial radiographs of target joints, including the hands, are useful in assessing disease progression.[1-3]

Patient education is essential early in the disease course and on an ongoing basis. Educational topics include the nature of the disease and its prognosis, vocational and avocational counseling, lifestyle and family counseling, enhancement of self-esteem, home modifications, and disease treatment. Patients are best served by a multidisciplinary approach with early referral to a rheumatologist and other specially trained medical personnel, including nurses, counselors, and occupational and physical therapists who are skilled and knowledgeable about RA. Appropriate medical care of people with RA encompasses attention to smoking cessation, immunizations, prompt treatment of infections, and management of comorbid conditions, such as diabetes, hypertension, and osteoporosis.[1-3]

DENTAL MANAGEMENT
Medical Considerations

Because patients may have multiple joint involvement with varying degrees of pain and immobility, dental appointments should be kept as short as possible, and the patient should be allowed to make frequent position changes as needed (Box 21-2). The patient also may be more comfortable in a sitting or semisupine position, as opposed to a supine one. Physical supports, such as a pillow or a rolled towel, may be used to provide support for deformed limbs, joints, or neck.

The most significant complications associated with RA are drug related (see Table 21-2). Aspirin and other NSAIDs can interfere with platelet function and cause prolonged bleeding; however, this generally is not found to be a significant clinical problem. A patient who is taking both aspirin and a corticosteroid may be at greater risk, and determination of pretreatment bleeding time may be advisable (bleeding time is very unreliable; the platelet function analyzer [PFA-100] should be used, if available; if not, then bleeding time should be used). Even when bleeding time is moderately prolonged (up to 20 minutes), the risk is not great, and patients usually can be treated, as long as curettage or surgery is performed conservatively in small segments with attention to good techniques.[8] Bleeding times longer than 20 minutes should be discussed with the physician (see Chapter 25).

Patients who are taking gold salts, penicillamine, sulfasalazine, or immunosuppressive agents are susceptible to bone marrow suppression that can result in anemia, agranulocytosis, and thrombocytopenia. As a rule, these patients should be followed closely by their physician for detection of this problem. If a patient has not undergone recent laboratory testing, a complete blood cell count

---

BOX 21-2

Dental Management of the Patient With Rheumatoid Arthritis

KEY POINTS
1. Short appointments
2. Ensurance of physical comfort
   a. Frequent position changes
   b. Comfortable chair position
   c. Physical supports as needed (pillows, towels, etc.)
3. Drug considerations
   a. Aspirin and NSAIDs—bleeding may be increased but usually is not clinically significant
   b. Gold salts, penicillamine, antimalarials, immunosuppressives—get complete blood cell count with differential, bleeding time; treat stomatitis symptomatically
   c. Corticosteroids—adrenal suppression possible
4. Joint prosthesis—prophylactic antibiotics are suggested by some authors (cephalosporin or clindamycin)
5. Technical treatment modification dictated by patient's disabilities
6. Temporomandibular joint pain/dysfunction—sudden occlusal changes possible
   a. Decrease jaw function
   b. Soft, nonchallenging diet
   c. Moist heat or ice to face/jaw
   d. Medication as directed by physician
   e. Occlusal appliance to decrease joint loading
   f. Consideration of surgery for persistent pain or dysfunction

---

with a differential white blood cell count and bleeding time should be ordered. Abnormal results should be discussed with the physician. If corticosteroids are used for prolonged periods, the potential for adrenal suppression exists. Management of this problem is discussed in Chapter 16. Corticosteroids may induce a number of adverse effects. These are presented in Table 21-2.

Prosthetic Joints. A potential long-term complication of chronic rheumatoid arthritis (also osteoarthritis [OA] and other types, including fractures that do not heal and avascular necrosis) is the ultimate destruction of particular joint structures to the degree that the joint must be replaced with synthetic materials. Patients with prosthetic joints (most commonly, hip and knee replacement, followed by shoulder, elbow, wrist, and ankle; excellent results are attained with hip, knee, and shoulder replacement, and more variable results with elbow, wrist, and ankle replacement) often are encountered in dental practice; when this occurs, a question arises concerning the need for antibiotic prophylaxis to prevent infection of the prosthesis. This is a legitimate concern; however, whether bacteremia resulting from dental procedures can cause prosthetic joint infection (PJI) is the primary issue. This issue has been debated for many years, although scientific data for decision making are lacking. Recommendations to place dental patients on prophylactic antibiotics have been made empirically by orthopedic surgeons, although little evidence suggests that dentally induced bacteremia may cause PJI.[9,10]

Although reports in the literature weakly associate PJI with dentally induced bacteremia, authors have questioned the validity of these reports. Examination of the microbiology of PJI is instructive. Pallasch and Slots[10] reviewed cumulative data from 281 isolates from 6 clinical studies of PJI caused by hematogenous bacterial spread. They found that two thirds of cases of PJI were the result of staphylococci, only 4.9% were caused by viridans streptococci of possible oral origin, and 2.1% were caused by *Peptostreptococcus* species. This suggests that wound contamination or skin infection is the source of the vast majority of infections. Even the few cases of PJI caused by presumably oral bacteria were more likely to result from physiologically occurring bacteremia or bacteremia caused by acute or chronic infection than from invasive dental procedures.[9,10]

In one study often cited as evidence of hematogenous PJI, an animal model demonstrated that PJI can result from bloodborne bacteria. To produce PJI, large inocula of staphylococci were injected into a group of rabbits, creating such an overwhelming septicemia that it caused the almost immediate death of one third of the animals. It also caused death within a few days in another one third; subsequently, 10 animals survived despite the development of PJI. This model is not applicable to usual clinical situations and thus does not provide support for any conclusion that related normal bacteremia to PJI. Unfortunately, however, many orthopedic surgeons have persisted in requesting that patients receive antibiotic prophylaxis for dental procedures.[9-11]

In an effort to clarify the issue, in 1997 and again in 2003, an advisory statement made jointly by the American Dental Association and the American Academy of Orthopedic Surgeons was published. This advisory statement, which is presented and debated in an article by Little,[9] concluded that scientific evidence does not support the need for antibiotic prophylaxis for dental procedures to prevent PJI. It further stated that antibiotic prophylaxis is not indicated for dental patients with pins, plates, and screws, nor is it routinely indicated for most patients with total joint replacement. The statement did indicate, however, that antibiotic prophylaxis should be considered for some "high-risk" patients who are at increased risk for infection and are undergoing dental procedures likely to cause significant bleeding (Box 21-3). No evidence suggests that even these "higher-risk" patients are at increased risk for dentally induced bacteremia, and in fact, the microbiology of PJI is the same as for other patients with PJI.

A more appropriate interpretation is that these patients are at increased risk for PJI from the usual sources such as wound contamination and acute infection from distant sites. The advisory statement also is clear that the final

---

BOX 21-3

High-Risk Patients With Prosthetic Joints

IMMUNOCOMPROMISED/IMMUNOSUPPRESSED PATIENTS
- Inflammatory arthropathies: rheumatoid arthritis; systemic lupus erythematosus; disease-, drug-, or radiation-induced immunosuppression

OTHER PATIENTS
- Insulin-dependent (type 1) diabetes
- First 2 years after joint replacement
- Previous prosthetic joint infections
- Malnourishment
- Hemophilia

BOX 21-4

Suggested Antibiotic Prophylaxis Regimens

PATIENTS NOT ALLERGIC TO PENICILLIN: CEPHALEXIN, CEPHADINE OR AMOXICILLIN
2 g orally 1 hour before the dental procedure

PATIENTS NOT ALLERGIC TO PENICILLIN AND UNABLE TO TAKE ORAL MEDICATIONS: CEPHAZOLIN OR AMPICILLIN
Cefazolin 1 g or ampicillin 2 g intramuscularly or intravenously 1 hour before the dental procedure

PATIENTS ALLERGIC TO PENICILLIN: CLINDAMYCIN
600 mg orally 1 hour before the dental procedure

PATIENTS ALLERGIC TO PENICILLIN AND UNABLE TO TAKE ORAL MEDICATIONS: CLINDAMYCIN
600 mg IV 1 hour before the dental procedure

---

decision on whether to provide antibiotic prophylaxis lies with the dentist, who must weigh perceived potential benefits against risks. The advisory statement provides suggested antibiotic regimens, should the practitioner elect to provide antibiotic prophylaxis (Box 21-4). The opinion of the authors of this is book is that no patient with a prosthetic joint requires antibiotic prophylaxis to prevent PJI caused by a dentally induced bacteremia. However, if by informed consent, the patient selects to be given prophylaxis, then one of the regimens shown in Box 21-4 can be used.[9-11]

Treatment Planning Modifications

Treatment planning modifications are dictated by the patient's physical disabilities. An individual with marked systemic disability or limited or painful jaw function due to TMJ involvement should not be subjected to prolonged or extensive treatment, such as complicated crown and bridge procedures. If replacement of missing teeth is desired, consideration should be given to a removable prosthesis because of the decreased chair time needed for mouth preparation and the ease of cleansability of the appliance. If a fixed prosthesis is desired, ease of cleansability must be a significant factor in design. Unpredictable, progressive, or abrupt changes in occlusion are possible because of erosion of the condylar head. Therefore, the dentist and the patient should take these potential occlusal changes into consideration when considering significant reconstructive treatment.

Disabled patients may have significant difficulty cleaning their teeth. Cleaning aids such as floss holders, toothpicks, irrigating devices, and mechanical toothbrushes may be recommended. Manual toothbrushes can be modified by placement of an acrylic or rubber ball on the handle to improve the grip.

RA is a progressive disease that ultimately may lead to severe disability and crippling in some patients, which can make providing dental care difficult. Therefore, the dentist should be aggressive in providing ongoing preventive care and should attempt to identify and treat or eliminate potential problems before the disease progresses.

Oral Complications and Manifestations

The most significant complication of the oral and maxillofacial complex in RA is TMJ involvement, which is found in up to 45% to 75% of patients with RA. This may present as bilateral preauricular pain, tenderness, swelling, stiffness, and decreased mobility of the TMJ, or it may be asymptomatic. Periods of remission and exacerbation may occur, as with other joint involvement. Fibrosis or bony ankylosis can occur. Clinically, patients may present with tenderness over the lateral pole of the condyle, crepitus, limited opening, and radiographic evidence of structural change. Radiographic changes initially may show increased joint space. Later, these changes are primarily erosive and can involve both the condyles and the fossa.

A particularly disturbing event is the development of an anterior open bite, caused by destruction of the condylar heads and loss of condylar height (Figure 21-4).

This sudden retrognathia and anterior open bite can be severe and has been reported to cause obstructive sleep apnea. Although palliative treatment such as interocclusal splints, physical therapy, and medication may prove to be helpful, surgical intervention often becomes necessary to decrease pain, improve appearance, or restore function.[12,13]

An additional complication that may be seen in patients with RA is severe stomatitis that occurs after the administration of drugs such as gold compounds, penicillamine, or immunosuppressive agents. This may be an indication of drug toxicity and should be reported to the physician. Palliative treatment for this problem may include bland mouth rinses, diphenhydramine elixir, or a topical emollient such as Orabase (see Appendix C).

OSTEOARTHRITIS

DEFINITION

Incidence and Prevalence

Osteoarthritis (OA, degenerative joint disease), another of the rheumatic diseases, is the most common form of arthritis. Almost everyone older than 60 years of age develops OA to some degree. Most people are minimally symptomatic; however, approximately 17 million people in the United States have OA to the extent that it results in pain. OA is the leading cause of disability among the elderly.[1]

OA, which is considered a regional disease, usually affects often used joints such as hips, knees, feet, spine, and hands. The TMJ also is affected. Women are afflicted twice as often as men; however, men are afflicted at an earlier age. It is generally a disease of middle to older age, first appearing after the age of 40. Racial differences have been noted in the prevalence of OA and in the pattern of joint involvement.[1]

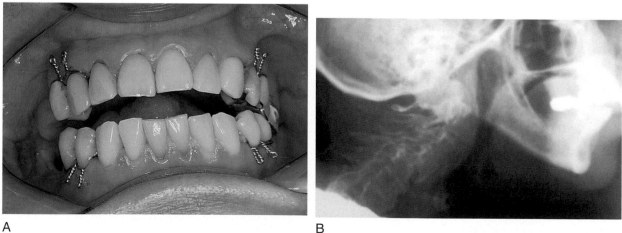

A   B

Figure 21-4. A, Anterior open bite resulting from progressive bilateral condylar resorption in a patient with advanced rheumatoid arthritis. **B,** Lateral skull film shows a swan-neck deformity. (From Quinn PD. Color Atlas of Temporomandibular Joint Surgery. St. Louis, Mosby, 1998.)

Etiology

Although the exact cause of OA is not known, it has been thought to result from normal wear and tear on joints over a long period. However, other factors are now believed to be of significance. Preexisting structural joint abnormalities, intrinsic aging, metabolic factors, genetic predisposition, obesity leading to overloaded joints, and macrotrauma or microtrauma are considered causative or contributory factors in the origin of the disease.[1]

Pathophysiology and Complications

In early stages of the disease, the articular cartilage actually becomes thicker than normal, and water content and the synthesis of proteoglycans are increased. This reflects a repair effort by the chondrocytes and may last for several years. Ultimately, however, the joint surface thins and proteoglycan concentration decreases, leading to softening of the cartilage. Progressive splitting and abrasion of cartilage down to the subchondral bone occur. The exposed bone becomes polished and sclerotic, resembling ivory (eburnation). Some resurfacing with cartilage may occur if the disorder is arrested or stabilized. New bone forms at the margin of the articular cartilage in the non–weight-bearing part of the joint, creating osteophytes (or spurs), often covered by cartilage, that augment the degree of deformity.[1]

In contrast to RA, OA has a more favorable prognosis and less serious complications, depending on the joint or joints involved. The two most important complications associated with OA are pain and disability. Although RA is a more serious disease, OA has a 30-fold greater economic impact, resulting in 68 million lost workdays per year compared with 2 million for RA. Conservative treatment often can retard the progress of the disease; however, surgery may be required to restore function and reduce pain.[1]

CLINICAL PRESENTATION

Signs and Symptoms

The primary symptom of OA is pain localized to one or two joints (see Table 21-1). The pain is described as a dull ache accompanied by stiffness that is typically worse in the morning or after a period of inactivity. The pain and stiffness usually last no longer than 15 minutes. Joint noises or grinding sounds (crepitus) may be detected with movement. Redness and swelling usually are not associated with OA.

The most common sign of OA is a painless bony growth on the medial and lateral aspects of the distal interphalangeal joints, called Heberden's nodes. When these enlargements occur on the distal interphalangeal joints, they are called Bouchard's nodes (Figure 21-5). On occasion, some pain may be associated with these nodes.

Depending on which joint or group of joints is involved, patients may experience varying degrees of

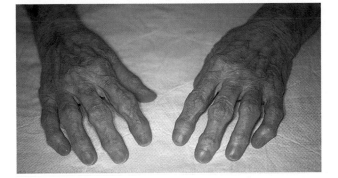

Figure 21-5. Heberden's nodes and Bouchard's nodes in osteoarthritis. (From Swartz MH. Textbook of Physical Diagnosis: History and Examination, 4th ed. Philadelphia, Saunders, 2002.)

incapacitation. Hip and knee joints are particularly troublesome and are a common source of disability.

One form of OA, called *primary generalized osteoarthritis*, is characterized by involvement of three or more joints or groups of joints. It occurs most often in women and affects hands, knees, hips, and spine.

Radiographic signs of OA include narrowing of the joint space, articular surface irregularities and remodeling, and osteophytes or spurs. In addition, subchondral sclerosis (eburnation) and ankylosis may be seen. Symptoms often are not well correlated with radiographic signs.[1]

Laboratory Findings

Laboratory findings in OA are essentially unremarkable. The erythrocyte sedimentation rate usually is normal, except for a mild elevation in primary generalized cases.

MEDICAL MANAGEMENT

The management of OA is palliative. For the most part, drug therapy is limited to analgesics. Acetaminophen frequently is effective in the management of OA and is recommended as a first-line drug. Aspirin or NSAIDs also are commonly employed when acetaminophen is not effective. Narcotic analgesics are generally used only for acute flares for short periods. Intra-articular steroid injections also may be used for acute flares for short periods. Intra-articular steroid injections may be used intermittently to reduce acute pain and inflammation. Patient education, physical therapy, mild exercise, weight reduction, and joint protection are all important aspects of management. Surgery, including joint replacement, may be required to improve function or relieve pain.[1] What about joint replacement?

DENTAL MANAGEMENT

Medical Considerations

Depending on which joints are involved, patients may not be comfortable in a supine position in the dental chair. Consideration should be given to providing a more

BOX 21-5

Dental Management of the Patient With Osteoarthritis

KEY POINTS
1. Short appointments
2. Physical comfort of patient
   a. Frequent position change
   b. Comfortable chair position
   c. Physical supports as needed (pillow, towel, etc.)
   d. Drug considerations
3. Aspirin and NSAIDs—bleeding may be increased but usually is not clinically significant
4. Joint prosthesis—generally, prophylactic antibiotics are not required unless diabetes mellitus or immunosuppression is present; if so, use cephalosporin or clindamycin
5. Technical treatment modifications dictated
6. Temporomandibular joint pain/dysfunction usually self-limiting
   a. Painless jaw function encouraged
   b. Soft, nonchallenging diet
   c. Moist heat or ice to face/jaw
   d. Acetaminophen, aspirin, or nonsteroidal anti-inflammatory drugs (NSAIDs) for analgesia
   e. Occlusal appliance to decrease joint loading
   f. Surgery consideration for persistent pain or dysfunction

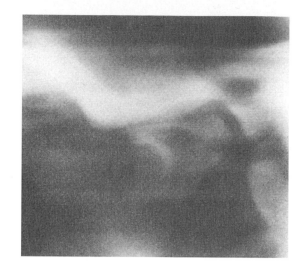

Figure 21-6. Osteoarthritic changes in the temporomandibular joint.

upright chair position, using neck, back, and leg supports, and scheduling short appointments (Box 21-5). Decreased platelet function caused by large doses of aspirin or other NSAIDs can lead to prolonged bleeding, but this is generally not a clinically significant problem. A pretreatment platelet function test or bleeding time can be obtained, if desired. Times elevated by 15 to 20 minutes do not pose a significant risk, as long as procedures that result in bleeding are kept to a minimum and other bleeding problems are not present (see Chapter 25). Grossly abnormal bleeding times (longer than 20 minutes) should be discussed with the physician.

Adrenal suppression generally is not a concern with occasional intra-articular injections of steroids. Patients with OA who have a joint prosthesis usually do not require antibiotic prophylaxis for dental treatment unless a concomitant condition, such as diabetes mellitus, exists, or the patient is otherwise immune suppressed. If this is the case, consideration of antimicrobial prophylaxis with cephalosporin or clindamycin as the drug of choice is recommended.[9]

Treatment Planning Modifications

As with RA, the technical modifications of dental treatment for OA are dictated by a patient's disabilities. For instance, severe disabilities of the hip, knee, or other joint or TMJ involvement may prevent lengthy appointments; therefore, extensive treatment such as reconstruction or a long surgical procedure may not be appropriate. Patients

with hand disabilities may have difficulty cleaning their teeth, and aids such as floss holders or electric toothbrushes may be helpful. Modified toothbrush handles also are recommended to facilitate cleaning.

Oral Complications and Manifestations

The TMJ may be affected by OA, and this may constitute a problem for the patient. As would be expected, most people older than 40 years of age show some degree of histologic and radiographic change in the TMJ, but most have no symptoms. Occasional TMJ pain caused by OA has been reported. The usual finding in patients with OA of the TMJ is insidious onset of unilateral preauricular aching and pain with stiffness after a period of inactivity that decreases with mild activity. Severe pain may be elicited on wide opening, and pain occurs with normal function and worsens during the day. Adjacent muscle splinting and spasm may occur. Crepitus is a common finding in the affected joint. In most cases, osteoarthritic pain in the TMJ resolves within 8 months of onset. Radiographic changes include decreased joint space, sclerosis, remodeling, and osteophytes (Figure 21-6). No correlation exists between TMJ symptoms and radiographic or histologic signs of OA.[14,15]

In the past, uncertainty was expressed about the relationship between disk displacement and OA. Reports of a 30-year longitudinal study have provided evidence that, for patients with reducing anterior disk displacement, about a 50% chance exists that no progression of the disorder will occur, nor will any significant radiographic changes happen in the TMJ hard or soft tissue structures. For the remaining 50%, progression to nonreducing disk displacement or dislocation (closed lock) is likely. These patients may experience a period of variable pain and dysfunction, but it appears to be self-limiting in most patients. Also, 86% of patients with nonreducing disks demonstrate significant radiographic changes in the condyle and fossa on plain films, along with disk changes on magnetic resonance imaging. These changes occur rapidly during the first 3 years; then, a stable, persistent, quiescent period is attained. Thus, most patients with disk displacement, whether reducing or nonreducing, can be treated successfully with conservative, reversible therapies.[14,15]

Treatment of OA of the TMJ consists of acetaminophen, aspirin or NSAIDs, muscle relaxants, approaches to limit jaw function, physical therapy (heat, ice, ultrasound, controlled exercise), and occlusal splints to decrease joint loading. Conservative therapy is successful in controlling symptoms in most cases; however, should pain or dysfunction be severe and persistent, TMJ surgery may be necessary.

SYSTEMIC LUPUS ERYTHEMATOSUS

DEFINITION

Lupus erythematosus has two forms: one that predominantly affects the skin (discoid, DLE) and a more generalized one that affects multiple organ systems (systemic, SLE). DLE is characterized by chronic, erythematous, scaly plaques on the face, scalp, or ears. Most patients with DLE do not have systemic manifestations, and the course tends to be benign. SLE involves the skin and many other organ systems and is the more serious form. This section focuses on SLE.

Incidence and Prevalence

SLE is a prototypical autoimmune disease that predominantly affects women of childbearing age, with a female/male ratio of 5:1; it is more common and severe among African Americans and Hispanics than whites. A defining feature of SLE is the almost invariable presence in the blood of antibodies directed against one or more components of cell nuclei; certain manifestations of the disease are associated with the presence of one or more of these different antinuclear antibodies.[16]

Etiology

The etiology of SLE is unknown, although it is clearly an autoimmune disease. A strong familial aggregation exists, with a much higher frequency noted among first-degree relatives of patients. Studies of patients with SLE suggest that the disease is caused by genetically determined immune abnormalities that can be triggered by exogenous and endogenous factors. Among these triggering factors are infectious agents, stress, diet, toxins, drugs, and sunlight.[16]

Pathophysiology and Complications

The production of pathogenic antibodies and immune complexes and their deposition with resultant inflammation and vasculopathy is the basic abnormality that underlies SLE. Antibodies are formed in response to some

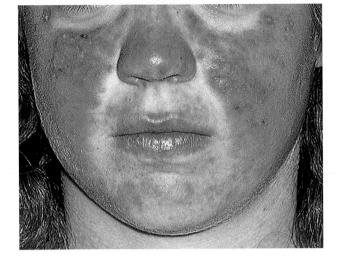

Figure 21-7. Female patient with butterfly-shaped rash of systemic lupus erythematosus. (From Habif TP. Clinical Dermatology: A Color Guide to Diagnosis and Therapy, 4th ed. Philadelphia, Mosby, 2004.)

antigenic stimulus, and the reaction between antigen and circulating antibodies forms antigen/antibody complexes, which are deposited in a wide variety of tissues and organs, including the kidney, skin, blood vessels, muscles and joints, heart, lung, brain, gastrointestinal tract, lymphatics, and eye. Clinical expression of the disease reflects the organs or tissues involved and the extent of that involvement.[16]

Despite advances in diagnosis and management, complications attributable to SLE or its treatment continue to cause substantial morbidity. Among hospitalizations for SLE, one third occurred because of neurologic or psychiatric involvement, whereas infection, coronary artery disease, and osteonecrosis were other major reasons.

Several studies have documented substantial improvement in the survival of patients with SLE, with 5-year survival rates of 90% or greater and 10-year survival rates of greater than 80%. The leading causes of death in patients with SLE are infectious complications and clinical manifestations related to lupus itself, such as acute vascular neurologic events, renal failure, and cardiovascular or pulmonary involvement.[17,18]

CLINICAL PRESENTATION

Signs and Symptoms

Because of the widespread systemic involvement of SLE, multiple manifestations are observed in many tissues and organs. Although malaise, overwhelming fatigue, fever, and weight loss are nonspecific manifestations that affect most patients at some time in their disease course, the classic picture of SLE is that of a young woman with polyarthritis and a butterfly-shaped rash across the nose and cheeks (Figure 21-7). The presentation of

SLE, however, varies widely from mild to severe and depends largely on the extent and selection of organ involvement.[19]

Arthritis, the most common manifestation of SLE, is seen in as many as 76% of patients. It affects the small joints and is migratory, and the pain typically is out of proportion to the signs. The classic butterfly rash of the nose and cheeks is found in only about one third of patients with SLE; a rash on the upper trunk or areas of exposed skin is more common. Recurrent noninfectious pharyngitis and oral ulcerations also are common.[19]

Serious renal abnormalities occur in less than one third of patients with SLE, although most show some abnormality on renal biopsy. Renal failure, one of the most serious problems, is the best clinical indicator of a poor prognosis.[17,18]

Neuropsychiatric symptoms are common and include organic brain syndrome, psychosis, seizures, stroke, movement disorders, and peripheral neuropathy. Thromboembolism associated with antiphospholipid antibody is an important cause of abnormalities in the central nervous system.[17,18]

Pulmonary manifestations include pleuritis, infection, pulmonary edema, pneumonitis, and pulmonary hypertension. Cardiac involvement is common and consists of pericarditis, myocarditis, endocarditis, and coronary artery disease. Valvular abnormalities can be identified by echocardiography in 25% of patients but rarely result in serious valvular dysfunction. However, Libman-Sacks endocarditis (nonbacterial verrucous endocarditis) is found at autopsy in 50% of patients with SLE. Unfortunately, this is not always demonstrated by echocardiography or by clinical examination findings. This condition is thought to predispose patients to infective endocarditis. A retrospective study of 313 patients with SLE suggested that the risk for bacterial endocarditis was similar to that in patients with rheumatic heart disease and prosthetic heart valves. A clinically detectable heart murmur found in 18.5% of patients required further investigation for determination of its significance. Approximately 4% of patients had cardiac valve abnormalities that placed them in the moderate risk group for endocarditis. However, no cases demonstrated a relationship between endocarditis and SLE.[20] On the basis of 2007 American Heart Association guidelines, none of these patients are recommended for antibiotic prophylaxis for invasive dental procedures (see Chapter 2).

A study by Rhodus[21] indicated that patients with SLE may have greater potential for arrhythmias and electrocardiographic abnormalities. The diagnosis of SLE is based on criteria suggested by the American Rheumatism Association. Although these criteria were primarily intended for research purposes, they are nevertheless clinically useful; at least 4 of 11 criteria must be met before the condition can be diagnosed.

Laboratory Findings

The antinuclear antibody test is the best screening test for SLE because it is positive in 95% of patients. This positivity also occurs in patients with other rheumatic diseases. Anti-DNA assays—double helix and single helix—also are elevated in 65% to 80% of patients with active untreated SLE.[19]

Hematologic abnormalities include hemolytic anemia, leukopenia, lymphopenia, and thrombocytopenia. Leukopenia in SLE usually is not associated with recurrent infection. Autoimmune thrombocytopenia occurs in as many as 25% of patients with SLE and may be severe in 5% of these. Patients with severe thrombocytopenia are at risk for bleeding spontaneously or after trauma. This event is rare, however, if the platelet count is greater than $50,000/mm^3$.[22]

A variety of clotting abnormalities may be seen; the most common of these is the lupus anticoagulant, which is associated with elevated partial thromboplastin time (PTT). This can result in thromboembolic events rather than increased bleeding, and invasive surgery may be performed without correction of this laboratory abnormality. The erythrocyte sedimentation rate often is elevated, but this does not reflect disease activity. With active nephritis, proteinuria is present, as are hematuria and cellular or granular casts. Other abnormalities include false-positive serologic tests for syphilis.[22]

MEDICAL MANAGEMENT

No cure for SLE is known; thus, all treatment is of a symptomatic or palliative nature. Patients with SLE are advised to avoid sun exposure because this may trigger onset or exacerbation of the disease. Many of the drugs used to treat patients with rheumatoid arthritis also are used in the management of SLE (see Table 21-2). These include aspirin and NSAIDs for mild disease, antimalarials for dermatologic disease, glucocorticoids for more severe symptoms, and cytotoxic agents for symptoms unresponsive to other therapies or as adjuncts in severe disease. Several experimental approaches to therapy, including plasmapheresis, lymph node irradiation, cyclosporine injection, sex hormone therapy, and immune gamma globulin, are under investigation.[19]

DENTAL MANAGEMENT
Medical Considerations

Because SLE is such a varied disease with so many potential problems caused by the disease or its treatment, pretreatment consultation with the patient's physician is advised (Box 21-6). As in rheumatoid arthritis, drug considerations and adverse effects in SLE are of major importance. Table 21-2 lists the dental and oral considerations associated with the use of these drugs. The leukopenia that is common in SLE usually is not associ-

BOX 21-6

Dental Management of Patient With Systemic Lupus Erythematosus

KEY POINTS
1. Consultation with physician
   a. Patient status and stability
   b. Extent of systemic manifestations (i.e., kidney, heart)
   c. Hematologic profile (complete blood cell count [CBC] with differential, prothrombin time [PT], partial thromboplastin time [PTT], bleeding time [BT])
   d. Drug profile
2. Drug considerations
   a. Aspirin and nonsteroidal anti-inflammatory drugs (NSAIDs)—bleeding may be increased but is not usually clinically significant; if patient is concurrently taking corticosteroids, bleeding is more likely—suggest obtaining pretreatment bleeding time (<20 minutes)
   b. Gold salts, antimalarials, penicillamine, and cytotoxic drugs may cause leukopenia and thrombocytopenia; also, severe stomatitis—treat symptomatically
   c. Corticosteroids may cause adrenal suppression
3. Hematologic considerations
   a. Leukopenia with corticosteroids or cytotoxic drugs may predispose patient to infection; use of postoperative antibiotics can be considered with surgical procedures
   b. Platelet count <50,000/mm^3 may result in severe bleeding—consultation with physician
   c. Elevated PTT associated with lupus anticoagulant usually does not cause increased bleeding—surgery can be performed
4. Infective endocarditis is a potential problem—antibiotic prophylaxis is not recommended by the American Heart Association.

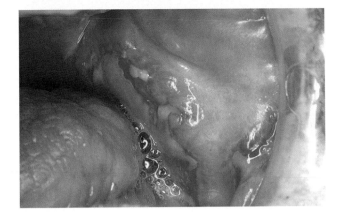

Figure 21-8. Systemic lupus erythematosus ulcerations of the buccal mucosa. (From Neville BW, et al. Oral and Maxillofacial Pathology, 2nd ed. Philadelphia, Saunders, 2002.)

ated with a significant increase in infection; however, when combined with corticosteroids or cytotoxic drugs, the likelihood of infection is increased. Therefore, in patients who are taking corticosteroids or cytotoxins who also have leukopenia, the use of prophylactic antibiotics for periodontal and oral surgical procedures may be considered. Patients who are taking corticosteroids also may develop significant adrenal suppression and could require supplementation, especially for surgical procedures or in cases of extreme anxiety (see Chapter 16).

Abnormal bleeding due to thrombocytopenia is a potential problem in some patients with SLE. A coagulation profile that especially notes the platelet count, PFA-100, bleeding time, and PTT, should be obtained. Bleeding times shorter than 20 minutes and a platelet count greater than 50,000/mm^3 are indications of adequate platelet activity. Other abnormalities should be discussed with the physician. As was previously mentioned, an elevated PTT associated with the lupus anticoagulant is not a risk factor for increased bleeding.

Cardiac valvular abnormalities are found in 25% to 50% of patients with SLE and often are not clinically detectable, the potential exists for bacterial endocarditis resulting from physiologic bacteremia. The American Heart Association 2007 Guidelines for endocarditis prevention do not recommend antibiotic prophylaxis for patients with valvular disease associated with SLE when receiving invasive dental procedures. Finally, patients with SLE-associated renal failure have the potential for altered drug metabolism, hematologic disorders, and infection (see Chapter 13 for management recommendations).

Treatment Planning Considerations

No specific treatment planning modifications are required. However, consideration should be given to physical disabilities related to arthritis and myalgia. Additionally, systemic complications such as renal impairment and cardiac problems such as arrhythmia and valvular defects may occur. For patients with SLE, the establishment and maintenance of optimal oral health are of paramount importance.

Oral Complications and Manifestations

Oral lesions of the lips and mucous membranes have been reported to occur in up to 5% to 25% of patients with SLE. These lesions are rather nonspecific and may be erythematous with white spots or radiating peripheral lines; they also may occur as painful ulcerations (Figure 21-8). Lesions frequently resemble lichen planus or leukoplakia. When they occur on the lip, a silvery, scaly margin, similar to that seen on the skin, may develop. Skin and lip lesions frequently are noted after exposure to the sun. Treatment of these lesions is symptomatic, and future sun exposure is avoided (see Appendix B). Other oral manifestations of SLE may include xerostomia and hyposalivation, dysgeusia, and glossodynia. The dentist should always remain alert to oral eruptions and lesions associated with any of a variety of medications used to treat patients with SLE; they may be a sign of toxicity. Similarly, some medications (hydralazine) have been associated with lupuslike eruptions.[23]

LYME DISEASE

DEFINITION

Lyme disease is a multisystemic inflammatory disease caused by the tickborne spirochete *Borrelia burgdorferi*. The disease was first identified in the United States in 1975 during an outbreak around Lyme, Connecticut, of an inflammatory condition presumed to be juvenile rheumatoid arthritis. The classical pattern of Lyme disease is a characteristic macular skin rash (erythema migrans) that appears within a month after the tick (*Ixodes dammini*) bite. Several different manifestations, including neurologic, articular, and cardiac manifestations, may follow.[19]

Incidence and Prevalence

Lyme disease has been reported in North America, Europe, and Asia. In the United States, more than 90% of all cases of Lyme disease have been reported in only eight states (New York, Connecticut, Pennsylvania, Massachusetts, Rhode Island, New Jersey, Wisconsin, and Minnesota). Differences in the organism and in the immunogenetics of the affected population may explain the differences in clinical presentation of Lyme disease.[24]

Pathophysiology and Complications

Precisely how *B burgdorferi* causes Lyme disease is not clear. The organism does not make toxins or cause tissue damage. It may activate proteolytic enzymes and induce spirochetemia. Local inflammation results from host response mechanisms. Vasculitis has been implicated in some cases of peripheral neuropathy, and a vascular lesion resembling endarteritis obliterans has been identified in the meninges and synovium of patients with Lyme disease.[24]

The clinical manifestations of Lyme disease can be divided into three phases: early localized, early disseminated, and late disease. Patients with a diagnosis of Lyme disease may not be identified until later stages of the disease. Early localized disease includes erythema migrans and associated findings. Erythema migrans occurs in 50% to 80% of infected patients within 1 month of the tick bite. Only about 30% of patients can recall an associated tick bite. Erythema migrans presents as a "target" or "bull's eye" lesion that typically appears in or near the axilla or belt line, because ticks like warm, moist areas of the human body (Figure 21-9). Most often, the lesion is asymptomatic, although it may itch, burn, or hurt. The lesion typically expands and enlarges over the course of a few days. Some sources have reported that 50% of patients have multiple lesions of erythema migrans

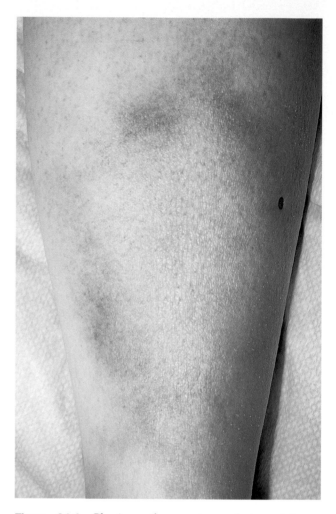

Figure 21-9. Classic erythema migrans lesion of Lyme disease. (From Habif TP. Clinical Dermatology: A Color Guide to Diagnosis and Therapy, 4th ed. Philadelphia, Mosby, 2004.)

because of spirochetemia. Patients also may have an acute viremia-like syndrome with fever, malaise, nausea, myalgia, fatigue, headache, and athralgias.[24]

The next phase of clinical presentation is early disseminated disease, which may occur within a few days to a few months after the tick bite, possibly without preceding erythema migrans. The primary clinical manifestations of this phase are cardiac and neurologic problems. In the absence of treatment, about 8% of patients infected with Lyme disease manifest some cardiac problems, including heart block and myopericarditis. In most cases, the carditis begins to resolve, even without antibiotic therapy. Neurologic damage occurs in approximately 10% of untreated patients with Lyme disease. Primary manifestations include lymphocytic meningitis, cranial nerve palsy (especially of the facial nerve), and radiculoneuritis. In the late disease stage, which may occur months to years after the infection and may not be preceded by the earlier manifestations, musculoskeletal problems are the primary manifestation. Intermittent, migratory episodes of polyarthritis that mimic the "juvenile arthritis" originally described in cases of Lyme disease occur in approximately 50% of patients. Chronic arthritis of the knee is common, along with erosion of bone and cartilage. Chronic inflammatory joint disease may last for 5 to 8 years.[24]

Late neurologic manifestations of Lyme disease, called *tertiary neuroborreliosis*, consist of encephalopathy, neurocognitive dysfunction, and peripheral neuropathy. Symptoms may be subtle and may be reported as headache and fatigue, in addition to cognitive, mood, and sleep disturbances. Neuropsychological testing may be useful in confirming the diagnosis. Patients also may manifest distal neuropathies. Fibromyalgia is common in patients with Lyme disease.[24]

Laboratory Findings

Although the diagnosis of Lyme disease is based on clinical findings, serologic testing may prove useful. Current practice is to confirm all enzyme-linked immunosorbent assay (ELISA) results with Western blot analysis. Many other conditions (e.g., Epstein-Barr virus [EBV] infections, SLE, infective endocarditis) may mimic Lyme disease; therefore, laboratory testing should be performed for a more precise, definitive diagnosis. Serologic testing has not been standardized between various laboratories; this may be problematic. Antibody responses may be undetectable in infections of less than 6 weeks duration, and early antibiotic therapy based on symptoms may render the infected patient seronegative. Most patients with late disease manifestations are strongly seropositive.[19]

MEDICAL MANAGEMENT

Antibiotic therapy is effective for the treatment of patients with *B burgdorferi* infection. Prompt antibiotic therapy when early symptoms are reported usually prevents progression to later stages of Lyme disease. Oral doses of 100 mg of doxycycline given twice daily for 3 to 4 weeks provide first-line treatment for early infection. Alternatively, tetracycline or amoxicillin (250 to 500 mg 4 times daily) may be given for the same duration. In the late disseminated stages of Lyme disease, intravenous antibiotics may be necessary. Third-generation cephalosporins (ceftriaxone 2 g 4 times daily, or cefotaxime 3 g twice daily), penicillin G (20 million units in 6 divided doses), or chloramphenicol (50 mg/kg/day in 4 divided doses) may be used. Some physicians treat all pregnant women only through the intravenous (IV) route. Some patients with arthritis are refractory to antibiotic therapy. These patients may benefit from intra-articular corticosteroid injections or hydroxychloroquine. Adequate therapy for neurologic damage is elusive, and recovery may be very slow.[25]

DENTAL MANAGEMENT
Medical Considerations

The major dental consideration in Lyme disease is the identification of unusual symptoms in the absence of a clear medical condition. Symptoms of fatigue, malaise, arthralgia, neuritis, or neuralgia, including facial palsy, may indicate the possibility of Lyme disease and the need for referral for proper medical diagnosis. Numerous reports have described facial nerve palsy that closely resembles Bell's palsy caused by Lyme disease. The presentation of this facial palsy may be combined with other neurologic deficits or may stand alone. Involvement of the parotid glands (acute parotitis) has been reported. Cases also have been identified during pregnancy. Along with facial nerve palsy, facial and dental neuralgia and temporomandibular joint symptoms have been reported to occur with Lyme disease.[26]

SJÖGREN'S SYNDROME
DEFINITION

Sjögren's syndrome (SS) is an autoimmune disease complex classified among the many rheumatic diseases that causes exocrinopathy and affects the salivary and lacrimal glands. SS is characterized by a triad of clinical conditions that consists of keratoconjunctivitis sicca, xerostomia, and a connective tissue disease (usually, rheumatoid arthritis). SS presents in two different forms: primary SS and secondary SS. Primary SS (SS-1) clinically manifests with the primary ocular complication of keratoconjunctivitis sicca; in the oral cavity, it presents as various levels of salivary gland dysfunction (xerostomia). Secondary SS (SS-2) manifests as the presence of keratoconjunctivitis sicca or xerostomia in the presence of a diagnosed systemic connective tissue disease. The connective tissue disorder from which SS develops most commonly is rheumatoid arthritis; SLE, primary biliary cirrhosis, fibromyalgia, mixed connective tissue disease, polymyositis, Raynaud's syndrome, and several others are among the associated inflammatory conditions.[27]

Incidence and Prevalence

According to the World Health Organization, the prevalence of SS is unknown. It has been estimated that its prevalence in the adult population is around 2.7%. Today, the prevalence of SS in the United States is estimated at more than 1 million. Originally named for an ophthalmologist from Sweden, SS has been reported in nearly every major country, and the geographic distribution of cases, although accurate data are lacking, appears to be relatively uniform. SS is primarily a disease of women, as more than 90% of all patients with SS are female.[1,21]

SS typically presents during the fourth or fifth decade of life, although the condition usually progresses insidiously over several years, often remaining unrecognized. Therefore, some individuals may begin developing SS at a much earlier age than when it is actually diagnosed. Isolated cases of SS have been reported in children.[1,21]

Etiology

The precise cause of SS, as of many of the autoimmune rheumatic disorders, is unknown, although several contributing factors have been identified. One theory is that the disease results from complications of viral infection with EBV. Exposure to or reactivation of EBV elicits expression of the HLA (human lymphocyte antigen) complex; this is recognized by the T-cell (CD4+) lymphocytes and results in the release of cytokines (tumor necrosis factor [TNF], interleukin [IL]-2, interferon [IFN]-γ, and others). Chronic inflammation, infiltration of lymphocytes, and ultimate destruction of exocrine gland tissue follow.[1,21]

Pathophysiology and Complications

SS is a chronic, progressive autoimmune disorder that is characterized by exocrinopathy and generalized lymphoproliferation that primarily affect the salivary and lacrimal glands. A genetic marker, HLA-DR4, has been identified as specific for SS.[19]

Labial salivary gland histopathology almost universally has been accepted as the prima facie diagnostic indicator for definitive diagnosis of SS. The classic histopathology of the minor salivary glands in SS is seen as lymphocytic infiltration that includes benign lymphosialadenopathy (focal lymphocytic sialadenitis or benign lymphoepithelial lesion in the major salivary glands). This benign lymphosialadenopathy may manifest as parotid hypertrophy, particularly in patients with primary SS. Small clusters of intralobular ducts enlarge to replace the acinar epithelial parenchyma. The lesion comprises primarily CD4+ T-cell lymphocytes, along with polyclonal B cells and plasma cells that are acquired late. Among the lymphocytic foci, approximately 75% are T cells and 5% to 10% are B cells. As the inflammatory process progresses, fibrosis and atrophy of the salivary glands occur, and hyposalivation progresses. Progression to lymphoma is a possibility in SS and is discussed in the patient management section.[19]

CLINICAL PRESENTATION

Signs and Symptoms

The oral clinical manifestations of SS typically include hyposalivation, glossitis, mucositis, parotid gland hypertrophy, angular cheilosis, dysgeusia (taste dysfunction), secondary infection, and a significantly increased caries rate (Table 21-3).[27]

Salivary Gland Dysfunction and Hyposalivation

Saliva in normal quantity and composition is rich in constituents that have potent antimicrobial, antacid, lubricative, and homeostatic properties. Saliva contains approximately 60 important protective constituents, including immunoglobulins, electrolytes, buffers, antimicrobial enzymes, digestive enzymes, and many others, all of which make saliva an essential contributor to the health and homeostasis of the oral cavity. Obviously, when saliva is diminished in quantity or altered in composition, as in

TABLE 21-3

Clinical Manifestations (with approximate frequency) of Subjects With Sjögren's Syndrome (SS)*

Clinical Manifestation	Prevalence, % of Patients With SS
Orcheilosis/angular cheilitis	75
Glossitis	60
Mucositis	30
Glossodynia	45
Dysgeusia	75
Dysphagia	45
Candidiasis	75
Dental caries	100
Periodontitis	60-100

Data published in part in Rhodus NL. Xerostomia and glossodynia in patients with autoimmune disorders. Ear Nose Throat J 1989;68:791-794; and Rhodus NL, et al. Quantitative assessment of dysphagia in patients with primary and secondary Sjögren's syndrome. Oral Surg Oral Med Oral Pathol Oral Radiol Endod 1995;79:305-310.
*From 62 consecutive patients with SS who presented to the University of Minnesota Xerostomia Clinic.

SS, deterioration of oral soft and mineralized tissues may occur.[27]

Patients with SS also demonstrate increased levels of dysphagia as compared with controls. Studies have shown that patients with SS have difficulty tasting, tolerating, and swallowing certain foods. These patients may have resultant nutritional intake inadequacies.[27]

Among its many beneficial constituents, saliva has been shown to be rich in proteins that have potent antifungal properties; thus, it plays an important role in host defense and protection from yeasts such as *Candida* species. Therefore, with reduced salivary flow in SS, *Candida* infections are very common.[27]

Results of a recently published study indicate that the presence and density of *Candida albicans* in subjects with SS were extremely high at baseline; this was evidenced by clinical signs in most subjects (especially those with the highest counts). This study also found that the prevailing clinical manifestation of infection with *C albicans* (before *and* after pilocarpine HCl administration) was erythema (63% and 25%, respectively). A few recent studies also have shown that patients with SS more frequently exhibit periodontal disease, especially loss of clinical attachment.[28]

Diagnosis

Precise diagnostic criteria for SS remain controversial, although specific laboratory tests are available for the major diagnostic categories of salivary and tear production, histopathologic changes, and serologic inflammatory markers. Five sets of published criteria are available for the diagnosis of SS; several common characteristics and some variations and modifications are notable (Box 21-7).

Diagnostic Criteria (European Criteria) for Sjögren's Syndrome* Used at the University of Minnesota

Ocular Symptoms (1:3)	Ocular Signs (1:2)
Daily dry eyes >3 mo	+Shirmer's test
Sand or gravel sensitivity	(<5 mm/5 min)
Use of tear substitutes	Rose Bengal score
(>3 times daily)	(>4 vBs)
Oral symptoms (1:3)	Salivary function (1:3)
Daily dry mouth >3 mo	+Scintigraphy
Swollen salivary glands	+Sialography
Need fluids to swallow	WUSF <1.5 mL/15 min
food	(0.1 mL/min)
Labial SG histology	Autoantibodies (1:2)
Focus scope biopsy	anti–SS-Ro
>1/4 mm	
>50 mononuclear cells in the field	anti–SS-La

*Subjects must meet 4 of 6 criteria; labial biopsy or serology must be performed.
vBs, von Blisterberg score for eyes; WUSF, whole unstimulated saliva flow.

Laboratory Findings

Serologically, hypergammaglobulinemia is the most frequent laboratory finding (80%) among patients with SS. Hyperactivity of B lymphocytes results in increased rheumatoid factor antibodies, antinuclear antibodies (ANA), and antibodies against organ-specific antigens, such as salivary duct epithelia or thyroid tissue. ANA make up the SS-A (Ro), which is present in approximately 70% of patients with SS-1 and 15% to 90% with SS-1 and SS-B (La) antibodies, which are present in approximately 50% of patients with SS-1 and 5% to 30% with SS-2. These ANA also may be found in other autoimmune disorders. Elevated erythrocyte sedimentation rate (ESR), mild anemia (approximately 25%), and leukopenia (approximately 10%) also are found in patients with SS. The laboratory tests used to diagnose SS are summarized in Box 21-7.[29]

Sialometry. Sialometry is useful as an initial screening tool for hyposalivation associated with SS and as an assessment for the level of severity of SS. To be valuable as a diagnostic technique, salivary flow collection must be performed precisely according to the type of gland and over a period of at least 5 minutes (often up to 15 minutes).[27]

Imaging. Radiographic findings may appear in advanced stages of fibrosis of the salivary glands. Sialograms are performed with injection of a radiocontrast dye into the salivary ductal system before conventional radiography. Sialograms may reveal punctate radiopaque calcifications or, if more advanced, larger, lobular calcifications. Sialectasis may occur in portions of the ductal system, or these portions may appear dilated or to have areas of absent acinar parenchyma. Magnetic resonance imaging (MRI)

sialography has been shown to be much more accurate in demonstrating levels of salivary gland destruction in SS.[69] Salivary scintigraphy with 99m technetium pertechnetate (sodium pertechnetate, a radioisotope of technetium) can be performed to assess the function of the salivary glands through measurement of the rate and density of technetium uptake.[27]

DENTAL MANAGEMENT

Medical Considerations

No cure for SS is known. Patient management for SS traditionally has been palliative and preventive. Relief of the primary symptoms of dryness (oral and ocular) and the secondary burning and discomfort is the main goal. Restoration and maintenance of a normal homeostatic oral environment is a secondary goal.[27]

Therapy for the oral component of SS may be classified into three major categories:
1. Provision of moisture and lubrication by stimulation or simulation
2. Treatment of secondary mucosal conditions (such as mucositis or candidiasis)
3. Prevention of oral disease, provision of maintenance and general support (such as nutrition)

These therapeutic strategies are outlined in Table 21-4.

Moisture and Lubrication

Patients with SS are quite thirsty and should be counseled to drink plenty of water (8 to 10 glasses per day) and to avoid diuretics such as caffeine, tobacco, and alcoholic beverages. Obviously, certain medications (more than 400) may contribute to and compound the xerostomia, so some may need to be modified or avoided, if possible. Any changes in the patient's medication must be coordinated with the patient's physician. Although salivary substitutes, oral moisturizers, and artificial salivas may provide some relief for the xerostomia experienced by patients with SS, by and large, they are inadequate. Most are compounds of carboxymethylcellulose or hydroxymethylcellulose and are too viscous or not viscous enough for most patients. The retentivity or longevity of their effect is very short-lived, and they provide little more relief than water. To date, these simulated salivas appear to provide little benefit to the patient with SS. Some artificial salivas from Europe (including Saliva Orthana) seem to be effective. On the other hand, pharmacologic stimulation of the salivary glands can be quite successful. Recently, the FDA approved the use of pilocarpine HCl (Salagen) and cevimeline HCL (Evoxac) for the treatment of patients with SS with signs and symptoms of hyposalivation.[27]

Systemic administration of pilocarpine or cevimeline effectively stimulates only the salivary acinar tissue, which remains functional. Therefore, patients with SS who have lost most of the salivary acinar tissue capable of fluid production benefit little from this drug. Conversely, those

TABLE **21-4**
Management of Salivary Dysfunction*

MOISTURE AND LUBRICATION (CONTINUOUS, AS NEEDED)

General	*Specific**
Drink (sip water, liquids)	Oral balance (especially at night)
Use sugarless candy or gum	Pilocarpine hydrochloride, 2% (Salagen 5 mg, 3 times daily)
Avoid ethanol	*or*
Avoid tobacco	Cevimeline hydrochloride (Evoxac 30 mg caps, 3 times daily)
Avoid coffee, tea, and other caffeinated beverages	Mouthkote (artificial saliva)
	MedOral (artificial saliva)
	Oasis (artificial saliva)
	Salivart (artificial saliva)
	Sodium carboxymethylcellulose, 05% sin

SOFT TISSUE LESIONS AND SORENESS (TREATMENT AND MAINTENANCE)

General	*Specific**
Oral balance	Benadryl + Maalox + nystatin elixir[†]
Biotene mouthwash	(Carafate, optional)
	(Lidocaine 2%, optional, for acute lesions)
	Decadron 0.5 mg/5 mL elixir[‡] (for acute lesions)
	Triamcinolone 0.1% (in Orabase) (for acute lesions)
	Orabase-HCA (for acute lesions)
	Mycelex 60-mg troches (for candidiasis)
	Mycolog II ointment (lips and tongue)

PREVENTION OF CARIES AND PERIODONTAL DISEASE (CONTINUOUS)

General	*Specific**
Meticulous perioral hygiene	Biotene toothpaste (neutral sodium fluoride, 1.0%, trays)
Avoid acids	Prevident, 5000 ppm[§]
Regular hygiene and prophylaxis recalls	(Optional) Peridex (chlorhexidine gluconate)
Sodium bicarbonate rinses (optional)	Waterpik

Published in part by Rhodus NL. Diagnosis and treatment of Sjögren's syndrome. Quintessence International, 1999,30:689-699.
*Specific treatments are dependent on the diagnosis.
[†]Benadryl, 25 mg/10 mL + Maalox, 64 mL + nystatin, 100,000 IU/mL = 16 mL.
[†]Decadron elixir, 0.5%/5 mL. Dispense 100 mL. To be swished and expectorated, 5 mL 3 times daily.
[§]Prevident neutral sodium fluoride, 1.0%, to be applied in trays 2 times daily.
Manufacturers: Oral Balance, Laclede Pharmaceuticals; Salagen, MGI Pharmaceuticals; Mouthkote, Parnell Pharmaceuticals; Optimoist, Colgate-Hoyt; Salivart, Gebauer; Biotene, Laclede Pharmaceuticals; Benadryl, Parke-Davis; Maalox, Novartis Pharmaceuticals; Carafate, Hoechst, Marion, Roussel Pharmaceuticals; Decadron, Merck & Co. Pharmaceuticals; Orabase, Colgate-Palmolive; Mycelex, ALZA Prevident, Colgate-Hoyte; Peridex, Procter & Gamble; Waterpik, Teledyne.

patients with functional tissue remaining experience an increase in salivary secretion after the administration of pilocarpine relative to the ability of the tissue to become stimulated. The dosage of pilocarpine ranges from 2.5 to 15 mg administered from 2 to 6 times daily. The dosage of cevimeline is 30 mg given 2 to 4 times daily.[27]

Other pharmacologic sialogogues, such as bethanechol chloride, bromhexine, and anethole trithione, have been shown to stimulate salivary flow, but none has withstood extensive clinical evaluation of safety and efficacy in the United States, and none has been approved by the FDA as of the time of this writing. Very recently, clinical trials have been undertaken to study the safety and efficacy of human IFN-α for the treatment of patients with SS. This NSAID appears to have significant promise as a new therapy for SS.[27]

Oral Complications and Manifestations

Among the oral symptoms most commonly associated with SS, aside from xerostomia, is glossodynia (burning tongue). The tongue often becomes depapillated and fissured and develops a scrotal appearance (Figure 21-10). The dorsal epithelium often is atrophic or eroded, erythematous, and potentially secondarily infected. Pain and burning may be spontaneous or may be elicited with acidic or spicy foods, such as those containing ascorbic or acetic acid. The tongue is commonly infected (in as many as 83%) with *C albicans* in patients with SS. Not only must the acute candidal infection be treated, but some type of maintenance therapy must be provided to prevent recurrence of the fungal infection. As long as the oral environment is adversely affected by hyposalivation,

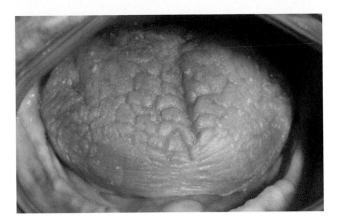

Figure 21-10. Dry and fissured tongue in a patient with Sjögren's syndrome. (Courtesy Dr. David Schaffner. In Neville BW, et al. Oral and Maxillofacial Pathology, 2nd ed. Philadelphia, Saunders, 2002.)

susceptibility to recurrence of the oral infection and continued deterioration occur. Atrophy of the epithelium in the dry environment may render the tissue susceptible to painful excoriation and ulceration. Therefore, clinical follow-up and some phased maintenance therapy may be necessary. Generally, these oral mucosal conditions are treated as if they occurred independently (i.e., with antifungal agents, topical anti-inflammatory agents including corticosteroids, analgesics, or anesthetics as indicated) (see Table 21-4).[27,30]

Prevention and Maintenance

The patient with SS may have less than 5% of the normal quantity of saliva to protect the oral cavity. The risk for caries as well as enamel erosion then is extremely high. Of particular risk is the cervical/cementoenamel junction portion of the tooth. Meticulous oral hygiene with minimally abrasive fluoridated dentifrices and irrigation devices is paramount. In the xerostomic environment, abrasion of the tooth surface should be minimized as much as possible. Frequent professional hygiene recall intervals are also extremely important.

Frequent application of concentrated fluorides delivered as a direct brush-on treatment or with custom-made trays is imperative, to prevent the rapid progression of caries. Over-the-counter fluoride rinses are inadequate; 5000 ppm sodium fluoride is preferred because of the unpleasant metallic taste of stannous fluoride, which also may cause some burning symptoms in the xerostomic patient and staining of the enamel. Special dentifrices have been found to be well accepted by patients with SS (see Table 21-4).[23]

Lymphoma. Most lymphomas occur in cases of SS-1. The prevalence is approximately 5%. Kassan and associates[19] in 1983 predicted the relative risk in patients with SS to be 44 times normal and even higher (67 times) in those patients with SS-1 with chronic parotid enlarge-

ment; whether patients had other cancers or had undergone irradiation therapy or chemotherapy (then the relative risk may be as high as 100 times) was considered. Progression to lymphoma in patients with SS is thought to be related to chronic inflammatory challenge, as in the case of *Helicobacter pylori* in gastric cancer. In the presence of continued and chronic inflammation (mediated first by type 1 cytokines—TNF-α, IL-2, IFN-γ—then later, by type 2 cytokines—IL-4, IL-6, and IL-10), B cells undergo oligoclonality and sometimes eventually monoclonality. Patients with SS may then manifest non-Hodgkin's lymphoma. B-cell monoclonality seems to be predictive of the occurrence of lymphoma outside the salivary glands.[31]

Clinical findings associated with lymphoma include anemia, cryoglobulinemia, lymphopenia, cutaneous vasculitis, and peripheral neuropathy. Lymphadenopathy is common (86%) and is associated with enlarged cervical and axillary nodes. Evidence suggests that initial transformation to lymphoma occurs in the salivary glands, and that the presence of B-cell monoclonality in labial minor salivary gland (LMSG) tissue is associated with progression to malignancy.[31]

The most common type of lymphoma in patients with SS involves mucosa-associated lymphoid tissue; 70% of cases are low-grade, nonaggressive lymphomas, and 15% are the high-grade lymphoblastic type. IL-6 and TNF-α are associated with lesions that go on to transform to lymphoma.[31]

REFERENCES

1. Arthritis Foundation. Primer on the Rheumatic Diseases, vol 12. Atlanta, GA, Arthritis Foundation, 2005, p 684.
2. Koopman WJ, Moreland LW (eds). Arthritis and Allied Conditions, vol 1, 15th ed. Philadelphia, Pa, Lippincott, Williams and Wilkins, 2005, p 1448.
3. Wordsworth WL. Rheumatoid arthritis: Etiology. In Klippel JH, Dieppe PA (eds). Rheumatology. London, Mosby-Year Book, 1994, p 998.
4. Danhauer SC, Miller CS, Rhodus NL, Carlson CR. Impact of criteria-based diagnosis of burning mouth syndrome on treatment outcome. J Orofac Pain 2002; 16:305-311.
5. Lipsky PE, van der Heijde DM, St. Clair EW, et al. Infliximab and methotrexate in the treatment of rheumatoid arthritis. Anti–Tumor Necrosis Factor Trial in Rheumatoid Arthritis With Concomitant Therapy Study Group. N Engl J Med 2000;343:1594-1602.
6. Bathon JM, Martin RW, Fleischmann RM, et al. A comparison of etanercept and methotrexate in patients with early rheumatoid arthritis. N Engl J Med 2000;343: 1586-1593.
7. Bradley JD, Brandt KD, Katz BP, et al. Comparison of an antiinflammatory dose of ibuprofen, an analgesic dose of ibuprofen, and acetaminophen in the treatment of patients with osteoarthritis of the knee. N Engl J Med 1991;325:87-91.

8. Amrein PC, Ellman L, Harris WH. Aspirin-induced prolongation of bleeding time and perioperative blood loss. JAMA 1981;245:1825-1828.

9. Little JW. Patients with prosthetic joints: Are they at risk when receiving invasive dental procedures? Spec Care Dent 1997;17:153-160.

10. Pallasch TJ, Slots J. Antibiotic prophylaxis and the medically compromised patient. Periodontology 1996; 10:107-138.

11. ADA/AAOS. Antibiotic prophylaxis for dental patients with total joint replacements. J Am Dent Asso 2003; 134:895-897.

12. Celiker R, Gokce-Kutsal Y, Eryilmaz M. Temporomandibular joint involvement in rheumatoid arthritis: Relationship with disease activity. Scand J Rheumatol 1995; 24:22-25.

13. Pepin JL, Della Negra E, Grosclaude S, et al. Sleep apnea syndrome secondary to rheumatoid arthritis. Thorax 1995;50:692-694.

14. Kreutziger KL, Mahan PE. Temporomandibular degenerative joint disease. Part I. Anatomy, pathophysiology and clinical description. Oral Surg Oral Med Oral Pathol 1995;40:165-172.

15. de Leeuw R, Boering G, Stegenga B, de Bont LG. Radiographic signs of temporomandibular joint osteoarthrosis and internal derangement 30 years after nonsurgical treatment. Oral Surg Oral Med Oral Pathol Oral Radiol Endod 1995;79:382-392.

16. Boumpas DT, Fessler BJ, Austin HA 3rd. Systemic lupus erythematosus: Emergency concepts. Part 2: Dermatologic and joint disease, the antiphospholipid antibody syndrome, pregnancy and hormone therapy, morbidity and mortality, and pathogenesis. Ann Intern Med 1995;123:42-53.

17. Petri M, Genovese M. Incidence of and risk factors for hospitalizations in systemic lupus erythematosus: A prospective study of the Hopkins Lupus Cohort. J Rheumatol 1992;19:1559-1565.

18. Seleznick MJ, Fries JF. Variables associated with decreased survival in systemic lupus erythematosus. Semin Arthritis Rheum 1991;21:73-80.

19. Kassan SS, Thomas TL, Moutsopoulos HM. Increased risk of lymphoma in sicca syndrome. Ann Intern Med 1978;89:888-892.

20. Hiser DG, Egan RM, Miller CS, et al. Risk of infective endocarditis in patients with systemic lupus erythematosus. Oral Surg Oral Med Oral Pathol Oral Radiol Endod 1995;80:423-425.

21. Rhodus NL, Little JW, Johnson DK. Electrocardiographic examination of dental patients with systemic lupus erythematosus. Spec Care Dentist 1990. 10(2): p. 46-50.

22. Gladman DD. Systemic lupus erythematosus: Clinical features. In Schumacher HR Jr (ed). Primer on Rheumatic Diseases, 10th ed. Atlanta, Ga, Arthritis Foundation, 1995.

23. Rhodus NL, Johnson DK. The prevalence of oral manifestations of systemic lupus erythematosus. Quintessence Int 1990;21:461-465.

24. Rhodus NL, Falace DA. Oral concerns in Lyme disease. Northwest Dent 2002;81:17-18.

25. Dotevall L. Successful oral doxycycline treatment of Lyme disease and associated facial palsy and meningitis. Clin Infect Dis 2000;28:569-572.

26. Centers for Disease Control and Prevention. Racial/ethnic disparities in diagnoses of HIV/AIDS—33 states, 2001-2004. MMWR Morb Mortal Wkly Rep 2006;55: 121-125.

27. Rhodus NL. Sjogren's syndrome. Quintessence Int 1999;30:689-699.

28. Rhodus NL, Michalowicz BS. Periodontal status and sulcular *Candida albicans* colonization in patients with primary Sjogren's syndrome. Quintessence Int 2005;36:228-233.

29. Fox RI. Sjogren's syndrome. Lancet 2005;366:321-331.

30. Rhodus NL. Xerostomia and glossodynia in patients with autoimmune disorders. Ear Nose Throat J 1989; 68:791-794.

31. Jordan RC, Speight PM. Lymphoma in Sjögren's syndrome: From histopathology to molecular pathology. Oral Surg Oral Med Oral Pathol Oral Radiol Endod 1996;81:808-820.

Organ and Bone Marrow Transplantation

CHAPTER 22

More than 26,500 solid organ transplantations occurred in the United States in 2004—an increase of nearly 1000 donors (7%) over 2003. During this time, the number of living donors increased by about 3% (7000), and the number of deceased donors grew by 11% to more than 19,000—the largest annual increase in deceased donors in the previous 10 years.[1] According to the Organ Procurement and Transplantation Network (OPTN), these numbers represent an increase of 6% in total number of organs transplanted during a single year. This increase in donors led to an additional 2240 deceased donor organs recovered for transplantation from the previous year—a significant increase. Some of this increase can likely be attributed to specific efforts—such as the Organ Donation Breakthrough Collaborative, which started in the fall of 2003—that focus on increasing the supply of organs for transplantation.[1]

Between 1990 and 2000, more than 200,000 solid organ transplantations were performed in the United States. In 2005, more than 85,000 patients were on waiting lists for organ transplants. This figure will continue to increase.[2]

Key outcomes after transplantation include survival of transplant recipients and function of transplanted grafts. One-year patient survival rates are highest for kidney and pancreas recipients (95% to 98%); the median survival for renal transplantation from living donors has increased from 17 years in 1988 to nearly 38 years at the present time. Corresponding survival rates for liver, intestine, and heart recipients were approximately 86% to 88%; rates were about 83% for lung and were lowest for the small number of heart/lung recipients, with around 58% surviving at 1 year.[1,3]

Therefore, because more organ and bone marrow transplants are being performed successfully, and because technology will continue to improve in this area and more posttransplantation patients are surviving longer, the number of these patients who will be seeking dental care will also increase. Because no precise guidelines are based on evidence-based clinical trials for the dental management of organ transplant patients, the dentist will need to apply a number of principles in assessing the dental patient before, during, and after the solid organ transplant process. This chapter reviews epidemiology, pathophysiology, process, complications, and dental management recommendations for these patients.[4]

DEFINITION

Organ transplants are common today and may be performed in several organ systems, depending on the mix of recipients and donors. Heart, liver, kidney, pancreas, heart/lung, bone marrow, and other transplants may be available for the appropriate recipient. The ideal combination involves transplantation of an organ from an identical twin to the other twin (syngeneic). The next best match for organ survival is transplantation of an organ from one living relative to another (allogeneic). This is followed by transplantation of an organ between living nonrelated individuals (xenograft). Each of these combinations, however, is limited by the fact that unless two organs are present, the donor may not survive. Thus, these types of matches are basically limited to kidney and bone marrow donors. Nevertheless, recent studies have reported success with transplantation of a portion of a liver or pancreas from living donors. The largest organ pool for transplantation is cadaver organs, but the match is poorest in this group.[5-9]

Incidence and Prevalence

Dr. Joseph E. Murray, a Nobel laureate, performed the first successful human organ transplantation in Boston in 1954, using a kidney donated by the patient's identical twin brother. Then, Murray performed the first successful kidney allograft transplant in 1959, applying total body irradiation as immunosuppression, and the first successful human kidney cadaver transplant in 1962, introducing azathioprine (Imuran) as an immunosuppressive drug. Before these early transplant procedures, patients with renal failure, hypertension, and azotemia were undergoing renal dialysis, which was not nearly as successful. Since those early days, more than a half-million kidney transplant procedures have been performed in the United States.[6]

Since 1987, all organ transplant procedures performed in the United States have been reported to the United Network for Organ Sharing (UNOS), and renal transplants have occurred at an average annual rate of more than 10,000 nationwide. At the University of Minnesota Hospital, more than 300 renal transplants are performed each year. Approximately this number of procedures is performed annually in about 20 other transplant centers around the United States. Nearly 600 medical centers perform kidney transplants in the United States. Improvements in preparation of the patient before the transplant, along with the use of better immunosuppressive techniques, have enhanced the success rate of this procedure and have extended the longevity of the transplant recipient. The 1-year survival rate of the renal transplant patient is greater than 97%, and the 5-year survival rate is greater than 90%[1] (Table 22-1).

The first human heart transplantation was performed in 1967. During 1968, 102 heart transplants were performed, and overall 1-year survival was only 22%. More than 85% of all heart transplantations performed worldwide have occurred since 1985. To date, more than 70,000 heart transplants have been performed, and the annual rate is approximately 3400 at more than 250 U.S. hospitals. The 1-year survival rate is higher than 87%, and 5-year survival is greater than 70% (see Table 22-1).[1]

The first orthotopic liver transplantation was performed in 1963. However, the first transplant that resulted in an extended survival of 13 months did not occur until 1967. By 1980, only 300 liver transplants had been performed, and the 1-year survival rate was only 28%. During 1988 and 1989, some 3343 patients received their first orthotopic liver transplant, as reported to UNOS. Most patients received a single liver graft; however, some patients received multiple liver grafts. From 1988 to 1989, the number of liver transplantations increased by 25%. Currently, more than 6000 liver transplants are performed each year, and about the same number of patients are on the waiting list for a liver transplant. A total of more than 100,000 liver transplant procedures have been performed in the United States. Survival rates for patients receiving transplants in 1988 were 75.5% at 1 year and 68.6% at 2 years after the operation. Survival rates have increased to approximately 80% for 1 year and 70% for 5 years.[9,10]

The first pancreas transplant, along with transplantation of a duodenum and a kidney, was performed in 1966 by Kelly and Lillehei at the University of Minnesota in a patient with diabetic nephropathy. Now, more than

TABLE 22-1
Numbers of Transplants* and 1- and 5-Year Patient Survival by Organ

KIDNEY: *13,000

Deceased Donor	Living Donor
1-year survival = 94.6%	97.9%
5-year survival = 81.1%	90.2%

PANCREAS ALONE: *1000
1-year survival = 96.2%
5-year survival = 90.6%

PANCREAS AFTER KIDNEY: *1000
1-year survival = 95.5%
5-year survival = 84.4%

KIDNEY/PANCREAS:*1000
1-year survival = 95.3%
5-year survival = 85.9%

LIVER: *6500

Deceased Donor	Living Donor
1-year survival = 86.8%	87.7%
5-year survival = 73.1%	77.4%

INTESTINE:*160
1-year survival = 85.7%
5-year survival = 53.5%

HEART:*2100
1-year survival = 87.5%
5-year survival = 72.8%

LUNG:*2000
1-year survival = 83.0%
5-year survival = 49.3%

HEART/LUNG:*30
1-year survival = 57.9%
5-year survival = 40.2%

Data from: 2005 OPTN/SRTR Annual Report.
Total: 26,000 solid organ transplants per year; approximate numbers based on 2004 statistics.

1000 pancreas transplantations are performed each year, and the 5-year survival rate is nearly 90%. Recently, pancreatic islet cell transplants have shown considerable success.[10]

By 1990, only five lung transplant procedures had been performed. Since that time, more than 10,000 lungs have been transplanted at 119 centers, most within the past 5 years. The first heart/lung combination transplantation was performed in 1981. Since that time, more than 1000 such procedures have been performed, and the 1-year survival rate is almost 60%.[10]

To date, only a few small bowel transplantations have been performed (some combined with liver transplants) at only a few transplant centers (Cambridge, England; London, Ontario; Pittsburgh, Pennsylvania; and Omaha,

Nebraska). However, much progress is being made in this area for the treatment of end-stage intestinal failure, and the current 1-year survival rate is approximately 70%.[10]

The modern era of bone marrow transplantation (BMT) was ushered in by the seminal experiments of Jacobsen (1950) and Lorenz (1951) and their colleagues, who showed that mice could be protected from lethal radiation that was used to treat severe aplastic anemia or leukemia by shielding of the spleen or intravenous infusion of bone marrow.[5] By 1956, several laboratories had demonstrated that protective effects against otherwise lethal doses of total body irradiation were caused by colonization of recipient bone marrow by infused donor cells.

In 1957, E. Donnell Thomas[5] described the clinical technique by which large quantities of marrow were safely and effectively infused intravenously into patients with leukemia; Thomas also reported on the performance of transient BMT in humans. In 1958, BMT was performed in six victims of a radiation accident.[7]

Most early BMTs were performed in terminally ill patients, and the effectiveness of the grafts could not be evaluated because patients did not live long enough. The few successful allogeneic graft procedures were followed by the lethal immunologic reaction of graft-versus-host disease (GVHD). Research conducted over many years in rodents, then dogs and monkeys, paved the way for the ultimate success of BMT in humans. Recent advances in histocompatibility typing, in the prevention of GVHD, and in the provision of supportive measures for the patient have resulted in greater success and more frequent BMTs.[7]

The International Bone Marrow Transplant Registry reported that more than 20,000 patients had received allogenic bone marrow transplants between 1955 and 1987. More than 50% of these procedures were performed during the years between 1985 and 1987. By 1991, that figure had doubled, and through 1999, nearly 90,000 BMTs had been performed. BMT is the treatment of choice for patients with aplastic anemia and chronic myelogenous leukemia, for those in whom conventional therapy for acute leukemia is ineffective, and for patients in whom a variety of immune deficiency disorders are diagnosed.

Etiology

With the development of effective immunosuppressive agents, improvement in surgical techniques (including percutaneous biopsy of solid transplanted organs to monitor rejection), and acceptance of the concept of "brain death" as a determinant of death in potential donors, major advances in organ transplantation and resultant successes have occurred.[11-13]

Transplantation of the heart, liver, or kidney is no longer considered an experimental procedure and is available as a treatment option for selected patients with end-organ disease. Transplantation of the pancreas is considered a major treatment option for uremic diabetic patients who are receiving a kidney transplant. BMT is

an indicated treatment for patients with myelogenous leukemia and other blood dyscrasias[6,8,9] (see Table 22-1).

The most common indications for heart transplantation are cardiomyopathy and severe coronary artery disease. The most common diseases in adults for which liver transplantation is indicated are primary biliary cirrhosis, chronic hepatitis, sclerosing cholangitis, fulminant hepatic failure, and metabolic disorders. In children, most liver transplantations are performed for extrahepatic biliary atresia or metabolic disorders. Common indications for kidney transplantation are bilateral chronic disease and end-stage renal disease. Glomerulonephritis, pyelonephritis, diabetic nephropathy, and congenital renal disorders are the conditions that most frequently lead to end-stage renal disease. The most common indication for pancreas transplantation is severe diabetes that leads to end-stage renal disease. Diabetic patients who are going to receive a kidney transplant also are good candidates for pancreas transplantation. The most common indications for BMT are acute and chronic myelogenous leukemia, acute lymphoblastic leukemia, aplastic anemia, and immune deficiency syndromes.[8,9]

Pathophysiology and Complications

All candidates for heart, liver, and bone marrow transplantation have severe end-stage organ disease and would die without transplantation. Patients with end-stage renal disease can be kept alive by hemodialysis. However, the quality of their lives can be greatly improved by renal transplantation. Patients with severe diabetes may be kept alive with daily insulin injections, but their lives also may be greatly improved by pancreas transplantation.[8,9]

CLINICAL PRESENTATION

Signs and Symptoms

Signs and symptoms of the diseases for which transplantation is necessary are discussed in the chapters indicated:

- Advanced cardiac disease: Chapters 4, 5, and 6
- End-stage renal disease: Chapter 13
- Advanced liver disease: Chapter 11
- Advanced diabetes mellitus: Chapter 15
- Bone marrow transplantation: Chapters 23 and 24

Laboratory Findings

Laboratory findings of particular importance to the dentist who may be involved with patients before transplantation include bleeding time, differential white blood cell count, prothrombin time, hematocrit, partial thromboplastin time, blood urea nitrogen, aspartate aminotransaminase, serum creatinine, specific gravity of urine, platelet count, white blood cell (WBC) count, serum bilirubin, alkaline phosphatase, and testing of urine for proteins. Elevations in aspartate aminotransaminase, alkaline phosphatase, prothrombin time, and serum bilirubin would suggest advanced liver disease. Increased

TABLE 22-2
Screening Laboratory Tests Used to Evaluate Status of Kidney, Liver, Pancreas, and Bone Marrow Function*

Test	Normal Range	Abnormal Result	Organ Affected
COMPLETE BLOOD COUNT			
White blood cell count	4400 to 11,000/mL	Decreased	Bone marrow
Hematocrit (male)	41.5% to 50.4%		
Hematocrit (female)	35.9% to 44.6%		
Hemoglobin (male)	13.5 to 17.5 g/dL		
Hemoglobin (female)	12.3 to 15.3 g/dL		
Platelet count	150,000 to 450,000/μL		
DIFFERENTIAL BC			
Neutrophils	43% to 47%	Decreased	Bone marrow
Lymphocytes	17% to 47%		
Monocytes	0% to 9%		
Platelet count	150,000 to 450,000/μL	Less than 80,000/μL	
HEMOSTASIS			
PFA–100†	Closure < 175 seconds	Prolonged	Bone marrow, kidney
Prothrombin Time (PT)	10 to 13 seconds		
aPTT‡	25 to 35 seconds		
Thrombin Time (TT)	9 to 13 seconds		
SERUM CHEMISTRY			
Glucose (fasting)	70 to 110 mg/dL	>126 mg/dL	Pancreas
Glucose	<180 mg/dL	>200 mg/dL	Pancreas
Blood urea nitrogen (BUN)	8 to 23 mg/dL	Elevated	Kidney
Creatinine	0.6 to 1.2 mg/dL	Elevated	Kidney
SERUM ELECTROLYTES			
Sodium	136 to 142 mEq/L	Elevated	Kidney
Potassium	3.9 to 5.0 mEq/L		
Chloride	95 to 103 mEq/L		
SERUM ENZYMES			
Alkaline phosphatase	20 to 130 IU/L	Elevated	Liver
Alanine aminotransferase	4 to 36 μ/L	Elevated	Liver
Aspartate aminotransferase	8 to 33 μ/L	Elevated	Liver
Amylase	16 to 120 Somogyi units/dL	Elevated	Pancreas
URINALYSIS			
Specific gravity	1.0003 to 1.03	Elevated	Kidney
pH	4.8 to 7.5	Decreased	
Protein	None	Present	
Blood	None	Present	

Data compiled from McPherson RA, Pincus MR. Henry's Clinical diagnosis and management by laboratory methods, ed 21, Philadelphia, 2007, Saunders Elsevier, pp 1404-1418.
*Normal values may vary depending on the techniques used.
†Platelet function analyzer 100 (PFA – 100).
†Activated partial thromboplastin time (aPTT).

bleeding time, low platelet count, decreased WBC count, and decreased hematocrit are associated with many of the blood dyscrasias. Elevations in serum creatinine and blood urea nitrogen and increased specific gravity of urine and proteinuria are associated with advanced renal disease. In addition, a low hematocrit value, prolonged partial thromboplastin time, and decreased WBC count may be found in patients with advanced renal disease. Depending on which organ is involved, these patients may be potential bleeders, may be prone to infection, and may build up toxic levels of drugs that are metabolized by the liver or kidney (Table 22-2).[6,7,14]

MEDICAL AND SURGICAL MANAGEMENT
Immunosuppression

The immunosuppressive agents now used for most heart, liver, kidney, and pancreas transplantations are cyclospo-

TABLE **22-3**
Current Immunosuppressive Agents for Early Posttransplant Protocols[13]

Agent	Class	Mechanism of Action
Prednisone	Corticosteroid	Blocks cytokine gene transcription
Cyclosporine	Calcineurin inhibitor	Inhibits IL-2 gene transcription
		Reduces activation of T cells
Tacrolimus	Calcineurin inhibitor	Inhibits IL-2 gene transcription
		Reduces activation of T cells
Azathioprine	Nucleoside inhibitor	Impairs DNA synthesis
		Inhibits B-cell proliferation
Mycophenolate mofetil	Nucleoside inhibitor	Impairs DNA synthesis
		Inhibits B-cell proliferation
Rapamycin (sirolimus)	TOR inhibitor	Inhibits tyrosine kinase
Everolimus (RAD)	TOR inhibitor	Inhibits tyrosine kinase

IL, Interleukin; TOR, transplanted organ rejection.

rine, azathioprine, mycophenolate mofetil, prednisone, tacrolimus, sirolimus, everolimus, and an antilymphocyte agent (Table 22-3).[13]

Since the 1980s, cyclosporine has been the standard immunosuppressive drug used to prevent organ graft rejection. Antilymphocyte agents include the Minnesota antilymphocyte globulin, equine antithymocyte globulin, rabbit antithymocyte globulin, and Orthoclone monoclonal antibody. The best clinical results are attained with triple-drug immunosuppressive therapy—cyclosporine, prednisone, and azathioprine or mycophenolate mofetil (MMF). Antilymphocyte agents are used at the time of induction of immunosuppression and for acute rejection episodes. Tacrolimus is a xenobiotic immunosuppressive drug that has proved effective in the prevention of graft rejection. It is now used in organ transplantation recipients as a primary immunosuppressive drug or as a rescue drug in cases of therapy-resistant acute rejection. It seems to produce fewer adverse effects than other forms of immunosuppressive therapy. Immunosuppression regimens vary from center to center in terms of dosage, timing, and duration of use of the various agents. After transplantation, doses of the immunosuppressive agents are reduced as much as possible to prevent rejection of the graft.[3,8,9,14]

The anti–interleukin-2 antibodies (IL-2 R-α) daclizumab (humanized anti–IL-2 R-α) and basiliximab (chimeric anti–IL-2 R-α) have proved successful in furthering immunosuppression. Two other important new drugs are rapamycin (sirolimus) and everolimus (RAD), which are macrocyclic lactones that block IL-2 receptors and impair DNA synthesis and B-cell proliferation. Organ rejection and the need for antilymphocyte globulin have been reduced by sirolimus and everolimus.[3,13]

Total body irradiation (1000 cGy) has been the most effective means of conditioning a bone marrow graft recipient. Cyclophosphamide usually is used in the immunosuppressive phase before (4 to 5 days) transplantation. Busulfan also has been used for conditioning the graft recipient. Cyclosporine, prednisone, and methotrexate are used after marrow transplantation to prevent or ameliorate GVHD.[7]

Surgical Procedure

Heart Transplantation. Heart transplantation involves surgical removal of the heart from the donor by one surgical team and removal of the recipient's diseased heart and attachment of the donor's heart to the major vessels of the recipient's heart by a second surgical team (Figure 22-1). In addition to the immunosuppressive agents given to the recipient, other medications are given at the time of transplantation. These include agents such as dipyridamole (for platelet suppression), trimethoprim-sulfamethoxazole (to prevent infection), and nystatin (Mycostatin) (*Candida* prophylaxis). Surveillance right ventricular endomyocardial biopsies are performed after transplantation to check for signs of acute or chronic rejection. Starting 1 year after transplantation, coronary angiography often is performed to look for evidence of coronary artery disease.[8]

Heart/Lung Transplantation. In addition to the surgical protocol for cardiac transplantation, the lungs are generally combined in patients with primary pulmonary hypertension, pulmonary fibrosis, cystic fibrosis, certain congenital heart conditions, and primary cardiac disease accompanied by secondary pulmonary hypertension. Heart/lung transplantation involves surgical removal of the heart and lungs from the donor by one surgical team and removal of the recipient's diseased heart and lungs and attachment of the donor's heart and lungs to anastomotic sites at the trachea, the right atrium, and the aorta by the second surgical team (Figure 22-2). Typical immunosuppressive agents are used, as in heart transplantation.[8,15]

An additional complication, however, that may be seen in heart/lung combination transplantation is the implantation response. This particular complication most commonly occurs between 4 and 21 days after transplantation. It is a reversible condition that is characterized by fever, tachypnea, diffuse pulmonary infiltrates on chest radiography, decreased arterial oxygen pressure (pO_2), and increased arterial carbon dioxide pressure (pCO_2). This complication is caused by lymphatic interruption, ischemia, denervation, and surgical trauma. The patient may

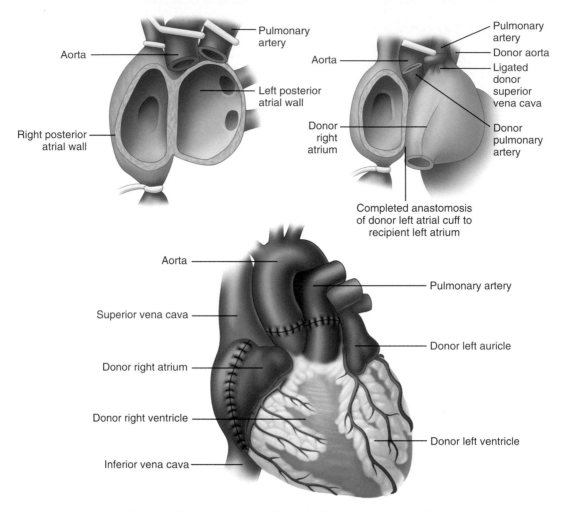

Figure 22-1. Orthotopic heart transplant. Through this procedure, a patient's atria and ventricles are completely replaced. (Redrawn from Am J Nurs 1980;80:1786.)

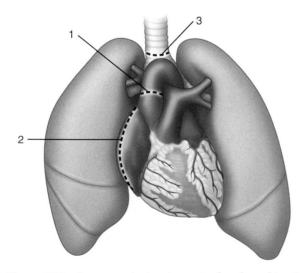

Figure 22-2. Anastomotic sites in a completed combination heart/lung transplantation. *1,* aorta; *2,* right atrium; *3,* trachea.

need short-term mechanical ventilation. Acute rejection of transplanted organs is a major complication and the most common cause of death within the first year.[8,15]

Liver Transplantation. Liver transplantation involves excision of the diseased recipient's liver, along with reconstruction of the vena cava, portal vein, and biliary tree (Figures 22-3 and 22-4). The transplant procedure is commonly divided into three phases[9]:

1. Dissection, during which the recipient's liver is dissected free of surrounding structures
2. Anhepatic phase, when blood flow through the vena cava, portal vein, and hepatic artery is interrupted (during this time, the recipient's liver is resected and the donor liver revascularized)
3. Reperfusion, by which the implanted donor's liver is filled with blood

The final step is biliary anastomosis.[12,15]

Liver transplantation has been performed in patients with hemophilia, and their factor VIII deficiency has been corrected. Therefore, factor VIII is produced by the liver and not by endothelial cells.

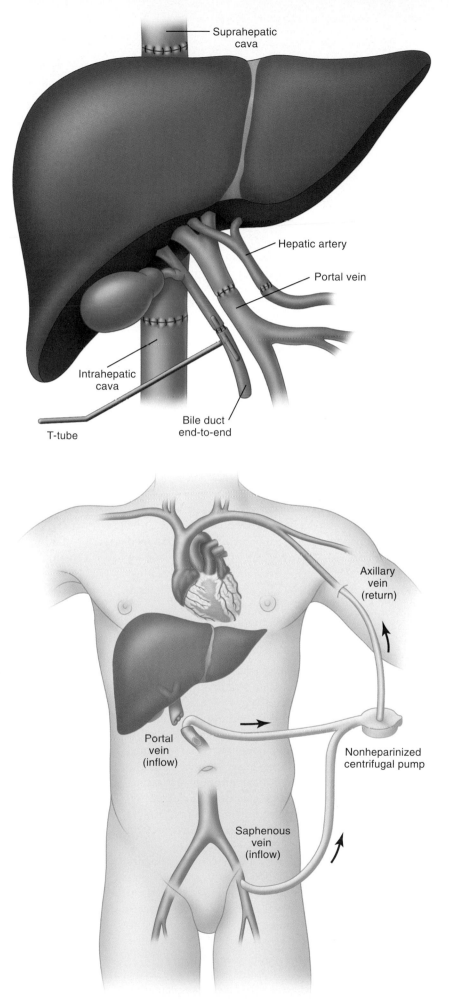

Figure 22-3. Completed liver transplant. Vascular anastomoses include the suprahepatic vena cava, infrahepatic vena cava, portal vein, and hepatic artery. A choledochocholedochostomy biliary reconstruction is depicted. (Redrawn from Howard TK, et al. Liver Transplantation. In Kaplowitz N [ed]. Liver and Biliary Diseases. Baltimore, Md, Williams & Wilkins, 1992.)

Suprahepatic cava

Hepatic artery

Portal vein

Intrahepatic cava

Bile duct end-to-end

T-tube

Figure 22-4. Venovenous bypass. The portal vein is divided, and devascularization of the liver is completed. Then, the portal vein is cannulated, and a second cannula is placed inside the iliac vein via the saphenous vein. The blood is pumped by a centrifugal pump through a nonheparinized system and is returned to the patient via a cannula placed in the axillary vein. Flows of 2 to 5 L/min are commonly attained. Flow must be maintained at above 700 to 1000 mL/min to prevent thrombosis. (Redrawn from Howard TK, et al. Liver Transplantation. In Kaplowitz N [ed]. Liver and Biliary Diseases. Baltimore, Md, Williams & Wilkins, 1992.)

Axillary vein (return)

Portal vein (inflow)

Nonheparinized centrifugal pump

Saphenous vein (inflow)

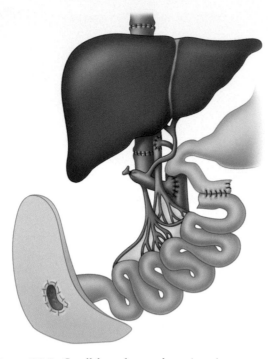

Figure 22-5. Small-bowel transplantation. Anastomoses are at the superior end of the small intestine at the jejunum, and the terminus is exteriorized in a stoma. Here, the liver also has been transplanted. (Redrawn from Asfar S, Zhong R, Grant D. Surg Clin North Am 1994;74:1197-1207.)

Small-Bowel Transplantation. Few small-bowel transplantations (SBTs) have been performed. Because of its quasi-experimental nature, SBT currently is performed only in patients with end-stage intestinal failure for whom conventional treatment has been unsuccessful. Intestinal failure is characterized by the inability to maintain a balance between nutrition and intestinal fluids and electrolytes. Several causes of this condition have been identified, the most common of which is massive small-bowel resection and the "short gut syndrome," which causes rapid intestinal transit without proper absorption of nutrients. This condition is diagnosed in nearly 2 million patients per year in the United States. SBT is commonly performed in conjunction with liver transplantation. The small bowel is unique among solid organ transplant grafts because of the large amount of lymphoid tissue contained in the mesenteric lymph nodes, Peyer's patches, and the lamina propria, and the heavy colonization that occurs with microorganisms and large quantities of antigens on the surface of the intestinal epithelium. These factors contribute to high rates of GVHD, graft rejection, and sepsis.[16]

The surgical technique for SBT is shown in Figure 22-5. The transplanted small bowel has anastomotic sites at the superior end of the native gastrointestinal tract at the jejunum, and at its distal end, a stoma is created exteriorly. The superior mesenteric artery is attached to the native aorta below the renal arteries.[16]

Kidney Transplantation. Patients who have a living related donor who is available for kidney transplantation

---

BOX 22-1

Signs of Overimmunosuppression in Posttransplantation Patients

- Viral infections (HSV, CMV, HBV, HIV)
- Bacterial infections (respiratory, wound, etc.)
- Fungal infections (candidiasis, pulmonary, etc.)
- Delayed healing
- Excessive bleeding
- Hypertension
- Cushingoid reaction (edema, ascites, etc.)
- Addison's reaction (adverse reaction to stress, etc.)
- Diabetes mellitus
- Anemia
- Osteoporosis
- Tumors

HSV, Herpes simplex virus, CMV, cytomegalovirus; HBV, hepatitis B virus; HIV, human immunodeficiency virus.

---

usually are admitted to the hospital 2 days before transplantation. When a kidney recipient is to receive a cadaver kidney, the patient is admitted to the hospital on an urgent basis. Current preservation techniques allow kidney storage for up to 72 hours.[17]

Indications for renal transplantation generally include chronic renal disease and end-stage renal disease (ESRD). ESRD is a progressive, bilateral deterioration of kidney nephrons that results in uremia and, ultimately, death. ESRD is associated with glomerulonephritis, nephrosclerosis, pyelonephritis, diabetic nephropathy, congenital renal disorders, drug-induced nephropathy, obstructive uropathy, and hypertension.[18]

Accompanying hypertension, diabetes, congestive heart failure, infection, volume depletion, urinary tract obstruction, hypercalcemia, and hyperuricemia must be constantly managed. After conservative care (e.g., drug therapy, dietary restrictions, treatment of underlying disease) provided to control waste products, fluid balance, and electrolyte levels becomes inadequate, renal dialysis is the next step. As renal disease progresses and more nephrons are destroyed, azotemia cannot be controlled, and the patient's blood must be artificially filtered. Thus, peritoneal dialysis or hemodialysis begins.[6,18]

More than 80,000 patients in the United States are currently being maintained on hemodialysis. Hemodialysis treatment must be provided every 2 to 3 days, and 4 to 5 hours is required for each treatment. The costs in terms of time, money, inconvenience, and so forth are enormous and extremely confining (see Chapter 13). An alternative to dialysis is transplantation of a kidney from a living donor or from a cadaver. Transplantation frees the patient from the burden of dialysis and from most of the chronic consequences of ESRD. Renal transplantation has become a standard surgical procedure in most major hospitals.[6,18]

As with all major transplant procedures, the major problem in renal transplantation is rejection of the graft. Recipients of a kidney transplant require immunosuppressive preparation so that they will not reject the graft.

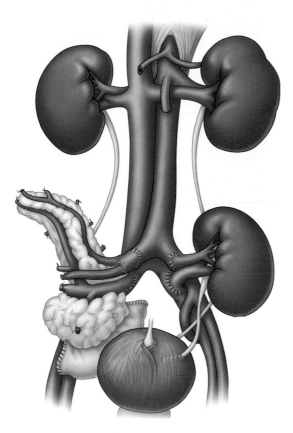

Figure 22-6. Pancreaticoduodenocystostomy. Combined kidney and pancreas transplants. (Redrawn from Groshek M, Smith VL. In Norris MK, House MA [eds]. Organ and Tissue Transplantation. Philadelphia, FA Davis, 1991, p 159.)

The type of preparation provided depends on the nature of the underlying renal disease. Intensive chemotherapy is commonly used. Chemotherapy with cytotoxic agents (azathioprine) or steroids (prednisone) and administration of antilymphocytic globulin (ALG) are effective. However, greater success has been attained when cyclosporine is used instead of prednisone or azathioprine.[6,18]

With immunosuppression, the patient is rendered susceptible to infection and poor wound healing. Sepsis is a major complication in renal transplant recipients. Adrenal function may be suppressed, as is endogenous cortisol production (Box 22-1).

In addition to immunosuppressive medications, the patient receives a bladder injection of antibiotic solution by means of a Foley catheter and a second generation cephalosporin. The donor renal artery usually is anastomosed to the aorta and the renal vein to the vena cava in children. In adults, the renal artery is anastomosed to the internal or the external iliac artery. After the kidneys have been reperfused, urethral implantation is performed. Antibiotics that were begun just before surgery are stopped 3 days after surgery, and the patient is given trimethoprim-sulfamethoxazole (Bactrim) daily for as long as the graft is functioning. Acyclovir and nystatin usually are given for the first 3 months to prevent herpes simplex virus (HSV), cytomegalovirus (CMV), and *Candida* infection.[6,18]

Pancreas Transplantation. Pancreas transplantation can be done:
- Simultaneously with kidney transplantation (Figure 22-6)
- After kidney transplantation
- As a separate procedure (Figures 22-7 and 22-8).

Living related donor grafts usually are used for recipients of pancreas transplants alone or of a pancreas transplant after a previous kidney transplant. However, cadaver grafts may be transplanted to all recipient categories. Cadaver donor pancreas grafts can be preserved by cold storage in a silica gel–filtered plasma solution for about 10 to 24 hours. In most grafts, the pancreatic duct is drained into the bladder. Urine amylase levels (25% reduction) are used in bladder-drained patients to monitor for rejection. Decreased urinary amylase activity precedes hyperglycemia as a manifestation of rejection. In patients who simultaneously receive kidney and pancreas transplants, an increase in serum creatinine indicates the possible onset of rejection before changes in urinary amylase are detected.[19]

A relatively new and revolutionary technique that may have far-reaching implications for the management of diabetes is transplantation of islet cells from a donor's pancreas into the liver of the recipient. Patient response to transplanted beta cells has helped in many cases of diabetes. One impediment to the success of this technique has been the occurrence of immune attacks from the recipient on transplanted donor cells. However, this technique certainly holds much promise for the future.[20]

Bone Marrow Transplantation. Patients who are going to undergo BMT are prepared with the use of different preoperative regimens, in accordance with the level of disease. The greatest chance for successful BMT occurs in patients with chronic myelogenous leukemia. Commonly, patients with aplastic anemia, lymphoma, Hodgkin's disease, neuroblastoma, or genetic diseases (e.g., immunodeficiency, Hurler's syndrome) undergo BMT as well. Chronic myelogenous leukemia is 100% fatal without BMT, but BMT is approximately 60% to 70% successful. Acute myelogenous leukemia is 40% to 60% curable, and acute lymphoblastic leukemia has a 20% to 25% cure rate. Cyclophosphamide and total body irradiation or busulfan may be used for patients with leukemia. Patients with a lymphoma may be given cyclophosphamide and total body irradiation, busulfan and cyclophosphamide, or busulfan alone. Patients with aplastic anemia may be given cyclophosphamide alone. The preoperative regimens start 7 to 10 days before transplantation. At transplantation, the donor's marrow is infused into the recipient.

The recipient of a syngeneic marrow graft (from an identical twin) requires no immunosuppressive preparation. Similarly, the patient with severe immunologic deficiency requires no immunosuppressive preparation because of the very nature of the disease. However, all other recipients of BMT must undergo some form of immunosuppressive therapy so that they will not reject

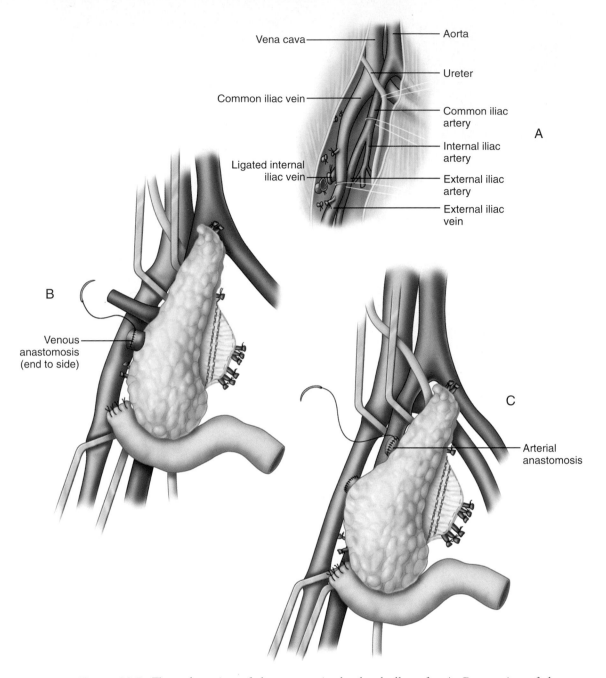

Figure 22-7. Transplantation of the pancreaticoduodenal allografts. **A,** Preparation of the recipient vessels. Note that all deep branches of the common and external iliac veins are ligated and divided. The vein is brought lateral to the artery. The ureter is mobilized and is brought medial to the artery. **B,** The venous anastomosis is performed end-to-side, with the portal vein of the pancreas graft anastomosed to the proximal external or distal common iliac vein. **C,** The arterial anastomosis is performed after the venous anastomosis and is placed superior to the venous anastomosis. The common iliac artery of the recipient is used as the site of the arterial anastomosis. (Redrawn from Brayman KL, et al. In Cameron JL [ed]. Current Surgical Therapy, 4th ed. St. Louis, Mosby, 1992, p 466.)

the graft. The type of preparation depends on the nature of the underlying disease. BMT is not a cure for cancer. Intensive chemotherapy or total body irradiation kills the cancer. However, these treatments also may kill the patient, so BMT may be used to "rescue" the patient from the lethal effects of chemoradiation therapy. Marrow is harvested from the donor's iliac bones through numer-

ous needle aspirations with the patient under spinal anesthesia in an operating room environment. The typical quantity of marrow obtained per needle aspiration is 1 to 3 mL (between 400 and 800 mL is required).[21] Generally, the procedure is well tolerated and involves few complications. In nonmalignant conditions (e.g., aplastic anemia), preparation of the recipient can be directed

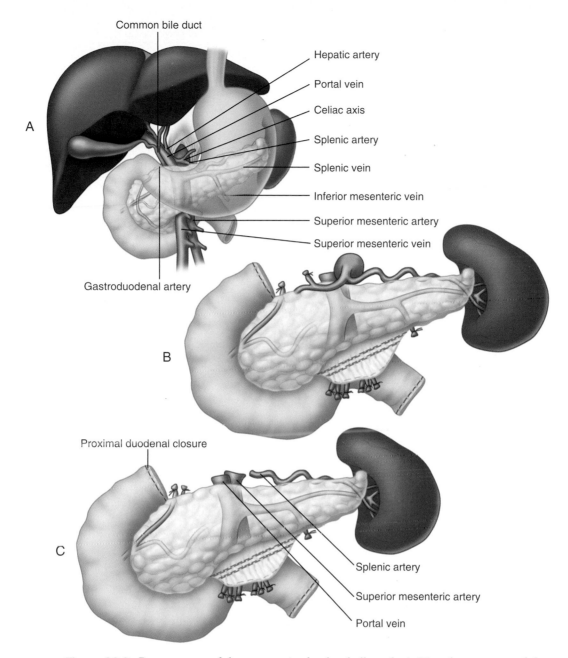

Figure 22-8. Procurement of the pancreaticoduodenal allograft. **A,** Vascular anatomy of the liver and pancreas. Note the gastroduodenal artery, which is divided during simultaneous procurement of the liver and the pancreas but not during procurement of the pancreas alone. **B,** Pancreaticoduodenal allograft following procurement (nonliver donor). Note that the proximal duodenum has been divided with the gastrointestinal anastomosis (GIA) stapler. The mesentery of the small intestine inferior to the pancreas also has been ligated and divided following placement of two parallel rows of TA 90 staples. **C,** Pancreaticoduodenal allograft after procurement from a donor whose liver also was procured. Note the splenic and superior mesenteric arteries, which require ex vivo reconstruction. (Redrawn from Brayman KL, et al. In Cameron JL [ed]. Current Surgical Therapy, 4th ed. St. Louis, Mosby, 1992, p 461.)

solely toward the problem of immunosuppression without worry about destruction of cancerous cells. In malignant disorders, however, specifically, acute myelogenous leukemia, preparation of the recipient must accomplish immunosuppression while killing all or nearly all of the malignant leukemic cells. Total body irradiation (1000 cGy) has been the most effective means of conditioning a bone marrow graft recipient. Cyclophospha-mide (50 mg/kg) is used during the immunosuppressive phase prior (4 to 5 days) to transplantation.[21]

Histocompatibility. Matching of blood type and human lymphocyte antigens (HLAs) with tissue compatibility tests usually results in longer graft and patient survival. The best matching occurs in identical twins; however, with appropriate screening tests, acceptable matches can be found for other potential organ recipients and living or cadaver donors.

Syngeneic or isogeneic human marrow transplantation involves donors and recipients who carry the same tissue antigens, as occurs in identical twins. Consequently, no immunologic barrier exists to transplantation. An autologous marrow graft refers to transplantation of the patient's own marrow, which has been harvested from the same patient and set aside before intense chemotherapy or total radiation therapy, until it is used for transplantation. An allogeneic marrow graft involves a donor and a recipient of different genetic origin within the same species (usually 50% to 70% of transplants). Siblings are the best candidates for a partial match (haploidentical), or parents may donate the marrow (they provide usually 30% to 50% of BMTs). Allogeneic grafts also may involve unrelated donors (usually 10% to 15%). These transplants involve moderate to severe histoincompatibility and present a bidirectional immunologic barrier to transplantation. The recipient may react adversely to the donated marrow and reject it, or infused marrow cells from the donor transplant, which contain immunologically competent cells, may react against the host to produce GVHD.[21,22]

In humans, the major histocompatibility complex (H-2) involves two closely associated serologically detected loci—the first, or "LA" locus, and the second, or "4" locus (HLA-A4). Marrow grafts between unrelated humans carry a high probability of major histocompatibility problems because of the complex polymorphism of the histocompatibility complex. Members of the same family, however, simplify the situation considerably, because only four haplotypes may be involved. HLA typing of the family can therefore reveal the most ideal donor.[7,21,22]

Before the grafting procedure begins, almost all marrow recipients undergo a period of no marrow function because of their underlying disease and immunosuppressive preparation. After the transplant, 10 to 20 days elapse before the transplanted marrow begins to function. Naturally, this is a critical period for the patient's recovery and for success of the BMT. The posttransplant period consists of three phases of recovery: the pancytopenic phase (absolute neutrophil count greater than 500 for 4 to 6 weeks), the immune recovery phase (3 to 12 months), and the long-term immunocompetent phase (1 to 3 years). Most patients are given cyclosporine, methotrexate, or steroids after transplantation. Patients who test positive for HSV are given prophylactic intravenous (IV) acyclovir. Patients usually are given an antifungal medication such as IV miconazole to prevent *Candida* infection. These medications are continued after bone marrow transplantation throughout the critical period needed for the transplanted marrow to begin functioning. This critical period may last up to 20 days or longer. Once the transplanted marrow starts to function, the risk of infection is decreased. However, long-term therapy with broad-spectrum antibiotics such as Bactrim is needed to reduce the risk of infection. Patients who develop evidence of GVHD are treated with methotrexate.[7,21,22]

BOX 22-2

Major Medical Complications Associated With Transplantation

- Excessive immunosuppression
- Infection
- Tumors
- Delayed healing
- Rejection of allograft
- Graft failure—heart, kidney, liver, pancreas
- Increased risk for excessive bleeding—liver, kidney, bone marrow
- Overdosage—if drugs are metabolized or excreted by kidney or liver, they are administered in normal amounts
- Death or retransplantation—heart, liver, bone marrow
- Insulin, hemodialysis, or retransplantation—kidney, pancreas
- Adverse effects caused by immunosuppressive agents
- Hypertension
- Diabetes mellitus
- Infection
- Excessive bleeding
- Anemia
- Osteoporosis
- Adrenal crisis (significant stress from surgery, trauma)
- Special organ complications
- Heart transplants—accelerated coronary artery atherosclerosis, cardiac valvulopathy
- Bone marrow transplants—graft-versus-host disease

Complications

Complications associated with organ transplantation generally consist of technical problems involving the surgical procedure, problems related to immunosuppression, and special problems specific to the organ transplanted. Discussion of surgical complications is beyond the scope of this text and would seldom apply to the dentist's management of such patients (Box 22-2).

Immunosuppression

Excessive immunosuppression increases the risk for infection and must be avoided. Invasive (biopsy) and noninvasive techniques are used to assess patients for signs of excessive immunosuppression. Clinical evidence of such immunosuppression consists of opportunistic infection and tumors known to be related to these agents. When evidence of excessive immunosuppression is found, dosages of immunosuppressant drugs must be reduced (see Table 22-3). This of course must be done only in collaboration with the patient's physician.

Of course, signs of overimmunosuppression may occur in all types of transplant patients. These signs include infection, delayed healing, hypertension, diabetes, Addison's reactions, cushingoid reactions (e.g., edema, ascites,

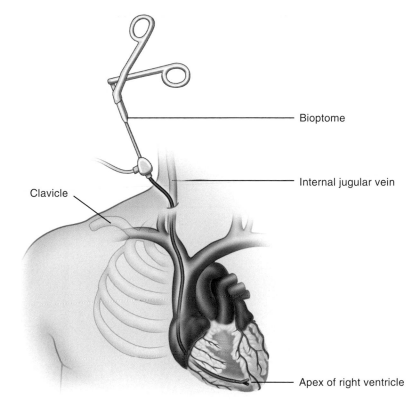

Figure 25-9. Endomyocardial biopsy technique showing the bioptome in place in the right ventricle. (Redrawn from Copeland JG, Stinson EB. Curr Probl Cardiol 1979;4:1-5.)

Bioptome

Internal jugular vein

Clavicle

Apex of right ventricle

buffalo hump, moon facies), increased susceptibility to infection, weakness, and fatigue (see Box 22-1).

Rejection

Rejection of the transplanted organ is apparent when signs and symptoms of organ failure begin to occur. Organ biopsies are used to confirm the rejection reaction (Figure 22-9). When evidence of acute rejection is found, dosages of immunosuppressive agents usually are increased.

Chronic rejection occurs insidiously and is progressive. It cannot be reversed through intensified therapy. Chronic rejection of the organ graft is associated with signs and symptoms of organ failure. Classic evidence of chronic rejection is found by means of biopsy.

Drug Adverse Effects

Agents used for immunosuppression have several important adverse effects. A major adverse effect of azathioprine is bone marrow suppression with resultant leukopenia, thrombocytopenia, and anemia. These changes place the patient at greater risk for infection and excessive bleeding. Cyclosporine has replaced azathioprine as the key agent for immunosuppression in transplant patients because it does not suppress the bone marrow. However, cyclosporine does have important adverse effects. It may cause severe kidney and liver changes, which can lead to hypertension, bleeding problems, and anemia; it also may potentiate renal injury caused by other agents. Cyclosporine also is related to an increased incidence of gingival hyperplasia, hirsutism, gynecomastia, and cancer of the skin and cervix. Antithy-

mocyte globulin (ATG) and ALG both act as lymphocyte-selective immunosuppressants. Important adverse effects associated with these agents include fever, hemolysis, leukopenia, thrombocytopenia, tumor development, and increased risk for infection.[6-9,14]

Prednisone has important adverse effects, including hypertension, diabetes mellitus, osteoporosis, impaired healing, mental depression, psychoses, and increased risk for infection (see Chapter 16 for adverse effects of corticosteroids). In addition to these adverse effects, prednisone therapy may cause adrenal gland suppression. If adrenal suppression occurs, the patient is unable to produce and release increased amounts of steroids needed to deal with the stress of infection, trauma, surgery, or extreme anxiety.[21]

An increased incidence of certain cancers is seen in immunosuppressed patients. Overall, approximately 6% of these patients develop various forms of cancer. Cancers commonly seen in the general population (carcinomas of lung, breast, prostate, and colon) show no change in occurrence in immunosuppressed patients. However, two types of cancer found commonly in the general population are found with increased frequency in immunosuppressed patients: squamous cell carcinoma of the skin and in situ carcinoma of the uterine cervix. Cancers that are uncommon in the general population but that occur with increased frequency in immunosuppressed patients are lymphoma, lip carcinoma, Kaposi's sarcoma, carcinoma of the kidney, and carcinoma of the vulva and perineum (Table 22-4). Cancer is a complication of intense immunosuppression per se and is not related to the use of any particular agent.

TABLE 22-4
Cancer Development in the General Population and in Transplant Patients

Tumor	General Population, %	Transplant Patients, %
Lymphoma	<5.3	20
Lip carcinoma	<0.3	28
Kaposi's sarcoma	<0.1	26
Carcinoma of kidney	2.1	25
Carcinoma of vulva and perineum	<0.6	2

From Najarian JS, Sutherland DER. Transplant Proc 1992;24: 1293-1296.

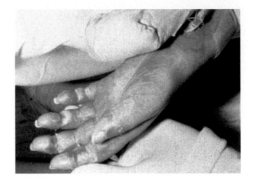

Figure 22-11. Graft-versus-host disease (GVHD) in a bone marrow transplant patient. Note areas of necrosis. (Courtesy Norma Ramsay, University of Minnesota Hospital.)

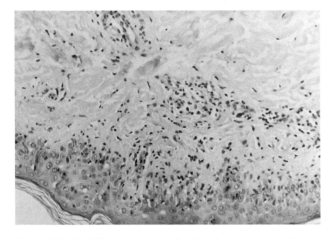

Figure 22-10. Photomicrograph of graft-versus-host disease (GVHD) in a post–bone marrow transplantation (BMT) patient.

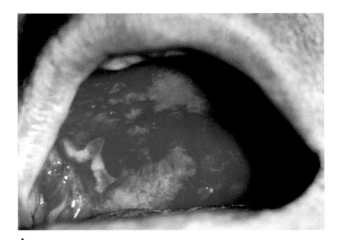

A

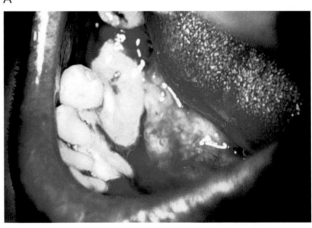

B

Figure 22-12. Oral mucositis/candidiasis in bone marrow transplantation (BMT). **A,** Hard and soft palate. **B,** Gingiva and floor of the mouth. (Courtesy Norma Ramsay, University of Minnesota Hospital.)

However, certain agents may play a more direct role. Cyclosporine is one of these agents, as are monoclonal antibodies. Both of these agents are associated with a higher incidence of lymphoma. Such lymphomas tend to occur earlier and to show greater nodal involvement.[21,23]

Special Organ Complications

Major specific organ complications of immunosuppression involve the heart and bone marrow. Recent improvements in immunosuppressant agents have not altered the development of graft coronary artery disease. In one study, the incidence of coronary artery disease in transplanted patients was 10% at 1 year, 25% at 3 years, and 36% at 5 years. Coronary artery disease was responsible for 60% of late deaths.[6-9] Cardiac valvulopathy may occur in transplanted hearts (see Chapter 2).

GVHD is an important and often lethal complication of allogeneic bone marrow transplantation. Acute GVHD occurs within the first 2 months after transplantation and is characterized by skin, liver, and gastrointestinal tract involvement (Figures 22-10, 22-11, and 22-12). Chronic GVHD occurs later and is characterized by skin changes similar to scleroderma, sicca syndrome, malabsorption, and features of autoimmunity. Cyclosporine appears to be more effective than methotrexate in preventing GVHD in HLA-identical siblings who have received a bone marrow transplant for severe aplastic anemia. Methotrexate appears to be more effective for acute leukemia.[6-9]

DENTAL MANAGEMENT
Pretransplant Medical Considerations

A number of significant medical problems must be considered during the dental treatment of patients who are being prepared for transplantation. First, the patient will have significant end-organ disease from the organ system, which is necessitating the transplant. The problems associated with advanced coronary artery disease, significant cardiac arrhythmias, and congestive heart failure are discussed in Chapters 4, 5, and 6. Medical considerations that affect the dental treatment of patients with renal failure and end-stage liver disease are discussed in Chapters 11 and 13. Medical considerations that affect dental treatment for patients with severe diabetes who are being considered for pancreas and kidney transplantation are covered in Chapters 13 and 15. Therefore, the dentist must treat the pretransplant patient as indicated for severe medical complications from the particular organ system.[6-9]

Secondly, a thorough dental evaluation will be necessary and required by most transplant centers for diagnosis and treatment of any existing dental disease, particularly any infection or oral condition that could result in an infection or in the need for oral surgery during the immediate posttransplant phase, when the patient will be immunocompromised and highly susceptible to infection. Immediately post transplant and for several weeks thereafter, the patient will be extremely immunosuppressed from induction immunosuppression, which will be directed to prevent graft rejection. Therefore, the potential for morbidity is extremely high and could result in devastating consequences.[14]

Obviously, a consultation with the transplant surgeon and/or team will be important for precise determination of the patient's physical status and details of the procedure, as well as the likelihood of posttransplant complications such as infection. Infection is a very serious concern in the transplant patient, and any potential source of infection during the posttransplant period must be identified and eliminated. Because protocols vary from one transplant center to another, no standard protocol applies. In many instances, transplant physicians and medical insurance request that the dental evaluation be performed as medically necessary and as an "inpatient" service.

Further, it is best to avoid the need for any dental treatment for about 6 months post transplant because of the many potential complications aside from infection, such as fatigue, medication interactions, and adverse effects, as well as inadvertent saliva aspiration leading to aspiration pneumonia.[14] The patient who is a candidate for a bone marrow transplant is generally very ill and prone to infection, bleeding, and delayed healing because of thrombocytopenia and leukopenia (see Chapter 24).

Dental treatment may be a very difficult process because patients preparing to undergo an organ or bone marrow transplant may have poor dental health and/or a history of infrequent dental visits. The ideal treatment plan should restore the patient to optimal oral health prior to surgery; therefore, it may need to be expeditious in that the transplant surgery may be imminent (less than 1 week away). Past dental history, as well as prognosis and attitudes toward maintenance of oral health, may strongly influence the scenario of aggressive treatment prior to

transplantation. Other factors that may affect the treatment plan include financial concerns, the patient's ability to tolerate dental procedures and to access dental care post transplant, the patient's general medical stability, and the constraints of the organ donor. Priority must be given to the patient's overall medical status and the ultimate success of the transplant.[14]

Posttransplant Medical Considerations

Medical considerations of importance to the dentist in management of the transplanted patient fall into three stages:
1. Immediate posttransplant period
2. Stable transplant period
3. Chronic rejection period[6-9]

During the immediate posttransplant period, which is generally the first 3 months after transplantation, the patient is started on immunosuppressive therapy to prevent cytotoxic T cells from destroying the graft. This is the time that the patient is at greatest risk for technical complications, acute rejection, and infection. The length of this period will vary, depending on a number of factors. Cyclosporine, prednisone, and other immunosuppressive agents (e.g., azathioprine, antilymphocyte globulin) have great benefit in enhancing survival and preventing rejection in posttransplant patients. However, these agents also have significant major adverse effects and place the patient at substantial risk for infection. Also, many drugs exist that may adversely interact with cyclosporine and other immunosuppressive agents, including several used by dentists (e.g., erythromycin, ketoconazole, carbamazepine, phenytoin). The dentist must consult with the patient's physician to confirm the patient's status and the level and severity of immunosuppression, and to determine whether the patient has progressed beyond this critical stage.

Medical complications are relatively common during the immediate posttransplant period. The patient may have acute respiratory distress syndrome; viral, bacterial, and fungal infections of varying types and severity; bleeding problems; hypertension; acute renal and or hepatic failure; acute pancreatitis; and other problems. For these reasons, during the first 3 months after organ transplantation, the patient should undergo only emergency dental treatment, and elective procedures should be postponed. Even emergency dental treatment must be provided in close association with the patient's physician(s). Antibiotic prophylaxis may be used during this time because of immunosuppression and the increased risk for infection. The types of agents and the regimen for this antibiotic prophylaxis are special for transplant patients and are presented in Table 22-5.[6-9]

The next stage is the period when the graft is stable and functional. In most cases, this occurs approximately 3 months post transplantation. The patient has undergone graft healing and the new organ should be functioning nearly normally. In most cases, coagulation factors, susceptibility to bleeding, and blood chemistry profiles will have returned to normal limits, although this should be confirmed by the patient's physician. Medical

TABLE **22-5**

Recommended Standard Prophylactic Regimen for Dental/Oral Procedures in the Posttransplant Patient (only when prophylactic antibiotics are indicated*)

Medication	Regimen
Amoxicillin	2 g orally 1 hour before the procedure
plus metronidazole, Amoxicillin-penicillin allergy*	500 mg orally 1 hour before procedure
Vancomycin 1 g IV	Infused slowly over 1 hour preoperatively
or	
Imipenem 1 g IV	Infused slowly over 1 hour preoperatively
Unable to take oral medication	
Ampicillin	2 g intravenously 1 hour before procedure
plus metronidazole	500 mg intravenously 1 hour before procedure

*For the prevention of spontaneous bacterial peritonitis.
Note: Clindamycin should not be used in most organ transplant patients because of acute liver toxicity.

considerations during this stage relate to the effects of immunosuppressive agents. The patient will continue to be susceptible to infection, but now, the major concern is overimmunosuppression, which increases the risk for infection, and underimmunosuppression, which increases the risk for acute rejection. If rejection of the graft occurs, the organ begins to fail, and the problems associated with end-stage heart, liver, kidney, and pancreas failure will have to be considered and managed when present.

Adverse effects of immunosuppressive agents may present significant medical problems during any of the stages after transplantation. However, those occurring during the stable graft stage are of greatest concern to the dentist. These adverse effects may increase the risk for infection; excessive bleeding; bone fracture; circulatory collapse after significant emotional, physical, or surgical stress; hypertension; diabetes mellitus; and anemia.[6-9,14]

Posttransplant patients are also particularly susceptible to fungal infection, especially with *Candida albicans*. Therefore, prevention and aggressive management with antifungal agents should be considered. Special organ complications observed in heart and bone marrow transplant recipients must be considered during the stable graft period. Symptomatic coronary artery disease develops in many heart transplantation patients. However, one important clinical feature of coronary insufficiency or myocardial infarction is missing in these patients. The transplanted heart has no nerve supply; thus, pain is not associated with angina or infarction.

BMT patients may develop GVHD after undergoing transplantation. Acute GVHD occurs during the immediate posttransplant period, whereas the chronic form of the disease may appear during the stable period. The patient is particularly susceptible to community-based infection, such as influenza and pneumonia, so precautions such as vaccination should be taken to prevent those from occurring.

The chronic rejection period begins with signs and symptoms usually associated with organ failure, along with histologic findings on biopsy indicating chronic rejection of the graft. This reaction is not reversible and will lead to retransplantation or death in heart and liver recipients. Kidney patients will require dialysis or retransplantation. Pancreas patients will require insulin or retransplantation.[6-9,14]

TREATMENT PLANNING CONSIDERATIONS

Pretransplant Patients

Patients who are being prepared for transplantation should be referred for an evaluation of their dental status. Whenever possible, patients found to have active dental disease should receive indicated dental care before the transplant operation. Patients with advanced periodontal disease may best be advised to have their teeth extracted and dentures constructed. The same consideration would be involved for patients who have extensive caries and have demonstrated little interest in improving, or ability to improve, their level of oral hygiene or to modify their diet.

Patients who have a very good level of dental health should be encouraged to keep their teeth, but they must be advised of the risks and problems involved if significant dental disease were to develop after transplantation. The need for effective preventive dental procedures and more frequent recall visits to the dentist after transplantation must be pointed out to the patient.

Recommendations concerning retention of teeth for patients who have a dental status that falls between the extremes of poor and very good are more difficult to make. The risks involved regarding infection, the steps needed to prevent these complications, and associated costs must be discussed with the patient and the transplant surgeon. Patients with poor oral hygiene who have failed to become motivated to improve their level of home care should be encouraged to consider extraction of teeth and construction of dentures.[6-9,14]

Before transplantation, all nonrestorable teeth and teeth with advanced periodontal disease should be extracted in those patients who decide to retain their dentition. Nonvital teeth should be endodontically treated or extracted, and all active carious lesions should be restored

TABLE **22-6**

Common Dental Drugs Metabolized Primarily by the Liver and Kidney That Therefore Should Be Avoided or Adjusted Before Dental Treatment

Drug Dosage	OK to Use Normal	Dose Adjustment
Lidocaine (Xylocaine)	Yes	Increase interval between doses (avoid if possible)
Acetaminophen (Tylenol)	No	Increase interval between doses (avoid if possible)
Ibuprofen (Motrin)	Yes	n/a
Propoxyphene (Darvon)	Yes	n/a
Codeine	Yes	n/a
Meperidine (Demerol)	Yes	n/a
Penicillin V	No	Increase interval between doses
Erythromycin	Yes	n/a
Cephalexin (Keflex)	No	Increase interval between doses
Tetracycline (Doxycycline)	No	Increase interval between doses (avoid if possible)
Diazepam (Valium)	Yes	n/a

Modified from Bennet WM, et al. Am J Kidney Dis 1983;3:155-176.

in these patients. Preventive dentistry techniques, including toothbrushing and flossing, diet modification, and the use of topical fluorides, should be initiated, reviewed, and implemented. The importance of using effective hygiene procedures, including antiseptic mouth rinses such as chlorhexidine or Listerine, and the need for maintenance of good oral hygiene must be emphasized.[14]

Before invasive dental procedures are performed on the patient, before transplantation, the dentist must consult with the patient's physician to establish the degree of organ dysfunction, the need for prophylactic antibiotics to prevent local or distant infection, the ability of the patient to tolerate dental treatment, and the need to obtain other management suggestions. In most cases, the earlier that most dental treatment is performed before the transplantation, the better.[6-9,14]

No data exist to show that prophylactic antibiotics are indicated in the dental management of patients with advanced heart, liver, kidney, and pancreatic disease unless patients are otherwise subject to endocarditis or endarteritis (heart or kidney patients on hemodialysis) (see Chapter 2). Although another group of patients are immunosuppressed, that is, those with acquired immunodeficiency syndrome (AIDS), no data suggest that prophylactic antibiotics are indicated. The need for prophylactic antibiotic treatment for invasive dental procedures in patients with advanced heart, liver, kidney, or bone marrow disease (or any immunosuppressed patient) should be discussed with the patient's physician before treatment is provided.[6-9,14]

Results of selective screening tests shown in Table 22-2 should be reviewed. If they are not available through medical consultation, they should be ordered before any invasive dental procedure is performed. If the screening tests reveal significant alterations in bleeding time and/or coagulation status (prothrombin time, thrombin time, and activated partial thromboplastin time), the dentist should consider using antifibrinolytic agents, fresh frozen plasma, vitamin K, and platelet replacement. Selection of

the approach should be based on consultation with the patient's physician. The physician also should be consulted regarding drug selection and dosage modification.[6-9,14]

To prevent increased or unexpected effects in patients with end-stage liver or kidney disease, the dentist should not use drugs that are metabolized by these organs or for which the dosage is reduced (Table 22-6). Patients with severe diabetes mellitus must be managed as described in Chapter 15. If infection is present, an increase in insulin dosage may be required. Again, the dentist should consult with the patient's physician to confirm the patient's current status and specific management needs (Box 22-3).

Posttransplant Patients

Dental management of the patient after transplantation can be divided into three phases (Box 22-4):

1. Immediate posttransplant period
2. Stable graft period
3. Chronic rejection period or, in bone marrow transplants, the onset of significant GVHD

Immediate Posttransplant Period. During this phase, when operative complications and acute rejection of the graft are the major medical concerns, no routine dentistry is indicated. Only emergency dental care should be provided, after medical consultation, and it should be as noninvasive as possible.[6-9,14]

Stable Posttransplant Period. Once the graft has healed and the acute rejection reaction has been controlled, the patient is considered to be in the stable phase. This period should be confirmed by medical consultation with the transplant surgeon. Usually, any indicated dental treatment can be performed during this period if the procedures shown in Box 22-4 are adhered to completely. Many of the dental management problems with stable graft patients are similar, regardless of the organ that was transplanted. However, some problems are unique to patients with specific transplanted organs.[6-9,14]

BOX 22-3

Dental Management of the Patient Being Prepared for Transplantation

- Consultation with physician(s)

KEY POINTS

Complete dental evaluation
1. Poor dental status—consider extractions and dentures
2. Good dental status—maintain dentition
3. Other—decide on individual patient basis

Patients maintaining their dentition
1. Extract all nonrestorable teeth
2. Extract all teeth with advanced periodontal disease
3. Perform endodontic treatment or extraction of nonvital teeth
4. Adjust dentures (if needed)
5. Provide dental prophylaxis
6. Perform elective dental treatment as time and necessity permit
7. Initiate an active, effective oral hygiene program
   a. Toothbrushing, flossing
   b. Diet modification, if indicated
   c. Topical fluorides
   d. Plaque control, calculus removal
   e. Chlorhexidine or Listerine mouthwash (daily)

Patients receiving dental treatment, including dental prophylaxis
1. Medical consultation
   a. Degree of organ failure
   b. Current status of patient
   c. Need for antibiotic prophylaxis (white blood cell [WBC] count depressed)
   d. Need to modify drug selection or dosage (kidney or liver failure)
   e. Need to take special precautions to avoid excessive bleeding
   f. Other special management procedures that may be required
2. Laboratory tests (surgical procedures planned)
   a. Access to current international normalized ratio (INR; PT), activated partial thromboplastin time (aPTT), BT, platelet count
   b. Access to WBC count and differential

INR, International normalized ratio; PT, prothrombin time; aPTT, activated partial thromboplastin time; BT, bleeding time; WBC, white blood cell.

BOX 22-4

Dental Management of the Patient With Transplanted Organs

IMMEDIATE POSTTRANSPLANT PERIOD (6 MO)
- Consultation with physician(s)

Key points
1. Avoid routine dental treatment
2. Continue oral hygiene procedures
3. Provide emergency dental care as needed (eliminate infection)
   a. Medical consultation
   b. Conservative selection of treatment

STABLE GRAFT PERIOD
- Consultation with physician(s)

Key points
1. Maintain effective oral hygiene procedures
2. Initiate active recall program every 3 to 6 months
3. Schedule medical consultation regarding patient status and management
4. Treat all new dental disease
5. Use universal precautions in controlling infection
6. Have staff vaccinated against hepatitis B virus (HBV) infection
7. Avoid infection
   a. Medical consultation—need for antibiotic prophylaxis (no evidence that it is needed)
   b. Screening tests—white blood cell (WBC) count, differential, CD4 and CD8 counts
   c. American Heart Association (AHA) standard regimen may be indicated for heart transplant

patients with cardiac valvulopathy (see Chapter 2)
8. Avoid excessive bleeding
   a. Screening tests—BT, international normalized ratio (INR; PT), activated partial thromboplastin time (aPTT), platelet count
   b. Special precautions
9. Alter drug selection, or reduce dosage
   a. Liver or kidney failure
   b. Avoid drugs that are toxic to liver or kidney (i.e., nonsteroidal anti-inflammatory drugs [NSAIDs])
10. Establish need for steroid supplementation, and be able to identify and deal with acute adrenal crisis, should it occur
11. Examine for oral signs and symptoms of overimmunosuppression or graft rejection
12. Monitor blood pressure for patients taking cyclosporine or prednisone; if blood pressure increases above baseline established, refer for medical evaluation

CHRONIC REJECTION PERIOD
Key points
- Consultation with physician(s)
1. Render immediate or emergency dental treatment (especially for infection)
2. Follow recommendations for patients with stable grafts, if dental treatment is needed

INR, International normalized ratio; PT, prothrombin time; aPTT, activated partial thromboplastin time; BT, bleeding time.

TABLE 22-7
Potential Posttransplantation Infections

Viral Infections	Time of Onset After Surgery	Susceptibility Period
Hepatitis B	Immediate	4 to 5 weeks
Hepatitis C	3 to 4 weeks	Continuous
HIV	3 to 4 weeks	Continuous
HSV	3 to 4 weeks	8 to 10 weeks
CMV	4 to 5 weeks	Continuous
BACTERIAL INFECTIONS		
Staphylococcal wound	Immediate	4 to 5 weeks
Staphylococcal pneumonia	Immediate	4 to 5 weeks*
Urinary tract infection (bacteremia/pyelonephritis)	Immediate	4 to 5 weeks
Tuberculosis, *Pneumocystis carinii* pneumonia, toxoplasmosis	4 to 5 weeks	25 to 30 weeks
FUNGAL INFECTIONS	4 to 5 weeks	Continuous

Modified from Rubin RH, et al: Am J Med 70:405-411, 1981.
HIV, Human immunodeficiency virus; HSV, herpes simplex virus; CMV, cytomegalovirus.
*Community-acquired pneumonia may occur/recur after approximately 6 months.

Risk of infection. Many posttransplantation infections may occur (Table 22-7). The health care professional must be aware of the clinical appearance, signs, and symptoms of these various infections. In some cases, specific prophylaxis may be indicated.

Increased risk for infection in the immunosuppressed transplant patient makes stronger the case for use of prophylactic antibiotics. Many transplant centers recommend prophylactic coverage for all dental procedures that can produce transient bacteremia in these patients. The rationale for this practice is based on the increased risk for local and systemic infection that results from suppression of the immune system. Again, no data are available to indicate whether this practice is effective or necessary for all immunosuppressed transplant patients. To further complicate the situation, the oral flora in these patients is altered by immunosuppressive therapy, making selection of the best antibiotics for prophylaxis difficult for the clinician. In addition, repeated antibiotic prophylaxis itself may alter the oral flora. Patients who have shown evidence of rejection and are receiving an increased dose of immunosuppressive agents are considered to be at greater risk for infection. A stronger case for the use of prophylactic antibiotics could be made for these patients.[6-9,14]

Because of the lack of scientific information indicating any benefit from antibiotic prophylaxis in the prevention of local or systemic infection in organ transplant patients undergoing invasive dental procedures, antibiotic use should be determined on an individual patient basis. Thus, the decisions about whether to use antibiotic prophylaxis and the appropriate regimen to follow should be made in consultation with the patient's transplant physician. Patients in excellent to good dental health whose grafts are stable and who are not undergoing extensive dental procedures do not require prophylaxis. In contrast, patients who need an increased dosage of immunosuppressants and those with active dental infection (chronic periodontitis) may best be managed with antibiotic prophylaxis for invasive dental procedures (see Table 22-5).

Recommendations for antibiotic prophylaxis in posttransplant patients are somewhat different from those for prevention of infective endocarditis. Part of the rationale for this is the susceptibility of posttransplant patients to subacute bacterial peritonitis. The basic prophylactic regimen consists of amoxicillin 2 g 1 hour before the dental procedure plus metronidazole 500 mg 1 hour before the dental procedure. In patients who are allergic to amoxicillin, vancomycin or imipenem 1 g infused slowly over 1 hour should be given before the dental procedure is performed. Clindamycin may be toxic to the liver and kidneys and therefore should not be used in most posttransplant patients. In patients who cannot take a drug by the oral route, intravenous ampicillin 1 g should be given with metronidazole 500 mg 1 hour before the dental procedure is performed[6-9,14] (see Table 22-5).

Immunosuppressive agents used in the transplant patient may mask the early signs and symptoms of oral infection, making diagnosis of the problem very difficult. When acute infection does occur, it often is more advanced and severe than that found in other patients. The dentist should look carefully for any evidence of acute infection in all transplant patients. The overimmunosuppressed patient may be more prone to oral infection, as is the patient with bone marrow suppression caused by the adverse effects of azathioprine, ALG, or ATG.[24,25]

Viral infection. Posttransplant patients may be especially susceptible to viral infection, including herpes simple virus (HSV), Epstein-Barr virus (EBV), cytomegalovirus (CMV), hepatitis B and hepatitis C viruses (HBV, HCV), and human immunodeficiency virus (HIV). The most common infection in these patients is CMV. Effective infection control procedures must be followed when transplant patients receive dental treatment. Patients who receive a transplant because of chronic complications of hepatitis may still be infected with HBV or HCV. In addition, during transplant surgery, additional blood is used, thereby increasing the risk of infection with HBV or HCV. A few transplant patients also become HIV infected (see Table 22-7). Excessively immunosuppressed patients may become infected with HSV, CMV, EBV, or other microorganisms that could be transmitted to dental staff or other patients. Patients also are at increased risk for infection transmitted to them in the dental operatory. The use of barrier techniques and the practice of universal precautions (recommended for all patients who are treated in the dental office) are considered adequate for management of transplantation patients with stable grafts. In addition, hepatitis B vaccine should be administered to all dental staff to protect against infection from HBV.[24,25]

Excessive bleeding. Liver transplantation patients may be taking anticoagulants to prevent recurrence of hepatic vein thrombosis. Heart transplantation patients may be taking anticoagulants to prevent thrombosis of the coronary vessels. Transplantation patients who are taking anticoagulants may need to have the dosage reduced by their physician before any dental surgical procedures are performed. If the level of anticoagulation (international normalized ration [INR]) is greater than 3.5, the patient's physician may have to reduce the dosage of medication (see Chapter 25). At least 3 to 4 days is required for the effect of the reduced dosage to lower the INR. When the patient's INR has been appropriately reduced, surgery can be performed. If the INR is greater than 3.5 the surgery may have to be delayed. After surgery has been performed, the dentist must be prepared to deal with excessive bleeding, if it should occur, with the use of splints, thrombin, antifibrinolytic agents, and so forth.

Liver, kidney, and bone marrow transplantation patients who are not taking anticoagulants still could be potential bleeders if rejection of the graft or GVHD and significant organ dysfunction occur. Therefore, before any dental surgical procedure is undertaken, the patient's physician should be consulted about the patient's current status. If necessary, selected screening tests (e.g., activated partial thromboplastin time [aPTT], INR, PT, bleeding time) should be ordered.[6-9,14]

Adverse reactions to stress. Transplantation patients who are receiving steroids may not be able to adjust to the stress of various dental surgical procedures because of adrenal suppression and may require additional steroids before and after these surgical procedures to protect against an acute adrenal crisis (see Chapter 16). The need for supplemental steroids should be established by medical consultation. If steroid supplementation is recommended, dosage and timing in relation to the dental procedure should be confirmed with the patient's physician. Dental treatment such as surgery or extensive appointments may require supplementation. If postoperative pain or com-

plications are anticipated, the need for supplementation is increased. Patients who are taking a very large daily dose of prednisone usually do not require supplementation (see Chapter 16). Also, many routine dental procedures, such as examinations, orthodontics, prophylaxis, simple restorations, and even minor oral surgery, may not require supplementation.

Even though precautions are taken and patients are managed through increased steroid levels, the dentist should remain alert to the possibility of an acute adrenal crisis. Signs and symptoms of acute adrenal insufficiency include hypotension, weakness, nausea, vomiting, headache, and, frequently, fever. Immediate treatment of this complication is required and consists of 100 mg of hydrocortisone (SoluCortef), given intravenously or intramuscularly, and emergency transportation to a medical facility (see Chapter 16).[6-9,14]

Hypertension. An important adverse effect of cyclosporine is renal damage and associated hypertension. Prednisone also can cause hypertension. The dentist must determine, through medical consultation once the graft is stable, what the "baseline" blood pressure is for each patient treated with cyclosporine or prednisone. During each visit to the dentist, the patient's blood pressure should be measured, and, if it becomes elevated to above the patient's baseline level, the patient's physician should be consulted immediately.[14,26]

Chronic Rejection Period. The third posttransplant period begins when significant signs and symptoms of chronic rejection of the graft or GVHD are noted. This phase should be established by medical consultation. In general, only emergency or immediate dental needs should be treated during this period.

Oral Complications and Manifestations

Oral complications associated with advanced heart, liver, and kidney disease are discussed in Chapters 4, 5, 6, 11, and 13. Oral complications noted in patients with blood dyscrasias are covered in Chapter 24. Oral complications reported in patients with organ transplants usually are caused by the following:
- Rejection
- Overimmunosuppression
- Adverse effects of immunosuppressive agents
- GVHD (after bone marrow transplantation)

Oral findings associated with graft rejection are the same as those found in patients with organ failure before transplantation. If lesions are found by the dentist that could be associated with organ failure, the patient immediately should be referred to the transplant physician for evaluation of possible organ rejection (Figure 22-12). Management of ulcerative or infectious lesions is described in Appendix C.[6-9,14]

Oral findings that may indicate overimmunosuppression include mucositis, herpes simplex infection, herpes zoster, CMV, candidiasis, large and slow-to-heal aphthous ulcers and other ulcerations, unusual alveolar bone loss, and, on occasion, lymphoma, Kaposi's sarcoma, squamous cell carcinoma of the lip, and hairy leukoplakia.[6-9,14]

In addition, the potential exists for progressive gingival and periodontal disease. The presence of any of these lesions may indicate that the transplant patient is overimmunosuppressed.

Oral complications associated with adverse effects of the immunosuppressive agents include infection, bleeding, poor healing, and tumor formation. Azathioprine may cause bone marrow suppression, and, when this occurs, patients may develop oral ulceration, petechiae, and bleeding. ATG and ALG may cause bone marrow suppression, thus increasing the risk for bleeding and infection. Cyclosporine may cause poor healing, increase the risk for infection, and produce gingival hyperplasia. The increased incidence of lymphoma in transplant patients is related to immunosuppression in general but also is related to the adverse effects of cyclosporine and antilymphocyte monoclonal antibodies. Oral ulcerations after liver transplantation were found to decrease once the dosage of the immunosuppressive agent (tacrolimus) had been reduced. After conducting proper investigation, the transplant physician may need to reduce the dosage of immunosuppressant agents.[6 9,14]

REFERENCES

1. U.S. Department of Health and Human Services. 2006 Annual Report of the U.S. Organ Procurement and Transplantation Network and the Scientific Registry for Transplant Recipients: Transplant data 2002-2005. Washington, DC, U.S. Department of Health and Human Services, 2006.
2. Guggenheimer J, Mayher D, Eghtesad B. A survey of dental care protocols among U.S. organ transplant centers. Clin Transplant 2005;19:15-18.
3. Cecka JM, Terasaki PI. Clinical Transplants. Los Angeles, Calif, UCLA Immunogenetic Center, 1999.
4. Henderson W (ed). Complications of Immunosuppression in Organ Transplants: Transplant Surgery. New York, NY, Elsevier, 1988.
5. Thomas ED, Lochte HL, Lu WC. Intravenous infusion of bone marrow patients receiving chemotherapy. N Engl J Med 1957;257:491-496.
6. Rhodus NL, Little JW. Dental management of the renal transplant patient. Compendium 1993;14:518-524,526, 528 passim; Quiz 532.
7. Rhodus NL, Little JW. Dental management of the bone marrow transplant patient. Compendium 1992;13: 1040,1042-1050.
8. Little JW, Rhodus NL. Dental management of the heart transplant patient. Gen Dent 1992;40:126-131.
9. Little JW, Rhodus NL. Dental treatment of the liver transplant patient. Oral Surg Oral Med Oral Pathol 1992;73:419-426.
10. Hornick P, Rose ML. Transplantation Immunology: Methods and Protocols. Clifton, NJ, Humana Press, 2006, p 429.
11. Thomas ED. Bone marrow transplantation. N Engl J Med 1975;292(16):835-839.
12. Ozaki CF. Liver transplants in horizons in organ transplantation. Surg Clin North Am 1994;74:1197-1209.
13. Frazier OH. Heart transplants in horizons in organ transplantation. Surg Clin North Am 1994;74:1169-1189.
14. Guggenheimer J, Eghtesad B, Stock DJ. Dental management of the (solid) organ transplant patient. Oral Surg Oral Med Oral Pathol Oral Radiol Endod 2003;95:383-389.
15. Frazier OH. Heart transplants in horizons in organ transplantation. Surg Clin North Am 1994;74:1169-1181.
16. Asfar S, Zhong R, Grant D. Small bowel transplants in horizons in organ transplantation. Surg Clin North Am 1994;74:1197-1207.
17. O'Connor KJ, Delmonico FL. Increasing the supply of kidneys for transplantation. Semin Dial 2005;18:460-462.
18. Browne BJ. Renal transplants in horizons in organ transplantation. Surg Clin North Am 1994;74:1097-1111.
19. Sollinger HW. Pancreas transplants in horizons in organ transplantation. Surg Clin North Am 1994;74:1183-1193.
20. Lacy P. Treating diabetes with transplanted islet cells. Sci Am 1995;89:50-55.
21. Kahan BC. Immunosuppressive drugs in horizons in organ transplantation. Surg Clin North Am 1994;74:1015-1027.
22. Heimdahl A, Mattsson T, Dahllof G, et al. The oral cavity as a port of entry for early infections in patients treated with bone marrow transplantation. Oral Surg Oral Med Oral Pathol 1989;68:711-716.
23. King GN. Increased prevalence of dysplastic and malignant oral lesions in renal transplant recipients. N Engl J Med 1995;332:677-681.
24. Morimoto Y, Niwa H, Imai Y, Kirita T. Dental management prior to hematopoietic stem cell transplantation. Spec Care Dentist 2004;24:287-292.
25. Cawley MM, Benson LM. Current trends in managing oral mucositis. Clin J Oncol Nurs 2005 Oct; 9:584-592.
26. Golla K, Epstein JB, Cabay RJ. Liver disease: Current perspectives on medical and dental management. Oral Surg Oral Med Oral Pathol Oral Radiol Endod 2004;98:516-521.

PART EIGHT

Hematologic and Oncologic Disease

Disorders of Red Blood Cells

isorders of the red blood cells (RBCs), which in large part consist of the anemias, are important to the dentist and to the health of the patient for several reasons. First, the dentist serves an important role in detecting patients with anemia through history, clinical examination, and results of screening laboratory tests. These screening procedures should lead to early referral to a physician and finalization of the diagnosis. This, in turn, can significantly affect morbidity and mortality because anemia often occurs as an underlying condition that requires attention and medical treatment. Also, the diagnosis of anemia is important because anemia is an independent risk factor for the development of adverse cardiovascular outcomes (i.e., acute myocardial infarction and death) in a variety of patient populations (e.g., chronic kidney disease, acute coronary syndrome, old age)[1-4]; therefore, preventive measures should be considered when one is performing stressful dental procedures.

ANEMIA

DEFINITION

Anemia, which is defined as a reduction in the oxygen-carrying capacity of the blood, is usually associated with a decreased number of circulating RBCs or an abnormality in the Hb contained within the RBCs. Anemia is not a disease but rather a symptom complex that may result from one of three underlying causes: (1) decreased production of RBCs (iron deficiency, pernicious anemia, folate deficiency), (2) blood loss, or (3) increased rate of destruction of circulating RBCs (hypersplenism, autoimmune destruction).

Erythropoiesis

About 1% of the circulating erythrocyte mass is generated by the bone marrow each day. Precursors of RBCs are reticulocytes, which account for 1% of the total red cell count. The normal red cell is about 33% hemoglobin by volume. Hemoglobin (Hb), the oxygen-carrying molecule of erythrocytes, consists of two pairs of globin chains (i.e., α plus β, δ, or γ) that form a shell around four oxygen-binding heme groups. Healthy adults have about 95% HbA (α2β2) and small amounts of HbA2 (α2δ2) and HbF (α2γ2). Genes on chromosome 16 encode α globin chains; β chains are encoded on chromosome 11.[5] Oxygen demand (hypoxia) serves as the stimulus for erythropoiesis. The kidney serves as the primary sensor for determining the level of oxygenation. If the level is low, the kidney releases erythropoietin, a hormone that stimulates the bone marrow to release RBCs. About 95% of erythropoietin is produced by cortical cells in the kidney. The other 5% is produced by the liver.[5,6]

EPIDEMIOLOGY

Approximately 4% of men and 8% of women in the United States have anemia, defined as Hb values below 13 g/dL for men and below 12 g/dL for women.[7] In the United States, iron deficiency anemia is the most common type.[8] The average dental practice that treats 2000 patients has about 12 men and 24 women who are anemic. In most of these patients, the condition may be undiagnosed.

Etiology

Anemia has numerous causes (Table 23-1). A partial list includes genetic disorders that produce aberrant RBCs that result in RBC destruction (hemolysis), nutritional disorders that limit the production of RBCs, immune-mediated disorders that result in attacks on RBCs, bleeding disorders that cause loss of RBCs, chronic diseases (rheumatoid arthritis), infections, and diseases of bone marrow. This chapter discusses select examples relevant to the practice of dentistry to demonstrate the clinical problems involved in the management of patients with anemia.

TABLE 23-1
Types of Anemia

Classification by Size and Shape of RBC	Cause
MICROCYTIC (MCV < 80 μm³)	
Iron deficiency anemia	Decreased production of RBCs
Thalassemias	Defective hemoglobin synthesis
Lead poisoning	Inhibition of hemoglobin synthesis
NORMOCYTIC (MCV 80-100 μm³)	
Hemolytic anemia	Increased destruction of RBCs
Sickle cell anemia	
Glucose-6-phosphate dehydrogenase deficiency	
Aplastic anemia	Decreased production of RBCs
Renal failure	Decreased production of RBCs
Anemia of chronic disease	Decreased production of RBCs
MACROCYTIC (MCV > 100 μm³)	
Pernicious anemia	Decreased production of RBCs
Folate deficiency	Decreased production of RBCs
Hypothyroidism	Decreased production of RBCs

RBC, Red blood cell; MCV, mean corpuscular volume.

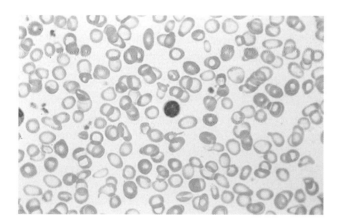

Figure 23-1. Microcytic anemia associated with iron deficiency. Peripheral blood smear shows red blood cells (RBCs) that are small and have marked hypochromic central pallor.

TYPES OF ANEMIA

Iron Deficiency Anemia

Iron deficiency anemia is a microcytic anemia (Figure 23-1) that can be caused by excessive blood loss, poor iron intake, poor iron absorption, or increased demand for iron. Blood loss may be caused by menses or bleeding from the gastrointestinal tract. Poor intake is more common in children who live in developing countries, where cereals and formula fortified with iron are not readily available. Malabsorption of iron can result from gastrectomy or intestinal disease that reduces absorption of iron from the duodenum and the jejunum. Increased demand is associated with chronic inflammation (autoimmune disease).

In women, menstruation and pregnancy contribute to the development of iron deficiency anemia. The repeated loss of blood associated with menses can lead to depletion of iron, resulting in a mild state of anemia. During pregnancy, the expectant mother experiences an increased demand for additional iron and vitamins to support the growth of her fetus, and unless sufficient amounts of these nutrients have been provided in some form, she may become anemic. Approximately 20% of pregnant women have iron deficiency anemia.[9] Also, 30% to 60% of individuals who have rheumatoid arthritis (more commonly, women) have this type of anemia.[10]

In contrast, mild anemia in men usually indicates the presence of a serious underlying medical problem (e.g., gastrointestinal bleeding, malignancy). Under normal physiologic conditions, men lose little iron, and because iron can be stored for months, iron deficiency anemia is rare in men. Therefore, any man who is found to be anemic should be promptly referred for medical evaluation.

Folate Deficiency Anemia and Pernicious Anemia

Vitamin B$_{12}$ (cobalamin) and folic acid are needed for red blood cell formation and growth within bone marrow. Vitamin B$_{12}$ is a cofactor in methionine-associated enzymatic reactions required of protein synthesis and thus in the maturation of RBCs. Folate is needed for enzymatic reactions required for the synthesis of purines and pyrimidines of deoxyribonucleic acid (DNA) and ribonucleic acid (RNA) and thus for the synthesis of proteins. A deficiency in daily intake (as in chronic alcoholism) or absorption (because of celiac disease or tropical sprue) of these vitamins can result in anemia.

Folate is found in fruits and leafy vegetables. It is not stored in the body in large amounts; thus, a continual dietary supply of this vitamin is needed. Its absorption and metabolism are interfered with by alcohol consumption and certain drugs (methotrexate, dilantin). Risk factors for folate deficiency include poor diet (seen frequently in the poor, the elderly, and individuals who do not eat fresh fruits or vegetables), alcoholism, history of malabsorption disorders, and pregnancy (third trimester). Folate deficiency anemia occurs in about 4 of 100,000 people.

Pernicious anemia is caused by a deficiency of intrinsic factor, a substance secreted by the stomach parietal cells that is necessary for absorption of vitamin B_{12} (cobalamin). Because vitamin B_{12} may be stored for several years, this form of nutritional deficiency is rare and usually does not develop until late adulthood. Most often, it occurs in 40-year-old to 70-year-old northern Europeans of fair complexion, with one notable exception. Early onset in black American women, 21% of whom were under the age of 40, has been observed.[11] Most patients with pernicious anemia have chronic atrophic gastritis with decreased intrinsic factor and hydrochloric acid secretion. Antibodies against parietal cells and intrinsic factor also are found in the sera of most patients.[12] This finding strongly suggests that the disease involves an autoimmune process.

Early symptoms of pernicious anemia include weakness, fatigue, palpitations, syncope, tingling of the fingers and toes (paresthesias), numbness, and uncoordination. However, many patients with pernicious anemia are asymptomatic, even with low Hb levels (<10 g/dL). Long-term patients with pernicious anemia are at increased risk for gastric carcinoma, myxedema, rheumatoid arthritis, and neuropsychiatric and neuromuscular abnormalities; the latter are due to a defect in myelin synthesis.[11]

Deficiencies of vitamin B_{12} and folic acid are associated with macrocytic anemia and the presence of hypersegmented polymorphonuclear leukocytes in the peripheral blood smear (Figure 23-2). Measures of serum methylmalonic acid and homocysteine levels and serologic testing for parietal cell and intrinsic factor antibodies are used to further screen for the deficiency.[12] Use of the serum cobalamin assay followed by the Schilling test helps to establish the diagnosis of pernicious anemia.[11,13,14] When the Schilling test is performed, after fasting, the patient receives a small oral dose of radioactive vitamin B_{12}, then a larger dose of nonradioactive vitamin B_{12}, as a parenteral flush. At 24 hours, the amount of radioactive cyanocobalamin in the urine is measured. About 7% of the radioactive B_{12} dose is excreted during the first 24 hours; however, those with pernicious anemia excrete less than 3%.[13]

Hemolytic Anemia

Hemolytic anemias are caused by immune attack, extrinsic factors (infection, splenomegaly, drugs, eclampsia), disor-

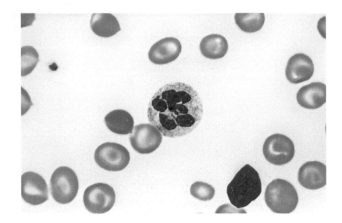

Figure 23-2. Megaloblastic anemia. Peripheral blood smear shows a hypersegmented neutrophil with a six-lobed nucleus. (From Kumar V, Abbas A, Fausto N. Robbins & Cotran Pathologic Basis of Disease, 7th ed. Philadelphia, WB Saunders, 2005. Courtesy Dr. Robert W. McKenna, Department of Pathology, University of Texas Southwestern Medical School, Dallas, Tex.)

ders of the RBC membrane (spherocytosis), enzymopathies (glucose-6-phosphate dehydrogenase deficiency), and hemoglobinopathies (sickle cell anemia, thalassemia). Glucose-6-phosphate dehydrogenase deficiency and sickle cell anemia are discussed here to illustrate the problems presented by the hemolytic anemias.[14]

Hemolytic Anemia: Glucose-6-Phosphate Dehydrogenase Deficiency

The search during World War II for a substitute quinine led to the use of newer antimalarial drugs and the discovery of deficiency of glucose-6-phosphate dehydrogenase (G-6-PD), an enzyme that helps the RBC to turn carbohydrates into energy. This discovery occurred after several persons who were given primaquine developed hemolytic anemia because they lacked G-6-PD, an enzyme needed for the hexose monophosphate shunt pathway.[11]

Glucose enters the RBC through a carrier mechanism, independent of insulin. About 90% of glucose is metabolized by the glycolytic pathway. The remaining glucose is metabolized by the hexose monophosphate shunt pathway. The by-product of the glycolytic pathway is adenosine triphosphate, which provides energy for the cell. The by-product of the hexose monophosphate shunt pathway is nicotinamide adenine dinucleotide phosphate (NADPH), which is used to reduce various cellular oxidants.[15] Blockage of the hexose monophosphate shunt pathway in individuals with G-6-PD deficiency allows accumulation of harmful oxidants within RBCs. These substances, which produce methemoglobin and denatured Hb, precipitate to form Heinz bodies, which attach to cell membranes. These alterations in cell membranes lead to hemolysis of the cell (hemolytic anemia).[16]

G-6-PD is deficient in more than 400 million persons worldwide, making this disorder the most common enzymopathy of humans.[17] At present, more than 350 G-6-PD variants have been identified. They are grouped into five classes (I to V), with class I being severely deficient, on the basis of level of enzyme deficiency.[18] The G-6-PD gene is located on the X chromosome; thus, disease inheritance is gender linked. G-6-PD A, the variant most commonly associated with hemolysis, is found in 11% of African Americans. G-6-PD MED, the second most common variant associated with hemolysis, occurs in ethnic groups from the Mediterranean, the Middle East, and Asia,[15] and is associated with sickle cell anemia.[19]

Clinical features of G-6-PD deficiency involve acute intravascular hemolysis, which may be severe. Jaundice, palpitations, dyspnea, and dizziness may result. Infection is the event that most commonly triggers hemolysis in G-6-PD A deficiency. Drugs are the most common trigger for hemolysis in G-6-PD MED deficiency.[17] Of more than 40 drugs that can induce hemolysis, those having dental significance include acetylsalicylic acid, acetophenetidin (phenacetin), dapsone, ascorbic acid, and vitamin K.[15] Fava bean ingestion is the most common dietary cause of hemolytic anemia in persons with G-6-PD deficiency.

Screening tests for Heinz bodies (hemoglobin precipitates; Figure 23-3) or NADPH may be used to detect individuals with G-6-PD deficiency. More sensitive tests use direct fluorescent measures of NADPH. Other tests used to detect this deficiency include the cyanide-ascorbate assay and the quantitative assay of G-6-PD.[13]

Sickle Cell Anemia

Sickle cell hemoglobin (HbS) was the first Hb variant of the more than 600 inherited human Hb variants (hemoglobinopathies) to be recognized. Of these, more than 90% have single amino acid substitutions in the Hb chain. HbS is the result of substitution of a single amino acid—valine for glutamic acid—at the sixth residue of the β chain. In contrast, the thalassemias, another type of hemoglobinopathy, are caused by deletions or mutations of the α or β globin gene that result in a defect in globin synthesis (reduced or absent synthesis of one or more globin chains).[20] The hemoglobinopathies are more commonly found in regions of malarial endemicity and in populations who have migrated from these regions, because the mutated gene(s) confer advantages against infection by *Plasmodium falciparum* (i.e., malaria). Hemoglobinopathies such as sickle cell anemia are inherited as autosomal recessive traits.[21,22]

Sickle cell disorders are distinguished by the number of globin genes affected. The two most common types are **sickle cell trait** and **sickle cell (disease) anemia**. **Sickle cell trait** is the heterozygous state in which the affected individual carries one gene for HbS. Approximately 8% to 10% of African Americans carry the trait. In central Africa, up to 25% of the population may be carriers. **Sickle cell anemia** is the homozygous state. A gene from each parent contributes to formation of the

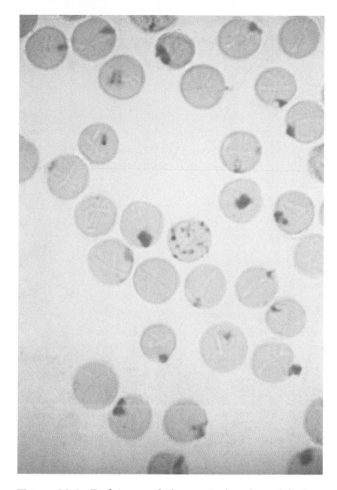

Figure 23-3. Deficiency of glucose 6-phosphate dehydrogenase: Peripheral blood film shows Heinz bodies in red cells and a single reticulocyte. (Supravital new methylene blue stain.) (From Hoffbrand AV, Pettit JE. Color Atlas of Clinical Hematology, 3rd ed. London, Mosby, 2000.)

HbS molecule responsible for the disease. The RBC in sickle cell anemia becomes sickle shaped when blood experiences lowered oxygen tension or decreased pH, or when the patient becomes dehydrated.[22-24] About 50,000 African Americans (about 0.003% to 0.15%), or 1 in 600, have sickle cell anemia.[21,24-27]

Distortion of the RBC into a sickled shape results from deoxygenation or decreased blood pH, causing partial crystallization of HbS, polymerization, and realignment of the defective Hb molecule (Figure 23-4). Cellular rigidity and membrane damage occur, and irreversible sickling is the final result. The net effects of these changes consist of erythrostasis, increased blood viscosity, reduced blood flow, hypoxia, increased adhesion of RBCs, vascular occlusion, and further sickling.[21,24] Sickling crises are rare in individuals with the sickle cell trait.[21]

In patients with sickle cell anemia, more than 80% of the Hb is HbS. Clinical signs and symptoms of sickle cell anemia are the result of chronic anemia and small blood vessel occlusion. They include jaundice, pallor, dactylitis (hand and foot warmth and tenderness), leg ulcers, organomegaly, cardiac failure, stroke, attacks of abdominal and bone pain (aseptic necrosis), and delays in growth development (Figure 23-5). Aplastic crisis, an acute illness wherein production of red cells stops and severe anemia occurs, may develop from infection, hypersensitivity reactions, hypoxia, systemic disease, acidosis, dehydration, or trauma. Diagnosis requires use of red cell indices and tests in which deoxygenating agents are used (Sickledex). Confirmatory tests use electrophoresis and/or high-performance liquid chromatography.[13]

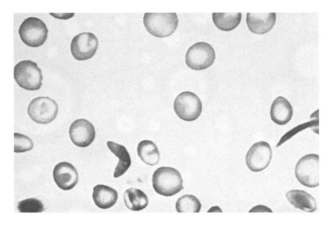

Figure 23-4. Sickle cell anemia. Peripheral blood smear shows abnormal sickle-shaped red blood cells (RBCs) in sickle cell anemia.

Individuals with the sickle cell trait generally have no symptoms unless they are placed in situations in which abnormally low concentrations of oxygen are present (e.g., in an unpressurized airplane, through the injudicious administration of general anesthesia). Patients with sickle cell trait are much more resistant to sickling stimuli because only 20% to 45% of their Hb is HbS. Patients with sickle cell trait are not at risk during dental treatment unless severe hypoxia, severe infection, or dehydration occurs.[21,24-27]

Renal Disease

The kidney produces the hormone erythropoietin, which stimulates RBC production by the bone marrow. If significant renal damage occurs, lack of production of this hormone results in anemia. Patients who have chronic renal failure and are on dialysis often have anemia and low erythropoietin levels. Erythropoietic drug therapy is offered to these patients.

Organ Transplantation

Patients who undergo organ (kidney, liver, bone marrow) transplantation and acquire immunosuppression develop anemia as a result of bone marrow suppression.

CLINICAL PRESENTATION

Signs and Symptoms

Symptoms of anemia occur in proportion to the rate of development of anemia; rapidly developing anemia has

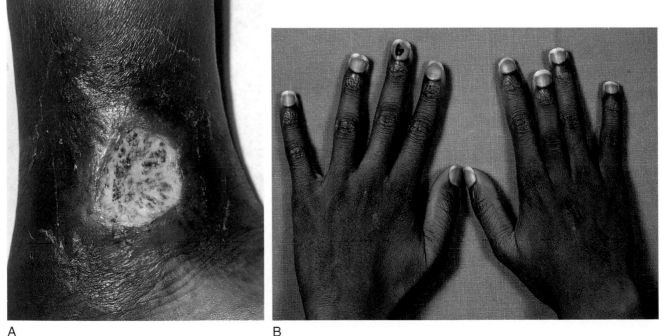

A B

Figure 23-5. Sickle cell anemia. **A,** Leg ulcer, and **B,** growth deformation of the middle finger from vaso-occlusive attack and dactylitis of the growth plate. (A and B from Hoffbrand AV, Pettit JE. Color Atlas of Clinical Hematology, 3rd ed. London, Mosby, 2000.)

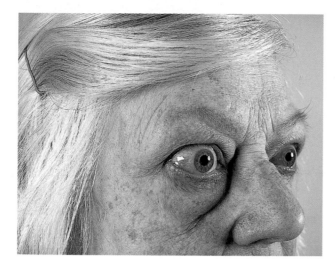

Figure 23-6. Pernicious anemia. This 38-year-old man shows premature graying and has blue eyes and vitiligo—three features that are more common in patients with pernicious anemia than in control subjects. (From Hoffbrand AV, Pettit JE. Color Atlas of Clinical Hematology, 3rd ed. London, Mosby, 2000.)

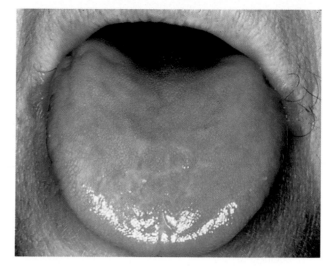

Figure 23-7. Smooth red tongue and angular cheilitis in a patient found to have iron deficiency anemia.

more profound features than slowly developing anemia. Because most patients develop anemia slowly, most have few symptoms until the condition worsens. Usual symptoms include fatigue, palpitations, shortness of breath, abdominal pain, bone pain, tingling of fingers and toes, and muscular weakness. Specific to iron deficiency anemia are features of ice chewing, calf cramps, and diminished capability to perform muscular work.

Signs of anemia may include jaundice, pallor, cracking, splitting and spooning of the fingernails, increased size of the liver and spleen, lymphadenopathy, and blood in the stool. Premature graying of hair and yellowing of the skin (due to jaundice) have been reported with pernicious anemia (Figure 23-6).[28] Patients with anemia may also describe a sore or painful tongue (glossitis), a smooth tongue, or redness of the tongue or cheilosis (Figure 23-7). Some patients may complain of loss of taste sensation.

Screening Laboratory Tests

If the dentist identifies a patient with signs or symptoms suggestive of anemia, this patient should be sent to a commercial laboratory for a complete blood count and differential, or referred to a physician for evaluation. Hb level, hematocrit, and RBC indices (mean corpuscular volume [MCV], mean corpuscular hemoglobin [MCH], and mean corpuscular hemoglobin concentration [MCHC]) are tests that are used to screen the patient. In addition, total white blood cell (WBC) count and platelet count should be obtained to determine whether a generalized bone marrow defect has occurred and to inspect for hypersegmented neutrophils (see Chapter 1). Anemia is generally defined as Hb < 12 g/dL for women

and < 13 g/dL for men.[13] In accordance with the size of RBCs, anemia is classified as microcytic (MCV < 80 μm³), macrocytic (MCV > 96 μm³), or normocytic (MCV, 80 μm³ to 96 μm³).[11] A reticulocyte count less than 1% indicates inadequate RBC production in the bone marrow, whereas a value greater than 1% indicates increased production in response to bleeding or destruction. To further distinguish the various types of anemias, key laboratory tests, as shown in Table 23-2, are performed.

All African American patients should be questioned about the presence of sickle cell disease in their family histories. If the history does not include an individual who was screened for sickle cell disease, the dentist should arrange for the patient to be tested. This can be done in the dental office with the Sickledex test (distributed by Johnson & Johnson), in a commercial clinical laboratory, or by a physician.

MEDICAL MANAGEMENT

The goal of treatment is to eliminate the underlying cause. Management protocols for several types of anemia are discussed in the following paragraphs.

In microcytic anemia (iron deficiency), the physician should look for a source of bleeding. Iron deficiency associated with pregnancy often resolves after childbirth. In children, iron supplements (ferrous sulfate, 2 to 6 mg/kg/day) are recommended to arrest motor and cognitive impairment brought on by iron deficiency.[29] In patients who have undergone a gastrectomy, iron supplements (ferrous sulfate or ferrous gluconate) are provided on a long-term basis. In men, management often involves treatment of the underlying cause (e.g., peptic ulcer disease, gastrointestinal malignancy).

Folate deficiency is managed by administering folic acid supplements and by increasing the intake of green,

TABLE **23-2**
Laboratory Assessments to Aid in the Diagnosis of Anemia*

	Type	Tests to Discriminate Types of Anemia
Microcytic anemia	Iron deficiency	Serum iron, ferritin, total iron binding capacity (TIBC), transferrin saturation, bone marrow aspirate. Also, stool examination for occult blood
Macrocytic anemia	Folate deficiency	CBC, serum folate level
Macrocytic anemia	Pernicious anemia	CBC, serum vitamin B_{12} (cobalamin) assay levels, Schilling's test, serum antiparietal cell, and intrinsic factor antibodies
Normocytic anemia	G-6-PD	Staining peripheral blood smear with methyl or crystal violet, cyanide-ascorbate assay, qualitative (fluorescent spot) test and quantitative test for G-6-PD, reticulocyte count, indirect bilirubin levels
Normocytic anemia	Sickle cell anemia	Sickledex, high-performance liquid chromatography, hemoglobin electrophoresis, reticulocyte count, indirect bilirubin levels
Normocytic anemia	Aplastic anemia	Erythropoietin levels, bone marrow aspirate

CBC, Complete blood count; G-6-PD, glucose-6-phosphate dehydrogenase.
MCV (mean corpuscular volume), MCH (mean corpuscular hemoglobin), and MCHC (mean corpuscular hemoglobin concentration) have been assessed, and values indicate that anemia is present.
*These tests are ordered after the initial CBC and differential, including red cell indices.

leafy vegetables and citrus fruits. In the case of poor intestinal absorption, replacement therapy with folic acid may be lifelong. Cyanocobalamin injections are used to treat patients with pernicious anemia. Injections generally are given daily for the first week, then are tapered eventually to once a month, as needed.

Management of sickle cell anemia is based on routine prophylactic penicillin for infants and the early use of antibiotics to prevent severe infection.[19] If contemporary health care is not provided, 50% of persons with sickle cell anemia will die before the age of 30 years. Because folic acid deficiency may play a role in the causes of crises, folic acid dietary supplements are given daily to most patients with sickle cell anemia. In addition, penicillin prophylaxis is used for at least the first 5 years of life. Therapeutic strategies include the use of hydroxyurea (with or without erythropoietin), which induces production of HbF and thus prevents formation of HbS polymers.[21,30,31] Once a crisis occurs, high doses of folic acid, analgesics for pain, hydration, and blood transfusions are used to treat the patient.[19,21] Bone marrow transplantation (BMT) has been used in children with sickle cell anemia and has met with moderate success (25% to 30% cure rate) but is associated with mortality.[32]

Treatment of patients with chronic renal failure often requires dialysis and long-term use of recombinant erythropoietin (see Chapter 13). Erythropoietic growth factors may be used when hemoglobin levels are <9.5 g/dL, or when Hb = 9.5 to 11.0 g/dL and symptoms of anemia are present.[33] Long-term use of erythropoietin is associated with hypertension and prothrombotic and inflammatory states.[34]

Anemic patients may require hospitalization if the hematocrit value is less than 20%. Transfusion with RBCs is reserved for patients who are actively bleeding and for those with severe and symptomatic anemia who have underlying disease.

DENTAL MANAGEMENT
Medical Considerations

The dentist should obtain a careful history to identify conditions associated with anemia. Inclusion of questions concerning dietary intake, malnutrition, alcohol or drug use, use of nonsteroidal anti-inflammatory drugs, menstrual blood loss, pregnancies, hypothyroidism, jaundice, gallstones, splenectomy, bleeding disorders and abnormal Hb, and organ transplantation is important. Historical information concerning family members is also important for identifying hereditary risk for hemolytic anemias.

In children, questions should assess normal growth. When the history of a woman is taken, questions that reveal the onset, nature, and regularity of the patient's menstruation cycle may be important. Women with a history of regular periods but with heavy flow may be anemic and should receive medical advice and treatment. A patient with a change in the pattern, onset, length, or rate of menstrual flow should be encouraged to seek medical evaluation. Patients who stopped having periods long before expected should be referred for medical evaluation, as should those who have had bleeding between regular periods. In addition, several historical questions should be posed to women who are pregnant or who recently experienced childbirth. For example, the dentist should establish whether the patient had excessive bleeding during pregnancy, and whether the patient has other children and when they were born, because the closer together the pregnancies were, the greater is the risk for developing iron deficiency anemia. Once the baby is born, the mother may lose additional iron during delivery and breast feeding.

The dentist should be keen to identify signs and symptoms of anemia in patients who are seen for dental treatment. A patient with classic signs or symptoms of anemia should be referred directly to a physician and screened by appropriate laboratory tests (see Table 23-2). Screening tests should include complete and differential blood counts, a smear for cell morphologic study, Hb or hematocrit count, a Sickledex test (for African Americans), and platelet count. If screening tests are ordered by the dentist and results of one or more are abnormal, the patient should be referred for medical evaluation and treatment.

Patients with anemia may have a serious underlying disease such as peptic ulcer or carcinoma, for which early detection may be lifesaving. Patients with sickle cell anemia may be in grave danger if the disease is not detected before dental treatment is started. Thus, it is important for the dentist to attempt to identify these patients through history and clinical examination before starting any treatment.

Assessment of the severity of a patient's anemia is important for preventing complications. First and foremost, the dentist should ensure that the patient's underlying condition is under therapeutic control before proceeding with routine dental treatment. In many cases, anemia is associated with chronic illness; thus, treatment may be provided in the presence of anemia. For minimal medical complications, the patient's Hb should be above 11 g/dL and the patient should be free from symptoms. Patients who are short of breath and who have Hb < 11 g/dL, an abnormal heart rate, or an oxygen saturation less than 91% (as determined by pulse oximetry) are considered unstable, and routine treatment should be deferred until their health status improves.

Patients with G-6-PD deficiency have an increased incidence of drug sensitivity, with sulfonamides (sulfamethoxazole), aspirin, and chloramphenicol being the prime offenders.[11,32] Penicillin, streptomycin, and isoniazid also have been linked to hemolysis in these patients. Dental infection may accelerate the rate of hemolysis in patients with this type of anemia.[25,35] Thus, dental infections should be avoided, and, if they occur, they must be dealt with effectively. The astute clinician will realize that febrile illness and elevated bilirubin are features of this condition. The drugs listed previously should not be used in these patients.

African Americans with sickle cell anemia can receive routine dental care during noncrisis periods; however, long and complicated procedures should be avoided. Good dental repair and preventive dental care are important because oral infection can precipitate a crisis. If infection occurs, it must be treated expeditiously through local and systemic measures such as incision and drainage, heat, high doses of appropriate antibiotics, pulpectomy, and/or extraction. If cellulitis develops, the patient's physician must be consulted and hospitalization considered.[24,25] Adequate fluid intake is important for avoiding dehydration. Dental management considerations for the patient with sickle cell anemia are summarized in Box 23-1.

BOX 23-1

Dental Management of the Patient With Sickle Cell Anemia

1. Confirm with patient's physician that the condition is stable.
2. Arrange short appointments.
3. Avoid long and complicated procedures.
4. Maintain good dental repair.
5. Institute aggressive preventive dental care.
   a. Oral hygiene instruction
   b. Diet control
   c. Toothbrushing and flossing
   d. Fluoride gel application
6. Avoid oral infection; treat aggressively when present.
7. Use pulse oximeter, maintain O_2 saturation above 95%.
8. Use local anesthetic without epinephrine for routine dental care. For surgical procedures, use 1:100,000 epinephrine in local anesthetic.
9. Avoid barbiturates and strong narcotics; sedation may be attained with diazepam (Valium).
10. Use prophylactic antibiotics for major surgical procedures.
11. Avoid liberal use of salicylates; control pain with acetaminophen and codeine.
12. Use nitrous oxide–oxygen with greater than 50% oxygen, high flow rate, and good ventilation.

For routine dental care, appointments should be short (to reduce stress) for patients with sickle cell anemia. The use of a local anesthetic is acceptable (avoid general anesthesia); however, inclusion of small amounts of epinephrine in the local anesthetic is controversial in that some authors believe it may impair circulation and cause vascular occlusion. Smith and colleagues[24] suggest that a local anesthetic should be used without a vasoconstrictor for routine dental care. When a surgical procedure must be performed, they recommend use of a local anesthetic with epinephrine 1:100,000 to attain hemostasis and profound anesthesia. If required, nitrous oxide–oxygen (N_2O-O_2) should be used for short periods with at least 50% oxygen concentration provided.[36,37]

Intravenous (IV) sedation must be used with extreme caution in patients who have a history of sickle cell anemia. Barbiturates and narcotics should be avoided because suppression of the respiratory center by these agents leads to hypoxia and acidosis, which may precipitate an acute crisis. Light sedation can be provided with diazepam (Valium) or nalbuphine hydrochloride.[18] Additional oxygen provided by nasal cannula and liberal use of IV fluids during sedation are advised.[31] General anesthesia is not recommended when the Hb level falls below 10 g/dL. High doses of salicylates should be avoided because the "acid" effect can cause a crisis. Pain control may be attempted with acetaminophen and small doses of codeine.[24,37]

Prophylactic antibiotics are recommended for sickle cell anemia when major surgical procedures are performed to prevent wound infection or osteomyelitis. Penicillin is the drug of choice in nonallergic patients. Intramuscular or IV antibiotics should be considered for use in sickle cell anemic patients who have an acute dental infection. Dehydration must be avoided during surgery and the postoperative period. Consultation with the patient's physician is a must before any surgical procedure. The dentist must establish the patient's current status, and, if blood transfusion is indicated, must correct severe anemia or its complications before surgery.[24]

Treatment Planning Modifications

Delays in dental treatment may be required for patients who have anemia due to severe underlying conditions. Treatment planning modifications are directed primarily toward individuals who have severe anemia or sickle cell anemia. Elective surgical procedures are best avoided in patients with sickle cell anemia. Routine dental care can be rendered for patients with sickle cell trait and for those whose disease is in a noncrisis state. Special emphasis should be placed on oral hygiene procedures to avoid dental caries, gingival inflammation, and infection that can lead to osteomyelitis. Adequate oxygenation should be provided during nitrous oxide inhalation procedures. Pulse oximetry monitoring is prudent during dental treatment of all patients with anemia.

Oral Complications and Manifestations

Oral findings in patients with anemia usually relate to the underlying cause of the anemia. The oral mucosa often appears pale. Patients with nutritional causes of anemia (e.g., vitamin B_{12} or iron deficiency) may show loss of papillae from the tongue and atrophic changes in the oral mucosa (see Figure 23-7). Angular cheilitis and aphthae may be found. Patients also may report a burning or sore tongue. Some patients with iron deficiency anemia develop Plummer-Vinson syndrome (Figure 23-8), which is characterized by a sore mouth, dysphagia (resulting from muscular degeneration in the esophagus with esophageal stenosis or "webbing"), and an increased frequency of carcinoma of the oral cavity and pharynx. Patients with this syndrome should be followed closely for any oral or pharyngeal tissue changes that might be early indicators of carcinoma.[25,38,39]

Patients with hemolytic anemia (e.g., sickle cell anemia) may show pallor and oral evidence of jaundice caused by hyperbilirubinemia caused by excessive erythrocyte destruction. The trabecular pattern of the bone on dental radiographs may be affected because of hyperplasia of marrow elements in response to increased destruction of RBCs. Therefore, dental radiographs may show enlarged bone marrow (medullary) spaces associated with bone marrow hyperplasia, increased widening and decreased numbers of trabeculations, and generalized osteoporosis (thinning of the inferior border of the mandible). Because of compensatory marrow expansion, the

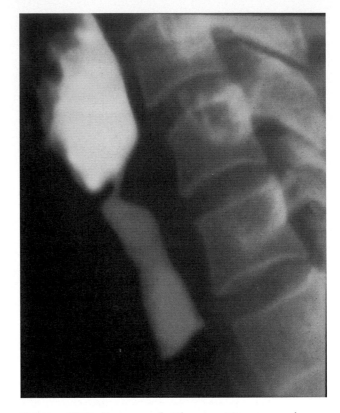

Figure 23-8. Feature of Plummer-Vinson syndrome. Barium contrast radiograph demonstrates esophageal webbing. (From Bricker SL, Langlais RP, Miller CS. Oral diagnosis, oral medicine, and treatment planning, ed 2. Hamilton, Ontario, BC Decker, 2002. Courtesy Dr. Thomas J. Vaughan.)

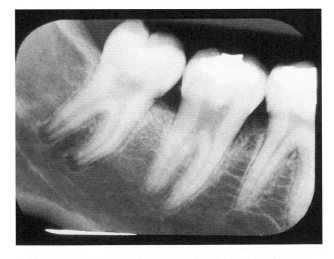

Figure 23-9. Periapical radiograph of the mandible in a patient with sickle cell anemia. Note the prominent horizontal trabeculations and the dense lamina dura.

bone appears more radiolucent with prominent lamellar striations.[25,38] Specifically, the trabeculae between teeth may appear as horizontal rows or as a "stepladder" (Figure 23-9). This can also manifest as frontal bossing and/or "hair on end" in the cortical regions of a skull film (Figure 23-10). Vaso-occlusive events can promote asymptomatic

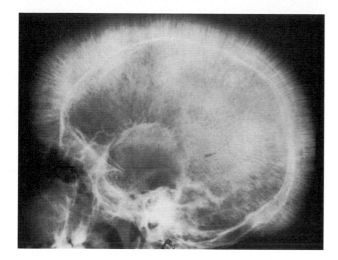

Figure 23-10. Skull film in a patient with hemolytic anemia shows new bone formation on the outer table, producing perpendicular radiations or "hair on end" appearance. (From Kumar V, Abbas A, Fausto N. Robbins & Cotran Pathologic Basis of Disease, 7th ed. Philadelphia, Saunders, 2005. Courtesy Dr. Jack Reynolds, Department of Radiology, University of Texas Southwestern Medical School, Dallas, Tex.)

pulpal necrosis, osteomyelitis, ischemic necrosis within the mandible, and peripheral neuropathy. Patients with sickle cell anemia often have delayed eruption of teeth and dental hypoplasia.[24,25,38,39]

REFERENCES

1. Cavusoglu E, Chopra V, Gupta A, et al. Usefulness of anemia in men as an independent predictor of two-year cardiovascular outcome in patients presenting with acute coronary syndrome. Am J Cardiol 2006;98:580-584.
2. Walker AM, Schneider G, Yeaw J, et al. Anemia as a predictor of cardiovascular events in patients with elevated serum creatinine. J Am Soc Nephrol 2006;17:2293-2298.
3. Penninx BW, Pahor M, Woodman RC, Guralnik JM. Anemia in old age is associated with increased mortality and hospitalization. J Gerontol A Biol Sci Med Sci 2006;61:474-479.
4. Swaak A. Anemia of chronic disease in patients with rheumatoid arthritis: Aspects of prevalence, outcome, diagnosis, and the effect of treatment on disease activity. J Rheumatol 2006;33:1467-1468.
5. Clarke GM, Higgins TN. Laboratory investigation of hemoglobinopathies and thalassemias: Review and update. Clin Chem 2000;46:1284-1290.
6. Adamson JW. Iron deficiency and other hypoproliferative anemias. In Kasper DL, Fauci AS, Hauser SL, Longo DL (eds). Harrison's Principles of Internal Medicine, 16th ed. New York, NY, McGraw-Hill, 2005; 586-592.
7. Frith-Terhune AL, Cogswell ME, Khan LK, et al. Iron deficiency anemia: Higher prevalence in Mexican American than in non-Hispanic white females in the Third National Health and Nutrition Examination Survey, 1988-1994. Am J Clin Nutr 2000;72:963-968.
8. Looker AC, Dallman PR, Carroll MD, et al. Prevalence of iron deficiency in the United States. JAMA 1997; 277:973-976.
9. Suresh L, Radfar L. Pregnancy and lactation. Oral Surg Oral Med Oral Pathol Oral Radiol Endod 2004;97: 672-682.
10. Wilson A, Yu HT, Goodenough LT, et al. Prevalence and outcomes of anemia in rheumatoid arthritis: A systematic review of the literature. Am J Med 2004;(suppl 7A):50S-57S.
11. Babior BM. Folate, cobalamin and megaloblastic anemias. In Lichtman MA, Beuter E, Kipps TJ, et al (eds). Williams Hematology. New York, NY, McGraw-Hill, 2006.
12. Oh R, Brown DL. Vitamin B12 deficiency. Am Fam Physician 2003;67:979-986.
13. Elghetany MT, Banki K. Erythrocytic disorders. In McPherson RA, Pincus MR (eds). Henry's Clinical Diagnosis and Management by Laboratory Methods, 21st ed. Philadelphia, Saunders Elsevier, 2007.
14. Aster JC. Red blood cell and bleeding disorders. In Kumar VK, Abbas AK, Fausto N (eds). Robbins and Cotran Pathologic Basis of Disease, 7th ed. Philadelphia, Elsevier Saunders, 2005.
15. Beck WS, Tepper RI. Hemolytic anemias. IV. Metabolic disorders. In Beck WS (ed). Hematology, 5th ed. Cambridge, Mass, MIT Press, 1991.
16. Berliner N. Disorders of red blood cells. In Andreoli TE, Carpenter CCJ, Griggs RC, Loscalzo J (eds). Cecil Essentials of Medicine, 6th ed. Philadelphia, WB Saunders, 2004.
17. Beutler E. Glucose-6-phosphate dehydrogenase deficiency. N Engl J Med 1991;324:169-174.
18. Ruwende C, Hill A. Glucose-6-phosphate dehydrogenase deficiency and malaria. J Mol Med 1998;76:581-588.
19. Steinberg MH. Management of sickle cell disease. N Engl J Med 1999;340:1021-1030.
20. Olivieri NF. The β-thalassemias. N Engl J Med 1999; 341:99-109.
21. Bunn HF. Hemoglobin. II. Sickle cell anemia and other hemoglobinopathies. In Beck WS (ed). Hematology, 5th ed. Cambridge, Mass, MIT Press, 1991.
22. May DA. Dental management of sickle cell anemia patients. Gen Dent 1991;39:182-184.
23. Ashley-Koch A, Yang Q, Olney RS. Sickle hemoglobin (HbS) allele and sickle cell disease: A HuGE review. Am J Epidemiol 2000;151:839-845.
24. Smith HB, McDonald DK, Miller RI. Dental management of patients with sickle cell disorders. J Am Dent Assoc 1987;114:85-87.
25. DeRossi SS, Garfunkel A, Greenberg MS. Hematologic diseases. In Lynch MA (ed). Burket's Oral Medicine: Diagnosis and Treatment, 10th ed. Hamilton, Ontario, BC Decker, 2003.
26. Bsoul SA, Flint DJ, Terezhalmy GT, Moore WS. Sickle cell disease. Quintessence Int 2003;34:76-77.
27. Hoffman R, Benz EJ, Shattil SJ, et al (eds). Hematology: Basic Principles and Practice, New York, Churchill Livingstone, 2000.

28. Forbes CD, Jackson WF. Color Atlas and Text of Clinical Medicine, 3rd ed. St. Louis, Mosby, 2003.

29. Centers for Disease Control and Prevention. Recommendation to prevent and control iron deficiency in the United States. MMWR Recomm Rep 1998;47:1-29.

30. Charache S, Terrin ML, Moore RD, et al. Effect of hydroxyurea on the frequency of painful crises in sickle cell anemia. Investigators of the Multicenter Study of Hydroxyurea in Sickle Cell Anemia. N Engl J Med 1995;332:1317-1322.

31. Davies SC, Gilmore A. The role of hydroxyurea in the management of sickle cell disease, Blood Rev 2003;17:99-109.

32. Davies SC, Roberts IA. Bone marrow transplant for sickle cell disease—An update. Arch Dis Child 1996;75:3-6.

33. Dubois RW, Goodnough LT, Ershler WB, et al. Identification, diagnosis, and management of anemia in adult ambulatory patients treated by primary care physicians: Evidence-based and consensus recommendations. Curr Med Res Opin 2006;22:385-395.

34. Agarwal R. Overcoming barriers that inhibit proper treatment of anemia. Kidney Int 2006;101:S9-S12.

35. Drug Information for the Health Care Professional. Taunton, Mass, Thomson Micromedex, 2006.

36. Ogundipe O, Pearson MW, Slater NG, et al. Sickle cell disease and nitrous oxide–induced neuropathy. Clin Lab Haematol 1999;21:409-412.

37. Sansevere JJ, Milles M. Management of the oral and maxillofacial surgery patient with sickle cell disease and related hemoglobinopathies. J Oral Maxillofac Surg 1993;51:912-916.

38. Shafer WG, Hine MK, Levy BM. A Textbook of Oral Pathology, 4th ed. Philadelphia, WB Saunders, 1983.

39. Neville BW, Damm DD, Allen CM, Bouquot JE. Oral and Maxillofacial Pathology, 2nd ed. Philadelphia, WB Saunders, 2002.

Disorders of White Blood Cells

CHAPTER

24

Disorders of white blood cells (WBCs) can greatly influence dental treatment because WBCs provide the primary defense against microbial infections and are critical for mounting an immune response (Box 24-1). Defects in WBCs can manifest as delayed healing, infection, or mucosal ulceration and, in some cases, may be fatal. To ensure the health of the patient, the dentist should be able to detect WBC abnormalities through history, clinical examination, and screening laboratory tests and should provide prompt referral to a physician for diagnosis and treatment before invasive dental procedures are performed. Patients with known life-threatening disorders who are under medical care should not receive dental care until after the dentist has consulted with the patient's physician.

Three groups of WBCs are found in the peripheral circulation: granulocytes, lymphocytes, and monocytes. Of the granulocyte population, 90% is composed of neutrophils; the remainder consists of eosinophils and basophils. Circulating lymphocytes are of three types: T lymphocytes (thymus mediated), B lymphocytes (bursa derived), and natural killer cells. Lymphocytes are subdivided by the surface markers they exhibit and by the cytokines they produce.[1]

The primary function of neutrophils is to defend the body against certain infectious agents (primarily bacteria) through phagocytosis and enzymatic destruction. Eosinophils and basophils are involved in inflammatory allergic reactions and mediate these reactions through release of their cytoplasmic granules. Eosinophils also combat infection by parasites. T lymphocytes (T cells) are involved with the delayed, or cellular, immune reaction, whereas B lymphocytes (B cells) play an important role in the immediate, or humoral, immune system involving the production of plasma cells and immunoglobulins (IgA, IgD, IgE, IgG, IgM). Monocytes have diverse functions that include phagocytosis, intracellular killing (especially of mycobacteria, fungi, and protozoa), and

mediating of the immune and inflammatory response through the production of more than 100 substances, such as cytokines and growth factors that increase the activity of lymphocytes. In addition, monocytes serve as antigen-presenting cells and migrate into tissues. In tissue, these antigen-presenting cells are known as dendritic cells (in lymph nodes) or Langerhans cells (in skin/mucosa). Monocytes in tissue that phagocytose microbes are known as macrophages.[1]

Most WBCs are produced primarily in the bone marrow (granulocytes and monocytes), and these cells form several "pools" in the marrow: (1) the mitotic pool, which consists of immature precursor cells; (2) a maturing pool, which consists of cells undergoing maturation; and (3) a storage pool of functional cells, which can be released as needed.

WBCs released by the bone marrow that circulate in the peripheral blood account for only 5% of the total WBC mass and form two pools of cells: a marginal one and a circulating one. Cells in the marginal pool adhere to vessel walls and are readily available. When infection threatens the body, the storage and marginal pools can be called on to help fight the invading organisms.

Growth-promoting substances called *colony-stimulating factors (CSFs)* are responsible for the growth of committed granulocyte-monocyte stem cells. The major function of CSFs is to amplify leukopoiesis rather than recruit new stem cells into the granulocyte-monocyte differentiation pathway. Thus, through the local release of CSFs, the bone marrow can increase the production of granulocytes and monocytes. This process occurs in response to infection.[2]

Lymphocytes localize primarily in three regions: lymph nodes, the spleen, and mucosa-associated lymphoid tissue (MALT; lining of the respiratory and gastrointestinal tracts). At these sites, microbial antigens are trapped and presented to B or T lymphocytes (cells). Antigens bind B cells via cell surface immunoglobulin,

Classification and Features of White Blood Cell (WBC) Dyscrasias

Leukocytosis—Increased number of circulating WBCs
Leukopenia—Decreased number of circulating WBCs
Myeloproliferative disorders
(1) Acute myeloid leukemia—Immature neoplastic malignancy of myeloid cells
(2) Chronic myeloid leukemia—Mature neoplastic malignancy of myeloid cells
Lymphoproliferative disorders
(1) Acute lymphoblastic leukemia—Immature neoplastic malignancy of lymphoid cells
(2) Chronic lymphocytic leukemia—Mature neoplastic malignancy of lymphoid cells
(3) Lymphomas
  (a) Hodgkin's disease—Malignant growth of B lymphocytes, primarily in lymph nodes
  (b) Non-Hodgkin's lymphoma—B- or T-cell malignant neoplasms, many types and locations; most are of B-cell lineage
    (i) Burkitt's lymphoma—Non-Hodgkin's B-cell lymphoma involving bone and lymph nodes
(4) Multiple myeloma—Overproduction of malignant plasma cells involving bone

whereupon B cells are activated, proliferate, and produce large amounts of immunoglobulin to aid in opsonization. Antigens are presented to CD4+ (helper) T cells via major histocompatibility complex (MHC) class I molecules, and to CD8+ T cells via MHC class II molecules. CD4+ T cells activate B cells and macrophages by producing cytokines and through direct contact. CD8+ T cells kill virus-infected cells.

LEUKOCYTOSIS AND LEUKOPENIA

The number of circulating WBCs normally ranges from 4400 to $11,000/mm^3$ in adults.[3] The differential WBC count is an estimation of the percentage of each cell type per cubic millimeter of blood. A normal differential count consists of neutrophils, 50% to 60%; eosinophils, 1% to 3%; basophils, less than 1%; lymphocytes, 20% to 34%; and monocytes, 3% to 7%. The term *leukocytosis* is defined as an increase in the number of circulating WBCs (lymphocytes or granulocytes) to more than $11,000/mm^3$, and *leukopenia* as a reduction in the number of circulating WBCs (usually to $<4400/mm^3$).

Many causes of leukocytosis are known. Exercise, pregnancy, and emotional stress can lead to increased numbers of WBCs in the peripheral circulation. Leukocytosis resulting from these causes is called *physiologic leukocytosis*. Pathologic leukocytosis can be caused by infection, neoplasia, and necrosis. Pyogenic infections induce a type of leukocytosis that is characterized by an increased number of neutrophils. If excessive numbers of

immature neutrophils (stab cells) are released into the circulation in response to a bacterial infection, a shift to the left is said to have occurred. Tuberculosis, syphilis, and viral infections produce a type of leukocytosis that is characterized by increased numbers of lymphocytes. Protozoan infections often produce a type of leukocytosis that increases the numbers of monocytes. Allergies and parasitic infections caused by certain helminths increase the numbers of circulating eosinophils. Cellular necrosis increases the numbers of circulating neutrophils. Leukemia (cancer of the WBCs) is characterized by a great increase in the numbers of circulating immature leukocytes. Carcinoma of glandular tissues may cause an increase in the number of circulating neutrophils. Acute bleeding also can result in leukocytosis.

Many causes of deficient numbers of leukocytes ($<4400/mm^3$) in the blood are evident. Leukopenia may occur in the early phase of leukemia and lymphoma as a result of bone marrow replacement through excessive proliferation of WBCs. Leukopenia also occurs during agranulocytosis (reduction of granulocytes) and pancytopenia (decreased WBCs and RBCs) that result from toxic effects of drugs and chemicals. Leukopenia is a common complication that results from the use of chemotherapeutic (anticancer) drugs.

Cyclic Neutropenia

An important form of leukopenia involving the cyclic depression of circulating neutrophils is a disorder called *cyclic neutropenia*. In this condition patients have a periodic decrease (at least a 40% drop) in the number of neutrophils (about every 21 to 28 days). During the period in which few circulating neutrophils are present, the patient is susceptible to infection and oral manifestations (see Oral Complications and Manifestations in this chapter).[4,5] Familial and chronic idiopathic forms of neutropenia also contribute.[6]

Patients with leukocytosis or leukopenia may have bone marrow abnormalities that can cause thrombocytopenia. Examination of the patient's bone marrow aspirate is important for making the final diagnosis. Infectious diseases that can cause leukocytosis and leukopenia are discussed in Chapters 9, 14, and 19.

LEUKEMIA AND LYMPHOMA

The remainder of this chapter focuses on leukemia and malignancies of lymphoid cells (lymphoma and multiple myeloma), with focused discussion of those types that are common and/or have head and neck manifestations.

Leukemia and lymphoma account for about 8% of all new malignancies each year in the United States, which amounts to approximately 101,000 cases per year.[7,8] These patients become gravely ill if they are not properly identified and do not receive appropriate medical care. In addition, patients are usually immunosuppressed as a result of the disease itself or because of the treatment used to control it. Hence, they are prone to develop serious infection and often bleed easily because of thrombocytopenia. A dental practice that manages 3000 patients is predicted to have 1 patient who develops leukemia or a malignancy of lymphoid cells.

Leukemia

Leukemia is cancer of the WBCs that affects the bone marrow and circulating blood. It involves exponential proliferation of a clonal myeloid or lymphoid cell and occurs in both acute and chronic forms. Acute leukemia is a rapidly progressive disease that results from accumulation of immature, functionless WBCs in the marrow and blood. Chronic leukemias have a slower onset, which allows production of larger numbers of more mature (terminally differentiated), functional cells. This section focuses on four types of leukemia: (1) acute lymphocytic, (2) acute myeloid, (3) chronic lymphocytic, and (4) chronic myeloid.

Leukemia occurs in all races, at any age, at an incidence of 10.4 per 100,000.[7] Approximately 35,000 new cases are diagnosed per year in the United States.[7-9] The incidence of leukemia has remained somewhat stable in the United States since about 1956. The mortality rate also has remained rather stable, at about 8.2 deaths per 100,000 population per year, with 50% to 60% of deaths caused by acute leukemia. All types of leukemia are somewhat more common in men. The male/female ratio for acute leukemia is about 3:2, and for chronic leukemia, it is about 2:1.

Acute leukemias are more common than chronic leukemias, accounting for 55% of all leukemias. Leukemia is 9 times more common in adults than in children, with more than half of all cases occurring after age 65 years. The most common types of leukemia in adults are acute myelogenous leukemia (AML), with an estimated 11,960 new cases this year, and chronic lymphocytic leukemia (CLL), with some 10,020 new cases this year. Chronic myelogenous leukemia (CML) is estimated to affect about 4600 persons this year. The most common form of leukemia among children younger than 19 years of age is acute lymphocytic leukemia (ALL). It accounts for about 3930 cases this year. Other unclassified forms of leukemia account for the remaining 4550 cases.[8]

The cause of leukemia remains unknown. Increased risk is associated with large doses of ionizing radiation, certain chemicals (benzene), and infection with specific viruses (e.g., Epstein-Barr virus [EBV], human lymphotropic virus [HTLV]-1).[9,10] Cigarette smoking and exposure to electromagnetic fields also have been proposed to be causative. Box 24-2 lists various factors that have been implicated as causes of human leukemia.

ACUTE MYELOGENOUS LEUKEMIA
DEFINITION

AML is a neoplasm of myeloid (immature) WBCs that demonstrate uncontrolled proliferation in the bone

---

BOX 24-2

Etiology of the Leukemias

1. Host factors
   a. Heredity
      (1) Generally not an inherited disease
      (2) High concordance among identical twins if one twin develops the disease early
      (3) A few leukemic families have been reported
   b. Chromosomal abnormalities—Increased risk in patients with the following:
      (1) Down syndrome
      (2) Turner's syndrome
      (3) Klinefelter's syndrome
      (4) Fanconi's anemia
   c. Immunodeficiency syndromes (hereditary types)
   d. Chronic bone marrow dysfunction
2. Environmental factors
   a. Ionizing radiation
      (1) Radiation therapy
      (2) Occupational exposure
      (3) Atomic bomb survivors
   b. Chemical and drugs
      (1) Benzene (organic solvents)
      (2) Chloramphenicol
      (3) Phenylbutazone
      (4) Arsenic pesticides
      (5) Alkylating chemotherapeutic agents
   c. Viruses
      (1) HTLV-I (adult T-cell leukemia)
      (2) HTLV-II (atypical hairy cell leukemia)

HTLV, Human T lymphotropic virus.

---

marrow space and subsequently appear in the peripheral blood.

EPIDEMIOLOGY

AML accounts for 32% of all leukemias and has an incidence of 4.6 per 100,000 persons in the United States. Incidence increases with age and rises exponentially after age 40. Incidence is 35 per 100,000 by age 90. The mean age of persons with AML in the United States is 63 years.[11]

Etiology

AML arises de novo in younger adults or secondarily in the elderly because of myelodysplasia. Environmental or genetic factors (e.g., translocation and rearrangement of chromosomes) may cause cytogenetic abnormalities that affect transcriptional cascades of myeloid precursor cells and uncontrolled proliferation of these cells.

Pathophysiology and Complications

AML has a sudden onset and leads to death in 1 to 3 months if left untreated.[12] It involves increased numbers of immature myeloid WBCs in the bone marrow space and peripheral circulation (Figure 24-1). As a result, patients are susceptible to excessive bleeding, anemia,

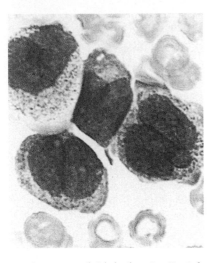

Figure 24-1. Acute myeloid leukemia. Peripheral blood smear shows many myeloid cells with large nuclei and azurophilic granules. (From Hoffbrand AV, Pettit JE. Color Atlas of Clinical Hematology, 3rd ed. London, Mosby, 2000. Courtesy Prof. J. M. Chessells.)

poor healing, and infection after surgical procedures.[12] Hemorrhage and infection, frequent complications of chemotherapy, are the chief causes of death.

CLINICAL PRESENTATION

Signs and Symptoms

AML produces a leukemic infiltration of marrow and organs that causes cytopenia and diverse nonspecific signs and symptoms, including fatigue, easy bruising, and bone pain. Anemia and thrombocytopenia usually manifest as malaise, pallor, dyspnea on exertion, and bleeding and small hemorrhage (petechiae, ecchymoses) in the skin and mucous membranes (Figure 24-2, *A*).[13] Because of granulocytopenia, at least one third of patients have recurrent infections (nonhealing wounds), oral ulcerations, and fever. Enlargement of the tonsils, lymph nodes, spleen, and gingiva (Figure 24-2, *B*) occurs as a result of leukemic infiltration of these tissues. Infiltration of the central nervous system (CNS) and the skin as a raised, nonpruritic rash is referred to as *leukemia cutis*.

Laboratory Findings

The diagnosis of leukemia is made through examination of peripheral blood and bone marrow stained with Wright-Giemsa. Cytochemical staining, immunophenotyping, and cytogenetic analyses are used to characterize the type and subtype, to allow for specific treatment approaches, and to detect residual disease after therapy is provided. Granulocytopenia and thrombocytopenia are common.

The diagnosis of AML is made when at least myeloblasts are found in the bone marrow or peripheral blood at a rate of 20%. Myeloblasts stain positive for myeloperoxidase and are immunotype positive for several of the following markers: CD13, CD33, CD34, CD65, and CD117.[14] The French-American-British classification categorizes AML into eight subtypes (Table 24-1). The

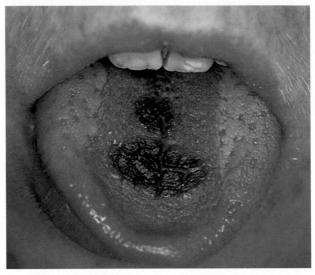

A

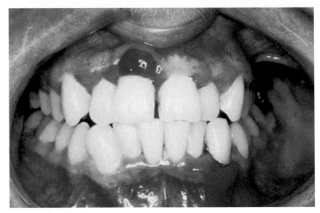

B

Figure 24-2. A, Acute myeloid leukemia presenting as bleeding and ecchymosis of the tongue in a 14-year-old. **B,** Gingival leukemia infiltrate in a patient with acute myeloid leukemia.

WHO classification describes four subtypes that differ in terms of genetic abnormalities, evolution, and response to therapy.[15]

ACUTE LYMPHOID LEUKEMIA

DEFINITION

ALL is the result of uncontrolled monoclonal proliferation of immature lymphoid cells in the bone marrow and peripheral blood. These neoplastic cells may also expand in the lymph nodes, liver, spleen, or CNS.

EPIDEMIOLOGY

ALL occurs at an incidence of 1.7 in 100,000 and typically occurs in children. It accounts for about 25% of all neoplasms in children and 80% of leukemias in children.[8] A remarkable peak of incidence occurs in children who are 2 to 4 years old, with 75% of cases reported in this age group. Boys are affected slightly more often than girls.

TABLE **24-1**

Classification of Acute Leukemias and Associated Clinical,* Cytologic, and Immunologic Abnormalities

| FAB Subtype | Common Name (% of Cases) | Results of Staining | | | Cell Surface Markers | Chromosomal Abnormalities |
		Myelo-peroxidase and Sudan Black	Nonspecific Esterase	PAS		
ACUTE MYELOID LEUKEMIAS (AMLS)						
M0	Acute myeloblastic leukemia with or without differentiation (3%)	–	–	–	HLADR, Anti-CD13, CD33, CD33, CD34, CD117	inv and t
M1	Acute myeloblastic leukemia with little maturation (15%-20%)	+	±	–	HLADR, Anti-CD13, CD33, CD33, CD34, CD65, CD117	Various
M2	Acute myeloblastic leukemia with differentiation (25%-30%)	+	±	+	HLADR, Anti-CD14, CD15, CD33, CD34, CD65, CD117	t(8;21)
M3	Acute promyelocytic leukemia (APML) (5%-10%)	+	+	+	Anti-CD13, CD15, CD33, CD65	t(15;17)
M4	Acute myelomonocytic leukemia (20%)	+	+++	++	Anti-CD13, CD15, CD33, CD34, CD65	inv and t
M5	Acute monocytic leukemia (2%-9%)	+	+++	++	HLADR, Anti-CD13, CD15, CD33, CD34, CD36, CD65	t(9;11)
M6	Acute erythroleukemia (3%-5%)	+	–	++	Antiglycopherin antispectrin, Anti-CD13, CD33, CD36, CD65	
M7	Acute megakaryocytic leukemia (3%-12%)	–	±	+	CD33, CD36, CD41,	t
ACUTE LYMPHOBLASTIC LEUKEMIAS (ALLS)						
L1, Childhood variant	Small, uniform blasts, nucleoli indistinct	–	–	+++	About 80% react with anti-CD10; 20% with T-Cell phenotype: anti-CD1, 2, 3, 5, or 7	t(9;22), t(4;11), and t(1;9)
L2, Adult variant	Larger, more irregular nucleoli present	–	–	++		
L3, Burkitt's-like	Large, with strong basophilic cytoplasm and vacuoles	–	–	–	Anti-CD19, 20	t(8;14)

Modified from Appelbaum FR. Acute myeloid leukemia in adults. In Abeloff MD, Armitage JO, Niederhuber JE, et al (eds). Clinical Oncology, 3rd ed. Philadelphia, Elsevier, 2004.

*Clinical signs of leukemia: Pallor, lymphadenopathy, petechiae, ecchymoses, gingival enlargement, oral ulcerations, loose teeth, pulpal abscess, enlarged tonsils, gingival bleeding, recurrent infections.

Clinical symptoms of leukemia: Dyspnea, palpitations, fever, weakness, weight loss, sore throat, bone and organ pain.

Note: The WHO classifies AML into four major categories: acute myeloid leukemia with recurrent genetic abnormalities (four subtypes), acute myeloid leukemia with multilineage dysplasia (two subtypes), acute myeloid leukemia and myelodysplastic syndromes (two subtypes), acute myeloid leukemia, and not otherwise categorized (11 subtypes).

Etiology

Although environmental, infectious, and genetic factors are considered likely causes of the disease, causal links for ALL have not been established. The disease is 20-fold more common in patients with Down syndrome (trisomy 21). Cytogenetic studies frequently display the Philadelphia chromosome, a shortened chromosome 22, as a result of translocation of genes between the long arms of chromosomes 9 and 22. Other chromosomal anomalies are also common and result in 50 to 65 chromosomes (e.g., hyperdiploidy).[14,16,17]

Pathophysiology and Complications

Similar to AML, ALL results in suppression of normal hematopoiesis, leaving patients susceptible to excessive bleeding, anemia, poor healing, and infection after

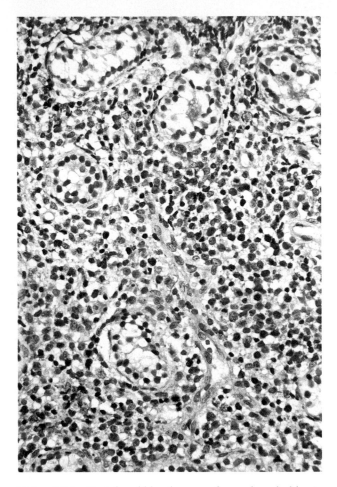

Figure 24-3. Peripheral blood smear of acute lymphoblastic leukemia. (From Hoffbrand AV, Pettit JE. Color Atlas of Clinical Hematology, 3rd ed. London, Mosby, 2000.)

surgical procedures have been performed.[14,18] Treatment of children results in remission rates that exceed 90% and cure rates above 70%. In adults, long-term survival from ALL occurs at rates of only about 30% to 40%.

CLINICAL PRESENTATION
Signs and Symptoms

The clinical presentation of ALL can be acute or insidious. Presenting signs and symptoms relate to anemia, thrombocytopenia, fever, and neutropenia. Frequently, bone and joint pain have effects on walking, bruisability, and infection. A higher propensity toward CNS disease occurs with ALL compared with AML. Patients may present with cranial nerve deficiencies.

Laboratory Findings

The diagnosis of ALL is made when massive replacement of the bone marrow space with leukemic blast cells is observed (Figure 24-3). A correspondingly high number of lymphoblasts are detected in the peripheral blood smear and levels of Hb, hematocrit, and platelets are depressed, reflecting large replacement of marrow by lymphoblasts. Immunotyping and flow cytometry is the preferred method of lineage assignment and assessment of cell maturation. Detection of a nuclear enzyme, terminal deoxynucleotidyl transferase (Tdt), along with (B cell) antigen (CD10, originally designated CALLA) and CD19, CD22, and HLA-DR, allows histologic classification of ALL.[5,14]

According to the French-American-British Cooperative Group, three distinct subtypes are based on type and size of neoplastic lymphocytes: L1 (cells small and homogenous), L2 (cells pleomorphic and often large in size), and L3 (cells homogenous of medium size with dispersed chromatic).[14,19]

MEDICAL MANAGEMENT OF ACUTE LEUKEMIA

The ability to cure a patient of acute leukemia is related to tumor burden and the rapid elimination of malignant WBCs. Normal bone marrow consists of 0.3% to 5% blast cells. Patients with acute leukemia have 100-fold more (about a trillion) blast cells. Once effective chemotherapy has been given, the number of blast cells is reduced from trillions to billions, leukemic cells can no longer be detected, and the patient is said to be in remission. With a 5-day generation time for the remaining undetectable leukemic cell mass, 10 doublings in 50 days could restore the leukemic cell mass to a trillion cells, and the patient would again show signs and symptoms of leukemia. This would constitute a short remission with relapse.[20]

Chemotherapy for acute leukemia consists of three phases. The purpose of the first phase (induction) is to hit hard and induce a state of remission by killing tumor cells with cytotoxic agents. Agents used to treat the acute leukemias are shown in Table 24-2. The second phase (consolidation or intensification) focuses on consolidating the kill of remaining leukemic cells. During the third phase (remission), maintenance therapy is provided to prevent expansion of any remaining leukemic cell mass. During induction and consolidation, myeloid growth factors (granulocyte colony-stimulating factor [G-CSF] and granulocyte-monocyte colony-stimulating factor [GM-CSF]) are administered at some institutes to shorten the duration of neutropenia and reduce the incidence of severe infection.

Patients are cured of leukemia when no leukemic cells remain. Long-term survival occurs when the leukemic cell mass is greatly reduced and is kept from increasing over a long period. In general, once a patient relapses, a second remission is more difficult to induce, and, if it occurs, it will be of a shorter duration. Bone marrow transplantation (BMT) is generally reserved for those younger than 45 years of age and for children and young adults who relapse when a suitable sibling match is available (allogeneic).[10,14] The marrow transplant or, more recently, the peripheral blood stem cell transplant, is preceded by high-dose chemotherapy (including busulfan) and radiation therapy.

TABLE 24-2
Classes of Drugs Used to Treat Leukemia

Class of Drug	Chemotherapeutic Agents	Mechanism of Action
Alkylating agents	Busulfan, carmustine, cyclophosphamide, dacarbazine, lomustine nitrogen mustard. Derivative: chlorambucil	Produce alkyl radicals, causing cross-linking of DNA and inhibition of DNA synthesis in rapidly replicating tumor cells
Antibiotics	Bleomycin, daunorubicin, doxorubicin, idarubicin, mitomycin C	Disrupt cellular functions, such as RNA synthesis, or inhibit mitosis
Antimetabolites	Folic acid analogs: Methotrexate Purine analogs: Cladribine, fludarabine, fluorouracil 6-mercaptopurine, thioguanine Pyrimidine nucleoside analogs: Arabinosyl cytosine (Ara-C, cytarabine)	Disrupt enzymatic processes or nucleic acid synthesis
Biologicals	Interferon alfa Monoclonal antibodies (e.g., rituximab [Rituxan]) All-trans retinoic acid (tretinoin)	Causes a direct antiproliferative effect on CML progenitor cells Binds antigen target on malignant lymphocyte Induces differentiation and apoptosis of malignant promyelocytes in APML
Enzymes	Asparaginase	Inhibits synthesis of asparagines, which is required for protein synthesis in leukemic lymphoblasts
Mitotic inhibitors	Vincristine, vinblastine Etoposide	Act as mitotic spindle inhibitors causing metaphase arrest Topoisomerase II inhibitor
Steroid	Prednisone	Hormone that has anti-inflammatory and antilymphocytic properties

APML, Acute promyelocytic leukemia; CML, chronic myelogenous leukemia.

Another concern related to treatment of patients with acute leukemia is that leukemic cells can migrate to areas in the body where chemotherapeutic agents cannot reach them. These areas are called *sanctuaries*, and they require special treatment. The most important sanctuary in patients with ALL is the CNS. Thus, patients with ALL are treated with intrathecal methotrexate plus high-dose systemic chemotherapy. Another important sanctuary (in males) is the testes.[10,14]

Treatment of patients with AML involves chemotherapy (see Table 24-2), BMT, or, in specific cases (e.g., M3, acute promyelocytic leukemia [APML]), tretinoin (vitamin A analog) and chemotherapy. The prognosis of AML in adults who are 60 years or older is poor. Chemotherapy can produce remission in 60% to 80% of these older patients, but the duration is short (Table 24-3). Additional adverse prognostic factors include previous chemotherapy for AML, WBC greater than 20,000/mm^3, elevated serum lactate dehydrogenase, and development of preleukemia syndrome.[21] In contrast, complete remission occurs in 70% to 80% of adults younger than 60 years of age who undergo intensive treatment and in more than 90% of those with promyelocytic leukemia who are treated with tretinoin.

ALL is treated with multiagent, dose-intensive chemotherapy. Vincristine, daunorubicin, and corticosteroids are the primary agents used. The prognosis for children with ALL is very good, with cure now being attained in more than 70% of cases. The prognosis is worse in those older than 30 years of age, with a blast count greater than 50,000/mm^3, with mature B-cell ALL phenotype, multiorgan involvement, and chromosomal translocations t(9;22) and t(4;11). In these patients, remission can be achieved with chemotherapy; however, the duration of remission is short. Overall long-term survival (cure) for adults is less than 20%.[10] Relapse can result in second remission in 75%, but less than 30% of these patients are cured.

Oral Manifestations of Acute Leukemia

Leukemic patients are prone to develop gingival enlargement, ulceration, and oral infection. Localized or generalized gingival enlargement is caused by inflammation and infiltration of atypical and immature WBCs (see Figure 24-2). It occurs in up to 36% of those with acute leukemia (most frequently with the acute myelomonocytic types) and in about 10% of those with chronic leukemia.[6] The gingiva is boggy and bleeds easily, and multiple tooth sites are typically affected. Generalized gingival enlargement is more common and is particularly prevalent when oral hygiene is poor and in patients who have AML (particularly the monocytic type [M5; see Table 24-1]). The combination of poor oral hygiene and gingival enlargement contributes to gingival bleeding and fetor oris. Gingival bleeding is exacerbated by the presence of thrombocytopenia. Plaque control measures,

TABLE 24-3
Clinical Factors in Acute and Chronic Leukemias

Factor	ALL	AML	CLL	CML
		Type of Leukemia		
Age	Children (75%)	Adults (85%)	Over 40 years	30-50 years
Prognosis	Very good	Poor	Good	Poor
Survival, mean	—	2 years	Stage I (19 months)	3-4 years
			Stage IV (12 years)	—
Remissions	90%	60%-80%	—	—
Duration	Usually long term	9-24 months	—	—
Cures	50%-70%	10%-30%	—	—
	ALL	**AML**	**CLL**	**CML**
Age	Adults (25%)	Children (15%)	Children (rare)	Children (rare)
Prognosis	Poor	Poor	—v	—
Survival, mean	26 months	—	—	—
Remissions	50%-70%	56%-66%	—	—
Duration	10-19 months	8-12 months	—	—
Cures	20%	20%-40%	—	—

Modified from Wetzler M, Byrd JC, Bloomfield CD. Acute and chronic myeloid leukemia. In Kasper DL, et al (eds). Harrison's Principles of Internal Medicine, 16th ed. New York, McGraw-Hill, 2005; Armitage JO, Longo DL. Malignancies of lymphoid cells. In Kasper DL, et al (eds). Harrison's Principles of Internal Medicine, 16th ed. New York, McGraw-Hill, 2005.
ALL, Acute lymphocytic leukemia; AML, acute myelogenous leukemia; CLL, chronic lymphocytic leukemia; CML, chronic myelogenous leukemia.

chlorhexidine, and chemotherapy promote resolution of the condition.

A localized mass of leukemic cells (in the gingiva or other sites) is specifically known as a *granulocytic sarcoma* or *chloroma*. These extramedullary tumors have been observed in the maxilla and the palate.[22]

CHRONIC MYELOID LEUKEMIA
DEFINITION

Chronic myeloid leukemia (CML) is a neoplasm of mature myeloid WBCs.

EPIDEMIOLOGY

CML has an incidence of 2 cases per 100,000 population, or about 4600 cases per year, in the United States.[7,8] It accounts for 15% of all leukemias and is less common than CLL in the United States. Most patients with CML are older than 60 years of age. Men are more commonly affected (2:1) than women. CML causes 3% of childhood leukemias.

Etiology

The etiology is unknown, but radiation exposure increases risk for the disease. The genetic defect consists of translocation of the cellular oncogene ABL from chromosome 9 to the BCR gene of chromosome 22 and a reciprocal translocation of part of BCR from chromosome 22 to the ABL gene in chromosome 9. A shortened chromosome 22, the Philadelphia (Ph) chromosome, results from the

translocations and is evident in more than 90% of cases of CLL.[5] The Philadelphia chromosome is also present in ALL. Translocation contributes to increased tyrosine kinase activity and myeloid proliferation.[23]

Pathophysiology and Complications

CML progresses slowly through a chronic phase for 3 to 5 years, then on to an accelerated phase followed by a blast phase (or crisis). During the indolent phase of CML, leukemic cells are functional; thus, infection is not a major problem. However, once transformation to the blastic stage has occurred, the leukemic cells are immature and nonfunctional. As a result, anemia, thrombocytopenia, and infection become problems. About 25% of patients with CML patients per year undergo transformation to the blast phase of the disease 6 to 12 months after diagnosis. The blast phase consists of 30% or more leukemic cells in the peripheral blood or marrow.[24] More than 85% of patients with CML die in the blast phase, and patients without the Philadelphia chromosome have a worse prognosis. The overall prognosis for CML is poor, and survival from the time of diagnosis is about 3.5 years.[5,25,26]

CLINICAL PRESENTATION
Signs and Symptoms

In nearly 90% of patients, CML is diagnosed during the chronic phase. Up to half of these patients are asymptomatic, and diagnosis is based on their complete blood count. Common symptoms are fatigue, weakness, abdom-

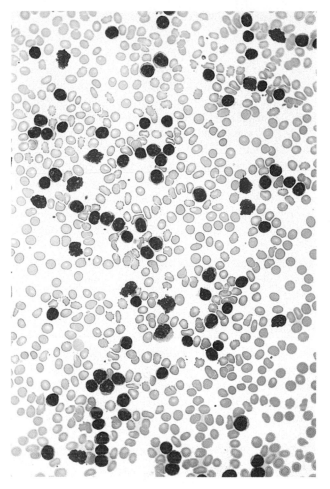

Figure 24-4. Chronic myeloid leukemia. Peripheral blood smear shows myeloblasts, promyelocytes, and segmented neutrophils. (From Hoffbrand AV, Pettit JE. Color Atlas of Clinical Hematology, 3rd ed., London, Mosby, 2000.)

inal (upper left quadrant) pain, abdominal fullness, weight loss, night sweats due to anemia, an enlarged and painful spleen (splenomegaly), and altered hematopoiesis. Hyperviscosity of the blood may cause a stroke.

Laboratory Findings

Patients are identified by marked elevation of their WBC count during routine examination (Figure 24-4). WBC count is usually above 50,000/mm³ at the time of diagnosis, and basophilia and eosinophilia are present. Cytogenetic analysis, a part of the standard diagnostic workup, reveals the Ph chromosome in more than 90% of cases. Serum chemistry reveals elevated levels of lactate dehydrogenase (LDH) and low levels of leukocyte alkaline phosphatase. The bone marrow is markedly hypercellular.

MEDICAL MANAGEMENT

Patients with CML were historically treated during the chronic phase with hydroxyurea or busulfan; this resulted in good symptom and blood count control, along with significant toxicity (see Table 24-2). Interferon-α or ima-

tinib mesylate (Gleevec), an inhibitor of tyrosine kinase, is widely used today.[26] Stem cell transplantation has resulted in remission in more than 55% of patients at 5 years when treatment is provided prior to transformation to the blastic stage.[25,26] Stem cell transplants are generally recommended for younger patients who have an adequate human leukocyte antigen (HLA) match.

Oral Manifestations

Chronic forms of leukemia are less likely to demonstrate oral manifestations than are acute forms of leukemia. Generalized lymphadenopathy, pallor of the oral mucosa, and soft tissue infection may be present.

CHRONIC LYMPHOCYTIC LEUKEMIA

DEFINITION

Chronic lymphocytic leukemia (CLL) is a neoplasm of mature clonal CD5+ B lymphocytes.

EPIDEMIOLOGY

CLL is the most common type of leukemia in adults.[27] It occurs at an incidence of 5.3 cases per 100,000 population. Patients with CLL are older; median age is older than 60 years. It is more common in Jewish people from Russian or Eastern European ancestry. This disease is rare in Asia and in children throughout the world.

Etiology

The etiology of CLL is unknown, and risk factors are more related to familial inheritance than to exposure to harmful environmental agents. Neoplastic B cells have various genetic aberrations, most commonly, gene deletions (e.g., on chromosome 11, 13, or 17) that lead to loss of cell cycle control.[27,28] The specific genetic defect dictates the course of the disease. A trisomy 12 chromosomal abnormality is present in the leukemic cells of 40% of patients. In most cases, low levels of expression of monoclonal immunoglobulin are demonstrated on the cell surface.

Pathophysiology and Complications

The pathophysiology of CLL relates directly to the slow lymphocytic infiltration of the bone marrow. This eventually results in marrow failure and anemia, hepatosplenomegaly, hypogammaglobulinemia, which contributes to poor wound healing, and risk for infection. Although the course of the disease is variable, median survival is 4 to 6 years.[5]

CLINICAL PRESENTATION

Signs and Symptoms

Most patients with CLL are asymptomatic at presentation. When symptoms occur, fatigue, anorexia, and

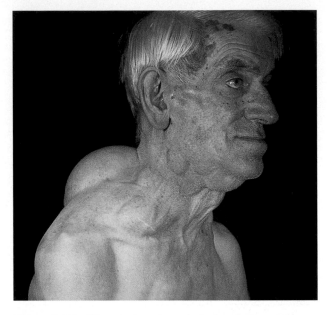

Figure 24-5. Chronic lymphocytic leukemia in a 65-year-old man with bilateral cervical lymphadenopathy. (From Hoffbrand AV, Pettit JE. Color Atlas of Clinical Hematology, 3rd ed. London, Mosby, 2000.)

TABLE 24-4
Comparison of Acute and Chronic Leukemias

Parameter	Acute	Chronic
Clinical onset	Sudden	Insidious
Course (untreated)	<6 months	2-6 years
Leukemic cells	Immature	Mature
Anemia	Mild to severe	Mild
Thrombocytopenia	Mild to severe	Mild
White blood cell count	Variable	Increased
Organomegaly	Mild	Prominent
Age	Adults and children	Adults

Modified from Perkins ML. Clinical Hematology and Fundamentals of Hemostasis. Philadelphia, FA Davis, 1992, pp 266-292.

weight loss are the most common complaints. Patients have an enlarged spleen, lymphadenopathy (Figure 24-5), and decreased serum immunoglobulin levels (hypogammaglobulinemia) that contribute to susceptibility to infection. Less frequently, patients with CLL develop autoantibodies against red blood cells (RBCs) or platelets that produce hemolytic anemia or thrombocytopenia. In about 15% of patients, CLL evolves into a more aggressive malignancy with increasing lymphadenopathy, hepatosplenomegaly, fever, abdominal pain, weight loss, progressive anemia, and thrombocytopenia. Second malignancies occur because of immune defects associated with the disease. Survival after this transformation lasts less than 1 year.[29] A comparison of the features of chronic and acute leukemias is provided in Table 24-4.

Laboratory Findings

CLL requires the presence of more than 5000 mature lymphocytes per cubic millimeter in the peripheral blood smear. Also evident in the smear are numerous small, round lymphocytes with scant cytoplasm. Immunotyping reveals the neoplastic cells to be B lymphocytes that are positive for CD3, CD19, CD20, and CD23.

CLL is classified with the use of an international staging system. Three stages are identified: stage A (two or fewer lymph node groups, no anemia or thrombocytopenia); stage B (three or more lymph node groups, no anemia or thrombocytopenia); and stage C (anemia and thrombocytopenia, any number of lymph node groups). Lymph node groups include cervical, axillary, inguinal, liver, and spleen. Mean survival time for patients with stage A disease is longer than 10 years; with stage B, about 5 years; and with stage C, only about 2 years.

MEDICAL MANAGEMENT

CLL is not a curable disease, and treatment has little effect on survival times. Patients in the asymptomatic phase usually are not treated. Only moderate effectiveness has been reported for some treatments in reducing lymphocyte counts and alleviating symptoms. Fludarabine is the most active agent used for the treatment of CLL. Chlorambucil and cyclophosphamide have been used in the treatment of CLL with some benefit.[20,21,27] These agents are used when disease-related symptoms (e.g., fevers, chills, anemia, thrombocytopenia, hepatosplenomegaly) affect the patient's quality of life. Prednisone is used to treat autoimmune complications.

Oral Manifestations

Generalized lymphadenopathy and pallor of the oral mucosa are features of CLL. Oral soft tissue infection may become evident as the patient develops hypoglobulinemia.

Lymphomas

Lymphoma is cancer of the lymphoid organs and tissues that presents as discrete tissue masses. Lymphomas represent the seventh most common malignancy worldwide and affect 63,000 Americans each year.[8] Lymphomas are classified by cell type (B cell, T cell, MALT, plasma cell), appearance (small or large cell, cleaved or noncleaved nucleus), and clinical behavior (of low, intermediate, and high grade); higher grades have been noted to be more aggressive. Of more than 20 types, 3 common lymphomas (Hodgkin's disease, non-Hodgkin's lymphoma, and Burkitt's lymphoma) and a plasma cell malignancy (multiple myeloma) are considered in this section. These diseases are of importance to the dentist because initial signs often occur in the mouth (e.g., Waldeyer's ring) and in the head and neck region, and precautions must be taken before any dental treatment is provided.

HODGKIN'S DISEASE

DEFINITION

Hodgkin's disease is a neoplasm (uncontrolled growth) of B lymphocytes that was named for Thomas Hodgkin, the British pathologist who first described it. This neoplasm contains a characteristic tumor cell called *the Reed-Sternberg cell* that represents usually <1% of the cellular infiltrate in affected tissues.[5]

EPIDEMIOLOGY

Hodgkin's disease affects about 7800 Americans per year.[7,8,30] It is the most common lymphoma in young adults. Hodgkin's disease has two peaks of incidence—one in early adulthood and the other around the fifth decade of life.[30] Men are at higher risk for developing the disease (3:2 male/female ratio).

Etiology

The cause of Hodgkin's disease is unknown, but EBV is frequently present (40% of cases in the Western world) in malignant lymphocytes. This virus can immortalize B cells in vitro and encodes a protein known as "latent membrane protein 1" that has oncogenic potential.[31] Increased risk is associated with family members who have the disease and human immunodeficiency virus (HIV)-infected patients.[32]

Pathophysiology and Complications

Enlarging tumorous nodes may cause lung or vascular obstruction, and enlarging mediastinal nodes can cause cough, shortness of breath, or dysphagia. The disease spreads predictably over weeks to months, first to other lymphoid sites (other lymph nodes and spleen), then hematogenously to extranodal sites, including bone marrow, liver, and lung. Without treatment, death occurs as a result of complications from bone marrow failure or infection.

CLINICAL PRESENTATION

Signs and Symptoms

Hodgkin's disease presents most commonly as a painless mass or a group of firm, nontender, enlarged lymph nodes, often (i.e., in more than 50% of cases) affecting the mediastinal nodes or the neck nodes (Figure 24-6, *A*).[30] Enlarged lymph nodes in the underarm or groin are also common presentations. Fever, weight loss, and night sweats occur in about one third of patients.[23] Pruritus and fatigue develop and may precede the appearance of enlarging lymph nodes. Palpation of the lymph nodes reveals a rubbery consistency.

Laboratory Findings

The diagnosis of lymphoma is made on the basis of nodal biopsy or bone marrow aspirate. Microscopically, tumor-

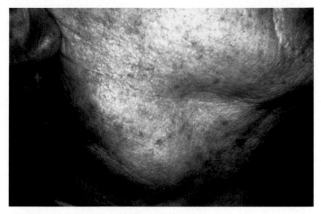

A

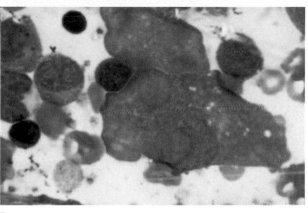

B

Figure 24-6. Hodgkin's disease. **A,** Cervical lymphadenopathy due to tumor infiltrate. **B,** Large Reed-Sternberg cells are shown in this bone marrow specimen.

ous tissue typically shows large, multinucleated Reed-Sternberg reticulum (monoclonal B) cells (Figure 24-6, *B*). Four pathologic variants have been described (nodular sclerosing, mixed cellularity, lymphocyte-depleted type, and lymphocyte-predominant type).

MEDICAL MANAGEMENT

Effective management requires accurate staging of the disease. Staging is performed on the basis of biopsies, medical history, physical examination findings, laboratory evaluation of the abdominal organs, and computed tomography (CT) and gallium scans that reveal the extent of disease (Figure 24-7). Poorer survival rates are associated with mixed cellularity and lymphocyte-depleted types, male sex, a large number of involved nodal sites, and bulky disease.

The current cure rate for Hodgkin's lymphoma is about 90%.[32] Historically, radiation (therapeutic dose >3.5 gray [Gy]) to involved sites was the primary mode of therapy. Contemporary strategies use a lower dose (<3.0 Gy) and more precise targeting of radiation (3-dimensional conformal radiotherapy intensity–modulated radiotherapy [IMRT]) to involved sites after disease volume has been reduced by chemotherapy with

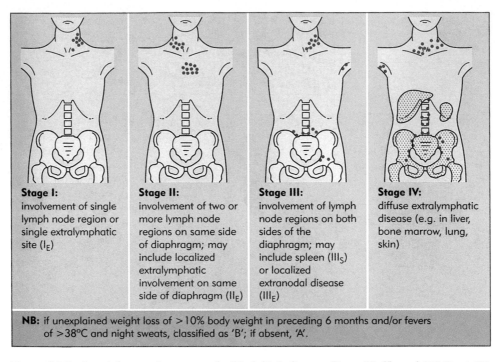

Stage I:
involvement of single lymph node region or single extralymphatic site (I$_E$)

Stage II:
involvement of two or more lymph node regions on same side of diaphragm; may include localized extralymphatic involvement on same side of diaphragm (II$_E$)

Stage III:
involvement of lymph node regions on both sides of the diaphragm; may include spleen (III$_S$) or localized extranodal disease (III$_E$)

Stage IV:
diffuse extralymphatic disease (e.g. in liver, bone marrow, lung, skin)

NB: if unexplained weight loss of >10% body weight in preceding 6 months and/or fevers of >38°C and night sweats, classified as 'B'; if absent, 'A'.

Figure 24-7. Ann Arbor staging system for Hodgkin's disease. (From Hoffbrand AV, Pettit JE. Color Atlas of Clinical Hematology, 3rd ed. London, Mosby, 2000. Originally modified from Hoffbrand AV, Pettit JE. Essential Haematology, 3rd ed. Oxford, Blackwell Science Publications, 1993.)

doxorubicin (Adriamycin), bleomycin, vinblastine, and dacarbazine (acronym ABVD). MOPP chemotherapy (mechlorethamine [an alkylating agent], vincristine [Oncovin], procarbazine, prednisone) is reserved for patients with preexisting cardiac disease. Increased risk for development of acute leukemia occurs in 3% to 10% of patients who receive alkylating agents as part of therapy,[33] and those receiving chest irradiation are at increased for breast cancer (women) and thyroid dysfunction (hypothyroidism).

Relapses, if they occur, generally occur within 2 years of therapy and seldom appear after 5 years. To prevent relapse, those who have received radiation therapy alone are provided subsequent ABVD chemotherapy (known as salvage therapy). If relapse occurs after standard radiation and/or chemotherapy, autologous peripheral stem cell transplantation is recommended.[34]

NON-HODGKIN'S LYMPHOMA
DEFINITION

Non-Hodgkin's lymphoma (NHL) comprises a large group of lymphoproliferative disorders classified as of B-cell or T-cell origin. More than 80% of these neoplasms are of B-cell origin.[5] The World Health Organization (WHO) classification system uses immunophenotype, cytogenetics, and epidemiologic/etiologic factors to distinguish the many types of NHL (Box 24-3). Four major categories of NHL are described: precursor (immature) B-cell neoplasms, peripheral (mature) B-cell neoplasms,

precursor (immature) T-cell neoplasms, and peripheral (mature) T-cell and natural killer (NK)-cell neoplasms.[5,23] Subcategories are based on pattern of distribution (diffuse or nodular), cell type (lymphocytic, histiocytic, mixed), and degree of differentiation of cells (good, moderate, poor). Of the more than 20 types of NHL that have been identified, diffuse large B-cell and follicular lymphomas account for about 60% of cases.[35]

EPIDEMIOLOGY

Each year, about 58,000 new cases are reported, and all races and age groups are affected. NHL is the sixth most common cancer in men and the fifth most common cancer in women in the United States.[8] NHL results in 25,000 deaths per year and is the seventh leading cause of death in the United States.[7,35,36] Median age at the time of diagnosis is 67 years.[36]

Etiology

The cause of NHL is unknown, but genetic factors, infectious agents, herbicides, radiation, and some forms of chemotherapy are increasingly recognized as causative agents. At the molecular level, malignant lymphocytes have chromosomal translocations or mutations in genes that regulate lymphocyte growth (*BCL6*) or survival (*BCL2*). Persistent inflammation from *Helicobacter pylori* infection of the stomach contributes to gastric lymphoma. Oncogenic viruses such as EBV, Kaposi's sarcoma herpes-virus (KSHV), and retroviruses are associated with several

WHO Classification of Non-Hodgkin's Lymphoma

B-CELL LYMPHOMAS
Precursor B-Cell lymphoma
• Precursor B lymphoblastic lymphoma/leukemia
Mature B-Cell lymphoma
• Chronic lymphocytic leukemia/small lymphocytic lymphoma
• Lymphoplasmacytic lymphoma
• Splenic marginal zone lymphoma
• Extranodal marginal zone B-cell lymphoma of mucosa-associated lymphoid tissue (MALT lymphoma)
• Nodal marginal zone B-cell lymphoma
• Follicular lymphoma
• Mantle cell lymphoma
• Diffuse large B-cell lymphoma
  • Mediastinal (thymic) large B-cell lymphoma
  • Intravascular large B-cell lymphoma
  • Primary effusion lymphoma
• Burkitt's lymphoma/leukemia

T/NK-CELL LYMPHOMA
Precursor T-Cell lymphoma
• Precursor T-cell lymphoblastic lymphoma
• Mature T/NK-cell lymphoma
• Adult T-cell lymphoma/leukemia
• Mycosis fungoides
• Sézary syndrome
• Primary cutaneous anaplastic large-cell lymphoma
• Anaplastic large-cell lymphoma
• Peripheral T-cell lymphoma, unspecified
• Angioimmunoblastic T-cell lymphoma
• Extranodal NK/T-cell lymphoma, nasal type
• Enteropathy-type T-cell lymphoma
• Hepatosplenic T-cell lymphoma
• Subcutaneous panniculitis-like T-cell lymphoma
• Blastic NK-cell lymphoma

Modified from Jaffe ES, et al. World Health Organization Classification of Tumours: Pathology & Genetics: Tumours of Haematopoietic and Lymphoid Tissues. Lyon, IARC, 2001.
WHO, World Health Organization; NK, natural killer.

types of NHL. Patients with autoimmune disease (Sjögren's syndrome) or immunodeficiency states (acquired immunodeficiency syndrome [AIDS], after chemotherapy) are at increased risk for the disease.[35]

Pathophysiology and Complications

The course of NHL varies from highly proliferative and rapidly fatal disorders to slowly progressing (indolent) malignancies that are tolerated for 10 to 20 years. Tumorous cells behave similarly to the cell of origin, tumorous B cells home to follicular regions of lymph nodes, and T cells have a propensity for paracortical T-cell zones. These neoplasms cause tumorous enlargements and abnormalities of the immune system. Tumors are often widespread at the time of diagnosis and more variable in location (to various organs such as liver and spleen) than

in Hodgkin's disease. Anemic and leukemic manifestations are common.

CLINICAL PRESENTATION
Signs and Symptoms

NHLs may occur at any age and are often marked by enlarged lymph nodes, fever, and weight loss. Different from Hodgkin's disease, which often begins with a single focus of tumor, NHL is usually multifocal when first detected.[30,55,36] The most prominent sign of NHL is a painless lymph node(s) swelling of longer than 2 weeks duration.[30,36] Additional signs and symptoms include persistent fever of unknown cause, weight loss, malaise, sweating, tender lymphadenopathy, abdominal or chest pain, and, on occasion, extranodal tumors.[36-38] Head, neck, and intra-abdominal manifestations occur fairly often.[45,46] Less frequently, an oral presentation (e.g., a firm swelling arising from the posterior hard palate) may be seen.

Laboratory Findings

The diagnosis of NHL is based on excisional biopsy of the involved lymph node. Tumorous cells are classified first by lineage (B, T, or NK cell) and second by level of differentiation. Immunologic and molecular genetic assays are performed to facilitate diagnosis. Proper staging of the patient requires complete blood count, chemistry screen, chest radiographs, CT scans, and bone marrow biopsy.

MEDICAL MANAGEMENT

Medical treatment of patients with the two most common NHLs (follicular and diffuse large B-cell lymphoma) is discussed. Follicular NHLs are radiosensitive, and the typical total dose is 35 Gy. Disease of more advanced stage (e.g., widespread lymphoid and organ involvement) requires the addition of chemotherapy. Survival is 80% at 15 years from the time of diagnosis.[35] Patients who have diffuse large B-cell lymphoma are treated with combination chemotherapy (cyclophosphamide, doxorubicin [Adriamycin], vincristine [Oncovin], and prednisone [CHOP]). Irradiation is added only if complete remission is not achieved. Those who have advanced disease who undergo radiotherapy and chemotherapy have a median survival of about 2 years.[44] Bone marrow transplants and monoclonal antibodies against antigens expressed by malignant lymphocytes (e.g., Rituxan), combined with chemotherapy, help patients who respond poorly to traditional therapies. Extranodal lymphomas in the oral/pharyngeal region have a poor prognosis. Table 24-5 compares the findings of Hodgkin's disease and NHL and emphasizes that disease-free survival with NHL is not very good.

Oral Complications and Manifestations

Patients with Hodgkin's disease or non-Hodgkin's lymphoma may present with cervical lymphadenopathy and

TABLE 24-5
Comparison of Non-Hodgkin's and Hodgkin's Lymphomas

Parameter	Non-Hodgkin's	Hodgkin's
Cellular derivation site	>80% B cell 10%-19% T cell or NK cell	B cell
Localized	Uncommon	Common
Waldeyer's ring	Commonly involved	Rarely involved
Extranodal	Common	Uncommon
Abdominal (mesenteric nodes)	Common	Uncommon
Mediastinal	Uncommon	Common
Bone marrow	Common	Uncommon
Symptoms (fever, night sweats, weight loss)	Uncommon	Common
Curability	<25%	>75%

Data from Armitage JO, Longo DL. Malignancies of lymphoid cells. In Kasper DL, et al (eds). Harrison's Principles of Internal Medicine, 16th ed. New York, McGraw-Hill, 2005.

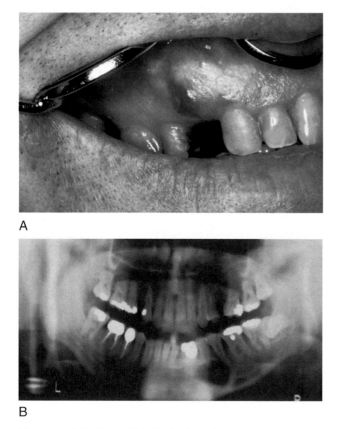

A

B

Figure 24-8. Non-Hodgkin's lymphoma presenting as **(A)** a gingival enlargement that also involved the underlying alveolar bone and **(B)** an osteolytic lesion of the mandible.

extranodal or intraoral tumors (Figure 24-8). This situation is of particular concern in immunosuppressed patients and individuals with Sjögren's syndrome who are at increased risk for the development of lymphoma. Patients should be periodically monitored for the development of orofacial neoplasia.[39]

Intraoral lymphoma most commonly involves Waldeyer's ring (soft palate and oropharynx)[40]; less often, the salivary glands and mandible are affected. Intraoral lymphomas appear as rapidly expanding (or chronic), unexplained swellings of the head and neck lymph nodes, palate, gingiva, buccal sulcus, or floor of the mouth. Enlargements may be painless or painful. Infrequently, patients experience deep "crateriform" oral ulcers and fever.[41] The presence of these orofacial abnormalities requires prompt evaluation by biopsy via needle, incisional, or excisional techniques.

Patients with lymphoma who have received medical treatment for their disease sometimes report that they have burning mouth symptoms, similar to those noted in patients with leukemia, that may be related to drug toxicity, xerostomia, candidiasis, or anemia[28] (see Appendix C for management regimens). Patients who have been given more than 30 Gy are susceptible to xerostomia and would benefit from salivary substitutes or pilocarpine.[52] Radiation also can damage taste buds, cause trismus of the masticatory muscles, and stunt craniomandibular growth and development. Osteoradionecrosis is a long-term risk associated with radiation doses to the jaws in excess of 50 Gy. The usual dose of irradiation to patients with lymphoma seldom puts them at risk for osteoradionecrosis, but they may develop xerostomia.[42] Protocols to reduce the risk of osteoradionecrosis have included the use of prophylactic antibiotics and/or hyperbaric oxygen, as well as antibiotics during the week of healing (see Chapter 26).[43]

BURKITT'S LYMPHOMA

DEFINITION

Burkitt's lymphoma is an aggressive B-cell (non-Hodgkin's) lymphoma that was originally described by Denis Burkitt.[44] The tumors are composed of mature B cells that express surface immunoglobulin (Ig)M.

EPIDEMIOLOGY

Burkitt's lymphoma is the most common lymphoma of childhood. It affects children and young adults at a rate of 0.05 cases per 100,000.[20,35] Two types are commonly described. Burkitt's lymphoma that is found most often in Central Africa is known as endemic Burkitt's lymphoma. Sporadic (nonendemic) Burkitt's lymphoma is more common in Western societies and affects slightly older children and adults in their 30s. A third aggressive type that occurs in HIV-infected individuals is also described.[5,20] Burkitt's lymphoma is more common among men.

Etiology

All Burkitt's lymphomas are associated with translocation of the *c-myc* gene (a gene involved in cellular proliferation) onto chromosome 8. In most cases, the immunoglobulin gene is translocated to chromosome 14 [t(8;14)], but it may also be translocated to chromosome 2 [t(2;8)] or 22 [t(8;22)]. These regions regulate immunoglobulin class (isotype) switching. All endemic tumors contain latent EBV. EBV is present in about 15% to 20% of sporadic lymphomas and in about 25% of HIV-associated tumors.

Pathophysiology and Complications

This malignancy is very aggressive and grows very rapidly. Tumors can double in size every 3 days; thus, obstruction of the airway, alimentary canal, and vasculature is possible. The tumor also has a propensity for spread to the central nervous system (CNS).

CLINICAL PRESENTATION

Signs and Symptoms

Most Burkitt's lymphomas arise at extranodal sites. The endemic form shows a predilection for tumors of the jaw and for involvement of select abdominal organs, particularly the kidneys, ovaries, and adrenal glands. Jaw involvement is more common in patients younger than 5 years of age than among those older than age 10 (Figure 24-9). Nonendemic Burkitt's lymphoma often presents as an abdominal mass that involves the lymph nodes of the intestine and peritoneum, with jaw lesions being less common. Tumors that enlarge as abdominal masses are accompanied by fluid buildup, pain, and, possibly, vomiting. The bone marrow is infrequently involved.

Laboratory Findings

The diagnosis is based on radiographic features and a histologic pattern of numerous small, noncleaved atypical B (CD10+) lymphocytes interspersed with lightly stained histiocytes ("starry sky" pattern) (Figure 24-10). Histologically, tumor cells are darkly stained and have small prominent nucleoli and a high mitotic index (feature of malignancy).[5] Intraoral radiographs of tumors of the endemic type reveal osteolytic jaw lesions with ill-defined margins and tooth displacement (floating teeth). Usually these develop distal to the last mandibular molar.

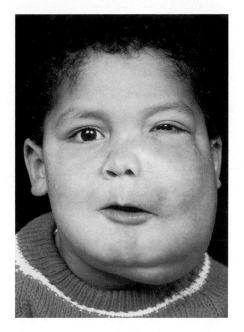

Figure 24-9. Burkitt's lymphoma showing characteristic facial swelling caused by extensive tumor involvement of the mandible and surrounding soft tissues. (From Hoffbrand AV, Pettit JE. Color Atlas of Clinical Hematology, 3rd ed. London, Mosby, 2000. Courtesy Prof. J. M. Chessells.)

MEDICAL MANAGEMENT

The disease responds well to high-dose chemotherapy. Tumors are particularly sensitive to cyclophosphamide. Combination chemotherapy with vincristine, doxorubicin, methotrexate, or cytarabine has achieved remission in more than 90% of patients. Those who live beyond 2 years often enjoy long-term remission.[45]

Oral Complications and Manifestations

Endemic Burkitt's lymphoma often presents as a rapidly expanding tumorous mass in the posterior region of the maxilla or mandible. Rapid growth pushes adjacent teeth, causing the teeth to become mobile and abnormally positioned. Pain and paresthesia accompany the condition. Radiographically, the tumor produces an osteolytic lesion with poorly demarcated margins, erosion of the cortical plate, and soft tissue involvement.

MULTIPLE MYELOMA

DEFINITION

Multiple myeloma (MM) is a lymphoproliferative disorder that results from overproduction of cloned malignant plasma cells that results in multiple tumorous masses scattered throughout the skeletal system. Malignant plasma cells secrete monoclonal immunoglobulins and various cytokines.

EPIDEMIOLOGY

About 16,000 new cases of MM occur each year; these account for more than 10% of hematologic malignancies.[36,42]

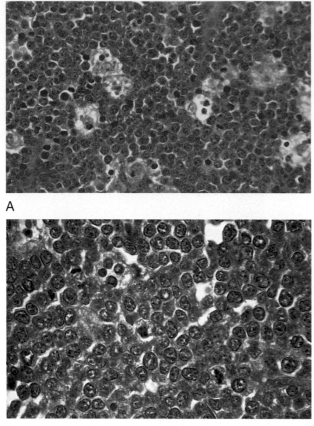

A

B

Figure 24-10. Burkitt's lymphoma. **A,** At low power, numerous pale macrophages are evident, interspersed among the tumor cells, producing a "starry sky" appearance. **B,** At high power, tumor cells are seen to have multiple small nucleoli and a high mitotic index. (**A** and **B** from Kumar V, Abbas A, Fausto N. Robbins & Cotran Pathologic Basis of Disease, 7th ed. Philadelphia, Saunders, 2005. **B,** Courtesy of Dr. Jose Hernandez, Department of Pathology, University of Texas Southwestern Medical School, Dallas, Tex.)

Men are affected slightly more often than women (male/female ratio is 1.5:1), and most cases occur after 65 years of age.[46] The disease is rarely diagnosed before the patient reaches 40 years of age.

Etiology

The etiology of MM is unknown but involves uncontrolled division of a clonal cell that produces daughter cells of the same genetic makeup. Chromosomal translocations that frequently involve the immunoglobulin heavy chain locus (IgH; 14q32) are common. The translocated gene is placed under transcriptional control of potent IgH enhancers, thus resulting in their overexpression. Various cytokines (interleukin [IL]-1α and RANKL [receptor activator for nuclear factor κ B ligand]) are also overproduced. Production of IL-6 by neoplastic plasma cells and normal stromal cells aids in the proliferation of tumor cells.[5] Additional cytokines act as osteoclast-activating factors that stimulate osteoclasts to resorb bone.[47,48]

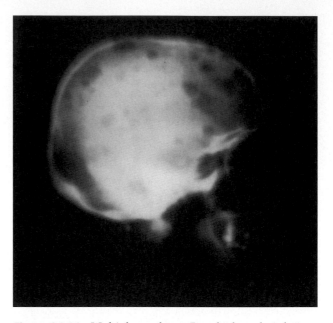

Figure 24-11. Multiple myeloma. Punched-out lytic lesions in the skull containing malignant plasma cells.

Pathophysiology and Complications

The disease consists of plasma and myeloma cell proliferation, immunoglobulin production, bone resorption at tumor sites, and bone marrow replacement. Resorption of bone leads to release of calcium and serum hypercalcemia. Bone marrow replacement leads to anemia, leukopenia, thrombocytopenia, and, eventually, a decrease in plasma immunoglobulins. During the early to middle stages of disease, increased plasma viscosity contributes to altered platelet function, excessive bleeding, renal impairment, and neuropathy. Renal failure results from tubular damage caused by excretion of light chains (of immunoglobulin) or by glomerular deposition of amyloid, hyperuricemia, recurrent pyelonephritis, or local infiltration of tumor cells. Infections are common because of diffuse hypogammaglobulinemia (an immune deficiency state) that is caused by decreased production of normal antibodies. Infection is a primary cause of death in MM. Renal failure is the second most common cause of death.

CLINICAL PRESENTATION
Signs and Symptoms

The most prominent feature of MM is observed radiographically. This disease produces multiple "punched-out" lesions or mottled areas, which represent areas of tumor that appear in the spine, ribs, and cortical regions of the skull (Figure 24-11). Osteolytic lesions of the jaw occur in up to 30% of patients. Amyloid deposition is seen in various soft tissues (heart, liver, nervous system). Because of the hypogammaglobulinemia, pneumonia and pyelonephritis commonly develop.

The most prominent symptom is persistent bone pain. The sites most commonly affected are the spine, ribs, and sternum. As bone marrow is replaced, anemia develops, along with associated features of weakness, weight loss, and recurrent infection. Headache and peripheral neuropathy are associated with hypercalcemia. Tumor destruction of bone may cause pathologic fracture.

Laboratory Findings

Osteolytic bone lesions, elevated serum calcium, increased immunoglobulins in the blood, abnormal immunoglobulin light chains (Bence-Jones proteins) in the urine, and anemia (normocytic and normochromic) are features of MM. The diagnosis is typically confirmed by protein electrophoresis of serum or urine that shows the presence of the myeloma or monoclonal (M) protein band. The immunoglobulin most commonly detected is IgG, followed by IgA and IgM. Tumor biopsy reveals sheets of plasmacytoid cells. Bone marrow aspirates show monoclonal plasma cells that constitute more than 30% of the marrow cellularity.

MEDICAL MANAGEMENT

Patients with MM are treated with high doses of chemotherapeutic agents (alkylating agents with prednisone); this treatment is followed by BMT or autologous stem cell transplantation for patients younger than 65 years of age.[49] Thalidomide and proteasome inhibitors (Bortezomib) are also used. Thalidomide is a potent inhibitor of angiogenesis and immune response (it inhibits secretion of tumor necrosis factor-α and IL-6). Proteasome inhibitors block proteases required for the accumulation of regulatory proteins important in cell cycle control. Radiation therapy is used as palliative treatment.

Interventions are provided to manage anemia, to prevent infection, and to treat or prevent bone disease. Usually, anemia is controlled with recombinant erythropoietin. Intravenous immunoglobulins and/or antibiotics are given selectively to prevent infection. Bisphosphonates are used to maintain bone strength and to reduce bone pain in early-stage and advanced disease.[50]

According to the International Myeloma Foundation, median survival can be predicted on the basis of serum beta$_2$-microglobulin and serum albumin levels. Those with low levels of beta$_2$-microglobulin (<3.5 mg/L) and high albumin levels (>3.5 mg/dL) have an estimated survival of 62 months from the time of diagnosis, whereas patients with high beta$_2$-microglobulin levels (>3.5 mg/L) have a median survival of 29 months.[51]

Oral Complications and Manifestations

Patients with MM may have jaw lesions, soft tissue lesions, and soft tissue deposits of amyloid. Bone and soft tissue lesions often are painful.[42] Dental radiographs may show "punched-out" lesions or mottled areas that represent areas of tumor. These osteolytic lesions are more common in the posterior body of the mandible and may be associated with cortical plate expansion. Extramedullary plasma cell tumors can occur in the oral pharynx. An amyloid-like protein is found sometimes in oral soft tissues (e.g., tongue) as a result of MM, and these areas may be swollen and painful. Biopsy and special amyloid stains can be used for diagnosis.[42]

Up to 80% of patients in whom MM is newly diagnosed present with osteopenia, osteolysis, and pathologic fractures. Patients are often treated with bisphosphonates—drugs that inhibit osteoclast activity. An infrequent adverse effect of bisphosphonates is osteonecrosis of the jaws.[52] Greatest risk is associated with intravenous bisphosphonates (pamidronate and zoledronic acid) used for at least 1 year and orally administered nitrogen-containing bisphosphonate (alendronate therapy [Fosamax], risedronate [Actonel], ibandronate [Boniva]) administered for 5 or more years.[52-54] The condition is often triggered by the extraction of a painful tooth or teeth. The typical presenting lesion is a severely painful and unexpected nonhealing extraction socket or exposed area of bone. However, the necrotic bone may be asymptomatic for weeks and may be noticed only on routine examination. Treatment is directed toward controlling and limiting progression by means of local debridement (bone and wound irrigation with antiseptics), together with long-term or intermittent courses of penicillin-type antibiotics (erythromycins or tetracyclines if penicillin allergic).[53,54] To minimize the likelihood that osteonecrosis will develop in these patients, the following recommendations should be followed: (1) Treat infections (periapical pathoses, sinus tracts, purulent periodontal pockets, severe periodontitis, and active abscesses) early; (2) nonsurgical approaches are preferable to surgical approaches; (3) if surgery or extractions are required, conservative surgical techniques should be used (limit the procedure to as few teeth as possible and to one sextant); (4) wait 2 months before performing surgery/extraction in a different sextant; and (5) be aware of and discuss the risks of osteonecrosis (including implant bone preparation) with the patient who is considering undergoing surgery.[54]

DENTAL MANAGEMENT

Recognition of Disorders of White Blood Cells and Medical Considerations

The dentist should search for evidence of WBC disorders in patients who are seen for dental treatment. This is critical because patients with leukemia or lymphoma may be in grave danger if the disease is not detected before dental treatment is started. Undetected leukemic patients may experience serious bleeding problems after any surgical procedure, may have problems with healing of surgical wounds, and are prone to postsurgical infection. Thus, it is important for the dentist to attempt to identify these patients through history and clinical examination before starting any treatment.

Physical evaluation requires a consistent approach by which important medical, historical, and clinical information is attained from the patient. Specific questions regarding blood disorders and cancer in family members, weight loss, fever, swollen or enlarged lymph nodes, and bleeding tendencies should be asked. In addition, the dentist should emphasize the importance of routine annual physical examinations that will provide screening of the patient's blood for potential abnormalities.

After the history is complete, clinical examination is mandatory. Examination of the head, neck, and mouth should include a thorough inspection of the oropharynx, head, and cervical and supraclavicular lymph nodes. The dentist should be cognizant that an enlarged supraclavicular node is highly suggestive of malignancy. Cranial nerve examination is important for identifying abnormalities suggestive of invasive neoplasms. Panoramic films also provide insight into potential osteolytic lesions associated with WBC disorders (see Figure 24-8).

A patient who has the classic signs or symptoms of leukemia, lymphoma, or MM (see Table 24-5) should be referred directly to a physician. Patients with signs and symptoms suggestive of these disorders should be screened by appropriate laboratory tests and/or biopsy of soft tissue and osseous lesions. Referral to a surgeon for excisional biopsy of a lymph node may be required. Screening laboratory tests can be conducted at a commercial clinical laboratory or in a physician's office. Screening tests should include total and differential WBC counts, a smear for cell morphologic study, Hb or hematocrit count, and platelet count. If screening tests are ordered by the dentist and one or more are abnormal, the patient should be referred for medical evaluation and treatment. Biopsy specimens that contain WBCs should be immunophenotyped with the use of a panel of monoclonal antibodies. Immunophenotyping allows determination of the cell of origin (B or T cell or nonlymphoid). Accurate diagnosis also requires culturing of WBCs for analyses of the chromosomes through cytogenetic methods.

Treatment Planning Modifications

Dental management of patients in whom a WBC disorder is diagnosed requires consideration of the three phases of medical therapy. Planning involves (1) pretreatment assessment and preparation of the patient, (2) oral health care during medical therapy, and (3) posttreatment management, including long-term considerations and possible remission.

Pretreatment Evaluation and Considerations. The dentist must be aware of the diagnosis and severity of the disorder, the type of treatment selected for the patient, and whether the WBC disorder can be controlled through consultation with the physician. Full knowledge of this information is required for effective decision making regarding dental treatment. For example, a patient who is receiving only palliative treatment is not a good candidate for extensive restorative or prosthodontic procedures that require months for completion.

For the patient in whom leukemia or lymphoma has been recently diagnosed, the dentist should become involved early—during the treatment planning stages of cancer therapy.[2] Guidance regarding the health of the oral cavity and jaws can help prevent severe oral infection. Accordingly, pretreatment assessment should include a thorough extraoral and intraoral examination, panoramic film, and review of blood laboratory findings, with the overall goal of minimizing and/or eliminating oral disease prior to the start of chemotherapy. Inspection of radiographs for undiagnosed or latent disease, retained root tips, impacted teeth, and latent osseous disease is important for clearing the oral cavity of disease.

Pretreatment care should include oral hygiene instructions that emphasize the importance of meticulous plaque removal. Caries and infection should be eliminated, if possible, before chemotherapy is begun, and treatment should be directed first toward acute needs (e.g., periapical disease, large lesions treated before small carious lesions). If pulpal disease is present, the dentist may recommend root canal therapy or extraction of teeth prior to chemotherapy. Dental attention is given to oral hygiene procedures, including using fluoride gels, encouraging a noncariogenic diet, eliminating mucosal and periodontal disease, eliminating sources of mucosal injury, and protecting salivary glands (with lead-lined stents or drugs) if head and neck radiation is planned.[2,55] Extraction should be considered if periodontal pocket depths are greater than 5 mm, periapical inflammation is present, the tooth is nonfunctional or partially erupted (third molar), or the patient is noncompliant with oral hygiene measures and routine dental care.[52]

Guidelines for extraction in patients before chemotherapy include scheduling a minimum of 10 to 14 days (3 weeks preferable) between the time of extraction and initiation of chemotherapy or radiotherapy, attaining primary closure, avoiding intra-alveolar hemostatic packing agents, avoiding invasive procedures if the platelet count is less than 50,000/mm^3, and transfusing if the platelet count is less than 40,000.[2,55,56] It is important to note that chemotherapy is initiated in many cases of acute leukemia within a few days of diagnosis, so dental treatment may have to be provided promptly before the patient becomes neutropenic as a result of chemotherapy.

Patients who are neutropenic should not undergo invasive dental procedures without special precautions. After necessary treatment is cleared with the patient's physician, the use of prophylactic antibiotics is dictated by WBC and neutrophil counts. Prophylactic antibiotics are recommended if the WBC count is less than 2000, or the neutrophil count is less than 500 (or 1000 at some institutions).[56] Antibiotic regimens are empiric. Penicillin VK 2 g given 1 hour before the procedure and 500 mg given 4 times daily for 1 week is a reasonable selection, when needed.

Oral Health Care and Oral Complications During Medical Therapy. Patients who are undergoing chemotherapy or radiotherapy are susceptible to many oral complications, including mucositis, neutropenia, infection, excessive bleeding, graft-versus-host disease, and alterations in growth and development. Fortunately, improved therapy protocols over the past 2 decades have resulted in a decline in the incidence (to about 30% of patients) of oral complications.[18]

Mucositis. Mucosae of the mouth and gastrointestinal tract grow rapidly and are likely to be affected by cancer therapy. Thus, these patients often develop mucositis, which usually begins 7 to 10 days after initiation of chemotherapy and resolves after cessation of chemotherapy. Cytotoxic agent treatments affect epithelial cells that have high replication rates.[57] Thus, younger persons have a greater prevalence of mucositis and nonkeratinized sites (ventral tongue, labial and buccal mucosae, floor of mouth) and are more severely affected.[58] Affected mucosa becomes red, raw, and tender. Breakdown of the epithelial barrier produces oral ulcerations that may become secondarily infected and can serve as a source of systemic infection. Oral hygiene should be maintained to minimize infection complications. A bland mouth rinse can be used to clean the surface of the ulcer (commercial mouth rinses are not recommended because they contain alcohol and tend to irritate ulcerated tissues). After the bland mouth rinse, use of a topical anesthetic and systemic analgesics makes the mouth more comfortable. Various solutions of antihistamines (benzydamine) that have local anesthetic properties are effective, and a thin layer of Orabase is useful in protecting ulcers from surface irritation. (See Appendix C for suggested regimens.[59]) This protocol can be repeated 4 to 6 times a day. In addition, removal of sharp edges of teeth and restorations is palliative. Antiseptic and antimicrobial rinses (e.g., chlorhexidine) are recommended to promote healing of oral ulcerations and to prevent oral infection.[4,60,61] Additional novel cytoprotective agents (e.g., amifostine, keratinocyte growth factor [Palifermin]) may provide some benefit in specific situations.[58]

Neutropenia and infection. Patients may present with neutropenia alone, neutropenia combined with leukemia or lymphoma, or neutropenia that results from medical treatment (chemotherapy or drug induced) (Figure 24-12). Patients who have neutropenia are unable to provide a protective response against oral microbes. Accordingly, these individuals develop acute gingival inflammation and mucosal ulcerations. Chronic neutropenia contributes to severe destruction of the periodontium with loss of attachment when oral hygiene is less than optimal. Periodontal therapy that includes instruction on oral hygiene, frequent scaling, and antimicrobial therapy can reduce the adverse effects associated with this disorder.[6]

Oral infection is less of a problem in patients with chronic leukemia than in those with acute leukemia because the cells are more mature and functional in chronic leukemia. However, in the later stages of both CML and CLL, infection can become a serious compli-

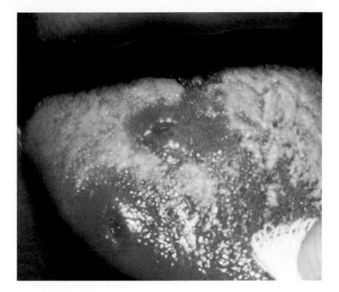

Figure 24-12. Oral ulcers due to neutropenia.

cation. Splenectomy due to massive splenomegaly may also increase the risk of infection.

Because of neutropenia, signs of infection are often masked in patients with leukemia. The swelling and erythema usually associated with oral infection are often less marked. In these patients, severe infection can occur with minimal clinical signs, which can make clinical diagnosis more difficult. Infections often develop in the presence of neutropenia as the result of invasion by unusual oral pathogens (i.e., bacteria that do not cause oral infection in most patients seen by the dentist). Unusual infections may be caused by *Pseudomonas*, *Klebsiella*, *Proteus*, *Escherichia coli*, or *Enterobacter*. Often, these infections present as oral ulcerations. When oral infection develops in such patients, a specimen of exudate should be sent for culture, diagnosis, and antibiotic sensitivity testing. If a bacterial infection is suspected, penicillin therapy should be started (if the patient is not allergic to penicillin). If the clinical course shows little or no improvement in several days, laboratory data should be used to select a more appropriate antimicrobial agent, and referral to a physician should be considered.

Opportunistic infections (bacterial, fungal, and viral) are common in leukemic patients because (1) malignant leukocytes are immature, (2) chemotherapy induces an immunocompromised state, and (3) use of broad-spectrum antibiotics produces selective antimicrobial killing. A common opportunistic infection is acute pseudomembranous candidiasis. When this complication occurs, the patient should be treated with one of the antifungal medications listed in Appendix C. Infrequently, unusual oral fungal infections (torulopsis, aspergillosis, mucormycosis) occur, or fungal septicemia may originate from the oral cavity. These patients require potent systemic antifungal agents such as fluconazole or amphotericin B.[62]

Another common infection in patients receiving chemotherapy is recurrent herpes simplex virus (HSV)

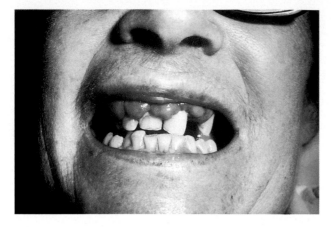

Figure 24-13. Leukemic gingival enlargement in a patient who has acute myeloid leukemia. Enlargement is due to leukemic infiltrations in the gingival tissue. (From Hoffbrand AV, Pettit JE. Color Atlas of Clinical Hematology, 3rd ed. London, Mosby, 2000.)

infection.[63,64] Herpetic lesions tend to be larger and take longer to heal than herpetic lesions found in nonleukemic patients. Generally, to prevent recurrence, antiviral agents (acyclovir, valacyclovir, famciclovir) are prescribed to HSV antibody–positive patients who are undergoing chemotherapy. In patients in whom HSV infection develops, diagnosis can be made rapidly with use of an enzyme-linked immunoassay.[65] Immunocompromised leukemic patients also are susceptible to varicella-zoster and cytomegalovirus infections. Lesions in the oral cavity have been reported.[57]

Bleeding. Small or large areas of submucosal hemorrhage may be found in the leukemic patient (see Figure 24-2, *A*). These lesions result from minor trauma (e.g., tongue biting) and are related to thrombocytopenia. Leukemic patients also may report spontaneous and severe gingival bleeding that is aggravated by poor oral hygiene. Enlarged and boggy gingiva (Figure 24-13) bleeds easily, especially if significant thrombocytopenia is present. The dentist should make efforts to improve oral hygiene and should use local measures to control bleeding. A gelatin sponge with thrombin or microfibrillar collagen can be placed over the area, or an oral antifibrinolytic rinse may be used. If local measures fail, medical help will be needed and may involve platelet transfusion.[60] Platelet counts should be at least 50,000/mm³ prior to performance of invasive dental procedures.

Graft-versus-host disease. Graft-versus-host disease (GVHD) is a common sequela of patients who undergo BMT or stem cell transplantation. It occurs when immunologically active donor T cells react against histocompatibility antigens of the host. The acute stage develops within the first 100 days (median, 2 to 3 weeks) and is marked by rash, mucosal ulcerations, elevated liver enzymes, and diarrhea. The chronic stage occurs at between 3 and 12 months and produces features that

mimic Sjögren's syndrome and scleroderma, including thickening and lichenoid changes of the skin and mucosa, arthritis, xerostomia, xerophthalmia, mucositis, and dysphagia. Damage to the liver, esophagus (stricture), and immune system may result in recurrent and life-threatening infections. To prevent this complication, patients who are preparing for BMT typically undergo T-cell depletion of the graft and prophylactic treatment with immunosuppressive agents, such as corticosteroids, cyclosporine, methotrexate, or tacrolimus.

Adverse drug effects. A small number of leukemic patients describe paresthesias that result from leukemic infiltration of the peripheral nerves or as adverse effects of chemotherapy (vincristine). An adverse effect of cyclosporine use in BMT patients is gingival overgrowth.

Growth and development. Chemotherapy during childhood can affect growth and development of the teeth and facial bones. This effect is not observed in adults. Restricted growth of the jaws leads to micrognathia, retrognathia, and/or malocclusion. Damage to the teeth that occurs at the time of chemotherapy can manifest as shortened or blunted roots, dilacerations, calcification abnormalities, pulp enlargement, microdontia, and hypodontia.

Posttreatment Management. Patients who have WBC disorders and are in a state of remission can receive most indicated dental treatment (Box 24-4). Patients who have advanced disease and a limited prognosis, as occurs in many cases of leukemia and MM, should receive emergency care only. Complex restorative procedures, extensive dental restorations, and other procedures usually are not indicated.

If invasive (scaling) or surgical procedures are planned for a patient who has a WBC disorder that is under good medical control, platelet count or bleeding time should be obtained on the day of the procedure. This is done to ensure that an adequate number of platelets are present and are functioning properly. The number of platelets can be depressed in these patients by the leukemic process or by agents used to treat the patient. If the platelet count is low, or the bleeding time abnormal, the procedure should be delayed until the patient's physician is consulted. In patients whose disease is under good control but who are still thrombocytopenic, platelet replacement by the physician can be instituted if a dental procedure must be done. Dental management of the patient receiving radiation or chemotherapy is discussed further in Chapter 26.

In Hodgkin's disease, the patient's spleen may be involved and surgically removed. These patients are at risk for bacterial infection. Greatest risk is reported to occur during the first 6 months after splenectomy.[65] McKenna[65] suggests that antibiotic prophylaxis should be provided for invasive procedures during the first 6 months after splenectomy. The need for prophylaxis after 6

BOX 24-4

Dental Management of the Leukemic Patient

1. Detection
   a. History
   b. Examination
   c. Screening laboratory tests
      (1) White cell count
      (2) Differential white cell count
      (3) Smear for cell morphologic study
      (4) Hemoglobin or hematocrit level
      (5) Platelet count
2. Referral
   a. Medical diagnosis
   b. Treatment
3. Consultation before any dental care is rendered
   a. Current status
   b. Review of dental treatment needs
   c. Dental management plan
4. Routine dental care
   a. None for patient with acute symptoms
   b. Once disease is under control, patient may receive indicated dental care
   c. Scaling and surgical procedures
      (1) Platelet count on day of procedure: if normal, proceed; if <50,000, avoid invasive procedures, if possible; if <40,000, provide platelet replacement
      (2) Prophylactic antibiotic therapy to prevent postoperative infection (if severe neutropenia is present)
5. Emergency dental care
   a. Treatment of oral ulcers (see Appendix B)
      (1) Antibiotics
      (2) Bland mouth rinse
      (3) Antihistamine solutions
      (4) Orabase
   b. Oral candidiasis—Treat with antifungal medication (see Appendix B)
   c. Conservative management of pain and infection
      (1) Antibiotic sensitivity testing
      (2) Antibiotics, heat for infection
      (3) Strong analgesics for pain

months has not been defined.[65,66] The antibiotic regimen is empirical. Penicillin VK 2 g given 1 hour before the procedure and 500 mg given 4 times daily for 1 week is a reasonable selection, when needed.[67]

REFERENCES

1. Roit I, Brostoff J, Male D. Immunology, 5th ed. Edinburgh, Mosby, 2001.
2. Sciubba J, Beckert CS, Curro FA, et al. National Institutes of Health consensus development conference statement: Oral complications of cancer therapies: Diagnosis, prevention, and treatment. J Am Dent Assoc 1989;119:179-183.
3. Viswanatha DS, Larson RS. Molecular diagnosis of hematopoietic neoplasms. In McPherson RA, Pincus MR (eds). Henry's Clinical Diagnosis and Management by Laboratory Methods, 21st ed. Philadelphia, Saunders Elsevier, 2007.
4. DeRossie SS, Garfinkel A, Greenberg MS, et al. Hematologic diseases. In Greenberg MS, Glick M (eds). Burket's Oral Medicine: Diagnosis and Treatment, 10th ed. Hamilton, Ontario, BC Decker, 2003.
5. Aster JC. Diseases of white blood cells, lymph nodes, spleen and thymus. In Kumar VK, Abbas AK, Fausto N (eds). Robbins and Cotran Pathologic Basis of Disease, 7th ed. Philadelphia, Elsevier Saunders, 2005.
6. Kinane D. Blood and lymphoreticular disorders. Periodontology 2000;21:84-93.
7. Greenlee RT, Murray T, Bolden S, Wingo PA. Cancer statistics, 2000. Cancer 2000;50:7-33.
8. Leukemia & Lymphoma Society. Non-Hodgkin lymphoma facts and statistics. Available at: http://www.leukemia-lymphoma.org/all_page?item_id=8965. Accessed April 26, 2007.
9. Perkins ML. Introduction to leukemia and the acute leukemias. In Harmening DM (ed). Clinical Hematology and Fundamentals of Hemostasis, 2nd ed. Philadelphia, FA Davis, 1992.
10. Wang ES, Berliner N. Clonal disorders of the hematopoietic stem cell. In Andreoli TE, Carpenter CCJ, Griggs RC, Loscalzo J (eds). Cecil Essentials of Medicine, 6th ed. Philadelphia, WB Saunders, 2004.
11. Linet MS, Devesa SS. Descriptive epidemiology of the leukemias. In Henderson ES, Lister TA (eds). Leukemia, 5th ed. Philadelphia, WB Saunders, 1990.
12. Wetzler M, Byrd JC, Bloomfield CD. Acute and chronic myeloid leukemia. In Kasper DL, Braunwald E, Fauci AS, et al (eds). Harrison's Principles of Internal Medicine, 16th ed. New York, NY, McGraw-Hill, 2005.
13. Lowenberg B, Downing JR, Burnett A. Acute myeloid leukemia. N Engl J Med 1999;30:1051-1062.
14. Appelbaum FR. Acute myeloid leukemia in adults. In Abeloff MD, Armitage JO, Niederhuber JE, et al (eds). Clinical Oncology, 3rd ed. Philadelphia, Elsevier, 2004.
15. Vardiman JW, Harris NL, Brunning RD. The World Health Organization (WHO) classification of the myeloid neoplasms. Blood 2002;100:2292-2302.
16. Micallef-Eynaud PD, Eden OB, Grace E, Ellis PM. Cytogenetic abnormalities in childhood acute lymphoblastic leukemia. Pediatr Hematol Oncol 1993;10:25-30.
17. Robison LL, Nesbit ME Jr, Sather HN, et al. Down syndrome and acute leukemia in children: A 10 year retrospective survey from Children's Cancer Study Group. J Pediatr 1984;105:235.
18. Childers NK, Stinnett EA, Wheeler P, et al. Oral complications in children with cancer. Oral Surg Oral Med Oral Pathol 1993;75:41-47.
19. Bennett JM, Catovsky D, Daniel MT, et al. Proposals for the classification of the acute leukemias: French-American-British cooperative group. Br J Haematol 1976;33:451-458.
20. O'Mura GA. The leukemias. In Rose LF, Kaye D (eds). Internal Medicine for Dentistry, 2nd ed. St. Louis, Mosby, 1990.
21. Geller RB, Dix SP. Oral chemotherapy agents in the treatment of leukaemia. Drugs 1999;58(suppl 3):109-118.

22. Ficarra G, Silverman S Jr, Quivey JM, et al. Granulo-cytic sarcoma (chloroma) of the oral cavity: A case with aleukemic presentation. Oral Surg Oral Med Oral Pathol 1987;63:709-714.

23. Keating MJ. Chronic leukemias. In Goldman L, Bennett JC (eds). Cecil Textbook of Medicine, 21st ed. Philadelphia, WB Saunders, 2000.

24. Faderl S, Talpaz M, Estrov Z, et al. The biology of chronic myeloid leukemia. N Engl J Med 1999;341:164-172.

25. Adamson JW. The myeloproliferative diseases. In Wilson JD, Braunwald E, Isselbacher KJ, et al (eds). Harrison's Principles of Internal Medicine, 12th ed. New York, NY, McGraw-Hill, 1991.

26. Druker BJ, Goldman JM. Chronic myeloid leukemia. In Abeloff MD, Armitage JO, Niederhuber JE, et al (eds). Clinical Oncology, 3rd ed. Philadelphia, Elsevier, 2004.

27. Chesan BD. Chronic lymphoid leukemias. In Abeloff MD, Armitage JO, Niederhuber JE, et al (eds). Clinical Oncology, 3rd ed. Philadelphia, Elsevier, 2004.

28. Wierda WG, Kipps TJ. Chronic lymphocytic leukemia. Curr Opin Hematol 1999;6:253-261.

29. Yee KW, O'Brien SW. Chronic lymphocytic leukemia: Diagnosis and treatment. Mayo Clin Proc 2006;81:1105-1129.

30. Armitage JO, Longo DL. Malignancies of lymphoid cells. In Kasper DL, Braunwald E, Fauci AS, et al (eds). Harrison's Principles of Internal Medicine, 16th ed. New York, NY, McGraw-Hill, 2005.

31. Knecht H, Berger C, Rothenberger S, et al. The role of Epstein-Barr virus in neoplastic transformation. Oncology 2001;60:289-302.

32. Küppers R. Molecular biology of Hodgkin's lymphoma. Adv Cancer Res 2002;84:277-312.

33. Moormeir JA, Williams SF, Golomb HM. The staging of Hodgkin's disease. Hematol Oncol Clin North Am 1989;3:237-251.

34. Kuppers R, Yahalom J, Josting A. Advances in biology, diagnostics, and treatment of Hodgkin's disease. Biol Blood Marrow Transplant 2006;12:66-76.

35. Lister TA, Coiffier B, Armitage JO. Non-Hodgkin's lymphoma. In Abeloff MD, Armitage JO, Niederhuber JE (eds). Clinical Oncology, 3rd ed. Philadelphia, Elsevier, 2004.

36. U.S. National Cancer Institute. Cancer stat fact sheets, 2006. Available at: http://seer.cancer.gov/statfacts/. Accessed April 26, 2007.

37. Eisenbud L, Sciubba J, Mir R, Sachs SA. Oral presentations in non-Hodgkin's lymphoma: A review of thirty-one cases. Oral Surg Oral Med Oral Pathol 1983;56:151-156.

38. Eisenbud L, Sciubba J, Mir R, Sachs SA. Oral presentations in non-Hodgkin's lymphoma: A review of thirty-one cases. Part II. Fourteen cases arising in bone. Oral Surg Oral Med Oral Pathol 1984;57:272-280.

39. Kassan SS, Thomas TL, Moutsopoulos HM, et al. Increased risk of lymphoma in sicca syndrome. Ann Intern Med 1978;89:888-892.

40. Kaugars GE, Burns JC. Non-Hodgkin's lymphoma of the oral cavity associated with AIDS. Oral Surg Oral Med Oral Pathol 1989;67:433-436.

41. Raut A, Huryn J, Pollack A, Zlotolow I. Unusual gingival presentation of post-transplantation lymphoproliferative disorder: A case report and review of the literature. Oral Surg Oral Med Oral Pathol Oral Radiol Endod 2000;90:436-441.

42. Silverman S (ed). Oral Cancer, 5th ed. Hamilton, Ontario, BC Decker, 2003.

43. Maxymiw WG, Wood RE, Liu FF. Postradiation dental extractions without hyperbaric oxygen. Oral Surg Oral Med Oral Pathol 1991;72:270-274.

44. Burkitt DP. The discovery of Burkitt's lymphoma. Cancer 1983;51:1177-1286.

45. Kasamon YL, Swinnen LJ. Treatment advances in adult Burkitt lymphoma and leukemia. Curr Opin Oncol 2004;16:429-435.

46. Dispenzieri A, Kyle RA. Multiple myeloma: Clinical features and indications for therapy. Best Pract Res Clin Haematol 2005;18:553-568.

47. Sezer O, Zavrski I, Kuhne A, et al. RANK ligand and osteoprotegerin in myeloma bone disease. Blood 2003;101:2094-2098.

48. Tosi P, Gamberi B, Giuliani N. Biology and treatment of multiple myeloma. Biol Blood Marrow Transplant 2006;12(1 suppl 1):81-86.

49. Child JA, Morgan GJ, Davies FE, et al. High-dose chemotherapy with hematopoietic stem-cell rescue for multiple myeloma. N Engl J Med 2003;348:1875-1883.

50. Barosi G, Boccadoro M, Cavo M, et al. Management of multiple myeloma and related disorders: Guidelines from the Italian Society of Hematology (SIE), Italian Society of Experimental Hematology (SIES) and Italian Group for Bone Marrow Transplantation (GITMO). Haematologica 2004;89:717-741.

51. Greipp PR, San Miguel J, Durie BG, et al. International staging system for multiple myeloma. J Clin Oncol 2005;23:3412-3420.

52. Migliorati CA, Siegel MA, Elting LS. Bisphosphonate-associated osteonecrosis: A long-term complication of bisphosphonate treatment. Lancet Oncol 2006;7:508-514.

53. Marx RE. Pamidronate (Aredia) and zoledronate (Zometa) induced avascular necrosis of the jaws: A growing epidemic. J Oral Maxillofac Surg 2003;61:1115-1117.

54. American Dental Association Council on Scientific Affairs. Dental management of patients receiving oral bisphosphonate therapy: Expert panel recommendations. J Am Dent Assoc 2006;137:1144-1150.

55. Semba SE, Mealey BL, Hallmon WW. Dentistry and the cancer patient: Part 2: Oral health management of the chemotherapy patient. Compendium 1994;15:1378-1388.

56. Peterson DE. Prevention of oral complications in cancer patients. Prev Med 1994;23:763-765.

57. Sonis S. Oral complications of cancer chemotherapy. In Peterson D, Sonis S (eds). Epidemiology, Frequency, Distribution, Mechanisms and Histopathology. The Hague, Martinus Nijhoff, 1983.

58. Scully C, Sonis S, Diz PD. Oral mucositis. Oral Dis 2006;12:229-241.

59. McGuire DB, Correa ME, Johnson J, Wienandts P. The role of basic oral care and good clinical practice princi-

ples in the management of oral mucositis. Support Care Cancer 2006;14:541-547.

60. Greenberg MS. Leukemia, dental correlations. In Rose LF, Kaye D (eds). Internal Medicine for Dentistry, 2nd ed. St. Louis, Mosby, 1990.

61. Ferretti GA, Ash RC, Brown AT, et al. Chlorhexidine for prophylaxis against oral infections and associated complications in patients receiving bone marrow transplants. J Am Dent Assoc 1987;114:461-467.

62. Myoken Y, Sugata T, Kyo TI, Fujihara M. Pathological features of invasive oral aspergillosis in patients with hematologic malignancies. J Oral Maxillofac Surg 1996;54:263-270.

63. Barrett AP. A long-term prospective clinical study of orofacial herpes simplex virus infection in acute leuke-

mia. Oral Surg Oral Med Oral Pathol 1986;61:149-152.

64. Redding SW. Role of herpes simplex virus reactivation in chemotherapy-induced oral mucositis. NCI Monogr 1990;9:103-105.

65. McKenna SJ. Immunocompromised host and infection. In Topazian RG, Goldberg MH, Hupp JR (eds). Oral and Maxillofacial Infections, 4th ed. Philadelphia, Elsevier, 2002.

66. Scully C, Cawson RA. Immunodeficiencies other than HIV/AIDS. In Scully C, Cawson RA (eds). Medical Problems in Dentistry, 5th ed. Edinburgh, Elsevier, 2005.

67. DeRossi SS, Glick M. Dental considerations in asplenic patients. J Am Dent Assoc 1996;127:1359-1363.

Bleeding Disorders

CHAPTER 25

A number of procedures that are performed in dentistry may cause bleeding. Under normal circumstances, these procedures can be performed with little risk to the patient; however, the patient whose ability to control bleeding has been altered by drugs or disease may be in grave danger unless the dentist identifies the problem before performing any dental procedure. In most cases, once the patient with a bleeding problem has been identified, steps can be taken to greatly reduce the risks associated with dental procedures.

DEFINITION

Bleeding disorders are conditions that alter the ability of blood vessels, platelets, and coagulation factors to maintain hemostasis. Inherited bleeding disorders are genetically transmitted. Acquired bleeding disorders occur as the result of diseases that affect vascular wall integrity, platelets, coagulation factors, drugs, radiation, or chemotherapy for cancer.

Most bleeding disorders are iatrogenic. Every patient who receives coumarin to prevent recurrent thrombosis has a potential bleeding problem. Most of these patients are receiving anticoagulant medication because they have had a recent myocardial infarction, a cerebrovascular accident, or thrombophlebitis. Patients who have atrial fibrillation; who have had open heart surgery to correct a congenital defect, replace diseased arteries, or repair or replace damaged heart valves; or who have had recent total hip or knee replacement also may be receiving long-term anticoagulation therapy. Some individuals treated with aspirin for cardiovascular disorders or chronic illnesses, such as rheumatoid arthritis, have potential bleeding problems.

In a dental practice of 2000 adults, about 100 to 150 patients may have a possible bleeding problem. This is a rough estimate and the number could be higher.

Epidemiology: Incidence and Prevalence

Patients on low-intensity warfarin therapy (international normalized ratio [INR], 2.0 to 3.0) for prophylaxis of venous thromboembolism have a risk of major bleeding of less than 1% and about an 8% risk for minor bleeding. Patients on high-intensity warfarin therapy (INR, 2.5 to 3.5) have up to a fivefold greater risk for bleeding.[1]

The most common inherited bleeding disorder is von Willebrand's disease (vWD). It affects about 1% of the population in the United States. The disease usually is inherited as an autosomal dominant trait. Hemophilia A, factor VIII deficiency, is the most common of the inherited coagulation disorders. It occurs in about 1 of every 5000 male births. More than 20,000 individuals in the United States have hemophilia A.[2] Because of its genetic mode of transfer, certain areas of the United States, such as North Carolina, are found to contain many more persons with hemophilia than other areas. Hemophilia B (Christmas disease), a factor IX deficiency, is found in about 1 of every 30,000 male births.[2] About 80% of all genetic coagulation disorders are hemophilia A, 13% are hemophilia B, and 6% are factor XI deficiency.[3]

Patients with acute or chronic leukemia may have clinical bleeding tendencies because of thrombocytopenia, which may result from overgrowth of malignant cells in the bone marrow that leaves no room for red blood cells or platelet precursors. In addition, leukemic patients may develop thrombocytopenia from the toxic effects of the various chemotherapeutic agents used to treat the disease. The incidence of leukemia is discussed in Chapter 24.

It is difficult to obtain accurate information about the incidence of other systemic conditions, such as liver disease, renal failure, thrombocytopenia, and drug-induced vascular wall defects, that may render the patient susceptible to prolonged bleeding after injury or surgery. However, when the prevalence of drug-influenced or disease-produced

BOX 25-1

Classification of Bleeding Disorders

I. Nonthrombocytopenic purpuras
  a. Vascular wall alterations
    (1) Scurvy
    (2) Infection
    (3) Chemicals
    (4) Allergy
  b. Disorders of platelet function
    (1) Genetic defects (Bernard-Soulier disease)
    (2) Drugs
      (a) Aspirin
      (b) NSAIDs
      (c) Alcohol
      (d) Beta-lactam antibiotics
      (e) Penicillin
      (f) Cephalothins
    (3) Allergy
    (4) Autoimmune disease
    (5) von Willebrand's disease (secondary factor VIII deficiency)
    (6) Uremia
II. Thrombocytopenic purpuras
  a. Primary—idiopathic
  b. Secondary
    (1) Chemicals
    (2) Physical agents (radiation)
    (3) Systemic disease (leukemia)
    (4) Metastatic cancer to bone

    (5) Splenomegaly
    (6) Drugs
      (a) Alcohol
      (b) Thiazide diuretics
      (c) Estrogens
      (d) Gold salts
    (7) Vasculitis
    (8) Mechanical prosthetic heart valves
    (9) Viral or bacterial infections
III. Disorders of coagulation
  a. Inherited
    (1) Hemophilia A (deficiency of factor VIII)
    (2) Hemophilia B (deficiency of factor IX)
    (3) Others
  b. Acquired
    (1) Liver disease
    (2) Vitamin deficiency
      (a) Biliary tract obstruction
      (b) Malabsorption
      (c) Excessive use of broad-spectrum antibiotics
    (3) Anticoagulation drugs
      (a) Heparin
      (b) Coumarin
      (c) Aspirin and NSAIDs
    (4) Disseminated intravascular coagulation (DIC)
    (5) Primary fibrinogenolysis

NSAIDs, Nonsteroidal antiinflammatory drugs.

defects in the normal control of blood loss is considered, a busy dental practice will contain a large number of patients who may be potential "bleeders."

ETIOLOGY

A pathologic alteration of blood vessel walls, a significant reduction in the number of platelets, defective platelets or platelet function, a deficiency of one or more coagulation factors, the administration of anticoagulant drugs, a disorder of platelet release, or the inability to destroy free plasmin can result in significant abnormal clinical bleeding. This may occur even after minor injuries and may lead to death in some patients if immediate action is not taken.

The classification given in Box 25-1 is based on bleeding problems in patients with normal numbers of platelets (nonthrombocytopenic purpura), decreased numbers of platelets (thrombocytopenic purpura), and disorders of coagulation.

Infections, chemicals, collagen disorders, or certain types of allergy can alter the structure and function of the vascular wall to the point that the patient may have a clinical bleeding problem. A patient may have normal numbers of platelets, but they may be defective or unable to perform their proper function in the control of blood loss from damaged tissues. If the total number of circulat-

ing platelets is reduced to below 50,000/mm^3 of blood, the patient may be a bleeder. In some cases, the total platelet count is reduced by unknown mechanisms; this is called *primary* or *idiopathic thrombocytopenia*. Chemicals, radiation, and various systemic diseases (e.g., leukemia) may have a direct effect on the bone marrow and may result in secondary thrombocytopenia.[4]

Patients may be born with a deficiency of one of the factors needed for blood coagulation, for example, factor VIII deficiency (hemophilia A) or factor IX deficiency (hemophilia B or Christmas disease). Congenital deficiencies of the other coagulation factors have been reported but are rare. When congenital deficiency of a coagulation factor occurs, only a single factor is affected.[5,6]

Acquired coagulation disorders are the most common cause of prolonged bleeding. Liver disease and disseminated intravascular coagulation (DIC) can lead to severe bleeding problems. Many of the other acquired coagulation disorders may become apparent in patients only after trauma or surgical procedures. In contrast to the congenital coagulation disorders in which only one factor is affected, the acquired coagulation disorders usually have multiple factor deficiencies.[3,7]

The liver produces all of the protein coagulation factors; thus, any patient with significant liver disease may have a bleeding problem. In addition to a possible disorder in coagulation, the patient with liver disease who

398   Hematologic and Oncologic Disease   PART EIGHT

develops portal hypertension and hypersplenism may be thrombocytopenic as a result of splenic overactivity, which leads to increased sequestration of platelets in the spleen.[7]

Any condition that so disrupts the intestinal flora that vitamin K is not produced in sufficient amounts will result in a decreased plasma level of the vitamin K–dependent coagulation factors. Vitamin K is needed by the liver to produce prothrombin (factor II) and factors VII, IX, and X. Biliary tract obstruction, malabsorption syndrome, and excessive use of broad-spectrum antibiotics can lead to low levels of prothrombin and factors VII, IX, and X on this basis.[7]

Drugs, such as heparin and coumarin derivatives, can cause a bleeding disorder because they may disrupt the coagulation process. Aspirin, other nonsteroidal anti-inflammatory drugs (NSAIDs), penicillin, cephalosporins, and alcohol also may interfere with platelet function.[8]

Pathophysiology

The three phases of hemostasis for controlling bleeding are vascular, platelet, and coagulation. The vascular and platelet phases are referred to as primary, and the coagulation phase is secondary. The coagulation phase is followed by the fibrinolytic phase, during which the clot is dissolved (Box 25-2).

Vascular Phase. The vascular phase begins immediately after injury and involves vasoconstriction of arteries and veins in the area of injury, retraction of arteries that have been cut, and buildup of extravascular pressure by blood loss from cut vessels. This pressure aids in collapsing the adjacent capillaries and veins in the area of injury. Vascular wall integrity is important for maintaining the fluidity of blood. The smooth endothelial lining consists of a nonwettable surface that, under normal conditions, does not activate platelet adhesion or coagulation. In fact, the endothelial cells synthesize and secrete three potent anti-platelet agents: prostacyclin, nitric oxide, and certain adenine nucleotides.[9]

Vascular endothelial cells also are involved in anti-thrombotic and prothrombotic activities. The major anti-thrombotic activity consists of secretion of heparin-like glycosaminoglycans (heparin sulfate) that catalyze inactivation of serine proteases such as thrombin and factor Xa by antithrombin III. Endothelial cells also produce thrombomodulin, which combines with thrombin to form a complex that activates protein C. Activated protein C (APC) then binds to endothelially released protein S, causing proteolysis of factor Va and factor VIIIa that inhibits coagulation. Tissue-type plasminogen activator (tPA) is released by injured endothelial cells to initiate fibrinolysis.[9,10]

Vessel wall components contribute prothrombotic activities. Exposure of vessel wall subendothelial tissues, collagen, and basement membrane through chemical or traumatic injury serves as a tissue factor (old term was *tissue thromboplastin*) and initiates coagulation via the extrinsic pathway. An inducible endothelial cell pro-thrombin activator may directly generate thrombin. Injured endothelial cells release adenosine diphosphate (ADP), which induces platelet adhesion. Vessel wall injury also promotes platelet adhesion and thrombus formation through exposure of subendothelial tissues to von Willebrand factor (vWF). Endothelial cells also contribute to normal homeostasis and vascular integrity through synthesis of type IV collagen, fibronectin, and vWF.[9,10]

Platelet Phase. Platelets are cellular fragments from the cytoplasm of megakaryocytes that last 8 to 12 days in the circulation. About 30% of platelets are sequestered in the microvasculature or spleen and serve as a functional reserve. Platelets do not have a nucleus; thus, they are unable to repair inhibited enzyme systems through drugs such as aspirin. Aged or nonviable platelets are removed and destroyed by the spleen and liver.[4,11,12] Functions of platelets include maintenance of vascular integrity, formation of a platelet plug to aid in initial control of bleeding, and stabilization of the platelet plug through involvement in the coagulation process. About 10% of platelets are used to nurture endothelial cells, allowing for endothelial and smooth muscle regeneration.

Subendothelial tissues are exposed at the site of injury and, through contact activation, cause the platelets to become sticky and adhere to subendothelial tissues (vWF/glycoprotein Ib). ADP released by damaged endothelial cells initiates aggregation of platelets (primary wave), and when platelets release their secretions, a second wave of aggregation results. Binding with fibrinogen (glycoprotein IIb) that is converted to fibrin stabilizes the platelet plug. The result of the preceding processes is a clot of platelets and fibrin attached to the subendothelial tissue.[11,12] Box 25-3 summarizes the functions of platelets.

A product of platelets, thromboxane, is needed to induce platelet aggregation. The enzyme cyclooxygenase

---

BOX 25-2

Normal Control of Bleeding

1. Vascular phase
   a. Vasoconstriction in the area of injury
   b. Begins immediately after injury
2. Platelet phase
   a. Platelets and vessel wall become "sticky"
   b. Mechanical plug of platelets seals off openings of cut vessels
   c. Begins seconds after injury
3. Coagulation phase
   a. Blood lost into surrounding area coagulates through extrinsic and common pathways
   b. Blood in vessels in area of injury coagulates through intrinsic and common pathways
   c. Takes place more slowly than other phases
4. Fibrinolytic phase
   a. Release of antithrombotic agents
   b. Spleen and liver destroy antithrombotic agents

BOX 25-3

Platelet Functions and Activation

- Plasma membrane receptors
- Glycoprotein Ib reacts with von Willebrand factor, which attaches to subendothelial tissue
- Glycoproteins IIb and IIIa attach to fibrinogen or fibronectin
- Platelets contain three types of secretory granules
  - Lysosomes
  - Alpha granules—contain platelet factor 4, beta thromboglobulin, and several growth factors, including platelet-derived growth factor (PDGF), endothelial cell growth factor (PD-ECGF), and transforming growth factor-beta (TGF-β) Alpha granules also contain several hemostatic proteins, including fibrinogen, factor V, and von Willebrand factor
  - Dense bodies (electron-dense organelles)— contain adenosine triphosphate (ATP), adenosine diphosphate (ADP), calcium, and serotonin
- Platelets provide a surface for activation of soluble coagulation factors
- Activated platelets expose specific receptors that bind factors Xa and Va, thus increasing their local concentration and accelerating prothrombin activation
- Factor X is also activated by factors IXa and VIII on the surface of the platelet
- Platelets contain a membrane phospholipase C
- When activated, forms diglyceride
- Diglyceride is converted to arachidonic acid by diglyceride lipase
- Arachidonic acid is a substrate for prostaglandin synthetase (cyclooxygenase)
- Cyclooxygenase formation is inhibited by aspirin and nonsteroidal anti-inflammatory drugs
- The prostaglandin, endoperoxide PGG_2, is required for ADP-induced aggregation and release, as is thromboxane A_2. Formation of both of these agents is dependent on cyclooxygenase
  Functions of platelets include the following:
- Nurturing of endothelial cells
- Endothelial and smooth muscle regeneration
- Formation of a platelet plug for initial control of bleeding
- Stabilization of the platelet plug

Based on material from Shuman M. Hemorrhagic disorders: Abnormalities of platelet and vascular function. In Goldman L, Ausiello D (eds). Cecil Textbook of Medicine. Philadelphia, WB Saunders, 2004, pp 1060-1069.

is essential in the process for generation of thromboxane. Endothelial cells, through a similar process (also dependent on cyclooxygenase), generate prostacyclin, which inhibits platelet aggregation. Aspirin acts as an inhibitor of cyclooxygenase, and this causes irreversible damage to the platelets. However, endothelial cells can, after a short period, recover and synthesize cyclooxygenase; thus, aspirin has only a short effect on the availability of prostacyclin from these cells. The net result of aspirin therapy is to inhibit platelet aggregation. This effect can last for

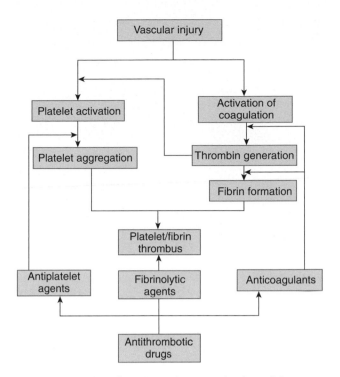

Figure 25-1. Vascular injury triggers activation of the coagulation system and activates platelet aggregation. These two systems lead to a platelet/fibrin clot or thrombus. Once the clot has served its role in the control of bleeding, plasminogen converted to plasmin promotes degradation of the clot. When thrombus formation must be inhibited, antithrombotic drugs (antiplatelet agents, fibrinolytic agents, and anticoagulants) are used. (From Weitz JI. Anticoagulant and fibrinolytic drugs. In Hoffman R, et al [eds]. Hematology: Basic Principles and Practices, 4th ed. Philadelphia, Churchill Livingstone, 2005.)

up to 9 days (time needed for all old platelets to be cleared from the blood).[4,11,12]

Coagulation Phase. The process of the fibrin-forming (coagulation) system is shown in Figure 25-1. The overall time involved from injury to a fibrin-stabilized clot is about 9 to 18 minutes. Platelets, blood proteins, lipids, and ions are involved in the process. Thrombin is generated on the surface of the platelets, and bound fibrinogen is converted to fibrin.[13-15] The end product of coagulation is a fibrin clot that can stop further blood loss from injured tissues (Figures 25-2 and 25-3).

Coagulation of blood involves the components shown in Table 25-1. Many of the coagulation factors are proenzymes that become activated in a "waterfall" or cascade manner—that is, one factor becomes activated, and it, in turn, activates another, and so on in an ordered sequence.[16] For example, the proenzyme (zymogen) factor XI is activated to the enzyme factor XIa through contact with injury-exposed subendothelial tissues in vivo to start the intrinsic pathway. In vitro, the intrinsic pathway is initiated by contact activation of factor XII. Coagulation proceeds through two pathways—the intrinsic and the extrinsic. Both use a common pathway to form the end

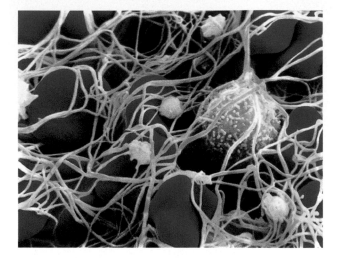

Figure 25-2. The end product of the coagulation system, which shows a fibrin clot or thrombus. White threads are fibrin, the structure with yellow on the surface is a white blood cell, platelets are green, and the red structures are red blood cells. (Reprinted with permission of CNRI/Photo Researchers, Inc.)

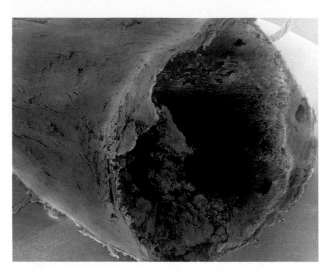

Figure 25-3. A colored scanning electron micrograph of a blood clot or thrombus inside the coronary artery of a human heart. (Reprinted with permission of P. M. Motta, G. Macchiarelli, S. A. Nottola/Photo Researchers, Inc.)

TABLE **25-1**
Blood Coagulation Components

Factor	Deficiency	Function
Factor II (prothrombin)	Congenital—Rare Acquired—Common	Protease zymogen
Factor X	Congenital—Rare Acquired—Common	Protease zymogen
Factor IX	Congenital—Rare Acquired—Common	Protease zymogen
Factor VII	Congenital—Very rare Acquired—Common	Protease zymogen
Factor VIII	Congenital—More common Acquired—Rare	Cofactor
Factor V	Congenital—Rare Acquired—Rare	Cofactor
Factor XI	Congenital—Rare Acquired—Common	Protease zymogen
Factor XII	Deficiency reported but does not cause bleeding, aPTT will be prolonged	Protease zymogen
Factor I (fibrinogen)	Congenital—Rare Acquired—Common	Structural
Von Willebrand factor	Congenital—Most common Acquired—Rare	Adhesion
Tissue factor	Not applicable	Cofactor initiator
Factor XIII	Congenital—Rare Will cause bleeding, but aPTT and PT normal	Fibrin stabilization
High molecular weight kininogen	Deficiency does not cause bleeding, will prolong aPTT	Coenzyme
Prekallikrein	Deficiency does not cause bleeding, will prolong aPTT	Coenzyme

From McVey JH. Coagulation factors. In Young NS, Gerson SL, High KA (eds). Clinical Hematology. St. Louis, Elsevier-Mosby, 2006, pp 103-123.
aPTT, Activated partial thromboplastin time; PT, prothrombin time.

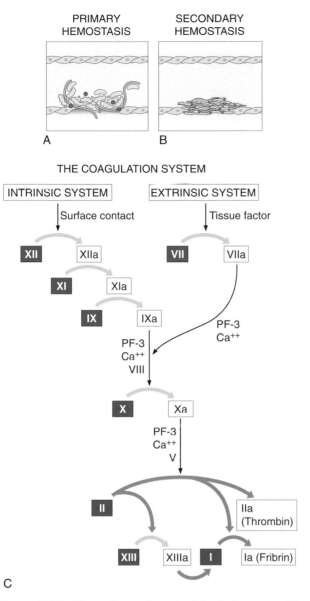

Figure 25-4. The primary (vascular/platelet) system **(A),** the secondary (coagulation) system for the control of bleeding **(B),** and the coagulation cascade **(C).** The intrinsic coagulation system is triggered by surface contact, the extrinsic system by release of tissue factor from injured tissues, and the common pathway by factor X. (From Ragni MV. The hemophilias: Factor VIII and factor IX deficiencies. In Young NS, Gerson SL, High KA [eds]. Clinical Hematology. St. Louis, Mosby, 2006.)

product, fibrin.[13-15] Figure 25-4 shows these coagulation pathways.

The (faster) extrinsic pathway is initiated through tissue factor (an integral membrane protein) and is released or exposed through injury to tissues; this process activates factor VII (VIIa). In the past, the trigger for initiating the extrinsic pathway was referred to as a tissue *thromboplastin.* It has since been shown that the real activator is the tissue factor (TF). The term *extrinsic pathway* continues to be used today, despite the fact that it is somewhat outdated. This is because TF is not always

extrinsic to the circulatory system but is expressed on the surface of vascular endothelial cells and leukocytes.[13,14]

Thrombin generated by the faster extrinsic and common pathway is used to accelerate the slower intrinsic and common pathway. Activation of factor XII acts as a common link between the component parts of the homeostatic mechanism: coagulation, fibrinolytic, kinin, and complement systems. As a result, thrombin is generated; in turn, fibrinogen is converted to fibrin, activates factor XIII, enhances factor V and factor VIII activity, and stimulates aggregation of additional platelets.[13-15]

Fibrinolytic Phase. The fibrin-lysing (fibrinolytic) system is needed to prevent coagulation of intravascular blood away from the site of injury and to dissolve the clot, once it has served its function in homeostasis (Figure 25-5). This system involves plasminogen, a proenzyme for the enzyme plasmin, which is produced in the liver, and various plasminogen activators and inhibitors of plasmin. The prime endogenous plasminogen activator is tPA, which is released by endothelial cells at the site of injury. Two other endogenous plasminogen activators are prourokinase (scu-PA) and urokinase (u-PA). Streptokinase (SK) acts as an exogenous plasminogen activator. Alpha$_2$ antiplasmin and three plasminogen activator inhibitors—PAI-1, PAI-2, and PAI-3—are present in plasma; their purpose is to inhibit plasminogen activators. The actions of plasmin are designed to destroy fibrin and fibrinogen-producing fibrin degradation products, destroy factors V and VIII, enhance conversion of factor XII to factor XIIa, amplify conversion of prekallikrein to kallikrein, and cleave complement (C3) into fragments. The fibrin-forming and fibrin-lysing systems are intimately related; activation of the fibrin-forming (coagulation) system also activates the fibrinolytic system. The tPA released by injured endothelial cells binds to fibrin as it activates the conversion of fibrin-bound plasminogen to plasmin. Circulating plasminogen (i.e., not fibrin bound) is not activated by tPA. Thus, tPA is efficient in dissolving a clot without causing systemic fibrinolysis.[14,17,18]

The effect of plasmin on fibrin and fibrinogen is to split off large pieces that are broken up into smaller and smaller segments. The final smaller pieces are called *split products.* These split products also are referred to as *fibrin-degradation products (FDPs).* These can be important clinically if they are allowed to accumulate. FDPs increase vascular permeability and interfere with thrombin-induced fibrin formation; this can provide the basis for clinical bleeding problems.[14,17,18] Box 25-4 summarizes the fibrin-lysing system.

Antiplasmin factors present in circulating blood rapidly destroy free plasmin but are relatively ineffective against plasmin that is bound to fibrin (Box 25-5). Thus, under normal conditions, once an injury has occurred, coagulation proceeds to the formation of fibrin. At the same time, bound plasminogen and free plasminogen become activated to plasmin. Free plasmin is rapidly

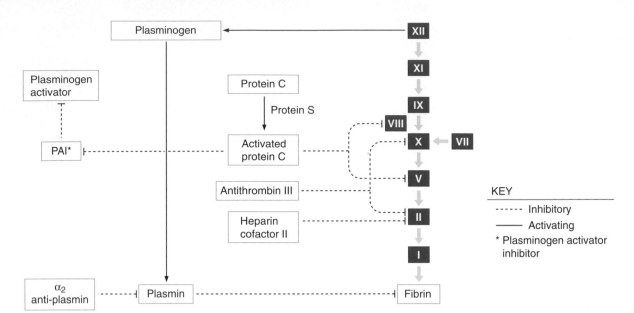

Figure 25-5. The coagulation and fibrinolytic pathways with inhibitors. (With permission from Bontempo FA. Hematologic abnormalities in liver disease. In Young NS, Gerson SL, High KA [eds]. Clinical Hematology. St. Louis, Mosby, 2006.)

BOX 25-4

Fibrin-Lysing (Fibrinolytic) System[2]

1. Activation of coagulation also activates fibrinolysis
2. Active enzyme: plasmin
3. Plasminogen activated to plasmin
   a. Tissue-type plasminogen activator (tPA)
   b. Prourokinase (scu-PA)
   c. Urokinase (u-PA), streptokinase
4. Tissue plasminogen activator (tPA)
   a. Produced by endothelial cells
   b. Released by injury
   c. Activates plasminogen bound to fibrin
   d. Circulating plasminogen not activated; t-PA will dissolve clot, will not cause systemic fibrinolysis
5. Action of plasmin
   a. Splits large pieces of alpha and beta polypeptides from fibrin
   b. Splits small pieces of gamma chains
   c. First product is X monomer
   d. Each X monomer splits into one E fragment and two D fragments
   e. Split products are called fibrin-split products (FSPs) and fibrin-degradation products (FDPs)
6. Action of fibrin-degradation products
   a. Increase vascular permeability
   b. Interfere with thrombin-induced fibrin formation

Based on material from McVey JH. Coagulation factors. In Young NS, Gerson SL, High KA (eds). Clinical Hematology. St. Louis, Elsevier-Mosby, 2006, pp 103-123.

BOX 25-5

Physiologic Antithrombotic Systems

- Normal endothelium promotes blood fluidity by inhibiting platelet activation
- Endothelium also plays a role in anticoagulation by preventing fibrin formation
- Antithrombin III
  - Major protease inhibitor of the coagulation system
  - Inactivates thrombin and other activated coagulation factors
- Heparin acts as an anticoagulant by binding to antithrombin and greatly accelerates the ability of antithrombin to inhibit coagulation proteases
- Heparin and heparin sulfate proteoglycans are naturally present on endothelial cells
- Activated protein C, with its cofactor protein S, acts as a natural anticoagulant by destroying factors Va and VIIIa
- Tissue factor pathway inhibitor (TFPI), a plasma protease inhibitor, inhibits factor VIIa and the extrinsic pathway
- The endogenous fibrinolytic system degrades any fibrin produced, despite the antithrombotic mechanisms listed above
- Inherited deficiency of antithrombin, protein C, or protein S is associated with a lifelong thrombotic tendency
- TFPI deficiency has yet to be related to clinical problems

Based on material from Esmon CT. Regulatory mechanisms in hemostasis: Natural anticoagulants. In Hoffman R, Benz EJJ, Shattil SJ, et al (eds). Hematology: Basic Principles and Practices, 4th ed. Philadelphia, Elsevier-Churchill Livingstone, 2005, pp 1961-1975.

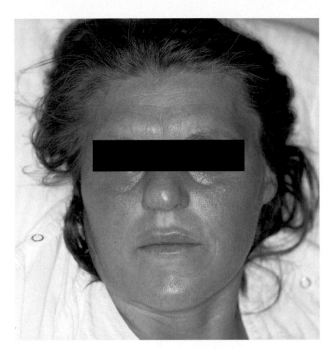

Figure 25-6. Jaundice of the skin in a patient with chronic liver disease.

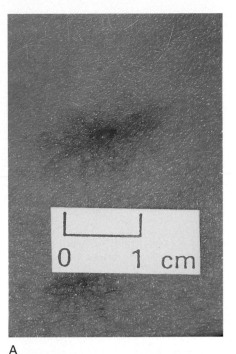

A

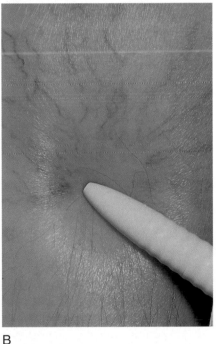

B

Figure 25-7. Spider angioma on the skin of a patient with chronic liver disease **(A)**. Note, on the right **(B)**, how the spider legs of the angioma blanch with pressure on the central arteriole. (From Forbes CD, Jackson WF. Color Atlas and Text of Clinical Medicine, 3rd ed. Edinburgh, Mosby Ltd., 2003.)

destroyed and does not interfere with the formation of a clot. Bound plasmin is not inactivated, and it is free to dispose of the fibrin clot after its function in homeostasis has been fulfilled. In a sense, the clot is "programmed" at the time of its formation to self-destruct.[14,17,18]

Timing of Clinical Bleeding. A significant disorder that may occur in the vascular or platelet phase leads to an immediate clinical bleeding problem after injury or surgery. These phases are concerned with controlling blood loss immediately after an injury and, if defective, will lead to an early problem. However, if the vascular and platelet phases are normal, and the coagulation phase is abnormal, the bleeding problem will not be detected until several hours or longer after the injury or surgical procedure. In the case of small cuts, for example, little bleeding would occur until several hours after the injury, and then a slow trickle of bleeding would start. If the coagulation defect were severe, this slow loss of blood could continue for days. Even with this "trivial" rate, a significant loss of blood might occur (0.5 mL per minute or ≈3 U per day).[14,19,20]

CLINICAL PRESENTATION

Signs and Symptoms

Signs associated with bleeding disorders may appear in the skin or mucous membranes or after trauma or invasive procedures. Jaundice (Figure 25-6), spider angiomas (Figure 25-7), and ecchymoses (Figure 25-8) may be seen in the person with liver disease. A fine tremor of the hands when held out also may be observed in these patients. In about 50% of persons with liver disease,

a reduction in platelets occurs because of hypersplenism that results from the effects of portal hypertension; these individuals may show petechiae on the skin and mucosa.[5,19,21,22]

The most common objective findings in patients with genetic coagulation disorders are ecchymoses, hemarthrosis, and dissecting hematomas.[5] The signs seen

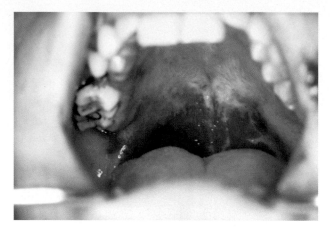

Figure 25-8. Ecchymoses on the mucosa of the hard and soft palate in a patient with chronic liver disease.

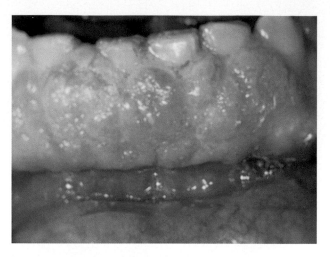

Figure 25-10. Hyperplastic gingiva in a patient with leukemia.

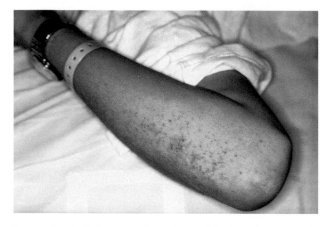

Figure 25-9. The arm of a patient with thrombocytopenia shows numerous petechiae.

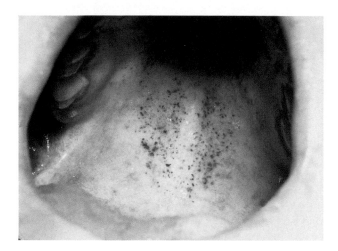

Figure 25-11. Palatal petechiae in a patient with leukemia. (From Hoffbrand AV. Color Atlas of Clinical Hematology, 3rd ed. St. Louis, Mosby, 2000.)

most commonly in patients with abnormal platelets or thrombocytopenia are petechiae (Figure 25-9) and ecchymoses.[4]

Patients with acute or chronic leukemia may reveal one or more of the following signs: ulceration of the oral mucosa, hyperplasia of the gingivae (Figure 25-10), petechiae of the skin or mucous membranes (Figure 25-11), ecchymoses of skin or mucous membranes, and lymphadenopathy. Chapter 24 discusses these findings in greater detail.

A number of patients with bleeding disorders may show no objective signs that suggest their underlying problem. Severe or chronic bleeding can lead to anemia with features of pallor, fatigue, and so forth. Anemia is discussed in detail in Chapter 23.

Laboratory Tests

Several tests are available to screen patients for bleeding disorders and to help pinpoint the specific deficiency. In general, screening is done in dentistry when the patient

reveals a history of a bleeding problem or a family member with a history of a bleeding problem, and/or when signs of bleeding disorders are found during the clinical examination. The dentist can order the screening tests, or the patient can be referred to a hematologist for screening. In medicine, routine screening is done for patients before major surgical procedures such as open heart surgery are performed.

Three tests are recommended for use in initial screening for possible bleeding disorders[20,23,24]: activated partial thromboplastin time (aPTT), prothrombin time (PT), and platelet count (Figure 25-12). If no clues are evident as to the cause of the bleeding problem, and the dentist is ordering the tests through a commercial laboratory, two additional tests can be added to the initial screen: platelet function analyzer (PFA-100) and thrombin time (TT).[23,24]

COAGULATION CASCADE

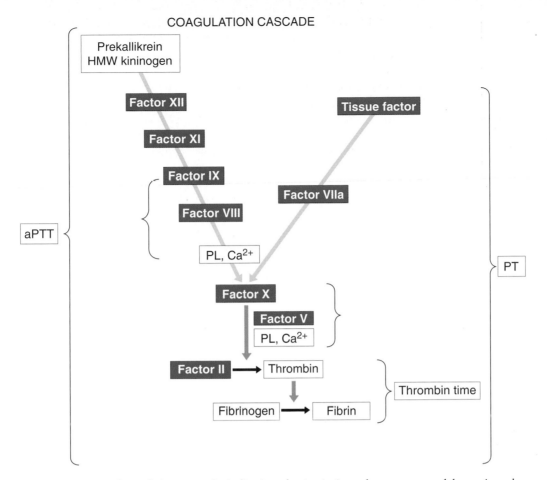

Figure 25-12. Coagulation cascade indicating the intrinsic pathway measured by activated partial thromboplastin time (aPTT), the extrinsic pathway measured by prothrombin time (PT), and the conversion of fibrinogen to fibrin, which is measured by thrombin time (TT). Other proteins—prekallikrein and high molecular weight (HMW) kininogen—participate in the contact activation phase but are not considered coagulation factors. Abbreviations: Ca^2, Calcium; PL, phospholipid. (From Rick ME. Coagulation testing. In Young NS, Gerson SL, High KA [eds]. Clinical Hematology. St. Louis, Mosby, 2006.)

Patients with positive screening tests should be evaluated further so the specific deficiency ca be identified and the presence of inhibitors ruled out. A hematologist orders these tests, establishes a diagnosis that is based on the additional testing, and makes recommendations for treatment of the patient who is found to have a significant bleeding problem.

Screening Tests.

Partial thromboplastin time. Partial thromboplastin time (PTT) is used to check the intrinsic system (factors VIII, IX, XI, and XII) and the common pathways (factors V and X, prothrombin, and fibrinogen). It also is the best single screening test for coagulation disorders. A phospholipid platelet substitute is added to the patient's blood to initiate the coagulation process. This material acts as a partial thromboplastin and cannot trigger the extrinsic pathway. For the PTT test, activation is accomplished by the glass wall of the test tube or by addition of a contact activator such as kaolin. When a contact activator is added, the test is referred to as *activated PTT (aPTT)*. A control must be run with the test sample, and results can be interpreted only if the control value falls within the normal range of results for the laboratory at which the test is performed.[20,23,24]

The aPTT varies from laboratory to laboratory; hence, the dentist must be aware of the normal range for the laboratory that is used. In general, aPTT ranges from 25 to 35 seconds, and results in excess of 35 seconds are considered abnormal or prolonged.

The aPTT screens for the following intrinsic pathway deficiencies: prekallikrein; high molecular weight (HMW) kininogen; and factors VIII, IX, XI, and XII. Deficiencies of factor XII, prekallikrein, and HMW kininogen result in a prolonged aPTT test, but these deficiencies do not cause clinical bleeding problems. The aPTT is prolonged in cases of mild to severe deficiency of factor VIII or IX. The test result is abnormal when a given factor is 15% to 30% below its normal value. In unusual cases with higher levels than normal with one of the intrinsic pathway coagulation factors, the aPTT is shortened (to less than 25 seconds).[20,23,24]

Prothrombin time. PT is used to check the extrinsic pathway (factor VII) and the common pathway (factors V and X, prothrombin, and fibrinogen). Three of these are vitamin K–dependent (factors VII and X and prothrombin) and are depressed by coumarin-like drugs. Thus, PT is used to evaluate the effects of coumarin-like drugs. For this test, tissue thromboplastin is added to the test sample to serve as the activating agent. Again, a control must be run, and results vary from one laboratory to another. In general, the normal range is 11 to 15 seconds, and results in excess of 15 seconds are considered abnormal or prolonged. PT is prolonged when the plasma level of any factor is below 10% of its normal value. When the test is used to evaluate the level of anticoagulation with coumarin-like drugs, the international normalized ratio (INR) format is recommended. INR, a method that standardizes PT assays, is defined later.[20,23,24]

Platelet count. Platelet count is used to screen for possible bleeding problems due to thrombocytopenia. Normal platelet count is 140,000 to 400,000/mm^3 of blood. Patients with a platelet count of between 50,000 and 100,000/mm^3 manifest excessive bleeding only with severe trauma. Patients with counts below 50,000/mm^3 demonstrate skin and mucosal purpura and bleed excessively with minor trauma. Patients with platelet counts below 20,000/mm^3 experience spontaneous bleeding. A peripheral blood smear is used to detect the presence of platelets.[17,23,24]

Ivy bleeding time. Ivy bleeding time (BT) has been used to screen for disorders of platelet function and thrombocytopenia. It has been found to be unreliable and is no longer used as a screening test. Some authorities still recommend use of the Ivy BT in screening for inherited disorders of platelet function in patients with a clinical history of mucocutaneous bleeding and normal screening results based on aPTT, PT, and platelet count.[20]

Platelet function analyzer 100 (PFA-100). An in vitro system for the detection of platelet dysfunction, PFA-100 is available in many laboratories. It provides a quantitative measure of platelet function in anticoagulated whole blood. The system consists of a microprocessor-controlled instrument and a disposable test cartridge that contains a biologically active membrane. Types of available cartridges include a standard cartridge that contains collagen/ADP and a collagen/epinephrine cartridge. The

instrument aspirates a blood sample under constant vacuum from the sample reservoir through a capillary and a microscopic aperture that is cut into the membrane. The presence of ADP or epinephrine and the high shear rates generated under standardized flow conditions result in platelet attachment, activation, and aggregation, which slowly build to a stable platelet plug of the aperture. The time required to attain full occlusion of the aperture is reported as "closure time" (normal < 175 seconds). The collagen/epinephrine cartridge is used to screen for aspirin effect. This instrument has been reported to be highly accurate in discriminating normal from abnormal platelet function.[23,25-27]

Thrombin time. In this test, thrombin is added to the patient's blood sample as the activating agent. It converts fibrinogen in the blood to insoluble fibrin, which makes up the essential portion of a blood clot. Again, a control must be run, and results vary from laboratory to laboratory. This test bypasses the intrinsic, extrinsic, and most of the common pathway. For example, patients with hemophilia A or factor V deficiency have a normal TT. Generally, the normal range for the TT test is 9 to 13 seconds, and results in excess of 16 to 18 seconds are considered abnormal or prolonged.[23,24] Abnormal test results are usually caused by excessive plasmin and/or fibrin-split products.

Diagnostic Tests Performed by the Hematologist. When one or more of the screening tests are found to be abnormal, the hematologist runs additional tests to pinpoint the specific defect of the bleeding disorder.

Platelet disorders. Platelet count is very effective for identifying patients with thrombocytopenia. It is not effective for identifying patients with disorders of platelet function such as vWD, Bernard-Soulier disease, Glanzmann's disease, uremia, and drug-induced platelet release defects. BT may be prolonged in these patients, but test results are inconsistent. Platelet aggregation tests, ristocetin-induced agglutination, platelet release reaction, and other tests may have to be performed for the nature of the clinical bleeding problem to become apparent.[20,23,24]

Additional laboratory tests are needed to establish the diagnosis and to identify the type of vWD. These consist of ristocetin cofactor activity, ristocetin-induced platelet aggregation, immunoassay of vWF, multimeric analysis of vWF, and specific assays for factor VIII.[20,23,24]

Disorders of the intrinsic pathway. Screening tests show prolonged aPTT, normal PT, and normal platelet count (except in some cases of vWD). The next step is to mix (mixing tests) the patient's blood with a sample of pooled plasma and repeat the aPTT. If this test is normal, then the specific missing factor is identified by specific assays. If the mixing test is abnormal, tests for inhibitor activity (antibodies to the factor) are performed. Some acquired coagulation disorders can produce prolonged aPTT along with normal PT. These include the Lupus inhibitor, antibodies to factor VIII, and heparin therapy.[20,23,24]

Disorders of the extrinsic pathway.

A normal aPTT and a prolonged PT suggest a factor VII deficiency, which is very rare, or inhibitors to factor VII. Factor VII deficiency is confirmed by specific assay. Mixing studies are used to rule out factor VII inhibitors.[20,23,24]

Disorders of the common pathway.

A prolonged aPTT and a prolonged PT in a patient with a history of a congenital bleeding disorder indicate a common pathway factor deficiency. Congenital deficiency of factors V and X, prothrombin, or fibrinogen is rare. When both of these tests are prolonged, an acquired common pathway factor deficiency is indicated. Often, multiple factors are found to be deficient. Conditions that can cause both tests to be abnormal are vitamin K deficiency, liver disease, and DIC. When both tests are prolonged in a patient with a history suggestive of a congenital bleeding problem, the next step is to exclude or identify an abnormality of fibrinogen in the laboratory. This involves measuring the plasma fibrinogen level and performing tests for D-dimer of fibrin-degradation products. Once a problem involving fibrinogen has been ruled out, the next step is to perform mixing studies to rule out inhibitor activity. If these studies are negative, then specific assays for deficiency of factor V or X or prothrombin are performed.[20,23,24]

Degradation products of fibrin or fibrinogen.

In patients with prolonged aPTT, PT, and TT, the defect involves the last stage of the common pathway, which is the activation of fibrinogen to form fibrin to stabilize the clot. The plasma level of fibrinogen is determined, and if it is within normal limits, then tests for fibrinolysis are performed. These tests, which detect the presence of fibrinogen and/or fibrin-degradation products, consist of staphylococcal clumping assay, agglutination of latex particles coated with antifibrinogen antibody, and euglobulin clot lysis time.[20,23,24]

Disorders with normal primary screening results.

Patients with vascular abnormalities that can cause clinical bleeding may not be identified through the use of recommended screening tests. BT is the only test that might be abnormal in these patients. However, it has clearly been shown that BT is inconsistent in these patients. Thus, this test is not reliable for identifying these patients. In most cases, the diagnosis must be based on history and clinical findings.[20]

Three known defects in the coagulation system do not affect PT, aPTT, or TT. These are rare and include factor XIII deficiency, alpha$_2$ plasmin inhibitor deficiency, and PAI-1 deficiency (major inhibitor of plasminogen activators). Patients with a strong clinical history of bleeding and normal coagulation test results (PT, aPTT, and TT) require additional testing, such as the use of 5M urea.[17]

Another small group of patients with a history of significant bleeding problems will have negative test results when screened by means of currently recommended methods. It appears that current methods are unable to reveal whatever disorder these patients may have. A clear-cut history of prolonged bleeding after trauma or surgical procedures is always more significant than negative laboratory data.[20]

MEDICAL MANAGEMENT

In this section, conditions that may cause clinical bleeding are considered. The emphasis is placed on detection of patients with a potential bleeding problem and management of these patients if surgical procedures are needed.

Disorders affecting the vascular, platelet, coagulation, and fibrinolytic phases are discussed. Hemophilia, vWD, Bernard-Soulier disease, DIC, disorders of platelet release, and primary fibrinogenolysis are described in some detail to show the nature of certain genetic and acquired bleeding disorders. These diseases reflect the roles of various factors involved in the control of excessive bleeding after injury, and they reveal what happens when these factors are defective. Table 25-2 summarizes the nature of the defects and the medical treatment available for excessive bleeding in patients with the disorders covered in this section. Table 25-3 lists the commercial products that are available to treat bleeding problems in these disorders.

Vascular Defects

Bleeding disorders caused by vascular abnormalities may be caused by structural malformation of vessels, hereditary disorders of connective tissue, and acquired connective tissue disorders.

Hereditary hemorrhagic telangiectasia (Osler-Weber-Rendu syndrome) is an autosomal dominant disorder that is characterized by multiple telangiectatic lesions involving the skin and mucous membranes. These lesions are associated with epistaxis and other bleeding complications. Bleeding occurs because of the inherent mechanical fragility of vessels. Lesions usually appear in affected individuals by the age of 40, and they increase in number with age.[28,29]

Ehlers-Danlos disease, osteogenesis imperfecta, pseudoxanthoma elasticum, and Marfan syndrome are hereditary disorders of connective tissue that may be associated with bleeding problems. In some patients with Ehlers-Danlos disease, an abnormal type III collagen, which leads to vessel wall weakness, is produced. These patients are prone to arterial aneurysms and bleeding from spontaneous rupture of vessels. Surgery should be avoided if at all possible. If surgery must be done, extreme care must be taken in manipulation of vascular tissues. In

TABLE 25-2
Medical Treatment of Bleeding Disorders

Condition	Defect	Medical Treatment
von Willebrand's disease	Deficiency or defect in vWF causing poor platelet adhesion and, in some cases, deficiency of F-VIII	DDAVP; EACA; F-VIII replacement that retains vWF
Hemophilia A	Deficiency or defect in F-VIII; some patients develop antibodies (inhibitors) to F-VIII	DDAVP; EACA; F-VIII; porcine F-VIII, PCC, aPCC, F-VIIa, and/or steroids for patients with inhibitors
Hemophilia B	Deficiency or defect in F-IX	F-IX
Primary thrombocytopenia (idiopathic thrombocytopenia)	Platelets destroyed by autoimmune processes	Prednisone; IV gamma globulin; platelet transfusion
Secondary thrombocytopenia	Deficiency of platelets due to accelerated destruction or consumption, deficient production, or abnormal pooling	Platelet transfusion
Bernard-Soulier disease	Genetic defect in platelet membrane; absence of glycoprotein Ib (GP-Ib) causes disorder in platelet adhesion	Platelet transfusion
Liver disease	Multiple coagulation factor defects; ` patients with portal hypertension may be thrombocytopenic	Vitamin K; replacement therapy only for serious bleeding or before surgical procedures; DDAVP provides some benefit
DIC	Multiple coagulation factor defects due to triggered consumption; formation of fibrin and fibrinogen-degradation products due to fibrinolysis; thrombocytopenia	Treatment of primary disorder; heparin; cryoprecipitate or fresh frozen plasma for replacement of fibrinogen; platelet transfusion; other blood product replacements lead to mixed results

aPCC, Activated prothrombin complex concentrate; DDAVP, desmopressin (1-desamino-8-D-arginine vasopressin); EACA, ε-aminocaproic acid; F-VIIa, activated factor VII; F-VIII, factor VIII; F-IX, factor IX; IV, intravenous; PCC, prothrombin complex concentrate; vWF, von Willebrand factor.

pseudoxanthoma elasticum, a genetic defect leads to calcification of elastic fibers. Bleeding can result when calcified vessels rupture. Bruising, epistaxis, and bladder, joint, and gastrointestinal bleeding are common.[28,29]

Acquired connective tissue disorders that may be complicated by bleeding include scurvy, small vessel vasculitis, and skin disorders. In scurvy, deficiency of vitamin C leads to lack of peptidyl hydroxylation of procollagen, resulting in weakened collagen fibers. The abnormal collagen results in defective perivascular supportive tissues, which can lead to capillary fragility and delayed wound healing. In patients on long-term use of steroids, thinning of connective tissues may result in bleeding after minor trauma.[28,29]

Small-vessel vasculitis may be caused by a variety of conditions that produce inflammation of small vessels, including arterioles, venules, and capillaries. Serum sickness can lead to purpura through immune complex deposits into vessel walls. Drugs such as penicillin, hydralazine, sulfonamides, and thiazides diuretics and hepatitis have been associated with serum sickness–like reactions.[28,29]

Platelet Disorders

von Willebrand's Disease. The most common inherited bleeding disorder is vWD, which is caused by an inherited defect involving platelet adhesion. Platelet adhesion is affected by a deficiency in vWF or a qualitative defect in the factor. The disease has several variants, depending on the severity of genetic expression. Most of the variants are transmitted as autosomal dominant traits (types 1 and 2). These variants of the disease tend to result in mild to moderate clinical bleeding problems. Type 1 disease involves a partial deficiency of vWF. Patients with type 2 variants (2A, 2B, 2M, and 2N) have various qualitative defects in vWF. In type 2N, vWF variants have a decreased affinity for factor VIII. Type 3 is transmitted as an autosomal recessive trait that leads to severe deficiency of vWF.[21,30,31]

vWF binds factor VIII in circulating blood. Unbound factor VIII is destroyed in the circulation. Thus, variants of vWD with a significant reduction in vWF or with a vWF that is unable to bind factor VIII may show signs and symptoms of hemophilia A, in addition to those associated with defective platelet adhesion. This is found in all cases of type 3 disease, in many cases of type 2N disease, and in some cases of type 1 disease. Reduction in factor VIII may occur in other variants of vWD, but when it occurs, it usually is not severe.[21,30,31]

Type 1 is the most common form of vWD. It accounts for about 70% to 80% of cases of vWD. The greater the deficiency of vWF in type 1 disease, the more likely it is

TABLE **25-3**

Factor VIII, Factor IX, Factor VIIa (Recombinant) Concentrates, and Other Blood Products Available in the United States

Factor	Product	Source of Factor	Risk of Infection With HIV and Hepatitis Viruses
Factor VIII (AHF) concentrates	Alphanate	Human plasma	No
	Hemofil M	Human plasma	No
	Humate-P	Human plasma	Yes (HBV, HCV)
	Koate-HP	Human plasma	No
	Monarc-M	Human plasma	No
	Monoclate-P	Human plasma	No
	Bioclate	Recombinant	No
	Helixate	Recombinant	No
	Kogenate FS	Recombinant	No
	Recombinate	Recombinant	No
	Hyate: C	Porcine plasma	No
	Antihemophilic Factor	Porcine plasma	No
Factor IX concentrates	AlphaNine SD	Human plasma	No
	Mononine	Human plasma	No
	BeneFix	Recombinant	No
Factor IX complex	Konyne-80 Factor IX Complex	Human plasma	Yes (low risk)
	Proplex T Factor IX Complex	Human plasma	Yes (low risk)
	Profilnine SD	Human plasma	Yes (low risk)
	Bebulin VH	Human plasma	Yes (hepatitis) Yes (low risk for HIV)
Activated factor IX complex	Autoplex T	Human plasma	Yes (low risk)
	FEIBA VH	Human plasma	Yes (low risk)
Factor VIIa concentrates	NovoSeven	Recombinant	No

Based on material from Kessler CM. Hemorrhagic disorders: Coagulation factor deficiencies. In Goldman L, Ausiello D (eds). Cecil Textbook of Medicine. Philadelphia, WB Saunders, 2004, pp 1069-1078; Lozier JN, Kessler GM. Clinical aspects and therapy of hemophilia. In Hoffman R, Benz EJJ, Shattil SJ, et al (eds). Hematology: Basic Principles and Practices, 4th ed. Philadelphia, Elsevier-Churchill Livingstone, 2005, pp 2047-2071; Ragni MV. The hemophilias: Factor VIII and factor IX deficiencies. In Young NS, Gerson SL, High KA (eds). Clinical Hematology. St. Louis, Elsevier-Mosby, 2006, pp 814-830.

HBV, Hepatitis B virus; HCV, hepatitis C virus; HIV, human immunodeficiency virus.

that signs and symptoms of hemophilia A will be found. Type 2A accounts for 15% to 20% of cases. The other variants of the disease are uncommon. In mild cases, bleeding occurs only after surgery or trauma. In the more severe cases—type 2N and type 3—spontaneous epistaxis or oral mucosal bleeding may be noted.[21,30,31]

The cause of platelet dysfunction in vWD is a deficiency or a qualitative defect in vWF, which is made from a group of glycoproteins. Megakaryocytes and endothelial cells produce these glycoproteins. They are formed into a single monomer that polymerizes into huge complexes, which are needed to carry factor VIII and to allow platelets to adhere to surfaces. As was stated earlier, non-bound factor VIII does not survive long in blood. Thus, a deficiency of vWF results in a similar decrease in plasma factor VIII levels. The complex of vWF and factor VIII attaches to the surface of circulating platelets, and it is from this location that the factors contribute to hemostasis.[21,30,31]

Clinical findings. Mild variants of vWD are characterized by a history of cutaneous and mucosal bleeding because platelet adhesion is lacking. In the more severe forms of the disease, in which factor VIII levels are low, hemarthroses and dissecting intramuscular hematomas are part of the clinical picture. Petechiae are rare in these patients. However, gastrointestinal bleeding, epistaxis, and menorrhagia are very common. Figure 25-13 shows the sites and frequency of bleeding in patients with type 1 von Willebrand disease. Serious bleeding can occur in these patients after trauma or surgical procedures. Patients with more severe forms of vWD may describe a family history of bleeding and also may report having had problems with bleeding after injury or surgery. Patients with mild forms of the disease may have a negative history for bleeding problems.

Laboratory. Laboratory investigation is needed to make the diagnosis. Screening laboratory tests may show prolonged PFA-100, prolonged aPTT, normal platelet count, normal PT, and normal TT. Additional laboratory tests are needed to establish the diagnosis and type of vWD. These consist of ristocetin cofactor activity, ristocetin-induced platelet aggregation, immunoassay of

CLINICAL BLEEDING SYMPTOMS ASSOCIATED WITH TYPE 1 VON WILLEBRAND DISEASE

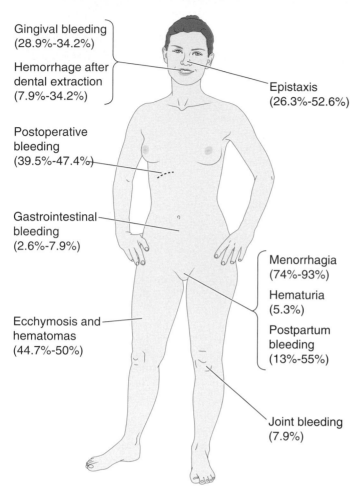

Gingival bleeding
(28.9%-34.2%)

Hemorrhage after
dental extraction
(7.9%-34.2%)

Epistaxis
(26.3%-52.6%)

Postoperative
bleeding
(39.5%-47.4%)

Gastrointestinal
bleeding
(2.6%-7.9%)

Menorrhagia
(74%-93%)

Hematuria
(5.3%)

Postpartum
bleeding
(13%-55%)

Ecchymosis and
hematomas
(44.7%-50%)

Joint bleeding
(7.9%)

Figure 25-13. Clinical bleeding symptoms by type and frequency (%) in patients with type 1 von Willebrand disease. (From Armstrong E, Konkle BA. Von Willebrand disease. In Young NS, Gerson SL, High KA [eds]. Clinical Hematology. St. Louis, Mosby, 2006.)

vWF, multimeric analysis of vWF, and specific assays for factor VIII.[3,21,23,31]

Treatment. Treatment depends on the clinical condition of the patient and the type of vWD that is diagnosed. Available treatment options include cryoprecipitate, factor VIII concentrates that retain HMW vWF multimers (Humate-P, Koate HS), and desmopressin (1-desamino-8-D-arginine vasopressin [DDAVP]). Before desmopressin is given, the patient must be tested for response to the agent. Desmopressin can be given parenterally or by nasal spray 1 hour before surgery. Parenterally, the dose of desmopressin is 0.3 μg/kg of body weight, with a maximum dose of 20 to 24 μg. The nasal spray, Stimate, contains 1.5 mg of desmopressin per milliliter and is given at a dose of 300 mg/kg. Usually, one dose is sufficient. If a second dose is needed, it is given 8 to 24 hours after the first dose. Desmopressin should be used with caution in older patients with cardiovascular

disease because of the potential risk of drug-induced thrombosis.[3,21,31,32]

Patients with type 1 vWD are the best candidates for desmopressin therapy. Desmopressin treatment must not be started without prior testing to determine which variant form of vWD is involved. It is not effective for type 3 vWD and most variants of type 2 vWD. These patients are treated with factor VIII replacement that retains the HMW vWF multimers (Humate-P or Koate HS). In patients with type 2 variants with qualitative defects in vWF, Humate-P or Koate HS supplies functional HMW vWF and factor VIII for those with decreased levels. In patients with type 3 vWD, these replacement agents supply deficient materials, vWF, and factor VIII. Women are often given oral contraceptive agents to suppress menses and avoid excessive physiologic loss of blood.[3,21,31,32]

Bernard-Soulier Disease. Bernard-Soulier disease represents a disorder of platelet adhesion; however, in this disease, the platelets are defective and unable to interact with vWF. The basic defect is the absence of glycoprotein Ib from the membrane of the platelet. Glycoprotein Ib appears to function as a receptor for vWF. Laboratory tests show a low platelet count, large platelets, faulty platelet adhesion, and poor aggregation with ristocetin. The only effective therapy for bleeding problems in patients with Bernard-Soulier disease is transfusion with normal platelets.[4]

Glanzmann's Thrombasthenia. Glanzmann's thrombasthenia is a disorder of platelet aggregation that is due to a genetic quantitative or qualitative abnormality of the platelet membrane complex glycoprotein IIb/IIIa. These platelets can adhere to the subendothelium but cannot bind to fibrinogen; thus, a total lack of platelet-to-platelet interaction is evident. Bleeding in this condition is very unpredictable. Treatment consists of platelet transfusions.[4]

Disorders of Platelet Release. Platelets participate directly in the clotting cascade by serving as constituents of factor X and prothrombin-converting complexes through the release of platelet factor 3 (PF3). The potency of this release effect is increased by increased participation of platelets in the clotting process. In some cases, platelets may fail to complete the release reaction of PF3. Sometimes, this is caused by defective production of thromboxane, other times by a deficiency in the production of dense-granule ADP.

Defective thromboxane production almost always results from the administration of anti-inflammatory drugs. The best example is aspirin, which inactivates cyclooxygenase, the first enzyme of the prostaglandin-thromboxane synthetic pathway. Other drugs that interfere with thromboxane formation include NSAIDs (indomethacin, phenylbutazone, ibuprofen, sulfinpyrazone), beta-lactam antibiotics; calcium channel blocking drugs (verapamil, diltiazem, and nifedipine), phenytoin, nitrates, phenothiazines, and tricyclic antidepressants. All platelet release defects produce about the same clinical picture.[4,8,33]

In otherwise healthy individuals, the impairment of platelet function that is produced by drugs usually is of no clinical significance. However, in patients with coagulation disorders, uremic or thrombocytopenic patients, and those receiving heparin or coumarin anticoagulants, drug-induced platelet dysfunction can result in serious bleeding. PFA-100 may be normal or prolonged, and platelet function studies often show an absence of secondary wave aggregation. Patients can be screened with standard screening tests; if these results are normal, surgical procedures can be performed. Surgery can still be performed in patients with a PFA-100 that is moderately prolonged if no other bleeding disorders are present.[4,33]

Uremia may interfere with platelet function. This effect can be severe with prolonged PFA-100 and grossly abnormal platelet function tests. Patients are in danger of bleeding to death if injury occurs or surgery is performed. They respond to dialysis, cryoprecipitate, or kidney transplant but not to platelet replacement. Although beta-lactam antibiotics (penicillin and cephalothins) may cause platelet dysfunction, usually no treatment is required. Alcohol can, in some undetermined way, impair platelet function; this effect may be severe enough to contraindicate surgery unless corrective measures are taken.[4,33,34]

Coagulation Disorders

Hemophilia A. The hemostatic abnormality in hemophilia A is caused by a deficiency or a defect of factor VIII. Factor VIII circulates in plasma bound to vWF. Unbound factor VIII is destroyed. Factor VIII was thought to be produced by endothelial cells and not by the liver, as most coagulation factors are. However, when disease was corrected by transplantation in several liver transplant patients with hemophilia, it became clear that liver parenchymal cells also produce factor VIII.[5,16,22]

Hemophilia A is an X-linked recessive trait. The defective gene is located on the X chromosome. An affected man will not transmit the disease to his sons; however, all of his daughters will be carriers of the trait because they inherit his X chromosome. A female carrier will transmit the disorder to half of her sons and the carrier state to half of her daughters. Severity of bleeding varies from kindred to kindred. Within a given kindred, the clinical severity of the disorder is constant, for example, relatives of severe hemophiliacs are likely to be affected severely. The mutation rate for the responsible gene is unusually high (up to 30%), which explains why a rare condition such as hemophilia A does not die out after several generations. Because of the high mutation rate of the responsible gene, a negative family history is of limited value in excluding the possibility of hemophilia A.[2,5,22]

The assay of factor VIII activity can be used to identify female carriers of the trait. About 35% of carriers will show a decrease in factor VIII (about 50% of normal factor VIII levels). Other carriers may have normal levels of factor VIII. Immunoassays for vWF can greatly improve the detection rate of carriers of hemophilia A. Polymorphic DNA probes are now available that are capable of detecting 90% of affected families and 96% or more of carriers.[3]

Hemophilia A can manifest in women. This occurs in a mating between an affected male and a female carrier. One half of the daughters of such a mating would inherit two abnormal X chromosomes—one from the affected father and one from the carrier mother. These daughters would have homozygous hemophilia. In addition, hemophilia may occur in a minority of heterozygous carriers. Rare cases of hemophilia in females have been reported because of a newly mutant gene.[2,5,22]

Normal homeostasis requires at least 30% factor VIII activity. Symptomatic patients usually have factor VIII levels below 5%. Severe forms of the disease occur when the level is less than 1% of normal. Patients with levels between 1% and 5% have moderate disease. Those with factor VIII levels between 5% and 30% have a mild form of the disease. About 60% of cases of hemophilia are severe.[2,5,22]

Clinical findings. Patients with severe hemophilia A bleed extensively from trivial injuries. However, the most characteristic bleeding manifestations associated with hemophilia A, such as hemarthrosis, often develop without significant trauma (Figure 25-14). The frequency and severity of bleeding problems in hemophiliac patients are generally related to the blood level of factor VIII. Patients with severe hemophilia (less than 1% of factor VIII) may experience severe, spontaneous bleeding. Hemarthrosis, ecchymoses, and soft tissue hematomas are common (Figures 25-15 and 25-16).

Gastrointestinal and genitourinary bleeding also is common in severe hemophilia. . Spontaneous bleeding from the mouth, gingivae, lips, tongue, and nose may occur in these patients. Those with moderate hemophilia (1% to 5% of factor VIII) have moderate bleeding with minimal trauma or surgery. Hemarthrosis and soft tissue hematomas occur less often. Individuals with mild hemophilia (5% to 30% of factor VIII) may develop mild bleeding with major trauma or surgery. Hemarthrosis and soft tissue hematomas are seldom found in these patients.[2,35]

Hemophiliac patients usually do not bleed abnormally from small cuts such as razor nicks. However, after larger injuries, bleeding out of proportion to the extent of injury is common. This bleeding may be massive and life threatening, or it may persist as a slow, continuous oozing for days, weeks, or months. The onset of excessive bleeding is usually delayed. At the time of surgery or injury, hemostasis appears to be normal. Bleeding of sudden onset and

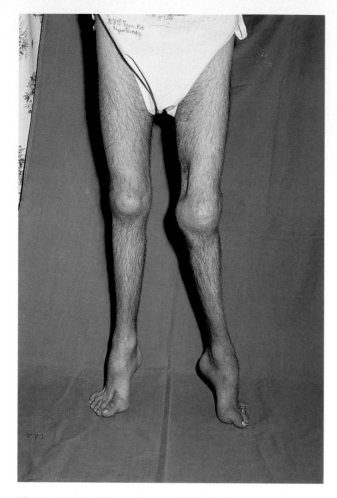

Figure 25-14. Hemarthrosis of the left knee in a patient with hemophilia. (From Hoffbrand AV. Color Atlas of Clinical Hematology, 3rd ed. St. Louis, Mosby, 2000.)

serious proportions may develop several hours or even several days later. Venipuncture, if skillfully performed, is of no danger to the hemophiliac patient because of the elasticity of the venous walls.[3]

Prognosis. The long-term survival of hemophiliac patients has been greatly affected by contamination of donated blood with human immunodeficiency virus (HIV) and hepatitis C virus (HCV). HIV has tripled the death rate in hemophiliac individuals and is currently responsible for more than 55% of all deaths related to hemophilia.[2] In contrast, the lifetime risk of death from intracranial hemorrhage is 2% to 8%. More than 75% of adults with hemophilia A and 45% of adults with hemophilia B are HIV positive. The anti-HIV protease inhibitors result in prolonged HIV disease survival among this group of patients. With the exception of HIV and HCV infection, life expectancy is related to the severity of hemophilia, and the mortality rate is 4 to 6 times higher in patients with severe disease than in those with mild to moderate disease. The mortality of patients with inhibitors is much greater than the mortality seen in those without inhibitors.[2]

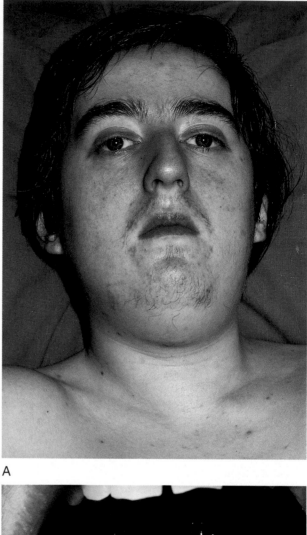

A

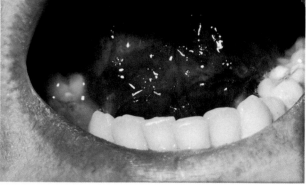

B

Figure 25-15. A, Note the swelling in the submandibular region in this patient with hemophilia caused by bleeding after intraoral trauma. **B,** The floor of the mouth has been elevated because of the bleeding. (From Hoffbrand AV. Color Atlas of Clinical Hematology, 3rd ed. St. Louis, Mosby, 2000.)

Replacement factors. Factor VIII replacement guidelines for the control of bleeding from trauma or surgical procedures in patients with severe hemophilia are as follows. For minor spontaneous bleeding or minor traumatic bleeding, 25% to 30% replacement of factor VIII is required. For treatment or prevention of severe

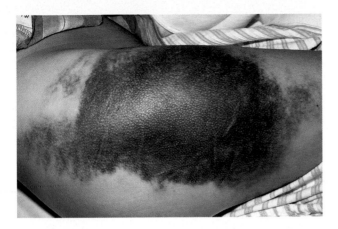

Figure 25-16. Large area of subcutaneous ecchymosis due to trauma in a patient with hemophilia. (From Hoffbrand AV. Color Atlas of Clinical Hematology, 3rd ed. St. Louis, Mosby, 2000.)

bleeding during procedures such as major dental surgery or maintenance replacement therapy after major surgery, 50% replacement or greater is needed. Treatment of life-threatening bleeding and limb-threatening bleeding during major surgery requires 80% to 100% replacement of factor VIII.[2]

The choice of which type of factor concentrate should be used is based on specific findings from the patient's management history and infectious disease exposure. The efficacy of replacement preparations, whether recombinant or plasma derived, is the same. Recombinant factor VIII concentrates are recommended for all patients with no history of factor concentrate treatment, for those who have received concentrates but are HCV and HIV seronegative, and after surgery or trauma for those with mild or moderate hemophilia that does not respond sufficiently to desmopressin therapy. Plasma-derived concentrates are recommended for patients who are HCV and HIV seropositive. High-purity products are preferred in regimens for immune tolerance induction and prophylaxis.[22]

Hemophiliacs without inhibitors. All types of general surgical procedures can now be performed in individuals without inducible inhibitors of factor VIII. The expected rate of postoperative bleeding problems is 6% to 23%; with orthopedic surgery on the knee, this rate increases to 40%. Patients with mild deficiency of factor VIII often undergo surgical procedures when desmopressin (1-deamino-8-d-arginine, DDAVP, vasopressin) is used alone or in combination with ε-aminocaproic acid (EACA). Desmopressin, which transiently increases the factor VIII level, can be given parenterally at a dose of 0.3 mg/kg or at an intranasal dose of 300 mg/kg. A second dose can be given if needed 8 to 24 hours after the first dose.[3,32,36,37]

EACA is a potent antifibrinolytic agent that can inhibit plasminogen activators present in oral secretions and stabilize clot formation in oral tissue. Patients with more severe anti–hemophilic factor (AHF) deficiency require

factor VIII replacement. EACA also is given to patients who are receiving factor replacement. Aspirin, aspirin-containing drugs, and NSAIDs, which impair platelet function and may cause severe bleeding, must not be used. Factor VIIa, a new recombinant product, is now used in some patients with severe hemophilia A with inducible inhibitors.[3,32,36,37]

Hemophiliac patients with inhibitors. A complication that poses great difficulties in the management of patients with hemophilia is the appearance of factor VIII inhibitors. These inhibitors are usually immunoglobulin G (IgG) antibodies. Factor VIII inhibitors develop in patients who have received multiple factor VIII replacement therapy. About 5% to 10% of individuals with hemophilia have factor VIII inhibitors. The increasing use of factor VIII concentrates increases the risk for development of factor VIII inhibitors; 20% to 30% of severe hemophiliac patients are affected. Patients who have low inhibitor levels of 5 Bethesda units (BU) or less that do not rise with further use of factor VIII concentrates are identified as low responders. About 40% of hemophiliac patients with inhibitors are low responders. Hemophiliac patients whose inhibitor levels rise with additional contact with factor VIII concentrates are called high responders; this situation is found in about 60% of hemophiliac patients with inhibitors. The medical management of hemophiliac patients is determined by the absence of inhibitors and low or high responder status. Patients who are most difficult to manage are high responders.[36]

Low responders with minor bleeding can be treated with human factor VIII concentrates. The dosage for these patients is larger than for those without inhibitors. Major bleeding in low responders is treated with human factor VIII concentrates but at a higher dosage and given by continuous infusion after an initial large bolus. Activated prothrombin complex concentrates may be used if needed in this group of patients. Also, porcine factor VIII can be used if low levels of cross-reactivity with this agent occur. For surgical or invasive procedures in low responders, any of these treatments may be used.

High responders with low or high titers and minor bleeding are treated with a bypassing agent such as factor VIIa, starting at a low dose (35 µg/kg); if this is ineffective, the dose should be increased to 90 µg/kg. Major bleeding in high responders with a low level of inhibitor titers (<5 BU) who are undergoing immune tolerance therapy can be treated with human factor VIII concentrates. Those with anti–human factor VIII titers greater than 5 BU but with anti–porcine factor VIII titers less than 5 BU can be treated with porcine factor VIII. High responders with high titers to both human and porcine factor VIII are treated with factor VIIa concentrates. Factor VIIa is used for surgery or invasive procedures in this group of patients.[36]

Gene therapy. Genes for factors VIII and IX have been cloned. Since 1998, five gene therapy studies have been initiated in the United States. These studies have been designed to prove that patients with hemophilia A or hemophilia B can benefit from this form of treatment. So far, these studies have shown undetectable to small increases in plasma clotting factors, but this increase has not been durable. However, many patients in these studies have reported fewer bleeds and reduced use of clotting factor concentrates. How much of this benefit might be due to placebo effect is not clear. Gene therapy for hemophilia will become practical when the limitations of gene transfer vectors are eliminated.[2,22]

Hemophilia B. In hemophilia B (Christmas disease), factor IX is deficient or defective. Hemophilia B is inherited as an X-linked recessive trait. Factor IX levels below 10% have been reported in a few women. Similar to hemophilia A, the disease manifests primarily in males. Severely affected patients (those with less than 1% of factor IX) are less common than in hemophilia A. Clinical manifestations of the two disorders are identical. Screening laboratory tests results are similar for both diseases. Specific factor assays for factor IX establish the diagnosis. Purified factor IX products (see Table 25-3) are recommended for the treatment of minor and major bleeding. Recombinant factor IX is now available for clinical use.[2,22]

Other Genetic Clotting Factor Deficiencies. Congenital deficiency of prothrombin occurs rarely. Factor V deficiency also is rare; only about 1 case per 1 million people is reported. Factor VII, which is inherited as an autosomal recessive trait, affects males and females equally; incidence is about 1 in 500,000. Factor X deficiency also is found in about 1 in 500,000 individuals. Factor XI deficiency most often occurs in Ashkenazi Jews, but also is seen in non-Jewish populations. Subjects with a deficiency of factor XII, prekallikrein, or HMW kininogen do not have clinical bleeding problems but do have prolonged aPTT. Another very rare clotting deficiency with significant bleeding problems involves factor XIII; this has been reported to occur in just over 100 patients. PT and aPTT test results are normal in these patients.[38]

Disseminated Intravascular Coagulation. DIC has been reported to occur in about 1 in 1000 hospital admissions. The syndrome is associated with a number of disorders such as infection, obstetric complications, cancer, and snakebites. In fact, worldwide, the most common cause of DIC is snakebites. DIC is a condition that results when the clotting system is activated in all or a major part of the vascular system. Despite widespread fibrin production, the major clinical problem is bleeding, not thrombosis. DIC is caused when large quantities of thromboplastic substances are introduced into the vascular system and "trip" the clotting cascade. Acute DIC may be caused by obstetric complications (abruptio placentae, missed abortion, amniotic fluid embolism), infection,

injuries and burns, antigen/antibody complexes, shock, and acidosis.[7,39,40]

Clinical findings. Symptoms of acute DIC include severe bleeding from small wounds, purpura, and spontaneous bleeding from the nose, gums, gastrointestinal tract, or urinary tract. Traumatic hemolytic anemia may occur because red blood cells are "sliced" by fibrin strands. On rare occasions, bilateral necrosis of the renal cortex has developed. Chronic DIC may occur in association with certain types of cancer. Malignant cells can release thromboplastic material as they die within the tumor mass. Antigen/antibody complexes associated with systemic lupus erythematosus may cause chronic DIC. In the chronic form of the disease, thrombosis is more common than bleeding.[7,37,39,40]

Treatment. Treatment of patients with DIC consists of an attempt to reverse the cause, control of the major symptom (bleeding or thrombosis), and a prophylactic regimen to prevent recurrence in cases of chronic DIC. Consumed coagulation factors need to be replaced, along with missing platelets. Fibrinogen levels must be restored. Cryoprecipitate is used if bleeding is the major problem. Fresh frozen plasma also may be used. If thrombosis is the major problem (early in the process), intravenous (IV) heparin is used. Long-term heparin infusion is used for prophylaxis in cases of chronic DIC.[7,37,39,40]

Fibrinolytic Disorders

Fibrinolysis and Fibrinogenolysis. Primary fibrinogenolysis may develop if active plasmin is generated in the circulation at a time when the clotting cascade is not in operation. It can occur in patients with liver disease, cancer of the lung, cancer of the prostate, or heatstroke. Severe bleeding results from the depletion of fibrinogen (split by plasmin) and the formation of fibrin-split products (with their anticoagulant properties) from fibrinogen.[41,42]

Laboratory test results are similar to those in DIC, with the following important exceptions:
- Platelet count is normal.
- Euglobulin lysis time is shortened in primary fibrinogenolysis and is normal in DIC (the euglobulin lysis test is a crude measurement of circulating plasmin).
- Fibrin-split products of primary fibrinogenolysis clump with the staphylococcal clumping assay (same for DIC), but no fibrin monomers can be released by paracoagulation with ethanol (in DIC, a loose complex of fibrin monomers is released from fibrin-split products and then polymerizes to form a gel).[23,37,42]

Fibrinogenolysis can be treated with EACA or tranexamic acid, which inhibits both plasmin and plasmin activators; however, these drugs may be dangerous if used in DIC because diffuse thromboses may result. Thus, exclusion of the diagnosis of DIC before antifibrinolytic agents are begun is very important. Use of a specific test such as D-dimer measurement can do this.[37,42]

Risk of Infection With Replacement Products

The use of cryoprecipitates, some factor VIII concentrates, and fresh frozen plasma carries several important risks. For example, transmission of hepatitis B virus (HBV), HCV, and HIV may occur.[3]

In the 1980s, more than 90% of multiply transfused hemophiliac patients became HIV positive and ultimately developed acquired immunodeficiency syndrome (AIDS). Many of these patients have died from the disease. The advent of sterile concentrates, together with rigid donor testing begun in 1985, and the availability of recombinant products have greatly reduced the risk of HIV infection through blood product administration. AIDS cases associated with hemophilia B have been less common, probably because of the rarity of this condition. A look at hemophilia mortality from 1900 to 1990 reveals the terrible impact of HIV infection. Survival increased from 1970, when factor VIII replacement first became available, to 1980, with a median life expectancy of 68 years. From 1980 to 1990, this decreased to 49 years. Most of this effect was caused by infection with HIV from contaminated blood products.[3]

During the 1970s and 1980s, more than 90% of patients treated with plasma-derived clotting factor concentrates became infected with HCV. This exposure rate has been greatly reduced on the basis of donor screening for HCV antibodies since the later 1980s, viral inactivation procedures started in 1985, and the use of ultrapure concentrates. However, as a result of the earlier contaminated blood pool, more than 80% of adult hemophiliac patients are infected with HCV. More than 25% of adult hemophiliac patients have biopsy-demonstrated cirrhosis, and HCV infection is the second leading cause of death in this population. Coinfection with HIV increases the risk for liver failure.[5,22]

Transmission of other infectious agents via blood products has occurred in the past. These agents have included various hepatitis viruses (HAV, HBV, HDV, and HGV) and parvovirus B19. Because of screening procedures and viral inactivation procedures, the hepatitis viruses (A, B, D, and G) have not been a major concern since 1985. Many hemophiliac patients who received multiple concentrate replacements prior to 1985 were infected with HBV. However, the rate of chronic infection was about 5% to 10%, and liver failure occurred late in some of these patients. Evidence of parvovirus B19 infection is found in 1 of every 1000 blood donors. About 80% of adult hemophiliac patients show evidence of infection with parvovirus B19, which occurs even in those who are given viral attenuated products. The long-term consequences of parvovirus B19 infection in hemophiliac patients have not been established.[5,22]

Screening of blood donors, viral inactivation procedures, ultrapure concentrates, and porcine factor VIII have eliminated or greatly reduced the risk of infection in hemophiliac patients with HIV, HCV, HBV, HGV, and other agents.[5,22]

Thrombosis and Antithrombotic Therapy

Thrombosis is the formation, from components of blood, of an abnormal mass within the vascular system. It involves the interaction of vascular, cellular, and humoral factors within a flowing stream of blood. Thrombosis and the complicating emboli that may result are one of the most important causes of sickness and death in developed countries. Thrombosis is of greater overall clinical importance in terms of morbidity and mortality than are all of the hemorrhagic disorders combined. Excessive activation of coagulation or inhibition of anticoagulant mechanisms may result in hypercoagulability and thrombosis. Injury to the vessel wall, alterations in blood flow, and changes in the composition of blood are major factors leading to thrombosis.[1,13-15]

Inherited thrombotic disorders may be caused by deficiency of antithrombin III, heparin cofactor II, protein C, protein S, thrombomodulin, plasminogen, tPA, activated protein C resistance (factor V Leiden), dysfibrinogenemia, and homocystinemia. Acquired deficiencies of most of these elements have been reported. Patients should be considered for laboratory evaluation for inherited thrombotic disorders if they are younger than 45 years of age and have recurrent thrombosis. In addition, patients who have experienced a single thrombotic event and have a family history of thrombosis should be tested.[1,46]

The pathologic basis for arterial thrombosis involves atherosclerotic vascular disease associated with platelet thrombi. Thrombin is a major mediator in this type of thrombosis. Drug therapy for arterial thrombi involves agents with antithrombin and antiplatelet activity. Venous thrombi usually occur in normal vessel walls; stasis and hypercoagulability are major predisposing factors. Drugs that prevent thrombin formation or lyse fibrin clots are the major agents used to treat venous thrombi.[1,45,47] Antidotes are available for overdosing of heparin (protamine) and warfarin (vitamin K); however, none is available for overdosing of the newer anticoagulant drugs.[47]

Anticoagulant Drugs

Heparin. Heparin is used in high doses to treat thromboembolism (IV bolus of 5000 U and IV infusion over a 5- to 10-day period) and in low-dose form as prophylaxis for thromboembolism. Heparin itself is not an anticoagulant. Plasma antithrombin III (ATIII) is the actual anticoagulant, and heparin serves as a catalyst. Patients older than 40 years of age who are about to undergo major surgery should receive prophylaxis with graded compression elastic stockings, low-dose heparin therapy, or intermittent pneumatic compression. If heparin prophylaxis is used, 5000 U is given subcutaneously (SQ) 2 hours before surgery and every 8 to 12 hours thereafter until the patient is ambulatory (Figure 25-17). Low molecular weight (LMW) heparin can be used instead of regular heparin and is rapidly becoming the treatment of choice. Patients

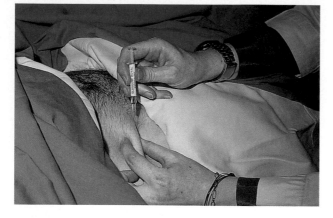

Figure 25-17. Subcutaneous heparin used to reduce the risk of deep vein thrombosis in medical and surgical procedures. (From Forbes CD, Jackson WF. Color Atlas and Text of Clinical Medicine, 3rd ed. Edinburgh, Mosby Ltd., 2003.)

who are about to undergo total hip or knee replacement should receive postoperative LMW heparin.[1,47]

Standard heparin consists of an unfractionated heterogeneous mixture of polysaccharide chains with a mean molecular weight of 12,000 to 16,000 Daltons. It inhibits factor Xa and thrombin equally. Treatment with standard heparin usually consists of IV infusion in a hospital setting and requires monitoring with aPTT. Standard heparin has a half-life of 1 to 2 hours. LMW heparin (LMWH) is prepared by depolymerization of unfractionated heparin chains, yielding heparin fragments with a mean molecular weight of 4000 to 6000 Da. LMWH preparations have greater activity against factor Xa than does thrombin. LMWHs exhibit less binding to plasma proteins, endothelial cells, and macrophages than is seen with standard heparin. Thus, they have better bioavailability when administered SQ, longer half-lives, and more predictable anticoagulant effects. LMWHs are administered SQ in the abdomen. The dosage is based on body weight, and no laboratory monitoring is needed. The half-life of the LMWHs is about 2 to 4 hours. Treatment with LMWHs may be provided on an outpatient basis.[47-49]

LMWH. LMWH preparations that are used commonly in North America for the treatment of deep vein thrombi and asymptomatic pulmonary embolism include dalteparin (Fragmin), enoxaparin (Lovenox), and tinzaparin (Innohep). Their mean molecular weight ranges from 4200 Da for enoxaparin to 6000 Da for dalteparin. Their anti-Xa/thrombin ratio varies from 1.9 for tinzaparin to 3.8 for enoxaparin.[47,48] Patients with deep vein thrombosis or pulmonary embolism are usually treated with IV heparin in dosages sufficient to prolong the aPTT to a range corresponding to a heparin level of 0.2 to 0.4 micro/mL (1.5 to 2.5 times control value). Heparin therapy is continued for 5 days or longer. Oral anticoagulation with warfarin is started early and should overlap heparin treatment for 4 to 5 days. Heparin treatment is stopped after 5 to 10 days, and warfarin treatment is

continued for at least 3 months. Complications with heparin treatment include thrombocytopenia and thrombosis. Starting warfarin therapy early after heparin is first started minimizes these complications. Overdosing of heparin can cause significant clinical bleeding.[1,47]

Synthetic Heparins. Two new synthetic heparin analogs are now available for anticoagulant use. Fondaparinux has been approved for thrombophylaxis in high-risk orthopedic patients; it also appears to provide a useful alternative to heparin or LMWH for the treatment of patients with established venous thromboembolism or pulmonary embolism (5 to 10 mg given once per day with warfarin). It is also given for prophylaxis for major orthopedic surgery at 2.5 mg once per day, starting 6 hours after surgery. The second agent, idraparinux, has a very long half-life (80 hours) and is administered SQ once per week; its efficacy and safety have not been established.[47,50]

Direct Thrombin Inhibitors. Heparin and LMWH are indirect inhibitors of thrombin because their activity is mediated by antithrombin. Direct thrombin inhibitors that do not require a plasma cofactor are now available for clinical use. Parenteral direct thrombin inhibitors now available include lepirudin, desirudin, argatroban, and bivalirudin. Lepirudin, desirudin, and bivalirudin are hirudins produced by recombinant DNA technology. Desirudin is given SQ to patients who are about to undergo hip replacement. Lepirudin is given IV to patients with history of heparin-induced thrombocytopenia (HIT) for treatment of deep venous thrombosis or for hip replacement. Bivalirudin is administered to patients about to undergo percutaneous coronary intervention. Argatroban may also be used in patients with a history of HIT. It is given by continuous infusion.[47,50]

Coumarin. Warfarin, the most widely used coumarin in the United States, is an oral anticoagulant that inhibits the biosynthesis of vitamin K–dependent coagulation proteins (factors VII, IX, and X and prothrombin). Warfarin is bound to albumin, metabolized through hydroxylation by the liver, and excreted in the urine. PT is used to monitor warfarin therapy because it measures three of the vitamin K–dependent coagulation proteins: factors VII and X and prothrombin. PT is particularly sensitive to factor VII deficiency. Therapeutic anticoagulation with warfarin takes 4 to 5 days.[1,47]

PT has been shown to be imprecise and variable. Little comparability has been seen of PT values obtained from different laboratories. These differences are caused by the source of thromboplastin (human brain, rabbit brain), the brand of thromboplastin, and the type of instrumentation used. This has caused problems with bleeding that results from a high degree of anticoagulation based on an artificially low PTT. International normalizing ratio (INR) is now used to monitor patients on warfarin therapy. The INR (INR = $[PTR]^{ISI}$; PTR = prothrombin time ratio; ISI = international sensitivity

TABLE **25-4**
Recommended Therapeutic Range for Warfarin Therapy

INR	Indication
INR 2.0 to 3.0, with target of 2.5	Prophylaxis of venous thrombosis (high-risk surgery)
	Treatment of pulmonary embolism
	Prevention of systemic embolism
	Tissue heart valves in aortic or mitral position for first 3 months
	Tissue heart valves with history of pulmonary embolism
	Tissue heart valves with atrial fibrillation
	Acute MI
	Atrial fibrillation
	Valvular heart disease
	Mitral valve prolapse with history of atrial fibrillation or embolism
INR 2.5 to 3.5, with target of 3.0	Mechanical prosthetic heart valves
	Prevention of recurrent myocardial infarction
	Treatment of thrombosis associated with antiphospholipid antibodies

Based on material from: Francis CW, Kaplan KL. Venous and arterial thrombosis. In Young NS, Gerson SL, High KA (eds). Clinical Hematology. St. Louis, Elsevier-Mosby, 2006, pp 1089-1106; Rodgers GM. Thrombosis and antithrombotic therapy. In Lee GR, Foerster J, Lukens J, et al (eds). Wintrobe's Clinical Hematology, 10th ed. Philadelphia, Lippincott Williams & Wilkins, 1999, pp 1781-1821. INR, International normalized ratio.

index for the thromboplastin used) ratio allows better comparison of PT values among different laboratories and minimizes the risk of bleeding due to artificially low PT values.[1,47] The recommended INR goal for a patient on low-intensity warfarin therapy is 2.5, with a range of 2.0 to 3.0. With a patient on high-intensity anticoagulation therapy, the INR goal is 3.0, with a range of 2.5 to 3.5. Table 25-4 shows the conditions for which warfarin therapy is recommended and the recommended INR.[1,51] Figure 25-18 shows a patient with deep venous thrombosis, which is one of the conditions for which warfarin treatment is required.

Antiplatelet Drugs

Platelets are an important contributor to arterial thrombi. Antiplatelet treatment has been reported to reduce overall mortality from vascular disease by 15% and to reduce nonfatal vascular complications by 30%. Aspirin, the prototypical antiplatelet drug, exerts its antithrombotic action by irreversibly inhibiting platelet cyclooxygenase, preventing synthesis of thromboxane A_2, and impairing platelet secretion and aggregation. Aspirin is the least expensive, most widely used, and most widely studied antiplatelet drug. NSAIDs such as ibuprofen and indobufen act as reversible inhibitors of cyclooxygenase and are used clinically to some extent. Dipyridamole, which increases cyclic adenosine monophosphate; ticlopidine and clopidogrel, which inhibit the fibrinogen receptor glycoprotein IIb/IIIa; abciximab, a monoclonal antibody (C7E3-Fab); and Integrilin, tirofiban, and lamifiban, which are peptide disintegrin inhibitors (platelet fibrinogen receptor inhibitors), are all used as antiplatelet agents. However, dipyridamole alone has been reported to be ineffective and now, when used, is given with aspirin.[1,44] The anticoagulant and antiplatelet drugs are summarized in Table 25-5.

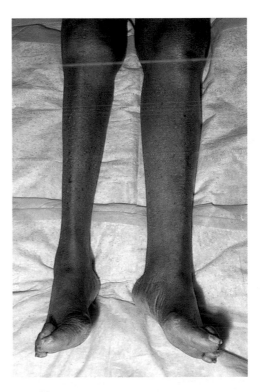

Figure 25-18. Deep vein thrombosis presenting as an acutely swollen left leg. (From Swartz MH. Textbook of Physical Diagnosis: History and Examination, 5th ed. Philadelphia, WB Saunders, 2006.)

PREOPERATIVE EVALUATION OF HEMOSTASIS

Most experts do not recommend routine preoperative screening for potential bleeding disorders in patients with a negative history and clinical findings who are scheduled for minor surgery such as dental extractions and biopsy procedures. It is recommended that patients

TABLE **25-5**
Current Antithrombotic Agents

Agent	Indications	Dosage	Monitoring	Complications
ANTICOAGULANTS				
Standard heparin, high-dose	Rx DVT Rx PE Prevention of DVT	IV bolus 5000-10,000 U, IV infusion at rate of 1300 U/hr over 5-10 days	aPTT 1.5 to 2.5 times the mean laboratory control value	Bleeding; thrombocytopenia
Standard heparin, low-dose	Prevention of DVT	Subcutaneously (SC), 5000 U 2 hours before surgery and every 8-12 hours until ambulatory	None	Bleeding; thrombocytopenia
Warfarin	Rx DVT, PE Prevention of DVT or thrombosis in AF MPHV Prevention of recurrent MI	Oral, 5-7 mg/day for 3 to 6 months Oral, 7-10 mg/day, long term	INR, 2.0-3.0 INR, 2.5-3.5	Bleeding intolerance Alopecia GI discomfort Rash Skin necrosis
Low molecular weight heparin (LMWH)	Prevention of DVT Prevention of PE	30 mg SC every 12 hours for up to 14 days (knee or hip), 40 mg SC once per day with first dose 2 hours prior to abdominal surgery	None None	Bleeding Thrombocytopenia Anemia Fever Peripheral edema
Enoxaparin* (Lovenox)	Rx DVT	1 mg/kg SC every 12 hours up to 5 days	Oral warfarin started within 72 hours	
Synthetic heparins Fondaparinux[†]	Prevention and treatment of DVT and PE	2.5 mg per day, 5-10 mg per day	None	Bleeding
Direct thrombin inhibitors Lepirudin[‡]	Used in patients with Hx of HIT, for prevention of DVT, Rx of DVT	0.4 mg/kg bolus, infusion 0.15 mg/kg	aPTT, 1.5-2.5 times laboratory normal test time	Bleeding Allergy Anaphylaxis
ANTIPLATELET DRUGS				
Aspirin	Prevention of recurrent MI, stroke, coronary thrombosis	Oral, 75 to 325 mg once per day	Usually none, but bleeding time can be used	GI bleeding Tinnitus Urticaria Bronchospasm
Aspirin plus dipyridamole (Aggrenox)	Stroke prevention (history of TIA)	Oral, 200 mg dipyridamole and 50 mg aspirin twice daily	Usually none	GI bleeding GI ulceration Urticaria Bronchospasm
NSAIDs Ibuprofen (Advil, Motrin)	Prevention of recurrent MI, stroke, coronary thrombosis	Oral, 400 mg once per day	Usually none	GI bleeding GI ulceration Rash, urticaria Tinnitus
ADP inhibitors: clopidogrel (Plavix), ticlopidine (Ticlid)	TIA, stroke and MI prevention	Oral, 75 mg once per day Oral, 250 mg twice daily	Usually none Complete blood count every 2 weeks	GI bleeding Thrombocytopenia Diarrhea
FRIs[§]: tirofiban (Aggrastat)	Prevention of recurrent MI, stroke, TIA	IV 0.4 µg/kg/min for 30 minutes, then 0.1 µg/kg/min until steady state	Usually none	GI bleeding GI ulceration Rash Neutropenia Thrombocytopenia

ADP, Adenosine diphosphate; AF, atrial fibrillation; aPTT, activated partial thromboplastin time; DVT, deep venous thrombosis; FRIs, fibrinogen receptor inhibitors; GI, gastrointestinal; HIT, heparin-induced thrombocytopenia; INR, international normalized ratio; IV, intravenous; MI, myocardial infarction; MPHV, mechanical prosthetic heart valve; NSAIDs, nonsteroidal anti-inflammatory drugs; PE, pulmonary embolus; TIA, transient ischemic attack.

*Other LMWHs—ardeparin (Normiflo), dalteparin (Fragmin), nadroparin (Fraxiparine), reviparin (Clivarin), and tinzaparin (Innohep).

[†]Other synthetic heparins—idraparinux.

[†]Other direct thrombin inhibitors—desirudin, argatroban, and bivalirudin.

[§]Other fibrinogen receptor (GP IIb-IIIa) inhibitors (FRIs)—abciximab (ReoPro), eptifibatide (Integrilin).

with a negative history for excessive bleeding who are scheduled for major surgery should be screened with use of platelet count and aPTT. Patients with an equivocal bleeding history who are scheduled for major surgery involving hemostatic impairment (heart bypass machine) should be screened with use of PT, aPTT, platelet count, factor XIII assay, and euglobulin clot lysis time. All patients with a positive bleeding history who are scheduled for minor or major surgery should be screened with use of PT, aPTT, platelet count, factor XIII assay, and euglobulin clot lysis time.[20] Our suggestions for dentistry are based on these recommendations. Patients with a significant history of a bleeding disorder should be referred to a hematologist for all screening and diagnostic testing. Patients with a history suggestive of a possible bleeding disorder may be screened by the dentist at a commercial laboratory or may be referred to a hematologist for screening. If the dentist orders screening tests we recommend that aPTT, PT, TT, platelet count, and PFA-100 should be used.

DENTAL MANAGEMENT

Patient Identification

The four methods by which the dentist can identify the patient who may have a bleeding problem are listed below. Skills acquired through application of these methods determine how well dentists can protect certain patients from the dangers of excessive bleeding after dental surgical treatment. These four methods consist of the following:

- A good history
- Physical examination
- Screening clinical laboratory tests
- Observation of excessive bleeding after a surgical procedure (Box 25-6)

History and Symptoms

The history provides the basis for the search for a potential bleeder in dental practice. To maximize the value of the patient's history in identifying the patient who may be a bleeder, several points must be considered.[19] Some healthy persons have been shown to consider their bleeding and bruising excessive; 23% in one study reported a positive bleeding history.[19] Patients with severe coagulation disorders may have dramatic abnormal bleeding histories but often do not volunteer this information unless asked. Patients with mild to moderate bleeding abnormalities may not have experienced excessive bleeding symptoms or may be unable to recognize subtle symptoms as abnormal. These patients, however, are at risk for excessive bleeding after more invasive procedures. Because of the high rate of false-positive bleeding histories and the low frequency of hemorrhagic disorders,[19] a good deal of clinical experience is required to distinguish patients with mild to moderate bleeding disorders from the normal population.

BOX 25-6

Detection of the Patient Who Is a "Bleeder"

1. History
   a. Bleeding problems in relatives
   b. Bleeding problems after operations and tooth extractions
   c. Bleeding problems after trauma (cuts, etc.)
   d. Medications that may cause bleeding problems
      (1) Aspirin
      (2) Anticoagulants
      (3) Long-term antibiotic therapy
      (4) Certain herbal preparations
   e. Presence of illnesses that may have associated bleeding problems
      (1) Leukemia
      (2) Liver disease
      (3) Hemophilia
      (4) Congenital heart disease
      (5) Renal disease—uremia
   f. Spontaneous bleeding from nose, mouth, ears, etc.
2. Examination findings
   a. Jaundice, pallor
   b. Spider angiomas
   c. Ecchymoses
   d. Petechiae
   e. Oral ulcers
   f. Hyperplastic gingival tissues
   g. Hemarthrosis
3. Screening laboratory tests
   a. PT
   b. aPTT
   c. TT
   d. PFA-100
   e. Platelet count
4. Surgical procedure—excessive bleeding after surgery may be first clue to underlying bleeding problem

aPTT, Activated partial thromboplastin time; PFA-100, platelet function analyzer; PT, prothrombin time; TT, thrombin time.

A search for objective evidence to support a history of excessive bleeding is important. This search should include a history of visits to other doctors for bleeding problems and any laboratory data that may be available; a history of transfusion of whole blood, packed red blood cells, plasma, platelets, or coagulation factor concentrates; a history of hospitalization for a bleeding problem; and a documented history of anemia or physician-prescribed iron therapy.[19]

A search for medications that may cause excessive bleeding is incomplete unless questions are asked regarding the use of aspirin, herbal remedies, dietary supplements, or over-the-counter medications that may affect coagulation or platelet function.[19] Patients who take oral anticoagulants should be asked whether they are taking vitamin tablets that contain vitamin K.[19]

In obtaining a good bleeding history, the dentist must go beyond a list of questions that the patient can respond to on a questionnaire. This involves an active process led by the dentist that is based first on the patient's initial responses on the questionnaire and is followed by hypothesis development with the construction of additional questions to be asked of the patient to test the hypothesis.[19] This process may lead to multiple hypotheses with follow-up questions that will allow the dentist to conclude that the patient is or is not a potential bleeder. Follow-up questions must be phrased in such a way that the patient can understand them.[19]

Often, multiple hemorrhagic symptoms suggest the cause of the disorder more effectively than any single symptom. A history of spontaneous hemarthroses and muscle hemorrhages is highly suggestive of severe hemophilia. In contrast, epistaxis, gingival bleeding, and menorrhagia are reported found in patients with thrombocytopenia, platelet disorders, or von Willebrand disease.[19] Several hemorrhagic symptoms are more specific for certain disorders, for example, a history of prolonged bleeding after extraction of teeth is more suggestive of von Willebrand disease or platelet disorders than of hemophilia. Patients with a history of bruising and bleeding but with normal coagulation tests and platelet count may be afflicted with blood vessel diseases such as hereditary hemorrhagic telangiectasias, Cushing's disease, scurvy, Ehlers-Danlos syndrome, or other similar conditions.[19] Dermatologic disorders must be considered in patients whose hemorrhagic symptoms are confined to the skin.

The history should include questions on the following six topics:

1. Presence of bleeding problems in relatives
2. Excessive bleeding after operations, surgical procedures, and tooth extractions
3. Excessive bleeding after trauma
4. Use of drugs for the prevention of coagulation or chronic pain
5. Past and present illness
6. Occurrence of spontaneous bleeding

Bleeding Problems in Relatives

Male offspring of parents with a family history of hemophilia are at risk for the disease. Children of a parent with vWD type 1, are at risk; about 33% of them are affected. Children of parents with a hereditary disorder of connective tissue or hereditary hemorrhagic telangiectasia are at risk for a bleeding disorder. In rare cases of a family history of disorders of platelet function, such as Bernard-Soulier syndrome or Glanzmann's thrombasthenia, the bleeding disorder may be passed to offspring.

Bleeding Problems After Operations and Tooth Extraction. Each new patient should be questioned about excessive bleeding after major or minor operations. The number of individuals who have had an appendectomy, a tonsillectomy, periodontal procedures (surgery or root scaling), or tooth extraction is large. Usually, the extraction of molar teeth is more traumatic than the extraction of incisors. A patient who reports prolonged bleeding after tooth extraction or other dental procedures should be asked whether he or she had to return to the dentist for packing, suturing, or referral for transfusion of blood products.

Persons who have undergone major operations without a bleeding problem do not have a significant inherited coagulation disorder. However, although they did not have a significant acquired bleeding problem at the time the operative procedure was performed, this does not mean that they are free of such a problem that may have been acquired since the last surgery.

Establishing the length of prolonged bleeding and the amount of blood that was lost is important. For example, normally, a small amount of blood may ooze from an extraction site for several hours or so. Oozing of blood from an extraction site for several days is abnormal unless a local infection was present. Some blood may be found on a pillow on the day after an extraction, but a pillow soaked with blood would be abnormal. Another area to ask about is the need for blood replacement after surgery; this would be most important if it was required during the postoperative period. Another important question explores whether the patient required hospitalization for the bleeding problem.

The patient should be asked whether the excessive bleeding started soon after minor surgical procedures or whether it was delayed in its onset. When excessive bleeding has been reported after minor surgery, the patient should be asked whether he or she sought medical attention and treatment. If treatment was rendered, the dentist should attempt to establish what type of treatment was given. Recall patients should be asked about any surgical procedures that have been performed since the last dental visit, and whether excessive bleeding occurred.

Bleeding Problems After Trauma. All new dental patients and recall patients should be asked whether they have experienced any recent trauma and, if so, whether excessive bleeding followed it. The more severe the trauma (knife wounds, automobile accidents), the more likely it is that the presence of an underlying bleeding disorder will be exposed. Small cuts in patients with coagulation disorders may not cause excessive bleeding initially because the vascular and platelet phases may be sufficient to control blood loss, even if a defect in coagulation is found. However, small cuts in patients with platelet or vascular deficiencies usually result in excessive bleeding, and in patients with severe coagulation disorders, this may lead to bleeding several hours after the injury.

When excessive bleeding occurs after trauma in patients with coagulation disorders, it usually is delayed because immediate control of blood loss by vasoconstriction, extravascular pressure, and platelet plugging proceeds normally. However, when these effects begin to lessen, they are not replaced by the formation of a good clot of fibrin, as happens in normal coagulation. At this point, bleeding occurs in the patient who has a coagulation defect.

The most meaningful data are reported as a recent negative or positive history of excessive bleeding after a major hemostatic challenge. With a negative history, the patient is not a bleeder. In contrast, the patient with a positive history is a bleeder. A negative history of bleeding after minor insults in a patient with a mild bleeding diathesis does not rule out a problem with more severe surgical or traumatic events. Thus, the more recent and severe the surgical or traumatic event, the more accurate it will be in revealing the presence of a bleeding disorder.

Medications That May Cause Bleeding. All new and recall dental patients should be asked whether they are taking an anticoagulant drug such as heparin (IV), LMWH (SQ), dipyridamole, or a coumarin derivative. If the patient is receiving one of these drugs, the dentist should contact the patient's physician to find out what degree of anticoagulation is being maintained and the purpose for which the drug is being used. All patients should be asked whether they have been taking aspirin or drugs that contain aspirin. Patients also should be asked whether they have undergone recent treatment with a broad-spectrum antibiotic and about excessive use of alcohol. Some herbal preparations may cause excessive bleeding (see Appendix D), as may some over-the-counter medications. The dentist must inquire about the use of such medications, particularly in the patient with a bleeding history.

Presence of Illness With Associated Bleeding Problems. The past and current medical status of patients must be reviewed. Patients should be questioned regarding a history of liver disease, biliary tract obstruction, malabsorption problems, infectious diseases, genetic coagulation disorders, chronic inflammatory diseases, chronic renal disease, or leukemia or other types of cancer, and whether they undergone received radiation therapy or been exposed to large amounts of radiation. It must be determined whether patients with cancer are being treated with chemotherapy, because this can cause significant suppression of platelet production.

Spontaneous Bleeding. Each patient should be asked about a history of spontaneous bleeding, including gingival, nasal, urinary, rectal, gastrointestinal, oral, pulmonary, and vaginal sources of bleeding. If spontaneous bleeding has occurred, the frequency, amount of blood lost, appearance of the blood, and steps that were necessary to stop it should be determined. A history of gingival bleeding is given by as many as 5% of healthy men and 50% of healthy women.[19] This bleeding may be related to periodontal disease or to the use of stiff-bristled toothbrushes. It is important to establish the frequency of gingival bleeding and to determine whether it occurs spontaneously. Excessive gingival bleeding, when it occurs, is usually related to thrombocytopenia, platelet disorders, or von Willebrand's disease.

Physical Examination

The dentist should inspect the exposed skin and mucosa of the oral cavity and pharynx of the patient for signs that might indicate a possible bleeding disorder. These include petechiae, ecchymoses (bruises), spider angioma, telangiectasias, jaundice, pallor, and cyanosis (possible thrombocytopenia). When any of these signs are found by the dentist and cannot be explained by the history or other clinical findings, the patient should be referred for medial evaluation.

Screening Laboratory Tests

The dentist can use five clinical laboratory tests to screen patients for bleeding disorders (Box 25-7): platelet count, PFA-100, aPTT, PT, and TT. The platelet count is ordered to screen for thrombocytopenia. The PFA-100 is used to screen for functional defects of platelets. The aPTT test is used to measure the status of the intrinsic and common pathways of coagulation. This test reflects

---

BOX 25-7

Screening Laboratory Tests for the Detection of a Potential "Bleeder"

1. PT—Activated by tissue thromboplastin
   a. Tests extrinsic and common pathways
   b. Control should be run
   c. Normal (11-15 seconds, depending on laboratory)
   d. Control must be within normal range
2. aPTT—Initiated by phospholipid platelet substitute and activated by addition of contact activator (kaolin)
   a. Tests intrinsic and common pathways
   b. Control should be run
   c. Normal (25-35 seconds, depending on laboratory)
   d. Control must be within normal range
3. TT—Activated by thrombin
   a. Tests ability to form initial clot from fibrinogen
   b. Controls should be run
   c. Normal (9-13 seconds)
4. PFA-100
   a. Tests platelet function
   b. Normal if adequate number of platelets of good quality present
   c. Normal (< 175 seconds)
5. Platelet count
   a. Tests platelet phase for adequate number of platelets
   b. Normal (140,000-400,000/mm³)
   c. Clinical bleeding problem can occur if less than 50,000/mm³

aPTT, Activated partial thromboplastin time; PFA-100, platelet function analyzer; PT, prothrombin time; TT, thrombin time.

the ability of blood remaining within vessels in the area of injury to coagulate. It will be prolonged in coagulation disorders affecting the intrinsic and common pathways (hemophilia, liver disease) and in cases of excessive fibrinolysis.

The PT test is used to measure the status of the extrinsic and common pathways of coagulation. This test reflects the ability of blood lost from vessels in the area of injury to coagulate. It will be prolonged in cases of factor VII deficiency (which is rare) and in disorders affecting the common pathway and fibrinolysis. This test usually is normal in patients with intrinsic pathway defects (hemophilia).

The TT test uses thrombin as the test-activating agent; hence, it measures only the ability of fibrinogen to form an initial clot. Because fibrin-degradation products tend to prolong TT, this test becomes reasonably sensitive for fibrinolysis disorders. When performed along with PT and aPTT tests, it allows for the identification of coagulation disorders involving the last "stage" of the sequence, for example, if PT, aPTT, and TT were all prolonged, the problem in the coagulation system would occur at the point of conversion of fibrinogen to the initial clot.

If positive, the results of these screening tests direct the hematologist to the possible source of a bleeding disorder and allow for the selection of more specific tests to identify the nature of the defect.

Surgical Procedure

Prolonged bleeding after a surgical procedure may be the first indication of a bleeding problem in a patient with a negative history and clinical findings. The dentist should use the appropriate local procedures (shown in Table 25-6) in an attempt to control the bleeding. If these should fail, the dentist must consult with the patient's physician or a hematologist. Screening laboratory tests may be ordered to better identify the source of the problem prior to the consultation.

Medical Considerations

No surgical procedures should be performed on a patient who is suspected of having a bleeding problem on the basis of history and physical examination findings. Such a patient should be screened by the dentist through appropriate clinical laboratory tests or should be referred to a hematologist for screening. Patients screened by the dentist with abnormal test results should be referred to a hematologist for diagnosis, treatment, and management recommendations. Patients under medical care who may have a bleeding problem should not receive dental treatment until consultation with the patient's physician has taken place, and appropriate preparations have been made to avoid excessive bleeding after dental procedures.

Ten clinical situations often present the dentist with the problem of whether a given patient has a bleeding problem. Each of these situations is discussed in Box 25-8.

BOX 25-8

Selection of Screening Laboratory Tests for Detecting the Patient With a Potential Bleeding Problem Based on History and Examination Findings

1. No clinical or historical clues to bleeding problem: Excessive bleeding occurs after surgery
2. History or clinical findings or both suggest possible bleeding problem but no clues to cause:
   - PT
   - aPTT
   - TT
   - PFA-100
   - Platelet count
3. Aspirin therapy: PFA-100
4. Coumarin therapy: PT
   - Low molecular weight heparin: aPTT
5. Possible liver disease: Platelet count, PT
6. Chronic leukemia: Platelet count
7. Malabsorption syndrome or long-term antibiotic therapy: PT
8. Renal dialysis (heparin): aPTT
9. Vascular wall alteration: BT (results often inconsistent)
10. Primary fibrinogenolysis (active plasmin in circulation), cancers (lung, prostate): TT

aPTT, Activated partial thromboplastin time; BT, bleeding time; PFA-100, platelet function analyzer; PT, prothrombin time; TT, thrombin time.

No Clinical or Historical Clues to Bleeding Problem. A person with a potential bleeding problem may have no subjective or objective findings that suggest the condition. The first indication may be prolonged bleeding after a dental surgical procedure. For this, local measures should be taken to control the bleeding; if these fail, a hematologist may have to be consulted. Once the problem has been brought under control, the patient should be screened with the appropriate laboratory tests (PT, aPTT, platelet count, and TT) by the dentist through a commercial clinical laboratory, or by a hematologist.

History or Clinical Findings, or Both, Suggest a Possible Bleeding Problem But Not Clues to Its Cause. When no clues are evident regarding the cause of a potential bleeding problem in a patient, all five screening laboratory tests should be performed. The stronger the history of excessive bleeding, the more advantageous it is to refer the patient to a hematologist for screening and diagnosis. In other cases, the patient's physician can order these tests, or the dentist can order them through a clinical laboratory facility (see Box 25-7).

Aspirin Therapy. Patients who are receiving aspirin therapy may have a bleeding problem because of the drug's effect on platelets. Some of these patients may have been receiving high doses (20 g or more, or 4 or more tablets) of aspirin each day for a prolonged period (longer

TABLE **25-6**
Topical Hemostatic Agents Used to Control Bleeding

Product	Company/Dealer	Description	Indications and Features
Gauze		$2'' \times 2''$ sterile gauze pads; place over the wound and have the patient put pressure on it by closing or finger pressure	Bleeding immediately following extractions or minor surgical procedures
Gelfoam	Upjohn	Absorbable gelatin sponge made from purified gelatin solution; absorbs for 3-5 days	Useful for most patients taking an antithrombotic agent; helpful to place topical thrombin on Gelfoam; for extensive or invasive surgery, should consider placing inside a splint
Instat	Johnson & Johnson	Absorbable collagen made from purified and lyophilized bovine dermal collagen; can be cut or shaped; adheres to bleeding surfaces when wet, but does not stick to instruments, gloves, or gauze sponges	Mild to moderate bleeding is usually controlled in 2-5 minutes; more expensive than Gelfoam
Surgicel	Johnson & Johnson	Oxidized regenerated cellulose; exerts physical effect rather than physiologic; swells upon contact with blood with resultant pressure adding to hemostasis; thrombin ineffective with these agents because of inactivation as a result of pH factors	After 24-48 hours, it becomes gelatinous; can be left in place or removed; useful to control bleeding when other agents are ineffective
Oxycel	Becton-Dickinson		
Avitene	MedChem	Microfibrillar collagen hemostat; dry, sterile, fibrous, water insoluble HCl acid salt purified bovine corium collagen; MCH attracts platelets and triggers aggregation in fibrous mass	Thrombin ineffective with these agents because of inactivation as a result of pH factors; use for moderate to severe bleeding
Helistat	Marion Merrell Dow		
Colla-Cote Tape, Plug	Colla-tec, Inc. Marion	Absorbable collagen dressings from bovine; can be sutured into place, used under stents, dentures, or alone; fully resorbed in 10-14 days	Shaped according to intended use; Cote $^3/_4'' \times 1.5''$; tape $1'' \times 3''$, plug $^3/_8'' \times ^3/_4''$; all are superior hemostats for moderate to severe bleeding
Thrombostat	Parke-Davis	Topical thrombin; directly converts fibrinogen to fibrin; derived from bovine sources	One 5000-U vial dissolved in 5 mL saline can clot equal amount of blood in less than 1 second; useful in severe bleeding
Thrombinar	Jones Medical		
Thrombogen	J & J/Merck		
Cyklokapron	KabiVitrum	Tranexamic acid; works as a competitive inhibitor of plasminogen activation; used as a rinse	Useful over short term for preventing hemorrhage after dental extractions; not available in the United States at this time
Amicar	Wyeth-Ayerst	ε-Aminocaproic acid; works as a competitive inhibitor of plasminogen activation; used as a rinse	Useful over short term to prevent bleeding
Beriplast	Behringwerke	Fibrin/tissue glue	Not available in United States at this time

than a week). Others have been taking 1 tablet a day or 1 tablet every other day to prevent coronary thrombosis. Even this low dosage of aspirin is enough to inhibit platelet thromboxane production and platelet aggregation. Although these effects are nonreversible, they may or may not be clinically significant.[37] If the PFA-100 is moderately prolonged in these patients, they will not experience excessive bleeding with minor surgery unless some other bleeding disorder is present.

The best screening test for aspirin effect is the PFA-100. Although aspirin affects platelets and the coagulation process through its effects on platelet release, this does not usually lead to a significant bleeding problem unless the PFA-100 is greatly prolonged. If surgery must be performed under emergency conditions, and the PFA-100 is greatly prolonged, DDAVP can be used to shorten the PFA-100. This should be done in consultation with the patient's physician or hematologist.[37] On a less urgent basis, with approval from the physician, aspirin may be discontinued for 3 days; this allows for arrival of a sufficient number of new platelets into the circulation.

NSAIDs can also inhibit platelet cyclooxygenase, thereby blocking the formation of thromboxane A_2. These drugs produce a systemic bleeding tendency by impairing thromboxane-dependent platelet aggregation and thus prolonging the PFA-100. However, they inhibit cyclooxygenase reversibly, and the duration of their action depends on the specific drug dose given, the serum level, and the half-life. Generally, if the clinician waits for 3 half-lives of the drug to pass, levels will be sufficiently eliminated to allow for return of normal platelet function. It should be remembered that the clinical risks of bleeding with aspirin or nonaspirin NSAIDs are enhanced by the use of alcohol or anticoagulants and by associated conditions such as advanced age, liver disease, and other coexisting coagulopathies.[52]

Coumarin Therapy. The major concern when one is performing surgical or invasive dental procedures on patients who are taking warfarin (Coumarin) is the potential for excessive bleeding. In contrast, if the anticoagulant is discontinued in preparation for the dental procedure, the major medical concern is thrombosis, which could be life threatening. The literature clearly supports the continuation of warfarin anticoagulation therapy for minor oral surgery and other similarly invasive dental procedures if the INR is 3.5 or less.[53-60] It is estimated that for every increase of 1.0 in the INR over 3.5, the risk for bleeding doubles.[47] For major oral surgery, the literature is less clear on management of the warfarin level. If other bleeding problems, such as liver disease and renal disease, are present, or if other drugs (e.g., aspirin, antibiotics, NSAIDs) are being taken, management of the patient will have to be planned on an individual basis. Before performing surgical or invasive dental procedures, the dentist should obtain medical consultation for all patients who are taking warfarin.

If acute infection is present, surgery should be avoided until the infection has been treated. When the patient is free of acute infection and the INR is 3.5 or less, minor surgery can be performed. The procedure should be done with as little trauma as possible.

The American College of Chest Physicians and the American Heart Association/American College of Cardiology also recommend that warfarin therapy should not be interrupted for invasive dental procedures, and that a tranexamic acid (Cyklokapron) or EACA (Amicar) mouthwash should be applied during the first 2 postoperative days to help control excessive bleeding.[57,61] Tranexamic acid rinses are used in other countries and are not readily available in the United States. For stability and sterility reasons, the Amicar solution can be prepared in the dental clinic on the day it is to be used.[62] A 5-g vial for injection (20 mL, contains 5 g of Amicar and 0.9% benzyl alcohol preservative) may be diluted with sterile water to a total volume of 100 mL. The patient is instructed to hold 10 mL of the Amicar solution (1.00 g of Amicar) in the area of the dental or surgical procedure for 2 minutes just before the procedure and every 1 to 2

hours after the procedure until all of the solution is gone. The patient is instructed not to "shish" to avoid dislodging a clot. Activities such as sucking on a straw or candy should be avoided because negative pressure may dislodge the clot.[62]

If excessive postoperative bleeding occurs after an extraction, Gelfoam with thrombin may be placed in the socket to control it. In addition, primary closure over the socket is desirable. Oxycel, Surgicel, or microfibrillar collagen may be used in place of Gelfoam. However, thrombin should not be used in combination with these agents because it is inactivated as a result of pH factors, thus representing an additional cost with no real benefits. An inhibitor of fibrinolysis (tranexamic acid or EACA) also can be applied.[63-65]

If excessive bleeding cannot be controlled by the local methods listed earlier, the dentist should consult the patient's physician. Available options include discontinuation of warfarin, which would take several days before an effect on bleeding would occur; administration of vitamin K; and administration of fresh frozen plasma or a prothrombin concentrate. Vitamin K can be given by the IV route (rapid response but slight risk of anaphylaxis), subcutaneously (response is unpredictable and sometimes delayed), or orally (predictable response, effective, convenient, safe, and effect seen within 24 hours). Fresh frozen plasma carries a risk of infection, and prothrombin concentrate is associated with a risk of thromboembolic complications. Another option is to administer recombinant factor VIIa.[38,47,50,66]

Box 25-9 summarizes appropriate dental management of the patient who is taking warfarin or Coumadin. If the dosage of anticoagulant must be adjusted, the patient's physician should instruct the patient. It will take 3 to 5 days before the effect of the dose reduction is reflected in the lower INR. On the day of surgery, the INR should be checked again to determine whether the desired reduction has occurred. If no excessive bleeding occurs on the day after the dental procedure is performed, the patient's physician can direct the patient to return to his or her usual warfarin dosage.

Patients who are about to undergo have major oral surgery and are receiving warfarin therapy should have input from their physician regarding the INR level that would be indicated. An INR of above 3.0 may need to be adjusted by the physician. Again, it will take 3 to 5 days for any effective reduction of the INR to occur.

Another option for these patients is to have the patient's physician discontinue warfarin therapy 4 days before major oral surgery and to begin a series of 30-mg subcutaneous enoxaparin (LMWH) injections every 12 hours (9 AM and 9 PM) on an outpatient basis, starting 3 days before the surgery is to be performed.[67] Through discontinuation of warfarin, the INR is allowed to normalize, and enoxaparin provides anticoagulation. The last enoxaparin injection is given at 9 PM on the evening before surgery. The INR should be checked on the morning of surgery and, if within normal values (1.0), the surgery can

BOX 25-9

Dental Management of the Patient Taking Warfarin or Coumadin for Whom Invasive Procedures Are Planned

PREOPERATIVE
- Medical consult
- Confirmation of diagnosis
- Status of medical condition
- Confirmation of INR level
- Type of surgery or invasive procedures planned
- Need for dosage reduction
- Based on level of anticoagulation
- Based on amount of expected bleeding

Dental
- Free of acute infection—If infection is present, treat prior to providing elective dental care
- Good oral hygiene
- Level of anticoagulation and need to alter dosage to avoid excessive bleeding
- INR, 2.0-3.0—Dosage does not have to be altered
- INR, 3.0-3.5—Dosage may be altered, usually will be altered for major oral surgery
- INR greater than 3.5—Delay invasive procedure until dosage is decreased
- Decision is made to alter dosage of anticoagulation medication
- Physician will reduce patient's dosage
- Effect of reduced dosage takes 3-5 days

- Dental appointment must be scheduled within 2 days, once desired reduction in INR has been confirmed

OPERATIVE
- Confirmation of status of INR on day of surgery
- Use of good surgical technique
- Control of bleeding by local means (see Table 25-6)

POSTOPERATIVE
- Avoid aspirin and NSAIDs
- Acetaminophen can be used with reduced dosage and can be combined with codeine
- Tell patient to call if bleeding occurs during first 24-48 hours
- See patient within 48-72 hours, and observe for the following:
  - Healing
  - Infection—Treat, if present
  - Bleeding—Use local means (see Table 25-6) to control, if present
- Patients whose anticoagulant dosage was reduced
  - If free of complications, call patient's physician and have patient returned to normal anticoagulation dosage
  - If not free of complications, treat and then call patient's physician to start normal dosage

INR, International normalized ratio; NSAIDs, nonsteroidal anti-inflammatory drugs.

be performed.[67] Enoxaparin injections are started again on the evening after the surgery; oral warfarin therapy is also restarted that evening. After 3 days, the postoperative enoxaparin injections are stopped.[67] A potential problem with this approach is that a temporary hypercoagulable state may occur when warfarin therapy is stopped.

The dentist must be aware that certain drugs will affect the action of warfarin (Coumadin). Drugs the dentist may use that potentiate the anticoagulant action of warfarin include acetaminophen, metronidazole, salicylates, broad-spectrum antibiotics, erythromycin, and the new cyclooxygenase (COX)-2–specific inhibitors (celecoxib and rofecoxib). Other drugs that have the same effect are cimetidine, chloral hydrate, phenytoin, propranolol, and thyroid drugs. Drugs that the dentist may use that will antagonize the anticoagulant action of warfarin are barbiturates, steroids, and nafcillin. Other drugs that have the same effect are carbamazepine, cholestyramine, griseofulvin, rifampin, and trazodone.[1,68]

Postoperative pain control can be attained with the use of minimal doses of acetaminophen with or without codeine. Aspirin and NSAIDs must be avoided. When used at the indicated dosage, COX-2–specific inhibitors (celecoxib and rofecoxib) do not affect platelet count, PT, and PPT and do not inhibit platelet aggregation. However, they can increase PT and INR in patients who are taking warfarin; if used, the dosage should be reduced. With recent concerns over the possible role that COX-2

inhibitors may play in increasing the risk of myocardial infarction, it may be best to avoid these agents, even though they would be used only for a short time.

Heparin Therapy. Most patients treated with standard heparin are hospitalized and will be prescribed warfarin once discharged. Dental emergencies in these patients during hospitalization should be treated as conservatively as possible, with avoidance of invasive procedures, if possible. Patients treated with hemodialysis are given heparin. The half-life of heparin is only 1 to 2 hours; thus, if they wait until the day after dialysis, these patients can receive invasive dental treatment. The dental management of these patients is presented in Chapter 13.

The dentist may see patients who are being treated on an outpatient basis with an LMWH, including patients with recent total hip or knee replacement and those being treated on an outpatient basis for deep vein thrombi or asymptomatic pulmonary embolism. Elective surgical procedures can be delayed until the patient is taken off the LMWH, which, in most cases, will occur within 3 to 6 months. If an invasive procedure must be performed, the dentist has several options. First, the dentist should consult with the patient's physician regarding the need for and the type of surgery. The half-life of the LMWHs is less than 1 day. Thus, the physician could suggest that the drug be stopped and the surgery be performed within 1 to 2 days. The other option is to go ahead with the surgery and deal with any bleeding complications on a local basis. It appears that these patients can undergo minor surgical procedures with little risk for any serious bleeding complications.[65,69]

Possible Liver Disease. A patient with a history of jaundice or heavy alcohol use may have significant liver disease. Most coagulation factors are produced in the liver; therefore, if enough liver damage has occurred, the patient could have a serious bleeding problem because of a defect in the coagulation phase. In addition, about 50% of patients with significant liver disease (with portal hypertension present) will be thrombocytopenic as a result of sequestration of platelets in the spleen. Alcohol also can have a direct effect on homeostasis by interfering with platelet function. The PT test can be used to screen for a defect in the coagulation phase in patients with a history that indicates liver disease (see Chapter 11 for blood tests indicative of alcoholism). A platelet count should be obtained to see if the platelet phase has been affected. The amount of liver damage that has occurred may not be great enough to affect the coagulation phase, but the effect on the platelet phase could be severe enough to lead to a serious bleeding problem. If both the PT and the platelet count are normal, surgery can be performed on these patients with little risk of a postoperative bleeding problem. If results of both tests are abnormal, then the dentist should consult with the patient's physician regarding management of the patient prior to surgery. This may involve vitamin K administration, platelet replacement, or other special physician-directed procedures.

Chronic Leukemia. Chapter 24 describes the management of patients with leukemia.

Malabsorption Syndrome or Long-Term Antibiotic Therapy. In patients with malabsorption syndrome and in those receiving long-term antibiotic therapy, bacteria in the intestine that produce vitamin K may be adversely affected. The liver needs vitamin K for the production and function of prothrombin (factor II) and related coagulation factors (factors VII, IX, and X). The PT test can be ordered to screen for a possible bleeding problem; if results are normal, surgery can be performed on these patients without risk of a bleeding problem. The patient's physician should be consulted regarding the patient's health status before surgery, because complicating factors may occur, in addition to the possible bleeding problem that would contraindicate surgery. Parenteral vitamin K may have to be administered in some of these cases.

End-Stage Renal Disease and Renal Dialysis. Management of patients with end-stage renal disease (ESRD) and those on renal dialysis is covered in Chapter 13.

Vascular Wall Alteration. In patients with autoimmune disease, infectious disease, structural malformation of vessels, hereditary disorders of connective tissue, scurvy,

steroid therapy, small-vessel vasculitis, or deposits of paraproteins, alterations of the vessel wall can result in excessive bleeding after surgical procedures. No reliable screening tests can detect those patients who will be bleeders. The Ivy BT test can be used in an attempt to identify potential bleeders, but, as stated earlier, this is not a reliable test. The dentist must rely on the medical history (questions related to excessive bleeding problems), clinical findings, and consultation with the patient's physician to identify these patients.

Management of the Patient With a Serious Bleeding Disorder

Dental treatment of patients with hemophilia A and with vWD and thrombocytopenia is used here to show how patients with serious bleeding disorders can be managed to avoid significant bleeding complications.

Before any dental treatment is performed for a patient with a bleeding disorder, the dentist must consult with the patient's physician to determine the severity of the disorder and the need for special preparations for dental treatment. Patients with significant bleeding disorders are at increased risk for spontaneous gingival bleeding or excessive bleeding after minor trauma to the oral tissues. They can be at even greater risk if surgical procedures are performed without special preparations.

Hemophilia. The patient with hemophilia A (factor VIII deficiency) can be used to illustrate some of the management problems involved in dealing with a serious coagulation disorder. Consultation with a hematologist is necessary. The hematologist first establishes the diagnosis and determines the degree of factor VIII deficiency, whether any factor VIII inhibitors are present, if the patient is a low or a high responder, and whether hospitalization is needed. The type of replacement material is selected (Box 25-10; see Table 25-3), and the hematologist determines the dosage of replacement material that should be used.[20,37]

Patients with severe hemophilia A manifest signs and symptoms at a very early age. It is important that preventive dentistry practices be initiated early and maintained through adulthood for all hemophiliac patients. Dental caries and periodontal disease should be minimized in these patients. The use of fluorides and fissure sealants and dietary recommendations regarding refined carbohydrate restriction are important for minimizing tooth loss. Toothbrushing, flossing, and regular dental visits, including cleaning of the teeth, are important for prevention of caries and periodontal disease, which should be treated when detected. Through maintenance of good oral hygiene and dental repair, the need for dental procedures requiring factor VIII replacement can be minimized.

In general, block anesthesia, lingual infiltrations or injections into the floor of the mouth, and intramuscular injections must be avoided unless appropriate replacement factors have been used in patients with moderate to

BOX 25-10

Dental Management of the Patient With Hemophilia

PREOPERATIVE
- Hematology consult
- Confirmation of diagnosis and severity of disease
- Presence of inhibitors (antibodies to factor VIII)
- No inhibitors
- Low responder
- High responder
- Determination of treatment location
- Patients with mild to moderate hemophilia are usually treated in the dental setting
- Patients with severe hemophilia and those with inhibitors are usually treated in the hospital
- Also influenced by type of dental treatment—Surgery, extractions, operations
- The more invasive the procedure, the more likely the patient will be treated in the hospital
- Management recommendations
  - DDAVP 0.3 µg/kg (maximal dose, 20 to 24 µg), given parenterally, 1 hour before the procedure
  - EACA 6 g every 6 hours, orally, for 3 to 4 days
  - Factor VIII replacement—Loading, 0 or 30-40 U/kg, IV; maintenance, 10-40 U/kg, IV every 12 hours
- Porcine factor VIII, PCC, APCC, or factor VII and steroids (patients with inducible inhibitors)

Dental
- Treat any acute oral infection
- Establish good oral hygiene
- Construct splints for patients with moderate to severe hemophilia who are having multiple extractions

OPERATIVE
- Use good surgical technique
- Use pressure packs (mild cases)
- Use Gelfoam with thrombin to control bleeding and/or other agents (see Table 25-6)
- Place palatal splints (moderate and severe cases)
- Hematologist will monitor treatment of hospitalized patients

POSTOPERATIVE
- Patients treated in the dental office may require second dose of DDAVP or replacement factor
- Hospitalized patients will require additional doses of DDAVP, factor VIII, or other agents
- Patients given factor VIII replacement must be examined for signs of allergy
- Hospitalized patients—Hematologist will do this
- Dental office—Dentist needs to do this; any questions about findings, consult with hematologist
- Examine patient 24-48 hours after surgery for the following:
  - Signs of infection—Treat, if present
  - Bleeding—Use local measures to control (see Table 25-6); if not effective, use other systemic measures as indicated
  - Healing
- Avoid aspirin, aspirin-containing compounds, and NSAIDs
- Acetaminophen with or without codeine is suggested for most patients

APCC, Activated prothrombin complex concentration; DDAVP, 1-desamino-8-D-arginine vasopressin; EACA, ε-aminocaproic acid; IV, intravenous; NSAIDs, nonsteroidal anti-inflammatory drugs; PCC, prothrombin complex concentrate.

severe factor VIII deficiency. Complex restorative procedures usually require replacement therapy.

Infiltration anesthesia and intraligamentary injections usually can be given without replacement therapy. Simple restorative procedures often can be performed without replacement therapy, as can endodontic treatment of nonvital teeth. However, overinstrumentation and overfilling must be avoided. Some experts recommend topical application of 10% cocaine to exposed pulp when a pulpectomy is performed. Intracanal injection of a local anesthetic along with epinephrine will help to control bleeding. Topical application of 1:1000 epinephrine with paper points will also help to control bleeding until the pulp has been removed.[65]

Orthodontic treatment can be provided to hemophiliac patients, but sharp edges on appliances must be avoided. Sharp edges can injury the mucosa and cause significant bleeding in patients with severe and moderate hemophilia.

Periodontal surgery, root planning, extractions, dentoalveolar surgery, soft tissue surgery, and complex oral surgery usually require factor replacement in patients with moderate and severe factor VIII deficiency. When

mucoperiosteal flaps are required in the mandibular region, the buccal or labial approach is suggested. Also, the buccal approach is recommended for surgical removal of mandibular third molars. Trauma to mandibular lingual tissues increases the risk of bleeding that can lead to airway obstruction. Mandibular acrylic splints are not used as often as they were in the past because of problems with tissue trauma and infection.[65] If local bleeding occurs, one or more of the procedures listed in Table 25-6 can be used to control it.

Conservative periodontal procedures, including polishing with a prophy cup and supragingival calculus removal, often can be performed without replacement therapy, as long as injury to the gingival tissues is avoided. In children, primary teeth should be removed soon after they become loose. Patients with mild factor VIII deficiency and no inhibitors often can be managed in the dental office for less invasive procedures such as scaling, soft tissue surgery, and extractions without factor VIII replacement; desmopressin and EACA or tranexamic acid may be used. Patients with moderate factor VIII deficiency without inhibitors may require factor VIII replacement for less invasive dental procedures. Patients with moderate hemophilia and no inhibitors will require factor VIII replacement for major oral surgery. Patients with severe hemophilia will require factor VIII replacement for all invasive dental treatments.[5,22,65] One or more of the local procedures listed in Table 25-6 can be used as adjuncts to aid in the control of bleeding.

Hemophiliac patients with inhibitors who are low responders usually will require factor VIII replacement for any invasive dental procedure. Human, porcine, or ultrapure factor VIII replacements may be used, depending on the clinical situation. Hemophiliac patients who are high responders will require factor VIIa concentrate for all invasive dental procedures.

Hemophiliac patients who have undergone invasive dental procedures should be seen within 24 to 48 hours by the dentist to check on control of bleeding. If bleeding is occurring, the hematologist may have to give additional factor VIII replacement concentrates, and/or the dentist may need to apply one or more of the local procedures listed in Table 25-6. Patients who have received factor VIII replacements also must be examined within 24 to 48 hours after surgery, for any evidence of an allergic reaction to the concentrates, and to determine whether the wound is healing without complications.

Before surgery, the dentist can make splints, so that mechanical displacement of the clot in wounds healing by secondary intention is prevented. Care should be taken in the construction of the splints so that pressure is not placed on soft tissues; such pressure could lead to tissue injury, bleeding, and infection. For these reasons, mandibular acrylic splints may no longer be used. All extraction sites should be packed with microfibrillar collagen, and the wound should be closed with sutures for primary healing whenever possible. Endodontic procedures should be performed, rather than extractions, whenever possible because the risk for serious bleeding is lessened by this approach.

In many cases, the patient must be hospitalized for surgical procedures. This decision should be made according to the dental procedure planned and in consultation with the patient's hematologist. Patients who have a mild to moderate form of hemophilia without inhibitors can be managed on an outpatient basis with the use of desmopressin, EACA, or tranexamic acid, or with replacement therapy plus EACA. When replacement therapy is used, the dentist and the hematologist must observe the patient for any signs of allergic reaction and must be prepared to take appropriate action. Box 25-10 reviews the roles and functions of the hematologist and the dentist in managing the patient with hemophilia. Postoperative pain control can usually be obtained with the use of acetaminophen with or without codeine (see Box 25-10).

von Willebrand's Disease. Surgical procedures can be performed in patients with mild vWD (type 1 and some type 2 variants) with the use of desmopressin and EACA or tranexamic acid. Patients with more severe types of vWD will require factor VIII concentrates such as Humate-P that retain vWF multimers to replace the missing vWF and factor VIII. A study by Federici[63] reported the results of bleeding complications in 63 consecutive patients with vWD. Of these cases, 31 had type 1 vWD, 22 had type 2 variants of vWD, and 10 had type 3 vWD. All patients had undergone extractions or periodontal surgery. In all cases, tranexamic acid was given before and for 7 days after surgery. Fibrin glue (not available in the United States) was used as local therapy in several patients during surgery. Desmopressin or factor VIII concentrates with vWF were given systemically as indicated. Of these patients, 29 were treated with tranexamic acid and local measures and did not experience excessive bleeding. Desmopressin was given to 24 patients, and 6 received factor VIII with vWF. Excessive bleeding after surgery occurred in only 2 patients. The authors[63] concluded that tranexamic acid, fibrin glue, and desmopressin can prevent bleeding complications in the vast majority of patients with vWD (84%). Box 25-11 reviews the roles and functions of the hematologist and dentist in the management of patients with vWD.

Thrombocytopenia. Patients found to have severe thrombocytopenia may require hospitalization and special preparation for surgery. A hematologist should be involved with the diagnosis, presurgical assessment, preparation, and postsurgical management of these patients.

Infiltration and block injections of local anesthesia can be provided in patients with platelet counts above 30,000/mm³. Also, most routine dental procedures can be performed. If the platelet count is below this level, routine dental treatment involving minor tissue injury should be delayed. For urgent or emergency dental needs, platelet replacement is indicated. If the platelet count is above 50,000/mm³, extractions and dentoalveolar surgery can be performed. For more advanced surgery, the platelet count should be been 80,000/mm³ and 100,000/mm³ or higher. Patients with platelet counts below these levels will need platelet replacement before undergoing the planned procedures.[65,70]

Two types of platelet transfusions are used in the United States. Platelet concentrates are prepared from pooled donor whole blood through centrifugation, or pheresis devices are used to provide continuous centrifugation of blood donated by a single donor, thereby providing apheresis units of concentrated platelets. These products must be used within several days or must be cryopreserved for future use. Platelets from a single donor reduce the risk of infection. Lyophilization of platelets for replacement use is being clinically tested but has not yet been approved for general use.[70]

The need for platelet transfusions can be reduced through the use of local measures (see Table 25-6), along with desmopressin and EACA or tranexamic acid to

BOX 25-11

Dental Management of the Patient With von Willebrand's Disease

PREOPERATIVE
- Hematology consult
- Confirmation of diagnosis—Establish variant and treatment modality
- Type 1—Partial deficiency of vWF; DDAVP usually effective, factor VIII with vWF in a few cases
- Type 2—Qualitative defects in vWF; DDAVP usually effective, factor VIII with vWF in some cases
- Type 3—Severe deficiency of vWF; factor VIII with vWF in all cases
- Test for DDAVP response if use is planned (most type 1 and many type 2 patients)
- Establish dosage for factor VIII replacement and need for EACA
- Location—Most patients can be treated in the dental office; those with type 3 may be hospitalized

Dental
- Treat any acute oral infection
- Good oral hygiene
- Construct palatal splints for multiple extractions in patients with type 3 and type 2 N variants

OPERATIVE
- Hematologist/Dentist
- Treat with DDAVP prior to procedure
- Treat with EACA prior to procedure

- Factor VIII replacement prior to procedure—Humate-P or Koate-HP

Dental
- Use good surgical technique
- Control bleeding with the use of local measures (see Table 25-6)
- Place splint (palatal)

POSTOPERATIVE
- Hematologist/Dentist
- Examine for signs of bleeding within 24-48 hours
- Type 1 and type 2 patients—Additional doses of DDAVP and EACA as indicated
- Type 3 and some type 2 patients—Additional doses of factor VIII and EACA as needed
- Examine for signs of allergy to factor VIII

Dental
- Have patient call if prolonged bleeding occurs after surgery
- Examine for signs of bleeding, infection, or delayed healing within 24-48 hours
- If infection occurs, treat by local and systemic means
- Bleeding can be managed through local means (see Table 25-6); if these fail, additional systemic therapy may be needed
- Avoid aspirin and NSAIDs; acetaminophen with or without codeine may be used

DDAVP, 1-Desamino-8-D-arginine vasopressin (desmopressin acetate); EACA, ε-aminocaproic acid; NSAIDs, nonsteroidal anti-inflammatory drugs; vWF, von Willebrand factor.

control bleeding. Also, topical platelet concentrates can be applied.[65]

Patients who fail to respond to platelet replacement therapy have what is called *platelet transfusion refractoriness*. This may occur on an immune or a nonimmune basis. Platelet transfusion refractoriness presents management problems that are beyond the scope of this presentation. The hematologist who is involved with the patient will make recommendations on how to prepare the patient for surgical procedures.[70]

Treatment Planning Modifications

With proper preparation, most indicated dental treatment can be provided for patients with various bleeding problems. Patients with congenital coagulation defects must be encouraged to improve and maintain good oral health, because most dental treatment for these patients at present is complicated by the need for replacement of the missing factor. Dental treatment often requires hospitalization for patients with severe defects. Patients with bleeding problems related to diseases that may be in the terminal phase should, in general, be offered only conservative dental treatment. Aspirin and other NSAIDs

should not be used for pain relief in those who have known bleeding disorders or who are receiving anticoagulant medication. This includes the various compounds that contain aspirin, such as Anacin, Synalgos-DC, Fiorinal, Bufferin, Alka-Seltzer, Empirin with Codeine, and Excedrin.

Oral Complications and Manifestations

Patients with bleeding disorders may experience spontaneous gingival bleeding. Oral tissues (e.g., soft palate, tongue, buccal mucosa) may show petechiae, ecchymoses, jaundice, pallor, and ulcers. Spontaneous gingival bleeding and petechiae usually are found in patients with thrombocytopenia. Hemarthrosis of the temporomandibular joint (TMJ) is a rare finding in patients with coagulation disorders and is not found in patients with thrombocytopenia. Enlargement of the parotid glands may be associated with chronic liver disease that is most often seen in alcoholics (Figure 25-19). Individuals with leukemia may reveal generalized hyperplasia of the gingiva (Figure 25-20). Patients with neoplastic disease may show osseous lesions on radiographs, as well as oral ulcers or tumors. These patients also may have drifting

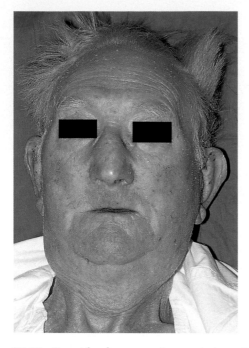

Figure 25-19. Parotid enlargement in association with cirrhosis is most common when alcohol is the cause of the cirrhosis. (From Forbes CD, Jackson WF. Color Atlas and Text of Clinical Medicine, 3rd ed. Edinburgh, Mosby Ltd., 2003.)

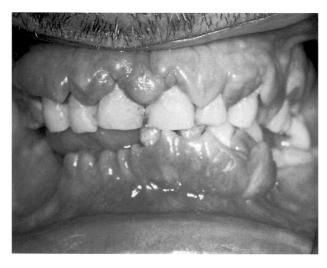

Figure 25-20. Generalized gingival hyperplasia in a patient with leukemia. (Courtesy of Dr. Edward V. Zegarelli. In Ibsen OAC, Phelan JA. Oral Pathology for the Dental Hygienist, 4th ed. St. Louis, Saunders, 2004.)

and loosening of teeth and may complain of paresthesias (e.g., burning of the tongue, numbness of the lip) (see Chapter 26).

REFERENCES

1. Rodgers GM. Thrombosis and antithrombotic therapy. In Lee GR, Foerster J, Lukens J, et al (eds). Wintrobe's Clinical Hematology, 10th ed. Philadelphia, Lippincott Williams & Wilkins, 1999, pp 1781-1821.

2. Kessler CM. Hemorrhagic disorders: Coagulation factor deficiencies. In Goldman L, Ausiello D (eds). Cecil Textbook of Medicine. Philadelphia, WB Saunders, 2004, pp 1069-1078.

3. Rodgers GM, Greenberg CS. Inherited coagulation disorders. In Lee GR, Foerster J, Lukens J, et al (eds). Wintrobe's Clinical Hematology, 10th ed. Philadelphia, Lippincott Williams & Wilkins, 1999, pp 1682-1733.

4. Bennett JS. Inherited and acquired disorders of platelet function. In Young NS, Gerson SL, High KA (eds). Clinical Hematology. St. Louis, Elsevier-Mosby, 2006, pp 767-781.

5. Ragni MV. The hemophilias: Factor VIII and factor IX deficiencies. In Young NS, Gerson SL, High KA (eds). Clinical Hematology. St. Louis, Elsevier-Mosby, 2006, pp 814-830.

6. Thompson AR. Congenital bleeding disorders from other coagulation protein deficiencies. In Young NS, Gerson SL, High KA (eds). Clinical Hematology. St. Louis, Elsevier-Mosby, 2006, pp 855-867.

7. Liebman HA, Weitz IC. Disseminated intravascular coagulation. In Hoffman R, Benz EJJ, Shattil SJ, et al (eds). Hematology Basic Principles and Practices, 4th ed. Philadelphia, Elsevier-Churchill Livingstone, 2005, pp 2169-2183.

8. George JN. Drug-induced thrombocytopenia. In Young NS, Gerson SL, High KA (eds). Clinical Hematology. St. Louis, Elsevier-Mosby, 2006, pp 791-802.

9. Rodgers GM. Endothelium and the regulation of hemostasis. In Lee GR, Foerster J, Lukens J, et al (eds). Wintrobe's Clinical Hematology, 10th ed. Philadelphia, Lippincott Williams & Wilkins, 1999, pp 765-774.

10. Karsan A, Harlan JM. The blood vessel wall. In Hoffman R, Benz EJJ, Shattil SJ, et al (eds). Hematology: Basic Principles and Practices, 4th ed. Philadelphia, Elsevier-Churchill Livingstone, 2005, pp 1915-1931.

11. Plow EF. The molecular basis for platelet function. In Hoffman R, Benz EJJ, Shattil SJ, et al (eds). Hematology: Basic Principles and Practices, 4th ed. Philadelphia, Elsevier-Churchill Livingstone, 2005, pp 1881-1889.

12. Stenberg PE, Hill RJ. Platelets and megakaryocytes. In Lee GR, Foerster J, Lukens J, et al (eds). Wintrobe's Clinical Hematology, 10th ed. Philadelphia, Lippincott Williams & Wilkins, 1999, pp 615-661.

13. Furie B, Furie BC. Molecular basis of blood coagulation. In Hoffman R, Benz EJJ, Shattil SJ, et al (eds). Hematology: Basic Principles and Practices, 4th ed. Philadelphia, Elsevier-Churchill Livingstone, 2005, pp 1931-1955.

14. Greenberg CS, Orthner CL. Blood coagulation and fibrinolysis. In Lee GR, Foerster J, Lukens J, et al (eds). Wintrobe's Clinical Hematology, 10th ed. Philadelphia, Lippincott Williams & Wilkins, 1999, pp 684-765.

15. Handin RI. Disorders of coagulation and thrombosis. In Kasper DL, Braunwald E, Fauci AS, et al (eds). Harrison's Principles of Internal Medicine. New York, NY, McGraw-Hill, 2005, pp 680-687.

16. McVey JH. Coagulation factors. In Young NS, Gerson SL, High KA (eds). Clinical Hematology. St. Louis, Elsevier-Mosby, 2006, pp 103-123.

17. Handin RI. Bleeding and thrombosis. In Kasper DL, Braunwald E, Fauci AS, et al (eds). Harrison's Online

Principles of Medicine, 16th ed. New York, NY, McGraw-Hill, 2005, pp 337-343.

18. Lijnen HR, Collen D. Molecular and cellular basis of fibrinolysis. In Hoffman R, Benz EJJ, Shattil SJ, et al (eds). Hematology: Basic Principles and Practices, 4th ed. Philadelphia, Elsevier-Churchill Livingstone, 2005, pp 1955-1961.

19. Coller BS, Schneiderman PI. Clinical evaluation of hemorrhagic disorders: The bleeding history and differential diagnosis of purpura. In Hoffman R, Benz EJJ, Shattil SJ, et al (eds). Hematology: Basic Principles and Practices, 4th ed. Philadelphia, Elsevier-Churchill Livingstone, 2005, pp 1975-2001.

20. Rodgers GM, Bithell TC. The Diagnostic approach to the bleeding disorders. In Lee GR, Foerster J, Lukens J, et al (eds). Wintrobe's Clinical Hematology, 10th ed. Philadelphia, Lippincott Williams & Wilkins, 1999, pp 1557-1578.

21. Armstrong E, Konkle BA. Von Willebrand disease. In Young NS, Gerson SL, High KA (eds). Clinical Hematology. St. Louis, Elsevier-Mosby, 2006, pp 830-842.

22. Lozier JN, Kessler GM. Clinical aspects and therapy of hemophilia. In Hoffman R, Benz EJJ, Shattil SJ, et al (eds). Hematology: Basic Principles and Practices, 4th ed. Philadelphia, Elsevier-Churchill Livingstone, 2005, pp 2047-2071.

23. Rand JH, Senzel L. Laboratory evaluation of hemostatic disorders. In Hoffman R, Benz EJJ, Shattil SJ, et al (eds). Hematology: Basic Principles and Practices, 4th ed. Philadelphia, Elsevier-Churchill Livingstone, 2005, pp 2001-2011.

24. Watzke HH. Evaluation of the acutely bleeding patient. In Young NS, Gerson SL, High KA (eds). Clinical Hematology. St. Louis, Elsevier-Mosby, 2006, pp 1169-1179.

25. Hezard N, Mctz D, Nazeyrollas P, et al. Use of the PFA-100 apparatus to assess platelet function in patients undergoing PTCA during and after infusion of cE3 Fab in the presence of other antiplatelet agents. Thromb Haemost 2000;83:540-544.

26. Homoncik M, Jilma B, Hergovich N, et al. Monitoring of aspirin (ASA) pharmacodynamics with the platelet function analyzer PFA-100. Thromb Haemost 2000;83: 316-321.

27. von Pape K, Aland E, Bohner J. Platelet function analysis with PFA-100(R) in patients medicated with acetylsalicylic acid strongly depends on concentration of sodium citrate used for anticoagulation of blood sample. Thromb Res 2000;98:295-299.

28. Rees MM, Rodgers GM. Bleeding disorders caused by vascular abnormalities. In Lee GR, Foerster J, Lukens J, et al (eds). Wintrobe's Clinical Hematology, 10th ed. Philadelphia, Lippincott Williams & Wilkins, 1999, pp 1633-1648.

29. Shuman M. Hemorrhagic disorders: Abnormalities of platelet and vascular function. In Goldman L, Ausiello D (eds). Cecil Textbook of Medicine. Philadelphia, WB Saunders, 2004, pp 1060-1069.

30. Ginsburg D, Wagner DD. Structure, biology, and genetics of von Willebrand factor. In Hoffman R, Benz EJJ, Shattil SJ, et al (eds). Hematology: Basic Principles and Practices, 4th ed. Philadelphia, Elsevier-Churchill Livingstone, 2005, pp 2111-2121.

31. White GCI, Sadler JE. Von Willebrand disease: Clinical aspects and therapy. In Hoffman R, Benz EJJ, Shattil SJ, et al (eds). Hematology: Basic Principles and Practices, 4th ed. Philadelphia, Elsevier-Churchill Livingstone, 2005, pp 2121-2136.

32. Shord SS, Lindley CM. Coagulation products and their uses. Am J Health-Syst Pharm 2000;57:1403-1417. Quiz 18-20.

33. Levine SP. Qualitative disorders of platelet function. In Lee GR, Foerster J, Lukens J, et al (eds). Wintrobe's Clinical Hematology, 10th ed. Philadelphia, Lippincott Williams & Wilkins, 1999, pp 1661-1682.

34. Zheng XL, Sadler JE. Thrombotic thrombocytopenic purpura and hemolytic-uremic syndrome. In Young NS, Gerson SL, High KA (eds). Clinical Hematology. St. Louis, Elsevier-Mosby, 2006, pp 802-814.

35. Shord SS, Lindley CM. Coagulation products and their uses. Am J Health-Syst Pharm 2000;57:1403-1418.

36. Feinstein DI. Inhibitors in hemophilia. In Hoffman R, Benz EJJ, Shattil SJ, et al (eds). Hematology: Basic Principles and Practices, 4th ed. Philadelphia, Elsevier-Churchill Livingstone, 2005, pp 2071-2081.

37. Grosset ABM, Rodgers GM. Acquired coagulation disorders. In Lee GR, Foerster J, Lukens J, et al (eds). Wintrobe's Clinical Hematology, 10th ed. Philadelphia, Lippincott Williams & Wilkins, 1999, pp 1733-1781.

38. Roberts HR, Escobar MA. Other clotting factor deficiencies. In Hoffman R, Benz EJJ, Shattil SJ, et al (eds). Hematology: Basic Principles and Practices, 4th ed. Philadelphia, Elsevier-Churchill Livingstone, 2005, pp 2081-2097.

39. Schafer AI. Hemorrhagic disorders: Disseminated intravascular coagulation, liver failure, and vitamin K deficiency. In Goldman L, Ausiello D (eds). Cecil Textbook of Medicine. Philadelphia, WB Saunders, 2004, pp 1078-1082.

40. Toh CH. Disseminated intravascular coagulation. In Young NS, Gerson SL, High KA (eds). Clinical Hematology. St. Louis, Elsevier-Mosby, 2006, pp 1134-1155.

41. Bontempo FA. Hematologic abnormalities in liver disease. In Young NS, Gerson SL, High KA (eds). Clinical Hematology. St. Louis, Elsevier-Mosby, 2006, pp 1073-1079.

42. LoRusso KL, Macik BG. Chronic bruising and bleeding diathesis. In Young NS, Gerson SL, High KA (eds). Clinical Hematology. St. Louis, Elsevier-Mosby, 2006, pp 1079-1089.

43. Crowther MA, Ginsberg JS. Venous thromboembolism. In Hoffman R, Benz EJJ, Shattil SJ, et al (eds). Hematology: Basic Principles and Practices, 4th ed. Philadelphia, Elsevier-Churchill Livingstone, 2005, pp 2225-2241.

44. Crowther MA, Ginsberg JS. Arterial thromboembolism. In Hoffman R, Benz EJJ, Shattil SJ, et al (eds). Hematology: Basic Principles and Practices, 4th ed. Philadelphia, Elsevier-Churchill Livingstone, 2005, pp 2241-2249.

45. Francis CW, Kaplan KL. Venous and arterial thrombosis. In Young NS, Gerson SL, High KA (eds). Clinical Hematology. St. Louis, Elsevier-Mosby, 2006, pp 1089-1106.

46. Bauer KA. Hypercoagulable states. In Hoffman R, Benz EJJ, Shattil SJ, et al (eds). Hematology: Basic Principles

and Practices, 4th ed. Philadelphia, Elsevier-Churchill Livingstone, 2005, pp 2197-2225.

47. Warkentin TE, Crowther MA. Anticoagulant and thrombolytic therapy. In Young NS, Gerson SL, High KA (eds). Clinical Hematology. St. Louis, Elsevier-Mosby, 2006, pp 1114-1134.

48. Elliott G. Concise review: Low-molecular-weight heparin in the treatment of acute pulmonary embolism. In Fauci AS, Braunwald E, Isselbacher KJ, et al (eds). Harrison's Principles of Internal Medicine, 14th ed. New York, NY, McGraw-Hill, 2000, pp 1-4.

49. Gould MK. Concise review: Efficacy and cost-effectiveness of low-molecular-weight heparins in acute deep venous thrombosis. In Fauci AS, Braunwald E, Isselbacher KJ, et al (eds). Harrison's Principles of Internal Medicine, 14th ed. New York, NY, McGraw-Hill, 2000, pp 1-5.

50. Weitz JI. Anticoagulant and fibrinolytic drugs. In Hoffman R, Benz EJJ, Shattil SJ, et al (eds). Hematology: Basic Principles and Practices, 4th ed. Philadelphia, Elsevier-Churchill Livingstone, 2005, pp 2249-2269.

51. Dalen JE, Albers GW, Ezekowitz MD, Hyers TM. Update on the Fifth ACCP Consensus Conference on Antithrombotic Therapy. Paper presented at: ACCP Consensus Conference, 1999, Tucson, Arizona.

52. Schafer AI. Effects of nonsteroidal antiinflammatory drugs on platelet function and systemic hemostasis. J Clin Pharmacol 1995;35:209-219.

53. Blinder D, Manor Y, Martinowitz U, Taicher S. Dental extractions in patients maintained on oral anticoagulant therapy: Comparison of INR value with occurrence of postoperative bleeding. Int J Oral Maxillofac Surg 2001;30:518-521.

54. Blinder D, Martinowitz U, Ardekian L, et al. [Oral surgical procedures during anticoagulant therapy]. Harefuah 1996;130:681-683,727.

55. Akopov S. Withdrawal of warfarin prior to a surgical procedure: Time to follow the guidelines? Cerebrovasc Dis 2005;19:337-342.

56. Devani P, Lavery K, Howell C. Dental extractions in patients on warfarin: Is alteration of anticoagulant regime necessary? Br J Oral Maxillofacial Surg 1998;35:107-111.

57. Hirsh J, Fuster V, Ansell J, Halperin JL. American Heart Association/American College of Cardiology Founda-tion guide to warfarin therapy. J Am Coll Cardiol 2003;41:1633-1652.

58. Wahl M. Dental surgery in anticoagulated patients. Arch Intern Med 1998;158:1610-1616.

59. Wahl MJ. Myths of dental surgery in patients receiving anticoagulant therapy. J Am Dent Assoc 2000;131:77-81.

60. Zanon E, Martinelli F, Bacci C, et al. Safety of dental extraction among consecutive patients on oral anticoagulant treatment managed using a specific dental management protocol. Blood Coagul Fibrinolysis 2003;14:27-30.

61. Ansell J, Hirsh J, Dalen J, et al. Managing oral anticoagulant therapy. Chest 2001;119(1 suppl):22S-38S.

62. Bussey HI. Should I stop my patient's warfarin prior to a dental procedure, 2005; available at http://www.clotcare.com, accessed May 10, 2006.

63. Federici AB, Sacco R, Stabile F, et al. Optimising local therapy during oral surgery in patients with von Willebrand disease: Effective results from a retrospective analysis of 63 cases. Haemophilia 2000;6:71-77.

64. Zanon E, Martinelli F, Bacci C, et al. Proposal of a standard approach to dental extraction in haemophilia patients: A case-control study with good results. Haemophilia 2000;6:533-536.

65. Scully C, Cawson RA. Medical Problems in Dentistry, 5th ed. Edinburgh, Elsevier, 2005.

66. Furie B, Furie BC. Vitamin K: Metabolism and disorders. In Hoffman R, Benz EJJ, Shattil SJ, et al (eds). Hematology: Basic Principles and Practices, 4th ed. Philadelphia, Elsevier-Churchill Livingstone, 2005, pp 2136-2143.

67. Johnson-Leong C, Rada RE. The use of low-molecular-weight heparins in outpatient oral surgery for patients receiving anticoagulation therapy. J Am Dent Assoc 2002;133:1083-1087.

68. Hylek EM, Heiman H, Skates SJ, et al. Acetaminophen and other risk factors for excessive warfarin anticoagulation [see comments]. JAMA 1998;279:657-662.

69. Little JW, Miller CS, Henry RG, McIntosh BA. Antithrombotic agents: Implications in dentistry. Oral Surg Oral Med Oral Path Oral Radiol Endod 2002;93:544-551.

70. Kickler TS. Principles of platelet transfusion therapy. In Hoffman R, Benz EJJ, Shattil SJ, et al (eds). Hematology: Basic Principles and Practices, 4th ed. Philadelphia, Elsevier-Churchill Livingstone, 2005, pp 2433-2441.

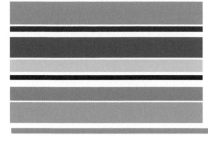

Cancer and Oral Care of the Patient

CHAPTER

26

Improvements in health care and sanitation have contributed to an increasing life span among persons worldwide. Concordant with increased longevity, the incidence of cancer has increased over the past 50 years. Cancer is a major public health problem in the United States and other developed countries. Currently, one in four deaths in the United States is due to cancer. In 2006, the probability of developing cancer from birth to death in the United States in men was 46% and in women 38%.[1]

A total of 1,399,790 new cancer cases and 564,830 deaths from cancer were expected in the United States in 2006. When deaths are aggregated by age, cancer is seen to have surpassed heart disease as the leading cause of death for those younger than age 85 since 1999.[1]

Between 2002 and 2003, the actual number of recorded cancer deaths decreased by 778 in men but increased by 409 in women, resulting in a net decrease of 369—the first decrease in the total number of cancer deaths since national mortality record keeping was instituted in 1930. The death rate from all cancers combined has decreased by 1.5% per year since 1993 among men and by 0.8% per year since 1992 among women. The mortality rate has also continued to decrease for the three most common cancer sites in men (lung and bronchus, colon and rectum, and prostate) and for breast and colon and rectum cancers in women. Lung cancer mortality among women continues to increase slightly. In analyses by race and ethnicity, African American men and women have 40% and 18% higher death rates from all cancers combined than white men and women, respectively. Cancer incidence and death rates are lower in other racial and ethnic groups than in whites and African Americans for all sites combined and for the four major cancer sites. However, these groups generally have higher rates for stomach, liver, and cervical cancers than whites. Furthermore, minority populations are more likely to be diagnosed with advanced-stage disease than are whites. Progress in reducing the burden of suffering and death from cancer can be enhanced by application of existing cancer control knowledge across all segments of the population.[1]

Because patients in whom cancer is diagnosed are experiencing increased survival as a result of improved diagnostics and advances in antineoplastic therapy, an increased likelihood exists that dentists will treat patients at various phases of cancer therapy. For optimal oral health, the dentist should be included as an integral part of the cancer patient's health care team. Knowledge of cancer progression, treatment modalities, the location of available cancer therapy (hospital or outpatient facility), and likely outcomes all affect the dental treatment plan. Maintenance of proper oral hygiene is critical for reducing local and systemic complications associated with chemotherapy, radiation therapy, and marrow and stem cell transplantation. In addition, dentists have the unique opportunity to reduce the risk of cancer by providing advice regarding cancer screening, a healthy diet, counseling regarding smoking cessation, and risks associated with alcohol consumption, and by performing cancer screening procedures.

This chapter focuses on common cancers that may affect patients who require dental care. The text does not attempt to address all cancers but instead provides an overview of cancer, a discussion of common cancers, and oral considerations of these patients. A discussion of lymphoma and leukemia is found in Chapter 24.

DEFINITION

Cancer is a condition that is characterized by uncontrolled growth of aberrant neoplastic cells. Cancerous cells kill by destructive invasion of tissues, that is, by direct extension and spread to distant sites by metastasis through blood, lymph, or serosal surfaces. Malignant cells arise from genetic and acquired mutations, chromosomal translocations, and overexpression or

Estimated new cases*

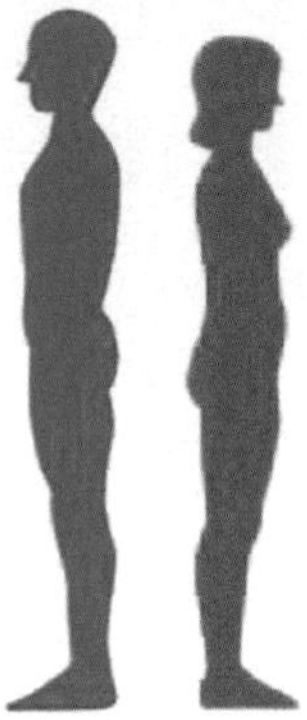

		Males	Females		
Prostate	234,460	33%	Breast	212,920	31%
Lung and bronchus	92,700	13%	Lung and bronchus	81,770	12%
Colon and rectum	72,800	10%	Colon and rectum	75,810	11%
Urinary bladder	44,690	6%	Uterine corpus	41,200	6%
Melanoma of the skin	34,260	5%	Non-Hodgkin lymphoma	28,190	4%
Non-Hodgkin lymphoma	30,680	4%	Melanoma of the skin	27,930	4%
Kidney and renal pelvis	24,650	3%	Thyroid	22,590	3%
Oral cavity and pharynx	20,180	3%	Ovary	20,180	3%
Leukemia	20,000	3%	Urinary bladder	16,730	2%
Pancreas	17,150	2%	Pancreas	16,580	2%
All sites	**720,280**	**100%**	**All sites**	**629,510**	**100%**

Estimated deaths

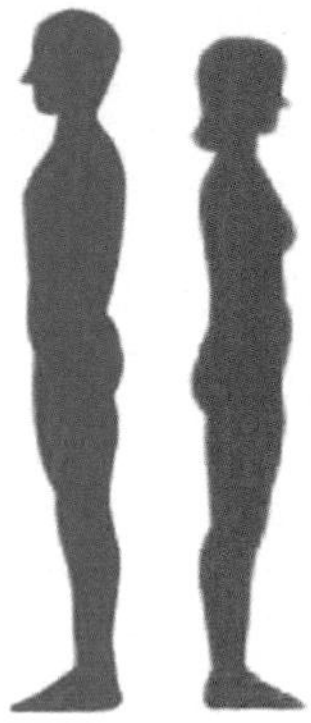

		Males	Females		
Lung and bronchus	90,330	31%	Lung and bronchus	72,130	26%
Colon and rectum	27,870	10%	Breast	40,970	15%
Prostate	27,350	9%	Colon and rectum	27,300	10%
Pancreas	16,090	6%	Pancreas	16,210	6%
Leukemia	12,470	4%	Ovary	15,310	6%
Liver and intrahepatic bile duct	10,840	4%	Leukemia	9,810	4%
Esophagus	10,730	4%	Non-Hodgkin lymphoma	8,840	3%
Non-Hodgkin lymphoma	10,000	3%	Uterine corpus	7,350	3%
Urinary bladder	8,990	3%	Multiple myeloma	5,630	2%
Kidney and renal pelvis	8,130	3%	Brain and other nervous system	5,560	2%
All sites	**291,270**	**100%**	**All sites**	**273,560**	**100%**

Figure 26-1. Ten leading cancer types of estimated new cancer cases and deaths, by gender, United States, 2006. This indicates the most common cancers that were expected to occur in men and women in 2006. Among men, cancers of the prostate, lung and bronchus, and colon and rectum account for more than 56% of all newly diagnosed cancers. Prostate cancer alone accounts for about 33% (234,460) of incident cases in men. On the basis of cases diagnosed between 1995 and 2001, an estimated 91% of new cases of prostate cancer were expected to be diagnosed at local or regional stages, for which relative 5-year survival approaches 100%. (From Jamal A, Siegel R, Ward E, et al. Cancer statistics, 2006. CA Cancer J Clin 2006;56:106-130. © 2006 The American Cancer Society.)

underexpression of factors (oncogenes, growth factor receptors, signal transducers, transcription factors) that cause cells to lose their ability to regulate deoxyribonucleic acid (DNA) synthesis and the cell cycle. Cellular abnormalities of malignancy result in three common features: uncontrolled proliferation, ability to recruit blood vessels (i.e., neovascularization), and ability to spread. Cancer is a major public health problem in the United States and in other developed countries. Currently, one in four deaths in the United States is due to cancer.[1]

Epidemiology: Incidence and Prevalence

Each year, about 1.2 million new cases of cancer are diagnosed in the United States, and about 560,000 persons die of the disease (Table 26-1). In 1998, for the first time, the total number of new cancer cases and cancer death rates in the United States declined. However, when deaths are aggregated by age, cancer has surpassed heart disease as the leading cause of death for those younger than age 85.[1]

Figure 26-1 indicates the most common cancers expected to occur in men and women in 2006. Among men, cancers of the prostate, lung and bronchus, and colon and rectum account for more than 56% of all newly diagnosed cancers. Prostate cancer alone accounts for about 33% (234,460) of cases in men. On the basis of cases diagnosed between 1995 and 2001, an estimated 91% of new cases of prostate cancer are expected to be diagnosed at local or regional stages, for which 5-year relative survival approaches 100%.[1]

Etiology and Prevention

Carcinogenesis is a complex multistep process that involves the accumulation of mutations and the loss of

TABLE **26-1**
Estimated New Cancer Cases and Deaths According to Gender, United States, 2006*

	Estimated New Cases			Estimated Deaths		
	Both Genders	**Male**	**Female**	**Both Genders**	**Male**	**Female**
ALL SITES	1,399,790	720,280	679,510	564,830	291,270	273,560
ORAL CAVITY AND PHARYNX	30,990	20,180	10,180	7,430	5,050	2,380
Tongue	9,040	5,870	3,170	1,780	1,150	630
Mouth	10,230	5,440	4,790	1,870	1,100	770
Pharynx	8,950	6,820	2,130	2,110	1,540	570
Other oral cavity	2,770	2,050	720	1,670	1,260	410
DIGESTIVE SYSTEM	263,060	137,630	125,430	136,180	75,210	60,970
Esophagus	14,550	11,260	3,290	13,770	10,730	3,040
Stomach	22,280	13,400	8,880	11,430	6,690	4,740
Small intestine	6,170	3,160	3,010	1,070	560	510
Colon	106,680	49,220	57,460	55,170	27,870	27,300
Rectum	41,930	23,580	18,350	—	—	—
Anus, anal canal, and anorectum	4,660	1,910	2,750	660	220	440
Liver and intrahepatic bile duct	18,510	12,600	5,910	16,200	10,840	5,360
Gallbladder and other biliary organs	8,570	3,720	4,850	3,260	1,280	1,980
Pancreas	33,730	17,150	16,580	32,300	16,090	16,210
Other digestive organs	5,980	1,630	4,350	2,320	930	1,390
RESPIRATORY SYSTEM	186,370	101,900	84,470	167,050	93,820	73,230
Larynx	9,510	7,700	1,810	3,740	2,950	790
Lung and bronchus	174,470	92,700	81,770	162,460	90,330	72,130
Other respiratory organs	2,390	1,500	890	850	540	310
BONES AND JOINTS	2,760	1,500	1,260	1,260	730	530
SOFT TISSUE (INCLUDING HEART)	9,530	5,720	3,810	3,500	1,830	1,670
SKIN (EXCLUDING BASAL AND SQUAMOUS)	68,780	38,360	30,420	10,710	6,990	3,720
Melanoma, skin	62,190	34,260	27,930	7,910	5,020	2,890
Other nonepithelial, skin	6,590	4,100	2,490	2,800	1,970	830
BREAST	214,640	1,720	212,920	41,430	460	40,970
GENITAL SYSTEM	321,490	244,240	77,250	56,060	28,000	28,060
Uterine cervix	9,710	—	9,710	3,700	—	3,700
Uterine corpus	41,200	—	41,200	7,350	—	7,350
Ovary	20,180	—	20,180	15,310	—	15,310
Vulva	3,740	—	3,740	880	—	880
Vagina and other genit1al, female	2,420	—	2,420	820	—	820
Prostate	234,460	234,460	—	27,350	27,350	—
Testis	8,250	8,250	—	370	370	—
Penis and other genital, male	1,530	1,530	—	280	280	—
URINARY SYSTEM	102,740	70,940	31,800	26,670	17,530	9,140
Urinary bladder	61,420	44,690	16,730	13,060	8,990	4,070
Kidney and renal pelvis	38,890	24,650	14,240	12,840	8,130	4,710
Ureter and other urinary organs	2,430	1,600	830	770	410	360
EYE AND ORBIT	2,360	1,230	1,130	230	110	120
BRAIN AND OTHER NERVOUS SYSTEM	18,820	10,730	8,090	12,820	7,260	5,560
ENDOCRINE SYSTEM	32,260	8,690	23,570	2,290	1,020	1,270
Thyroid	30,180	7,590	22,590	1,500	630	870
Other endocrine	2,080	1,100	980	790	390	400
LYMPHOMA	66,670	34,870	31,800	20,330	10,770	9,560
Hodgkin's lymphoma	7,800	4,190	3,610	1,490	770	720
Non-Hodgkin's lymphoma	58,870	30,680	28,190	18,840	10,000	8,840

TABLE 26-1
Estimated New Cancer Cases and Deaths According to Gender, United States, 2006*

	Estimated New Cases			Estimated Deaths		
	Both Genders	**Male**	**Female**	**Both Genders**	**Male**	**Female**
Multiple myeloma	16,570	9,250	7,320	11,310	5,680	5,630
Leukemia	35,070	20,000	15,070	22,280	12,470	9,810
• Acute lymphocytic leukemia	3,930	2,150	1,780	1,490	900	590
• Chronic lymphocytic leukemia	10,020	6,280	3,740	4,660	2,590	2,070
• Acute myeloid leukemia	11,930	6,350	5,580	9,040	5,090	3,950
• Chronic myeloid leukemia	4,500	2,550	1,950	600	300	300
• Other leukemia	4,690	2,670	2,020	6,490	3,590	2,900
Other and unspecified primary sites	27,680	13,320	14,360	45,280	24,340	20,940

From Jamal A, Siegel R, Ward E, et al. Cancer statistics, 2006. CA Cancer J Clin 2006;56:106-130. © 2006 The American Cancer Society.

*Excludes basal and squamous cell skin cancers and in situ carcinoma, except urinary bladder. Estimates are rounded to the nearest 10.

Note: Percentage may not total 100% owing to rounding.

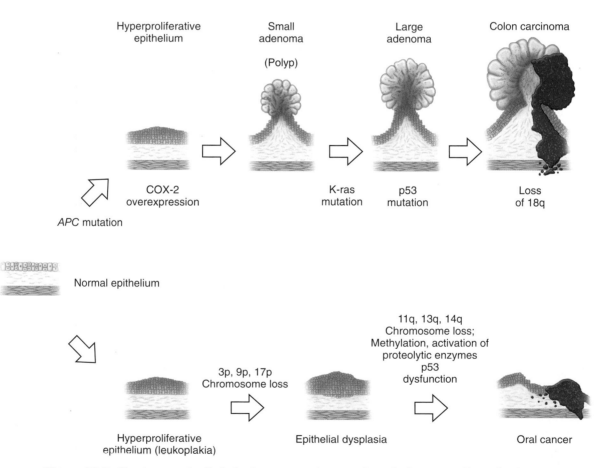

Figure 26-2. Carcinogenesis: Pathologic sequence in gastrointestinal mucosa. Examples in colon and oral mucosa. (Redrawn from Jänne PA, Mayer RJ. Chemoprevention of colorectal cancer. N Engl J Med 2000;342:1960-1968.)

regulatory control over cell division, differentiation, apoptosis, and adhesion (Figure 26-2). This process originates at the level of gene and cell cycle control through a hereditary mutation, an acquired mutation, or inappropriate expression of a transcription factor. At least three to six somatic mutations are needed for a normal cell to be transformed into a malignant cell. Acquired mutations may result from exposure to hazardous chemicals and pathogens that leads to activation of oncogenes, inactivation of tumor suppressor genes (*pRb* and *p53*), and chromosomal abnormalities (translocations, deletions, insertions). Accumulation of these abnormalities results in a cell that becomes functionally independent and aggressive. Natural killer cells provide surveillance for cancerous cells. Reduced numbers or functions of natural killer cells, which occur during immunosuppression, increase the risk for cancer.[2]

Research over several decades has focused on agents that prevent carcinogenesis at the cellular level. National efforts currently focus on the reduction or elimination of factors known to be associated with cancer. Recommendations from the American Cancer Society are to minimize exposure to tobacco smoke and to environmental and occupational carcinogens (e.g., asbestos fibers, arsenic compounds, chromium compounds, pesticides), to decrease intake of fat and exposure to ultraviolet light, to moderate intake of alcohol, to ensure an adequate intake of dietary fiber and antioxidants (vitamins C and E, selenium), and to perform moderate levels of physical activity.[2]

Pathophysiology and Complications

Loss of regulatory control in a cell destined to become a cancer cell results in a series of pathologic changes that include hyperproliferative epithelium, dysplasia, and, finally, carcinoma. Dysplastic tissue is characterized by atypical cell proliferation, nuclear enlargement, failure of maturation, and differentiation short of malignancy. Malignant cells exhibit antigenic, karyotypic, biochemical, and membranous changes that cause loss of contact inhibition, changes in chromosomal morphology, and increased permeability. Malignant tumors lack cell cycle control and replicate rapidly, becoming clinically detectable after about 30 cell doublings when the mass contains about 10^9 cells (1 g). A three-log increase to 10^{12} cells produces a tumor that weighs 1 kg and is often lethal. After reaching clinically detectable size, tumors slow in growth as they reach anatomic boundaries and begin to outgrow their blood supply. Malignant tumors overcome the limitation of anatomic boundaries by losing cell adherence and by metastasizing. Metastasis is a distinct form of cancerous spread that occurs when malignant cells enter blood or lymphatic vessels and travel to distant sites. Metastasis is related to factors produced by tumor cells that allow individual cells to invade tissues and endothelium. It often results in end-organ failure and death.[2]

CLINICAL PRESENTATION

Signs and Symptoms

Cancer often presents as a palpable mass that increases in size over time. Preceding development of the tumor, subtle changes occur that are dependent on the anatomic site involved and the cell type of origin. Initial features may include a change in surface color, a lump, enlarged lymph nodes, or altered organ function. Symptoms include pain and paresthesia. Tumors permitted to increase in size often result in a reddened epithelial surface (caused by increased blood vessels) that ulcerates.[3]

BOX 26-1

International TNM System of Classification and Staging of Oral Carcinomas

- T—Size of tumor
  - T_{IS}, Carcinoma in situ
  - T_1, Tumor <2 cm in size
  - T_2, Tumor >2 cm to <4 cm in size
  - T_3, Tumor >4 cm in size
  - T_4, Massive tumor with deep invasion into bone, muscle, skin, etc.
- N—Regional lymph node involvement
  - N_0, No palpable nodes
  - N_1, Single, homolateral palpable node <3 cm in diameter
  - N_2, Single, homolateral palpable node, 3-6 cm, *or* Multiple, homolateral nodes, none >6 cm
  - N_3, Single or multiple, homolateral nodes, one >6 cm, *or* Bilateral nodes (stage each side of neck), *or* Contralateral nodes
- M—Metastases
  - M_0, No known distant metastasis
  - M_1, Distant metastasis—PUL (pulmonary), OSS (osseous), HEP (liver), BRA (brain)

STAGE CLASSIFICATION
- 0 (carcinoma in situ) T_{IS}, N_0, M_0
- I T_1, N_0, M_0
- II T_2, N_0, M_0
- III T_3, N_0, M_0, or T_1, T_2, or T_3, N_1, M_0
- IVA T_4, N_0, M_0, or T_4, N_1, M_0, or Any T, N_2, M_0
- IVB   Any T, N_3, M_0
- IVC   Any T, any N, M_1

T, Tumor; N, node; M, metastasis.

Staging

Most cancers are assigned a stage (I, II, III, or IV) by the medical team on the basis of the size of the tumor and how far it has spread. Generically speaking, Stage I is localized and is confined to the organ of origin. Stage II is regional in nearby structures. Stage III is extensive beyond the regional site, crossing several tissue planes, and Stage IV is widely disseminated. This system often is supplemented by detailed and specific staging systems developed for particular cancers and generally does not apply to leukemia because leukemia is a disease of the blood cells that does not usually form a solid mass or tumor. The TNM system is frequently employed, whereby *T* stands for tumor size, *N* represents nodal involvement, and *M* indicates metastases (Box 26-1). The prognosis of patients depends in large part on the stage of disease at the time of diagnosis.[3]

Laboratory Findings

The diagnosis of cancer is based on microscopic examination of an adequate sample of tissue taken from the lesion (Box 26-2). Tissue can be obtained by cytologic smear, needle biopsy, or incisional or excisional biopsy. Cells may be subjected to flow cytometry, chromosomal analyses, in situ hybridization, or other molecular procedures for identification of specific cancer markers, ploidy, and DNA analysis. Serum tumor markers such as carcinoembryonic antigen (CEA) for colorectal carcinoma (CA 15-3 or CEA in breast cancer and CA 125 for ovarian cancer) have low sensitivity for the detection of early-stage cancers but are useful in monitoring disease progression and response to therapy.

MEDICAL MANAGEMENT

Treatment strategies for patients with cancer are based on elimination of fast multiplying cancer cells without

killing of the host. Therapeutic modalities include surgery; radiation (external beam or implants); cytotoxic, chemotherapeutic, and endocrine drugs; and possibly, stem cell or bone marrow transplantation. Surgery often is used when anatomy permits for debulking of a tumor, or if the cancer is limited in size. Radiation (often greater than 50 Gray[4]), which kills cells by damaging cancer cell DNA and chromosomes needed for cell replication, is used when tissue cannot be excised, and when cells are most susceptible to this form of therapy. Chemotherapeutic agents are most effective against rapidly growing tumors because they adversely affect DNA synthesis or protein synthesis of cancerous cells. A wide range of cancer chemotherapeutic compounds exist. They are divided into several categories: alkylating agents, antimetabolites, hormones, antibiotics, mitotic inhibitors, and miscellaneous drugs (Table 26-2). Tumoricidal efficacy is gained from use of chemotherapeutic drugs in combination. High-dose multidrug protocols are employed in hospital settings to induce myelosuppression for patients with leukemia, lymphoma (see Chapter 24), and, more recently, breast cancer who are scheduled to undergo bone marrow transplantation. Opportunistic infections are a matter of major concern during the myelosuppressive period. Patients who receive outpatient chemotherapy are administered a lower-dose regimen on a 3- to 4-week schedule and are at lower risk for opportunistic infection.[4]

BOX 26-2

Microscopic Criteria of Malignancy

- **Cytoplasm:** Scant cytoplasm, increased nucleus-to-cytoplasm ratio, tight molding of cytoplasmic membrane around nucleus
- **Nucleus:** Enlargement with variation in size, irregular membrane with sharp angles, hyperchromasia, irregular chromatin distribution with clumping, prominent nucleoli, abundant or abnormal mitotic figures
- **Relationships:** Variation in cell size and shapes, abnormal stratification, decreased cohesiveness

---

TABLE **26-2**
Chemotherapy Drugs of Choice for Common Cancers

Cancer	Drugs of Choice
Breast	*Risk reduction:* Tamoxifen
	Adjuvant: Doxorubicin + cyclophosphamide ± fluorouracil followed by paclitaxel; cyclophosphamide + methotrexate + fluorouracil; tamoxifen for receptor positive and hormone responsive
	Metastatic: Doxorubicin + cyclophosphamide ± fluorouracil; cyclophosphamide + methotrexate + fluorouracil
	Tamoxifen or toremifene for receptor positive and/or hormone responsive
	Paclitaxel + trastuzumab for tumors that overexpress HER2 protein
Cervix	*Locally advanced:* Cisplatin ± fluorouracil
	Metastatic: Cisplatin; ifosfamide with mesna; bleomycin + ifosfamide with mesna + cisplatin
Colorectal	*Adjuvant:* Fluorouracil + leucovorin
	Metastatic: Fluorouracil + leucovorin + irinotecan
Head and neck	Cisplatin + fluorouracil or paclitaxel
Kaposi's sarcoma	Liposomal doxorubicin or daunorubicin; doxorubicin + bleomycin + vincristine
Leukemia and lymphoma	See Table 24-2
Liver	Hepatic intra-arterial floxuridine, cisplatin, doxorubicin or mitomycin
Lung	
Non–small cell	Paclitaxel + cisplatin or carboplatin; cisplatin + vinorelbine; gemcitabine + cisplatin; cisplatin or
Small cell	carboplatin + etoposide (PE)
Melanoma	*Adjuvant:* Interferon alfa
	Metastatic: Dacarbazine
Multiple myeloma	Melphalan or cyclophosphamide + prednisone; vincristine + doxorubicin + dexamethasone (VAD)
Prostate	Gonadotropin-releasing hormone (GnRH) agonists (leuprolide or goserelin) ± antiandrogen (flutamide, bicalutamide, or nilutamide)
Renal	Interleukin-2

Modified from Drugs for Cancer. Med Lett Drugs Ther 2000;42:83-92.

Breast Cancer

Breast cancer is the most common type of cancer in the United States; 98% of cases occur in women. In 2005, approximately 214,000 cases of breast cancer were reported in the United States, and more than 41,000 persons died of the disease during that year. The incidence of breast cancer increases with age. Risk factors include early menarche, late menopause, and nulliparity (women who do not bear children). All breast cancers are the result of somatic genetic abnormalities. The most important risk factor for breast cancer is family history of the disease; 5% to 10% of cases arise in high-risk families. The most common mutations identified in breast cancer cells occur in the *BRCA1* and *BRCA2* genes. These mutations confer a 50% to 85% lifetime risk of breast cancer. Abnormalities also have been identified in genes (*bcl-2*, *c-myc*, *c-myb*, and *p53*) and gene products (Her2/*neu* and cyclin D1) that regulate the cell cycle and DNA replication. Gonadal steroid hormones, growth factors, and various chemokines (interleukin [IL]-6) influence the behavior and dissemination of the disease. Cancer in one breast increases the risk for cancer development in the other.[4-6]

Breast cancer often is detected as a lump in the breast with or without nipple discharge, breast skin changes, and breast pain. Mammography detects the mass in only 75% to 85% of patients (Figure 26-3). In a small percentage of patients, the first sign is an axillary mass. Diagnosis is made from a tissue core biopsy of breast tissue. Most breast cancers are infiltrating ductal carcinomas, whereas a smaller percentage of breast cancers are infiltrating lobular carcinomas, medullary carcinomas, mucinous carcinomas, or tubular carcinomas. Metastasis, primarily to regional lymph nodes and within the chest wall, bone, lung, and liver, occurs after the cancer becomes clinically detectable.[7]

Treatment selected for breast cancer depends on the histologic type and stage of cancer. Cellular markers such as the Her2/*neu* molecule (target of drug Herceptin) and the sodium/iodide symporter (NIS) aid in diagnosis and treatment planning. Lumpectomy (when the tumor is smaller than 5 cm) or lumpectomy plus radiotherapy is preferred to radical mastectomy. Axillary node dissection is performed if the regional sentinel node is positive. Hormone therapy (tamoxifen) or chemotherapy combined with local therapy is recommended when invasive carcinoma exceeds 1 cm in diameter, or when axillary lymph nodes are positive. The combination of fluorouracil, doxorubicin, and cyclophosphamide usually is administered for 4 to 6 months and is given at 3- to 4-week intervals. At present, metastatic breast cancer is incurable. Accordingly, the American Cancer Society recommends a mammogram and a professional clinical examination every year for women 40 years of age and older (Boxes 26-3 and 26-4). Women 20 to 29 years of age should have a professional breast examination at least every 3 years. Women 20 years of age and older should

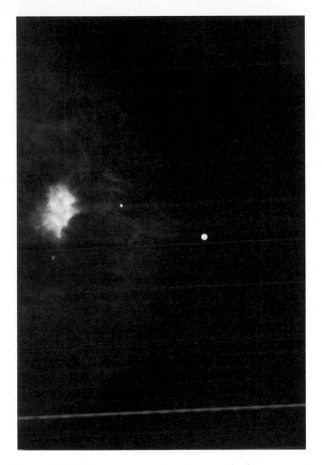

Figure 26-3. Mammogram showing a radiodense area in the breast, suggestive of a malignancy. A specimen should be sent for biopsy. (Courtesy A. R. Moore, Lexington, Ky.)

perform a breast self-examination every month. The American Geriatrics Society recommends mammography every 2 or 3 years for healthy women between the ages of 65 and 85 years.[7]

Cervical Cancer

Cancer of the uterine cervix occurred in nearly 10,000 women in the United States in 2005, and 3700 women died of the disease.[1] Cervical cancer is relatively uncommon in developed countries because of intensive screening programs that are in place. Since the use of screening Papanicolaou (Pap) smears that detect asymptomatic cancerous precursor lesions at early stages became widespread, the incidence of cervical cancer has decreased dramatically from 32 cases per 100,000 women in the 1940s to 8.3 cases per 100,000 women in the 1980s. However, approximately 30% of these patients die of the disease within 5 years, and the death rate for African Americans is more than twice the national average.[8]

Human papillomaviruses (HPVs), which are epitheliotropic sexually transmitted DNA viruses, are the major causative factor in cervical carcinogenesis (Figure 26-4). These viruses dysregulate the cell cycle and tumor suppressor genes (*p53* and *pRb*) via overexpression of viral early genes E6 and E7. Certain HPV strains (HPV16, 18,

BOX 26-3

Screening Recommendations of the American Cancer Society

BREAST
- Self-examination (age ≥20 y)—Every month
- Clinical examination (age 20-40 y; >40 y)—Every 3 years; every year
- Mammography (age 40-49 y; ≥50 y)—Every 1-2 y; every year

COLON
- Sigmoidoscopy (age ≥50 y)—Every 3-5 y
- Fecal occult blood test (age ≥50 y)—Every year
- Digital rectal examination (age ≥40 y)—Every year

CERVICAL
- Papanicolaou test (women, age ≥18 y, and every year* sexually active)—Every year
- Pelvic examination—Every year

PROSTATE
- Prostate examination (men, age ≥50 y)—Every year
- Blood tests for prostate-specific antigen (PSA)— Every year
  Health counseling and cancer checkups[†] (men and women, age >40 y)—Every year

*If 3 or more consecutive satisfactory normal annual examinations, screening may be performed less frequently.
[†]To include examination for cancers of the thyroid, testes, prostate, ovaries, lymph nodes, oral region, and skin.
These recommendations are often applied 5 to 10 years earlier for specific cancers in persons with a family history of cancer, and when specific racial populations (e.g., African American) are at increased risk.

BOX 26-4

American Cancer Society Recommendations for Early Breast Cancer Detection

- Women age 40 years and older should have a screening mammogram every year and should continue to do so for as long as they are in good health.
- Women in their 20s and 30s should have a clinical breast examination (CBE) as part of a periodic (regular) health examination performed by a health care professional preferably every 3 years. After age 40, women should undergo breast examination by a health care professional every year.
- Breast self-examination (BSE): Women at increased risk should talk with their doctors about the benefits and limitations of starting mammograms when they are younger and of undergoing additional tests (e.g., breast ultrasound, magnetic resonance imaging [MRI]) or more frequent examinations.
- All women are at risk for breast cancer, and this risk increases as women get older, especially after age 40. Some women possess certain factors that increase their likelihood of developing breast cancer. Available evidence for women at increased risk is sufficient only in providing general guidance for women and their doctors to allow them to make informed decisions about finding breast cancer early. Women should discuss with their doctor what approach is best for them.

45, 56) are classified as high-risk types because they are associated with most reported cases (see Figure 26-4). HPV types 30, 31, 33, 35, 39, 51, 52, 58, and 66 are classified as intermediate oncogenic risk. In addition to viral infection, chronic cigarette smoking, multiple sexual partners, and immunosuppression increase risks for cervical cancer.[9,10]

Cervical cancer typically involves a long asymptomatic period before the disease becomes clinically evident. This cancer classically presents in women who are between 40 and 60 years of age. The earliest preinvasive changes are diagnosed by Pap smear. Further evaluation is made with the use of colposcopy and colposcopically directed biopsy. If neoplastic cells penetrate the underlying basement membrane of the uterine cervix, widespread dissemination may occur. Metastases often affect renal tissues, resulting in ureteral obstruction and azotemia. Treatment is based on disease stage and involves hysterectomy in the early stages and radiation therapy for disease that extends to or invades local organs. The 5-year survival rate is relatively high (see Table 26-1) but drops to below 50% when the cancer extends to and beyond the pelvic wall.[10]

The American Cancer Society recommends that a Pap smear and a professional pelvic examination be performed in women at the onset of sexual activity or at 18 years of age. Because immunosuppression is associated with cervical cancer, the Centers for Disease Control and Prevention (CDC) advises all women with human immunodeficiency virus (HIV) to undergo semiannual screening, beginning the first year after diagnosis. Health care providers may elect to screen less often when three annual examinations in a row are negative.[11]

Colorectal Cancer

Cancer of the large bowel (colon and rectum) is the most common malignancy of the gastrointestinal tract and overall is the fourth most common cancer of persons living in the United States. This cancer was diagnosed in approximately 141,000 persons in the United States in 2005, and nearly 56,000 people died.[1] Colorectal cancer accounts for about 10% of all cancer in the United States and has a 5-year survival rate of 61%. Over the past 2 decades, mortality has decreased for white women and men but has increased in African American men and women.[12]

The vast majority of colorectal cancers are adenocarcinomas (Figure 26-5). Inherited predisposition and environmental factors contribute to their development. Genetic abnormalities in chromosome 5 (in familial ade-

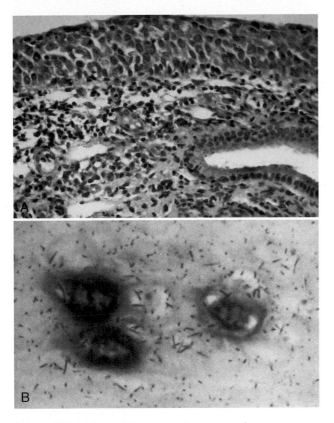

Figure 26-4. A, A biopsy specimen revealing cancerous epithelium of the uterine cervix (hematoxylin and eosin). **B,** Human papillomavirus DNA detected in cervical epithelium by in situ hybridization. (Courtesy M. Cibull, Lexington, Ky.)

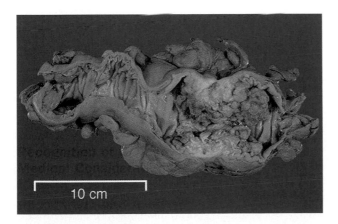

Figure 26-5. Destructive effects of colon cancer. (From Klatt EC. Robbins and Cotran Atlas of Pathology. Philadelphia, Saunders, 2006.)

nomatous polyposis), chromosome 17 (*p53* gene), and chromosome 18 (DCC gene) are contributory. An initiating and probably obligatory event is the oncogenic activation of the adhesion protein, beta-catenin, caused by its overexpression, or loss of its negative regulator, the adenomatous polyposis cancer protein (APC). These abnormalities result in an upregulation in cell cycle signaling. Patients with chronic inflammation (ulcerative

colitis) have approximately 10 to 20 times the risk of colorectal cancer as the general population. This risk increases with a high-fat diet (40% of total calories), low dietary fiber intake, and cigarette smoking for 20 years or longer. By contrast, the use of nonsteroidal anti-inflammatory drugs (NSAIDs) and folate reduces the risk for colorectal cancer. Colonic adenomas (polyps) have malignant potential; however, less than 5% develop into carcinoma. The exception to this rule is seen in Gardner's syndrome, through which virtually all affected patients develop malignant polyposis by age 40 unless treated.[13-15]

Colorectal cancer is not often seen until age 40, and it increases in incidence after age 50. Risk rises sharply by age 60 and doubles every decade until it peaks at age 75 years. Spread occurs by direct extension through the bowel wall and invasion of adjacent organs by lymphatics and the portal vein to the liver. Major signs and symptoms of colorectal cancer include rectal bleeding, abdominal pain, and change in bowel habits (constipation). Presenting symptoms may include those related to invasion of adjacent organs (kidney, liver, vagina).[13-15] Screening for colorectal cancer as recommended by the American Cancer Society is described in Boxes 26-3 and 26-5.

Colonoscopy is the preferred approach for evaluating a patient for colorectal cancer. This technique permits tissue and brush biopsies to be performed. Staging of the patient is aided by endoscopic ultrasonography and computed tomography (CT) scanning. Surgical excision is the treatment of choice for lesions encroaching on the distal 5 cm of the colon; this results in colostomy. Radiation therapy is used for rectal and anal cancer. Chemotherapy (fluorouracil and leucovorin for up to 6 months or, more recently, topoisomerase I inhibitors [camptothecins] and oxaliplatin) is used when metastatic spread occurs. Liver metastases have been treated with hepatic arterial therapy through implantable pumps and injection ports that deliver chemotherapeutic agents.[13-15]

The poor prognosis associated with advanced colorectal cancer (Stage III or IV) emphasizes the need for annual screening of at-risk adults. Digital rectal examination, fecal occult blood test, stool DNA testing, sigmoidoscopy, colonoscopy, and barium enema with air contrast are the screening procedures used for colorectal cancer. The American Cancer Society recommends that screening should start at age 50 for both men and women, and even earlier if a family history is reported, especially involving first-degree relatives with colorectal cancer, present inflammatory bowel disease, a personal history of colorectal cancer or adenomatous polyp, or a family history of hereditary colorectal cancer syndromes (e.g., familial adenomatous polyposis, Peutz-Jeghers, Gardner's syndrome). Digital rectal examination and a test for occult blood should be performed once a year. It is recommended that sigmoidoscopy be performed every 5 years, and colonoscopy every 10 years. A barium enema can be done in place of sigmoidoscopy and colonoscopy.[16]

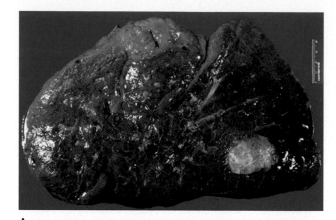

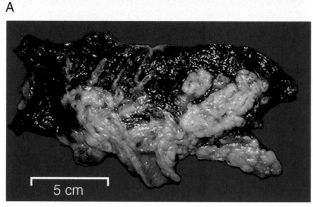

5 cm

B

Figure 26-6. A, A large cell anaplastic carcinoma of the liver. **B,** A small cell anaplastic (oat cell) carcinoma of the liver. (From Klatt EC. Robbins and Cotran Atlas of Pathology. Philadelphia, Saunders, 2006.)

Lung Cancer

Lung cancer is the cause of 14% of cancer cases and is the leading cause of cancer deaths (almost 175,000 deaths annually) in the United States (see Table 26-1).[1] Although it maintains a similar incidence with breast and prostate cancer, the number of deaths caused by lung cancer exceeds that of the two combined. The number of new cases reported in men has been declining since 1984; by contrast, the incidence in women increased in the 1980s and 1990s and only recently declined. Lung cancer is more prevalent in industrialized countries, but increased incidence in nonindustrialized countries has resulted from the introduction of cigarettes into these regions. Overall, more than 85% of cases are related to tobacco smoking, and the effect is dose dependent. In 60% of human lung cancers, the *p53* tumor suppressor gene is mutated. Current evidence suggests that polycyclic aromatic hydrocarbons (e.g., benzopyrene metabolite) of tobacco smoke form adducts within the *p53* gene that contribute to an abnormally functioning *p53*. Deletions in chromosomes 3p and 9p and overexpression of the *ras* and *myc* oncogenes and growth factor receptor c-erbB-2 appear to be important malignant steps. Risk of lung cancer increases in persons who are exposed to certain inorganic minerals (asbestos and crystalline silica), metals (arsenic, chromium, and nickel), and ionizing radiation (e.g., radon).[7]

Histologically, lung cancers are divided into two groups. About 80% are non–small cell lung cancers (large cell undifferentiated, 10%; squamous cell carcinoma [SCC], 30%; and adenocarcinoma, 40%), and 20% are small cell lung cancers (i.e., oat cell carcinomas) (Figure 26-6). Small cell cancers have a rapid growth rate and metastasize early.[17]

Lung cancer is a clinically silent disease until late in its course. Tumors that grow locally can produce a cough or change the nature of a chronic cough. Cancers that invade adjacent structures can produce chest pain and dyspnea or hemoptysis or may cause syndromes (e.g., Horner's syndrome) from disruption of nerves in the chest and neck, or endocrine, cutaneous, or neurologic manifestations.[17] Metastases to the brain, bone, adrenal gland, and liver produce features associated with malfunction of these organs and lymphadenopathy. During advanced disease, patients present with anorexia, weight loss, weakness, and profound fatigue.[17]

Unfortunately, so far, no lung cancer screening test has been shown to prevent people from dying of this disease. The use of chest x-rays and sputum cytology (to microscopically evaluate phlegm for abnormal cells) has been studied for several years. Recently updated studies have not yet yielded any value in the early detection of lung cancer. Lung cancer screening is not recommended, even for high-risk individuals such as smokers.

The diagnosis of lung cancer is made via imaging studies, bronchoscopy, bronchial washings, brush and tissue biopsies, and histologic examination of cells and tissue. Stages I and II non–small cell lung cancers are treated by surgical resection. Radiotherapy is used for more advanced non–small cell lung cancers and for patients with Stage I or II disease who refuse to undergo or are medically unfit for surgery. Chemotherapy comprising two or three agents (e.g., cisplatin, carboplatin, etoposide, vinblastine, vindesine) is employed in combination with radiotherapy for Stage III and IV non–small cell lung cancers and is the mainstay of treatment for small cell lung cancer. Adjuvant radiotherapy is used in patients with limited disease. Stage I lung cancer and Stage II squamous cell lung cancers are associated with 5-year survival rates of more than 50%. The 5-year survival rate for all stages of lung cancer, at present, is just 14%. Despite the poor prognosis, national recommendations have not been made in the United States to deploy diagnostic image screening for the detection of lung cancer, even in high-risk persons.[17]

Prostate Cancer

Prostate cancer is the second most common cancer (approximately 234,000 cases per year) and the most common cancer among men in the United States (see Table 26-1). It is the second leading cause of cancer death among men (nearly 28,000 per year).[1] Prostate cancer develops in approximately 9% of white and 11% of African American men. Family history and race (African Americans) are definitive risk factors for development of this disease.[18]

At present, causes of prostate cancer remain unknown. High dietary fat intake and mutations in chromosome 1 (1q24-25) and X (Xq27-28) appear to increase risk for prostate cancer. Overexpression of the c-*myc* oncogene also is commonly detected in solid tumors such as prostate cancer.[18]

More than 90% of all prostate carcinomas are adenocarcinomas. They typically arise at multiple locations within the gland. Cancer of the prostate produces few signs and symptoms other than problems in urination (hesitancy, decreased force of urination) that, if present, occur late in the course of the disease. Thus, screening procedures are paramount to the successful management of this disease. Methods used to screen for prostate cancer include digital rectal examination (DRE) in combination with blood tests for prostate-specific antigen (PSA) and

---

BOX 26-6

American Cancer Society Recommendations for the Early Detection of Prostate Cancer

Men at higher risk (because they have several first-degree relatives who had prostate cancer at an early age) could begin testing at age 40. Depending on the results of this initial test, further testing might not be needed until age 45.

PERCENT-FREE PROSTATE-SPECIFIC ANTIGEN
Percent-free prostate-specific antigen (PSA) occurs in two major forms in the blood. In one form, it is attached to blood proteins, and in the other, it circulates free (unattached). The percent-free PSA test indicates how much PSA is circulating free compared with total PSA level. The percentage of free PSA is lower in men who have prostate cancer than in men who do not.

PSA results in the borderline range (4-10 ng/mL) combined with a low percent-free PSA (<10%) indicate that the likelihood that a patient has prostate cancer is about 50%, and that a biopsy is indicated. PSA velocity is not a separate test. It indicates how fast PSA rises over time. Even when the total PSA value is not greater than 4 ng/mL, a high PSA velocity suggests that cancer may be present, and a biopsy should be considered.

DIGITAL RECTAL EXAMINATION
The clinician should palpate for any irregular or firm area that might be a cancer. Although digital rectal examination (DRE) is less effective than the PSA blood test in detecting prostate cancer, it can sometimes be used to identify cancers in men with normal PSA levels. For this reason, the American Cancer Society guidelines recommend that when prostate cancer screening is done, both the DRE and the PSA blood test should be performed.

TRANSRECTAL ULTRASOUND
Transrectal ultrasound (TRUS) uses sound waves to make an image of the prostate. TRUS is useful in other situations as well. It can be used to measure the size of the prostate gland; this information can reveal PSA density and may affect treatment options.

---

endorectal ultrasound (Box 26-6; see Box 26-3). Nonbound or free PSA (expressed as percent of total PSA) and PSA velocity (change in PSA level over time) are helpful in the diagnosis of this disorder. The upper level of normal for PSA is 4 ng/mL. Transrectal ultrasound–guided needle biopsy is recommended when the patient has the following[18]:

- PSA value >10 ng/mL
- Positive DRE (palpable nodule or abnormality); even if PSA value is <4 ng/mL, a positive DRE represents about 25% of all prostate cancers
- PSA value between 4 ng/mL and 10 ng/mL, negative DRE, and free PSA value <25%

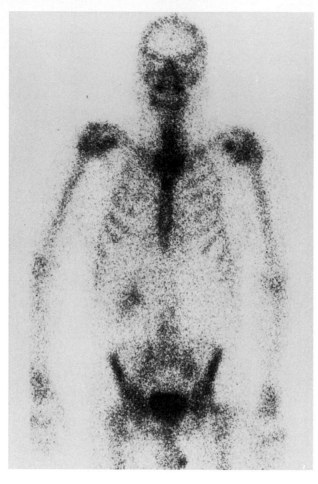

Figure 26-7. Radionuclide scan showing increased uptake of technetium at sites of bony metastasis from prostate cancer. (Courtesy Dale Miles, Lexington, Ky.)

- PSA value <4 ng/mL, negative DRE, and PSA value that has increased from 1 year to the next by 0.75 ng/mL (PSA velocity) or more
- PSA value between 2 ng/mL and 4 ng/mL, negative DRE, and free PSA level <25%

To determine the extent of disease, radionuclide scanning or pelvic magnetic resonance imaging (MRI) is recommended for men in whom prostate cancer has been diagnosed who have a PSA value greater than 10 ng/mL. Metastasis occurs by lymphatic or hematogenous dissemination. Lymphatic spread usually occurs to thoracic and pelvic regions, and hematogenous spread is usually to bone. Bony metastasis is often identified in the pelvis, spine, and femur (Figure 26-7).

Treatment options include radical prostatectomy, external beam radiation, interstitial seed radiation, and cryosurgery. Androgen deprivation therapy is offered in cases of more advanced disease. Prognosis correlates with histologic grade and stage of the tumor; persons who have limited disease (Stage I) have the best prognosis.

Skin Cancer

Of the three primary types of skin cancer, basal cell carcinoma is the most common type, followed by SCC (dis-

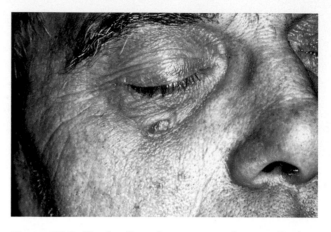

Figure 26-8. Basal cell carcinoma presenting as a "rodent ulcer."

cussed under oral cancer) and melanoma. About 70,000 new cases of basal cell carcinoma occur annually in the United States. These are slow-growing, locally invasive tumors that arise in the basal layer of epithelium, generally as the result of chromosomal changes caused by chronic exposure to ultraviolet (UV) light (particularly UVB radiation). Evidence suggests that mutation and inactivation of the human "patched" gene located in chromosome 9 (9q22.3) is probably a requirement for the development of basal cell carcinoma.

Basal cell carcinomas are more common in older persons with lighter skin and blond and red hair. However, diagnosis during the second and third decades is becoming more common. About 85% of lesions appear on sun-exposed surfaces of the head and neck (including the lip). Four types of basal cell carcinomas are recognized: nodular, superficial, sclerosing (morpheaform), and pigmented forms. Each type presents as a gradual local growth. Classically, the nodular basal cell carcinoma is a pearly papule with telangiectasias, a rolled waxy border, and a central ulceration ("rodent ulcer") (Figure 26-8). A history of intermittent encrustation and bleeding is common. Less common types appear reddish, pigmented, or scarlike. Basal cell carcinomas are readily removed through cryotherapy and surgical excision. Contemporary therapy results in a cure rate of over 95%. Because basal cell carcinomas are locally invasive and destructive, preventive measures that include reduced sun exposure and frequent examination of sun-exposed skin by a health care provider are important in preventing recurrence. Inadequate treatment results in spread to deeper structures, but rarely do these tumors metastasize.[19]

Melanoma is a malignant neoplasm that arises from melanocytes. This cancer occurs primarily in skin but can occur at any site where melanocytes are found, including the oral cavity. The incidence of melanoma is increasing faster than that of any other cancer; approximately 70,000 new cases of melanoma are reported annually in the United States.[1] Ultraviolet light sun exposure is the major causative factor. Because of increased time spent outdoors and thinning of the atmosphere, the rate of melanoma

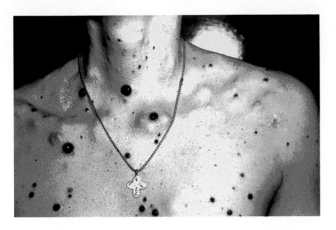

Figure 26-9. Malignant melanoma. The arms, face, and neck are visible surfaces to be examined by the dentist.

has increased from 1 in 1500 persons in 1935 to 1 in 75 persons in 2000. Increased risk also is associated with light skin type, severe sunburns as a child, overall nevus count greater than 50, light and red hair color, and extensive freckling. Men are more commonly affected, as are persons over the age of 50. Cytogenetic studies have implicated chromosomes 1p and 9p as possible locations for genetic alterations that predispose a person to melanoma.[20,21]

Approximately 30% of melanomas arise from previously existing pigmented lesions, particularly those associated with a history of trauma. Clinical features of melanoma are characterized by A, B, C, and D, that is, *A*symmetry, irregular *B*order, *C*olor variegation, and *D*iameter greater than 6 mm. The color is usually deep and may be brown, gray, blue, or jet black (Figure 26-9). Multiple colors provide a prominent sign. Bleeding, ulceration, firmness, and satellite lesions are characteristic of established lesions. Early diagnosis and complete resection are critical to long-term survival; cure rates approach 100% for persons who have a melanoma with a depth of 0.75 mm or less. In contrast, a depth of 1.6 mm or greater confers only a 20% to 30% 10-year survival. Vaccine therapies for melanoma are currently under clinical investigation.[21]

Prevention of skin cancer is attained through the use of sun protection measures (sunscreens and clothing) and periodic screening. The American Cancer Society recommends self-examination once a month with use of a full length mirror and a hand mirror for visualization of the back and other areas of the body that are difficult to see. The skin should be professionally examined every 3 years in persons 20 to 40 years of age; after 40 years of age, it should be examined every year.[21]

Oral Cancer

Oral cancer includes a variety of malignant neoplasms that occur within the mouth (Box 26-7). More than 90% of cases are attributed to SCC. About 9% are carcinomas that arise from salivary gland tissue and other tissue types such as sarcoma and lymphoma. The remaining 1% or so are metastatic from elsewhere in the body, most commonly from lung, breast, prostate, and kidney. In the year 2005, the American Cancer Society reported almost 31,000 cancers of the oral cavity and pharynx and 7500 deaths due to this disease in the United States.[3]

Oropharyngeal cancer accounts for about 3% of all cancers in the United States. The vast majority of oral cancers occur in patients older than 45 years of age; incidence increases with each decade after age 40 for men and women until age 65. Cancer in African American men and women is increasing faster than in whites and other racial groups. Over the past 20 years, little change has occurred in incidence and 5-year survival rates (see Table 26-1). Five-year survival rates for all stages of oral cavity and pharyngeal cancer (53%) remain lower for African Americans (34%) than for whites (56%).[22]

The biochemical factors of oral SCC have not been fully elucidated. At least 80% of cases are associated with multiple cellular abnormalities that result from chronic and excessive exposure to carcinogens found in smoking tobacco, alcohol (including mouthwashes with high alcohol content), smokeless tobacco, and betel leaf that contains areca nut. Ultraviolet light exposure and immunodeficiency (e.g., HIV infection, solid organ transplant recipients) are associated with approximately 10% of cases, particularly those involving the lip. HPV (high-risk types) infection can be detected in about 30% of cases. Plummer-Vinson syndrome and vitamin A deficiency also increase the risk of cancer of the oral cavity and oropharynx. Other factors suggested to play a minor role in the cause of oral cancer include arsenic compounds used in the treatment of syphilis, nutritional deficiencies, heavy

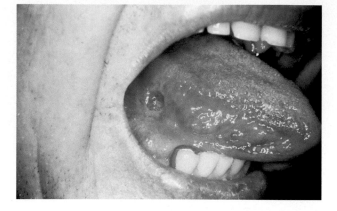

Figure 26-10. A clinical cause for this tongue lesion could not be identified, and its appearance was not highly suggestive of cancer. Nevertheless, it was diagnosed as early squamous cell carcinoma (SCC) through histopathology. In such cases, it would be appropriate for the dentist to request a biopsy of the lesion.

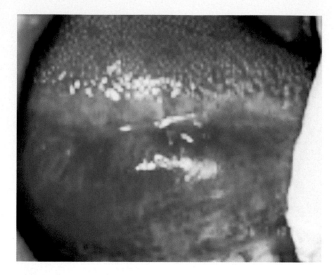

Figure 26-11. Squamous cell carcinoma (SCC) appearing as erythroleukoplakia (a red patch in a diffuse white lesion).

exposure to materials such as wood and metal dusts, and *Candida* infection.[3,22]

Cellular changes and contributory processes that result in SCC are shown in Figure 26-2. At the subcellular level, chronic exposure of mucosal cells to carcinogens results in activation of oncogenes and gene mutations and deletions. The most common deletion in smoking tobacco–related oral SCCs (66% of SCCs of the aerodigestive tract) occurs in chromosome 9 (9p21-22). The most frequently detected mutation occurs in *p53*.[3,22]

Overexpression of epidermal growth factor receptor (EGFR) and activation of the *ras* and c-*myc* oncogenes play contributory roles. Involvement of HPV appears to occur as the result of its early gene (E6 and E7) products, which increase degradation of the p53 protein and protect cells from p53-induced apoptosis/tumor suppression. As a result of these processes, a normal cell is transformed into a dysplastic cell that eventually develops increased DNA content, functional independence, and loss of adherence. Eventually, these cells also promote angiogenesis (i.e., a malignant cell).[3,22]

Oral SCC has a variable appearance. It may occur as a white or red patch, an exophytic mass, an ulceration, a granular raised lesion, or combinations of these (Figures 26-10 and 26-11). White lesions that cannot be scraped off and are clinically nonspecific, called *leukoplakia*, are potential precursors lesions. About 19% of leukoplakias are dysplastic, and about 4% are considered SCC at initial biopsy. Leukoplakias that are not cancerous when they are first biopsied have about a 6% chance of developing into cancer over time. Thus, the overall incidence of SCC in oral leukoplakia is approximately 10% (Table 26-3). Malignant transformation rates for homogeneous and mixed leukoplakias are higher (as high as 17.5%). The histologic diagnosis of epithelial dysplasia carries an even greater likelihood of becoming SCC (as high as 42%, if severe).[3] Leukoplakias with areas of erythema

TABLE 26-3
Color Characteristics of Oral Squamous Cell Carcinomas (SCCs)*

Color	Total SCCs, %
Only white lesions	24.8
White lesions with erythroplakia	60.0
Only erythroplakia (red) lesions	33.3
Other	1.9

Modified from Mashberg A, Samit A. Early diagnosis of asymptomatic oral and oropharyngeal squamous cancers. CA Cancer J Clin 1995;45:328-351.
*From 207 asymptomatic intraoral SCCs.

have a 3 to 5 times greater chance of being cancerous at initial biopsy or developing into cancer than do homogeneous leukoplakias. Nonspecific red lesions involving the oral mucosa (erythroplakia), although less common than white lesions (see Table 26-3), are malignant at initial biopsy in more than 60% of cases.[3,22]

Most early carcinomas are asymptomatic and have an erythroplastic component (see Table 26-3). Advanced lesions are more often ulcerated, with raised margins and induration (Figure 26-12). Pain is often absent until late in the course of the disease. High-risk sites include the floor of the mouth, lateral (posterior) and ventral (anterior) surfaces of the tongue (Figure 26-13), the soft palate, and surrounding tissues. These areas are less keratinized and are more susceptible to carcinogens. The buccal mucosa and gingivae also are common sites, especially in regions where social oral habits result in placement of carcinogens in close proximity to these tissues. Carcinomas of the upper lip and the dorsum of the tongue (e.g., caused by use of arsenic compounds) are rare.[3,22]

Oral SCC spreads by local infiltration into surrounding tissues or by metastasis to regional lymph nodes

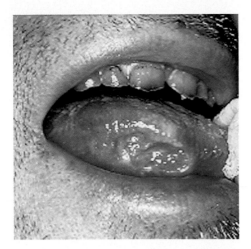

Figure 26-12. Squamous cell carcinoma (SCC) appearing as an ulcerated lesion with induration and raised margins.

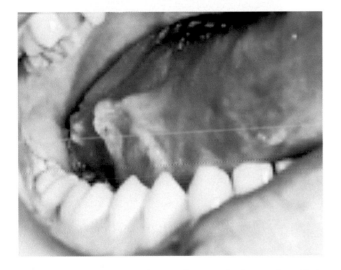

Figure 26-13. A tongue lesion that, on the basis of its clinical appearance (size, margins, induration), may be cancerous. Direct referral to a cancer treatment center for diagnosis and therapy is indicated. This lesion was diagnosed as squamous cell carcinoma (SCC).

through lymphatic channels. Spread to local structures results in induration, fixation, and lymphadenopathy. Routes of lymph node metastasis pass through first-station drainage nodes (buccinator, jugulodigastric, submandibular, and submental), and then second-stage nodes (parotid, jugular, and the upper and lower posterior cervical nodes). Distant metastasis is rare but occurs more commonly to the lung, liver, and bone. Lesions of the floor of the mouth, tongue, and posterior sites tend to metastasize earlier than carcinomas located in anterior oral sites such as the lip. Moreover, about 40% of patients with SCC of the tongue and floor of the mouth lack evidence of metastasis at the time of treatment but develop metastatic disease later. Lesions in the maxillary region have a greater tendency to metastasize than do those in the mandibular region. Oral cancer can lead to death caused by the following[3,22]:

- Local obstruction of the pathway for food and air
- Infiltration into major vessels of the head and neck (resulting in significant blood loss)
- Secondary infection
- Impaired function of other organs caused by distant metastases
- General wasting
- Complications of therapy

In advanced cases of oral carcinoma, the patient may report weight loss and difficulty in breathing, or nerve involvement that may cause local musculature to become atrophic or that may result in unilateral paralysis (e.g., loss of the gag reflex when the soft palate is involved). Other symptoms include hoarseness, dysphagia, intractable ulcers, bleeding, numbness, loosening of teeth, difficulty opening, and a change in the fit of a denture. The diagnosis of oral cancer is made on the basis of microscopic examination of tissues or cells taken from the lesion. Vital staining with toluidine blue can aid in identification of the location from which to obtain a biopsy specimen. The international TNM system of classification and staging is used to evaluate and classify the status of a tumor (see Box 26-1).[3,22]

Most early oral SCCs are amenable to surgery, whereas Stage III or IV cancers (and those involving bone, vascular structures, and multiple lymph nodes) are usually treated by mean of combination therapy (irradiation and surgery). Radiation is provided by interstitial, implantation, or, more commonly, external beam methods, usually within 6 weeks of surgical resection. The tumoricidal dose of external beam radiation ranges from 5000 to 7000 Centigray (cGy), given in separate doses of 150 to 200 cGy over a 6- to 7-week period, with 4 or 5 treatment days followed by 2 or 3 nontreatment days. Hyperfractionation requires slightly lower daily doses and is delivered twice a day. "Prophylactic" neck dissection is performed to minimize the development of metastases after the primary tumor has been treated. Radiosensitizers, topical 5-fluorouracil, laser surgery photodynamic therapy (PDT) with a photosensitizing drug (Photofrin II), and 630-nm light from an argon dye laser also have been used as alternative treatment methods. A combination of radiotherapy and chemotherapy (cisplatin, 5-fluorouracil, or taxanes) is reserved for patients for whom the chance of cure is poor. Selective intra-arterial infusion of a chemotherapeutic agent (cisplatin) has been used successfully in a select group of patients.[23]

The overall 5-year survival rate (53%) of oral SCC has remained virtually unchanged for 30 years. Higher survival rates are associated with early diagnosis, younger age, early cancers (Stages I and II), anterior sites, cancer depth of 5 mm or less, and carcinomas that do not infiltrate bone. Recurrences are frequent, especially if patients fail to stop using tobacco and alcohol products.[3,24]

Bisphosphonate-Associated Osteonecrosis

Recently, a new oral complication of cancer treatment was identified—bisphosphonate-associated osteonecrosis (BON).

Bisphosphonates, synthetic analogs of inorganic pyrophosphate that have a high affinity for calcium, are also potent inhibitors of osteoclastic activity. All bisphosphonate compounds accumulate over extended periods in mineralized bone matrix. Depending on the duration of the treatment and the specific bisphosphonate prescribed, the drug may remain in the body for years.[24-26]

Bisphosphonates are used to treat osteoporosis, Paget's disease of bone, and hypercalcemia of malignancy. In patients with osteoporosis, it is expected that bisphosphonates will arrest bone loss and increase bone density, decreasing the risk of pathologic fracture caused by progressive bone loss. Bisphosphonates are given to patients with cancer to help control bone loss caused by metastatic skeletal lesions. They reduce skeletal events associated with multiple myeloma (such as fractures) and metastatic solid tumor (such as breast, lung, and prostate cancers) in the bone. The physician's decision regarding which type of bisphosphonate to use depends on the type of medical condition that is being treated and the potency of the drug required. For example, orally administered bisphosphonates often are used in patients with osteoporosis, but injectable bisphosphonates are used in patients with cancer who develop primary lesions of bone or skeletal metastasis.[25] BON can occur with the oral administration of bisphosphonates but is rare. In contrast, BON is a much more common complication of injected bisphosphonates. The exact mechanism that leads to the induction of BON remains unknown. However, risk factors have been recognized and may be classified as systemic or local. These involve use of intravenous bisphosphonates (i.e., etidronate [Didronel], pamidronate [Aredia], zoledronic acid [Zometa]), diabetes mellitus, overall cancer stage and tumor burden, overall systemic and immune health, immunosuppressive drug use, any periodontal or other oral infection, and history of radiation to the jaws.[24-26]

Bone remodeling is a physiologic function that occurs in normal bone. During bone remodeling, the drug is taken up by osteoclasts and internalized in the cell cytoplasm, where it inhibits osteoclastic function and induces apoptotic cell death. It also inhibits osteoblast-mediated osteoclastic resorption and has antiangiogenic properties. As a result, bone turnover becomes profoundly suppressed and, over time, the bone shows little physiologic remodeling. The bone becomes brittle and unable to repair physiologic microfractures that occur in the human skeleton as the result of daily activity. In the oral cavity, the maxilla and the mandible are subjected to constant stress from masticatory forces.[24,25]

Physiologic microdamage and microfractures occur daily in the oral cavity. It is theorized that in a patient who is taking a bisphosphonate, resultant microdamage is not repaired, thus setting the stage for oral osteonecrosis to occur. Therefore, BON results from a complex interlay of bone metabolism, local trauma, increased demand for bone repair, infection, and hypovascularity.[25]

In the early stages of oral BON, no radiographic manifestations may be seen. Patients usually are asymptomatic but may develop severe pain because of the fact that

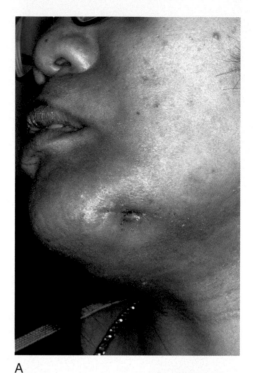

A

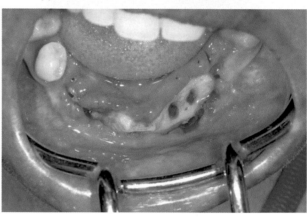

B

Figure 26-14. Bisphosphonate-associated osteonecrosis of the mandible in a patient with metastatic breast cancer.

necrotic bone becomes infected secondarily after it has been exposed to the oral environment. Osteonecrosis often is progressive and may lead to extensive areas of bony exposure and dehiscence. When tissues are acutely infected, patients may report severe pain and lack of sensory sensation (paresthesia). This may be an indication of peripheral nerve compression (Figure 26-14).[25,26]

In patients who develop BON spontaneously, the most common initial complaint is the sudden presence of intraoral discomfort and roughness that may progress to traumatization of the oral soft tissues surrounding the area of necrotic bone. Therefore, the diagnosis of BON is based on the medical and dental history of each patient, as well as on observation of clinical signs and symptoms of this pathologic process.[26]

Treatment strategies that would yield consistent resolution and healing of BON are needed. In fact, many cases have had poor outcomes in spite of therapy, progressing to extensive dehiscence and exposure of bone. Treatment strategies have included local surgical debridement, bone curettage, local irrigation with antibiotics, and hyperbaric oxygen therapy. However, none of these therapeutic modalities has proved successful. Therefore, an inability to manage lesions of BON compromises the oncologic, nutritional, and oral management of affected patients. Prevention of this condition is of paramount importance for these patients, so that they receive the anticancer therapies necessary for the best possible outcome of their neoplastic disease.[25]

The dentist should manage patients who are taking oral bisphosphonates in the following ways:

1. Medical consultation should be obtained to determine medical diagnoses and types of drugs taken.
2. Protocol for prevention of complications from cancer chemotherapy or radiation therapy:
   a. Comprehensive examination
   b. Excellent periodontal health (eradicate infection or inflammation)
   c. Immediate extraction of all nonrestorable or questionable teeth
   d. Elimination of dental caries
   e. Excellent oral hygiene and oral health maintenance
3. Routine dental care can and should be provided, with the use of routine local anesthetics.
4. All procedures should be performed as atraumatically as possible with little tissue trauma, bleeding, and risk for postoperative infection.
5. Should BON occur, only sharp edges of exposed bone should be removed; minimal surgery should be performed. No definitive treatment for BON is available at this time.
6. In case of any infection, aggressive use of systemic antibiotics is indicated.[24-26]

DENTAL MANAGEMENT

Recognition of Cancer and Medical Considerations

The dentist has an important role in the management of the patient with cancer. A primary role is early recognition of the disease. Accordingly, dentists are advised to use a consistent approach in ascertaining pertinent medical, historical, and clinical information related to the patient. The dentist should question the patient carefully for signs and symptoms of cancer, particularly those in the head and neck region. Matters involving cancer can be approached by asking the patient questions such as, "Have you experienced any change in your health since your last visit?" or "Are you aware of a lump or bump developing under your arm or in your neck for no apparent reason, a lesion changing color, pain in any body region, or abnormal bleeding from any site, such as blood in the stool?" Such questions encourage patients to recall events and situations pertinent to the pathogenesis of disease and may permit them to discuss the condition with you. Questions about the social history regarding overall health, exercise, diet, vitamin intake, tobacco and alcohol use, and cancer in family members are also important and allow the dentist to globally assess the risk of cancer in the patient. The dentist also is in a prime position to discuss the benefits of cancer screening of organ systems (e.g., breast, colon, rectum, cervix, mouth, ovary, prostate, skin) and its impact on survival. Some medical centers and programs offer free cancer screening, and patients should be encouraged to take advantage of these services.

After the interview has been completed, clinical examination is mandatory to reveal clues of underlying cancer. A head and neck and intraoral soft tissue examination should be performed on each dental patient as he or she enters the practice. This examination, which may be lifesaving in the patient with an early cancerous lesion, should be repeated on a regular basis as often as possible, but at least during dental recall visits. It is important to remember that the early stages of cancer are often subtle, and cancer is most amenable to treatment when the lesion is small or asymptomatic and has not spread. The dentist also should remember that clinical features vary with the type and location of cancer. Lesions clinically suspicious for cancer and those that fail to heal within 14 days despite measures to alleviate them should be biopsied by a skilled clinician. In addition, patients with hard, fixed, and/or matted lymph nodes should be referred directly to a head and neck surgeon or a cancer treatment center. Each patient should be advised of the concern in a frank and open manner. In patients with other signs and symptoms suggestive of cancer, laboratory tests and imaging studies should be performed. Screening laboratory tests can be obtained by sending the patient to a hospital, a commercial clinical laboratory, or a physician's office. Blood tests should include a total red blood cell (RBC) and white blood cell (WBC) count, a differential white cell count, a smear for cell morphologic study, hemoglobin, hematocrit count, and platelet count. If screening tests are ordered by the dentist, and one or more test results are abnormal, the patient should be referred for medical evaluation and treatment.

Treatment Planning Modifications

Dental treatment planning for the patient with cancer begins with establishment of the diagnosis. Planning involves the following:

- Pretreatment evaluation and preparation of the patient
- Oral health care during cancer therapy, which includes hospital and outpatient care
- Posttreatment management of the patient, including long-term considerations

Cancers that are amenable to surgery and that do not affect the oral cavity require few treatment plan modifications. However, some cancers affect oral health directly because of surgery or indirectly through chemotherapy or immunosuppression. The remainder of this chapter focuses on those treatments and complications that may affect the oral cavity.

Pretreatment Evaluation and Considerations. The dentist should be aware of the type of treatment selected for the patient and whether the cancer stands a good chance of being controlled. A patient who is to receive palliative therapy may not want replacement of missing teeth; however, this patient must be free of active dental disease that could worsen during cancer therapy. By contrast, a patient who has cancer in Stage I or II and no evidence of regional spread can be managed for future dental care as a normal patient, except that the dentist should consider recalling this patient for more frequent examinations for evidence of metastases, recurrence of the lesion, or presence of a new cancer. This is particularly important for patients with oral cancer who are at increased risk for a second primary cancer in the respiratory system, upper digestive tract, or oral cavity. The risk for a second oral cancer in smokers whose habits remain unchanged is about 30%, as compared with 13% for those who quit.[3,24]

A pretreatment oral evaluation is recommended for all patients with cancer before cancer therapy is initiated to attain the following:

- Rule out oral disease that may worsen during cancer therapy.
- Provide a baseline for comparison and monitoring of sequelae of radiation and chemotherapy damage.
- Detect metastatic lesions.
- Minimize oral discomfort during cancer therapy.

This evaluation should include a thorough clinical and radiographic examination and review of blood laboratory findings. Edentulous regions should be surveyed so that impacted teeth, retained root tips, and latent osseous disease that may worsen during immunosuppressive cancer therapy can be ruled out. A panoramic film is acceptable; however, supplemental bitewing and periapical films may be required for adequate visualization of dental and osseous structures.[3,24]

Pretreatment care should include oral hygiene instructions, encouragement of a noncariogenic diet, calculus removal, prophylaxis and fluoride treatment, and elimination of all sources of irritation and infection. In children undergoing chemotherapy, mobile primary teeth and those expected to be lost during chemotherapy should be extracted, and gingival opercula should be evaluated for surgical removal to prevent entrapment of food debris. Orthodontic bands should be removed before chemotherapy is begun.

If head and neck radiation and immunosuppressive chemotherapy are scheduled, the following recommendations should be considered[3,24]:

- Reduction in radiation exposure to noncancerous tissues (salivary glands) with lead-lined stents, beam-sparing procedures, or the use of anticholinergic (biperiden) or parasympathomimetic (pilocarpine HCl [Salagen]) drugs during and after radiotherapy should be discussed with the radiation oncologist and the patient.
- Nonrestorable teeth with poor or hopeless prognosis, acute infection, or severe periodontal disease that

may predispose the patient to complications (e.g., sepsis, osteoradionecrosis) should be extracted; sharp, bony edges trimmed and smoothed; and primary closure obtained (Box 26-8). Chronic inflammatory lesions in the jaws and potential sources of infection should be examined and treated or eradicated before radiation or chemotherapy.

Adequate time for wound healing should be provided for extractions and surgical procedures before radiation therapy or myelosuppressive chemotherapy is induced (see Box 26-8).

Symptomatic nonvital teeth should be endodontically treated at least 1 week before initiation of head and neck radiation or chemotherapy. However, dental treatment of asymptomatic teeth even with periapical involvement may be delayed.

One should prioritize treatment of infections and extractions, periodontal care, and treatment of irritations before providing treatment of carious teeth, root canal therapy, and replacement of faulty restorations. Temporary restorations may be placed and some types of treatment (e.g., cosmetic, prosthodontic, endodontic) can be delayed when time is limited.

To optimize oral health and reduce the risk of oral complications such as mucositis and infection, tooth scaling and prophylaxis should be provided before cancer therapy is initiated. Removable prosthodontic appliances should be removed during therapy.

Patients who will be retaining their teeth and undergoing head and neck radiation therapy must be informed about problems associated with decreased salivary function, which include xerostomia, the increased risk of oral infection, including radiation caries, and the risk for osteoradionecrosis (Box 26-9).

Dental preparation of the patient with cancer who is about to undergo surgical treatment is not as critical as for the patient about to undergo head and neck radiation and chemotherapy. However, active oral infection should be treated, teeth that are broken down should be removed, and teeth that may be used for retention of a prosthetic appliance can be restored as needed. The better the dental health of the patient, the lower is the risk that dental infection may complicate the healing process. For the patient with oral cancer, the dentist should consider consultation with the maxillofacial prosthodontist, so that proper coordination of the patient's dental and tooth replacement needs can be ensured during the presurgical and postsurgical phases of treatment.

Oral Care During Cancer Therapy. The oral health of the patient with cancer must be maintained during cancer therapy because oral complications develop in a significant number of patients (more than 400,000) who receive cancer radiation and chemotherapy. Oral infections and potential problems should be eliminated before cancer therapy is provided to patients who are undergoing head and neck radiation and inpatient chemotherapy; routine dental care should be delayed until after cancer

---

BOX 26-8

Guidelines for Tooth Extraction in Patients Scheduled to Receive Radiation Treatment to the Head and Neck (Including the Mouth) or Chemotherapy

INDICATORS OF EXTRACTION
- Pocket depths are 6 mm or greater, mobility is excessive, purulence is seen on probing
- Periapical inflammation is noted
- Tooth is broken down, nonrestorable, nonfunctional, or partially erupted; patient is noncompliant with oral hygiene measures
- Patient has no interest in saving tooth/teeth
- Tooth is associated with an inflammatory (e.g., pericoronitis), infectious, or malignant osseous disease

EXTRACTION GUIDELINES
- Perform extraction with minimal trauma
  - At least 2 weeks before initiation of radiation therapy*

- Ideally 3 weeks before initiation of radiation therapy
- At least 5 days (in maxilla) before initiation of chemotherapy
- At least 7 days (in mandible) before initiation of chemotherapy
- Trim bone at wound margins to eliminate sharp edges
- Obtain primary closure
- Avoid intra-alveolar hemostatic packing agents that can serve as a nidus of microbial growth
- Transfuse if the platelet count is less than $50,000/mm^3$
- Delay if the white blood count is less than $2000/mm^3$ or the absolute neutrophil is less than $1000/mm^3$ or is expected to be this level within 10 days; alternatively, prophylactic antibiotics (cephalosporin) may be used with extractions that are mandatory

Modified in part from Rankin KV, Jones DL. Oral Health in Cancer Therapy. Austin, Tex, Texas Cancer Council, 1999.
*In *select* circumstances when healing will not be compromised, a minimum of 10 days can be used. Biological modifiers that promote healing (e.g., vitamin C) may be useful in these circumstances. Alternatively, if these time recommendations cannot be met before initiation of chemotherapy, a root canal may be performed to reduce the number of viable microbes; then, the extraction can be performed after the white blood cell count returns to an acceptable level.

BOX 26-9

Complications of Head and Neck Radiotherapy and Myelosuppressive Chemotherapy

- Nausea and vomiting (acute onset)
- Mucositis—Starts about second week
- Ulceration (C)
- Taste alteration—Starts about second week
- Xerostomia (R)—Starts about second week
- Secondary infection (fungal, bacterial, viral)
- Bleeding (C)
- Radiation caries (R) (delayed onset)
- Hypersensitive teeth (acute and delayed onset)
- Muscular dysfunction (R) (delayed onset)
- Osteoradionecrosis (R) (delayed onset [more common in mandible, less common in maxilla])
- Pulpal pain and necrosis (delayed onset [R]—Orthovoltage, not found with cobalt-60)

(C), Limited to, or more prominent with, chemotherapy; (R), limited to, or more prominent with, radiotherapy.

therapy has been completed. Patients given outpatient chemotherapy require provision of dental treatment at appropriate times between cycles. This section discusses oral complications that occur during and after chemotherapy and irradiation of head and neck structures that may require modifications in oral health care management.[27]

Management of Complications of Radiation and Chemotherapy. General management considerations for radiation and chemotherapy are presented in Box 26-10. Acute toxicity reactions are seen during and immediately after radiation and chemotherapy. Acute toxicities are directly proportionate to the amount of radiation or cytotoxic drug to which tissues are exposed and are more evident in rapidly dividing cells. Delayed toxicities may occur several months to years after radiation therapy is provided.

Radiation therapy induces cell necrosis, microvascular damage, and parenchymal and stromal damage. Production of oxygen-free radicals from ionizing radiation is one of the leading causes of cell damage. Cells that have rapid turnover are more susceptible to damage. For this reason, hypoxic cells and slowly replicative cells are more resistant to radiation than are those that are well oxygenated and mitotically active. Box 26-11 lists the effects of radiotherapy on various oral tissues.

Most chemotherapeutic agents cause alopecia, breakdown of the mucous membranes (mucositis), depression of the bone marrow (infection, bleeding, anemia), gastrointestinal changes (diarrhea, malabsorption), and altered nutritional status; they may also induce cardiac and pulmonary dysfunction. Bone marrow suppression and mucositis associated with chemotherapy are predictable, dose dependent, and usually manageable. Patients receiving chemotherapy may manifest erythema and ulceration of the oral mucosa, infection of the surrounding tissues, excessive bleeding with minor trauma, xerostomia, anemia, and neurotoxicity.

Mucositis. Mucositis, inflammation of the oral mucosa, results from the direct cytotoxic effects of radiation or antineoplastic agents on rapidly dividing oral epithelium and the upregulation of proinflammatory cytokine expression (see Appendix C). Mucositis occurs in up to 40% of patients who are undergoing chemotherapy and

BOX 26-10

Management of the Patient With Oral Complications of Radiotherapy and Chemotherapy

MUCOSITIS
- Eliminate infection and irritation; establish good oral hygiene.
- Use mouth rinse (three choices are similar in controlling mucositis[108]).
- Recommend a salt and sodium bicarbonate mouthwash (1 tsp of each in 1 pint of water).
- Provide elixir of diphenhydramine (Benadryl) or viscous lidocaine 0.5% in Milk of Magnesia, Kaopectate, or sucralfate.
- Use chlorhexidine 0.12% (can be formulated in water by a pharmacist).
- Prescribe antiinflammatory agents (e.g., topical steroids, kamillosan liquidim).
- Use protectants (e.g., Orabase).
- Avoid tobacco, alcohol, and carbonated drinks.
- Follow a soft diet; maintain hydration.
- Use a humidifier or vaporizer.
- Consider topical and systemic antimicrobials, if severe.
- Use biologic response modifiers (under investigation).

XEROSTOMIA
- Recommend sugarless lemon drops, sorbitol-based chewing gum, buffered solution of glycerine and water, or salivary substitutes.

RADIATION CARIES
- Educate patients about associated risks, and motivate them to maintain optimal oral hygiene.
- For daily application of fluoride, use custom trays that are constructed of soft, flexible mouthguard material.

Trays hold 5 to 10 drops of a 1% to 2% acidulated fluoride gel that should be applied for 5 minutes each day. If the 1% to 2% acidulated gel is found to be irritating to the tissues, 0.5% neutral sodium fluoride gel may be substituted. *Alternative:* A single brush-on application of 5000 ppm fluoride (PrevDent) may be more effective for some patients.
- Ensure frequent dental recall.
- Confirm patient compliance through monthly recalls during the first year.
- Restore early carious lesions.

SECONDARY INFECTION
- Use culture, cytologic study, antibiotics, antifungal agents, and antiviral agents.

SENSITIVITY OF TEETH
- Give topical fluorides.

LOSS OF TASTE
- Provide zinc supplementation.

OSTEORADIONECROSIS
- Caution with surgery.
- May need hyperbaric oxygen therapy.

MUSCULAR DYSFUNCTION
- Insert tongue blade to ensure maximal opening of jaws and access to the oral cavity.

See Appendix B for medications, dosage, and duration of use.

BOX 26-11

Radiation Effects on Normal Tissues in the Path of the External Beam

MUCOSA AND LAMINA PROPRIA
- Epithelial changes (atrophy), mucositis, vascular changes, intimal thickening, luminal stenosis, obliteration, decreased blood flow

MUSCLE
- Fibrosis, vascular changes

BONE
- Decreased numbers of osteocytes and osteoblasts, decreased blood flow

SALIVARY GLANDS
- Atrophy of acini, vascular changes, fibrosis

PULP
- Necrosis (orthovoltage)

is often a dose-limiting factor for chemotherapy and a cause of dose interruption in radiation therapy. It develops more often in nonkeratinized mucosa (buccal and labial mucosa, ventral tongue) and adjacent to metallic restorations by the end of the second week of radiation therapy (if the dose is 200 cGy per week; Figure 26-15). Mucositis develops most often between the seventh and fourteenth days after chemotherapy is provided (especially VP16, epotoside, methotrexate) when effects of the drugs produce an extremely low WBC count (nadir). It generally subsides 1 to 2 weeks after completion of treatment. Young patients with cancer who have higher division rates have a greater prevalence of chemotherapy-induced mucositis than do older patients with cancer.[28]

Mucositis produces red, raw, and tender oral mucosa with epithelial sloughing similar to that seen in a severe oral burn. Oral ulcerations may result from breakdown of the epithelial barrier and from infection by viral, bacterial or fungal organisms. Patients typically report ulceration, pain, dysphagia, loss of taste, and difficulty in

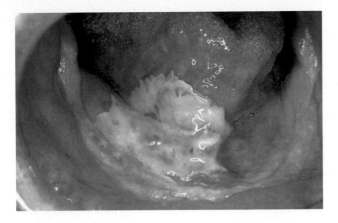

Figure 26-15. Squamous cell carcinoma after initiation of radiation therapy. Note the large, irregular area of epithelial necrosis and ulceration of the anterior floor of the mouth on the patient's right side. (From Neville BW, Damm DD, Allen CW, et al: Oral and Maxillofacial Pathology, ed 2, St. Louis, 2002, Saunders.)

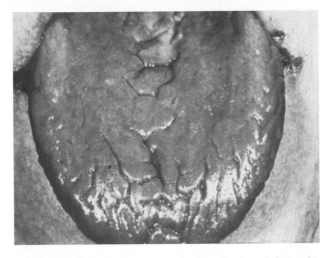

Figure 26-16. Severe xerostomia that developed from the effects of radiation on the oral mucosa. Note the angular cheilitis.

eating, which increases the risks for oral and systemic infection. If the major salivary glands have been irradiated, xerostomia (Figure 26-16) may occur after the onset of mucositis. Complications of mucositis and xerostomia make the patient extremely uncomfortable and increase the difficulty associated with maintaining proper nutritional intake.[27,28]

During this acute phase, the goals are to maintain mucosal integrity and to promote oral hygiene. Patients are generally treated in the following ways:
- A bland mouth rinse (salt and soda water) to keep ulcerated areas as clean as possible
- Topical anesthetics (viscous lidocaine 0.5%) and/or an antihistamine solution (benzydamine HCl [Tantum rinse], diphenhydramine [Benadryl], promethazine [Phenergan]) that can provide pain control or that may be combined with milk of magnesia (Maalox), Kaopectate, or sucralfate to serve as a coating agent (for protection of ulcerated areas)
- Antimicrobial rinses such as chlorhexidine
- Anti-inflammatory agents (kamillosan liquidim or topical steroids [dexamethasone])
- Adequate hydration
- A diet consisting of soft foods, protein, and vitamin supplementation at therapeutic levels
- Oral lubricants and lip balms containing a water base, a beeswax base, or a vegetable oil base (e.g., Surgi-Lube)
- Humidified air (humidifiers or vaporizers)
- Avoidance of alcohol, tobacco, and irritating foods (e.g., citrus fruits and juices, hot, spicy dishes; see Box 26-10 and Appendix C)

Dentures should not be worn until the acute phase of mucositis has resolved. Dentures should be cleaned and soaked with an antimicrobial solution daily for the prevention of infection.[29]

Secondary infections. During radiation and chemotherapy, patients are prone to secondary infection. Because of the quantitative decrease that occurs in actual salivary flow, and because of compositional alterations in saliva, several organisms (bacterial, fungal, and viral) may opportunistically infect the oral cavity. Moreover, if the patient is immunosuppressed as the result of chemotherapy, and if the WBC count falls to below 2000 cells/mm^3, the immune system is less able to manage these infections. Opportunistic infections are also common in patients who receive chemotherapy and broad-spectrum antibiotics.

The organism that most frequently opportunistically infects the oral cavity in individuals undergoing cancer therapy (who have hyposalivation and immunosuppression) is *Candida albicans*. Cytologic study, potassium hydroxide (KOH) staining, microscopic examination, and *Candida*-specific cultures are often performed to establish a definitive diagnosis. Candidal infections may produce pain, burning, taste alterations, and intolerance to certain foods, especially acidic citrus fruits or spicy foods. They present clinically in four different forms, ranging from denuded epithelium to hyperplastic lesions. During cancer therapy, the most common type is pseudomembranous candidiasis, which produces white plaques that are easily scraped off, leaving behind tiny petechial hemorrhages (Figure 26-17). Slightly less prevalent is the erythematous, atrophic form, which manifests as a red patch accompanied by a burning sensation (see Appendix C). Other forms of candidiasis (i.e., angular cheilosis and the less common hypertrophic form, which presents as a thick, white plaque that cannot be scraped off) are more commonly detected in patients with chronic hyposalivation.

Candidiasis is best managed with the use of topical oral antifungal agents. These include nystatin (oral

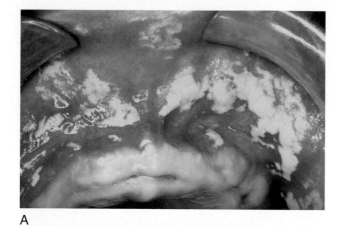

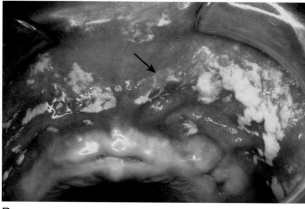

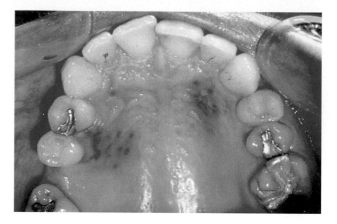

Figure 26-18. Recurrent herpes simplex virus infection presenting as a large ulcer on the palate of a patient undergoing chemotherapy.

Figure 26-17. Pseudomembranous candidiasis. **A,** Classic "curdled milk" appearance of the oral lesions of pseudomembranous candidiasis. This patient had no apparent risk factors for candidiasis development. **B,** Removal of one of the pseudomembranous plaques *(arrow)* reveals a mildly erythematous mucosal surface. (From Allen CM, Blozis GG: Oral mucosal lesions. In Cummings CW, Fredrickson JM, Harker LA, et al (eds): Otolaryngology: head and neck surgery, ed 3, St. Louis, 1998, Mosby.)

suspension 100,000 international units [IU]/mL 4 to 5 times daily), clotrimazole (Mycelex lozenges 10 mg 5 times day), and other preparations (e.g., vaginal topical antifungal agents). Prophylactic use of antifungal agents may be required in patients undergoing chemotherapy who have frequent recurrent infections. Ketoconazole (Nizoral), fluconazole (Diflucan), or itraconazole (Sporanox) may be used if systemic therapy is warranted, or if patients develop unusual oral fungal infections (Torulopsis, aspergillosis, mucormycosis) or fungal septicemia (possibly from the oral cavity). Alternatively, the physician may place the patient on granulocyte (monocyte) colony-stimulating factor (G[M]-CSF) that elevates the neutrophil count to normal levels and can contribute to resolution of the lesions.[29]

Bacteria or viruses may be the cause of other secondary infections. Oral bacterial infections may appear with typical signs of swelling, erythema, and fever. Alternatively, these features may be masked in patients with low

WBC counts due to chemotherapy. In immunosuppressed patients, a shift occurs in the oral flora to Gram-negative organisms that normally inhabit the gastrointestinal or respiratory tract, such as *Pseudomonas, Klebsiella, Proteus, Escherichia coli,* or *Enterobacter.* The most common presentation is an oral ulceration. Thus, dentists should culture all nonhealing oral ulcerations in such patients, and these specimens should be sent for diagnosis and antibiotic sensitivity testing. If a bacterial infection is suspected, appropriate antibacterial therapy should be initiated. Antimicrobial sensitivity data are important for the selection of an effective antibiotic when the clinical course shows little or no improvement over several days.

Recurrent herpes simplex virus (HSV) eruptions occur often during chemotherapy if antiviral agents are not prophylactically prescribed. They are infrequent during radiation therapy. Herpes recurrences in patients with cancer who are undergoing chemotherapy tend to be larger and to take longer to heal than herpetic lesions found in nonimmunocompromised patients (Figure 26-18). Antiviral agents (e.g., acyclovir, famciclovir, valacyclovir) are recommended prophylactically for HSV antibody–positive patients who are undergoing chemotherapy, to prevent recurrence. A daily dose of at least 1 g acyclovir/equivalent is needed to suppress HSV recurrences. Because these ulcers mimic the appearance of aphthous and may occur on nonkeratinized mucosa in immunocompromised patients with cancer, culture or use of an enzyme-linked immunoassay is important for accurate diagnosis. Laboratory tests also help to distinguish the infection from other oral herpes virus infections such as varicella zoster and cytomegalovirus that can occur in these patients. Antiviral sensitivity testing should be considered for patients with unresolving or extensive infection and for those in poor general health.[30]

Bleeding. Patients with cancer who undergo total body irradiation or high-dose chemotherapy, or who have bone marrow involvement due to disease, are also susceptible to thrombocytopenia. Gingival bleeding and submucosal hemorrhage as a result of minor trauma (e.g., tongue biting, toothbrushing) can occur when the platelet count drops to below 50,000 cells/mm³. Palatal petechiae, purpura on the lateral margin of the tongue, and gingival bleeding/oozing are common features. Gingival hemorrhage is aggravated by poor oral hygiene. When gingival tissues bleed easily and the platelet count is severely reduced, the patient should avoid vigorous brushing of the teeth and should begin using softer devices such as toothettes or gauze wrapped around a finger and dampened in warm water or an antimicrobial solution (chlorhexidine in water, prepared by the pharmacist). During this stage, patients should be instructed not to use toothpicks, water-irrigating appliances, or dental floss. To control gingival bleeding, local measures, such as pressure applied with a gelatin sponge along with thrombin or microfibrillar collagen placed over the area or an oral antifibrinolytic rinse (aminocaproic acid [Amicar] syrup, 250 mg/mL) placed in a soft vinyl mouthguard, can be used to control bleeding. If local measures fail, medical help should be obtained and platelet transfusion considered.

Neural and chemosensory changes. Many patients who are receiving radiation therapy experience a diminished sense of taste, probably as a result of damage to the microvilli of the taste cells. Patients who are given chemotherapeutic agents complain of bitter tastes, unpleasant odors, and conditioned aversions to foods. To minimize sensory stimulation, the dentist should avoid wearing cologne or perfume when in contact with patients who are undergoing radiation/chemotherapy.

In most patients, the ability to taste is restored within 3 to 4 months after completion of radiotherapy. In cases of chronic loss of taste, zinc supplementation has been reported to improve taste perception. Silverman[29] recommends 220 mg of zinc 2 times per day for patients with severe chronic loss of taste. However, currently, no effective treatment is available that completely restores damaged taste.[29]

Neurotoxicity is an adverse effect of chemotherapeutic agents, particularly vincristine and vinblastine. Although this complication commonly arises in the peripheral nerves, patients may experience odontogenic pain that mimics irreversible pulpitis caused by these agents. Pain is more common in the molar region and can be bilateral. Proper diagnosis requires the clinician to be familiar with the chemotherapeutic drug regimen and is aided by the absence of clinical or radiographic abnormalities.

OTHER CONSIDERATIONS

Patients with cancer have indwelling catheters (Hickman catheters or ports) that are susceptible to infection. However, these infections are not related to dental treatment bacteremias (see Chapter 2). Prosthetic implants (breast, penile, oral) that have been placed to restore esthetics or function lost as the result of cancerous tissue

---

> **BOX 26-12**
>
> **Recommendations for Invasive Oral Procedures in the Cancer Patient Undergoing Chemotherapy in an Outpatient Setting**
>
> Provide routine care when
> - The patient feels best—generally, 17 to 20 days after chemotherapy
> - Granulocyte count* >2000 cells/mm³
> - Platelet count*† >50,000 cells/mm³

*Consultation with a physician is recommended when values are lower than indicated here, and there is a need for antibiotic prophylaxis.
†Platelet values lower than 50,000 may cause significant bleeding.

---

or cancer treatment are not considered at risk for bacterial seeding from oral invasive procedures and do not require antibiotic coverage.[32]

Whether a patient is receiving inpatient or outpatient chemotherapy, the dentist should be familiar with the patient's WBC count and platelet status before providing dental care. In general, routine dental procedures can be performed if the granulocyte count is greater than 2000/mm³, the platelet count is greater than 50,000/mm³, and the patient feels capable of withstanding dental care. For outpatient care, this is generally the case 17 days after chemotherapy or a few days before the start of the next chemotherapy cycle (Box 26-12). If urgent care is needed and the platelet count is below 50,000/mm³, consultation with the patient's oncologist is required. Platelet replacement may be indicated if invasive or traumatic dental procedures are to be performed; topical therapy that includes the use of pressure, thrombin, microfibrillar collagen, and splints may be required (see Chapter 25).[32]

If urgent dental care is needed and the granulocyte count is less than 2000 cells/mm³, consultation with the physician is recommended and antibiotic prophylaxis should be provided. The dentist should be aware that use of prophylactic antibiotics for these patients is rational, although scientific evidence of effectiveness is lacking. The potential adverse effects of antibiotics should be kept in mind when one is making a decision about whether to use them. No standard antibiotic regimen is recommended for prophylaxis. The drug(s), duration, and dosage to be used for prophylaxis should be established in consultation with the patient's oncologist. Penicillin V 500 mg every 6 hours, starting at least 1 hour before any invasive procedure that involves bone, pulp, or periodontium and continuing for at least 3 days, is a reasonable regimen. Patients with periodontal infection and those who are allergic to penicillin will require alternative antibiotics.[27-29]

Post–Cancer Treatment Management

After cancer therapy has been provided, consultation with the physician is recommended to determine whether the patient is cured, in remission, or completing palliative care. If cancer therapy has been completed and remission or cure is the outcome, the patient with cancer should be placed on an oral recall program. Usually, the patient is seen once every 1 to 3 months during the first 2 years and at least every 3 to 6 months thereafter. After 5 years, the patient should be examined at least once per year. This recall program is important for the following reasons:

- A patient with cancer tends to develop additional lesions
- Latent metastases may occur
- Initial lesions may recur
- Complications related to therapy can be detected and managed

The usual long-term complications associated with cancer and its therapy include chronic xerostomia, loss of taste, altered bone, and related problems. Recall appointments are also important to ensure that the dentate patient continues to maintain good oral hygiene (including daily brushing, flossing, and continued use of daily fluoride gel applications); detection of oral soft tissue and hard tissue disease can occur early, before inflammation and infection involve the underlying bone, leading to necrosis. Patients who have completed palliative care should be afforded preventive oral care and dental procedures that they desire and can withstand.

Hyposalivation and Its Sequelae. Salivary gland tissue is moderately sensitive to radiation damage. Because of this, acinar tissue that is within the field of radiation can be permanently damaged during head and neck radiation therapy, resulting in hyposalivation. The degree of hyposalivation that occurs is directly related to the radiation field and dose (i.e., the dose delivered to the major salivary glands) and to baseline salivary function. Dosages in excess of 3000 cGy are the most damaging, especially if shielding or medication is not provided to the patient during radiation. Irradiated salivary glands become dysfunctional owing to acinar atrophy, vascular alterations, chronic inflammation, and loss of salivary parenchymal tissue. Usually, a 50% to 60% reduction in salivary flow occurs during the first week after irradiation therapy is provided. After radiation therapy has been given, saliva is reduced in volume and altered in consistency, pH, and immunoglobulin concentration. It becomes mucinous, thick, sticky, and ropy because serous acini are more sensitive than mucous acini to radiation. Unfortunately, pathologic changes often progress several months after radiotherapy has ceased, and radiation-induced salivary gland damage and dysfunction are permanent. In most cases, no salivary gland function is recovered.[27]

The direct effects of hyposalivation include extreme dryness of the oral mucosa. Of major significance are the discomfort, inconvenience, and substantial diminution of quality of life that accompany oral dryness. Clearly, saliva is an important host defense mechanism against oral disease, and it serves a variety of important functions in

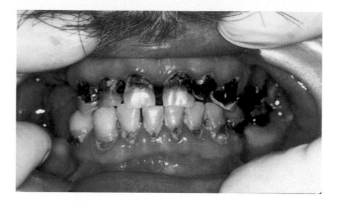

Figure 26-19. Note the extensive cervical caries in a patient who received radiotherapy. (Courtesy R. Gorlin, Minneapolis, Minn.)

the oral cavity. In a healthy mouth, copious saliva containing essential electrolytes, glycoproteins, immunoglobulins, hydrolytic enzymes (amylase), antimicrobial enzymes, and a number of other important factors continually lubricates and protects the oral mucosa. Saliva in normal quantities and composition serves to cleanse the mouth, clear potentially toxic substances, regulate acidity, buffer decalcifying acids, neutralize bacterial toxins and enzymes, destroy microorganisms, and remineralize enamel with inorganic elements (e.g., calcium, phosphorus), thus maintaining the integrity of the teeth and soft tissues.[27]

When the normal environment of the oral cavity is altered because of a decrease in or total absence of salivary flow or because of alterations in salivary composition, a healthy mouth becomes susceptible to painful deterioration and decay. Dry, atrophic, and fissured oral mucosa and soft tissues usually result from the hyposalivary condition, along with accompanying ulcers and desquamation, opportunistic bacterial and fungal infections, inflamed and edematous tongue, caries, and periodontal disease. Extreme difficulty in lubricating and masticating food (sticking to the tongue or hard palate) and in swallowing food (dysphagia) is common; this is among the most devastating and potentially most systemically damaging manifestations of hyposalivation in these individuals. Additionally, lack of or altered taste perception (i.e., hypogeusia or dysgeusia) and tolerance for certain acidic foods (e.g., citrus fruits, acetic acid, vinegar) are substantially altered in these individuals. As a result, nutritional intake may be impaired.[33]

Manifestations of salivary hypofunction in patients who have undergone irradiation therapy for head and neck cancer include severe xerostomia (less than 0.2 mL/min unstimulated salivary flow), mucositis, cheilitis, glossitis, fissured tongue, glossodynia, dysgeusia, dysphagia, and a severe form of caries called *radiation caries* (Figure 26-19). Radiation caries is estimated to occur 100 times more often in patients who have received head and neck radiation than in normal individuals. It can progress within months, advancing toward pulpal tissue and resulting in periapical infection that extends to surrounding irradiated bone. Extensive infection and necrosis may

BOX 26-13

Management of Salivary Dysfunction*

1. MOISTURE/LUBRICATION
   General
   a. Drink—Sip water, other liquids (that lack fermentable carbohydrate and carbonic acid).
   b. Avoid ethanol, tobacco, coffee, tea, and hot spicy foods.
   c. Use sugarless candy/gum.

   Over-the-Counter (OTC) products
   • Oral balance: Apply $1/2$ tsp 5 to 6 times daily.

   Prescription (Rx) products
   • Pilocarpine HCl 2% (Salagen)[†] 5 mg 3 or 4 times daily
   • Anethole trithione (Sialor)[†] 25 mg 3 times daily
   • Bethanechol chloride (Urecholine)[†] 25 mg 3 times daily
   • Cevimeline (Evoxac)[†] 30-mg caps 3 times daily
   • Artificial salivas: Glandosane Spray, Moi-Stir, Mouthkote, Optimoist, Roxane Saliva Substitute, Salivart Spray, Salix Lozenges, or generic (sodium carboxymethylcellulose 0.5% aqueous solution)

2. SOFT TISSUE LESIONS/SORENESS
   OTC
   • Oral balance
   • Biotene mouthwash

   Rx
   • Diphenhydramine (Benadryl) + Maalox nystatin elixir[†] (±sucralfate) (±0.5% viscous lidocaine)
   • Dexamethasone (Decadron Elixir) 0.5 mg/5 mL[§]
   • Triamcinolone 0.1% (in hydrocortisone acetate [Orabase], Orabase-HCA)
   • Clotrimazole (Mycelex) 60-mg troches
   • Nystatin and triamcinolone ointment (Mycolog II, Tristatin II, Mytrex)

3. PREVENTION OF CARIES/PERIODONTAL DISEASE
   General
   a. Practice meticulous personal oral hygiene.
   b. Avoid acidic drinks.
   c. Use toothpaste (Biotene).
   d. Attend regular hygiene recalls, and comply with dental prophylaxis.
   e. Use mechanical brushes (Waterpik) and sodium bicarbonate (NaHCO$_4$) rinses.

   Rx products
   • Neutral NaF 1.0%, trays (Prevident 5000)
   • Chlorhexidine gluconate (Peridex, Periguard)

*Salivary gland dysfunction, hyposalivation, or xerostomia should be managed in accordance with the diagnosis and signs, symptoms, and severity of manifestations within the oral cavity. Decreases in the quantity, and alterations in the composition, of beneficial constituents of saliva render the patient subject to many problems. Strategies for management vary from individual to individual in terms of severity and are divided into the three major areas discussed in this table.

†Caution should be used in patients who have chronic obstructive pulmonary disease (COPD) and in those at risk for myocardial infarction (MI).

‡Rx: Benadryl 25 mg/10 mL; nystatin 100,000 IU/mL; Maalox 4 mL; Eq 15 mL.

§Rx: Decadron Elixir 0.5 mg/5 mL. Dispense 100 mL. Sig 1 tsp 3 times daily swish-swallow.

result. A prescription for concentrated fluoride toothpaste (5000 ppm) should be provided to these patients for use in custom trays or brush-on application (Box 26-13), and salivary flow should be assessed.[25,30]

After a proper diagnostic assessment that determines levels of unstimulated and stimulated salivary flow, xerostomia is managed according to the three categories delineated in Box 26-13. First is the provision of additional moisture and lubrication to the oral cavity and oropharynx. This may be accomplished by simulation of oral fluids or stimulation of endogenous saliva. Several artificial salivas are available, some of which provide a modicum of symptomatic relief from oral dryness.

However, synthetic saliva solutions alone do not appear to be satisfactory for relief of the complaints associated with chronic xerostomia. Generally, they are compounded from carboxymethylcellulose or hydroxymethylcellulose. Some contain fluoride and supersaturated calcium and phosphate ions. An artificial saliva that has been particularly effective but is found only in Europe is Saliva-Orthana, which contains some natural animal mucins. Mouthkote contains a plant glycoprotein that reproduces the lubricating mucosal protection normally provided by saliva. Xero-Lube, Optimoist, Glandosane, and Salivart are other examples of artificial salivas that primarily are compounds of carboxymethylcellulose and may be effective. A gel form of artificial saliva that provides long-lasting relief, especially at night, is Oral Balance. This contains two antimicrobial enzymes (lactoperoxidase and glucose oxidase) that normally are found in saliva.

Patients should be encouraged to drink plenty of water and other fluids, with the exception of diuretics such as coffee or tea. Ethanol and tobacco should be avoided or minimized because these dry the oral mucosa. Also, post–radiation treatment patients who sip drinks constantly to keep the oral mucosa moist should avoid sipping drinks that contain a fermentable carbohydrate or carbonic acid because exposed cementum and dentin break down rapidly (in less than 6 months), resulting in radiation caries. Sugarless mints, candies, and chewing gum are beneficial in producing some additional moisture.[34]

Considerable research has been performed on various sialogogue drugs such as pilocarpine HCl (Salagen), anethole trithione (Sialor), and, recently, cevimeline (Evoxac). Pilocarpine is the prototype parasympathomimetic drug that has been derived from the pilocarpus plant. It is an alkaloid, muscarinic/cholinergic agonist that is known to stimulate smooth muscle and exocrine secretions. Pilocarpine has been extensively tested in safety and efficacy trials, and it appears to be very promising as a sialogogue. Parasympathomimetic drugs appear to be effective for stimulating salivary flow in most patients who have some residual salivary acinar function. However, certain adverse effects occur, and patients have to be carefully screened (i.e., for cardiovascular disease, diabetes, concomitant medications) before being placed on these drugs. Of particular note is that approximately 50% of patients who use pilocarpine and experience increased salivary flow notice symptomatic improvement in their dry mouth. Although the drug promotes salivary flow and provides endogenous beneficial constituents to the oral cavity, patients may need adjunctive artificial salivas to feel more comfortable.[34,35]

Fungal Infection. Opportunistic infection with *C albicans* is prevalent in postirradiation patients, with more than 80% of these individuals exhibiting infection with the fungus if proper diagnostic testing is used (see Secondary Infections, earlier).

Tooth Sensitivity. During and after radiotherapy, the teeth may become hypersensitive; this event may be related to decreased secretion of saliva and the lowered pH of secreted saliva. Topical application of a fluoride gel should be of benefit in reducing these symptoms.

Muscle Trismus. Radiation therapy of the head and neck can cause damage to the vasculature of muscles (obliterative endarteritis) and thus trismus of the masticatory muscles and joint capsule. To minimize the effects of radiation on muscles around the face and muscles of mastication, a mouth block should be placed when the patient is receiving external beam irradiation. The patient also should perform daily stretching exercises to improve trismus and should apply warm, moist heat. One exercise

requires the patient to place a given number of tongue blades inside the mouth at least 3 times a day for 10-minute intervals. With a slow increase in the number of tongue blades, muscle stretching occurs and improved function ensues.

Prosthodontics. Patients should avoid wearing their dentures during the first 6 months after completion of radiotherapy because mild trauma to the altered mucosa can result in ulceration and possible necrosis of underlying bone (see Osteoradionecrosis, later). Once patients start to wear their dentures, they must be told to come to the dentist if any sore spots develop, so dentures can be adjusted. Ill-fitting dentures should be replaced by new ones. In severe cases of chronic xerostomia, a small amount of petrolatum can be applied to the mucosal surface of the denture to enhance adhesion. Implants may be placed 12 to 18 months after radiation therapy has been provided, but clinician knowledge of tissue irradiation fields, degree of healing, and vascularity of the region is required because, for example, implants placed in the maxilla and the anterior mandible present less of a risk for osteoradionecrosis than those placed in the posterior mandible.

Osteoradionecrosis. Osteoradionecrosis (ORN) is a condition that is characterized by exposed bone that fails to heal (present for 6 months) after high-dose radiation to the jaws. ORN results from radiation-induced changes (hypocellularity, hypovascularity, and ischemia) in the jaws. Most cases result from damage to tissues overlying the bone rather than from direct damage to the bone. Accordingly, soft tissue necrosis usually precedes ORN and is variably present at the time of diagnosis. Risk is greatest in posterior mandibular sites for patients whose jaws have been treated with in excess of 6500 cGy, who continue to smoke, and who have undergone a traumatic (e.g., extraction) procedure. Risk is greater for dentate patients than for edentulous patients, and periodontal disease enhances risk. Nonsurgical procedures that are traumatic (e.g., curettage) or that cause a reduction in blood supply to the region (e.g., use of vasoconstrictors) can result in ORN. Spontaneous ORN also occurs. This risk continues throughout a patient's lifetime.[36,37]

If the dentist is unsure of the amount of radiation that was received and if invasive procedures are planned, the radiation oncologist should be contacted to determine the total dose given to the head and neck region before care is initiated. Clinicians should be aware that risk of ORN increases with increasing dose to the jaws (e.g., 7500 cGy presents a greater risk than 6500 cGy). Patients determined to be at risk should be provided appropriate preventive measures. Protocols to reduce the risk of ORN include selection of endodontic therapy over extraction, use of nonlidocaine local anesthetics that contain no or low concentrations of epinephrine, atraumatic surgical procedures (if surgery is necessary), pro-

BOX 26-14

Recommendations for Preventing Osteoradionecrosis in the Head and Neck–Irradiated Patient

1. Extract teeth with questionable and hopeless prognosis at least 2 weeks before radiotherapy.
2. Avoid extractions during radiotherapy.
   - The mandible is at greater risk than the maxilla.
   - Posterior sites are at greater risk than anterior sites.
3. Minimize infection.
   - Use prophylactic antibiotics.
   - Give 2 g penicillin VK orally 1 hour before the surgical procedure.
   - After surgery, continue with penicillin VK 500 mg 4 times daily for 1 week.
4. Minimize hypovascularity after radiotherapy.
   - Use nonlidocaine local anesthetic (e.g., Prilocaine plain or forte) for dental procedures.
   - Minimize or avoid vasoconstrictor use; if necessary, consider low-concentration epinephrine (1:200,000 or less).
   - Consider hyperbaric oxygen.*
5. Minimize trauma.
   - Endodontic therapy is preferred over extraction (assuming the tooth is restorable).
   - Follow atraumatic surgical technique.
   - Avoid periosteal elevations.
   - Limit extractions to two teeth per quadrant per appointment.
   - Irrigate with saline, obtain primary closure, and eliminate bony edges or spicules.
6. Maintain good oral hygiene.
   - Use oral irrigators.
   - Use antimicrobial rinses (chlorhexidine).
   - Use daily fluoride gels.
   - Eliminate smoking.
   - Attend frequent postoperative recall appointments.

*Alternatives include referral of a patient in need of extraction to an oral and maxillofacial surgeon who has experience with these patients and discussion of the use of hyperbaric oxygen (HBO) with a medical specialist. HBO treatments often consist of 20 preextraction dives and 10 postsurgical dives.

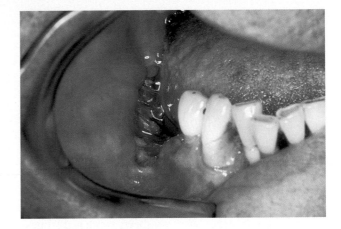

Figure 26-20. Osteoradionecrosis. Exposed necrotic bone in the posterior mandible edentulous ridge of a patient who previously received radiation therapy to the head and neck region.

phylactic antibiotics plus antibiotics during the week of healing (penicillin VK for 7 days), and hyperbaric oxygen administered before invasive procedures are performed (Box 26-14). Hyperbaric oxygen involves sequential daily dives under 2 atmospheres of oxygen pressure in a chamber.[37]

The use of prophylactic antibiotics to prevent infection after surgical procedures in post–radiation treatment patients minimizes bacterial invasion of the surgical site.[31] However, the effectiveness of such coverage may be greatly reduced by altered blood flow to the affected bone. The dentist should be aware that reduction in blood flow after radiotherapy is much greater in the mandible than in the maxilla because of the limited source

and lack of collateral circulation; this accounts for the greater frequency and severity of ORN in the mandible. The use of hyperbaric oxygen treatment at the time of extraction is gaining support but is costly and cannot be repeated later with the same effect.[37]

Once necrosis occurs, conservative management usually is indicated. Exposed bone (Figure 26-20) should be irrigated with a saline or antibiotic solution, and the patient should be directed to use oral irrigating devices to clean the involved area. However, extreme pressures should be avoided when these devices are prescribed. Bony sequestra should be removed to allow for epithelialization. If swelling and suppuration are present, broad-spectrum antibiotics are used. Severe cases benefit from hyperbaric oxygen treatment (60- to 90-minute dives 5 days per week, for a total of 20 to 30 dives). Cases that do not respond to conservative measures may require surgical resection of involved bone.[37]

Bisphosphonate-Associated Osteonecrosis. As was mentioned previously, bisphosphonate-associated osteonecrosis (BON) is potentially a very serious oral complication of cancer therapy. In patients who develop BON spontaneously, the most common initial complaints are the sudden presence of intraoral discomfort and the presence of roughness that may progress to traumatization of oral soft tissues surrounding the area of necrotic bone. Therefore, the diagnosis of BON is based on the medical and dental history of each patient, as well as on the observation of clinical signs and symptoms of this pathologic process.[26]

Treatment strategies that would yield consistent resolution and healing of BON have not yet been developed. In fact, many cases have had poor outcomes in spite of therapy and have progressed to extensive dehiscence and exposure of bone. Treatment strategies have included local surgical debridement, bone curettage, local irrigation with antibiotics, and hyperbaric oxygen therapy.

However, none of these therapeutic modalities has proved successful. Therefore, the inability to manage lesions of BON compromises the oncologic, nutritional, and oral management of affected patients. Prevention of this condition is of paramount importance for these patients, so that they can receive the anticancer therapies so necessary for the best possible outcome of their neoplastic disease.[25,26]

Carotid Atheroma. Patients who have received neck irradiation (more than or equivalent to 45 Gy) are more likely to develop carotid artery atheroma (calcified atherosclerotic plaque) after treatment than are risk-matched control patients who have not been irradiated. These lesions may be detected by panoramic radiography and represent a risk factor for stroke that warrants referral of the patient to a physician for evaluation.[38]

REFERENCES

1. Jamal A, Siegel R, Ward E, et al. Cancer statistics, 2006. CA Cancer J Clin 2006;56:106-130.
2. Simone EA. Oncology. In Goldman L, Ausiello D (eds). Cecil Textbook of Medicine, 22nd ed. Philadelphia, Saunders, 2004, p 1498.
3. Rhodus NL. Oral cancer: Leukoplakia and squamous cell carcinoma. Dent Clin North Am 2005;49:143-165, ix.
4. Hortobagyi GN. Treatment of breast cancer. N Engl J Med 1998;339:974-984.
5. McKenzie K, Sukumar S. Molecular genetics of human breast cancer. Prog Clin Biol Res 1997;396:133-145.
6. Chu KC, Tarone RE, Kessler LG, et al. Recent trends in U.S. breast cancer incidence, survival, and mortality rates. J Natl Cancer Inst 1996;88:1571-1579.
7. D'Angelo PC, Galliano DE, Rosemurgy AS. Stereotactic excisional breast biopsies utilizing the advanced breast biopsy instrumentation system. Am J Surg 1997;174:297-302.
8. Canavan TP, Doshi NR. Cervical cancer. Am Fam Physician 2000;61:1369-1376.
9. Southern SA, Herrington CS. Differential cell cycle regulation by low- and high-risk human papillomaviruses in low-grade squamous intraepithelial lesions of the cervix. Cancer Res 1998;58:2941-2945.
10. zur Hausen H. Papillomaviruses in human cancers. Proc Assoc Am Physicians 1999;111:581-587.
11. Centers for Disease Control. Guidelines for treatment of sexually transmitted diseases. MMWR Morb Mortal Wkly Rep 1998;47:101-111.
12. Fox RI. Clinical features, pathogenesis, and treatment of Sjögren's syndrome. Curr Opin Rheumatol 1996;8:438-445.
13. Hill MJ. Molecular and clinical risk markers in colon cancer trials. Eur J Cancer 2000;36:1288-1291.
14. Fuchs CS, Giovannucci EL, Colditz GA, et al. Dietary fiber and the risk of colorectal cancer and adenoma in women. N Engl J Med 1999;340:169-176.
15. Chao A, Thun MJ, Jacobs EJ, et al. Cigarette smoking and colorectal cancer mortality in the cancer prevention study II. J Natl Cancer Inst 2000;92:1888-1896.
16. Ahlquist DA, Skoletsky JE, Boynton KA, et al. Colorectal cancer screening by detection of altered human DNA in stool: Feasibility of a multitarget assay panel. Gastroenterology 2000;119:1219-1227.
17. Hoffman PC, Mauer AM, Vokes EE. Lung cancer. Lancet 2000;355:479-485.
18. Ozen M, Pathak S. Genetic alterations in human prostate cancer: A review of current literature. Anticancer Res 2000;20:1905-1912.
19. Green A, Whiteman D, Frost C, et al. Sun exposure, skin cancers and related skin conditions. J Epidemiol 1999;9(suppl 6):S7-S13.
20. Rigel DS, Friedman RJ, Kopf AW. The incidence of malignant melanoma in the United States: Issues as we approach the 21st century. J Am Acad Dermatol 1996;34:839-847.
21. Parker WA. Skin diseases of general importance. In Goldman L, Ausiello D (eds). Cecil Textbook of Medicine, 22nd ed. Philadelphia, Saunders, 2004, 556-568.
22. Brennan JA, Boyle JO, Koch WM, et al. Association between cigarette smoking and mutation of the *p53* gene in squamous cell carcinoma of the head and neck. N Engl J Med 1999;332:712-717.
23. Suntharalingam S. Principles and complications of radiation therapy. In Ord RA, Blanchaert RH (eds). Oral Cancer: The Dentist's Role in Diagnosis, Management, Rehabilitation, and Prevention. Chicago, Quintessence Publishing, 2000, 186-188.
24. Melo MD, Obeid G. Osteonecrosis of the jaws in patients with a history of receiving bisphosphonate therapy. J Am Dent Assoc 2005;136:1675-1681.
25. Migliorati CA. Bisphosphonate-associated osteoradionecrosis: Position statement. J Am Dent Assoc 2005;136:12.
26. Markiewicz MR, Margarone JE 3rd, Campbell JH, Aguirre A. Bisphosphonate-associated osteonecrosis (BON) of the jaws: A review. J Am Dent Assoc 2005;136:1669-1676.
27. Eisbruch A, Rhodus N, Rosenthal D, et al. The prevention and treatment of radiotherapy-induced xerostomia. Semin Radiat Oncol 2003;13:302-308.
28. Dodd MJ, Dibble SL, Miaskowski C, et al. Randomized clinical trial of the effectiveness of 3 commonly used mouthwashes to treat chemotherapy-induced mucositis. Oral Surg Oral Med Oral Pathol Oral Radiol Endod 2000;90:39-47.
29. Silverman S Jr. Oral Cancer, 4th ed. Hamilton, Ontario, BC Decker Inc., 1998.
30. Miller CS, Redding SW. Diagnosis and management of orofacial herpes simplex virus infections. Dent Clin North Am 1992;36:879-895.
31. Baddour LM, Bettmann MA, Bolger AF, et al. Nonvalvular cardiovascular device-related infections. Circulation 2003;108:2015-2031.
32. Robbins MA. Oral care of the patient receiving chemotherapy. In Ord RA, Blanchaert RH (eds). Oral Cancer: The Dentist's Role in Diagnosis, Management, Rehabilitation, and Prevention. Chicago, Quintessence Publishing, 2000, 120-131.
33. Rhodus NL, Moller K, Colby S, Bereuter J. Dysphagia in patients with three different etiologies of salivary gland dysfunction. Ear Nose Throat J 1995;74:39-42, 45-48.

34. Rhodus NL. Dysphagia in post-irradiation therapy head and neck cancer patients. J Cancer Res Ther Control 1994;4:49-54.

35. LeVeque FG, Montgomery M, Potter D, et al. A multicenter, randomized, double-blind, placebo-controlled, dose-titration study of oral pilocarpine for treatment of radiation-induced xerostomia in head and neck cancer patients. J Clin Oncol 1993;11:1124.

36. McKenzie MR, Wong FL, Epstein JB, Lepawsky M. Hyperbaric oxygen and postradiation osteonecrosis of the mandible. Eur J Cancer B Oral Oncol 1993;29B: 201-207.

37. Epstein J, van der Meij E, McKenzie M, et al. Postradiation osteonecrosis of the mandible: A long-term follow-up study. Oral Surg Oral Med Oral Pathol Oral Radiol Endod 1997;83:657-662.

38. Freymiller EG, Sung EC, Friedlander AH. Detection of radiation-induced cervical atheromas by panoramic radiography. Oral Oncol 2000;36:175-179.

PART NINE

Neurologic, Behavioral, and Psychiatric Disorders

Neurologic Disorders

CHAPTER
27

Five of the more common and significant neurologic diseases (i.e., epilepsy, stroke, Parkinson's disease, Alzheimer's disease, and multiple sclerosis) are discussed in this chapter. Cerebrospinal fluid shunts also are discussed because of concern for bacterial seeding after an invasive dental procedure.

EPILEPSY

DEFINITION

Epilepsy is a term that refers to a group of disorders characterized by chronic recurrent, paroxysmal changes in neurologic function (seizures), altered consciousness, or involuntary movements caused by abnormal and spontaneous electrical activity in the brain. Seizures may be convulsive (i.e., accompanied by motor manifestations) or may occur with other changes in neurologic function (i.e., sensory, cognitive, and emotional).[1] In the past, much confusion surrounded the nature and classification of epilepsy, but recent efforts have enhanced our understanding of these disorders.

In the 1800s, Hughlings Jackson's discourse on epilepsy concluded that "a convulsion is but a symptom, and implies only that there is an occasional, an excessive, and a disorderly discharge of nerve tissue." This has proved accurate but only in a limited way, in that epilepsy occurs in many forms besides the tonic-clonic generalized convulsion. Many epileptic events are focal, limited, and nonconvulsive.

Today, epilepsy denotes a group of chronic conditions whose major manifestation is the occurrence of epileptic seizures.[1] Seizures are characterized by discrete episodes that tend to be recurrent and are often unprovoked, in which movement, sensation, behavior, perception, and consciousness are disturbed. Symptoms are produced by excessive temporary neuronal discharging, which results from intracranial or extracranial causes.

Although seizures are required for the diagnosis of epilepsy, not all seizures imply epilepsy. Seizures may occur during many medical or neurologic illnesses, including stress, sleep deprivation, fever, alcohol or drug withdrawal, and syncope.[1]

The currently accepted classification of epilepsy (Box 27-1) was developed by the International League Against Epilepsy.[2] This classification is based on clinical behaviors and electroencephalographic changes and consists of two major groups: partial and generalized. Partial seizures are limited in scope (to a part of the cerebral hemisphere) and clinical manifestations, and involve motor, sensory, autonomic, or psychic abnormalities. Partial seizures are subdivided as simple, when consciousness is preserved, and complex, when consciousness is impaired. Generalized seizures are more global in scope and manifestation. They begin diffusely, involve both cerebral hemispheres, alter consciousness, and frequently produce abnormal motor activity. Discussion in this section is limited to generalized tonic-clonic seizures (idiopathic grand mal) because these represent the most severe expression of epilepsy that the dentist is likely to encounter.

EPIDEMIOLOGY

Incidence and Prevalence

Approximately 10% of the population will have at least one epileptic seizure in a lifetime, and 2% to 4% will have recurrent seizures at some time during their lives. The overall incidence of seizures is 0.5%.[1] Seizures are most common during childhood, with as many as 4% of children having at least one seizure during the first 15 years of life. Most children outgrow the disorder. About 4 in 1000 children do not outgrow the disorder and require medical care. Seizures also are common in the elderly, with an estimated annual incidence of 134 per 100,000.[3,4] Cerebrovascular disease is the most common factor underlying seizures in the elderly. An average dental

BOX 27-1

Classification of Epileptic Seizures

I. PARTIAL (FOCAL, LOCAL)
- Simple partial seizures
- Complex partial seizures
- Partial seizures evolving to secondarily generalized seizures

II. GENERALIZED (CONVULSIVE OR NONCONVULSIVE)
- Absence seizures (petit mal)
- Myoclonic seizures
- Tonic-clonic seizures (grand mal)
- Tonic seizures
- Atonic seizures

III. UNCLASSIFIED EPILEPTIC SEIZURES

Data from Commission on Classification and Terminology of the International League Against Epilepsy. Proposal for revised clinical and electroencephalographic classification of epileptic seizures. Epilepsia 1981;22:489-501.

practice of 2000 adult patients is predicted to have between 2 and 5 patients who experience seizures.

Etiology

The cause of epilepsy is idiopathic in more than half of all patients. Vascular (cerebrovascular disease) and developmental abnormalities (cavernous malformation), intracranial neoplasms (gliomas), and head trauma are causative in about 35% of adult cases. Other common causes include hypoglycemia, drug withdrawal, infection, and febrile illness (e.g., meningitis, encephalitis). Seizures occur with genetic conditions such as Down syndrome, tuberous sclerosis, and neurofibromatosis and are associated with several genetic abnormalities that result in neuronal channel dysfunction.

Seizures sometimes can be evoked by specific stimuli. Approximately 1 of 15 patients reports that seizures occurred after exposure to flickering lights, monotonous sounds, music, or a loud noise. Of interest have been reports[5] of epileptic seizures in youngsters exposed to flickering lights and geometric patterns while playing video games. Syncope and diminished oxygen supply to the brain also are known to trigger seizures.

Pathophysiology and Complications

The basic event underlying an epileptic seizure is an excessive focal neuronal discharge that spreads to thalamic and brainstem nuclei. The cause of this abnormal electrical activity is not precisely known, although a number of theories have been put forth.[1,6] These include altered sodium channel function, altered neuronal membrane potentials, altered synaptic transmission, diminution of inhibitory neurons, increased neuronal excitability, and decreased electrical threshold for epileptic activity. During the seizure, blood becomes hypoxic, and lactic acidosis occurs.

Approximately 60% to 80% of patients with epilepsy achieve complete control over their seizures within 5 years; the remainder achieve only partial or poor control.[6,7] A significant problem with epileptic patients is one of compliance (i.e., making sure that patients take their medication as directed). This problem is common to many chronic disorders, such as hypertension, because patients may have to take medication for the rest of their lives, even though they remain asymptomatic. Complications of seizures include trauma (as a result of falls) to the head, neck, and mouth and aspiration pneumonia. Also, frequent and severe seizures are associated with altered mental function, dullness, confusion, argumentativeness, and increased risk of sudden death (about 1 in 75 persons in this group die annually).[8]

Status Epilepticus. A serious acute complication of epilepsy (especially tonic-clonic) is the occurrence of repeated seizures over a short time without a recovery period, called *status epilepticus*. This condition is most frequently caused by abrupt withdrawal of anticonvulsant medication or an abused substance but may be triggered by infection, neoplasm, or trauma. Status epilepticus constitutes a medical emergency. Patients may become seriously hypoxic and acidotic during this event and suffer permanent brain damage or death. Patients with epilepsy also are at increased risk for sudden death and death due to accident.

CLINICAL PRESENTATION

Signs and Symptoms

The clinical manifestations of generalized tonic-clonic convulsions (grand mal seizure) are classic. An aura (a momentary sensory alteration that produces an unusual smell or visual disturbance) precedes the convulsion in one third of patients. Irritability is another premonitory signal. After the aura warning, the patient emits a sudden "epileptic cry" (caused by spasm of the diaphragmatic muscles) and immediately loses consciousness. The tonic phase consists of generalized muscle rigidity, pupil dilation, eyes rolling upward or to the side, and loss of consciousness. Breathing may stop because of spasm of respiratory muscles. This is followed by clonic activity that consists of uncoordinated beating movements of the limbs and head, forcible jaw closing, and head rocking. Urinary incontinence is common, but fecal incontinence is rare. The seizure (ictus) usually does not last longer than 90 seconds; then, movement ceases, muscles relax, and a gradual return to consciousness occurs, which is accompanied by stupor, headache, confusion, and mental dulling. Several hours of rest or sleep may be needed for the patient to fully regain cognitive and physical abilities.

Laboratory Findings

The diagnosis of epilepsy generally is based on the history of seizures and an abnormal electroencephalogram (EEG). Seizures produce characteristic spike and sharp wave patterns on EEG. Serial recordings of sleep deprivation that can induce seizures may help to establish the diagnosis. Other diagnostic procedures that are useful for ruling out other causes of seizures include computed axial tomography (CT), magnetic resonance imaging (MRI), single-photon emission computed tomography (SPECT), lumbar puncture, serum chemistry profiles, and toxicology screening.[6]

MEDICAL MANAGEMENT

The medical management of epilepsy usually is based on long-term drug therapy. Phenytoin (Dilantin), carbamazepine (Tegretol), and valproic acid are considered first-line treatments. Several other drugs are available for control of generalized tonic-clonic seizures (Table 27-1).[7-9] These drugs reduce the frequency of seizures by

TABLE 27-1
Anticonvulsants Used in the Management of Generalized Tonic-Clonic (Grand Mal) Seizures

Generic Name	Trade Name	Mechanism of Action	Dental Considerations
DRUGS OF CHOICE			
Phenytoin*	Dilantin	Blocks sodium channels	Gingival hyperplasia, increased incidence of microbial infection, delayed healing, gingival bleeding (leukopenia), osteoporosis, Stevens-Johnson syndrome
Carbamazepine*	Tegretol	Blocks sodium channels	Xerostomia, microbial infection, delayed healing, ataxia, gingival bleeding (leukopenia and thrombocytopenia), ataxia, osteoporosis, Stevens-Johnson syndrome. Drug interactions: Propoxyphene, erythromycin
Valproic acid*	Depakene, Depakote	γ-Aminobutyric acid (GABA) augmentation and N-methyl-d-aspartate (NMDA) receptor	Excessive bleeding and petechiae, decreased platelet aggregation, increased incidence of microbial infection, delayed healing, drowsiness, gingival bleeding (leukopenia and thrombocytopenia), hepatotoxicity. Drug interactions: Aspirin and nonsteroidal anti-inflammatory drugs (NSAIDs)
Lamotrigine*	Lamictal	Blocks sodium and calcium channels, reduces glutamate	Ataxia, may require help getting into and out of the dental chair, risk for developing Stevens-Johnson syndrome
ALTERNATIVES			
Clonazepam*	Klonopin	Augments inhibitory GABAergic system	Drug interactions: Central nervous system (CNS) depressants
Ethosuximide	Zarontin	Blocks sodium and calcium channels	Risk for developing Stevens-Johnson syndrome, blood dyscracias
Felbamate	Felbatol	Blocks sodium channels, reduces glutamate	Risks for aplastic anemia, Stevens-Johnson syndrome
Gabapentin	Neurontin	Modulates calcium channel; augments GABAergic system	Dizziness
Oxcarbazepine	Trileptal	Blocks sodium channels	Liver enzyme induction but less than carbamazepine
Phenobarbital*	Luminal	Blocks calcium channel; augments inhibitory GABAergic system	Sedation, liver enzyme induction. Drug interaction: CNS depressants
Primidone*	Mysoline	Blocks calcium channel; augments inhibitory GABAergic system	Ataxia, vertigo—increased risk of falls
Topiramate	Topemax	Blocks sodium channel; augments inhibitory GABAergic system	Impaired cognition
Vigabatrin	Sabril	Augments inhibitory GABAergic system	Drug interactions: CNS depressants

*Preexisting liver disease can exacerbate adverse effects associated with antiepileptics. Drugs of choice for absence (petit mal) seizures: Ethosuximide (Zarontin), valproate, lamotrigine, or clonazepam. Drugs of choice for status epilepticus: Lorazepam 4 to 8 mg, or diazepam 10 mg, intravenously.

elevating the seizure threshold of motor cortex neurons, depressing abnormal cerebral electrical discharge, and limiting the spread of excitation from abnormal foci. Phenytoin and carbamazepine are efficient at blocking sodium or calcium channels of motor neurons. Many of the other antiepileptic drugs augment gamma-aminobutyric acid (GABA), which inhibits glutamate activity—the major determinant of brain excitability. Adverse effects of phenytoin include anemia, ataxia, gingival overgrowth, cosmetic changes (coarsening of facial features, hirsutism, facial acne, gingival overgrowth), lethargy, skin rash, and gastrointestinal disturbances. Phenobarbital, which is considered a second-line drug,[10] can induce hepatic microsomal enzymes that promote the metabolism of concurrently used drugs. Several antiseizure medications (see Table 27-1) may cause drowsiness, sedation, ataxia, weight gain, cognitive impairment, and hypersensitivity reactions.[11] Adverse effects are more common at the start of therapy when drugs are administered rapidly or at high dose. For these reasons, and to facilitate compliance, single-drug therapy and a slow increase in dose are recommended. Unfortunately, the use of combination therapy is frequently necessary. Drug therapy is usually continued in children until a 1- to 2-year seizure-free period is attained, or until around age 16 years. Attempts to taper antiepileptic drug therapy are made thereafter.

Vagus nerve stimulation (VNS) is reserved for patients who have had unsatisfactory seizure control with several medications, and it is an option for some before brain surgery. VNS is similar to an implantable cardiac pacemaker, in which a subcutaneous pulse generator is implanted in the left chest wall and delivers electrical signals to the left vagus nerve through a bipolar lead.[12]

The stimulated vagus nerve provides direct projection to regions in the brain potentially responsible for the seizure. This device generally is used in combination with antiepileptic medications.

DENTAL MANAGEMENT
Medical Considerations

The first step in the management of an epileptic dental patient is identification (Box 27-2). This is best accomplished by the medical history and by discussion with the patient or family members. Once a patient with epilepsy has been identified, the dental practitioner must learn as much as possible about the seizure history, including the type of seizures, age at onset, cause (if known), current and regular use of medications, frequency of physician visits, degree of seizure control, frequency of seizures, date of last seizure, and any known precipitating factors. In addition, a history of previous injuries associated with seizures and their treatment may be helpful.

Fortunately, most epileptic patients are able to attain good control of their seizures with anticonvulsant drugs and are therefore able to receive normal routine dental care. In some instances, however, the history may reveal a degree of seizure activity that suggests noncompliance or a severe seizure disorder that does not respond to anticonvulsants. For these patients, a consultation with the physician is advised before dental treatment is rendered. A patient with poorly controlled disease may require additional anticonvulsant or sedative medication, as directed by the physician.

Patients who take anticonvulsants may suffer from the toxic effects of these drugs, and the dentist should be

---

BOX 27-2

Dental Management of the Epileptic Patient

1. Identification of patient by history
   a. Type of seizure
   b. Age at time of onset
   c. Cause of seizures (if known)
   d. Medications
   e. Frequency of physician visits (name and phone number)
   f. Degree of seizure control
   g. Frequency of seizures
   h. Date of last seizure
   i. Known precipitating factors
   j. History of seizure-related injuries
2. Provision of normal care: Well-controlled seizures pose no management problems
3. If questionable history or poorly controlled seizures, consultation with physician before dental treatment—may require modification of medications
4. Attention to adverse effects of anticonvulsants; these include:
   a. Drowsiness
   b. Slow mentation
   c. Dizziness

   d. Ataxia
   e. Gastrointestinal upset
   f. Allergic signs (rash, erythema multiforme)
5. Possibility of bleeding tendency in patients taking valproic acid (Depakene) or carbamazepine (Tegretol) as the result of platelet interference—Pretreatment platelet function analyzer (PFA)-100; if grossly abnormal, consultation with physician
6. Management of grand mal seizure
   a. Possible placement of a ligated mouth prop at the beginning of the procedure
   b. Chair back in supported supine position
7. Management of the seizure
   a. Clear the area
   b. Turn the patient to the side (to avoid aspiration)
   c. Do not attempt to use a padded tongue blade
   d. Passively restrain
8. After the seizure
   a. Examine for traumatic injuries
   b. Discontinue treatment, arrange for patient transport

aware of their manifestations. In addition to the more common adverse effects (see Table 27-1), allergy may be seen occasionally as a rash, erythema multiforme, or worse (Stevens-Johnson syndrome). Phenytoin, carbamazepine, and valproic acid can cause bone marrow suppression, leukopenia, and thrombocytopenia, resulting in an increased incidence of microbial infection, delayed healing, and gingival and postoperative bleeding.[13] Valproic acid can decrease platelet aggregation, leading to spontaneous hemorrhage and petechiae.[14]

Propoxyphene and erythromycin should not be administered to patients who are taking carbamazepine because of interference with metabolism of carbamazepine, which could lead to toxic levels of the anticonvulsant drug. Aspirin and nonsteroidal anti-inflammatory drugs (NSAIDs) (see Table 27-1) should not be administered to patients who are taking valproic acid because they can further decrease platelet aggregation, leading to hemorrhagic episodes.[13] No contraindication has been identified to the use of local anesthetics in proper amounts in these patients. Patients who have a VNS device implanted in their chest do not need antibiotic prophylaxis before undergoing invasive dental procedures.

Seizure Management. In spite of appropriate preventive measures taken by the dentist and by the patient, the possibility always exists that an epileptic patient may have a generalized tonic-clonic convulsion in the dental office. The dentist and staff should anticipate this occurrence and be prepared for it. Preventive measures include knowing the patient's history, scheduling the patient at a time within a few hours of taking the anticonvulsant medication, using a mouth prop, removing dentures, and discussing with the patient the urgency of mentioning an aura as soon as it is sensed. The clinician also should be aware that irritability is often a symptom of impending seizure. If sufficient time in the premonitory stage occurs, 0.5 to 2 mg of lorazepam can be given sublingually, or 2 to 10 mg diazepam can be given intravenously.[9,15]

If the patient has a seizure while in the dental chair, the primary task of management is to protect the patient and try to prevent injury. No attempt should be made to move the patient to the floor. Instead, the instruments and instrument tray should be cleared from the area, and the chair should be placed in a supported supine position (Figure 27-1). The patient's airway should be maintained patent. No attempt should be made to restrain or hold the patient down. Passive restraint should be used only to prevent injury that may result when the patient hits nearby objects or falls out of the chair.

If a mouth prop (e.g., a padded tongue blade between the teeth to prevent tongue biting) is used, it should be inserted at the beginning of the dental procedure. Trying to insert a mouth prop is not advised during the seizure, because doing so may damage the patient's teeth or oral soft tissue and may be nearly an impossible task. An exception would occur if the patient senses a pending seizure and can cooperate.

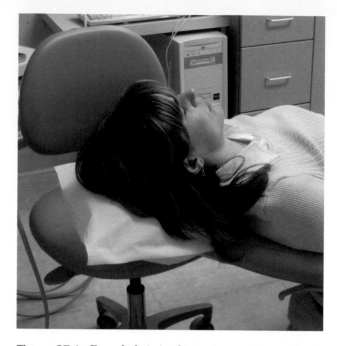

Figure 27-1. Dental chair in the supine position with the back supported by the operator's or by the assistant's stool.

Seizures generally do not last longer than a few minutes. Afterward, the patient may fall into a deep sleep from which he or she cannot be aroused. Oxygen (100%), maintenance of a patent airway, and mouth suction should be provided during this phase. Alternatively, the patient can be turned to the side to control the airway and to minimize aspiration of secretions. Within a few minutes, the patient gradually regains consciousness but may be confused, disoriented, and embarrassed. Headache is a prominent feature during this period. If the patient does not respond within a few minutes, the seizure may be associated with low serum glucose, and delivery of glucose may be needed.

No further dental treatment should be attempted after generalized tonic-clonic seizures, although examination for sustained injuries (e.g., lacerations, fractures) should be performed. In the event of avulsed or fractured teeth (Figure 27-2) or a fractured appliance, an attempt should be made to locate the tooth or fragments to rule out aspiration. A chest radiograph may be required to locate a missing fragment or tooth.

In the event that a seizure becomes prolonged (status epilepticus) or is repeated, intravenous lorazepam (0.05-0.1 mg/kg) 4 to 8 mg, or 10 mg diazepam, is generally effective in controlling it. Lorazepam is preferred by many experts because it is more efficacious and lasts longer than diazepam.[15,16] Oxygen and respiratory support should be provided because respiratory function may become depressed. If the seizure lasts longer than 15 minutes, the following should be provided: intravenous access, repeat lorazepam dosing, fosphenytoin administration, and activation of the emergency medical system (EMS).[9]

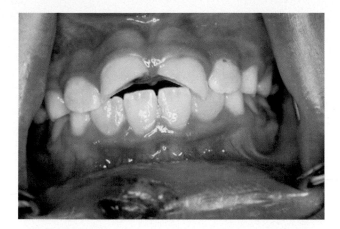

Figure 27-2. Fractured teeth and lacerated lower lip sustained during a grand mal seizure. (Courtesy G. Ferretti, Lexington, Ky.)

Treatment Planning Considerations

Because gingival overgrowth is associated with phenytoin administration, every effort should be made to maintain a patient at an optimal level of oral hygiene. This may require frequent visits for monitoring of progress. If significant gingival overgrowth exists, surgical reduction will be necessary. However, this must be accompanied by an increased awareness of oral hygiene needs and a positive commitment by the patient to maintain oral cleanliness.

A missing tooth or teeth should be replaced if possible to prevent the tongue from being caught in the edentulous space during a seizure (as commonly happens). Generally, a fixed prosthesis or implant is preferable to a removable one. (The removable prosthesis becomes dislodged more easily.) For fixed prostheses, all-metal units should be considered when possible to minimize the chance of fracture. When placing anterior castings, the dentist may wish to consider using three quarter crowns or retentive nonporcelain facings.

Removable prostheses are, nevertheless, sometimes constructed for epileptic patients. Metallic palates and bases are preferable to all-acrylic ones. If acrylic is used, it should be reinforced with wire mesh.

Oral Complications and Manifestations

The most significant oral complication seen in epileptic patients is gingival overgrowth, which is associated with phenytoin (Figure 27-3) and rarely with valproic acid[17,18] and vigabatrin.[19] The incidence of phenytoin-induced gingival overgrowth in epileptic patients ranges from 0% to 100%, with an average rate of approximately 42%.[20] A greater tendency to develop gingival overgrowth occurs in youngsters than in adults. The anterior labial surfaces of the maxillary and mandibular gingivae are most commonly and severely affected.

Meticulous oral hygiene is important for preventing and significantly decreasing its severity.[21-23] Good home care must always be combined with the removal of irritants, such as overhanging restorations and calculus.

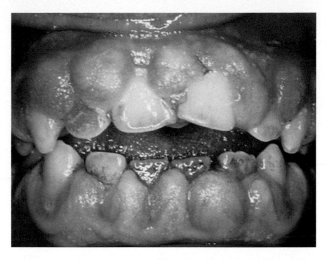

Figure 27-3. Phenytoin-induced gingival overgrowth. (Courtesy H. Abrams, Lexington, Ky.)

Frequently, enlarged tissues interfere with function or appearance, and surgical reduction may become necessary.

Traumatic injuries such as broken teeth, tongue lacerations, and lip scars also are common in patients who experience generalized tonic-clonic seizures. Stomatitis, erythema multiforme, and Stevens-Johnson syndrome are rare adverse effects associated with the use of phenytoin, valproic acid, lamotrigine, phenobarbital, and carbamazepine.[24,25] These complications are more common during the first 8 weeks of treatment.[25]

STROKE

DEFINITION

Stroke is a generic term that is used to refer to a cerebrovascular accident—a serious and often fatal neurologic event caused by sudden interruption of oxygenated blood to the brain. This in turn results in focal necrosis of brain tissue and possibly death. Even if a stroke is not fatal, the survivor often is to some degree debilitated in motor function, speech, or mentation. The scope and gravity of stroke are reflected in the fact that stroke is the leading cause of serious, long-term disability in the United States; 5% of the population older than 65 years of age has had one stroke.[26]

EPIDEMIOLOGY

Incidence and Prevalence

Although the incidence of stroke has declined, it remains one of the most significant health problems in the United States. Each year in the United States, about 700,000 people experience new or recurrent stroke.[26] This translates to the occurrence of one stroke about every minute, and 75% of persons survive their stroke. Approximately 4.5 million persons living in 2001 had survived a stroke.[26] Risk is associated with race; African Americans are at 38% greater risk of first stroke than are whites.[27] Also,

40,000 more women than men have a stroke each year.

Stroke is the third leading cause of death (behind heart disease and cancer) in the United States, with 275,000 Americans dying of stroke annually. African Americans and other racial minorities in the United States have higher stroke mortality than whites. The risk of death from stroke in African Americans aged 35 to 74 years is 2 to 3 times greater than in non-Hispanic whites. African American males and persons living in the South and Northwest are at greatest risk.[26,28] Native Americans and Native Alaskans are also at increased risk. Risk of stroke increases with age; however, on average, 28% of people who have a stroke are younger than 65 years. The chance of having a stroke before age 70 is 1 in 20 for both genders.[26] A total of 4.7 million stroke survivors live in the United States, and an average dental practice of 2000 adult patients will include about 31 patients who have or will experience a stroke.

Etiology

Stroke is caused by the interruption of blood supply and oxygen to the brain as a result of ischemia or hemorrhage. The most common type is ischemic stroke induced by thrombosis (60% to 80% of cases) of a cerebral vessel. Ischemic stroke can also result from occlusion of a cerebral blood vessel by distant emboli. Hemorrhage causes about 15% of all strokes and has a 1-year mortality greater than 60%.[29]

Cerebrovascular disease is the primary factor associated with stroke. Atherosclerosis and cardiac pathosis (myocardial infarction, atrial fibrillation) increase the risk of thrombolic and embolic strokes, whereas hypertension is the most important risk factor for intracerebral hemorrhagic stroke.[29] Approximately 10% of persons who have had a myocardial infarction will have a stroke within 6 years.[26] Additional factors that increase the risk for stroke include the occurrence of transient ischemic attacks, a previous stroke, high dietary fat, obesity and elevated blood lipid levels, physical inactivity, uncontrolled hypertension, cardiac abnormalities, diabetes mellitus, elevated homocysteine levels, elevated hematocrit, elevated antiphospholipid antibodies, heavy tobacco smoking, increasing age (risk doubles each decade after 65 years), and periodontal disease.[30-32] Increased risk for hemorrhagic stroke also occurs with use of phenylpropanolamine, an alpha-adrenergic agonist.[33] This has led to an order from the U.S. Food and Drug Administration that phenylpropanolamine must be removed from over-the-counter cold remedies and weight loss aids.[34] Intake of fruits and vegetables and moderate levels of exercise have a protective effect against stroke.[35,36]

Pathophysiology and Complications

Pathologic changes associated with stroke result from infarction, intracerebral hemorrhage, or subarachnoid hemorrhage. Cerebral infarctions are most commonly caused by atherosclerotic thrombi or emboli of cardiac origin. The extent of an infarction is determined by a

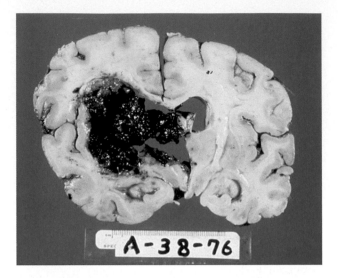

Figure 27-4. Cerebral infarction in an individual who had chronic hypertension.

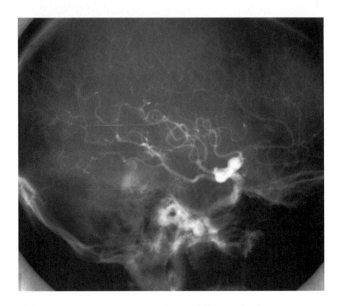

Figure 27-5. Aneurysm of the middle cerebral artery.

number of factors, including site of the occlusion, size of the occluded vessel, duration of the occlusion, and collateral circulation. The production and circulation of proinflammatory cytokines, the occurrence of clotting factors, and arterial inflammation contribute to platelet aggregation. Neurologic abnormalities result from excitotoxicity, free radical accumulation, inflammation, mitochondrial and DNA damage, and apoptosis of the region supplied by the damaged artery.[37]

The most common cause of intracerebral hemorrhage is hypertensive atherosclerosis, which results in microaneurysms of the arterioles (Figure 27-4). Vessels within the circle of Willis often are affected (Figure 27-5). Rupture of these microaneurysms within brain tissue leads to extravasation of blood, which displaces brain tissue and causes increased intracranial volume until resultant tissue compression halts bleeding. Hemorrhagic strokes also may be caused by subarachnoid hemorrhage. The most common cause of subarachnoid hemorrhage is rupture of a saccular aneurysm at the bifurcation of a major cerebral artery.

The most serious outcome of stroke is death, which occurs in 8% of those who experience ischemic strokes and 38% to 47% of those with hemorrhagic strokes within a month of the event. Overall, about 23% of patients die within 1 year.[26] Mortality rates are directly related to type of stroke,[29] with 80% of patients dying after an intracerebral hemorrhage, 50% after a subarachnoid hemorrhage, and 30% after occlusion of a major vessel by a thrombus. Death from stroke may not be immediate (sudden death) but rather may occur hours, days, or even weeks after the initial stroke episode.

If the victim survives, an excellent chance exists that a neurologic deficit or disability of varying degree and duration will remain. Of those who survive the stroke, 10% recover with no impairment, 50% have a mild residual disability, 15% to 30% are disabled and require special services, and 10% to 20% require institutionalization.[26,38] Approximately 50% of those who survive the acute period (the first 6 months) are alive 7 years later.[38,39]

The type of residual deficit that results from a stroke is directly dependent on the size and location of the infarct or hemorrhage. Deficits include unilateral paralysis, numbness, sensory impairment, dysphasia, blindness, diplopia, dizziness, and dysarthria. Return of function is unpredictable and usually takes place slowly, over several months. Even with improvement, patients frequently are left with some permanent residual problem, such as difficulty in walking, using the hands, performing skilled acts, or speaking. Dementia also is an outcome of stroke.

CLINICAL PRESENTATION

Signs and Symptoms

Familiarity with the warning signs and symptoms and the phases of stroke can lead to appropriate action that may be lifesaving. Four events associated with stroke are (1) the transient ischemic attack (TIA), (2) reversible ischemic neurologic deficit (RIND), (3) stroke-in-evolution, and (4) the completed stroke. These events are defined principally by their duration.

A TIA is a "mini" stroke that is caused by a temporary disturbance in blood supply to a localized area of the brain. A TIA often causes numbness of the face, arm, or leg on one side of the body (hemiplegia), weakness, tingling, numbness, or speech disturbances that usually last less than 10 minutes. Most commonly, a major stroke is preceded by one or two TIAs within several days of the first attack.[29]

A RIND is a neurologic deficit that is similar to a TIA but does not clear within 24 hours; eventual recovery occurs.[29]

Stroke-in-evolution is a neurologic condition that is caused by occlusion or hemorrhage of a cerebral artery

---

BOX 27-3

Differences Between Right-Sided Brain Damage and Left-Sided Brain Damage

Right-Sided Brain Damage

- Paralyzed left side
- Spatial/perceptual deficits
- Thought impaired
- Quick, impulsive behavior
- Patient cannot use mirror
- Difficulty performing tasks (toothbrushing)
- Memory deficits
- Neglect of left side

Left-Sided Brain Damage

- Paralyzed right side
- Language and speech problems
- Decreased auditory memory (cannot remember long instructions)
- Slow, cautious, disorganized behavior
- Memory deficits— language based
- Patients anxious

---

in which the deficit has been present for several hours and continues to worsen during a period of observation.[29] Signs of stroke include hemiplegia, temporary loss of speech or trouble in speaking or understanding speech, temporary dimness or loss of vision, particularly in one eye (may be confused with migraine), unexplained dizziness, unsteadiness, or a sudden fall.

Clinical manifestations that remain after a stroke vary in accordance with the site and size of residual brain deficits; these include language disorders, hemiplegia, and paresis, a form of paralysis that is associated with loss of sensory function and memory and weakened motor power. Box 27-3 presents the different behavioral patterns of right-sided brain damage versus left-sided brain damage. Of note, in most patients with stroke, the intellect remains intact; however, large, left-sided stroke has been associated with cognitive decline.[40]

Laboratory Findings

Patients suspected of having had a stroke usually receive a variety of laboratory and diagnostic imaging tests to rule out conditions that can produce neurologic alterations, such as diabetes mellitus, uremia, abscess, tumor, acute alcoholism, drug poisoning, and extradural hemorrhage.[29] Laboratory tests often include urinalysis, blood sugar level, complete blood count, erythrocyte sedimentation rate, serologic tests for syphilis, blood cholesterol and lipid levels, chest radiographs, and electrocardiogram. Various abnormalities may be disclosed by these test results, depending on the type and severity of stroke and its causative factors. A lumbar puncture also may be ordered by the physician in an effort to check for blood or protein in the cerebrospinal fluid (CSF) and for altered CSF pressure that would be suggestive of subarachnoid hemorrhage.[29,41] Doppler blood flow, EEG, cerebral angiography, CT (Figure 27-6), and MRI, including diffusion and perfusion studies of the brain, are important for determining the extent and location of arterial injury.

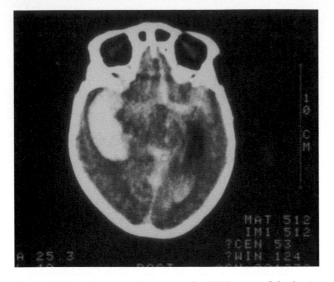

Figure 27-6. Computed tomography (CT) scan of the brain demonstrating a cerebrovascular accident that extended from the midbrain to the temporal lobe.

MEDICAL MANAGEMENT
Prevention

The first aspect of stroke management is prevention. This is accomplished by identifying risk factors in individuals (e.g., hypertension, diabetes, atherosclerosis, cigarette smoking) and attempting to reduce or eliminate as many of these as possible. Blood pressure lowering (see Chapter 3), antiplatelet therapy (see Chapter 25), and statin therapy are primary stroke prevention methods. Carotid endarterectomy is a secondary stroke prevention method.

The benefit of lowering blood pressure is evident in the fact that a reduction of systolic blood pressure by 10 mm Hg is associated with a one-third reduction in risk for stroke.[42] Aspirin, ticlopidine, and extended-release dipyridamole are accepted preventive therapies for ischemic stroke in patients who have experienced TIAs, or who have had a stroke. Aspirin dosed at 81 to 325 mg daily reduces the risk of stroke by about 25% in this at-risk population.[43] Similarly, statin therapy reduces risk by about 20%. Also, surgical intervention through endarterectomy reduces the risk by about 1% per year, such that one stroke is prevented for every 20 patients who undergo surgery over a 5-year period.[43]

Stroke Treatment

If an individual has a stroke, treatment is generally three-fold. The immediate task is to sustain life during the period immediately after the stroke. This is done by means of life support measures and transport to a hospital. The second task involves emergency efforts to prevent further thrombosis or hemorrhage, and to attempt to lyse the clot in cases of thrombosis or embolism. Thrombolysis and improved neurologic outcomes have been achieved with intravenous recombinant tissue-type plasminogen activator (rt-PA) and intra-arterial prourokinase.[44] Of the

two, intravenous administration of rt-PA within 3 hours of ischemic stroke onset is the only approved therapy in the United States.[44-47]

After the initial period, efforts to stabilize the patient continue with anticoagulant medications such as heparin, coumarin, aspirin, and dipyridamole combined with aspirin (Aggrenox) in cases of thrombosis or embolism. Heparin is administered intravenously during acute episodes, whereas coumarin, dipyridamole, aspirin, subcutaneous low molecular weight heparin, or platelet receptor antagonists (clopidogrel, abciximab, ticlopidine) are employed for prolonged periods to reduce risk of thrombosis (e.g., deep vein thrombosis). Corticosteroids may be used acutely after a stroke to reduce the cerebral edema that accompanies cerebral infarction. This can markedly lessen complications. Surgical intervention may be indicated for removal of a superficial hematoma or management of a vascular obstruction. The latter usually is accomplished by thromboendarterectomy or by bypass grafts in the neck or thorax. Valium, Dilantin, and other anticonvulsants are prescribed in the management of seizures that may accompany the postoperative course of stroke.

If the patient survives, the third and final task consists of institution of preventive therapy, administration of medications that reduce the risk of another stroke (statins and antihypertensive drugs), and initiation of rehabilitation. Rehabilitation generally is accomplished by intense physical, occupational, and speech therapy (if indicated). Although marked improvement is common, many patients are left with some degree of permanent deficit.

DENTAL MANAGEMENT
Medical Considerations

Some primary tasks of the dentist include stroke prevention and identification of the stroke-prone individual. Patients with a history or clinical evidence of hypertension, congestive heart failure, diabetes mellitus, previous stroke or TIA, and advancing age are predisposed to stroke, as well as to myocardial infarction. As these factors increase, so does the level of risk (Box 27-4).[48] The dentist should assess patient risk, encourage individuals to seek medical care, and eliminate or control all possible risk factors.

Assessment of risk aids in the decision-making process regarding the timing and type of dental care to be provided.[49] For example, a patient who has had a stroke or TIA is at greater risk for having another than a person who has not had one.[29,40] In fact, up to one third of strokes recur within 1 month of the initial event, and risk remains elevated for at least 6 months.[29] These individuals therefore should be approached with a degree of caution, and deferral of treatment is advised for 6 months. Although risk decreases after 6 months, it continues to be present; 14% of those who survive a stroke or TIA have a recurrence within 1 year.[26] In addition, patients who experience a TIA or RIND are unstable and should not undergo

---

BOX 27-4

Dental Management of the Patient With Stroke

1. Identify risk factors.
   a. Hypertension*
   b. Congestive heart failure*
   c. Diabetes mellitus*
   d. TIA or previous stroke*
   e. Increasing age ≥75 years*
   f. Elevated blood cholesterol or lipid levels
   g. Coronary atherosclerosis
   h. Cigarette smoking
   i. *Note:* Risk of stroke increases by a factor of 1.5 for each condition above indicated by*. Thus, having multiple risk factors listed above greatly increases the risk of a stroke.[48]
2. Encourage control of risk factors (referral to physician, if appropriate).
3. Obtain thorough history of stroke.
   a. Note date of event, current status, medical therapy, and any residual disabilities.
   b. Provide only urgent dental care during first 6 months after a stroke, TIA, or RIND.
   c. Avoid elective care in patients who have had recent TIAs or RINDs.
   d. Determine risk for bleeding problems in patients taking anticoagulant drugs, and minimize perioperative bleeding.
      (1) Aspirin ± dipyridamole (Aggrenox), clopidogrel (Plavix), abciximab (ReoPro), or ticlopidine (Ticlid); obtain pretreatment PFA-100.
      (2) Coumarin—Pretreatment INR ≤3.5. Higher levels require consultation with physician to reduce dose.
      (3) Heparin (IV)—Use palliative emergency dental care only, or 6 to 12 hours before surgery, discontinue heparin and start another anticoagulant (e.g., coumadin) with physician's approval. Then, restart heparin after clot forms (6 h later). Heparin (subcutaneous, low molecular weight)—generally, no changes required.
      (4) Use measures that minimize hemorrhage (atraumatic surgery, pressure, gelfoam, suturing), as needed.
      (5) Have available nonadrenergic hemostatic agents and devices (stents, electrocautery).
4. Schedule short, stress-free, midmorning appointments. Provide N_2O-O_2 inhalation as needed.
5. Monitor blood pressure and oxygen saturation.
6. Use minimum amount of anesthetic containing vasoconstrictor.
7. Avoid epinephrine in retraction cord.
8. Recognize signs and symptoms of a stroke, provide emergency care, and activate emergency medical support system.
9. A prior stroke may require assistance for patient transfer to the chair, effective oral evacuation and airway management, and rigorous oral hygiene measures delivered by a health care provider.

INR, International normalized ratio; IV, intravenous; PFA, platelet function analyzer; RIND, reversible ischemic neurologic deficits; TIA, transient ischemic attack.

---

elective dental care. Medical consultation and referral to a physician are mandatory.

A patient who takes coumarin or antiplatelet drugs is at risk for abnormal bleeding (see Box 27-4). The status of coumarin anticoagulation is monitored by assessment of the international normalized ratio (INR). An INR level of 3.5 or less is acceptable for performance of most invasive and noninvasive dental procedures. If the INR is greater than 3.5 and oral surgery is planned, significant bleeding may occur, and the physician should be consulted for a decrease in dosage of the anticoagulant. In these cases, a reduction in dose of the anticoagulant is recommended over interruption of anticoagulation therapy because the risk for significant adverse outcomes is minimized by this approach[50] (see Chapter 25). Also, metronidazole and tetracycline may increase the INR by inhibiting the metabolism of Coumadin; therefore, concurrent use of these drugs may have to be avoided.[51]

The effects of aspirin and dipyridamole on platelet aggregation are monitored by the platelet function analyzer (PFA)-100. Abnormal results should be discussed with the physician. Postoperative pain should be managed with acetaminophen-containing products.

Management of stroke-prone patients or patients with a history of stroke includes the use of short, midmorning appointments that are as stress free as possible. Assisted transfer to the dental chair may be needed. Do not overestimate the patient's abilities, especially because some stroke patients may be able to verbalize but do not realize the extent of paresis that is present. Dental care providers should move slowly around the patient and should speak clearly while facing the patient with the mask off. Effective communication techniques are listed in Box 27-5.

Blood pressure should be monitored to ensure good control. Pain control is important. Nitrous oxide–oxygen may be given if good oxygenation is maintained at all times. A pulse oximeter should be used to ensure that oxygenation is adequate. A local anesthetic with 1:100,000 or 1:200,000 epinephrine may be used in judicious amounts (≤ 4 mL).[52] Gingival retraction cord impregnated with epinephrine should not be used.

A patient who develops signs or symptoms of a stroke in the dental office should be provided oxygen, and the EMS should be activated. Transport to a medical facility should not be delayed (minutes count when one is treating patients with acute stroke). For ischemic stroke, thrombolytic agents should be administered within 3

Effective Communication Techniques for the Patient With Stroke

- Face the patient.
- Use a slower, more deliberate, less complex pattern of speech.
- Communicate at eye level.
- Be positive.
- Ask yes/no questions—Be simple and brief.
- Give frequent, accurate, and immediate feedback.
- Use simple drawings to explain procedures.
- Do not underestimate or overestimate abilities.
- Do not raise voice or use baby talk.
- Do not wear a mask when talking to the patient.
- Communicate also with significant other/personal care provider.

Data from Henry R. Personal communication, 1995; and Ostuni E. Stroke and the dental patient. J Am Dent Assoc 1994;125: 721-727.

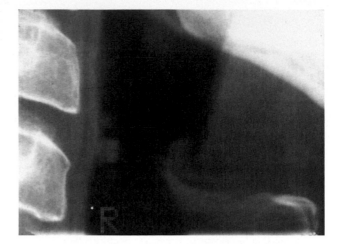

Figure 27-7. Carotid atheroma in an elderly patient at risk for stroke. The calcification is usually located near cervical vertebrae 3 and 4, generally at a 45° angle from the angle of the mandible.

hours if they are to be maximally effective in reestablishing arterial flow; the earlier subjects receive these agents, the better is the outcome.[44,45,53,54] The phrase "time is brain" emphasizes the immediacy of the situation. Finally, the dental staff should remember that patients who have had a stroke have feelings of grief, loss, and depression and should be treated with compassion.

Treatment Planning Modifications

Technical modifications may be required for patients with residual physical deficits who have difficulty practice adequate oral hygiene. For these patients, extensive bridgework is not a good choice. However, fixed prostheses may be more desirable than removable ones because of difficulties associated with daily placement and removal. Individualized treatment plans are important. All restorations should be placed with ease of cleansability in mind. Hygiene is often facilitated by an electric toothbrush, a large-handled toothbrush, or a water irrigation device. Flossing aids should be prescribed, and loved ones and personal care providers should be instructed on how and when these services should be provided. Frequent professional prophylaxis and the provision of topical fluoride and chlorhexidine are advisable.

Oral Complications and Manifestations

A stroke-in-evolution may become apparent through slurred speech, a weak palate, or difficulty swallowing. After a stroke, loss or difficulty in speech, unilateral paralysis of the orofacial musculature, and loss of sensory stimuli of oral tissues may occur. The tongue may be flaccid, with multiple folds, and may deviate on extrusion. Dysphagia is common, along with difficulty in managing liquids and solids. Patients with right-sided brain damage may neglect the left side. Thus, food and debris may accumulate around teeth, beneath the tongue, or in alveolar folds. Patients may need to learn to clean teeth or

dentures with only one hand, or they may require assistance to maintain oral hygiene; otherwise, caries, periodontal disease, and halitosis occur commonly.

Calcified atherosclerotic plaques have been demonstrated in the carotid arteries of elderly and diabetic patients on panoramic films (Figure 27-7).[55-57] This radiographic feature indicates a risk for stroke and warrants referral to the patient's physician for evaluation. Also of note, severe periodontal bone loss is associated with carotid artery plaques and increased risk for stroke.[58] However, the exact causative relationship between periodontal disease and stroke remains to be defined. Although periodontal treatment can reduce serum inflammatory markers potentially involved in stroke,[59,60] evidence that periodontal therapy reduces the risk for stroke is lacking.[61]

PARKINSON'S DISEASE

DEFINITION

Parkinson's disease, first described by James Parkinson[62] in 1817, is a progressive neurodegenerative disorder of neurons that produce dopamine. Loss of these neurons results in characteristic motor disturbances (resting tremor, muscular rigidity, bradykinesia, postural instability). Dopaminergic neurons are found in the nigrostriatal pathway of the brain. Approximately 80% of the dopamine in these neurons must be depleted before symptoms of the disease arise.[63] This disease is chronic and progressive.

EPIDEMIOLOGY

Incidence and Prevalence

Parkinson's disease is a common disease of the central nervous system (CNS) that affects about 1 million Americans, or 1 in 300 persons. Each year, this disease is diagnosed in 50,000 individuals. About 1% of the population

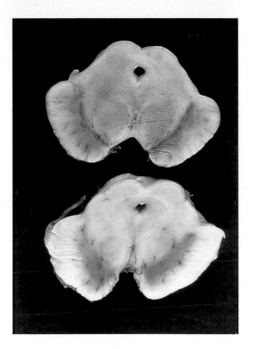

Figure 27-8. Parkinson's disease. Normal pigmentation of dopaminergic neurons in the substantia nigrans of a healthy patient *(top)*, in contrast with depleted and depigmented dopaminergic neurons of the substantia nigrans in a patient who has Parkinson's disease *(bottom)*.

older than 50 years of age and 2.5% of the population over age 70 have the disease. Given the aging phenomenon in the United States, a threefold to fourfold increase in Parkinson's disease frequency is predicted over the next 50 years.[64] Parkinson's disease has a peak age of onset between 55 and 66 years, but a particular form of the disease can strike teenagers. Men are affected slightly more often than women, and no racial predilection exists. An average dental practice of 2000 adult patients is predicted to include about 6 patients who have Parkinson's disease.

Etiology

Parkinson's disease is caused by death and depletion of dopaminergic neurons, which are manufactured in the substantia nigra (Figure 27-8) and released in the caudate nucleus and putamen (the nigrostriatal pathway). Although the cause of Parkinson's disease remains unknown, many factors have been identified that are associated with development of the disease. Genetic mutations (such as mutations in the alpha-synuclein gene or the Parkin gene, which contributes to protein degradation) contribute to less than 10% of cases.[65] Other causes include stroke, brain tumor, and head injury (e.g., boxing) that damage cells in the nigrostriatal pathway. Exposure to manganese (in miners and welders), mercury, carbon disulfide, certain agricultural herbicides (rotenone), and street heroin contaminated with a meperidine analog (1-methyl-4-phenyl-1,2,3,6-tetrahydropyridine) can be neurotoxic and give rise to Parkinson's disease symptoms.[63] Also, neuroleptic drugs (phenothiazines, butyrophenones) may cause Parkinson symptoms and rigidity.

Pathophysiology and Complications

Parkinson's disease is thought to be caused by environmental and genetic factors that trigger failure in proteasome-mediated protein turnover in susceptible neurons, resulting in accumulation of toxic proteins.[65] This leads to degeneration and loss of pigmented neurons primarily of the substantia nigra and destructive lesions in the circuitry to the limbic system, motor system, and centers that regulate autonomic functions. Damaged neurons display neuronal cytoskeleton changes, including eosinophilic intraneuronal inclusion bodies (called Lewy bodies)[66] and Lewy neurites in their neuronal processes. Inclusion bodies contain compacted aggregates of presynaptic protein alpha-synuclein.[67] The course of the disease is complicated by degeneration of other regions in the brain such as the cholinergic nucleus basalis, which can result in depression.

CLINICAL PRESENTATION

Signs and Symptoms

Parkinson's disease results in resting tremor (that is attenuated during activity), muscle rigidity, slow movement (bradykinesia, shuffling gait), and facial impassiveness (mask of Parkinson's disease) (Figure 27-9). The tremor, which is rhythmic and fine and is best seen in the extremity at rest, produces a "pill-rolling rest tremor" and handwriting changes. Cogwheel-type rigidity (decreased arm swing with walking and foot dragging), stooped posture, unsteadiness, imbalance (gait instability), and falls also are common features. In addition, pain, (musculoskeletal, sensory [burning, numbness, tingling], or akathisia—subjective feeling of restlessness—restless leg syndrome), orthostatic hypotension, and bowel and bladder dysfunction occur in approximately 50% of patients. Cognitive impairment of memory and concentration occurs to varying degrees, depending on the extent of destruction of the cortical–basal ganglia–thalamic neural loops. Mood disturbances (depression, dysthymia, apathy, anxiety), insomnia, and fatigue occur in approximately 40% of patients; dementia occurs in approximately 25% of patients.[68] Psychosis, related to dopaminergic medications, occurs in approximately 20% of patients.[69]

Laboratory Findings

Because no diagnostic test is available to detect Parkinson's disease, the diagnosis requires a thorough history, clinical examination, and specific tests and images to rule out diseases that can produce similar symptoms, such as Wilson's disease, arteriosclerotic pseudoparkinsonism, multiple stem atrophy, and progressive supranuclear palsy.

MEDICAL MANAGEMENT

Therapy is begun with the goal of increasing dopamine levels in the brain. Because no optimal drug treatment is available for Parkinson's disease, each person is treated

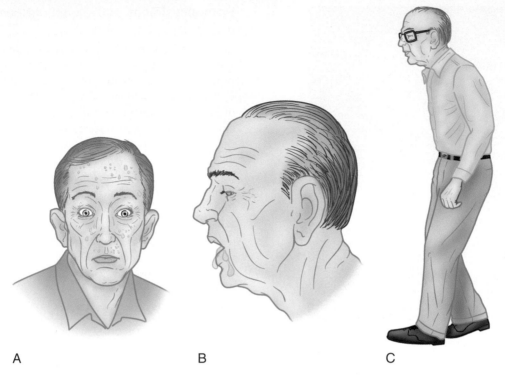

Figure 27-9. Characteristic features of Parkinson's disease. **A,** Masklike appearance, stare, and excessive sweating. **B,** Drooling with excess saliva. **C,** Gait with rapid, short, shuffling steps and reduced arm swinging. (From Seidel HM, Ball JW, Dains JE, et al. Mosby's Guide to Physical Examination, 6th ed. St. Louis, Mosby, 2006. Originally modified from Rudy EB. Advanced Neurological and Neurosurgical Nursing. St. Louis, Mosby, 1984.)

on an individual basis with a variety of drugs. The six classes of drugs used to manage the symptoms of Parkinson's disease are shown in Table 27-2.[70] Drug therapy generally is not initiated until lifestyle impairment such as slowness or imbalance occurs. Drug selection is based on anticipated adverse effects and complications and is initiated at the lowest effective dose.

The mainstay of treatment for advanced Parkinson's disease is carbidopa/levodopa (Sinemet), an immediate precursor of the neurotransmitter dopamine. Its use is generally reserved for later in the course of the disease because its activity wanes after about 5 to 10 years, and when given over the long term, it produces complicating adverse effects (dyskinesia—involuntary rapid, flowing movements of limbs, trunk, or head). Management of progressive disease requires a careful balance between the beneficial effects of Sinemet or controlled-release levodopa (Sinemet CR) and the use of adjunct medications such as (1) dopamine agonists and (2) catechol-O-methyltransferase (COMT) inhibitors (entacapone) used to diminish motor fluctuations, as well as (3) serotonin reuptake inhibitors used to manage depression and (4) acetylcholinesterase inhibitors given for dementia. Dosage adjustments are required when dyskinesias, immobility, psychosis, or other adverse effects occur. Physical therapy is important for providing patients with safe methods for rising from a chair, walking around a room, traversing stairs, and combating immobility and contractures.

If symptoms progress despite drug therapy, surgery involving replacement of dopamine neurons by grafting of fetal nerve tissue appears to be an encouraging alternative for those with advanced Parkinson's disease.[71] Newer modalities are focusing on halting neuronal loss with the use of antioxidants, or introducing (injecting) trophic factors through lentiviral delivery of a gene that encodes glial cell line–derived neurotrophic factor.[72] Deep brain stimulation of subthalamic nuclei, thalamotomy, or pallidotomy is reserved for advanced disease and severe disabling or intractable tremor.

DENTAL MANAGEMENT
Medical Considerations

The dentist who manages adult patients plays an important role in recognizing the features of Parkinson's disease and making a referral to a physician for thorough evaluation of patients who exhibit features of the disease. Once the diagnosis has been made, concerns in dental management are twofold: (1) minimizing the adverse outcomes of muscle rigidity and tremor, and (2) avoiding drug interactions.

Because the muscular defect and tremor can contribute to poor oral hygiene, the dentist should assess patients' ability to cleanse their dentition by demonstration. If a patient is unable to provide adequate home care, alternative solutions should be provided, such as the

TABLE **27-2**
Drugs Used in the Management of Parkinson's Disease

Class and Drug	Reason Used	Adverse Effects	Dental Consideration
ANTICHOLINERGIC	Blocks the effect of another brain neurotransmitter (acetylcholine) to rebalance its levels with dopamine		
Trihexyphenidyl HCl (Artane) Benztropine mesylate (Cogentin)		Sedation, urinary retention, constipation	Dry mouth
DOPAMINE PRECURSOR	Provides a drug that is metabolized into dopamine (dopamine replacement)		
Levodopa Carbidopa/levodopa (Sinemet CR, Madopar CR)		Dyskinesia, fatigue, headache, anxiety, confusion, insomnia, orthostatic hypotension	If choreiform movements, dyskinesias, or tremors present, may require sedation techniques to perform dentistry; caution when getting up from the dental chair
DOPAMINE AGONIST	Mimics the action of dopamine		
Bromocriptine mesylate (Parlodel)*		Dopaminergic effects: Psychosis (hallucinations, delusions), orthostatic hypotension, dyskinesia, nausea	Caution when getting up from the dental chair
Pramipexole (Mirapex)			Mirapex adversely interacts with erythromycin
Ropinirole HCl (Requip)			
CATECHOL-O-METHYLTRANSFERASE (COMT) INHIBITOR	Used along with levodopa. This medication blocks an enzyme (COMT), to prevent levodopa breakdown in the intestine, thus allowing more of levodopa to reach the brain		
Tolcapone (Tasmar)* Entacapone (Comtan)		Potentiate levodopa effects: Dyskinesia, psychosis, or orthostatic hypotension; nausea and diarrhea, abnormal taste	Caution with use of vasoconstrictors. Monitor vital signs during and after administration of first capsule; limit dose to 2 capsules containing 1:100,000 epinephrine (36 µg) or less, depending on vital signs and patient response; aspirate to avoid intravascular injection

TABLE **27-2**
Drugs Used in the Management of Parkinson's Disease—cont'd

Class and Drug	Reason Used	Adverse Effects	Dental Consideration
MONOAMINE OXIDASE B INHIBITOR	Prevents metabolism of dopamine within the brain		
Selegiline		Dizziness, orthostatic hypotension, nausea	Select adrenergic agents (i.e., amphetamine, pseudoephedrine, and tyramine) may cause increased pressor response. However, this does not appear to occur with epinephrine or levonordefrin
NEUROTRANSMITTER INHIBITOR	Has anticholinergic properties that enhance dopamine transmission		
Amantadine		Sedation, urinary retention, peripheral edema, nausea, constipation, confusion	

*May cause significant hepatic toxicity.
†Also has adverse vasoconstrictive properties.

introduction of the Collis curve toothbrush, mechanical toothbrushes, assisted brushing, or chlorhexidine rinses.

Drug interactions of concern to dentistry are outlined in Table 27-2. Although no adverse interactions have been reported between COMT inhibitors (tolcapone [Tasmar]; entacapone [Comtan]) and epinephrine at dosages typically used in dentistry, they can potentially interact, and it is advisable to limit the dose of epinephrine to 2 carpules containing 1:100,000 epinephrine (36 µg) in patients who take COMT inhibitors. Erythromycin should not be given to patients who take the dopamine agonist, pramipexole (Mirapex). The clinician should be aware that antiparkinsonian drugs can be CNS depressants, and a dentally prescribed sedative may have an additive effect.

Orthostatic hypotension and rigidity are common in patients who have Parkinson's disease. Orthostatic hypotension is an adverse effect associated with COMT inhibitors. To reduce the likelihood of a fall from the dental chair, the patient should be assisted to and from the chair. At the end of the appointment, the chair should be inclined slowly to allow for reequilibration.

Treatment Planning Modifications

The treatment plan for the patient with Parkinson's disease may require modification based on the patient's ability to cleanse the oral cavity. When communicating the treatment plan and other advice, the dentist should directly face the patient. This provides effective communication with a person who has the potential for cognitive impairment.

Patients should receive dental care during the time of day at which their medication has maximum effect (gen-erally, 2 to 3 hours after taking it). The presence of tremors or choreiform movements may dictate that the dentist use soft arm restraints or sedation procedures.

Oral Complications and Manifestations

Parkinson's disease is associated with staring, excess salivation and drooling, and decreased frequency of blinking and swallowing. Muscle rigidity makes repetitive muscle movement and maintenance of good oral hygiene difficult. In contrast, the drugs used to manage the disease (anticholinergics, dopaminergics, amantadine, and L-dopa) often result in xerostomia, nausea, and tardive dyskinesia. Dental recall visits should be more frequent for this population, and specific measures (specialized toothbrushes—e.g., Collis curve toothbrush, mechanical brushes) should be devised to maintain adequate oral hygiene. If the patient is experiencing xerostomia, then dysphagia and poor denture retention are likely. Salivary substitutes are beneficial in alleviating symptoms. Topical fluoride should be considered for use in dentate patients with xerostomia to prevent root caries. Personal care providers should be educated about their role in assisting and maintaining the oral hygiene of these patients.

DEMENTIA AND ALZHEIMER'S DISEASE

DEFINITION

Dementia consists of a slow, progressive, chronic decline in intellectual abilities that includes impairment in memory, abstract thinking, and judgment.[73] It is primarily a disease of aging; 1% of cases appear by age 60, and more than 40% of cases occur by age 85. Overall, the course of dementia is chronic in 65% of cases, partially treatable in 25% of cases, and reversible in only 10% of cases. The most common causes of dementia are Alzheimer's disease, vascular dementia, and dementia caused by Parkinson's disease. Other causes include hepatic encephalopathy, acid/base and electrolyte disturbances, hypoglycemia, thyroid disease (low or high), uremia, primary or metastatic brain lesions, acquired immune deficiency syndrome (AIDS), trauma, syphilis, multiple sclerosis, stroke, and drugs.

Because of its common prevalence, Alzheimer's disease serves as the prototype for a discussion of dementia in this chapter. This disease, which was first described by Alois Alzheimer in 1907, predominantly affects the elderly. However, the process may occur in younger adults as well.

EPIDEMIOLOGY

Incidence and Prevalence

Approximately 6 million to 8 million people in the United States experience dementia, and more than half of these cases are the Alzheimer's type. Alzheimer's disease occurs predominantly in persons over the age of 65 years, with about 11% of individuals over age 65 are affected. From age 70 years, prevalence doubles every 5 years. By age 85, more than 40% of individuals will have developed Alzheimer's disease.[74,75] Given the aging population in the United States, the prevalence of this disease is predicted to double by 2020. Women are at greater risk for developing the disease. An average dental practice of 2000 adult patients is predicted to include about 46 patients who experience Alzheimer's disease.

Etiology

The cause of Alzheimer's disease is unknown but appears to involve the loss of cholinergic neurons. Unidentified factors trigger the deposition of beta-amyloid plaques that initiate an inflammatory response, oxidative damage, progressive neuritic injury, and loss of cortical neurons. As a result, levels of neurotransmitters important for learning and memory decrease. Genetic predisposition contributes to less than 20% of all cases. In these cases, the disease appears to be inherited via the apolipoprotein E4 (ApoE4) allele located on chromosome 19. Three other chromosomes have been implicated to a lesser degree in the transmission of Alzheimer's disease—an amyloid precursor gene on chromosome 21, a presenilin-1 gene on chromosome 14, and a presenilin-2 gene on chromosome 1.[74,76] In as much as chromosome 21 contains a gene that expresses a cleavage product of the amyloid precursor protein, it is not surprising that adults with trisomy 21 (Down syndrome) consistently develop neuropathologic hallmarks of Alzheimer's disease if they survive beyond the age of 40 years. Numerous environmental factors such as aluminum, mercury, and viruses have been proposed as causes of Alzheimer's disease, but none has proved to play a role.[74,75] Risk factors for Alzheimer's disease comprise age, family history of dementia, and the presence of both ApoE4 alleles.[76]

Pathophysiology and Complications

Alzheimer's disease is characterized by beta-amyloid plaques and neuroinflammation that results in neurofibrillary tangles and loss of cortical neurons. The process begins in the hippocampus and the entorhinal cortex. Over time, it spreads to specific regions of the brain (temporal, parietal, and frontal lobes) that are important for learning and memory. Affected neurons make up part of the cholinergic system and use acetylcholine and glutamate as their primary neurotransmitters. These neurotransmitters are intimately involved in cognition. Progressive destruction of the neurons leads to atrophy of the cerebral cortex and enlargement of the ventricles. Motor, visual, and somatosensory portions of the cerebral cortex are typically spared. Resultant cognitive defects and associated memory loss cause significant impairment in social and occupational functioning.

CLINICAL PRESENTATION

Signs and Symptoms

The onset of Alzheimer's disease occurs subtly and insidiously; the first sign is loss of recent memory, orientation, or language, or a change in personality (apathy) or behavior. Slowly, cognitive problems at the early stage begin to interfere with daily activities such as keeping track of finances, following instructions on the job, driving, shopping, and housekeeping. Some patients remain unaware of these developing problems; others are aware of them and become frustrated and anxious. At the middle stage of the disease, the patient is unable to work, is easily lost and confused, and requires daily supervision. Patients may become lost while taking walks or driving. Social graces, routine conversation, and superficial conversation may be maintained for varying lengths of time. Language may be impaired, especially comprehension and naming of objects. Motor skills such as eating, dressing, or solving simple puzzles are eventually lost. Patients are unable to do simple calculations or to tell time. Loss of inhibitions and belligerence may occur, and nighttime wandering may become a problem with some patients. Anxiety and depression become more of a problem as the disease progresses. At the advanced stage of Alzheimer's disease, patients may become rigid, mute, incontinent, and bedridden, often requiring a nursing facility. Generalized seizures may occur. Death usually results from malnutrition, secondary infection, or heart disease. The typical duration of Alzheimer's disease is 5 to 15 years. However, the course of the illness can range from 1 to 20 years. Some patients have a steady downhill course; others may have prolonged plateaus without major deterioration.[74,75]

Laboratory Findings

Although the definitive diagnosis of Alzheimer's can be made only by brain biopsy or at autopsy, the clinical diagnosis of Alzheimer's disease can be made on the basis of patient history and clinical findings. Criteria for making this diagnosis include (1) progressive functional decline and dementia established by clinical examination and mental status testing, (2) the presence of at least two cognitive deficits, (3) normal level of consciousness at presentation, (4) onset between the ages of 40 and 90 years, and (5) absence of any other condition that could account for the deficits. The battery of tests useful in ruling out other correctable causes of dementia include a complete blood count, electrolyte panel, screening metabolic panel, thyroid function, vitamin B$_{12}$ and folate levels, tests for syphilis and human immunodeficiency virus (HIV) antibodies, urinalysis, electrocardiogram, chest radiograph, and noncontrast CT scan or MRI of the brain.

At autopsy, characteristic macroscopic changes include cerebral cortical atrophy and ventricular enlargement. Microscopic features include neurofibrillary tangles, neuritic plaques that contain beta-amyloid, and accumulation of beta-amyloid in the walls of cerebral vessels (amyloid angiopathy). On a biochemical level, a deficiency of acetylcholine and its associated enzymes exists.

MEDICAL MANAGEMENT

The management of Alzheimer's disease remains difficult. Standard medications used in the treatment of mild to moderate disease have been the cholinesterase inhibi-

tors. These drugs (donepezil [Aricept], rivastigmine [Exelon], galantamine [Reminyl], and Tacrine [Cognex]) increase acetylcholine levels in the brain by inhibiting hydrolysis of cholinesterase (Table 27-3). Clinical trials indicate that these agents perform better than placebo but have limited effectiveness in preventing disease progression and in reversing memory deficits. Less than 50% of patients appear to benefit from these medications.[76-79] Common adverse effects of the cholinesterase inhibitors include gastrointestinal disturbance and headache. Tacrine, the first of the cholinesterase inhibitors to be marketed, is infrequently prescribed today because it requires frequent dosing and can be hepatotoxic.

To slow the progression of disease, the American Academy of Neurology recommends that vitamin E be considered as an additional medication.[80] Studies have shown that vitamin E and selegiline (two antioxidants) separately delay the development of dementia in patients with Alzheimer's disease.[81]

For the management of moderate to severe Alzheimer's disease, only one medication—memantine (Axura), a N-methyl-D-aspartate (NMDA) receptor antagonist—has been approved by the U.S. Food and Drug Administration (FDA). This drug works by selectively blocking the excitotoxic effects of abnormal glutamate transmission. Initial studies suggest that it may preserve or improve memory and learning, and, when given with the cholinesterase inhibitors, appears to produce additive

TABLE 27-3
Drugs Used in the Management of Alzheimer's Disease

Class	Dental Management Considerations		Local Anesthetic/Vasoconstrictor
ACETYLCHOLINESTERASE INHIBITORS (ACHIS)			
Donepezil (Aricept)	1. Minor effect on CYP450 enzymes, with minor potential for increasing ketoconazole and erythromycin concentrations	2. Increased gastric acid secretion, which may pose greater risk for peptic ulcer in patients who take nonsteroidal anti-inflammatory drugs (NSAIDs)	No information to suggest that any special precautions are required
Galantamine (Reminyl)	1. Minor effect on CYP450 enzymes with minor potential for increasing ketoconazole, floxacin, and erythromycin concentrations	2. Increased gastric acid secretion, which may pose greater risk for peptic ulcer in those on NSAIDs	No information to suggest that any special precautions are required
Rivastigmine (Exelon)	—	Increased gastric acid secretion, which may pose greater risk for peptic ulcer in those on NSAIDs	No information to suggest that any special precautions are required
Tacrine (Cognex)	Greater effect on CYP450 enzymes than other AChIs. Potential for increasing concentrations of ketoconazole, floxacin, and erythromycin. Potentially hepatotoxic	Not commonly prescribed	No information to suggest that any special precautions are required

beneficial effects.[82,83] Memantine-related adverse effects are mild and include headache and confusion.

Noncognitive symptoms of Alzheimer's disease are manageable. Although efforts are made to use nonpharmacologic approaches to manage symptoms such as anxiety, depression, irritability, and sleep disturbances, medications inevitably are generally required. Antidepressants, sedative-hypnotics, and antipsychiatric agents are all used, with varying degrees of success. A small percentage of patients experience seizures and are treated with standard anticonvulsants.[74,75] Nursing home care is often provided during the latter stages of the disease.

DENTAL MANAGEMENT

Medical Considerations

Dental management requires knowledge of the stage of disease, medications taken, and the cognitive abilities of the patient. Patients with mild to moderate disease generally maintain normal systemic organ function and can receive routine dental treatment. As the disease progresses, antipsychotics, antidepressants, and anxiolytics are used frequently for behavioral disturbances. These medications contribute to xerostomia and increased risk for dental caries. Drug interactions associated with medications used in the management of Alzheimer's disease are listed in Box 27-3.

Treatment Planning Considerations

Patients with Alzheimer's are managed best through an understanding and empathetic approach. The dental team should communicate to the patient and family members a positive, hopeful attitude toward maintenance of the patient's oral health. The dental team should determine whether the patient is legally able to make rational decisions. This should be discussed with the patient and a loved one. Treatment planning often involves input and permission from a loved one, so that decisions can be made. A patient's attention should be sustained, and the dentist should explain what is going to happen before initiating treatment. The dentist should communicate using short words and sentences and should repeat instructions and explanations. Nonverbal communication can be very helpful. Facial motion and body posture of the dentist should show support—cues that the patient is understood and that the dentist cares for the patient. Positive nonverbal communication includes direct eye contact, smiling, touching the patient on the arm, and so forth. Patients with Alzheimer's disease should be placed on an aggressive preventive dentistry program, including 3-month recall, oral examination, prophylaxis, fluoride gel application, oral hygiene education, and adjustment of prostheses.[84-86]

In a patient with mild dementia, good oral health should be quickly restored because of the progressive nature of the disease. Subsequent care should concentrate on preventing dental disease as dementia progresses. A patient with moderate dementia may not be as amenable to dental treatment as a patient in earlier stages of the disease. For such patients, treatment consists of maintaining dental status and minimizing deterioration. Complex dental procedures should be performed, if at all, in such a patient before the disease has reached the moderate to advanced stage.

Patients with advanced dementia often are anxious, hostile, and uncooperative in the dental office and very difficult to treat. These patients likely require short appointments and noncomplex procedures, or sedation for more complex and tedious procedures. Sedative medication should be selected in consultation with the patient's physician. Chloral hydrate and benzodiazepines can be used to provide the level of sedation required for performance of routine dental procedures.

In advanced cases, removable prosthetic devices may have to be taken from the patient because of the danger of self-injury. All treatment should be provided with the knowledge that these patients have memory loss, lack of drive, and slowed thinking. Thus, their ability to maintain proper daily oral hygiene can become severely compromised.

Oral Complications and Manifestations

Patients with moderate to severe Alzheimer's disease may not have an interest in caring for themselves, and they may lack the ability to do so. Hence, oral hygiene is poor, and dental problems are increased. Most of the medications used to treat psychiatric disorders contribute to increased dental problems in such patients because xerostomia is one of their primary adverse effects. Patients with Alzheimer's disease have a greater incidence of dry mouth, mucosal lesions, candidiasis, plaque and calculus buildup, periodontal disease, and smooth surface (root) and coronal caries, along with an increased risk for aspiration pneumonia.[84-86] They often sustain oral injuries from falls and ulcerations of the tongue, cheeks, and alveolar mucosa as the result of accidents with forks or spoons, mastication, attrition and abrasion of teeth, missing teeth, and migration of teeth.[74] Edentulous patients with dementia may misplace or lose their dentures and at times may even attempt to wear the upper denture on the lower arch and vice versa.[85,86]

Antipsychotic drugs sometimes taken by these patients can cause agranulocytosis, leukopenia, or thrombocytopenia. Additional adverse effects of antipsychotic agents include muscular problems such as dystonia, dyskinesia, or tardive dyskinesia in the oral and facial regions.[86]

MULTIPLE SCLEROSIS
DEFINITION

Multiple sclerosis is the most common autoimmune disease of the nervous system. It is characterized by chronic and continuous demyelination of the corticospinal tract neurons in two or more regions of the brain; 85% of patients present with relapsing and remitting

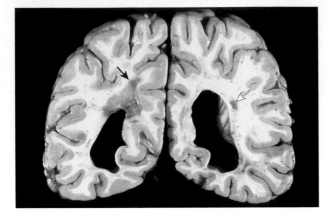

Figure 27-10. Multiple sclerosis. Large periventricular "demyelinated plaque" (*dark region above left ventricle, black arrow*) and smaller "demyelinated plaque" (*white arrow*) lateral to right ventricle shown in a coronal section of the brain of a patient who had multiple sclerosis. (Courtesy Daron G. Davis, Lexington, Ky.)

symptoms.[87] Demyelinated regions are limited to the white matter of the CNS and are randomly located and multiple (Figure 27-10). The peripheral nervous system is not affected.

EPIDEMIOLOGY

Incidence and Prevalence

Approximately 380,000 persons in the United States have multiple sclerosis; this represents a prevalence of about 1 per 850 persons.[76] The incidence of multiple sclerosis has been increasing during the past century. The disease affects young adults between 15 and 50 years of age, and women twice as often as men. Its prevalence is highest in the temperate regions of the world (i.e., northern and southern latitudes), and it is infrequently seen along the equator.[88] Dentists who manage 2000 adult patients can expect to have about 3 patients in their practice in whom this condition has been diagnosed.

Etiology

Multiple sclerosis involves autoimmune-mediated inflammation that leads to demyelination and axonal injury. The cause of multiple sclerosis remains unknown; however, it is widely held that the disease is triggered by an infectious agent. Initial support for this arises from cluster studies of multiple sclerosis outbreaks in small regions.[88] Over the past century, several microbes (e.g., rabies, measles, herpes viruses, *Chlamydia pneumoniae*) have been purported to be associated with multiple sclerosis. In recent years, human herpes virus type 6 has been identified in active demyelinated regions of the CNS in patients who have MS.[89,90] It is hypothesized that this neurotropic virus in combination with host genetic factors results in processes that cause immune-mediated attacks on myelin. However, not all persons who are infected with human herpes virus type 6 develop multiple sclerosis, suggesting that genetic factors and other environ-

mental factors are also important. Consistent with the role of genetic factor involvement, the concordance rate among monozygotic twins is 30%.[91,92] Risk is increased when human leukocyte antigen DR2 is carried by a northern European.[93]

Pathophysiology and Complications

Demyelination of multiple sclerosis occurs in scattered white matter regions in the brain. Myelin loss ranges in size from 1 mm to several centimeters in diameter. Affected regions show inflammatory demyelination and axonal damage with accumulation of macrophages, B and T lymphocytes, and plasma cells. Specifically, myelin-reactive type 1 helper T cells (T_h1) that produce lymphotoxin and interferon-gamma, but little interleukin 4 (IL-4), appear central to the pathogenesis of this disease.[94] As a result, inflammatory cytokines and antimyelin immunoglobulins accompany the acute multiple sclerosis lesion and influence macrophages to attack myelin. This results in tissue destruction, swelling, and breakdown of the blood–brain barrier.[95] Demyelinated disease areas or "plaques" are impaired in axonal conduction, thus producing the pathophysiologic defect. The most common demyelinated regions are the optic nerve, periventricular cerebral white matter, and cervical spinal cord.

A significant complication of the axonal damage associated with multiple sclerosis is that 50% of patients need help to walk within 15 years of onset of the disease.[96] Continued muscle atrophy can cause restriction to a wheelchair or a bed, thus increasing the chances for development of pneumonia. The life expectancy for patients with multiple sclerosis is calculated to be 82.5% of normal (approximately 58 years).[97]

CLINICAL PRESENTATION

Signs and Symptoms

The first clinical signs of multiple sclerosis often begin in young adulthood. Clinical signs vary according to which region of the CNS is involved (motor or sensory region) and what degree of disruption occurs in the myelin sheath. Disturbance in visual function (sometimes resulting in blindness) and abnormal eye movements (nystagmus and double vision) are the most common presenting symptoms. Motor disturbances that affect walking and use of the hands (incoordination, spasticity, difficulty in walking, loss of balance and vertigo, coordination or weakness, tremor or paralysis of a limb) and that cause bowel and bladder incontinence, spastic paresis of skeletal muscles (imprecise speech or tremor), and sensory disturbances, including loss of touch, pain, temperature, and proprioception (numbness, pins and needles sensations), are common. Fatigue is a major symptom (occurring in up to 90%), and worsening fatigue occurs in the afternoon. Symptoms are exacerbated by heat (hot baths, sun exposure) and dehydration and generally appear over a few days before stabilizing and improving a few weeks later. Problems with concentration also occur.

A typical presentation consists of attacks and relapses that recur for several years. The course is unpredictable and depends on the frequency of attacks and the extent of recovery. Four categories have been used to describe the course of the disease: relapsing-remitting (occurs in 85% of patients), primary progressive, secondary progressive, and progressive-relapsing. Recovery in most cases is temporary because remyelination is only transient. Repeated attacks can cause permanent physical damage; however, intellectual function remains intact. Depression and emotional instability are features that commonly accompany this disease.

Laboratory Findings

The diagnosis of multiple sclerosis usually is made on the basis of information derived from the history, clinical examination, CSF, sensory evoked potential, and magnetic resonance imaging (MRI) performed over time. Relapsing-remitting multiple sclerosis is diagnosed when two or more clinical attacks occur in a patient who has two or more affected CNS locations, or an MRI lesion newly appears after a second clinical attack.[98] The disease is also diagnosed after one clinical attack when a new MRI lesion appears. MRI scans typically reveal multiple hypodense demyelinated regions (plaques) in white matter, usually near the ventricles (see Figure 27-10), brainstem cerebellum, and optic nerves.[99] The CSF shows signs of low-grade inflammation, and protein and immunoglobulin levels are increased in 80% to 90% of patients. Antibodies to myelin basic protein can also be detected in the CSF. Myelin destruction causes slowing of conduction velocity. The conduction response to visual stimuli (visual evoked potential) or to somatosensory evoked stimuli is usually delayed and altered in amplitude.

MEDICAL MANAGEMENT

Patients who have relapses of multiple sclerosis are given anti-inflammatory medications in the form of intravenous corticosteroids (methylprednisolone) for acute attacks, interferon beta-1a (Avonex), or interferon beta-1b (Betaseron) injections.[99] The interferons reduce antigen presentation, proliferation of T cells, and production of tumor necrosis factor and have been shown to slow the progression of disease (Table 27-4). Corticosteroids have many anti-inflammatory functions, including the ability to block eicosanoid and cytokine release, and endothelial cell expression of intracellular and extracellular adhesion molecules (ICAMs and ELAMs, respectively) that attract neutrophils. Interferons and glatiramer acetate (Copaxone), a myelin-like polypeptide that suppresses T-cell attacks on the myelin sheath, are used during periods of remission to reduce the rate of clinical relapse.[99,100] Mitoxantrone, an antineoplastic medication that arrests cell cycle and reduces T_h1 cytokines, is reserved for patients who have aggressive disease and whose symptoms are worsening despite therapy. It is used on a short-term basis with Copaxone. However, mitoxantrone use is associated with cardiac complications and risk for leukemia.[101]

Many complications of multiple sclerosis require management with several drugs. Spasticity is managed with antispastic drugs such as baclofen (GABA agonist), benzodiazepines (GABA receptor activator), dantrolene (modifier of calcium release in muscle fibers), and tizanidine (Zanaflex; alpha$_2$-adrenergic agonist). An implantable pump for intrathecal administration of baclofen sometimes is used. Poor bladder control is managed with anticholinergics such as oxybutynin (Ditropan) or tolterodine tartrate (Detrol). Fatigue is managed with afternoon naps, exercise, and amantidine (Symmetrel) or modafinil. Paroxysmal events respond to carbamazepine, phenytoin, gabapentin, and pergolide. Serotonin reuptake inhibitors (fluoxetine [Prozac]) and tricyclic antidepressants are used to manage the depression that accompanies multiple sclerosis in about 50% of patients. Associated conditions (e.g., trigeminal neuralgia, headache, optic neuritis) are often managed by experts in chronic pain clinics.

DENTAL MANAGEMENT

Medical Considerations

The dentist can play an important role in directing the patient whose multiple sclerosis remains undiagnosed to

---

TABLE 27-4

Drugs Used in the Management of Multiple Sclerosis

Class (Drug)	Dental Management Consideration	Local Anesthetic/Vasoconstrictor
PRIMARY DRUGS		
Interferon (IFN)-β-1a (Avonex, Rebif) Injection	Transient flulike symptoms, anemia uncommon; may increase anticoagulant effects of warfarin	No information to suggest that any special precautions are required
IFN-β-1b (Betaseron) Injection	Transient flulike symptoms, anemia uncommon	No information to suggest that any special precautions are required
ALTERNATIVES		
Glatiramer acetate (Copaxone) Injection	Ulcerative stomatitis, lymphadenopathy, and salivary gland enlargement	No information to suggest that any special precautions are required
Mitoxantron (Vovantrone) Infusion	Leukopenia, risk for cardiac complications and leukemia, mucositis, and stomatitis	No information to suggest that any special precautions are required

the appropriate health care provider for diagnosis. Reports of abnormal facial pain (mimicking trigeminal neuralgia), numbness of an extremity, visual disturbance, or muscle weakness require the dentist to perform a neuromuscular examination to rule out multiple sclerosis. The disease should be suspected if onset is progressive over several days, the patient is between 20 and 35 years old, and afternoon fatigue is present. Referral to a neurologist is the next step in confirming the diagnosis.

Patients who experience relapse are unfit for routine dental care. Emergency dental care can be provided but is affected by the medications the patient takes. In particular, corticosteroids are immunosuppressive, and during stressful surgical procedures, the patient may require an increase in dose (see Chapter 16). The physician should be consulted before emergency dental care is provided to these patients.

The optimal time for treating patients with multiple sclerosis is during periods of remission. Dental care should be provided with the understanding that the medications these patients take can affect the practice of dentistry. In particular, the anticholinergics (oxybutynin [Ditropan], tolterodine tartrate [Detrol]) and tricyclic antidepressants can cause a dry or burning mouth that may require the use of salivary substitutes for relief. If additional relief is needed, the use of pilocarpine (see Appendix C) should be discussed with the physician.

Treatment Planning Modifications

Treatment planning changes are dictated by levels of motor impairment and fatigue. Patients with stable disease and little motor spasticity or weakness can receive routine dental care. Patients with more advanced disease may require help in transferring to and from the dental chair, may have difficulty maintaining oral hygiene, and may be poor candidates for reconstructive and prosthetic procedures. Because fatigue is often worse in the afternoon, short morning appointments are advised.

Oral Complications and Manifestations

Oral manifestations of multiple sclerosis are reported to occur in 2% to 3% of those affected. These features may serve as the first presenting symptoms of multiple sclerosis. The most common features include dysarthria, paresthesia, numbness of the orofacial structures, and trigeminal neuralgia. Dysarthria produces slow, irregular speech with unusual separation of syllables of words, referred to as *scanning speech*. During an attack, a patient's face may develop paresthesia, and muscles of facial expression (especially the periorbital) can undulate in the manner of waves. The term *myokymia* is used to describe the unusual muscle movement that resembles movement of a "bag of worms." Referral to a physician is advised if the condition has not been diagnosed.

Trigeminal neuralgia is 400 times more likely among individuals with multiple sclerosis than among the general population.[102] Relief of trigeminal neuralgic pain can be attained through the use of carbamazepine, clonazepam, amitriptyline, or surgery.

CEREBROSPINAL FLUID SHUNTS

Within the spectrum of neurologic disorders is the condition known as *hydrocephalus*, a disorder that is characterized by an increasing accumulation of CSF within the cerebral ventricles. This condition often requires placement of a shunt within cerebral ventricles and peripheral cavities to reduce increased cerebrospinal fluid pressure. Several types of shunts are used to reduce fluid pressure. Ventriculoperitoneal, ventriculoatrial, and lumboperitoneal are the most common types of shunts.[103-105] In the United States, around 75,000 cerebrospinal fluid shunts are placed each year.[106]

With respect to dentistry, the most significant concern is the risk of CSF shunt infection. Overall, shunt infection rates range from about 5% to 15%, with most infections resulting from wound contamination.[107] Almost 70% of infections are caused by skin flora staphylococcal organisms.[107] Cerebrospinal fluid shunt infections usually occur within 2 months after implantation.[108] The infection rate is higher for ventriculoperitoneal shunts than for ventriculoatrial shunts. However, other types of complications include thromboemboli, severe complications of infection, and shunt malfunctions.[103,105]

CSF shunts do not appear to increase the risk for infection produced by hematogenous seeding of bacteria after dental procedures.[103-105] Thus, the American Heart Association has issued a statement indicating that antibiotic prophylaxis is not recommended for patients with CSF shunts who are undergoing dental procedures.[109]

REFERENCES

1. Griggs RC. Epilepsy. In Goldman L, Ausiello D (eds). Cecil Textbook of Medicine, 22nd ed. St. Louis, Elsevier, 2004.
2. Commission on Classification and Terminology of the International League Against Epilepsy. Proposal for revised clinical and electroencephalographic classification of epileptic seizures. Epilepsia 1981;22:489-501.
3. Sander JW, Hart WM, Johnson AL, Shorvon SD. National General Practice Study of Epilepsy: Newly diagnosed epileptic seizures in a general population. Lancet 1990;336:1267-1271.
4. de la Court A, Breteler MM, Meinardi H, et al. Prevalence of epilepsy in the elderly: The Rotterdam study. Epilepsia 1996;37:141-147.
5. Dalquist N, Mellinger J, Klass D. Hazard of video games in patients with light-sensitive epilepsy. JAMA 1983;249:776-777.
6. Lowenstein DH. Seizures and epilepsy. In Kasper DL, Harrison DR (eds). Harrison's Principles of Internal Medicine, 16th ed. New York, McGraw-Hill, 2005.
7. Dichter M, Brodie M. New antiepileptic drugs. N Engl J Med 1996;334:1583-1590.

8. Sperling MR, Feldman H, Kinman J, et al. Seizure control and mortality in epilepsy. Ann Neurol 1999;46:45-50.

9. Guerrini R. Epilepsy in children. Lancet 2006;367:499-524.

10. Camfield P, Camfield C. Management guidelines for children with idiopathic generalized epilepsy. Epilepsia 2005;46(suppl 9):112-116.

11. Greenwood RS. Adverse effects of antiepileptic drugs. Epilepsia 2000;41(suppl 2):S42-S52.

12. George MS, Sackeim HA, Rush AJ, et al. Vagus nerve stimulation: A new tool for brain research and therapy. Biol Psychiatry 2000;47:287-295.

13. Drug Information for the Health Care Professional. Taunton, Mass, Thomson Micromedex, 2006.

14. Hassell TM, White GC 2nd, Jewson LG, Peele LC 3rd. Valproic acid: A new antiepileptic drug with potential side effects of dental concern. J Am Dent Assoc 1979;9:983-987.

15. Starreveld E, Starreveld A. Status epilepticus: Current concepts and management. Can Fam Physician 2000;46:1817-1823.

16. Leppik IE, Derivan AT, Homan RW, et al. Double-blind study of lorazepam and diazepam in status epilepticus. JAMA 1983;249:1452-1454.

17. Syrjanen S, Syrjanen K. Hyperplastic gingivitis in a child receiving sodium valproate treatment. Proc Finn Dent Soc 1979;75:95-98.

18. Anderson H, Rapley J, Williams D. Gingival overgrowth with valproic acid: A case report. J Dent Child 1997;64:294-297.

19. Katz J, Givol N, Chaushu G, et al. Vigabatrin-induced gingival overgrowth. J Clin Periodontol 1997;24:180-182.

20. Hassell T. Epilepsy and the oral manifestations of phenytoin therapy. In Myers H (ed). Monographs in Oral Science. Basel, S Karger, 1981.

21. Hall W. Dilantin hyperplasia: A preventable lesion? Compendium 1990;14(suppl):S502-S505.

22. Handin RI. Bleeding and thrombosis. In Kasper DL, Harrison DR (eds). Harrison's Principles of Internal Medicine, 16th ed. New York, McGraw-Hill, 2005.

23. Philstrom B. Prevention and treatment of dilantin-associated gingival enlargement. Compendium 1990;14(suppl):S506-S510.

24. Ryan M, Baumann RJ, Miller CS, Baker C. Valproate-associated stomatitis. J Child Neurol 2002;17:225-227.

25. Rzany B, Correia O, Kelly JP, et al. Risk of Stevens-Johnson syndrome and toxic epidermal necrolysis during first weeks of antiepileptic therapy: A case-control study. Study Group of the International Case Control Study on Severe Cutaneous Adverse Reactions. Lancet 1999;353:2190-2194.

26. American Heart Association. Heart Disease and Stroke Statistics, 2005 Update. Dallas, Tex, American Heart Association, 2005. Available at: http://www.americanheart.org/presenter.jhtml?identifier=2007

27. Rosamond WD, Folsom AR, Chambless LE, et al. Stroke incidence and survival among middle-aged adults: 9-Year follow-up of the atherosclerosis risk in communities (ARIC) cohort. Stroke 1999;30:736-743.

28. Centers for Disease Control and Prevention. Age-specific excess deaths associated with stroke among racial/ethnic minority populations—United States, 1997. MMWR 2000;49:94-97.

29. Feigin VL, Lawes CM, Bennett DA, Anderson CS. Stroke epidemiology: A review of population-based studies of incidence, prevalence, and case-fatality in the late 20th century. Lancet Neurol 2003;2:43-53.

30. Gillman MW, Cupples LA, Millen BE, et al. Inverse association of dietary fat with development of ischemic stroke in men. JAMA 1997;278:2145-2150.

31. Bostom AG, Rosenberg IH, Silbershatz H, et al. Non-fasting plasma total homocysteine levels and stroke incidence in elderly persons: The Framingham study. Ann Intern Med 1999;131:352-355.

32. Wu T, Trevisan M, Genco RJ, et al. Periodontal disease and risk of cerebrovascular disease: The First National Health and Nutrition Examination Survey and its follow-up study. Arch Intern Med 2000;160:2749-2755.

33. Kernan WN, Viscoli CM, Brass LM, et al. Phenylpropanolamine and the risk of hemorrhagic stroke. N Engl J Med 2000;343:1826-1832.

34. Abramowicz M (ed). Phenylpropanolamine and Other OTC Alpha-Adrenergic Agonists, vol 42. New Rochelle, NY, The Medical Letter, Inc., 2000.

35. Gillman MW, Cupples LA, Gagnon D, et al. Protective effect of fruits and vegetables on development of stroke in men. JAMA 1995;273:1113-1117.

36. Kiely D, Wolf PA, Cupples LA, et al. Physical activity and stroke risk: The Framingham study. Am J Epidemiol 1994;140:608-620.

37. Li Y, Chopp M, Jiang N, et al. Temporal profile of in situ DNA fragmentation after transient middle cerebral artery occlusion in the rat. J Cereb Blood Flow Metab 1995;15:389-397.

38. Ostuni E. Stroke and the dental patient. J Am Dent Assoc 1994;125:721-727.

39. Wolf PA, D'Agostino RB, Belanger AJ, Kannel WB. Probability of stroke: A risk profile from the Framingham study. Stroke 1991;22:312-318.

40. Smith WS, Johnstone SC, Easton JD. Cerebrovascular diseases. In Kasper DL, Harrison DR (eds). Harrison's Principles of Internal Medicine, 16th ed. New York, McGraw-Hill, 2005.

41. Kase CS, Wolf PA, Kelly-Hayes M, et al. Intellectual decline after stroke: The Framingham study. Stroke 1998;29:805-812.

42. Lawes CM. Blood pressure and stroke: An overview of published reviews. Stroke 2004;35:776-785.

43. Tonarelli SB, Hart RG. What's new in stroke? The top 10 for 2004/05. J Am Geriatr Soc 2006;54:674-679.

44. Furlan A, Higashida R, Wechsler L, et al. Intra-arterial prourokinase for acute ischemic stroke. The PROACT II study: A randomized controlled trial. Prolyse in Acute Cerebral Thromboembolism. JAMA 1999;282:2003-2011.

45. The National Institute of Neurological Disorders and Stroke rt-PA Stroke Study Group. Tissue plasminogen activator for acute ischemic stroke. N Engl J Med 1995;333:1581-1587.

46. Caplan L. Tissue plasminogen activator for acute ischemic stroke. N Engl J Med 1999;341:1240-1241.

47. Albers GW, Bates VE, Clark WM, et al. Intravenous tissue-type plasminogen activator for treatment of acute stroke: The Standard Treatment with Activase to Reverse Stroke (STARS) study. JAMA 2000;283:1145-1150.

48. Gage BF, Waterman AD, Shannon W, et al. Validation of clinical classification schemes for predicting stroke: Results from the National Registry of Atrial Fibrillation. JAMA 2001;285:2864-2870.

49. Fatahzadeh M, Glick M. Stroke: Epidemiology, classification, risk factors, complications, diagnosis, prevention, and medical and dental management. Oral Surg Oral Med Oral Pathol Oral Radiol Endod 2006;102:180-191.

50. Wahl M. Myths of dental surgery in patients receiving anticoagulant therapy. J Am Dent Assoc 2000;131:77-81.

51. Rice PJ, Perry RJ, Afzal Z, Stockley IH. Antibacterial prescribing and warfarin: A review. Br Dent J 2003;194:411-415.

52. Niwa H, Satoh Y, Matsuura H. Cardiovascular responses to epinephrine-containing local anesthetics for dental use: A comparison of hemodynamic responses to infiltration anesthesia and ergometer-stress testing. Oral Surg Oral Med Oral Pathol Oral Radiol Endod 2000;90:171-181.

53. Furlan AJ, Higashida R, Wechsler L, et al. PROACT II: Recombinant prourokinase (r-ProUK) in acute cerebral thromboembolism: Initial trial results. Stroke 1999;30:234.

54. Hacke W, Donnan G, Fieschi C, et al. Association of outcome with early stroke treatment: Pooled analysis of ATLANTIS, ECASS, and NINDS rt-PA stroke trials. Lancet 2005;363:768-774.

55. Friedlander A, Baker J. Panoramic radiography: An aid in detecting patients at risk of cerebrovascular accident. J Am Dent Assoc 1994;125:1598-1603.

56. Friedlander A, Friedlander I. Identification of stroke prone patients by panoramic radiography. Aust Dent J 1998;43:51-54.

57. Carter LC, Haller AD, Nadarajah V, et al. Use of panoramic radiography among an ambulatory dental population to detect patients at risk of stroke. J Am Dent Assoc 1997;128:977-984.

58. Joshipura KJ, Hung HC, Rimm EB, et al. Periodontal disease, tooth loss, and incidence of ischemic stroke. Stroke 2003;34:47-52.

59. D'Aiuto F, Casas JP, Shah T, et al. C-reactive protein (+1444C>T) polymorphism influences CRP response following a moderate inflammatory stimulus. Atherosclerosis 2005;179:413-417.

60. D'Aiuto F, Parkar M, Andreou G, et al. Periodontitis and systemic inflammation: Control of the local infection is associated with a reduction in serum inflammatory markers. J Dent Res 2004;83:156-160.

61. Dietrich T, Garcia RI. Associations between periodontal disease and systemic disease: Evaluating the strength of the evidence. J Periodontol 2005;76:2175-2184.

62. Parkinson J. An Essay on Shaking Palsy. London, Sherwood Neely and Jones, 1817.

63. Ebadi M, Pfeifer RF (eds). Parkinson's Disease. Boca Raton, Fla, CRC Press, 2005.

64. Tanner C, Ben-Shlomo Y. Epidemiology of Parkinson's disease. Adv Neurol 1999;30:153-159.

65. Eriksen JL, Wszolek Z, Petrucelli L. Molecular pathogenesis of Parkinson disease. Arch Neurol 2005;62:353-357.

66. Hughes A, Daniel SE, Kilford L, Lees AJ. Accuracy of clinical diagnosis of idiopathic Parkinson's disease: A clinico-pathological study of 100 cases. J Neurol Neurosurg Psychiatry 1992;55:181-184.

67. Braak H, Braak E. Pathoanatomy of Parkinson's disease. J Neurol 2000;247(suppl 2):II3-II110.

68. Marsh L. Neuropsychiatric aspects of Parkinson's disease. Psychosomatics 2000;41:15-23.

69. Weintraub D, Stern MB. Psychiatric complications in Parkinson disease. Am J Geriatr Psychiatry 2005;13:844-951.

70. Marshall FJ. Disorders of the motor system. In Goldman L, Ausiello D (eds). Cecil Textbook of Medicine, 22nd ed. St. Louis, Elsevier, 2004.

71. Hallett M, Litvan I. Evaluation of surgery for Parkinson's disease: A report of the Therapeutics and Technology Assessment Subcommittee of the American Academy of Neurology. The Task Force on Surgery for Parkinson's Disease. Neurology 1999;53:1910-1921.

72. Kordower JH, Emborg ME, Bloch J, et al. Neurodegeneration prevented by lentiviral vector delivery of GDNF in primate models of Parkinson's disease. Science 2000;290:767-773.

73. First MB, Tasman A (eds). DSM-IV-TR Mental Disorders: Diagnosis, Etiology, and Treatment. Hoboken, NJ, Wiley, 2004.

74. Bird TD, Miller BL. Alzheimer's disease and other dementias. In Kasper DL, Harrison DR (eds). Harrison's Principles of Internal Medicine, 16th ed. New York, McGraw-Hill, 2005.

75. Feinstein RE. Cognitive and mental disorders due to general medical conditions. In Cutler JL, Marcus ER (eds). Saunders Text and Review Series: Psychiatry. Philadelphia, WB Saunders, 1999.

76. Connelly PJ, James R. SIGN guideline for the management of patients with dementia. Int J Geriatr Psychiatry 2006;21:14-16.

77. Zimmermann M, Gardoni F, Di Luca M. Molecular rationale for the pharmacological treatment of Alzheimer's disease. Drugs Aging 2005;22(suppl 1):27-37.

78. Rogers SL, Farlow MR, Doody RS, et al. A 24-week, double-blind, placebo-controlled trial of donepezil in patients with Alzheimer's disease. Donepezil Study Group. Neurology 1998;50:136-145.

79. Wilkinson DG, Francis PT, Schwam E, Payne-Parrish J. Cholinesterase inhibitors used in the treatment of Alzheimer's disease: The relationship between pharmacological effects and clinical efficacy. Drugs Aging 2004;21:453-478.

80. Doody RS, Stevens JC, Beck C, et al. Practice parameter: Management of dementia (an evidence-based review). Report of the Quality Standards Subcommittee of the American Academy of Neurology. Neurology 2001;56:1154-1166.

81. Sano M, Ernesto C, Thomas RG, et al. A controlled trial of selegiline, alpha-tocopherol, or both as treat-

ment for Alzheimer's disease. The Alzheimer's Disease Cooperative Study. N Engl J Med 1997;336:1216-1222.

82. Doody RS. Refining treatment guidelines in Alzheimer's disease. Geriatrics 2005;(suppl):14-20.

83. Hartmann S, Mobius HJ. Tolerability of memantine in combination with cholinesterase inhibitors in dementia therapy. Int Clin Psychopharmacol 2003;18:81-85.

84. Rejnefelt I, Andersson P, Renvert S. Oral health status in individuals with dementia living in special facilities. Int J Dent Hyg 2006;4:67-71.

85. Steinberg BJ, Brown S. Dental treatment of the health compromised elderly: Medical and psychological considerations. Alpha Omegan 1986;79:34-41.

86. Friedlander AH, Jarvik LF. The dental management of the patient with dementia. Oral Surg 1987;64:549-553.

87. Murray TJ. Diagnosis and treatment of multiple sclerosis. BMJ 2006;332:525-527.

88. Ebers G, Sadovnick A. The geographic distribution of multiple sclerosis: A review. Neuroepidemiology 1993;12:1-5.

89. Griggs RC. Demyelingating and inflammatory disorders. In Goldman L, Ausiello D (eds). Cecil Textbook of Medicine, 22nd ed. St. Louis, Elsevier, 2004.

90. Knox KK, Brewer JH, Henry JM, et al. Human herpesvirus 6 and multiple sclerosis: Systemic active infections in patients with early disease. Clin Infect Dis 2000;31:894-903.

91. Ebers GC, Bulman DE, Sadovnick AD, et al. A population based study of multiple sclerosis in twins. N Engl J Med 1986;315:1638-1642.

92. Ebers GC, Sadovnick AD, Risch NJ. A genetic basis for familial aggregation in multiple sclerosis. Nature 1995;377:150-151.

93. Altmann D, Sansom D, Marsh S. What is the basis for HLA-DQ associations with autoimmune disease? Immunol Today 1991;12:267-270.

94. Frohman EM, Racke MK, Raine CS. Multiple sclerosis—The plaque and its pathogenesis. N Engl J Med 2006;354:942-955.

95. Steinman L. Multiple sclerosis: A coordinated immunological attack against myelin in the central nervous system. Cell 1996;85:299-302.

96. Weinshenker BG, Bass B, Rice GP, et al. The natural history of multiple sclerosis: A geographically based study. I. Clinical course and disability. Brain 1989;112:133-146.

97. National Center for Health Statistics: Vital Statistics of the U.S. 1992–Mortality. Washington, DC, U.S. Department of Health and Human Services, U.S. Government Printing Office, 1996.

98. Birnbaum G. Making the diagnosis of multiple sclerosis. Adv Neurol 2006;98:111-124.

99. Noseworthy JH, Lucchinetti C, Rodriguez M, Weinshenker BG. Multiple sclerosis. N Engl J Med 2000;343:938-952.

100. Fox RJ, Bethoux F, Goldman MD, Cohen JA. Multiple sclerosis: Advances in understanding, diagnosing, and treating the underlying disease. Cleve Clin J Med 2006;73:91-102.

101. Murray TJ. Diagnosis and treatment of multiple sclerosis. BMJ 2006;332:525-527.

102. Maloni HW. Pain in multiple sclerosis: An overview of its nature and management. J Neurosci Nurs 2000;32:139-144,152.

103. Fan-Havard P, Nahata MC. Treatment and prevention of infections of cerebrospinal fluid shunts. Clin Pharm 1987;6:866-880.

104. Fernell E, von Wendt L, Serlo W, et al. Ventriculoatrial or ventriculoperitoneal shunts in the treatment of hydrocephalus in children. Z Kinderchir 1985;40:12-14.

105. Gardner P, Leipzig T, Sadigh M. Infections of mechanical cerebrospinal fluid shunts. Curr Clin Top Infect Dis 1989;9:185-214.

106. Sugarman B, Young E. Infections associated with prosthetic devices: Magnitude of the problem. Infect Dis Clin North Am 1989;3:187-198.

107. Drucker MH, Vanek WW, Franco AA, et al. Thromboembolic complications of ventriculoatrial shunts. Surg Neurol 1984;22:444-448.

108. Aoki N. Lumboperitoneal shunt: Clinical applications, complications and comparison with ventriculoperitoneal shunt. Neurosurgery 1990;26:998-1003.

109. Baddour LM, Bettmann MA, Bolger AF, et al. Nonvalvular cardiovascular device–related infections. Circulation 2003;108:2015-2031.

Behavioral and Psychiatric Disorders (Anxiety, Delirium, and Eating Disorders)

CHAPTER 28

Problems may be encountered in dental practice that stem from a patient's behavioral patterns rather than from physical conditions. A good dentist/patient relationship can reduce the number of behavioral problems encountered in practice and can modify the intensity of emotional reactions. A positive dentist/patient relationship is based on mutual respect, trust, understanding, cooperation, and empathy. Role conflicts between the dentist and the patient should be avoided or should be identified and dealt with effectively. The anxious patient should be offered support that minimizes the damaging effects of anxiety, and the angry or uncooperative patient should be accepted and encouraged to share reasons for feelings and behavior, thus becoming a more peaceful and cooperative individual. Patients with emotional factors that contribute to oral or systemic diseases or symptoms and patients with more serious mental disorders can be managed in an understanding, safe, and empathetic manner.

The dentist may treat patients with a variety of behavioral and mental disorders. The fourth edition of *Diagnostic and Statistical Manual of Mental Disorders* (DSM-IV)[1] and the fourth edition of *Diagnostic and Statistical Manual of Mental Disorders, Text Revision* (DSM-IV-TR)[2] present a classification system with which the dentist should be familiar to be better able to understand psychiatric diagnoses and associated symptoms. This system consists of five axes (axis I through axis V), or categories, used to describe mental disorders. Table 28-1 lists the five specific areas used to evaluate a patient's psychosocial health. Box 28-1 lists the clinical conditions encountered in an axis I disorder.[1,2]

This chapter discusses anxiety disorders (panic, phobias, posttraumatic stress disorder, and generalized anxiety disorders), delirium, eating disorders, and behavioral reactions to illness (Box 28-2). Adverse reactions and drug interactions associated with drugs used to treat anxiety states are covered, with an emphasis on the dental

implications of these reactions. The dental management of the patient with anxiety and eating disorders is covered in detail. Chapter 29 is devoted to mood disorders (depression and bipolar disorders), somatoform disorders (conversion, hypochondriasis, pain, somatization), substance abuse (sedatives, opiates, stimulants, and cannabis), and schizophrenia. Dementia is discussed in Chapter 27. A dental practice of 2000 adults would have over 100 patients with a behavioral or psychiatric disorder.

ANXIETY DISORDERS

DEFINITION

Anxiety is a sense of psychological distress that may not have a focus. It is a state of apprehension that may involve an internal psychological conflict, an environmental stress, a physical disease state, a medicine or drug effect, or combinations of these. Anxiety can be purely a psychological experience with few somatic manifestations. In contrast, it can present as purely a physical experience with tachycardia, palpitations, chest pain, indigestion, headaches, and so forth, with no psychological distress other than concern about the physical symptoms. Why some individuals experience anxiety in a psychological way and others in a physical way is not clear.[3]

Epidemiology: Incidence and Prevalence

Anxiety disorders constitute the most frequently found psychiatric problem in the general population. Simple phobia is the most common of the anxiety disorders (10% of the population will experience a phobia); however, panic disorder is the most common anxiety disorder in people who seek medical treatment (lifetime prevalence of 1% to 3%).[4] About 33% of individuals with panic disorder will have recurrent attacks.[3] Posttraumatic stress disorder (PTSD) has a lifetime prevalence of 5% to 10%, with a point prevalence of 3% to 4%.[4,5]

TABLE 28-1
System for Classification of Psychosocial Health

Type	Description
Axis I	Clinical disorders
	Other conditions that may be the focus of clinical attention
Axis II	Personality disorders
	Mental retardation
Axis III	General medical conditions
Axis IV	Psychosocial and environmental problems
Axis V	Global assessment of functioning

Data from American Psychiatric Association. Diagnostic and Statistical Manual of Mental Disorders Text Revision, 4th ed. Washington DC, American Psychiatric Association, 2000, p 27.

A *phobia* is defined as an irrational fear that interferes with normal behavior. Phobias are fears of specific objects, situations, or experiences. The feared object, situation, or experience has taken on a symbolic meaning for the patient. Unconscious wishes and fears have been displaced from an original goal onto an external object.[3]

A *panic disorder* consists of a sudden, unexpected, overwhelming feeling of terror with symptoms of dyspnea, palpitations, dizziness, faintness, trembling, sweating, choking, flushes or chills, numbness or tingling sensations, and chest pains. The panic attack peaks in about 10 minutes and usually lasts for about 20 to 30 minutes.[6]

Panic disorder, phobic disorders, and obsessive-compulsive disorders occur more frequently among first-degree relatives of people with these disorders than among the general population.[3,6]

Etiology

Anxiety represents a threatened emergence into consciousness of painful, unacceptable thoughts, impulses, or desires (anxiety may result from psychological conflicts of the past and present). These psychological conflicts or feelings stimulate physiologic changes that lead to clinical manifestations of anxiety.[3,6] Anxiety disorders may occur in persons who are under emotional stress, in those with certain systemic illnesses, or as a component of various psychiatric disorders. Panic disorders tend to occur in families. If one first-degree relative has a panic disorder, other relatives have about an 18% chance of developing a panic disorder.[3,6]

The cause of panic disorder is unknown but appears to involve a genetic predisposition, altered autonomic responsivity, and social learning. Panic disorder shows a familial aggregation; the disorder is concordant in 30% to 45% of monozygotic twins, and genome-wide screens have identified suggestive risk loci on 1q, 7p15, 10q, 11p, and 13q. Acute panic attacks appear to be associated with increased noradrenergic discharges in the locus coeruleus.[5]

No single theory fully explains all anxiety disorders. No single biologic or psychological cause of anxiety has been identified. Psychosocial and biologic processes together may best explain anxiety. The locus coeruleus,

BOX 28-1

Axis I: Clinical Disorders, Other Conditions That May Be a Focus of Clinical Attention

- Disorders usually first diagnosed in infancy, childhood, or adolescence
- Delirium, dementia, and amnestic and other cognitive disorders
- Mental disorders caused by a general medical condition
- Substance-related disorders
- Schizophrenia and other psychotic disorders
- Mood disorders
- Anxiety disorders
- Somatoform disorders
- Factitious disorders
- Dissociative disorders
- Sexual and gender identity disorders
- Eating disorders
- Sleep disorders
- Psychological factors that affect medical conditions
- Impulse control disorders not elsewhere classified
- Adjustment disorders
- Other conditions that may be a focus of clinical attention

From American Psychiatric Association. Diagnostic and Statistical Manual of Mental Disorders, 4th ed. Washington DC, American Psychiatric Association, 1994, p 26.

a brainstem structure that contains most of the noradrenergic neurons in the central nervous system (CNS), appears to be involved in panic attacks and anxiety. Panic and anxiety may be correlated with dysregulated firing of the locus coeruleus caused by input from multiple sources, including peripheral autonomic afferents, medullary afferents, and serotonergic fibers.[3]

Other neurobiologic theories proposed to explain panic attacks and anxiety involve lactate infusion, benzodiazepine receptors, the amygdala, and synaptic responses in the brain. Lactate infusion causes peripheral somatic sensations that resemble those in natural panic attacks. Dysfunction of the benzodiazepine receptor may be responsible for some components of anxiety. The amygdala is a brain structure that influences fear, vigilance, and rage. Some think that the amygdala plays a role in anxiety through interaction with various hypothalamic and brainstem structures.[3]

Anxiety states also may be associated with organic diseases, other psychiatric disorders, use of certain drugs, hyperthyroidism, and mitral valve prolapse. Anxiety also is associated with mood disorders, schizophrenia, or personality disorders.[3,4]

CLINICAL PRESENTATION AND MEDICAL MANAGEMENT

From a psychological perspective, anxiety can be defined as emotional pain or a feeling that all is not well—a feeling of impending disaster. The source of the problem

BOX 28-2

Classification of Behavioral and Psychiatric Disorders

ANXIETY DISORDERS

Specifics
- Panic disorders
- Agoraphobia
- Phobias
- Obsessive-compulsive disorder*
- Posttraumatic stress disorder
- Acute stress disorder
- Generalized anxiety disorder
- Anxiety disorder due to a general medical condition
- Substance-induced anxiety disorder

MOOD DISORDERS

Specifics
- Depressive disorders
- Major depression
- Dysthymic disorder
- Depression not otherwise specified
- Bipolar disorders
- Bipolar I—Manic, mixed, depressed
- Bipolar II—Hypomanic, depressed
- Cyclothymic disorder
- Bipolar not otherwise specified

SOMATOFORM DISORDERS

Specifics
- Body dysmorphic disorder*
- Conversion disorder
- Hypochondriasis
- Somatization disorder
- Pain disorder

FACTITIOUS DISORDERS*

Specifics
- Predominantly psychological signs and symptoms
- Predominantly physical signs and symptoms
- Combined psychological and physical signs and symptoms

PSYCHOLOGICAL FACTORS THAT AFFECT MEDICAL CONDITIONS*

Specifics
- Mental disorder affecting medical condition
- Stress-related physiologic response affecting medical condition

SUBSTANCE ABUSE DISORDERS

Specifics
- Alcohol and other sedatives (barbiturates, benzodiazepines, and others)
- Opiates
- Stimulants (amphetamine, cocaine)
- Cannabis
- Hallucinogens (lysergic acid diethylamide [LSD], phencyclidine [PCP])
- Nicotine
- Others (steroids; inhalants such as paint, glue, and gasoline)

COGNITIVE DISORDERS

Specifics
- Delirium
- Dementia
- Primary (Alzheimer's type)
- Vascular
- Human immunodeficiency virus (HIV)
- Parkinson's disease
- Amnestic disorder

SCHIZOPHRENIA

Specifics
- Catatonic type
- Disorganized type
- Paranoid type
- Undifferentiated type

DELUSIONAL (PARANOID) DISORDER
- Erotomania, grandiosity, jealousy, persecution complex, somatic delusions*

Data from American Psychiatric Association. Diagnostic and Statistical Manual of Mental Disorders, Text Revision, 4th ed (DSM-IV-TR). Washington DC, American Psychiatric Association, 2002.
*Conditions not covered in Chapter 28 or 29.

usually is not apparent to persons with anxiety. The feeling is the same in anxious patients as that in patients with fear, but they are aware of what the problem is and why they are "fearful."[7]

Physiologic reactions to anxiety and to fear are the same and are mediated through the autonomic nervous system. Sympathetic and parasympathetic components may be involved. Symptoms of anxiety caused by overactivation of the sympathetic nervous system include increased heart rate, sweating, dilated pupils, and muscle tension. Symptoms of anxiety resulting from stimulation of the parasympathetic system include urination and diarrhea.

Most individuals experience some anxiety. Anxiety can be a strong motivator; low levels of anxiety can increase attention and improve performance. Anxiety leads to dysfunction when it is constant, or it may result in episodes of extreme vigilance, excessive motor tension, autonomic hyperactivity, and impaired concentration. Anxiety is part of the clinical picture in many patients with psychiatric disorders. Patients with mood disorders, dementia, psychosis, panic disorder, adjustment disorders, and toxic and withdrawal states often report feelings of anxiety.[3,8-10]

Phobias

Phobias consist of three major groups: agoraphobia, social, and simple. Agoraphobia is a fear of having distressful or embarrassing symptoms if one leaves home. It often accompanies panic disorder. Social phobias may be

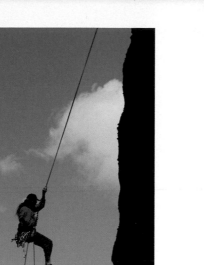

Figure 28-1. A specific phobia is acrophobia, the fear of heights.

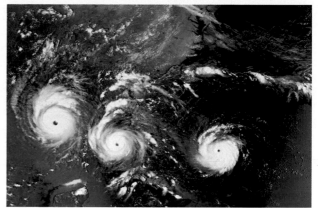

Figure 28-2. Time lapse photo of Hurricane Andrew, which hit southern Florida in August 1992. During past years, a number of major hurricanes hit the United States. Hurricane Katrina, which hit the Gulf Coast states in August 2005, was the most destructive in recent history in terms of number of deaths and extent of property damage.

specific, such as fear of public speaking, or general, such as fear of being embarrassed when with people. Simple phobias include fear of snakes, heights (Figure 28-1), flying, darkness, and needles. The two phobias that may affect medical or dental care are needle phobia and claustrophobia, during magnetic resonance imaging (MRI) or radiation therapy.[3] Dental "phobia" is more extreme than anxiety about going to the dentist.[11] Previous frightening dental experiences are cited as the major cause. Patients may fear the noise and vibration of the drill, the sight of the injection needle, and the act of sitting in the dental chair, and they exhibit muscle tension, fast heart rate, accelerated breathing, sweating, and/or stomach cramps. Patients with true phobic neurosis about dental treatment, however, are few.[11]

Panic Attack

About 15% of patients who are seen by cardiologists come to the doctor because of symptoms associated with a panic attack. Onset usually occurs between late adolescence and the mid 30s, but it may occur at any age. A key feature of panic is the adrenergic surge, which results in the fight-or-flight response. This response is an exaggerated sympathetic response (Table 28-2). Panic attacks may be cued or uncued. An example of a cued attack would be the individual who is fearful of flying. Many patients report that they are unaware of any life stressors preceding the onset of panic disorder. These attacks are classified as uncued. The major complication of repeated

panic attacks is a restricted lifestyle adopted to avoid situations that might trigger an attack. Some patients develop agoraphobia, an irrational fear of being alone in public places, which can cause them to be housebound for years. Sudden loss of social supports or disruption of important interpersonal relationships appears to predispose an individual to development of panic disorder.[3,6,9,10]

Generalized Anxiety Disorder

Some patients present with a persistent diffuse form of anxiety with symptoms of motor tension, autonomic hyperactivity, and apprehension (see Table 28-2). No familial or genetic basis for the disorder exists. It has a better outcome than panic disorder; however, it may lead to depression and substance abuse.[3,6,9,10]

Posttraumatic Stress Disorder

Posttraumatic stress disorder (PTSD) is a syndrome of psychophysiologic signs and symptoms that occur after exposure to a traumatic event outside the usual range of human experience, such as combat exposure, a holocaust experience, rape, or a civilian disaster such as a hurricane (Figure 28-2) or eruption of a volcano (Figure 28-3).[3,9,10] Most men with PTSD have been in combat (Figure 28-4), and most women give a history of sexual or physical abuse. The three cardinal features of PTSD are hyperarousal; intrusive symptoms, or flashbacks of the initial trauma; and psychic numbing.[6,7] PTSD may occur after traumatic events that are anticipated or not anticipated, constant or repetitive, natural or malevolent. PTSD happens when the onset of symptoms occurs at least 6 months after the trauma, or when the disorder lasts longer than 3 months (see Table 28-2). The traumatic event is outside the range of usual human experience. It may represent a serious threat to one's life or physical integrity; a serious threat to one's children, spouse, or other loved ones; or sudden destruction of

TABLE 28-2
Anxiety, Panic Attack, and Posttraumatic Stress Syndrome

Anxiety Disorder	Signs and Symptoms	Major Diagnostic Criteria
Anxiety	Motor tension • Trembling, twitching, or feeling shaky • Muscle tension, aches, or soreness • Restlessness • Easy fatigability Autonomic hyperactivity • Shortness of breath or smothering sensations • Palpitations or accelerated heart rate (tachycardia) • Sweating or cold, sweaty hands • Dry mouth • Dizziness or lightheadedness • Nausea, diarrhea, or other abdominal distress • Flashes (hot flashes) or chills • Frequent urination • Trouble swallowing or "lump in throat" Vigilance and scanning • Feeling keyed up or on edge • Exaggerated startle response • Difficulty concentrating or "mind goes blank" • Trouble falling or staying asleep • Irritability	Some of the signs and symptoms of anxiety may be noted in persons who are under the daily stresses of life. This form of anxiety can be helpful in the sense of focusing one's attention on a specific task, such as an exam, a driver's test, or an athletic event. Anxiety becomes a negative factor when signs and symptoms are present for longer periods and start having an effect on the emotional and physical well-being of a person.
Panic disorder	Sudden onset of intense fear, arousal, and cardiac and/or respiratory symptoms without provocation (panic attack); often confused with systemic medical illness such as angina pectoris or epilepsy Symptoms of anxiety listed above Fear of dying Fear of "going crazy" or doing something uncontrolled	One or more panic attacks have occurred that were unexpected and were not triggered by situations in which the person was the focus of another's attention. Either four attacks have occurred within a 4-week period, or one or more attacks have been followed by a period of at least 1 month of persistent fear of having another attack.
Generalized anxiety	At least six of the symptoms of anxiety listed above must be present over a period of 6 months or longer.	Presence of unrealistic or excessive worry and apprehension about two or more life circumstances, for a period of 6 months or longer, during which the person has been bothered more days than not by these concerns
Posttraumatic stress disorder (PTSD)	Symptoms of PTSD arise only after an exceptionally threatening event that is outside the normal range of experience (e.g., combat, rape, attempted murder or torture, acts of terrorism, natural disasters). Marked irritability Hyperarousal Hypervigilance Insomnia Secondary drug and alcohol abuse is common.	Repeated reliving of trauma as daydreams, intrusive memories, flashbacks, or nightmares Persistent numbness or emotional bloating Avoidance of thoughts about or reminders of the trauma, which may lead to marked detachment from personal involvement or relationships Symbols, anniversaries, or similar events often prompt exacerbation of symptoms.

Based on material from Schiffer RB. Psychiatric disorders in medical practice. In Goldman L, Ausiello D (eds). Cecil Textbook of Medicine, 22nd ed. Philadelphia, Saunders, 2004; Lucey JV, Corvin A. Anxiety disorders. In Wright P, Stern J, Phelan M (eds). Core Psychiatry, 2nd ed. Edinburgh, Elsevier, 2005.

one's home or community; or, it may result when one sees an accident or an act of physical violence that seriously injures or kills another person(s).[6]

Diagnostic criteria for PTSD consist of a history of a traumatic experience and reexperiencing of the event through intrusive memories, disturbing dreams, "flashbacks," and psychological or physical distress in response to reminders of the event; another criterion is avoidance of things associated with the trauma (see Table 28-2). Symptoms include sleep problems, irritability, trouble concentrating, hypervigilance, startle responses, and psychic numbing seen as detachment from others, reduced capacity for intimacy, and decreased interest in sex.[6,7]

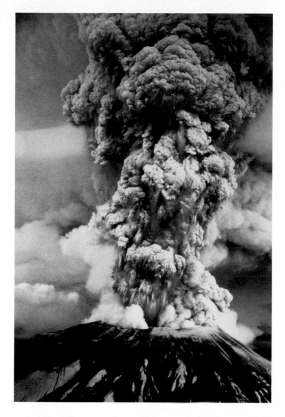

Figure 28-3. The eruption of Mount St. Helens on May 18, 1980 led to an increased incidence of posttraumatic stress disorder among residents of the Pacific North West.

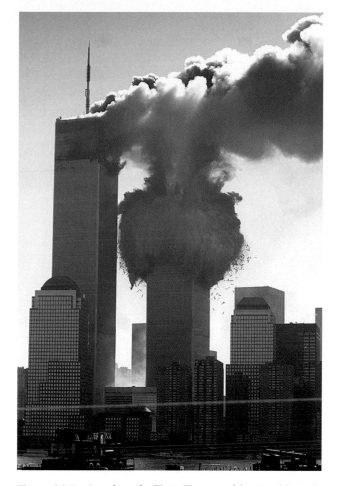

Figure 28-5. Attack on the Twin Towers of the World Trade Center in New York City on September 11, 2001. (Courtesy Getty Images.)

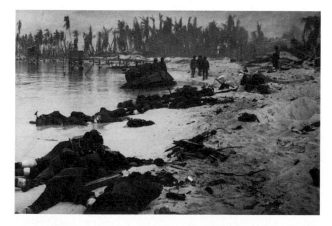

Figure 28-4. Combat during World War II on the island of Tarawa.

Recent terrorist attacks in the United States have affected the mental health status of individuals involved directly in the attacks, as well as others who were far away from the actual scene of the attack.[12-15] In a national survey of 560 adults conducted 3 to 5 days after the 2001 attacks on the World Trade Center (Figure 28-5) and the Pentagon, Schuster et al[15] found that 44% of adults displayed one or more substantial symptoms of stress. In a survey of 2273 adults performed 1 to 2 months after the attack, Schlenger et al[14] found that individuals in New York City displayed a prevalence for PTSD that was nearly 3 times that of respondents from the rest of the

country. In a survey of 414 residents of Lower Manhattan conducted from October 25, 2001 to November 2, 2001, 39.9% showed that they had the potential for PTSD.[16] A study of stress-related illnesses among New York City Fire Department rescue workers found that 1277 stress-related incidents were reported during the 11 months after the attacks, compared with 75 such incidents during the 11 months before the attacks.[17] A 2002 study found that workers at a high school and a college within 5 miles of the World Trade Center had much higher rates of depression and PTSD than did people with similar jobs who worked 5 or more miles from the World Trade Center.[18]

A study of survivors from the 1995 Oklahoma City bombing (Figure 28-6) examined 182 survivors 6 months after the bombing and 141 survivors 12 months later. Among survivors, 33% were given a diagnosis of PTSD 6 months after the bombing; all cases evaluated after 18 months were chronic.[13]

Although women are generally given the diagnosis of PTSD more often than men, the rate of PTSD is higher in male veterans than in female veterans; however, it is likely that the condition is underdiagnosed in female veterans.[19] Pereira[19] found that (1) men experienced higher levels of combat stress, (2) greater exposure to stress was

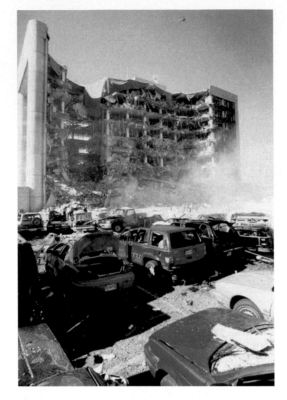

Figure 28-6. The bombing of the Alfred P. Murrah Federal Building in Oklahoma City on April 19, 1995, resulted in a greater than 33% incidence of posttraumatic stress disorder among survivors. (Courtesy NASA Ames Research Center, Disaster Assistance and Rescue Team, Mountain View, Calif.)

associated with increased symptoms of PTSD, (3) men and women exposed to similar levels of stress were equally likely to experience PTSD symptoms, and (4) men were more likely to be given the diagnosis of PTSD. Drug treatment of men and persons with combat trauma–induced PTSD (men and women) is less effective than that provided to other veteran women or women with civilian trauma–induced PTSD.[20] Data are few regarding the effectiveness of drug treatment among children with acute stress reaction or PTSD.[20]

Acute Stress Disorder

This is a new DSM-IV category of anxiety disorder. A patient with this disorder has been exposed to a traumatic event and has specific signs and symptoms that resemble those of PTSD. In acute stress disorder, symptoms are of shorter duration, and their onset occurs more rapidly after the trauma. The symptomatic reaction is limited to the time that the stressful event is occurring and its immediate aftermath.[4,6]

Treatment of Anxiety Disorders

Psychological, behavioral, and drug modalities are used to treat anxiety disorders. Psychological treatment involves psychotherapy, which, in general, is used in more severe cases. Behavioral treatment includes cognitive approaches (anxiety management, relaxation, and cognitive restructuring), biofeedback, hypnosis, relaxation imaging, desensitization, and flooding. Drug treatment includes the use of tricyclic antidepressants, selective serotonin reuptake inhibitors (SSRIs), monoamine oxidase inhibitors (MOIs), benzodiazepines, antihistamines, beta-adrenoreceptor antagonists, and sedative-hypnotics. The most commonly used drugs are the benzodiazepines, an SSRI, buspirone, or a combination of medications (Table 28-3). Most patients benefit maximally from a combination of therapies such as cognitive therapy plus medication.[3,5,21]

Systemic desensitization (whereby the patient is gradually exposed to the feared situation) and flooding (by which the patient is exposed directly to the anxiety-provoking stimulus) are used in the treatment of phobias. Claustrophobia associated with MRI can be managed with a low dose of benzodiazepines and behavioral therapy.[3,21,22]

First-line treatment for PTSD consists of psychotherapy (exposure therapy, group therapy, patient and family education), cognitive-behavioral therapy, and eye movement desensitization and reprocessing (EMDR).[23] EMDR is a newer, relatively novel treatment by which the patient focuses on movements of the clinician's finger while maintaining a mental image of the traumatic experience.[23]

Second-line treatment consists of a combination of psychotherapy and pharmacologic therapy.[23] In cases with comorbid psychiatric disorders or with especially severe symptoms of PTSD, a combination of psychotherapy and pharmacologic treatment is recommended as the first line of treatment. The U.S. Food and Drug Administration (FDA) has approved the SSRIs paroxetine and sertraline for the treatment of PTSD (see Table 28-3). Bupropion or other antidepressants are used when depression is a component of the clinical picture.

Benzodiazepines are used when anxiety is part of the symptom complex. Early intervention in patients with PTSD can shorten the duration and severity of anxiety.[23] In some cases, complex and treatment-resistant mood stabilizers such as valproate or carbamazepine are indicated.[23]

COGNITIVE DISORDERS— DELIRIUM AND AMNESTIC DISORDERS

DEFINITION

Cognitive disorders consist of dementia, delirium, and amnestic disorders. Dementia is covered in Chapter 27. Patients who experience delirium have an acute change in mental status.[24] Typical signs include confusion, periods of sleepiness alternating with periods of agitation, deficits in attention and memory, and failure to accurately perceive the outside world and to use and understand language. Amnesia is an impairment of memory that is out of proportion to other cognitive impairments.[24]

TABLE **28-3**
Drugs Used to Treat Patients With Anxiety and Panic

Drug Class	Drug	Trade Name	Initial Dose	Target Dose Range	Comments
Antihistamines	Diphenhydramine	Benadryl	25 mg PO qhs	50 mg	Most useful at bedtime
	Hydroxyzine	Atarax	50 mg PO qhs	100 mg	for associated sleep
Benzodiazepines	Lorazepam	Ativan	0.5 mg PO	2-10 mg tid dosing	Also effective for
	Diazepam	Valium	5 mg PO	5-10 mg bid	generalized anxiety
	Triazolam	Halcion	0.125 mg	0.25-0.5 mg hs	Abuse potential in many
	Chlordiazepoxide	Librium	5 mg bid	10-30 mg	
	Temazepam	Restoril	7.5 mg hs	15-30 mg	
	Alprazolam	Xanax	0.25 mg bid	2-8 mg/day	
	Clorazepate	Tranxene	7.5 mg hs	15-60 mg/day	Abuse potential
	Flurazepam	Dalmane	15 mg hs	30-60 mg	
	Oxazepam	Serax	10 mg bid	60-120 mg/day	
	Clonazepam	Klonopin	0.25 mg qd	1-3 mg/day	Long duration of action permits once-daily dosing
	Buspirone	Buspar	5 mg bid	20-30 mg/day	Most useful on an as-needed basis
	Zolpidem	Ambien	10 mg hs	10 mg hs	
SSRIs	Paroxetine	Paxil	20 mg	20-50 mg/day	Slower onset than the
	Sertraline	Zoloft	once/day 25 mg once/day	50 mg/day	benzodiazepines
Atypical	Bupropion	Wellbutrin	100 mg bid	300 mg/day, given tid	Slower onset than benzodiazepines
Beta blockers	Propranolol	Inderal	20 mg bid	Individualize 40-120 mg/day	Does not block the fear component of anxiety or panic
Sedative-hypnotics	Chloral hydrate	Noctel	500 mg	500-1000 mg	Seldom appropriate
	Meprobamate	Miltown	200 mg tid	1200-1600 mg	

From Schiffer RB. Psychiatric disorder in medical practice. In Goldman L, Ausiello D (eds). Cecil Textbook of Medicine, 22nd ed. Philadelphia, WB Saunders, 2004.
qhs, Every bedtime; PO, by mouth; tid, 3 times daily; bid, twice daily; hs, at bedtime; qd, every day; SSRIs, selective serotonin reuptake inhibitors.

Epidemiology: Incidence and Prevalence

Delirium is one of the most commonly encountered mental disorders in medical practice. It will affect up to 30% of hospitalized and elderly medically ill patients. Delirium often is mistaken as depression, anxiety, dementia, or personality disorder, or it may be overlooked completely.[25] Table 28-4 lists the prevalence, age of onset, course, and risk factors for delirium. Amnesia may occur as the result of a number of causes; however, few data are available to demonstrate its incidence and prevalence.[24]

Etiology

The impairment of attention and consciousness that are characteristic of delirium can develop over a short time and tend to fluctuate over the course of the day. Causes of delirium include systemic medical conditions (thyroid disease, hepatic failure, renal failure, primary brain tumor, metastatic lesion to the brain, lupus erythematosus, infection of the brain, and others), substance intoxication or withdrawal (alcohol or cocaine abuse), and multifactorial

conditions such as hyponatremia, hypoxia, anemia, and fever (see Table 28-4).[24,25]

Amnestic disorders may be caused by any illness or trauma that damages the deep brain structures associated with memory (see Table 28-4). These disorders are common in head trauma victims, with seizures, and in patients with thiamine deficiency (seen in alcohol abuse). Infection, neoplastic conditions, drugs (phencyclidine), and autoimmune disease such as vasculitis of the posterior cerebral artery may lead to amnestic disorders.[24]

CLINICAL PRESENTATION AND MEDICAL MANAGEMENT

Delirium, which has been defined as impaired consciousness with intrusive abnormalities of perception and affect,[24] is a transitory state that is primarily characterized by impaired attention and consciousness. Other cognitive changes, such as memory impairment, disorientation, language disturbance, and perceptual disturbance, may be present. Illusions are frequent, and vivid visual

TABLE 28-4
Delirium and Amnestic Disorders

Clinical Features	Delirium	Amnestic Disorders
DESCRIPTION	Consists of acute disorder of attention and cognitive function	Most clinical disorders of amnesia are specifically concerned with disturbed recent memory, or the inability to store new information.
ETIOLOGY	Usually has multifactorial cause: • Infections—Systemic, intracranial • Cardiovascular—Heart failure, myocardial infarction, pulmonary embolism, intracranial bleeding • Endocrine disorders—Diabetes, hypothyroidism, hyperthyroidism • Gastrointestinal disorders—Hepatic failure, pancreatitis • Intoxications—Alcohol, prescribed drugs, illicit drugs, carbon monoxide poisoning • Neurologic disorders—Head injury, meningitis, encephalitis, tumors Risk increases with age Family history increases the risk	Alcoholism with thiamine deficiency (Wernicke-Korsakoff syndrome) Malabsorption syndromes associated with carcinoma of the stomach Head injuries—Traumatic brain injury is another common cause of amnesia when temporolimbic structures are injured bilaterally. Herpes simplex encephalitis Infarction in posterior cerebral arteries Hypoxia Most focal amnesic syndromes involve lesions in the temporolimbic region. Anoxia and ischemia are common causes of residual memory impairment. Seizures and electroconvulsive therapy Often associated with the dementias
EPIDEMIOLOGY PREVALENCE	10% to 30% of hospitalized patients; one study showed that 13.5% of patients admitted to a general medical ward had delirium, and another 3% became delirious during hospitalization.	May be very common, as indicated by the incidence and prevalence of dementia (7% after age 65 and about 50% after age 85 worldwide) and alcoholism
SIGNS AND SYMPTOMS	In some cases, these are the only initial signs of an underlying life-threatening illness: • Clouding of consciousness • Disturbances of memory—Retention, recall • Easily distracted • Slowed thinking • Impaired reasoning • Disorganized and fragmented thought • Incoherence • Visual hallucinations • Delusions—Fleeting, with persecutory content • Fear and anxiety replaced by apathy • Arousal, agitation, and hypervigilance, followed by listlessness and hypoactivity • Disorientation in time and place	Patient may deny existence of memory problem. Often disoriented to time Lack of knowledge of current events Unable to store, retain, or retrieve a list of 4 or 5 words over several minutes. Patients may even forget that they were given a list. In some cases, unable to recall historical events
TREATMENT	Must determine the primary cause and then initiate the appropriate treatment Nonpharmacologic management should be used in all delirious patients: • family members sitting with patient for orienting influence, • lots of interpersonal contact and • communication, explanations and eye contact, involve patient in decision making • when ever possible, encourage self-care and independence, provide clocks and calendars • to assist in orientation, room and staff • changes should be kept to a minimum and a quiet environment with low-level lighting. If drug management is needed neuroleptics are the preferred agents, with haloperidol being the most widely used agent. The lowest dose for the shortest period of time should be selected.	Depends on the cause of amnesia. More effective drugs are now available for treating the early stages of Alzheimer's disease but none are effective in the later stages of the disease. In cases of head trauma the amnesia may clear without treatment. In cases caused by infection effective treatment of the infection may clear the amnesia.

TABLE **28-5**
Clinical Findings and Epidemiology of Eating Disorders

Condition	Clinical Findings	Epidemiology
ANOREXIA NERVOSA	Refusal to maintain body weight (less than 85% of expected) Fear of gaining weight Fear of becoming fat Disturbance in body image Amenorrhea Hypotension Dry skin Bradycardia Other arrhythmias may develop	Prevalence—0.5% to 1.0% Mean age at onset—bimodal 14 and 18 years Rare after 40 years of age Females, 90% to 95% of cases More common in women in higher socioeconomic groups and among white women Mortality—5% to 15% • Starvation • Suicide • Electrolyte imbalance
BULIMIA NERVOSA	Recurrent episodes of binge eating: • Large amounts of food • Discrete period of time • Lack control over eating Binge eating—At least 2 times per week over at least a 3-month period Inappropriate behavior, to prevent weight gain: • Self-induced vomiting • Laxatives • Diuretics • Enemas • Ipecac (induces vomiting, may cause myopathy) • Fasting • Excessive exercise Self-evaluation is unduly influenced by body shape and weight.	Prevalence—1% to 2% of women and 0.1% of men develop the condition during their lifetime. Average age of onset—Around 20 years Females, 90% to 95% of cases More than 30% abuse alcohol and stimulants. 50% have personality disorders. Rates are similar in high and lower income groups, but treatment is sought more often by women in higher income groups. Higher rate in white women, but more cases beginning to appear in ethnic minority groups Long-term outcome not known but appears to have a more optimistic prognosis than anorexia nervosa
EATING DISORDERS NOT OTHERWISE SPECIFIED	Fall short of the criteria for anorexia nervosa or bulimia nervosa For example, individual uses laxatives or induces vomiting but is not a binge eater	Difficult to establish the prevalence of this group of eating disorders

hallucinations are common. Delusions are also common and often are persecutory in nature. Patients with delirium may appear withdrawn, agitated, or psychotic.[24] Symptoms last hours to days and tend to change during the day. Recognition of delirium is important because it often leads to a diagnosis of underlying medical disease or drug use. Treatment of the medical disorder will in most cases correct the delirium. However, delirium has a high rate of mortality, with one study reporting that 25% of patients were dead within 6 months.[24] Agitated behaviors associated with delirium are managed with neuroleptics, benzodiazepines, or a combination of the two. Partial or complete restraints may be needed for some patients to prevent injury (see Table 28-4). Delirious patients should not drive or walk in areas with traffic.[21]

In most cases of amnesia, the ability to recall recent memory is affected, as is the ability to incorporate new information. Recovery is dependent on the cause of the memory problem (see Table 28-4). In some cases of amnesia caused by concussion or seizures, complete recovery may occur. However, in other cases, impairment may be permanent. Memory loss in some cases can be modestly improved through cognitive rehabilitation techniques. Medications and dietary substances have done little to improve memory.[26]

EATING DISORDERS
DEFINITION

The two major eating disorders are anorexia nervosa and bulimia nervosa (Table 28-5). Anorexia nervosa is characterized by severe restriction of food intake, leading to weight loss and the medical sequelae of starvation (Figure 28-7). Bulimia nervosa is characterized by attempts to restrict food intake, but in a different form than that seen in anorexia nervosa. In bulimia, attempts at restriction are interspersed with binge eating followed by various methods of trying to rid the body of food. These include induced vomiting (finger in the throat, syrup of ipecac), laxatives, and diuretics.[4,27,28]

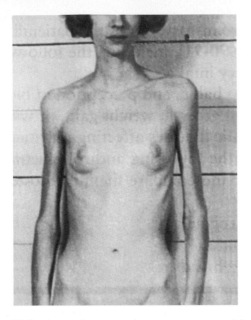

Figure 28-7. Anorexia nervosa in a young woman. Note the low body weight and the preservation of breast tissue. (From Ezrin C, Godden JO, Volpe R: Systemic endocrinology, ed 2, New York, 1979, Harper & Row.)

Epidemiology: Incidence and Prevalence

These disorders cause psychological and physical morbidity in women (90% to 95% of cases) and, to a much lesser extent, in men (5% to 10% of cases).[28,29] Anorexia nervosa affects an estimated 1% of women between 12 and 25 years of age.[28,29] It is more common in white women and women from higher socioeconomic groups (see Table 28-5). The overall incidence is 0.24 to 7.3 cases per 100,000 per year.[30] The mean age of onset of anorexia nervosa is bimodal at ages 14 and 18.[29] Bulimia nervosa is more common than anorexia nervosa. Its prevalence is estimated at 1% to 2% for most populations.[28,29] The average age of onset for bulimia nervosa is about 20 years. In contrast to anorexia nervosa, bulimia nervosa occurs at about the same rate in higher and lower income groups of women. It is more common in white women than in women of ethnic minority groups.[29]

Etiology

The cause of eating disorders is unknown. Genetic, cultural, and psychiatric factors appear to play a role in the origin of these disorders. In addition, primary dysfunction of the hypothalamus has been suggested to play a causative role in eating disorders. However, recognized hypothalamic abnormalities revert to normal with weight gain and thus appear to be secondary in nature.[30,31] Some evidence indicates that dysfunction in serotonin-mediated neurotransmission may contribute to the development of eating disorders.[28]

Family and twin studies suggest a weak genetic component in the causes of anorexia nervosa and bulimia nervosa. In anorexia nervosa, 50% concordance exists

in monozygotic twins, and 7% in dizygotic twins.[30] In bulimia nervosa, 23% concordance occurs in monozygotic twins and 9% in dizygotic twins.[30] With both disorders, first-degree relatives of probands are at increased risk for eating disorders, affective disorders, and substance abuse. A genetic predisposition indicates increased risk if the right cultural and psychological stresses are present.[30] Linkage studies have found an association of anorexia nervosa with chromosome 1, and an association of bulimia nervosa with chromosome 10.[28]

Cultural issues are important in the origin of eating disorders. The quest for health and slimness is a powerful force in modern society and may reinforce the fear of fatness in patients with an eating disorder or may tip the borderline case into overt disease. Certain hobbies and occupations (e.g., modeling, skating, gymnastics, wrestling, track, ballet dancing) that emphasize body shape, weight, and appearance may also play a role in eating disorders.[4,27,28]

CLINICAL PRESENTATION AND MEDICAL MANAGEMENT

Anorexia nervosa and bulimia nervosa are eating disorders that usually occur in young, previously healthy women who develop a paralyzing fear of becoming fat (Box 28-3). The population at risk consists largely of white women from middle-class backgrounds. These disorders rarely occur in African American or Asian American women, in the poor, or in men. The driving force is the pursuit of thinness, all other aspects of life being secondary. In anorexia nervosa, this aim is achieved primarily through radical restriction of food intake, the end result being emaciation. In bulimia, induced vomiting and excessive use of laxatives follow massive binge eating. Weight loss in bulimic subjects is not great, despite the obsession with food. Some authors consider the two disorders to be distinct illnesses; others classify bulimia as a variant of anorexia nervosa. Overlap syndromes exist in that emaciated patients who fulfill the criteria for true anorexia nervosa may exhibit bulimic behavior, and subjects with bulimia often pass through a phase of anorexia.[27,28,32]

The diagnosis of eating disorder is made on clinical grounds (see Box 28-3). In anorexia nervosa, amenorrhea is a consistent feature. The weight criterion for diagnosis is 85% or less than expected ideal weight. An expressed intense fear of gaining weight or becoming fat, even when underweight, and a disturbance in body image complete the diagnostic triad.[27,28,32] The diagnosis of bulimia is made with a history of binge eating without major weight gain, evidence of purging (induced vomiting or regular use of laxatives or diuretics), obsessive-compulsive behavior, and antisocial activity or self-mutilation.[27,28,32]

Anorexia nervosa usually begins around puberty but may appear later, usually by the middle 20s. Despite severe weight loss, patients deny hunger, thinness, or

BOX 28-3

Diagnosis of Anorexia Nervosa and Bulimia Nervosa (DSM-IV)

Criteria for Anorexia Nervosa

- Refusal to maintain body weight at or above minimally normal weight for age and height (body weight <85% expected)
- Intense fear of gaining weight or becoming fat, even though underweight
- Disturbed by body weight and shape of body; denial of the seriousness of current low body weight
- In postmenarchal women, amenorrhea (absence of at least three consecutive menstrual cycles)

SPECIFY TYPE

- *Restricting type:* During the current episode of anorexia nervosa, the person has not regularly engaged in binge eating or purging behavior (self-induced vomiting or misuse of laxatives, diuretics, or enemas)
- *Binge eating/purging type:* During the current episode of anorexia nervosa, the person has regularly engaged in binge eating or purging behavior (self-induced vomiting or misuse of laxatives, diuretics, or enemas)

Criteria for Bulimia Nervosa

- Recurrent episodes of binge eating; an episode of binge eating is characterized by both of the following:
  - Eating, within a discrete period (e.g., within a 2-hour period), an amount of food that is definitely larger than most people would eat during a similar period and under similar circumstances
  - A sense of lack of control over eating during these episodes (e.g., a feeling that one cannot stop eating or cannot control what or how much one is eating)
- Recurrent inappropriate compensatory behavior to prevent weight gain, such as self-induced vomiting; misuse of laxatives, diuretics, enemas, or other medication; fasting; or excessive exercise
- Binge eating and inappropriate compensatory behaviors occur, on average, at least twice a week for 3 months
- Self-evaluation is unduly influenced by body shape and weight
- The disturbance does not occur exclusively during episodes of anorexia nervosa

SPECIFY TYPE

- *Purging type:* During the current episode of bulimia nervosa, the person has regularly engaged in self-induced vomiting or the misuse of laxatives, diuretics, or enemas
- *Nonpurging type:* During the current episode of bulimia nervosa, the person has used other inappropriate compensatory behaviors, such as fasting or excessive exercise, but has not regularly engaged in self-induced vomiting or the misuse of laxatives, diuretics, or enemas

Based on material from West DS. The eating disorders. In Goldman L, Ausiello D (eds). Cecil Textbook of Medicine, 22nd ed. Philadelphia, WB Saunders, 2004, Tables 232-1 and 232-2, pp 1336-1338; Majid SH, Treasure JL. Eating disorders. In Wright P, Stern J, Phelan M (eds). Core Psychiatry, 2nd ed. Edinburgh, Elsevier, 2005, pp 217-241; American Psychiatric Association. Diagnostic and Statistical Manual of Mental Disorders, Text Revision, 4th ed (DSM-IV-TR). Washington DC, American Psychiatric Association, 2000.

fatigue. They are often physically active and participate in ritualized exercise. Constipation and cold intolerance are common. Amenorrhea usually accompanies or comes after weight loss. In advanced cases, bradycardia, hypothermia, and hypotension occur. Little or no body fat is evident, and bones protrude through the skin. Parotid glands may become enlarged. The skin may be dry and scaly and is often yellow because of carotenemia. Patients with eating disorders may show other dermatologic manifestations; alopecia, xerosis, hypertrichosis, and nail fragility occur as the result of starvation.[27,28,32]

Patients with bulimia ("ox-hunger") nervosa engage in episodic, compulsive ingestion of large amounts of food (see Box 28-3). They are aware that this eating is abnormal; they have a fear that they cannot stop eating and have feelings of depression at the completion of eating. Bulimic patients have a morbid fear of becoming fat. Secrecy about the eating/vomiting sequence is common. Episodes

of binge eating are followed by vomiting induced with the use of a finger, an object, or a drug such as ipecac, with or without subsequent ingestion of laxatives or diuretics. Bloating, constipation, esophagitis, abdominal pain, and nausea are common. Binge eating generally occurs daily; large amounts of food, usually high-carbohydrate foods such as ice cream, bread, candy, and doughnuts, are consumed. Dental caries becomes a problem because of the high carbohydrate content of the diet.[27,28,31,32]

Serum amylase has been reported to be elevated in 45% of bulimic patients.[33] In the same study, serum amylase was found to be elevated in pregnant women with hyperemesis but not in nonvomiting pregnant women. The authors of the study[33] concluded that vomiting, rather than binge eating, increases serum amylase in bulimic patients. They speculated that increased amylase came from the salivary gland. Another study[34] found that parotid gland size was enlarged in 36% of bulimic patients and was correlated with frequency of bulimic symptoms and with serum amylase concentrations.

Patients with anorexia nervosa are vulnerable to sudden death from ventricular tachyarrhythmias. The risk of death becomes greater when weight declines to below 35% of ideal weight. Complications of bulimia include aspiration of vomitus, esophageal or gastric rupture, hypokalemia with cardiac arrhythmias, pancreatitis, and ipecac-induced myopathy and cardiomypathy.[27,28,31,32]

The prognosis is better for anorexia nervosa than for bulimia nervosa. About 49% of patients with anorexia nervosa achieve normal weight, 20% improve but remain underweight, 20% continue to be anorexic, 5% become obese, and 6% or more die. Death is caused by cardiac arrhythmias associated with starvation or suicide. Patients with bulimia have poorer outcomes because of more severe psychiatric disturbances that lead to a higher suicide rate, and because of the medical complications of gorging. About 40% of treated patients remain bulimic after 18 months of treatment. Relapse occurs in about two thirds of patients within a year of recovery.[27,28,31,32]

The treatment of anorexia nervosa cannot proceed in a meaningful way in the absence of weight gain. The patient's nutritional status and medical stability are first evaluated. Patients with electrolyte disturbances or with abnormalities on electrocardiogram (ECG) may require hospitalization. Once the patient is medically stable, psychiatric treatment can begin. Behavior modification techniques are used to assist the patient in weight gain. The efficacy of psychotherapy has not been established. Drug therapy (antipsychotics, cyproheptadine, antidepressants) has not significantly improved the outcomes of patients with anorexia nervosa. The antidepressant fluoxetine has been shown to be useful in preventing relapse in patients who have gained back their weight.[28,30-32]

Antidepressant medication, cognitive-behavioral therapy, and interpersonal therapy all are effective in bulimia nervosa. Most patients are treated on an outpatient basis. Those patients with medical complications such as extreme electrolyte imbalance or severe bulimic symptoms may require hospitalization.[28,30] The supportive care of an understanding physician also may be helpful for the bulimic patient. Attempts should be made to stop the gorging/regurgitation cycle, or at least to limit the load of food ingested, to minimize the chance of aspiration or gastric rupture. Potassium supplementation may be needed in patients who vomit and in those who use laxatives.[28,30,31]

DRUGS USED TO TREAT ANXIETY DISORDERS

The benzodiazepines are used to treat various anxiety states (see Table 28-3). These drugs selectively but indirectly enhance gamma-aminobutyric acid neurotransmission. This may occur via the drugs' increasing neuronal receptor sensitivity to gamma-aminobutyric acid. The benzodiazepines are very effective for short-lived reactive states of tension and anxiety. They are the drugs of choice for generalized anxiety disorders. Tricyclics and MOIs are the drugs of choice for panic disorders. Benzodiazepines are used for the treatment of anticipatory anxiety associated with panic disorder. They also are used in the treatment of other forms of anxiety associated with panic disorders and for anxiety symptoms in patients with phobic disorder.[5,10,23]

Diazepam is the standard for antianxiety therapy. No other anxiolytic drug has shown better antianxiety efficacy. Treatment with anxiolytic drugs should continue only for a period of 4 weeks or less. To avoid the development of drug tolerance, these drugs often are given for 7 to 10 days; a 2- to 3-day period without the drug follows. An early sign of drug tolerance occurs when increased dosage is required. Symptoms of drug withdrawal include muscle aches, agitation, restlessness, insomnia, confusion, delirium, and, on rare occasions, grand mal seizures. Some patients may experience rebound anxiety after the drug has been stopped.[3,5,23,35,36]

Adverse effects of the benzodiazepines include daytime sedation, mild cognitive impairment, and aggressive and impulsive behavioral responses. The benzodiazepines, which can potentiate the CNS effects of opioids, barbiturates, and alcohol, are hazardous or are contraindicated in the following patients: those who drive or operate machinery, patients with depressive mood disorders or psychosis, and moderate to heavy drinkers, pregnant women, and the elderly. Tolerance and habitual and physical dependence may occur with therapeutic doses. Actions of the benzodiazepines are additive and usually synergistic with psychotropic agents. Drug interactions have been reported with cimetidine and erythromycin.[5,23,35,36]

Buspirone has mixed agonist/antagonist actions at serotonergic receptors that are thought to be involved in anxiety. It appears to have anxiolytic effects that are comparable with those of benzodiazepines, without sedative, anticonvulsant, or muscle relaxant effects. These anxiolytic effects are delayed in onset, taking up to 3 weeks before becoming clinical obvious. The drug is recommended for short-term use only. At this time, buspirone is not a first-line drug for the treatment of anxiety.[5,23,35,37]

Several tricyclics and other antidepressants have additional sedative or anxiolytic effects. They appear to be as effective as benzodiazepines in generalized anxiety, and superior in panic disorder and agoraphobia. SSRIs and MOIs also are effective in phobic states and panic disorders. Disadvantages of these drugs include their slow rate of onset, the fact that they may initially exacerbate anxiety symptoms, their toxicity in overdose, and numerous adverse effects.[5,23,35]

DENTAL MANAGEMENT
Patients' Attitudes Toward Dentists

Childhood experiences and learned social roles of patients are important factors in the development of patients' feelings and attitudes toward dentists. Children learn role expectations through the teachings of physicians, dentists, parents, and peers. The patient may come to believe that the physician and the dentist are powerful and dangerous, and thus may feel awe, envy, and wonder in their presence. Other emotions, attitudes, and actions associated with patients' relationships with their parents also may be transferred to the dentist. Those of respect and politeness can be helpful. However, those associated with a need for unending love, a demand for unceasing attention, and feelings of resentment and hate can be destructive. The more that dentists reveal themselves to patients from the first contact, the less likely it is that these attitudes and feelings will be encouraged. Unrealistic expectations and inappropriate behaviors should be open for discussion between the dentist and the patient if a solid relationship is to be developed and maintained.

Behavioral Reactions to Illness

The DSM-IV calls attention to the interplay of psychological and behavioral factors with medical illness under the diagnostic category of psychological factors that affect medical conditions. All patients with medical illness experience psychological reactions to being ill. A patient's reactions may vary according to the nature of the illness and the nature of the patient. Significant aspects of the illness include severity, chronicity, and the site and nature of symptoms. Relevant patient characteristics include age, level of maturity, character style, previous experience with illness, and social supports.[2,38]

Regression, denial, anxiety, depression, and anger are general responses to illness that are common to all human beings. These responses originate in the various meanings that people attribute to physical illness, the fears that are typically raised by being ill, and the means used to cope with illness.[38,39]

Depressive thoughts and feelings are common psychological reactions to medical illness. Being ill usually is perceived as a loss, which may be experienced as loss of physical abilities and loss of bodily integrity through the loss of organs or limbs. Feelings of loss of control are very common among hospitalized patients. Patients may feel that they cannot do some of the things they have always done that are an important part of their identities. These activities include being unable to fulfill family roles, taking care of professional responsibilities, and participating in recreational and social events. All medical patients experience loss of their sense of being healthy. Transient depressed thoughts and feelings are common in medically ill patients. Major depression in medically ill patients is not normal and must be aggressively identified and treated.[38,39]

Patients commonly experience anger about being ill. However, some patients become enraged; in an effort to feel less helpless, guilty, or afraid, they lash out at the people around them. These patients may become hostile, suspicious, and accusatory toward family members and health care providers. The most common causes of anger, irritability, and suspiciousness in medically ill patients are medications and substances of abuse. Some groups of patients are at high risk for paranoid reactions. These include elderly patients, those with depression or cognitive impairment, and those with a prior history of psychotic illness.[38,39]

Severe and chronic illnesses foster a type of dependency of the patient on others. Severely disabled patients have a greater need to relay on others. Some individuals cannot accept this dependency and become anxious and try to deny their need for help. Feelings of resentment, anger, and hostility may develop toward persons in contact with such a patient. Once again, an understanding of this process will allow individuals who care for such a patient to be empathetic and supportive.[38,39]

Sick people tend to view the world around them as small, and they develop a preoccupation with their sickness, needs, and fears. They may retreat to highly personal or magical notions about the cause of their illness. For example, cancer patients may believe that their illness is a punishment for swearing at their mother or for some "evil" thoughts they may have had.[38,39]

Patient Management

Generalized Anxiety. The dentist may detect anxiety in persons by observing their physical appearance, speech, and dress, and the presence of certain signs and symptoms.

The anxious person looks overly alert, displaying it in such ways as sitting forward in a chair; moving fingers, arms, or legs; getting up and moving; pacing around the room; checking certain portions of clothing; straightening ties or scarves; and so forth. On the other hand, sloppy dress habits and other signs—just the opposite of a concern with perfection—may be seen. Anxious persons may show signs of being watchful of possessions and always trying to keep them in sight.[7]

The anxious person may speak mechanically and rapidly and at times may seem to block out or not connect thoughts. The anxious person may respond quickly, often not allowing the dentist to finish a question.[7]

Sweating, tension in the muscles, increased breathing, and rapid heart rate may be seen. The patient may report an inability to sleep, may awaken at an early hour, and may not be able to go back to sleep. Attacks of diarrhea and increased frequency of urination may occur. In general, anxious persons are overly alert and tense, feel apprehensive, and have a sense of impending disaster that has no apparent cause. Insomnia, tension, and apprehension lead to fatigue, which makes it even more difficult for the individual to deal with anxiety.[7]

The dentist should talk with the patient and show personal interest. Verbal and nonverbal communication must be consistent (Table 28-6). The dentist should confront the patient with the observation that the patient appears anxious, then ask if the individual would like to talk about feelings, which may include the person's attitude toward the dentist. During these discussions,

TABLE 28-6
Dental Management of the Anxious Patient

Clinical Setting	Behavioral	Pharmacologic	Dosage
PREOPERATIVE	Establish effective communication. Be open and honest; let patients see who you are. Provide consistent verbal and nonverbal communication. Explain procedures and answer questions. Explain what you will do to make procedure "pain free." If discomfort is anticipated, explain this to the patient. Consider confronting the patient who appears anxious: • "You seem tense today." • "Would you like to talk about it?"	Oral sedation • Benzodiazepine selection • Fast-acting drug • As low a dose as can be effective • Night before appointment • Day of appointment	Alprazolam • Xanax 0.5-mg tab PO, 1 tab in the evening before bed, 1 tab 1 hour before appointment Diazepam • Valium 2-, 5-, or 10-mg tab, 1 tab PO, in the evening before bed, 1 tab 1 hour before appointment Triazolam • Halcion 0.125- or 0.25-mg tab, 1 tab in the evening before bed, 1 tab 1 hour before appointment
OPERATIVE	Allow patient to ask questions about what is happening. Let patient know if any discomfort is about to be felt. Reassure patient that the procedure is going well.	Effective local anesthesia Oral sedation (benzodiazepine) Inhalation sedation (nitrous oxide) Intramuscular (IM) sedation • Midazolam • Promethazine • Meperidine Intravenous (IV) sedation • Diazepam • Midazolam • Fentanyl	Midazolam • Versed IV, 2.5 mg or less over 2 minutes just before procedure Fentanyl • Sublimaze IV, 0.07 to 2.0 µg/kg, given minutes before procedure Meperidine • Demerol IM, 1 mg/kg, 30-90 minutes before procedure

POSTOPERATIVE	Explain what usually occurs after the procedure. Explain what the patient needs to do. Explain what the patient needs to avoid. Describe what complications can occur, such as:
	• Pain
	• Bleeding
	• Infection
	• Allergic reaction to medications prescribed
	Tell patient to contact you if any complication develops
	In cases of severe bleeding or allergic reaction, the patient should go to the nearest hospital emergency room.
		Effective postoperative pain control is essential.
		Select the most appropriate drug for pain control from the following:
		• Analgesics
		• NSAIDs, salicylates
		• Acetaminophen, codeine
		• Oxycodone, fentanyl
		• Morphine, others
		• Adjunctive medications
		  • Antidepressants
		  • Muscle relaxants
		  • Steroids
		  • Anticonvulsants
		  • Antibiotics
			Check on dosage for selected drug in other chapters of this book, *Physician's Desk Reference (PDR)*, or other reference sources.

NSAIDs, Nonsteroidal anti-inflammatory drugs.

tension-free pauses between ideas should be permitted, allowing a temporary state of regression to occur that will help the patient to restore a more anxiety-free state. Some patients may respond well to this approach without ever indicating why they were anxious.[7]

If the patient remains anxious in the dental situation, the dentist may plan to use hypnosis, oral or parenteral sedation agents or nitrous oxide, and oxygen to better manage the dental treatment (see Table 28-6).

Anxiety or a history of panic attacks also may be associated with mitral valve prolapse.[3,6,40] In the past patients with mitral valve prolapse and valvular regurgitation were given antibiotic prophylaxis for invasive dental procedures. Based on the 2007 AHA guidelines these patients no longer require prophylaxis (see Chapter 2).

Patients with uncontrolled hyperthyroidism also may have associated anxiety; these patients must avoid epinephrine, including even the small amounts used in local anesthetics (see Chapter 17). Patients who display signs and symptoms of hyperthyroidism should be referred for medical evaluation and treatment.[42]

PTSD. Veterans with PTSD may view the dentist as an authority figure who misled them and sent them to war.[7] They may associate dental treatment with loss of control; hence, the dentist must attempt to establish communication and trust with these patients. Patients with intravenous (IV) drug habits may be carriers of the hepatitis B virus (hepatitis B surface antigen [HBsAg] positive) and of human immunodeficiency virus (HIV). Those who are heavy drinkers may have liver and bone marrow involvement and may be at increased risk for infection, excessive bleeding, delayed healing, and altered drug metabolism. During the depressive stage of PTSD, patients often show a total disregard for oral hygiene procedures and are at increased risk for dental caries, periodontal disease, and pericoronitis. They may report atypical facial pain, glossodynia, temporomandibular joint (TMJ) disorder, and bruxism.[7]

Stress-Related Disorders. Oral diseases that are thought to have a psychological component in their clinical presentation (the older term was *psychophysiologic disorders*) include aphthous ulcers, lichen planus, TMJ dysfunction, myofascial pain, and geographic tongue. Examples of some of these lesions are shown in Figures 28-8, 28-9, and 28-10.

In these disorders, an identifiable lesion with an emotional component to the clinical presentation exists. The pathologic process is potentially dangerous to the patient. The disorder does not reduce the level of anxiety or depression but rather increases it, and increased anxiety or depression can aggravate the condition. These disorders can be treated through the regimen provided in Appendix C. The anxious patient can be sedated with the use of one of the agents shown in Table 28-6. Patients with atypical facial pain, TMJ dysfunction, or myofascial pain are often treated with an antidepressant medication.

Delirium. Patients with signs and symptoms of delirium should be referred for medical evaluation and treatment. These patients can receive routine dental treatment once the cause of delirium has been identified and corrected. If emergency dental care is needed, the dentist should consult with the patient's physician before treating, if possible.

Eating Disorders. The major role of the dentist in the management of patients with bulimia nervosa is to deal with the results of their diet (dental caries) and the effects

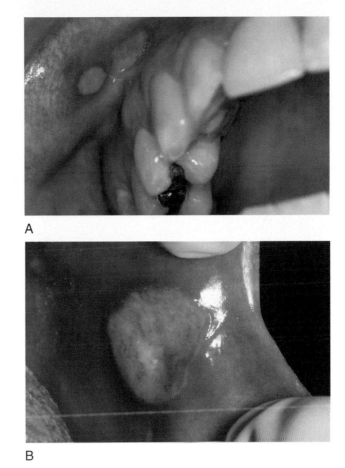

A

B

Figure 28-8. A, A single minor aphthous ulceration of the anterior buccal mucosa. **B,** A large major aphthous ulceration of the left anterior buccal mucosa. (From Neville BW, Damm DD, Allen CM, Bouquot JE. Oral and Maxillofacial Pathology, 2nd ed. Philadelphia, Saunders, 2002.)

of chronic vomiting on the teeth (erosion).[32] One study[43] found that the average pH of vomitus was 3.8; with chronic exposure, this can lead to severe erosion of teeth. The dentist's role as a case finder is important to the patient. The dentist may be the first person to become aware of the eating disorder by finding a pattern of erosion of the teeth that is consistent with regurgitation of stomach contents (Figure 28-11). This can lead to referral and medical diagnosis and treatment. However, patients often deny this is a problem. The erosive pattern involves the lingual surfaces of the teeth, primarily the maxillary teeth because the tongue protects the mandibular teeth. This particular type of erosion is known as *perimylolysis.* In some cases, erosion also can affect the occlusal surfaces of molar and premolar teeth, where the process can be accelerated by attrition.[43-45] Serious medical complications of bulimia nervosa (gastric rupture, esophageal tears, cardiac arrhythmia, and death) must be pointed out to the patient, along with the fact that these can be avoided with proper medical and psychological therapy.[28,30,31]

The diet of some bulimic patients is rich in carbohydrates and carbonated liquids and can lead to extensive

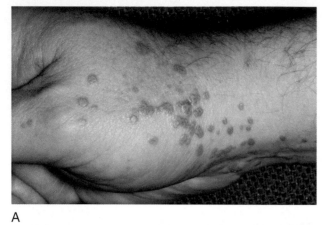

A

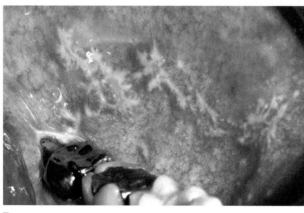

B

Figure 28-9. A, Lichen planus on the skin of the wrist. **B,** Lichen planus on the buccal mucosa. (From Neville BW, Damm DD, Allen CM, Bouquot JE. Oral and Maxillofacial Pathology, 2nd ed. Philadelphia, Saunders, 2002.)

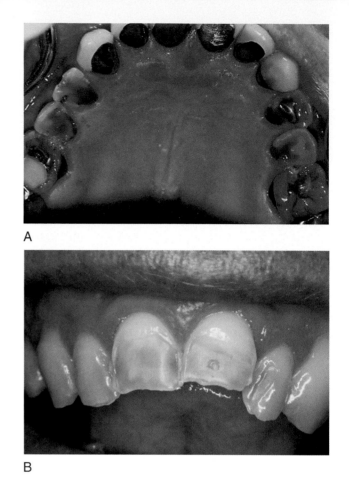

A

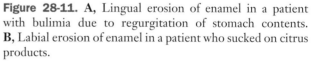

B

Figure 28-11. A, Lingual erosion of enamel in a patient with bulimia due to regurgitation of stomach contents. **B,** Labial erosion of enamel in a patient who sucked on citrus products.

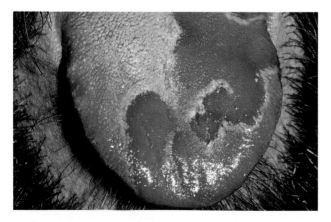

Figure 28-10. Geographic tongue (benign migratory glossitis, erythremia migrans) consists of erythematous well-demarcated areas of papillary atrophy, with a tendency to involve the lateral aspects of the tongue. (From Neville BW, Damm DD, Allen CM, Bouquot JE. Oral and Maxillofacial Pathology, 2nd ed. Philadelphia, Saunders, 2002.)

dental caries and additional erosion of the teeth. An increase in dental caries most often occurs in patients with poor oral hygiene. For these patients, the dentist's goal is to improve the patient's oral hygiene.[32] This involves providing instruction on toothbrushing, use of dental floss, and application of topical fluoride. The patient is instructed to use a baking soda mouth rinse and to brush the teeth after induced vomiting.[32] Tooth sensitivity can be managed with the use of desensitizing toothpastes, fluoride applications, and other means.[32]

Patients with anorexia nervosa may be difficult to identify and deal with in a dental practice. About 40% to 50% of patients with anorexia nervosa are also bulimic and may show dental signs of bulimia.[28,30] Young patients who appear to be anorexic should be confronted about the weight loss. If no symptoms or history of serious medical disease such as cancer or diabetes mellitus is noted, the possibility of self-starvation should be discussed with the patient. Serious medical complications of anorexia nervosa, including death (mortality rate is as high as 15% to 18%), must be discussed in a straightforward manner. Again, when young patients are involved, parents must be informed. Every attempt should be made to refer patients to a physician for evaluation and treatment.

Drug Interactions and Adverse Effects

Important drug interactions between benzodiazepines and barbiturates, opioids, psychotropic agents, cimetidine, and erythromycin may occur. In general, these agents potentiate the CNS depressant effects of benzodiazepines. Regarding the use of these agents, two situations are of concern to the dentist:

1. Barbiturates (not used often now in dentistry) and opioids used for dental sedation or pain control must be administered with caution in decreased dosages in patients who are taking a benzodiazepine for an anxiety disorder.
2. The dentist may prescribe a benzodiazepine for sedation to control dental-related anxiety, but care must be taken when dealing with the individual who is being treated with psychotropic agents for a psychiatric disorder.

Usually, the dosage of the medication can be reduced to avoid overdepression of the CNS. The dentist should consult with the patient's physician before using these drug combinations. During treatment, the patient can be monitored with the use of a pulse oximeter.[4,5,7,25]

Treatment Planning Considerations

Goals of treatment planning for patients with psychiatric disorders are to maintain oral health, comfort, and function, and to prevent and control oral disease. Without an aggressive approach to prevention, many of these patients will be susceptible to dental caries and periodontal disease. Susceptibility to such disease increases because of the adverse effects of xerostomia associated with most of these medications, and the fact that some of the psychiatric conditions for which these patients are being treated reduce interest in or the ability to perform oral hygiene procedures. Also, many of these patients' diets contain foods or drinks that increase the risk for dental disease.[7,46]

The dental treatment plan should contain the following elements: (1) Daily oral hygiene procedures must be identified, (2) the treatment plan must be realistic in terms of the patient's psychiatric disorder and physical status, and (3) the plan must be dynamic to take into account changes in the psychiatric disorder and in the patient's physical status.[47]

The dental team should communicate to the patient and family members a positive, hopeful attitude toward maintenance of the patient's oral health. The dental team should determine whether the patient is legally able to make rational decisions. This should be discussed with the patient and a loved one. Treatment planning often involves input and permission from a loved one, so that decisions can be made.[47]

The last aspect of the treatment plan deals with the selection of medications to be used in providing dental treatment to the patient. Some agents may have to be avoided; others may require a reduction in the usual dosage. Medical consultation is suggested to establish the patient's current status, confirm the medications the patient is taking, identify complications that may be present, and confirm dental medications and doses that will minimize possible drug interactions.[47]

For bulimic patients, treatment through complex restorative procedures should not be planned until the gorging and vomiting cycle has been broken. In a few cases, crowns may be required in an attempt to save teeth. Once the patient is stable and wants to have teeth with severe erosion restored, this can be done. The dentist and the patient must be aware that relapse is common and that complex restorations may fail with recurrence of chronic vomiting.[32]

Oral Complications and Manifestations

Patients with bulimia may present with severe erosion of the lingual and occlusal surfaces of the teeth (see Figure 28-11). Severe erosion can cause increased tooth sensitivity to touch and to cold temperature. Dental caries may be more prevalent in these patients. The amount of saliva produced may be decreased. Patients often report dry mouth. Those with poor oral hygiene have increased periodontal disease. The parotid gland may become enlarged, and patients with anorexia nervosa may have decreased salivary flow, dry mouth, atrophic mucosa, and an enlarged parotid gland.[32]

REFERENCES

1. American Psychiatric Association. Diagnostic and Statistical Manual of Mental Disorders, 2nd ed. Washington DC, American Psychiatric Association, 1994.
2. American Psychiatric Association. Diagnostic and Statistical Manual of Mental Disorders, Text Revision, 4th ed (DSM-IV-TR). Washington DC, American Psychiatric Association, 2000.
3. Vogel LR, Muskin PR. Anxiety disorders. In Cutler JL, Marcus ER (eds). Saunders Text and Review Series: Psychiatry. Philadelphia, WB Saunders, 1999, pp 105-127.
4. Reus VI. Mental disorders. In Kasper DL, Braunwald E, Fauci AS, et al (eds). Harrison's Online Principles of Medicine, 16th ed. New York, McGraw-Hill, 2005, pp 2547-2562.
5. Saver DF, Ferri FF, Pearson RL, et al. Anxiety. Available at: http://www.firstconsult.com/anxiety. Accessed Dec. 20, 2006.
6. American Psychiatric Association. Anxiety disorders. In Diagnostic and Statistical Manual of Mental Disorders, Text Revision, 4th ed (DSM-IV-TR). Washington DC, American Psychiatric Association, 2000, pp 429-485.
7. Little JW. Anxiety disorders: Dental implications. J Gen Dent 2003;51:562-570.
8. Pollack EF, Baustian GH, Jones RC, et al. Schizophrenia. St. Louis, Mo, Elsevier, 2006.
9. Scherger J, Sudak D, Alici-Evciment Y. Depression. Available at: http://www.firstconsult.com/depression. Accessed Dec. 20, 2006.
10. Schiffer RB. Psychiatric disorders in medical practice. In Goldman L, Ausiello D (eds). Cecil Textbook of

Medicine, 22nd ed. Philadelphia, WB Saunders, 2004, pp 2212-2222.

11. Scully C, Cawson RA. Medical Problems in Dentistry, 5th ed. Edinburgh, Elsevier (Churchill Livingstone), 2005.

12. Centers for Disease Control and Prevention. Psychological and emotional effects of the September 11 attacks on the World Trade Center: Connecticut, New Jersey, and New York, 2001. MMWR 2002;51:784-786.

13. North CS. The course of post-traumatic stress disorder after the Oklahoma City bombing. Mil Med 2001;166(12 suppl):51-52.

14. Schlenger WE, Caddell JM, Ebert L, et al. Psychological reactions to terrorist attacks: Reactions to September 11, 2001. JAMA 2002;288:581-588.

15. Schuster MA, Stein BD, Jaycox LH, et al. A national survey of stress reactions after the September 11, 2001 terrorist attacks. N Engl J Med 2001;345:1507-1512.

16. Centers for Disease Control and Prevention. Community needs assessment of Lower Manhattan residents following the World Trade Center attacks: Manhattan, New York City, 2001. MMWR 2002;51(special issue): 10-13.

17. Centers for Disease Control and Prevention. Injuries and illnesses among New York City Fire Department rescue workers after responding to the World Trade Center attacks. MMWR 2002;51(special issue):1-5.

18. Centers for Disease Control and Prevention. Impact of September 11 attacks on workers in the vicinity of the World Trade Center: New York City. MMWR 2002;51(special issue):8-10.

19. Pereira A. Combat trauma and the diagnosis of post-traumatic stress disorder in female and male veterans. Mil Med 2002;167:23-27.

20. Davis LL, English BA, Ambrose SM, Petty F. Pharmacotherapy for post-traumatic stress disorder: A comprehensive review. Expert Opin Pharmacother 2001;2: 1583-1595.

21. Goldberg RJ. Practical Guide to the Care of the Psychiatric Patient. St. Louis, Mosby, 1995.

22. Judd LL, Britton KT, Braff DL. Mental disorders. In Harrison TR, Isselbacher KJ (eds). Harrison's Principles of Internal Medicine, 13th ed. New York, McGraw-Hill, 1994, pp 2400-2420.

23. Kabongo ML, Jones RC, Stangler RS, et al. Posttraumatic stress disorder. Available at: http://www.firstconsult.com/posttraumaticstressdisorder. Accessed Dec. 20, 2006.

24. Wright P, Sigmundson T. Organic psychiatry and epilepsy. In Wright P, Stern J, Phelan M (eds). Core Psychiatry, 2nd ed. Edinburgh, Elsevier, 2005, pp 381-413.

25. Feinstein RE. Cognitive and mental disorders due to general medical conditions. In Cutler JL, Marcus ER (eds). Saunders Text and Review Series: Psychiatry. Philadelphia, WB Saunders, 1999, pp 81-104.

26. Cummings JL, Mendez MF. Alzheimer's disease and other disorders of cognition. In Goldman L, Ausiello D (eds). Cecil Textbook of Medicine, 22nd ed. Philadelphia, WB Saunders, 2004, pp 2248-2257.

27. American Psychiatric Association. Eating disorders. In Diagnostic and Statistical Manual of Mental Disorders, Text Revision, 4th ed (DSM-IV-TR). Washington DC, American Psychiatric Association, 2000, pp 583-597.

28. Majid SH, Treasure JL. Eating disorders. In Wright P, Stern J, Phelan M (eds). Core Psychiatry, 2nd ed. Edinburgh, Elsevier, 2005, pp 217-241.

29. West DS. The eating disorders. In Goldman L, Ausiello D (eds). Cecil Textbook of Medicine, 22nd ed. Philadelphia, WB Saunders, 2004, pp 1336-1338.

30. Devlin MJ. Eating disorders. In Cutler JL, Marcus ER (eds). Saunders Text and Review Series: Psychiatry. Philadelphia, WB Saunders, 1999, pp 170-185.

31. Foster DW. Anorexia nervosa and bulimia nervosa. In Fauci AS, Braunwald E, Isselbacher KJ, et al (eds). Harrison's Principles of Internal Medicine, 14th ed. New York, McGraw-Hill, 1998, pp 462-472.

32. Little JW. Eating disorders. Oral Surg Oral Med Oral Path Oral Radiol Endod 2002;93:138-144.

33. Robertson C, Millar H. Hyperamylasemia in bulimia nervosa and hyperemesis gravidarum. Int J Eat Disord 1999;26:223-227.

34. Metzger ED, Levine JM, McArdle CR, et al. Salivary gland enlargement and elevated serum amylase in bulimia nervosa. Biol Psychiatry 1999;45:1520-1522.

35. Ashton CH. Insomnia and anxiety. In Walker R, Edwards C (eds). Clinical Pharmacy and Therapeutics, 2nd ed. London, Churchill Livingstone, 1999, pp 393-408.

36. Pratt JP. Affective disorders. In Walker R, Edwards C (eds). Clinical Pharmacy and Therapeutics, 2nd ed. London, Churchill Livingstone, 1999, pp 409-425.

37. Horwath E, Courinos F. Schizophrenia and other psychotic disorders. In Cutler JL, Marcus ER (eds). Saunders Text and Review Series: Psychiatry. Philadelphia, WB Saunders, 1999, pp 64-80.

38. Caligor E. Psychological factors affecting medical conditions. In Cutler JL, Marcus ER (eds). Saunders Text and Review Series: Psychiatry. Philadelphia, WB Saunders, 1999, pp 221-246.

39. American Psychiatric Association. Diagnostic and Statistical Manual of Mental Disorders, Text Revision, 4th ed (DSM-IV-TR). Washington DC, American Psychiatric Association, 2000, pp 13-24.

40. Friedlander AH, Gorelick DA. Panic disorder: Its association with mitral valve prolapse and appropriate dental management. Oral Surg Oral Med Oral Pathol 1987; 63:309-312.

41. Dajani AS, Taubert KA, Wilson W, et al. Prevention of bacterial endocarditis: Recommendations by the American Heart Association. JAMA 1997;22:1794-1801.

42. Little JW. Thyroid disorders: Part I, Hyperthyroidism. Oral Surg Oral Med Oral Path Oral Radiol Endod 2006;101:276-284.

43. Milosevic A, Brodie DA, Slade PD. Dental erosion, oral hygiene, and nutrition in eating disorders. Int J Eat Disord 1997;21:195-199.

44. Milosevic A. Eating disorders and the dentist. Br Dent J 1999;186:109-113.

45. Scheutzel P. Etiology of dental erosion—Intrinsic factors. Eur J Oral Sci 1996;104(2 Pt 2):178-190.

46. Little JW. Dental implications of mood disorders. J Gen Dent 2004;52:442-450.

47. Little JW. Alzheimer's disease. J Gen Dent 2005;53: 289-298.

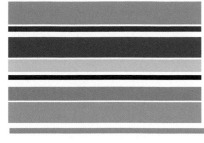

Psychiatric Disorders

CHAPTER
29

Mental disorders are common in today's society. Approximately one third of the population in the United States will have at least one psychiatric disorder during their lifetime, and 20% to 30% of adults in the United States will experience one or more psychiatric disorders during a 1-year period. About 10% of the adult population has a serious drug abuse or dependency problem; about 5% of the population suffers from serious affective or mood disorders. Schizophrenic disorders are reported in 1.1%.[1-6]

Psychiatric problems, which affect the course and outcomes of patients with various medical illnesses, increase length of treatment, decrease the functional level of patients, and have a negative impact on overall prognosis and outcome. Disorders related to smoking, drinking, and drug use account for a significant portion of the health care dollar. In the elderly population, a high prevalence of psychiatric complications is associated with medical illness. About 11% to 15% experience depressive symptoms, and between 10% and 20% have anxiety disorders, including phobias. Phobia is the most common psychiatric disorder in women older than 65 years of age. Approximately 20% of the elderly have a substance abuse disorder.[7,8]

This chapter provides a discussion of mood disorders, somatoform disorders, substance abuse (alcohol abuse is covered in Chapter 11, and nicotine abuse in Chapter 8), and schizophrenia. The emphasis here is on drugs used to treat these conditions and their significant adverse reactions and interactions with drugs used in dentistry. The dental management of these patients is described in detail.

MOOD DISORDERS

DEFINITION

Mood disorders represent a heterogeneous group of mental disorders that are characterized by extreme exaggeration and disturbance of mood and affect. These disorders are associated with physiologic, cognitive, and psychomotor dysfunction. Mood disorders, which tend to be cyclic, include depression and bipolar disorder.[2,3,9]

EPIDEMIOLOGY

Incidence and Prevalence

About 5% of the adults in the United States have a significant mood disorder. Mood disorders are more common among women (Table 29-1). Major depression may begin at any age, but the prevalence is highest among the elderly, followed by 30- to 40-year-old people and, in recent years, an increased number of 15- to 19-year-old individuals.[10] Between 20% and 25% of adult women and between 7% and 12% of adult men at some time experience a major depressive episode. Prevalence for major depression is 4.5% to 9.3% among women and 2.3% to 3.2% in men. After 55 years of age, depression starts to occur more commonly in men.[10] About one third of depressed individuals require hospitalization; 30% follow a chronic course with residual symptoms and social impairment.[2-4,10]

The prevalence of major depression is somewhat consistent across races and cultures. However, it is greater among recent immigrants and the displaced.[10] No evidence suggests significant geographic variability, except in seasonal affective disorder, which is due to limited exposure to the sun during the winter in the northern states. No clear association with social class has been found, but major depression is associated with poverty and unemployment as significant stressors.[10]

The lifetime prevalence of dysthymia, a chronic, milder form of depression, is 2.2% in women and 4.1% in men.[1,4] Approximately 0.4% to 1.6% of adults in the United States have bipolar disorder.[1,4] In contrast to major depression, which is more than twice as common in women as in men, bipolar disorder occurs with equal frequency between both sexes.[2] Bipolar disorders are much less common than major depression and occur equally in both sexes (see Table 29-1).

Etiology

Several theories have been presented to explain the origin of mood disorders. Reduced brain concentrations of norepinephrine and serotonin (neurotransmitters) for some time have been believed to cause depression. Increased levels of these neurotransmitters have contributed to the onset of mania. The causes of depression and mania now appear to be complex. Current research focuses on the interactions of norepinephrine and serotonin with a variety of other brain systems and on abnormalities in the function or quantity of receptors for these transmitters.[1,2,11] Thyrotropin release of thyroid-stimulating hormone and cortisol release by corticotropin-releasing factor and adrenocorticotropin over a long period may be associated with the development of depression. This model suggests that depression is the result of a stress reaction that has gone on too long.[1,2,11]

Evidence for a genetic predisposition to bipolar disorder is significant. The concordance rate for monozygotic twin pairs approaches 80%, and segregation analyses are consistent with autosomal dominant transmission. Multiple genes are likely to be involved, with strongest evidence for loci on chromosomes 18p, 18q, 4p, 4q, 5q, 8p, and 21q.[2]

Positron emission tomography (PET) studies show decreased metabolic activity in the caudate nuclei and frontal lobes in depressed patients that returns to normal with recovery. Single-photon emission computed tomography (SPECT) studies show comparable changes in blood flow.[2]

Psychosocial theory focuses on loss as the cause of depression in vulnerable individuals. Mania receives

---

TABLE **29-1**
Epidemiology of Mood Disorders

Variable	Depressive Disorders	Bipolar Disorders
PREVALENCE	MAJOR DEPRESSION • Point Men: 2.3 % to 3.2% Women: 4.5% to 9.3% Older adults: 11% to 15% • Lifetime Men: 7.0% to 12.0% Women: 20% to 25% • More common in divorced or separated individuals *Dysthymia* • Lifetime Men: 4.1% Women: 2.2%	Bipolar I lifetime: 0.4 % to −1.6% Bipolar II lifetime: 0.5% More common in upper socioeconomic classes Equal in sex and race High rates of divorce Cyclothymia lifetime: 0.4% to −1.0%
AGE OF ONSET	Late 20s or 30s Childhood possible May have much later onset Higher rate and earlier onset for individuals born after 1940 than for those born before	Late teens or early 20s Childhood possible Cyclothymia may precede late onset of overt mania or depression.
FAMILY AND GENETIC STUDIES	Unipolar patients tend to have relatives with major depression and dysthymic disorder and fewer with bipolar disorder Early onset, recurrent course, and psychotic depression appear to be heritable	Bipolar patients have many relatives with bipolar disorder, cyclothymia, unipolar depression, and schizoaffective disorder
TWIN STUDIES	Concordance in monozygotic twins • Recurrent depression: 59% • Single episode only: 33% Concordance rates for identical (monozygotic) twins is 4 times greater than that found in fraternal (dizygotic) twins	72% concordance in monozygotic twins, 19% in same sex dizygotic twins

From Kahn DA. Mood disorders. In Saunders Text and Review Series: Psychiatry. Philadelphia, Saunders, 1999, p 35. Also based on information from Schiffer RB. Psychiatric disorders in medical practice. In Goldman L, Ausiello D (eds). Cecil Textbook of Medicine. Philadelphia: Saunders, 2004, pp 2212-2222.

much less attention because it is thought to be more of a biologically caused disorder. The psychoanalytic hypothesis suggests that unconscious mental conflicts and incomplete psychological development are important factors in the development of some mental disorders, including depression. The interpersonal hypothesis states that social losses in a patient's current life contribute to depression, and improved interpersonal relations may reduce or eliminate depression. The cognitive hypothesis proposes that depression results from distorted thinking, which leads to unrealistically pessimistic and negative views of oneself and the world.[4]

CLINICAL PRESENTATION AND MEDICAL MANAGEMENT

Depressive Disorders

The *Diagnostic and Statistical Manual of Mental Disorders, 4th Edition* (DSM-IV) lists three types of depressive disorders: major depression, dysthymic disorder, and depression not otherwise specified (NOS). Major depression (unipolar) is one of the primary mood disorders. Patients with major depression are depressed most of the day, show a marked decrease in interest or pleasure in most

activities, have a marked gain or loss in weight, and manifest insomnia or hypersomnia (Box 29-1). These symptoms must be present for at least 2 weeks before a diagnosis of major depression can be made. About 50% to 80% of individuals who have had a major depressive episode will have at least one more depressive episode; 20% of these individuals will have a subsequent manic episode and should be reclassified as bipolar. A major depression usually will last about 8 to 9 months if the individual is not treated. Dysthymia represents a chronic, milder form of depression with symptoms that last at least 2 years (see Box 29-1). Depression NOS is a form of depression that falls short of the diagnostic criteria for major depression and has been too brief for dysthymic disorder.[4,10,12] A form of depression called *seasonal affective disorder* may occur in areas of the country that have limited amounts of sunlight during the winter.[10]

Bipolar Disorder

The DSM-IV lists four types of bipolar disorder: bipolar I, bipolar II, cyclothymic, and bipolar disorder NOS (Figure 29-1). Bipolar I disorder consists of recurrences of mania and major depression or mixed states that occur at different times in the patient, or a mixture of symptoms

---

BOX 29-1

Diagnostic Criteria for Depressive Disorders

Major Depressive Episode

At least five of the following symptoms have been present during the same 2-week period (one of the symptoms must be depressed mood or loss of interest or pleasure):
- Depressed mood most of the day
- Marked loss of interest or pleasure in most or all activities most of the day
- Significant weight gain or loss when not dieting, or change in appetite
- Insomnia or hypersomnia nearly every day
- Psychomotor agitation or retardation nearly every day: that is observable by others
- Fatigue or loss of energy nearly every day
- Feelings of worthlessness or excessive guilt feelings
- Inability to think or concentrate, or indecisiveness
- Recurrent thoughts of death, or suicidal ideation without a specific plan, or with a plan, or attempted

An organic factor did not initiate or maintain the disturbance

The disturbance is not a normal reaction to the death of a loved one

No delusions or hallucinations during symptoms or before the development of mood symptoms, developed or after they have remitted

Not superimposed on schizophrenia, schizophreniform disorder, delusional disorder, or psychotic disorder; no other specific diagnosis

Dysthymia

Depressed mood for most of the day for at least 2 years

Presence, while depressed, of two or more of the following:
- Poor appetite
- Insomnia or hypersomnia
- Low energy or fatigue
- Low self-esteem
- Poor concentration or difficulty making decisions
- Feelings of hopelessness

During the 2-year period, the person has never been without the symptoms for more longer than 2 months at a time

No major depressive episode has been present during the first 2 years of the disturbance

There has not been an intermixed manic episode

The disturbance does not occur during the course of a psychotic disorder

The symptoms are not caused by the physiologic effects of a substance

The symptoms cause significant distress or functional impairment

---

From Schiffer RB. Psychiatric disorders in medical practice. In Goldman L., Ausiello D (eds). Cecil Textbook of Medicine, Philadelphia: Saunders, 2004, Table 426-1.

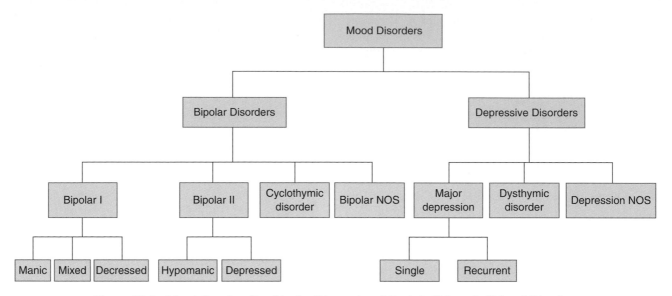

Figure 29-1. Mood disorders listed in the *Diagnostic and Statistical Manual of Mental Disorders,* 4th ed (DSM-IV). Patients with bipolar disorder have had at least one episode of mania or hypomania. Cyclothymic disorder consists of recurrent brief episodes of hypomania and mild depression. Major depression is usually recurrent but sometimes happens as a single lifetime episode. Dysthymic disorder is mild depression that lasts at least 2 years.

that occur at the same time. The essential feature of a manic episode is a distinct period during which the person's mood is elevated and expansive or irritable (Table 29-2). Associated symptoms of the manic syndrome include inflated self-esteem, grandiosity, a decreased need for sleep, excessive speech, flight of ideas, distractibility, psychomotor agitation, and excessive involvement in pleasurable activities. During a manic episode, the mood often is described as euphoric, cheerful, or "high." The expansive quality of the mood is characterized by unceasing and unselective enthusiasm for interacting with people. However, the predominant mood disturbance may be irritability and anger. Speech often is loud, rapid, and difficult to interpret, and behavior may be intrusive and demanding. Style of dress is often colorful and strange, and long periods without sleep are common. Poor judgment may lead to financial and legal problems. Drug and alcohol abuse often is seen.[2,4,10,12]

Bipolar II disorder consists of recurrences of major depression and hypomania (mild mania). Cyclothymic disorder comprises recurrent brief episodes of hypomania (see Table 29-2) and mild depression. Bipolar disorder NOS describes partial syndromes, such as recurrent hypomania without depression. Patients with bipolar disorder have at least one episode of mania or hypomania.[2,4,10,12]

The diagnosis of bipolar disorder is made as soon as a patient has one manic episode, even if that person has never had a depressive episode. Most patients who become manic will eventually experience depression. However, about 10% of patients in whom bipolar disorder is diagnosed appear to have only manic episodes.[4]

Men tend to have a greater number of manic episodes and women, more numerous depressive episodes.

Untreated individuals with bipolar disorder will have a mean of nine affective episodes during their lifetime. The length of each cycle tends to decrease, although the number of cycles increases with age (Figure 29-2). Each affective episode lasts about 8 to 9 months. Bipolar patients have a greater number of episodes, hospitalizations, divorces, and suicides compared with unipolar patients.[13]

Treatment of Mood Disorders

Table 29-3 shows commonly used antidepressants. The first-line medication is a selective serotonin reuptake inhibitor (SSRI) such as citalopram. Sertraline, venlafaxine, and bupropion are second-line drugs that may be used in patients who fail to achieve remission with citalopram.[14,15] These agents are primarily used to treat major depression, dysthymic disorder, depression NOS, and depression associated with bipolar disorder. Drug therapy is essential in bipolar disorder for achieving two goals: rapid control of symptoms in acute episodes of mania and depression, and prevention of future episodes or reduction of their severity and frequency. Mood disorders have a tendency to recur. Affective episodes may occur spontaneously or may be triggered by adverse events. Individuals with mood disorders and their families must become aware of the early signs and symptoms of affective episodes, so that treatment can be initiated. These individuals also must be made aware of the need for medication compliance and of the medication's adverse effects and possible complications.[1-3,11]

The mainstays of drug therapy are the mood-stabilizing drugs that generally act on both mania and depression. The three drugs used are lithium, valproate, and

TABLE **29-2**
Clinical Features of Hypomania and Mania

Feature	Hypomania	Mania
APPEARANCE	May be unremarkable Demeanor may be cheerful	Often striking Clothes may reflect mood state Demeanor may be cheerful Disordered and fatigued in severe states
BEHAVIOR	Increased sociability and loss of inhibition	Overactivity and excitement Social loss of inhibition
SPEECH	May be talkative	Often pressured with flight of ideas
MOOD	Mild elation or irritability	Elated or irritable Boundless optimism Typically, no diurnal pattern May be labile
VEGETATIVE SIGNS	Increased appetite Reduced need for sleep Increased libido	Increased appetite Reduced need for sleep Increased libido
PSYCHOTIC SYMPTOMS	Not present Thoughts may have an expansive quality	Thoughts may have an expansive quality Delusions and second-person auditory hallucinations may be present, often grandiose in nature Schneiderian First Rank (symptoms associated with schizophrenia) symptoms found in 10% to 20%
COGNITION	Mild distractibility	Marked distractibility More marked disturbances in severe states
INSIGHT	Usually preserved	Insight often lost, especially in severe states

From Mackin P, Young A. Bipolar disorders. In Wright P, Stern J, Phelan M (eds). Core Psychiatry, 2nd ed. Edinburgh: Elsevier, 2005, pp 295-319, Table 20-1.

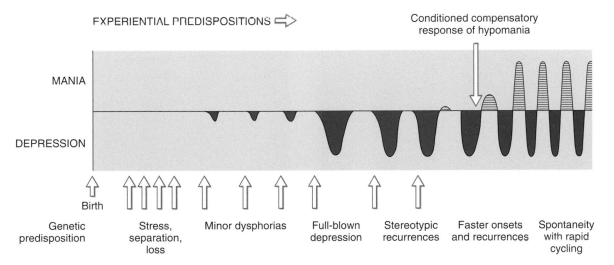

Figure 29-2. Natural history of recurrent mood disorders: An integrated model. Genetic factors and early environmental stress may predispose to development of a mood disorder. Early episodes are likely to be precipitated by environmental stress; later episodes are more likely to occur closer together and spontaneously, without precipitants.

carbamazepine. The most widely used mood stabilizer is lithium carbonate. Lithium is most helpful in patients with euphoric mania. When lithium is ineffective, or when medical problems prevent its use, one of the anticonvulsants (valproate or carbamazepine) is used. Electroconvulsive therapy is an effective antimanic treatment.

It may be used in cases of manic violence, delirium, or exhaustion. It is also appropriate for use with patients who do not respond to medication taken for many weeks. When antidepressant drugs are given for bipolar depression, they may cause a switch to mania or a mixed state, or they may induce rapid cycling. The most common

TABLE 29-3
Commonly Used Antidepressants (by structural group)

Drug	Trade Name	Initial Dose Range	Target Dose Range	Comments
TRICYCLICS				
Amitriptyline	Elavil	10-50 mg	150-300 mg	
Desipramine	Norpramin	10-75 mg	150-250 mg	
Doxepin	Sinequan	25-75 mg	75-300 mg	
Imipramine	Tofranil	10-75 mg	100-300 mg	
Nortriptyline	Pamelor	10-50 mg	75-150 mg	
Protriptyline	Vivactil	10-30 mg	20-50 mg	
HETEROCYCLICS				
Amoxapine	Asendin	25-75 mg	100-300 mg	
Clomipramine	Anaframil	10-75 mg	150-300 mg	
Maprotiline	Ludiomil	25-75 mg	100-300 mg	
SSRIs				
Citalopram	Celexa	10 mg/day	10-40 mg/day	
Fluoxetine	Prozac	10-20 mg/day	10-80 mg/day	
Fluvoxamine	Luvox	50 mg/day	50-300 mg/day	
Paroxetine	Paxil	20 mg/day	20-50 mg/day	
Sertraline	Zoloft	50 mg/day	50-200 mg/day	
MOIs				Patients taking MOIs must be on a tyramine-free diet
Isocarboxazid	Marplan	10-30 mg	10-30 mg	
Phenelzine	Nardil	15-45 mg	45-75 mg	
Tranylcypromine	Parnate	10-20 mg	20-30 mg	
SNRIs				SNRIs may be effective in the treatment of resistant depression; nefazodone is as effective as imipramine
Nefazodone	Serzone	100 mg bid	200-400 mg	
Venlafaxine	Effexor	25 mg tid	200-275 mg/day tid dosing	
ATYPICAL				
Bupropion	Wellbutrin	100 mg bid	300 mg/day tid	Bupropion may be used in atypical depression
Mirtazapine	Remeron	15 mg/day	30-45 mg	Mirtazapine increases at 1- to 2-wk intervals
Trazodone	Desyrel	25-75 mg/day in divided doses	300 mg/day in divided doses	Trazodone is helpful as a second drug for sleep disturbance
PSYCHOSTIMULANTS				Abuse potential must be considered
Dextroamphetamine	Dexedrine	2.5 gm	5-10 mg	
Methylphenidate	Ritalin	2.5 mg bid	10 mg tid	
Pemoline	Cylert	18.75 mg	37 mg bid	

From Schiffer RB. Psychiatric disorders in medical practice. In Goldman L, Ausiello D (eds). Cecil Textbook of Medicine. Philadelphia: Saunders, 2004, based on Table 426-2.
bid, Twice daily; MOIs, monoamine oxidase inhibitors; SNRIs, serotonin and noradrenergic reuptake inhibitors; SSRIs, selective serotonin reuptake inhibitors; tid, 3 times daily.

treatment for bipolar depression is an antidepressant combined with a mood stabilizer to prevent a manic switch or rapid cycling.[1-3,11]

It takes about 7 to 10 days for lithium to reach full therapeutic effectiveness. With most antidepressant drugs, a delay (10 to 21 days) is noted before full therapeutic benefits are achieved.[2,3,11]

Patients who have had two or three episodes of bipolar disorder, including depressive episodes, usually are treated indefinitely because of the near certainty of relapse. Prevention targets both manic and depressive episodes. Lithium is the treatment of choice. About one third of patients will not have additional episodes and are considered cured. Another one third of those who take lithium will have less frequent or less severe episodes and will function well. The remaining third of patients will continue to have frequent and severe episodes with ongoing disability.[4]

TABLE 29-4
Somatoform Disorders

Somatoform Disorders	Features
SOMATIZATION DISORDER	Chronic multisystem disorder characterized by complaints of pain, and gastrointestinal and sexual dysfunction. Onset is usually early in life, and psychosocial and vocational achievements are limited. Rarely affects men. Diagnostic criteria include four pain symptoms plus two gastrointestinal symptoms, plus one sexual/reproductive symptom, plus one pseudoneurologic symptom.
CONVERSION DISORDER	Syndrome of symptoms or deficits mimicking neurologic or medical illness, in which psychological factors are judged to be of etiologic importance. Patients report isolated symptoms that have no physical cause (blindness, deafness, stocking anesthesia) and that do not conform to known anatomic pathways or physiologic mechanisms. When a group of these patients is followed over time, a physical disease process will become apparent in 10% to 50%.
PAIN DISORDER	Clinical syndrome characterized predominantly by pain in which psychological factors are judged to be of etiologic importance
HYPOCHONDRIASIS	Chronic preoccupation with the idea of having serious disease. This preoccupation is usually poorly amenable to reassurance. May consist of a morbid preoccupation with physical symptoms or bodily functions. Can be described as "illness is a way of life."
BODY DYSMORPHIC DISORDER	Preoccupation with an imagined or exaggerated defect in physical appearance
Other Somatoform-Like Disorders	**Features**
FACTITIOUS DISORDER	Intentional production or feigning of physical or psychological signs when external reinforcers (e.g., avoidance of responsibility, financial gain) are not clearly present. Voluntary production of symptoms without external incentive. More common in men and seen in health care workers more often. Skin lesions more common than oral (oral lesions cannot be seen). Oral lesions include self-extraction of teeth, picking at the gingiva with fingernails, nail file gingival injury, and application of caustic substances to the lips.
MALINGERING	Intentional production or feigning of physical or psychological signs when external reinforcers (e.g., avoidance of responsibility, financial gain) are present
DISSOCIATIVE DISORDERS	Disruptions of consciousness, memory, identity, or perception judged to be due to psychological factors

From Schiffer RB. Psychiatric disorders in medical practice. In Goldman L, Ausiello D (eds). Cecil Textbook of Medicine. Philadelphia: Saunders, 2004, based on Table 426-7. Material added from Scully C, Cawson RA. Medical Problems in Dentistry, 5th ed. Edinburgh: Elsevier Churchill Livingstone, 2005, p 612.

An estimated 30,000 suicides occur each year in the United States. About 70% of these involve individuals with major depression. The physician must consider suicidal lethality in the management of patients with depression. In general, the risk for suicide is increased in the following situations: alcoholism, drug abuse, social isolation, being an elderly male, terminal illness, and undiagnosed/untreated mental disorders. Patients at greatest risk are those with a history of previous suicide attempts, drug or alcohol abuse, recent diagnosis of a serious condition, loss of a loved one, recent retirement, living alone, or having poor social support. Patients with a plan and the means to carry out that plan are at greatest risk of suicide. Once medical control is attained in the patient with a mood disorder, insight-oriented psychotherapy often is initiated as an adjunct for management of the patient's condition.[9,16,17]

SOMATOFORM DISORDERS

DEFINITION

Individuals with somatoform disorders have physical complaints for which no general medical cause is present. Associated unconscious psychological factors contribute to the onset, exacerbation, or maintenance of physical symptoms. The following conditions are regarded as somatoform disorders: somatization, conversion disorder, pain disorder, and hypochondriasis (Table 29-4). Patients with a somatization disorder experience multiple, unexplained somatic symptoms that may last for years.[2,18]

EPIDEMIOLOGY

Incidence and Prevalence

The prevalence of somatoform disorders is 5%.[2] Most of these occur in women. Patients with symptoms that do not meet the full criteria for somatization disorder are much more common. Conversion disorder, pain disorder, and hypochondriasis appear to be more common than somatization disorder.[2]

Etiology

In this group of disorders, physical symptoms suggest a physical disorder for which no underlying physical basis can be found. Symptoms are linked to psychological factors. Somatization therefore is defined as the manifestation of psychological stress in somatic symptoms.

A conversion reaction results when a psychological conflict or need is expressed as an alteration or loss of physical function, suggesting a physical disorder. A person who views a traumatic event, for example, but has a conflict about acknowledging that event may develop a conversion disorder of blindness. In this case, the symptom of blindness has symbolic value and is a representation of and a partial solution to the underlying psychological conflict. In contrast, patients with hypochondriasis or a factitious (self-inflicted) disorder are aware of the nature of their problem but may be unable to control it. Many patients with pain disorder describe a history of a physical injury that precedes later onset of pain. This onset of pain is accompanied by environmental stress or emotional conflict.[2-4,18]

CLINICAL PRESENTATION AND MEDICAL MANAGEMENT

Somatization Disorder

Somatization consists of multiple symptoms and usually begins before the age of 30 years. Patients experience multiple, unexplained somatic symptoms, which may include pain, diarrhea, bloating, vomiting, sexual dysfunction, blindness, deafness, weakness, paralysis, or coordination problems. This is a serious psychiatric illness. Many patients have concurrent anxiety, depression, or personality disorder.[2,3,18]

Conversion Disorder

Conversion disorder is a monosymptomatic somatoform disorder that affects the individual's voluntary motor system or sensory functions. The patient may experience blindness, deafness, paralysis, or an inability to speak or to walk. Symptoms suggest a physical condition, but the cause is psychological. The symptom, which is not intentionally produced, typically is a symbolic representation that relieves an underlying emotional conflict.[2,3,18]

Pain Disorder

Pain disorder causes the patient significant distress in important areas of functioning such as social and occupational activities. In patients with pain disorder, no organic disease can be identified. Often, a stressful event precedes the onset of pain. Pain often results in secondary gain in the form of increased attention and sympathy from others.[2,3,18]

Hypochondriasis

Patients with hypochondriasis are preoccupied with the fear or belief that they have a serious disease. Their misinterpretations of normal bodily functions are generally to blame.[2,3,18]

Factitious Disorder

Factitious disorder consists of intentional self-harm that is produced by infliction of physical, chemical, or thermal injury to one's self. It involves the voluntary production of signs and symptoms (physical injury or psychological symptoms) without external incentives such as avoidance of responsibility or financial gain. Factitious disorder is more common among men and occurs more often in health care workers. The skin is the most common site for injury.

Treatment

Treatment of patients with somatoform disorders often requires multiple therapeutic modalities, including psychotherapy for their interpersonal and psychological problems. Medication for the treatment of underlying depressive disorder also may be needed. Group therapy is beneficial in some cases. Unneeded medical or surgical treatment must not be rendered and will not correct the problem. It is costly and may lead to significant associated complications.[2,3,18]

SUBSTANCE-RELATED DISORDERS

DEFINITION

Substance-related disorders consist of symptoms and maladaptive behavioral changes associated with the regular use of psychoactive substances that affect the central nervous system (CNS). These disorders involve substance dependence, abuse, and tolerance, as well as withdrawal symptoms.[19-21]

EPIDEMIOLOGY

Incidence and Prevalence

In 2004, about 66% of the U.S. population aged 16 to 24 years had taken an illicit drug.[22] Cannabis is the most commonly abused drug in the United States, with about 3 million individuals (11% of those aged 16 to 59 years) using the drug in 2004.[22] More than 75 million Americans have used marijuana during their lifetime.[23] It is also the most commonly used illicit drug in the world.[23] Abuse of class A drugs occurs in about 8% of the adult population.[22] The level of drug use is highest among the 20- to 24-year-old segment of the U.S. population.[22]

The lifetime prevalence of stimulant abuse or dependence is estimated at 1.7% in the United States.[24] This includes use of cocaine, amphetamine, and various analogs of amphetamine such as methamphetamine and MDMA (ecstasy; 3,4-methylylenedioxymethamphetamine).[22,74] About 900,000 Americans use cocaine for the first time each year, and more than 30 million have used the drug at least once.[23] Cocaine use increased from 2003 to 2004.[22]

Methamphetamine is a synthetic drug that is easily manufactured; its use is spreading across the United States from the West coast at alarming rates. A recent survey of 500 law enforcement agencies in 45 states reported that 58% of these agencies indicated that methamphetamine is their biggest drug problem.[25] States that reported the greatest "meth" problem were located along the West Coast and the Upper Midwest. In the Northeast, on the other hand, only 4% of these agencies rated methamphetamine or "speed" as their biggest drug problem.[25]

Etiology

A complex, unique set of variables influence the addictive behavior of individuals with alcohol or drug problems. Evidence suggests that genetic transmission is involved in alcoholism. Psychological factors such as depression, self-medication (used to treat psychic distress), personality disorder, poor coping skills, and others appear to be involved in addictive behavior. Social factors that may be involved include interpersonal, cultural, and societal influences.[21]

CLINICAL PRESENTATION AND MEDICAL MANAGEMENT

Substance dependence occurs when an individual takes a substance in larger amounts or over a longer period than was originally intended. A great deal of time may be spent in activities needed to get the substance, take it, or recover from its effects. The person gives up important social, occupational, and recreational activities because of substance use. Marked tolerance to the substance may develop (>50% increase); hence, larger amounts are needed to achieve intoxication or to produce the desired effect. The person with this disorder continues to take the substance, despite persistent or recurrent social, psychological, and physical problems that result from its use.[21]

Substance abuse denotes substance use that does not meet the criteria for dependence (Box 29-2). This diagnosis is most likely to be applicable to individuals who have just started to take psychoactive substances. Examples of substance abuse may include the following: a middle-aged man who repeatedly drives his car while intoxicated (the man has no other symptoms) and a woman who keeps drinking even though her physician has warned her that alcohol is responsible for exacerbating the symptoms of a duodenal ulcer (she has no other symptoms).[20,21] Table 29-5 lists the physical complaints (symptoms) and possible physical findings (signs) noted in individuals with chronic substance use.

Withdrawal occurs when the person with substance dependence stops or reduces intake of the substance. Withdrawal symptoms vary in accordance with the substance involved. Physiologic signs of withdrawal are common after prolonged use of alcohol, opioids, sedatives, hypnotics, and anxiolytics. Such signs are less obvious in withdrawal from cocaine, nicotine, amphetamines, and cannabis.[19-21]

BOX 29-2

Diagnostic Criteria for Dependence and Drug Abuse

Dependence (3 or more needed)

- Tolerance
- Withdrawal
- The substance is often taken in larger amounts over a longer period than intended
- Any unsuccessful effort or a persistent desire to cut down or control substance use
- A great deal of time is spent in activities necessary to obtain the substance or to recover from its effects
- Important social, occupational, or recreational activities given up or reduced because of substance use
- Continued substance use despite knowledge of having had persistent or recurrent physical or psychological problems that are likely to be caused or exacerbated by the substance

Abuse (2 or more for 12 months)

- Recurrent substance use resulting in failure to fulfill major role obligations at work, school, and home
- Recurrent substance use in situations in which it is physically hazardous
- Recurrent substance-related legal problems
- Continued substance use despite having persistent or recurrent social or interpersonal problems caused or exacerbated by the effects of the substance
- Never met criteria for dependence

From Samet JH. Drug abuse and dependence. In Cecil Textbook of Medicine, Goldman L., Ausiello D (eds). Cecil Textbook of Medicine, 22nd edition. Philadelphia: Saunders, 2004, Table 30-1.

TABLE **29-5**
Chronic Substance Use

Substance	Related Physical Complaints	Possible Physical Findings
ALCOHOL	Frequent injuries; abdominal pain, nausea, and vomiting (gastritis, pancreatitis); diarrhea; headaches; vague physical complaints; erectile dysfunction; convulsions; palpitations; insomnia	Hypertension; injuries (e.g., bruises, cigarette burns, unexplained burns); enlarged liver; cutaneous stigmas, stigmata of liver disease (spider angioma, palmar erythema); ecchymoses on legs, arms, or chest; smell of alcohol on breath; myopathy; peripheral neuritis; congestive heart failure
COCAINE	Fatigue, sinusitis, sore throat, hoarseness, persistent fever, chest pain, sexual problems, bronchitis, weight loss, nausea and vomiting, headaches, muscle jerks and spasms, convulsions, arrhythmia	*Cocaine:* rhinitis, rash around nasal area, perforation of nasal septum, hypertension, tachycardia *Crack cocaine:* hoarseness; parched lips, tongue, and throat; singed eyebrows or eyelashes; stigmas stigmata of IV use
METHAMPHETAMINE	Insomnia, weight loss, vomiting or diarrhea, headaches, aggressive behavior, psychosis, hypertension, arrhythmias, stroke, heart failure, convulsions, coma	Worn-down teeth (from tooth grinding), scratches, skin ulcers, dyskinesia, "meth" mouth (xerostomia, caries, periodontal disease), severe anxiety
INHALANTS (HYDROCARBONS)	Weight loss, breathing difficulties, fatigue, nosebleeds, weakness, stomach upset, intellectual changes	Halitosis, rash around nose or mouth, mental status changes
CANNABIS	Chronic dry cough, bronchitis, sinusitis, pharyngitis, laryngitis	Conjunctival suffusion; distinct odor of burnt leaves on breath and clothes; dilated, poorly reactive pupils
OPIOIDS	False complaints of severe pain made to obtain drugs; infections (especially cellulitis, abscess, pneumonia, SBE)	Needle track marks, skin lesions, constricted pupils, swollen nasal mucosa, thrombosis, lymphadenopathy
OTHER SEDATIVES	Insomnia, restlessness, convulsions, pneumonia	Slurred speech, needle track marks if IV user (especially with barbiturates), pupillary constriction with glutethimide
HALLUCINOGENS	Palpitations, chest pain (especially in older users), convulsions with PCP	Myopathy, renal failure with PCP

From Levin FR, Kleber HD. Alcohol and substance abuse disorders. In Cutler JL, Marcus ER (eds). Psychiatry: Review Series. Philadelphia: Saunders, 1999, p 140; Samet JH. Drug abuse and dependence. In Goldman L, Ausiello D (eds). Cecil Textbook of Medicine, 22nd ed. Philadelphia: Saunders, 2004, pp 145-152.

Sedative Use

The primary groups of psychoactive substances used as sedatives and hypnotics are benzodiazepines (diazepam, lorazepam, temazepam), barbiturates (phenobarbital, secobarbital, mephobarbital), chloral hydrate, and zolpidem. Drugs from each of these groups have a history of being abused. The benzodiazepines are now the most frequently abused of the sedative and hypnotic drugs, replacing the barbiturates, which are no longer extensively used in the clinical setting.[22,24]

The percentage of users of benzodiazepines who become dependent is a function of dose, type, and duration of use. Longer use is more likely to lead to dependence. Few people become dependent with periods of use shorter than 3 months.[22] Usage that lasts between 3 and 12 months leads to dependence in 10% to 20%. The rate of dependency increases to 20% to 45% when benzodiazepines are used for periods longer than a year.[22] Benzodiazepines should be avoided in high-risk, dependence-prone individuals and their use limited to no longer than 2 weeks when possible.[22] Patients who are dependent on benzodiazepines are managed by prescription of a regimen that ensures gradual dose reduction of the abused drug, or by substitution of another long-acting sedative-hypnotic with gradual reduction in dosage.[23]

Withdrawal symptoms produced by benzodiazepines are similar to those caused by withdrawal from alcohol.[26] They can occur after several weeks or longer of moderate use of the drug.[26] Symptoms of withdrawal from benzodiazepines include nausea and vomiting, weakness, autonomic hyperactivity (tachycardia and sweating), anxiety, orthostatic hypotension, tremor, loss of appetite and weight loss, tinnitus, delirium with delusions, and hallucinations.[26]

Opioid Use

The primary effects of the opioids (opiate-like drugs) are to decrease pain perception, cause modest levels of sedation, and produce euphoria. Drugs included in this category include heroin, morphine, codeine, and many nonsteroidal prescription analgesics. Semisynthetic drugs produced from morphine or thebaine molecules include hydromorphone, heroin, and oxycodone. Synthetic opioids include meperidine, propoxyphene, diphenoxylate, fentanyl, buprenorphine, methadone, and pentazocine. Tolerance to any single opioid is likely to generalize to other drugs in the group.[19,27]

Through direct effects on the CNS, opiates may produce nausea and vomiting, decreased pain perception, euphoria, and sedation. Additives in street drugs can cause permanent damage to the nervous system, including peripheral neuropathy and CNS dysfunction. Patients may experience constipation and anorexia. Respiratory depression occurs as the result of a decreased response of the brainstem to carbon dioxide tension. This effect is part of the toxic reaction to opiates that is described later, but it also can be significant in patients with compromised lung activity. Cardiovascular effects of the opiates are mild, and no direct effect on heart rhythm or myocardial contractility has been noted with their use. Orthostatic hypotension, probably caused by dilation of peripheral vessels, may occur. A major danger associated with intravenous (IV) use of these drugs involves the use of contaminated needles. This practice leads to increased risk for hepatitis B and C, bacterial endocarditis, and infection with human immunodeficiency virus (HIV).[20,27]

Dependence on opiates can be seen in at least three groups of patients. A minority of patients with chronic pain syndromes misuse their prescribed drugs. The second group at high risk consists of physicians, dentists, nurses, and pharmacists. These individuals have easy access to drugs with abuse potential. Members of the third group buy their drugs on the street to get high. Once persistent opiate use has been established, the outcome is often very serious. More than 25% of such users are likely to die after 10 to 20 years of active use. Death results from suicide, homicide, accidents, and infectious diseases such as hepatitis or acquired immunodeficiency syndrome (AIDS).[27]

Toxic reactions are seen with all opiates. These reactions are more frequent and dangerous with more potent drugs such as fentanyl, which is 80 to 100 times more powerful than morphine. IV overdose can lead immediately to slow, shallow respirations, bradycardia, a drop in body temperature, and lack of responsiveness to external stimulation. Emergency treatment includes support of vital signs with the use of a respirator and a reversal agent such as naloxone injected intramuscularly or intravenously.[20,27]

In contrast to sedative withdrawal, withdrawal from opiates is an unpleasant but not life-threatening experience. Gastrointestinal upset, muscle cramps, rhinorrhea, and irritability are the prominent symptoms. Opiate users with memory impairment or cognitive dysfunction should be assessed for HIV infection via evaluation of risk factors and blood screening of the patient after appropriate counseling has been provided.[20]

Cocaine Use

Cocaine is a stimulant and a local anesthetic with potent vasoconstrictor properties. The drug produces physiologic and behavioral effects when administered orally, intranasally, intravenously, or via inhalation by smoking. Cocaine has potent pharmacologic effects on dopamine, norepinephrine, and serotonin neurons in the CNS. Cocaine has a short plasma half-life of about 1 hour.[19,28]

Cocaine intoxication causes a sense of well-being, a heightened awareness of sensory input, anorexia, a decreased desire to sleep, restlessness, elation, grandiosity, agitation, and psychotic states (panic attack, paranoid ideation, delusions, and auditory and visual hallucinations). Physical findings of cocaine intoxication consist of tachycardia, cardiac arrhythmias, papillary dilation, and elevated blood pressure. Individuals in this condition may experience headache, as well as chills, nausea, and vomiting. Needle tracks ("skin popping") may be found on the arms of intravenous users of cocaine and heroin. Frequent or high-dose use of cocaine can produce psychiatric states similar to acute schizophrenic episodes. Pregnant women who are chronic users of cocaine or heroin may give birth to infants who are "addicted."[20,28]

Cocaine overdose can be life threatening. "Crack" cocaine, which is inhaled via "freebasing" or smoking, results in much higher blood levels of cocaine than are produced by "snorting" the drug. Myocardial infarction, arrhythmia, stroke, and symptoms consistent with neuroleptic malignant syndrome have been associated with cocaine use. Depression is common in cocaine addicts, particularly during periods of withdrawal, and under these conditions, the drug may be taken in an attempt to commit suicide.[20]

Cocaine abuse is treated via psychotherapy, behavioral therapy, and 12-step programs.[23] Acupuncture may be used for detoxification and prevention of relapse.[23] Treatment of cocaine overdose is a medical emergency that involves resuscitation in an intensive care unit. Intravenous diazepam has been shown to be effective for control of seizures. Ventricular arrhythmias can be managed by intravenous propranolol. Medication is not available that is both safe and effective for cocaine detoxification or for maintenance of abstinence.[28] IV cocaine abusers are at increased risk for hepatitis B, hepatitis C, and exposure to HIV. Some IV cocaine abusers develop a pruritic rash on the chest (allergic reaction to a benzoic acid ester), and ester-type local anesthetics must be avoided in these patients.[20,29]

Amphetamine Use

Amphetamines and related drugs are CNS stimulants. Their psychoactive effects last longer than those of cocaine. Their peripheral sympathomimetic effects also may be more potent than those of cocaine. Amphetamines are used to promote weight loss and for treatment of attention deficit disorder, narcolepsy, and treatment-resistant depression. Many people develop dependence when they first use amphetamines for their appetite suppressant effects in an attempt at weight control. Intravenous administration of amphetamine can lead to rapid development of dependence. Progressive tolerance is common in amphetamine dependence. Amphetamine use may result in the same symptoms and complications that are seen with cocaine abuse.[20,21]

Brand names of amphetamines used for medical purposes include Desoxyn, Pemoline, and Dexedrine.[30-33] Amphetamines were widely abused during the 1960s by individuals in the "counterculture movement." Amphetamine sulfate was known on the street as speed, whiz, blues, bennies, pep pills, uppers, or splash. It was inhaled, snorted, smoked, taken orally, or injected intravenously. In the 1980s and 1990s, cocaine became the drug of choice.[30-33]

Amphetamine analogs produce very similar signs and symptoms. Those associated with normal dosage include hyperalertness, euphoria, hyperactivity, and increased physical endurance. Higher doses of these drugs may cause dysphonia, headache, tachycardia, and confusion. When methamphetamine is introduced intravenously or by inhalation, a rapid, prolonged rush may result. When abused, "meth" can induce psychotic symptoms very similar to those associated with acute schizophrenia.[30-33]

Methamphetamine is a potent synthetic psychostimulant form of amphetamine.[23] It is highly addictive, and chronic use has been associated with violent behavior. On the street, methamphetamine is referred to as "speed," "crank," "go," and "zip." The smokeable form is called "ice" or "crystal." The biologic half-life of methamphetamine is much longer than that of cocaine. Symptoms of withdrawal from methamphetamine may be more intense than those associated with cocaine. Cessation after daily use may result in severe depression with suicidal or homicidal ideation, hypersomnia, or sleeping difficulty.[23,34]

Methamphetamine ("meth") and MDMA (Ecstasy) have undergone a major resurgence among adolescents and people in their early 20s. Methamphetamine was made illegal in 1971, and Ecstasy in 1985. Methamphetamine is widely used in California and in some Midwestern states, where it is synthesized in "home" laboratories.[35,36] Methamphetamine is the most widely illegally manufactured, distributed, and abused type of amphetamine. Its use in Japan has been rampant since the end of World War II.[31,37]

Medications that contain pseudoephedrine (over-the-counter [OTC] decongestants, such as Sudafed) are used by "home" laboratory operators to produce methamphetamine.

More than 44 states have passed laws to make it more difficult to purchase OTC medicines that contain pseudoephedrine.[38,39] Some states require individuals who purchase these medications to show identification and sign a ledger.[38,39] In other states, it is required that these medicines be placed behind the pharmacy counter. Oklahoma was the first state to impose restrictions, and during the first year, the sale of OTC medicines that contain pseudoephedrine was reduced by 16%. President Bush, in March of 2006, signed into law a bill that imposes strict standards on products made with pseudoephedrine. This bill requires that products be placed behind the counter; customers must show identification and must sign a log book, and limitations have been set on how much of the medicine can be sold at one time.[38,39]

Cannabis Use

Delta-9-tetrahydrocannabinol (THC) is the major psychoactive ingredient in substances that cause cannabis dependence. Several different preparations of marijuana are available. These preparations—bhang, charas, ganja, and hashish—are known to vary in potency and quality. They usually are smoked but can be taken orally and are sometimes mixed with food. Current marijuana supplies are much more potent than those that were available in the 1960s. Most users describe an altered sense of time and distance perception. Acute intoxication may result in anxiety and paranoid ideation or frank delusions. Marijuana can destabilize patients whose schizophrenia is in remission. Social and occupational impairment occurs but is less severe than that seen with alcohol and cocaine use.[20,21] An amotivational syndrome, consisting of loss of goal-directed behavior in young people, has been described with chronic use of marijuana.[23] Marijuana use rarely requires medical treatment. Anxiety reactions may require treatment with benzodiazepines.[23]

Alcohol Dependence

The behavioral and physiologic effects of alcohol vary according to the amount of intake, its rate of increase in plasma, the presence of other drugs or medical problems, and the individual's past experience with alcohol. The effects of alcohol are more dramatic with rising blood levels of the agent. Ethanol alone or with other drugs such as benzodiazepines is probably responsible for more toxic overdose deaths than any other agent.[27]

The DSM-IV defines alcohol dependence as repeated alcohol-related difficulties in at least three of seven areas of functioning. These include any combination of tolerance, withdrawal, taking larger amounts of alcohol over longer periods than intended, an inability to control use, giving up important activities to drink, spending a great deal of time pursuing alcohol use, and continued use of alcohol despite physical or psychological consequences. Thus, a clinical diagnosis of alcohol dependence rests on the documentation of a pattern of difficulties associated with alcohol use and is not based on the quantity and frequency of alcohol consumption.[27] Chapter 11 covers in detail alcohol abuse and dependence and the treatment of alcoholics.

Nicotine Addiction

Cigarette smoking is the main cause of preventable disease, disability, and premature death in the United States,[40] yet more than a million children and teenagers start smoking each year, and established smokers have difficulty in quitting. Nicotine is addictive and accounts for most of this public health problem. For effective treatment of patients, tobacco use must be viewed as an addiction and nicotine as the addictive drug. Nicotine use produces a compelling urge to smoke, provides pleasurable alterations in mood, and motivates chronic tobacco using behavior. Smokers regulate their nicotine dose to attain desired effects and to avoid withdrawal symptoms, which consist of a craving for tobacco products, depressed mood, insomnia, irritability, anxiety, restlessness, difficulty concentrating, and increased appetite.[40] Chapter 8 discusses the complications associated with smoking and nicotine and smoking cessation programs that can be incorporated into the dental practice.

SCHIZOPHRENIA

DEFINITION

Disordered thinking, inappropriate emotional responses, hallucinations, delusions, and bizarre behavior characterize schizophrenia. The lifetime prevalence rate for schizophrenic disorders is about 1% to 1.5% (this includes all cultures and both genders). Worldwide, the prevalence is 0.85%.[2] Onset usually occurs during adolescence or early adulthood. Studies have suggested an earlier onset in men than in women.[2]

EPIDEMIOLOGY

Etiology

The cause of schizophrenia is not known, but it appears to involve the interaction of genetic and environmental factors. Evidence for a genetic relationship has come from family, twin, and adoption studies. Family studies have shown a 13% risk for schizophrenia in children with one parent with schizophrenia. If both parents are schizophrenic, the risk increases to 46%.[41] The risk of developing schizophrenia for first-degree relatives is 5% to 10%, and for second-degree relatives, it is 2% to 4%. Concordance in twins for schizophrenia is 46% for identical twins and 14% for nonidentical twins. However, 89% of individuals with schizophrenia do not have a parent with the disease, and 81% do not have a parent or a sibling with the disease.[2,5,42] Despite evidence for a genetic causation, the results of molecular genetic linkage studies in schizophrenia are inconclusive. Major gene effects appear unlikely. Possible susceptibility genes include neuroregulin-1 at chromosome 8p21, dysbindin at 6p22.3, proline dehydrogenase at 22q11, and G72 at 13q34.[2]

The predominant biologic hypothesis for a neurophysiologic defect in schizophrenia is the dopamine hypothesis, which states that symptoms of schizophrenia are caused in part by a disturbance in dopamine-mediated neuronal pathways in the brain. This theory is supported by the blocking effect that most antipsychotics drugs have on postsynaptic dopamine receptors. The disease is more common among persons in lower socioeconomic classes. A separate risk factor is the chronic stress of poverty, which may have an adverse effect on the outcomes of the illness.[5,41]

Schizophrenia appears to be triggered by certain environmental events in a genetically predisposed individual. Drugs, medical illness, stressful psychosocial events, viral infection, and family situations characterized by conflicting and self-contradictory forms of communication have been reported to precipitate schizophrenia in susceptible individuals.[5,41]

CLINICAL PRESENTATION AND MEDICAL MANAGEMENT

According to the DSM-IV definition, schizophrenia can be diagnosed in patients who have two or more of the following symptoms for at least 1 month: hallucinations, delusions, disorganized speech, grossly disorganized or catatonic behavior, or negative symptoms such as affective flattening, alogia, or avolition. In addition, the patient's social or occupational functioning must have deteriorated.[42]

Patients with schizophrenia show psychotic symptoms consisting of delusions, hallucinations, incoherence, catatonic behavior, or flat or grossly inappropriate affect. Delusions and hallucinations are referred to as "positive" symptoms, and withdrawal and reduction of affect as "negative" symptoms. Delusions, such as thought broadcasting or being controlled by a dead person, usually are bizarre. Hallucinations are prominent and occur throughout the day for several days or several times a week for several weeks. The four types of schizophrenic disorders are catatonic, disorganized, paranoid, and undifferentiated. Patients with schizophrenic disorders show deterioration in their level of functioning regarding work, social relations, and self-care. They are often confused, depressed, withdrawn, anxious, and without emotion. Physically, they may grimace and pace about, or they may be rigid and catatonic. Vulnerability to a schizophrenic disorder is inherited, and life stresses appear to trigger the disorder.[5,41,42]

In schizophrenia, two types of thought disturbances are seen: formal thought disorder and disorder of thought content. Formal thought disorders affect relationships and associations among the words used to express thought. Thoughts may be strung together by incidental associations, or they may be completely unrelated. Thought blocking is common with psychotic patients. Disorders of thought content involve the development of delusions, which are fixed ideas that are based on incorrect perceptions of reality. Delusions, which are commonly paranoid or persecutory, also may be bizarre, somatic, grandiose, or referential (events that the patient believes have special significance). Perceptual disturbances in schizophrenic patients include auditory, visual, tactile, olfactory, and gustatory hallucinations. Auditory hallucinations consist of sounds heard by the patient in the absence of any real auditory stimulus. Patients may hear sounds of bells, whistles, whispers, rustlings and other noises. The most commonly heard sound is that of voices talking. Often, visual, tactile, or olfactory hallucinations occur.[5,41,42]

The most common emotional change in schizophrenia is a general "blunting" or "flattening" of affective expression. The patient seems to be emotionally detached or distant, may appear wooden and robotlike, and may lack warmth or spontaneity. Paranoid patients may feel frightened or enraged in response to a perceived threat or a delusion of persecution. They can be very hostile and guarded to any perceived slight.[5,41,42]

The long-term course of illness is variable. About 25% of patients have a full remission of symptoms. Another 25% have mild residual symptoms. The remaining 50% report moderate to severe symptoms.[5]

Drug treatment has had the most dramatic impact on control of symptoms and improvement in quality of life of patients with schizophrenia. Psychotherapy and other psychosocial treatments also are important because they provide patients with the human connection that helps them develop social skills, educates them about their illness and what to expect, and offers support throughout a long, difficult course of illness. Drug treatment of schizophrenic disorders consists of antipsychotic medications that act selectively against specific target symptoms. These drugs are effective for "positive" symptoms such as hallucinations and psychotic agitation but are non-effective for "negative" symptoms such as social withdrawal or anhedonia (inability to get pleasure from or find interest in activities). The newer atypical antipsychotic medications (clozapine, olanzapine, risperidone, and quetiapine) are effective for "positive" and "negative" symptoms of schizophrenia and have minimal movement adverse effects. Antipsychotic drugs are described later in this chapter.[5,41,42]

DRUGS USED TO TREAT PSYCHIATRIC DISORDERS
Antidepressant Medications

Tricyclics. The group of drugs that is primarily used to treat depression is tricyclics (see Table 29-3). The first tricyclic used to treat depression was imipramine. Tricyclics inhibit neural reuptake of norepinephrine and 5-hydroxytryptamine (5-HT), resulting in downregulation of their respective receptors. Tricyclics are all equally effective in the management of depression, but they differ in their associated adverse effects. Amitriptyline and doxepin are the most sedating, and this adverse effect is

put to advantage by patients who take these drugs just before bedtime. Two combinations of drugs are available for treating depression and other psychotic symptoms. Triavil (amitriptyline and perphenazine) is used to treat patients with depression and agitation or psychotic behavior. Limbitrol (amitriptyline and chlordiazepoxide) is used to treat patients with depression and anxiety.[1-3,43] Table 29-3 shows the drugs used to treat depression.

Adverse effects associated with tricyclics include dry mouth, constipation, blurred vision, cardiac dysrhythmias such as tachycardia, hypotension, blurred vision, allergic reactions, and important drug interactions (Table 29-6). Tricyclic drugs should be used with caution in patients with cardiac conditions because of the presence of risk for atrial fibrillation, atrial ventricular block, or ventricular tachycardia. Tricyclics can lower the seizure threshold and must be used with care in patients with a history of seizures. They can increase intraocular pressure in patients with glaucoma. Urinary retention may be increased if tricyclics are used in patients with prostate hypertrophy. Erectile or ejaculatory disturbances occur in up to 30% to 40% of patients. If used in some patients with bipolar disorder, tricyclics can reduce the time between episodes, induce manic episodes, and cause rapid cycling of episodes.[1-3,43]

Drug interactions reported with the use of tricyclics include the following: (1) tricyclics may potentiate the effects of other CNS depressants such as ethanol and benzodiazepines, (2) they may potentiate the actions of anticholinergic drugs such as antihistamines, (3) their levels are reduced by the use of oral contraceptives, alcohol, barbiturates, and dilantin, and (4) they may cause other drug interactions, including potentiation of the pressor effects of sympathomimetic agents such as epinephrine and levonordefrin, blockage of the antihypertensive effects of guanethidine, and induction of a hypertensive crisis if taken with or soon after a monoamine oxidase inhibitor (see Table 29-6). Overdosage with a tricyclic can cause death from cardiac arrhythmia or respiratory failure.[1-3,43]

Monoamine Oxidase Inhibitors. Traditional monoamine oxidase (MAO) inhibitors, which are both nonselective and irreversible, were the first effective drugs used for the treatment of depression. Only three drugs now on the market are included in the group of MAO inhibitors: phenelzine (Nardil), tranylcypromine (Parnate), and isocarboxazid (Marplan). These drugs act by inhibiting the two forms of MAO—type A and type B. Inhibition of type A MAO results in the antidepressant effects seen with MAO inhibitors. More than 80% of type A MAO must be bound to serum proteins before adverse effects can be seen clinically. Resynthesis of new enzymes takes 10 to 14 days. If a patient is changing from an MAO inhibitor drug to a tricyclic drug, 2 weeks or more must elapse after the MAO inhibitor is stopped and before the tricyclic is begun. Significant drug interactions may occur between MAO inhibitors and opioids and sympathomi-

TABLE 29-6
Adverse Effects and Drug Interactions of Antidepressant Drugs

Complications	Tetracyclics	MAO Inhibitors	SSRIs	SNRIs
ADVERSE EFFECTS	Dry mouth Nausea and vomiting Constipation Urinary retention Postural hypotension Nervousness Insomnia Drowsiness Sleepiness Reflux Anorgasmia (women) Erectile problems (men) Loss of libido Gynecomastia (men)	Dry mouth Nausea and vomiting Constipation Urinary retention Drowsiness Confusion Anorexia Weight gain Tremor Fatigue Insomnia Anorgasmia (women) Erectile problems (men)	Dry mouth Nausea and vomiting Diarrhea Anorexia Weight loss Blurred vision Insomnia Nervousness Sexual dysfunction Sweating Sedation (paroxetine) Akathisia	Dry mouth Nausea and vomiting Constipation Somnolence Weight loss/gain Blurred vision Dizziness Anorexia Impotence Loss of libido
SERIOUS ADVERSE EFFECTS	Mania Seizures Obstructive jaundice Leukopenia Tachycardia Arrhythmias Myocardial infarction Stroke	Mania Hypertensive crisis Orthostatic hypotension Peripheral edema Anemia Leukopenia Thrombocytopenia Agranulocytosis	Mania Seizures Orthostatic hypotension Anemia Bleeding (platelet effect) Hypothyroidism	Mania Hypertension (venlafaxine)
DRUG INTERACTIONS				
Barbiturates	CNS depression	CNS depression		
Benzodiazepines	CNS depression	CNS depression	CNS depression	
SSRIs	Dangerous—Do not use	Dangerous—Do not use		Serotonin syndrome Seizures
SNRIs	Dangerous—Do not use	Dangerous—Do not use	Dangerous—Do not use	
MAO inhibitors	Anticholinergic toxicity	Do not use two or more agents		Dangerous—Do not use
Heterocyclics	Dangerous—Do not use	Dangerous—Do not use		Dangerous—Do not use
Anticonvulsants	Interferes with action of anticonvulsants	Interferes with action of anticonvulsants		
Antihistamines	CNS depression	CNS depression		
Beta blockers	Anticholinergic toxicity	Sinus bradycardia	Bradycardia	
Warfarin	Warfarin metabolism inhibited—can lead to increased INR values		Warfarin metabolism inhibited—can lead to increase in INR values	
Cimetidine	Inhibits clearance—can lead to toxicity		Inhibits clearance—can lead to overdosage	
Erythromycin	Interferes with action of the antibiotic			
Opioid analgesics	Increase sedative effect			
Vasoconstrictors	Actions are enhanced	Actions are enhanced		
• Epinephrine	Use with caution	Use with caution		
• Levonordefrin		Best to avoid		
• Phenylephrine		Avoid		
FOODS AND BEVERAGES				
• Tyramine	Avoid	Hypertension/arrhythmias; must avoid these agents		
• Caffeine	Avoid			
• Ethanol	CNS depression	CNS depression		

CNS, Central nervous system; INR, international normalized ratio; MAO, monoamine oxidase; SNRIs, serotonin and noradrenergic reuptake inhibitors; SSRIs, selective serotonin reuptake inhibitors.

metic amines. MAO inhibitors potentiate the depressant activity of opioids. They can produce a hypertensive crisis if combined with specific sympathomimetic amines (see Table 29-6).[4,44]

Phenylethylamine and phenylephrine must not be given to patients who are taking MAO inhibitors. MAO metabolizes these agents, and their use with an MAO inhibitor could lead to significant potentiation of their pressor effects (see Chapter 4). These adverse effects are not seen with epinephrine and levonordefrin. Many OTC cold remedies contain phenylephrine and should not be prescribed for patients who are taking MAO inhibitors (see Table 29-6).

Tyramine is a naturally occurring amine that releases norepinephrine from sympathetic nerve endings. Dietary tyramine is deaminated by gastrointestinal MAO-A. In the presence of MAO inhibitors, dietary tyramine is rapidly absorbed into the circulation, and a hypertensive crisis may result. Patients must avoid foods that contain high concentrations of tyramine. Foods with high tyramine levels include aged foods such as cheeses, red wines, pickled fish, bananas, and chocolate.[4,44]

Second-Generation Antidepressant Drugs.

Selective serotonin reuptake inhibitors. The group of drugs known as selective serotonin reuptake inhibitors (SSRIs) includes fluoxetine (Prozac), sertraline (Zoloft), paroxetine (Paxil), and citalopram (Celexa); these agents now are considered first-line drugs for the treatment of depression. As a group, these drugs are just as effective as the tricyclics, but they are not more effective. These drugs are better tolerated than the tricyclics. The tricyclics are generally more lethal in overdose than the newer antidepressants. The SSRIs are considerably more expensive than the traditional tricyclic agents. Nausea, which occurs in up to 25% of patients who use these drugs, is the most frequent problem associated with their use. Higher doses of the SSRIs more often are associated with nervousness and insomnia (see Table 29-6). Many physicians consider SSRIs as first-line drugs for the treatment of depression.[1-3,43]

Other antidepressants. Amoxapine (Asendin), bupropion (Wellbutrin), trazodone (Desyrel), maprotiline (Ludiomil), nefazodone (Serzone), mirtazapine (Remeron), and venlafaxine (Effexor) are other nontricyclics that are used as antidepressants. Bupropion has a greater tendency to produce seizures than the other antidepressants. Nefazodone does not cause sexual adverse effects. Mirtazapine was one of the first antidepressants to have a significantly improved toxicity profile after overdose. However, blood dyscrasias have been reported with its use. Venlafaxine is a drug that belongs to the new class of antidepressants—the serotonin-noradrenaline reuptake inhibitors (see Tables 29-3 and 29-6). Venlafaxine has a similar adverse effect profile to the SSRIs. It also has been reported to increase blood pressure in

higher doses.[1-3,45] Table 29-3 shows the dosages of some of the second-generation antidepressant drugs.

Mood-Stabilizing Drugs

Lithium. Lithium has some antidepressant effects, but it is primarily used for the treatment of patients with bipolar disorder. Its mode of action is unclear. Lithium is used to treat acute manic episodes and to prevent manic episodes in patients with bipolar disorder. It is effective when used alone in 60% to 80% of classic bipolar patients. Lithium should not be used if renal disease is present. Lower doses must be used in older patients. The dose ranges from 600 to 3000 mg/day, and full therapeutic effect is attained in 7 to 10 days. The patient who is on maintenance therapy should be evaluated every 3 to 6 months for serum levels of lithium, sodium, potassium, creatinine, thyroxine (T_4), thyroid-stimulating hormone, and free T_4 index. Medical complications associated with long-term lithium use include nontoxic goiter and hypothyroidism, arrhythmia, T-wave depression, and vasopressin-resistant nephrogenic diabetes insipidus. All these complications are related to the effects of lithium on adenylate cyclase activity. Drugs that interact with lithium include erythromycin and nonsteroidal anti-inflammatory drugs (NSAIDs), which increase serum lithium levels, possibly leading to toxicity.[4,44,46]

Carbamazepine and Valproate. Carbamazepine, an anticonvulsant drug, has been successful in the treatment of manic episodes in bipolar patients who do not respond to lithium or who cannot take lithium because of associated complications. The dose is 600 to 1600 mg/day. Adverse effects include nausea, blurred vision, ataxia, leukopenia, and aplastic anemia. Valproate is an anticonvulsant drug that is used for the treatment of manic episodes. It has adverse effects that include thrombocytopenia.[2-4,46]

Antipsychotic (Neuroleptic) Drugs. The introduction of chlorpromazine in the 1950s revolutionized the practice of psychiatry. Other agents have been introduced since chlorpromazine, but none represents any real improvement beyond this prototypic agent. The popularity of these drugs is shown by the fact that two thirds of all prescriptions for antidepressant and antipsychotic (neuroleptic) drugs are written by physicians other than psychiatrists. Antipsychotic drugs appear to work by antagonizing the effects of dopamine in the basal ganglia and limbic portions of the forebrain. Because of significant adverse reactions associated with their use, these drugs should be used only when they are clearly the drugs of choice.[3,47,48]

Antipsychotic drugs sedate, tranquilize, blunt emotional expression, attenuate aggressive and impulsive behavior, and cause disinterest in the environment. They leave higher intellectual functions intact but ameliorate the bizarre behavior and thinking of psychotic patients.

TABLE 29-7
Commonly Used Antipsychotic Medications

Class	Generic Name	Trade Name	Acute Dose Per 24 Hours	Maintenance Dose
Phenothiazine Aliphatic	Chlorpromazine	Thorazine	25-1000 mg PO 25-400 mg IM	25-400 mg PO
Phenothiazine Piperazine	Perphenazine	Trilafon	8-64 mg PO 15-30 mg IM	12-24 mg PO
Piperazine	Fluphenazine	Prolixin	2.5-40 mg PO 5-20 mg IM	12.5-50 mg IM decanoate weekly
Piperazine	Trifluoperazine	Stelazine	1-5 mg PO	
Phenothiazine Piperidine	Thioridazine	Mellaril	25-800 PO	25-30 mg PO
Piperidine	Mesoridazine	Serentil	50-400 mg PO	200-400 mg PO
Butyrophenone	Haloperidol	Haldol	2-25 mg PO 6-30 mg IM	1-15 mg PO 25-200 mg IM decanoate monthly
Thioxanthene	Chlorprothixene	Taractan	30-100 mg PO	100-300 mg PO
	Thiothixene	Navane	2-5 mg PO	5-10 mg PO
Dibenzoxazepine				
Dihydroindole	Loxapine	Loxitane	50-250 mg PO	60-100 mg PO
Dihydroindole	Molindone	Moban	50-225 mg PO	20-200 mg PO
Benzisoxazole				
Dibenzodiazepine	Risperidone	Risperdal	2-4 mg PO	2-20 mg PO
Dibenzodiazepine	Olanzapine	Zyprexa	5-15 mg PO	5-10 mg PO
Dibenzodiazepine	Clozapine	Clozaril	200-400 mg PO	200-600 mg PO
Diphenylbutylpiperidine				
Phenylindole	Pimozide	Orap	10-30 mg PO	10-30 mg PO
Phenylindole	Quetiapine	Seroquel	25 mg bid	300-400 mg/day
Phenylindole	Ziprasidone	Geodon	40-80 mg bid	

From Schiffer RB. Psychiatric disorders in medical practice. In Goldman L, Ausiello D (eds). Cecil Textbook of Medicine. Philadelphia: Saunders, 2004, based on Table 426-10.
bid, Twice daily; IM, intramuscularly; PO, by mouth.

They all have significant anticholinergic adverse effects and produce dystonias and extrapyramidal symptoms. Commonly used antipsychotic drugs are shown in Table 29-7.[3,47,48]

Adverse effects of the antipsychotic drugs are numerous and often significant (Table 29-8). Patients become sedated, lethargic, and drowsy when first placed on these drugs; however, after several days, they develop a tolerance to these effects. The anticholinergic actions produced by these drugs include dry mouth, postural hypotension, constipation, and urinary retention. Other adverse effects observed are obstructive jaundice, retinal pigmentation, lenticular opacity, skin pigmentation, and male impotence.[3,5,15,16]

The extrapyramidal adverse effects (motor or movement disorders) include acute and chronic conditions. During the first 5 days of treatment with an antipsychotic agent, acute muscular dystonic reactions or a Parkinson-like syndrome may occur. Akathisia, or extreme motor restlessness, also may develop early in treatment. Symptoms consist of involuntary repetitive movements of the lips (lip smacking), the tongue (tongue thrusting), the extremities, and the trunk. This risk increases for patients over 60 years of age and for those with preexisting CNS disease (70% risk). Many of the acute extrapyramidal adverse effects are reversible if the drug is stopped, or if anticholinergic agents are given.[3,5,45,46]

Tardive dyskinesia is the most common late extrapyramidal adverse effect associated with the use of antipsychotic drugs. It usually occurs after antipsychotic medication has been used for several years. The chief sign is involuntary movement of the lips, tongue, mouth, jaw, upper and lower extremities, or trunk. Classic tardive dyskinesia affects the buccal, lingual, and masticatory muscles, leading to "flycatcher's tongue," "bonbon sign," grimaces, or chewing movements. Flycatcher's tongue refers to darting of the tongue into and out of the mouth. Bonbon sign is the pushing of the tongue against the cheek wall, so that it looks as though a piece of candy is pressed against the cheek. An early sign of tardive dyskinesia is wormlike movement of the tongue while it is at rest in the mouth. Tardive dyskinesia develops in about 20% of schizophrenic patients who are treated for years. Patients treated with antipsychotics who are followed longitudinally will develop tardive dyskinesia at the rate of about 4% per year. Elderly patients appear to have a much higher risk of developing tardive dyskinesia early in their treatment.[5,43,49]

Additional adverse effects of the anticholinergic antipsychotic drugs include hormonal effects, postural

TABLE **29-8**
Adverse Reactions of Antipsychotic Drugs Based on the Type of Neuroreceptor Affected

Neuroreceptor	Adverse Effects
ANTICHOLINERGIC	Dry mouth Urinary hesitancy Constipation Urinary retention Dry eyes Sexual dysfunction Blurred vision Mild tachycardia Closed angle glaucoma Impaired memory and confusion
ANTISEROTONERGIC	Weight gain (antihistaminergic mechanisms also proposed)
ANTIADRENERGIC	Dizziness Postural hypotension (may lead to fails falls and hip fractures in older patients) Sexual dysfunction
ANTIDOPAMINERGIC	Hyperprolactinemia (causes hypo-estrogenemia) • *In men:* Gynecomastia, impotence, loss of libido, impaired spermatogenesis • *In women:* Amenorrhea, altered ovarian function, loss of libido, risk for osteoporosis Extrapyramidal syndromes (least frequent with atypical drugs—olanzapine, quetiapine, risperidone, and ziprasidone) Acute dystonia • Parkinsonism • Akathisia • Tardive dyskinesia
COMBINATION OF RECEPTORS	Neuroleptic malignant syndrome—rigidity, fluctuating consciousness (delirium, stupor), and autonomic lability (hyperthermia, tachycardia, hypotension or hypertension, sweating, pallor, salivation, and urinary incontinence)
OTHER ADVERSE EFFECTS	Agranulocytosis Cholestatic jaundice Seizures Some agents increase risk of suicide suicidal behavior (during induction of drug)

From Wright P, Perahia D. Psychopharmacology. In Wright P, Stern J, Phelan M (editors.). Core Psychiatry, 2nd ed. Edinburgh: Elsevier, 2005. p 579-611, based on Table 38-2.

hypotension, and photosensitivity (see Table 29-8). These hormonal effects are primarily influenced by the effect of these drugs on prolactin. This may result in galactorrhea, missed menstrual periods, and loss of libido. Orthostatic hypotension is a potentially serious adverse effect, which is most common with low-potency agents. Dehydrated patients are at greatest risk for this complication.[5,49]

Several atypical antipsychotic drugs, including clozapine (Clozaril), risperidone (Risperdal), olanzapine (Zyprexa), and quetiapine (Seroquel), are available for the treatment of schizophrenia. Clozapine does not cause extrapyramidal adverse effects or risk of tardive dyskinesia. It also can be effective for improving the negative symptoms of schizophrenia. Unfortunately, a 1% to 2% incidence of agranulocytosis exists. Patients treated with clozapine must be monitored weekly with complete blood cell counts. Clozapine is effective in some schizophrenic patients who do not respond to standard antipsychotics drugs. Risperidone is a combined serotonin/dopamine antagonist. In contrast to the standard neuroleptics, which have little or no effect on the "negative" symptoms, risperidone is effective for both "negative" and "positive" symptoms of schizophrenia. All of the atypical antipsychotics have a lower affinity for binding to D2 receptors and a lower risk for extrapyramidal adverse effects.[3,5,47,48]

Important drug interactions may occur in patients who are being treated with antipsychotic drugs (Table 29-9). Antacids can diminish the absorption of neuroleptic drugs from the gut. Neuroleptic drugs can decrease blood levels of warfarin sodium. Neuroleptics and tricyclic antidepressants reduce the metabolism of each other, allowing for increased plasma concentrations of both drugs. Thioridazine can prevent the metabolism of phenytoin, allowing toxic blood levels to occur. Smoking can decrease the blood levels of antipsychotic agents. When neuroleptic drugs are used with tricyclic antidepressants or antiparkinsonian drugs, a powerful anticholinergic effect may result.[2,5,49]

TABLE **29-9**
Significant Drug Interactions With the Antipsychotic (AP) Agents

Interacting Drug or Class of Drugs	Complication
Alcohol	Increases risk of hypotension and respiratory depression
Anesthetics	Increase risk of hypotension
Antiarrhythmics	Increase risk of arrhythmias
Anticonvulsants	Reduce effects of AP drug
Tricyclic antidepressants	The AP will increase the serum level of the tricyclic drug
Antihypertensives	Increase the risk of hypotension
Anxiolytics	Increase risk of sedation
	Increase risk of respiratory depression
Cimetidine	Increases the antipsychotic effects of the AP drug
Opioids	Increase the sedative effects of the opioids
	Increase risk of respiratory depression
Erythromycin	Increases the serum level of the AP drug, risk of convulsions
Sympathomimetics (epinephrine)	Increase risk of hypotension

Malignant neuroleptic syndrome represents a rare but very serious adverse effect of antipsychotics drugs. This syndrome combines autonomic dysfunction, extrapyramidal dysfunction, and hyperthermia. The patient develops tachycardia, labile blood pressure, dyspnea, masked facies, tremors, muscle rigidity, catatonic behavior, dystonia, and marked elevation in temperature (106° F). The syndrome was first reported in 1960, and, since that time, more than 200 cases have been described. It occurs after neuroleptic drugs are given in therapeutic doses. Malignant neuroleptic syndrome is most common in young male adults with mood disorders. Symptoms continue 5 to 10 days after the drug has been stopped. The mortality rate is 10% to 20%. Treatment consists of stopping all neuroleptic medication, body cooling, rehydration, and treatment with bromocriptine (a dopamine agonist).[2,5,49]

DENTAL MANAGEMENT

Medical Considerations

Depression. During a deep depressive episode, significant impairment of all personal hygiene may occur, including a total lack of oral hygiene. Salivary flow may be reduced, and patients may report dry mouth, an increased rate of dental caries, and periodontal disease. In addition, complaints of glossodynia and various facial pain syndromes are common.[50]

Signs of low-grade chronic depression include tiredness even after getting enough sleep; difficulty getting up in the morning; restlessness; loss of interest in family, work, and sex; inability to make decisions; anger and resentment; chronic complaining; self-criticism; feelings of inferiority; and excessive daydreaming. Signs of more severe depression include excessive crying, change in sleeping habits, thoughts of food making one sick, weight loss without dieting, strong feelings of guilt, nightmares, thoughts about suicide, feeling unreal or in a "fog," and an inability to concentrate.[50]

Depressed patients often have poor oral hygiene because they lack interest in caring for themselves. The effects of poor oral hygiene may be compounded by xerostomia, which is an adverse effect of medications that the patient may be taking. Only small amounts of epinephrine should be used in local anesthesia because more concentrated forms of epinephrine can cause severe hypotension. Sedative medication may have to be given in reduced dosages to avoid overdepression of the CNS. No medical contraindication exists for dental treatment during a depressive episode. However, most depressed patients may be best managed when only their immediate dental needs are met during the depression. Once the patient has responded to medical treatment, more complex dental procedures can be performed (Table 29-10).[50]

Patients with severe depression must be referred for medical evaluation and treatment. If the patient is not responsive to this recommendation, the problem should be shared with a family member and every attempt made to get the individual in for medical attention. During severe depression, suicide is an ever possible outcome; however, medical treatment can reduce this possibility.[50]

Bipolar Disorder. From a dental standpoint, lithium, which is used to manage bipolar disorders, can cause xerostomia and stomatitis. However, no adverse drug interactions occur between lithium and other agents used in dentistry other than NSAIDs and erythromycin, which can cause lithium toxicity.[18]

Patients who do not respond to lithium and those who can no longer take lithium usually are treated with a phenothiazine type of drug. Phenothiazines can cause bone marrow suppression and fluctuations in blood pressure. The dentist must be aware of these adverse effects and must examine the patient for signs of thrombocytopenia and leukopenia (see Chapters 24 and 25) because serious problems with infection and/or excessive bleeding may occur. Phenothiazine drugs potentiate the sedative action of sedative medications, and serious respiratory depression may occur when these agents are used at their normal dosage. Therefore, if these agents must be used,

TABLE 29-10
Dental Management of Patients With Depression, Bipolar Disorder, and Schizophrenia

Clinical Setting	Clinical Findings	Action to Take
PREOPERATIVE	Examine for signs and symptoms of depression, mania, and schizophrenia; also for evidence of factitious injury	If present, refer for medical evaluation and treatment
		If present, these may indicate a severe adverse drug reaction
	Examine for signs of thrombocytopenia and leukopenia	Findings may be related taking
	Clinical examination reveals:	Request change of drug by physician
	• Xerostomia	Consult with patient's physician:
	• Excessive dental caries	Determine current status
	• Periodontal disease	Confirm medications
	For patients with a diagnosis of depression, mania, or schizophrenia:	Drugs to avoid or use in reduced dosage of drugs
	• Establish drugs being taken to control disease	Findings may indicate a diagnosis of patient with mania
	• When did the patient last see his/her physician?	Suicide is a risk for patients with severe depression, bipolar disease, and schizophrenia
	Excessive abrasion and gingival injury from excessive tooth brushing may be noted	Contact patient's physician and relative
	Ask the patient if suicidal thoughts have occurred, and if so, how often? Have they planned on how to commit suicide?	
OPERATIVE	A patient with severe mania, depression, or symptoms of schizophrenia	Defer dental treatment, difficult to manage, wait until better controlled if possible; compliance may be poor regarding appointments and treatment
	Patients taking antidepressants or antipsychotic (AP) drugs	Limit the use of epinephrine:
		• Anesthetic—1:100,000 epinephrine is okay
		• Limit of 2 cartridges
		• Avoid more concentrated forms
		• Retraction cord with epinephrine
		• 1:1000 epinephrine to control bleeding
		Avoid or use in reduced dosage:
		• Sedatives, hypnotics, narcotic agents
	Patients taking tricyclics and monoamine oxidase inhibitors (MOIs)	May cause postural hypotension; change chair position slowly and support patient getting out of chair
POSTOPERATIVE	Patients taking antidepressants or neuroleptic drugs	Avoid or use in reduced dosage:
	Patients taking lithium	• Sedatives
		• Narcotics
		• Hypnotics
		Avoid nonsteroidal anti-inflammatory drugs (NSAIDs), tetracycline, and metronidazole; can may cause lithium toxicity; also, avoid diazepam, which can may cause hypothermia
		May safely use aspirin, acetaminophen, codeine, and other antibiotics

the dosage must be reduced. The dentist should consult with the patient's physician regarding this point. Epinephrine used in normal amounts in local anesthetic solutions (1:100,000) usually will produce no adverse effects when given to patients who are taking phenothiazine-type drugs (see Table 29-10). The primary effect of epinephrine/phenothiazine interaction—hypotension—should be monitored.[7,48]

Somatoform Disorder. The characteristics of a somatoform disorder include the following: no identifiable lesion or pathologic condition can be found, the disorder or reaction has an emotional cause, it is not dangerous to the patient, and it is a defense for the patient in terms of reducing the level of anxiety. Reducing anxiety by converting it into a symptom is called *primary gain*. Patients also may have *secondary gains* as a result of their condition, for example, because of their symptoms, they may not be able to work, or they may receive increased attention from their family.

Following are examples of oral symptoms that can be produced by somatoform disorders: burning tongue, painful tongue, numbness of soft tissue, tingling sensations of oral tissues, and pain in the facial region. The diagnosis of a somatoform disorder should be made only under the following circumstances: (1) A thorough search from a clinical standpoint has failed to provide any evidence of a disease process that could explain the symptoms, (2) the symptoms have been present long enough that if they were related to a disease process, a lesion would have developed, (3) the symptoms have not followed known anatomic distribution of nerves, or (4) underlying systemic conditions that could produce the symptoms have been ruled out by laboratory tests or by referral to a physician. Systemic conditions that must be ruled out include anemia, diabetes, cancer, and a nutritional deficiency (vitamin B complex).[7,18]

The process of establishing the diagnosis of somatoform disorders is slow and time consuming. Dental treatment should not be provided on the basis of a patient's symptoms unless a dental cause can be found. Many patients have undergone needless extractions, root canals, and other procedures in an attempt to correct somatoform symptoms. Complex dental care should not be attempted until the somatoform problem has been managed. The diagnosis of a somatoform disorder should not be reached until a thorough search has been made over a period that fails to uncover pathologic findings that could explain the symptoms.

After the diagnosis of an oral somatoform disorder has been established, the patient may be managed as follows. First, the findings should be discussed with the patient in the presence of a close relative, husband, or wife. During this discussion, the dentist should point out that no organic source for the patient's problem could be found, that the patient does not have oral cancer, and that the pain or symptom is real to the patient. Next, the possibility that feelings of "unhappiness" are the source of the symptoms should be pointed out; this will be difficult for the patient to understand and accept, but it is important to establish this "groundwork." Complex or unnecessary dental procedures should not be performed, even if the patient demands them in the belief that this will cause the symptoms to disappear.

Dentists should pay close attention to their feelings toward the patient. Symptoms may be viewed only as a device to gain attention and sympathy, and this may cause feelings of hostility and anger on the part of the dentist, which will not enhance proper management of the patient. The dentist should try to feel empathy toward the patient and to understand the cause of the problem, and then should react in a positive manner.

An attempt should be made by the dentist to manage the patient with a mild somatoform disorder (mild in the sense that the patient is able to function at a reasonable level even with the symptom, the patient's emotional status appears to be "stable," and the patient has shown or expressed no suicidal tendencies). Such patients should be assured that they do not have a life-threatening disease such as cancer. A series of regular short appointments should be scheduled to reexamine the patient for possible signs of disease, to discuss symptoms, and to reassure the individual that no tissue changes are present. The patient should be charged for this time and told what the fee will be before the appointments are set up.

Patients with a severe somatoform disorder should be referred to a psychiatrist; however, once a patient has been referred, the dentist should be willing to continue to be involved. The patient may need to be reexamined and the psychiatrist consulted regarding the findings. If patients feel that the dentist only wants to get rid of them, the suggestion of referral will not be helpful or effective.

Substance Abuse. The dentist should be on the alert for signs and symptoms that may indicate substance abuse (see Table 29-5). Telltale cutaneous lesions often indicate parenteral abuse of drugs. These include subcutaneous abscesses, cellulitis, thrombophlebitis, skin "tracks" (chronic inflammation from multiple injections), and infected lesions. Skin tracks usually appear as linear or bifurcated erythematous lesions, which become indurated and hyperpigmented. An ill-defined febrile illness also may indicate a possible problem with parenteral drug abuse.[19,51]

Drug abusers may try to obtain drugs from dentists by demanding pain medication for a dental problem that they refuse to have treated. The opioid abuser may claim to be allergic to codeine in an attempt to obtain a stronger drug such as morphine or hydrocodone. The dentist should not let patients know where drugs are kept or leave prescription pads out where they can be taken, and the dentist should not use prewritten prescription forms.[51]

Drug abuse occurs more often in dentists than in the general population because of the ready availability of opioid analgesics and sedative-hypnotic drugs. Inhalation of nitrous oxide also is another form of drug abuse that is common among dentists.[51]

Cannabis. Chronic use of marijuana can lead to chronic bronchitis, airway obstruction, poor oral health due to neglect and xerostomia, and squamous metaplasia.[51] The autonomic effects of marijuana include tachycardia, reduced peripheral resistance, and, with large doses, orthostatic hypotension.[51] Thus, marijuana use by individuals with ischemic heart disease or cardiac failure may be harmful. Care should be taken in providing dental treatment to such patients, and, if such an association has been identified, dental treatment should be postponed until the patient is stable.

Cocaine. Patients who are "high" on cocaine should not receive any dental treatment for at least 6 hours after the last administration of cocaine.[52] Peak blood levels occur within 30 minutes and usually dissipate within 2 hours. The danger of significant myocardial ischemia and cardiac arrhythmia is the primary concern in patients who are high on the drug. Local anesthetics with epinephrine or levonordefrin must not be used during the 6-hour waiting period after cocaine administration because cocaine potentiates the response of sympathetically innervated organs to sympathomimetic amines, which could result in a hypertensive crisis, a cerebrovascular accident, or a myocardial infarction.[29]

Before treating a patient who is participating in a cocaine treatment program, the dentist should consult the patient's physician regarding medications that the patient may be taking and how best to manage the patient in pain. Patients with substance abuse should not be prescribed addictive substances.

Methamphetamine. Patients who are "high" on methamphetamine should not receive dental treatment for at least 8 hours after the last administration of a drug, and, to be safe, dental treatment should not occur until at least 24 hours after the last administration of the drug. Peak blood levels occur within 30 to 60 minutes and usually dissipate within 8 hours; however, with large doses, peak levels may last 24 hours.[32] Significant myocardial ischemia and cardiac arrhythmia are the primary concerns in patients who are high on the drug. Local anesthetics with epinephrine or levonordefrin must not be used during the 8-hour waiting period after methamphetamine administration because methamphetamine potentiates the response of sympathetically innervated organs to sympathomimetic amines, which could result in a hypertensive crisis, a cerebrovascular accident, or a myocardial infarction.[53]

Chronic methamphetamine use causes xerostomia and rampant caries, bad taste, bruxism (grinding of the teeth), and muscle trismus (jaw clenching).[30-33,54-56] Xerostomia significantly increases the risks for dental caries, enamel erosion, and periodontal disease. Neglect of personal oral hygiene, high intake of refined carbohydrates and sucrose, and increased acidity from gastrointestinal regurgitation, bulimia, or vomiting also contribute to exaggerated caries erosion problems in the meth patient.[53] The combination of these effects in meth abusers is referred to as "meth mouth."[53,55,57] Meth users are "wired" and have extremely high levels of energy and neuromuscular activity; this leads to parafunctional jaw activity and bruxism. Bruxism and muscle trismus can compound the effects of periodontal disease.[53]

Alcohol. Dental management of the patient at risk for or with alcohol abuse problems is presented in Chapter 11.

Pain control. Drug abusers often take their favorite drug to counteract dental fears and anxiety before dental appointments. If it is determined that this has occurred, the dental appointment should be rescheduled and the patient counseled to not use drugs before the next appointment. Tolerance to sedative drugs and local anesthetics may occur, particularly among parenteral drug abusers. The need for larger doses of these agents carries the risk of increased incidence of adverse effects. Treatment of pain and anxiety in the recovering or reformed substance abuser presents a problem to the dentist. Before beginning dental treatment for these patients, the dentist must establish the patient's attitude toward drug treatment. Many patients will refuse mood-altering drugs. In addition, the dentist should never administer a drug, or another of its class, that has been abused by the patient in the past. For control of anxiety in these patients, oral propranolol may be considered. NSAIDs can usually be used to manage postoperative pain.[51]

Nicotine. The dentist is in the unique position of being able to observe the oral effects of tobacco use and to use this information to try to motivate patients to stop the habit. Tobacco use counseling and cessation programs are important preventive services that dentists should provide to their patients (see Chapter 8). Cessation programs are incorporated easily into the dental practice. Patients must be informed of the medical problems associated with tobacco use (cardiovascular disease, chronic obstructive pulmonary disease, chronic bronchitis, gastric ulcers, low birth weight babies, spontaneous abortions, and cancer of the lung, larynx, esophagus, pancreas, bladder, colon, and oral cavity).

Schizophrenia. Consultation with the patient's physician is recommended before dental treatment is started, to establish the patient's current status, medications the patient is taking, and the ability of the patient to give a valid consent for treatment.[58] It is suggested that the dentist ask the psychiatrist's opinion regarding the patient's medicolegal competence to sign a consent form.[58] Also, the dentist should inquire about the ability of the patient to perform preventive hygiene procedures.[58] Routine dental treatment of the schizophrenic patient should not be attempted unless the patient is under medical management. Even then, these patients may be difficult to deal with. An attendant or family member should accompany the patient to maximize comfort and familiarity. Patients should be scheduled for morning appointments. Preventive dental education is important and is more difficult to convey to this group of patients. Oral instructions, modeled demonstrations (hygienist brushes and flosses his or her own teeth), and descriptive posters showing proper toothbrushing and flossing techniques can be used to communicate to the patient what needs to be done and how.[58] For patients who are not able to perform oral hygiene procedures, or who lack the motivation, a family member or attendant should be instructed on the procedures. The dentist may use artificial saliva products, antimicrobial agents (chlorhexidine gluconate), and fluoride mouth rinses to promote good oral hygiene.[58] Patients should be recalled at 3-month intervals for examination, oral prophylaxis, and application of a fluoride gel.[58]

Confrontation and an authoritative attitude on the part of the dentist should be avoided. If such an approach does not allow for proper dental management, the dentist should consider sedation or tranquilization, which should be provided in consultation with the patient's physician. Chlorpromazine (Thorazine), chloral hydrate, diazepam (Valium), or oxazepam may be considered.[52,59] Antipsychotic medications may add to or potentiate the actions of other CNS depressants such as narcotic analgesics, barbiturates, and others. When these agents are used, caution must be exercised to avoid excessive CNS depression, hypotension, orthostatic hypotension, and respiratory depression. Patients who are treated with clozapine can develop bone marrow suppression; the most recent white blood cell count should be reviewed before dental treatment is started.[58]

Suicidal Patient. Suicide is one of the leading causes of death among individuals younger than 45 years of age. It also is far too common in the elderly. Since 1980, a dramatic increase has occurred in the rate of suicide in persons 5 to 19 years of age and in persons 65 years or older. In fact, in some countries, the suicide rate has increased by 60% during the past 45 years.[16] Men are 3 times more successful in their suicide attempts than are women. However, women are 10 times more likely to attempt suicide. The most common methods of suicide include hanging, overdoses of medication or poison, carbon monoxide poisoning through car exhausts, jumping from a height (building, cliff), jumping in front of a moving vehicle, and the use of firearms (Figure 29-3).[16]

Physician-assisted suicide occurs when a physician administers an agent that will end the patient's life. The patient has given prior consent for the procedure and usually has a terminal condition such as advanced cancer that is not responding to treatment. Only a very few countries in the world and one state in the United States have endorsed this practice. Oregon made it lawful in 1997, the Netherlands in 2001, and Belgium in 2002.[16]

Patients with suicidal symptoms often say that they feel frustrated, helpless, or hopeless. They frequently are angry, self-punishing, and harshly self-critical. Suicide is a hazard for individuals who suffer from any of the following conditions: chronic physical illness, alcoholism, drug abuse, and depression. Suicide statistics show that men, adolescents, and the elderly are at greatest risk. A history of a previous suicide attempt greatly increases the risk. A history of recent psychiatric hospitalization also increases the risk. Recent diagnosis of a serious condition such as cancer or AIDS may increase the risk for suicide. The recent loss of a loved one or recent retirement may increase this risk as well. If any of these events occurs in the individual who lives alone or who has little or no social support, the risk for suicide increases. Patients who are at greatest risk are those who are perturbed, who state a plan for suicide, and who have the means to carry it out.[16,60]

The dentist should ask whether the very depressed patient has had any thoughts about suicide. Studies have

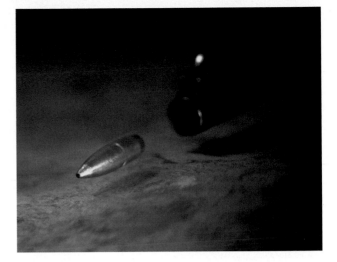

Figure 29-3. In the United States during 2001, about 55% of all suicides were committed with the use of firearms.

shown that questions about suicide do not prompt the act in these patients. Patients who state they have had these thoughts must be referred for immediate medical care. If possible, members of the family should get involved.[16,50]

Drug Interactions and Adverse Effects

Tricyclic Antidepressants. Many of the heterocyclic antidepressants can cause hypotension, orthostatic hypotension, tachycardia, and cardiac arrhythmia. When sedatives, hypnotics, barbiturates, and narcotics are used together with the heterocyclic antidepressants, severe respiratory depression may result. If these agents must be used, the dosage should be reduced. Atropine should be used with care in these patients because increased intraocular pressure may result. Small amounts of epinephrine (1:100,000) can be used in patients who are taking heterocyclic antidepressants if the dentist aspirates before injecting and injects the anesthetic slowly. No more than two cartridges should be injected at any appointment (see Table 29-10). Other, more concentrated forms of epinephrine must be avoided. Levonordefrin is contraindicated in patients who are taking tricyclics because of the possibility of an exaggerated hypertensive response.[10,43,61]

Monoamine Oxidase Inhibitors. Patients who are taking MAO inhibitors can receive small amounts of epinephrine in local anesthetics, as described previously. Other forms of epinephrine (retraction cord, topical for control of bleeding) are best avoided. Phenylephrine must not be used in patients who are taking MAO inhibitors. MAO inhibitors may interact with sedatives, narcotics, nonnarcotic analgesics, antihistamines, and atropine to prolong and intensify their effects on the CNS (see Table 29-6).[10,43,61]

Antipsychotic Drugs. Several important drug interactions may occur in patients who are taking neuroleptic drugs. Extreme care must be taken if sedatives, hypnotics, antihistamines, and opioids are used in patients who are taking neuroleptic agents because neuroleptic drugs increase the respiratory depressant effects of these agents. This can be dangerous, particularly in patients with compromised respiratory function. If these types of drugs must be used, the dosage must be reduced. The dentist must consult with the patient's physician before using these agents.[43,47,61]

Epinephrine must be used with great care in patients who are receiving a neuroleptic drug because a severe hypotensive episode may result. Small amounts of epinephrine (1:100,000) can be used in patients who are taking neuroleptic drugs if the dentist aspirates before injecting, injects the anesthetic solution slowly, and, in general, uses no more than two cartridges. Epinephrine in retraction cords or topically applied for control of bleeding is contraindicated (see Table 29-10).

Older patients who are taking antipsychotic drugs present several important problems in terms of drug usage. These patients usually have decreased levels of serum albumin; hence, many of them have a higher percentage of the drug in an unbound state. This increases the risk for toxic reactions. In addition, many of these patients have marginal liver function; hence, drugs metabolized by the liver may remain in the circulation for longer periods and in increased concentrations.

Treatment Planning Considerations

The goals of treatment planning for patients with psychiatric disorders are to maintain oral health, comfort, and function, and to prevent and control oral disease. Without an aggressive approach to prevention, many of these patients will be susceptible to dental caries and periodontal disease. Susceptibility to such diseases increases because of the adverse effect of xerostomia, which is associated with most of these medications, and the fact that some of the psychiatric conditions for which these patients are being treated reduce interest in performing or the ability to perform oral hygiene procedures. Also, many of these patients' diets contain foods or drinks that increase the risk for dental disease.[50]

The dental treatment plan should contain the following elements. Daily oral hygiene procedures must be identified. The treatment plan must be realistic for the patient's psychiatric disorder and physical status. The plan must be dynamic, to take into account changes in the status of the psychiatric disorder and the patient's physical status. An example of the need for a flexible, dynamic treatment plan is seen in patients with major depression or bipolar disorder. During affective episodes, emphasis should be placed on maintenance and prevention. Complex dental procedures should be performed only when the patient is in a stable condition in terms of the mood disorder. The treatment plan should minimize any stress associated with the dental visit. This can best be accomplished through effective patient management efforts and the use of nonverbal communication.

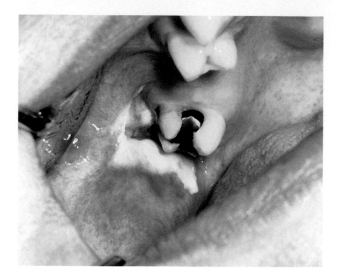

Figure 29-4. Agranulocytosis. The dentist should be aware that agranulocytosis may be associated with the drugs used to treat psychoses. (From Sapp JP, Eversole LR, Wysocki GP. Contemporary Oral and Maxillofacial Pathology, 2nd ed. St. Louis, Mosby, 2004.)

The dental team should communicate to the patient and family members a positive, hopeful attitude toward maintenance of the patient's oral health. The dental team should determine whether the patient is legally able to make rational decisions. This should be discussed with the patient and a loved one. Treatment planning often involves input and permission from a loved one, so that decisions can be made.

The last aspect of the treatment plan deals with selection of medications to be used in the dental treatment of the patient. Certain agents may have to be avoided, and others may require a reduction in their usual dosage. Medical consultation is suggested to establish the patient's current status, confirm medications the patient is taking, identify possible complications, and confirm dental medications and doses that will minimize possible drug interactions.

Oral Complications and Manifestations

Antipsychotic drugs may cause agranulocytosis, leukopenia, or thrombocytopenia. Oral lesions associated with these reactions may occur. If the dentist notes oral lesions, fever, or sore throat in patients who are taking antipsychotic drugs, the patient must be evaluated for possible agranulocytosis. The mood-stabilizing drugs—carbamazepine and valproate—also may cause agranulocytosis, leukopenia, or thrombocytopenia (Figure 29-4).

Patients who are taking antipsychotic agents may develop muscular problems (dystonia, dyskinesia, or tardive dyskinesia) in the oral and facial regions. If the dentist first observes symptoms of dysfunction, the patient should be referred to the patient's physician for evaluation and management.[47]

Patients with psychiatric disorders may engage in painful self-destructive acts. Acts of orofacial mutilation such as eye gouging, pushing sharp objects into the ear canal, lip biting, cheek biting, tongue biting, burning of oral tissues with the tip of a cigarette, and mucosal injury with a sharp or blunt object have been reported.

Patients with severe psychiatric disorders may not have an interest in caring or the ability to care for themselves. Hence, oral hygiene is poor, and increased dental problems develop. Most of the medications used to treat psychiatric disorders contribute to increased dental problems in such patients because xerostomia is one of their primary adverse effects. This may lead to an increased incidence of smooth surface caries and candidiasis. Stiefel et al[62] reported on the oral health of persons with and without chronic mental illness in community settings. Patients with chronic mental illness were found to have a significantly greater incidence of dry mouth, mucosal lesions, and coronal smooth surface caries, as well as increased severity of plaque and calculus buildup.

REFERENCES

1. Cleare A. Unipolar depression. In Wright P, Stern J, Phelan M (eds). Core Psychiatry, 2nd ed. Edinburgh, Elsevier, 2005, pp 271-295.
2. Reus VI. Mental disorders. In Kasper DL, Braunwald E, Fauci AS, et al (eds). Harrison's Online Principles of Medicine, 16th ed. New York, McGraw-Hill, 2005, pp 2547-2562.
3. Schiffer RB. Psychiatric disorders in medical practice. In Goldman L, Ausiello D (eds). Cecil Textbook of Medicine. Philadelphia, Saunders, 2004, pp 2212-2222.
4. Kahn DA. Mood disorders. In Cutler JL, Marcus ER (eds). Saunders Text and Review Series: Psychiatry. Philadelphia, Saunders, 1999, pp 34-63.
5. Horwath E, Courinos F. Schizophrenia and other psychotic disorders. In Cutler JL, Marcus ER (eds). Saunders Text and Review Series: Psychiatry. Philadelphia, Saunders, 1999, pp 64-80.
6. Vogel LR, Muskin PR. Anxiety disorders. In Cutler JL, Marcus ER (eds). Saunders Text and Review Series: Psychiatry. Philadelphia, Saunders, 1999, pp 105-127.
7. Goldberg RJ. Practical Guide to the Care of the Psychiatric Patient. St. Louis, Mosby, 1995.
8. Shah A, Tovey E. Psychiatry of old age. In Wright P, Stern J, Phelan M (eds). Core Psychiatry, 2nd ed. Edinburgh, Elsevier, 2005, pp 481-493.
9. American Psychiatric Association. Mood disorders. In Diagnostic and Statistical Manual of Mental Disorders, Text Revision, 4th ed (DSM-IV-TR). Washington DC, American Psychiatric Association, 2000, pp 345-428.
10. Scherger J, Sudak D, Alici-Evciment Y. Depression. Available at: http://www.firstconsult.com/depression. Accessed 2006.
11. Mackin P, Young A. Bipolar disorders. In Wright P, Stern J, Phelan M (eds). Core Psychiatry, 2nd ed. Edinburgh, Elsevier, 2005, pp 295-319.
12. American Psychiatric Association. Diagnostic and Statistical Manual of Mental Disorders, Text Revision, 4th ed (DSM-IV-TR). Washington DC, American Psychiatric Association, 2000.
13. Judd LL, Britton KT, Braff DL. Mental disorders. In Isselbacher KJ, Brauwald E (eds). Harrison's Principles of Internal Medicine, 13th ed. New York, McGraw-Hill, 1994, pp 2400-2420.
14. Rush AJ, Trivedi MH, Wisniewski SR, et al. Bupropion-SR, sertraline, or venlafaxine-XR after failure of SSRIs for depression. N Engl J Med 2006;354:1231-1242.
15. Trivedi MH, Fava M, Wisniewski SR, et al. Medication augmentation after the failure of SSRIs for depression. N Engl J Med 2006;354:1243-1252.
16. Srinath S. Suicide and deliberate self-harm. In Wright P, Stern J, Phelan M (eds). Core Psychiatry, 2nd ed. Edinburgh, Elsevier, 2005, pp 319-335.
17. Adelman SA, Scott ME. Depression. In Greene H, Fincher RE, Johnson WP, et al (eds). Clinical Medicine, 2nd ed. St. Louis, Mosby, 1996, pp 730-735.
18. American Psychiatric Association. Somatoform disorders. In Diagnostic and Statistical Manual of Mental Disorders, Text Revision, 4th ed (DSM-IV-TR). Washington DC, American Psychiatric Association, 2000, pp 485-513.
19. Samet JH. Drug abuse and dependence. In Goldman L, Ausiello D (eds). Cecil Textbook of Medicine. Philadelphia, Saunders, 2004, pp 145-152.
20. Levin FR, Kleber HD. Alcohol and substance abuse disorders. In Cutler JL, Marcus ER (eds). Saunders Text and Review Series: Psychiatry. Philadelphia, Saunders, 1999, pp 128-149.
21. American Psychiatric Association. Substance-related disorders. In Diagnostic and Statistical Manual of Mental Disorders, Text Revision, 4th ed (DSM-IV-TR). Washington DC, American Psychiatric Association, 2000, pp 191-296.
22. Winstock A. Psychoactive drug misuse. In Wright P, Stern J, Phelan M (eds). Core Psychiatry, 2nd ed. Edinburgh, Elsevier, 2005, pp 431-455.
23. Samet JH. Drugs of abuse: Cocaine and other psychostimulants. In Goldman L, Ausiello D (eds). Cecil Textbook of Medicine, 22nd ed. Philadelphia, Saunders, 2004, pp 148-152.
24. Moore D, Jefferson J. Handbook of Medical Psychiatry, 2nd ed. St. Louis, Mosby, 2004.
25. Counties NAo. Meth is top drug problem for most counties. MSNBC 2005.
26. Puri BK, Laking PJ, Treasaden IH. Textbook of Psychiatry. Edinburgh, Churchill Livingstone, 2003.
27. Schuckit MA. Alcoholism and drug dependency. In Fauci AS, Braunwald E, Isselbacher KJ, et al (eds). Harrison's Principles of Internal Medicine, 14th ed. New York, McGraw-Hill, 1998, pp 2503-2512.
28. Mendelson JH, Mello NK. Cocaine and other commonly abused drugs. In Fauci AS, Braunwald E, Isselbacher KJ, et al (eds). Harrison's Principles of Internal Medicine, 14th ed. New York, McGraw-Hill, 1998, pp 2512-2516.
29. Friedlander AH, Gorelick DA. Dental management of the cocaine addict. Oral Surg 1988;65:45-48.
30. Elsevier MDConsult. Patient handouts: Amphetamine dependence. Available at: http://home.mdconsult.com/methamphetamine/patienthandouts. Accessed 2004.
31. Goetz C. Exogenous acquired metabolic disorders of the nervous system: Toxins and illicit drugs. In Goetz C

(ed). Textbook of Clinical Neurology, 2nd ed. St. Louis, Elsevier, 2003, pp 866-869.

32. Henry JA. Amphetamines. In Ford M, Delaney K, Ling L, Erickson T (eds). Clinical Toxicology, 1st ed. Philadelphia, Saunders, 2001, pp 620-627.

33. Elsevier MDConsult. Clinical topics: Illicit drug abuse. Available at: http://home.mdconsult.com/ illicitdrugabuse. Accessed 2005.

34. Rakel R. Abuse of controlled substances. In Rakel R (ed). Textbook of Family Practice, 6th ed. Philadelphia, Saunders, 2002, p 1546.

35. Cho AK, Melega WP. Patterns of methamphetamine abuse and their consequences. J Addict Dis 2002;21: 21-34.

36. Cretzmeyer M, Sarrazin MV, Huber DL, et al. Treatment of methamphetamine abuse: Research findings and clinical directions. J Subst Abuse 2003;24:267-277.

37. Centers for Disease Control and Prevention. Increasing morbidity and mortality associated with abuse of methamphetamine. Morb Mortal Wkly Rep 1995;44:882-886.

38. Leinwand D. Drug makers take action to foil meth cooks. USA Today, 2005.

39. McIndoe J, Wagne MA, Doyle R. Pseudoephedrine Legislative Update and Market Impact and Opportunities. Information Resources Inc., 2005.

40. Holbrook JH. Nicotine addiction. In Fauci AS, Braunwald E, Isselbacher KJ, et al (eds). Harrison's Principles of Internal Medicine, 14th ed. New York, McGraw-Hill, 1998, pp 2516-2519.

41. Wright P. Schizophrenia and related disorders. In Wright P, Stern J, Phelan M (eds). Core Psychiatry, 2nd ed. Edinburgh, Elsevier, 2005, pp 241-267.

42. American Psychiatric Association. Schizophrenia and other psychotic disorders. In Diagnostic and Statistical Manual of Mental Disorders, Text Revision, 4th ed (DSM-IV-TR). Washington DC, American Psychiatric Association, 2000, pp 297-345.

43. Russakoff LM. Psychopharmacology. In Cutler JL, Marcus ER (eds). Saunders Text and Review Series: Psychiatry. Philadelphia, Saunders, 1999, pp 308-331.

44. Pratt JP. Affective disorders. In Walker R, Edwards C (eds). Clinical Pharmacy and Therapeutics, 2nd ed. London, Churchill Livingstone, 1999, pp 409-425.

45. Zanardi R, Franchini L, Serretti A, et al. Venlafaxine versus fluvoxamine in the treatment of delusional depression: A pilot double-blind controlled study. J Clin Psychiatry 2000;61:26-29.

46. Scherger JE, Baustian GH, O'Hanlon KM, et al. Bipolar disorders. Available at: http://www.firstconsult.com/ bipolardisorders. Accessed 2006.

47. Pollack EF, Baustian GH, Jones RC, et al. Schizophrenia. Available at: http://www.firstconsult.com/ schizophrenia. Accessed 2006.

48. Wright P, Perahia D. Psychopharmacology. In Wright P, Stern J, Phelan M (eds). Core Psychiatry, 2nd ed. Edinburgh, Elsevier, 2005, pp 579-611.

49. Branford D. Schizophrenia. In Walker R, Edwards C (eds). Clinical Pharmacy and Therapeutics, 2nd ed. London, Churchill Livingstone, 1999, pp 425-435.

50. Little JW. Dental implications of mood disorders. J Gen Dent 2004;52:442-450.

51. Abel PW, Bockman CS. Drugs of abuse. In Yagiela JA, Neidle EA, Dowd FJ (eds). Pharmacology and Therapeutics for Dentistry, 4th ed. St. Louis, Mosby, 1998, pp 656-670.

52. Scully C, Cawson RA. Medical Problems in Dentistry, 5th ed. Edinburgh, Elsevier (Churchill Livingstone), 2005.

53. Rhodus NL, Little JW. Methamphetamine abuse: Meth mouth. J Northwest Dent 2005;29-39.

54. Duxbury AJ. Ecstasy: Dental implications. Br Dent J 1998;175:38.

55. Shaner JW. Caries associated with methamphetamine abuse. J Mich Dent Assoc 2002;84:42-47.

56. Wynn RL. Dental considerations of patients taking appetite suppressants. Gen Dent 1997;45:330-331.

57. Increasing morbidity and mortality associated with abuse of methamphetamine—United States, 1991-1994. MMWR Morb Mortal Wkly Rep 1995;44:882-886.

58. Friedlander AH, Marder SR. The psychopathology, medical management and dental implications of schizophrenia. J Am Dent Assoc 2002;133:603-610; quiz 24-25.

59. Friedlander AH, Brill NQ. Dental management of patients with schizophrenia. Spec Care Dent 1986;6: 217-219.

60. Feinstein RE. Suicide and violence. In Cutler JL, Marcus ER (eds). Saunders Text and Review Series: Psychiatry. Philadelphia, Saunders, 1999, pp 201-221.

61. Felpel LP. Psychopharmacology: Antipsychotics and antidepressants. In Yagiela JA, Neidle EA, Dowd FJ (eds). Pharmacology and Therapeutics for Dentistry, 4th ed. St. Louis, Mosby, 1998, pp 151-168.

62. Stiefel DJ, Truelove EL, Menard TW, et al. A comparison of oral health of persons with and without chronic mental illness in community settings. Spec Care Dent 1990;10:6-12.

PART TEN

Geriatrics

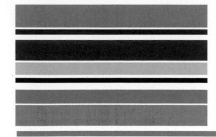

Dental Management of Older Adults

CHAPTER 30

After reaching the age of 40 years, people experience a progressive decline in homeostatic control and in the ability to respond to stress and change. The World Health Organization defines the population between 65 and 75 years as "elderly." The term "old" is used for individuals between 76 and 90 years and "very old" for those over age 90. Elderly and old individuals are often very different with respect to their physiologic function, burden of illness, and any associated disability.[1] This chapter uses the term "older adults" for individuals 65 years or older. It is interesting that of all of the people who have ever lived to age 65 years, more than half are alive today.[2] The organization of this chapter differs from that of the others because the content does not lend itself to the usual presentation. An average general dental practice would be expected to have about 260 or more patients 65 years of age or older.

EPIDEMIOLOGY

Incidence and Prevalence

More than 35 million individuals age 65 and older live in the United States. This represents about 13% of the population.[3] In 1900, just 3 million individuals age 65 and older accounted for less than 4% of the population.[3] By the year 2030, this group will represent about 20% of the population.[3] These significant increases in the older population in the United States are due to a dramatic increase in life expectancy over the past century, which is predicted to continue into the present century.[3] In 1900, at birth, men were expected to live 48 years and women 51 years.[3] By 1997, life expectancy had increased to 74 years for men and 79 years for women.[3]

Today, a significant number of years are lived after the age of 65 by a number of older adults.[3] In fact, the 85 and older age group is the most rapidly growing segment of the U.S. population.[4]

The leading causes of death in 1900 were pneumonia and influenza, tuberculosis, diarrhea, and enteritis, which accounted for 30% of all deaths in individuals 65 years or older.[3] In 1997, heart disease was the leading cause of death in older adults, followed by cancer and stroke; the three conditions were responsible for about 60% of all deaths among older adults.[3] In 1997, heart disease alone accounted for 40% of all deaths among persons age 85 years and older.[3]

Although heart disease and stroke remain leading causes of death in individuals 65 years and older, their death rates from 1980 to 1997 have declined by 30% for heart disease and by 36% for stroke.[3] Improved medical care, reduction in risk factors, and changes in lifestyle are responsible for these declines in death rates.[3] Death rates from cancer, pneumonia, and influenza increased slightly during this period. In contrast, the death rate for chronic obstructive pulmonary disease increased by 57%, and for diabetes mellitus by 32%.[3]

Cancer (lung, breast, prostate, and colon) is the second most common cause of death in older adults. Since 1940, a 20% increase in cancer deaths among persons 55 years of age or older has been documented. Statistics show that 37% of men and 22% of women aged 60 to 79 years will develop invasive cancer. The risk for invasive cancer from birth to death is 50% in men and 30% in women. The most marked increase has occurred in cancer of the lung in both men and women.[3,5]

The proportion of adults who report very good or excellent health decreases with increasing age. Very good or excellent health is reported by 82% of individuals aged 18 years, 68% of persons aged 18 to 64 years, and 39% of individuals aged 65 years and older.[3]

One primary cause for death in older adults is usually identified, but often, multiple contributing causes are revealed.[3] These contributing causes include sociodemographic characteristics, health habits, cardiovascular risk factors, clinical diseases, subclinical diseases, physical disability, and cognitive impairment.[3] When these risk factors and conditions are taken into account, age becomes less important as a predictor of mortality.[3] However, overall, the death rate increases with aging until patients are very old, at which time it slows down.[3]

Nearly 90% of all older adults have a chronic illness.[3,6] At present, 30% of individuals older than 65 years of age have three or more chronic illnesses and account for more than 33% of the costs paid for health care in the United States.[4] Illnesses most commonly found in older American adults are arthritis, hypertension, impaired hearing, heart disease, diabetes, and impaired vision, in that order.

Older patients differ in several important ways from young to middle-aged adults with the same disease.[3] Many older adults have two or more diseases at the same time. This comorbidity can result in added risk for adverse outcomes, such as death.[3] In addition, treatment for one disease, such as aspirin for stroke prevention, may adversely affect another disease such as peptic ulcer.[3] Some pairs of diseases significantly increase the risk of disability. For example, when arthritis or heart disease is found alone in an older adult, the risk for disability is increased by 3 to 4 times. However, when they occur at the same time (they coexist in 18% of older adults), the risk of disability increases by 14 times.[3] Another way that older adults differ from younger adults is that often the signs and symptoms associated with a disease are nonspecific. For example, the frequency of silent myocardial infarction increases with age.

Frailty, a condition that is primarily found in older adults, consists of a wasting syndrome with reduced muscle mass, weight loss, weakness, poor exercise tolerance, and low levels of physical activity, which, in late stages, can lead to death.[3] Cognitive impairment, which increases in frequency as people age, is a risk factor for falls, immobilization, dependency, institutionalization, and mortality.[3] Physical disability (i.e., being dependent on others for basic self-care, shopping, paying bills, etc.) is a serious and common outcome of chronic disease in older adults.

On the basis of the information provided here, a dramatic increase is expected in the number of older adults in this country and in the proportion with significant chronic illness and disability. These older adults will need increasing levels of dental care in the years to come. Dentists must be aware of the special management needed to treat this group of patients. For example, drug dosages and duration of treatment may have to be modified, some drugs may have to be avoided, antibiotic prophylaxis may have to be administered, and special precautions may have to be made before surgery is performed, to avoid excessive bleeding.

Etiology

Normal aging can be subdivided into successful and usual aging. Successful aging describes individuals who demonstrate minimal physiologic decline from aging alone. Healthful strategies such as exercise, modification of diet,

TABLE 30-1
Older Adults' Life Expectancy and Number of Years Free of Dependency in Activities of Daily Living

Age (yr)	Life Expectancy, Average		Disability-Free Years Remaining	
	Men	Women	Men	Women
65-69	13	20	9	11
70-74	12	16	8	8
75-79	10	13	7	7
80-84	7	10	5	5
≥85 and older	7	8	3	3

From Resnick NM. Geriatric medicine. In Fauci AS, et al (eds). Harrison's principles of internal medicine. New York, McGraw-Hill, 1998, p 39.

social and intellectual stimulation, and cessation of smoking enhance a person's quality of life and promote successful aging. Usual aging refers to the more common mode of aging. It is associated, for example, with an observed decline in renal, immune, visual, musculoskeletal, and hearing function.[7] Table 30-1 shows the estimated life expectancy and number of years free of dependency in activities of daily living for different age groups.

It is important to understand that with normal aging, many things do not change.[7] Many hormone levels, liver enzymes, electrolytes, body temperature, and basal glucose remain constant throughout life.[7] No age-related anemia has been reported (a slight decline does occur in hematocrit in men owing to decreasing testosterone levels).[7]

As individuals age, changes occur in their health and reaction to disease. These changes are due to variations in physiology that occur with aging, the presence of other diseases that develop over time, genetic predisposition for certain diseases, lifestyle factors (diet, exercise, exposure to medicines and toxins, smoking, alcohol taken in excess), and the variation intrinsic to diseases.[7]

Theories of Aging. No single hypothesis fully explains the process of aging. At the present time, two main theories have been presented to explain aging (Table 30-2). The first relates to programmed (genetic) causes, dominated by genetic theories, and the second involves random damage (stochastic or process-of-living theories).[2,7]

Programmed theories include programmed senescence (genes interfere with the ability of cells to reproduce), hormonal (biologic clock alters hormone secretion) and immunologic factors (T-cell function declines, with increasing risks for infection and cancer), and telomere shortening (shortening of telomeres in somatic cells reduces the ability of cells to divide).[2,7] Telomeres are regions of DNA that cap the ends of linear chromosomes.[8] In somatic cells, telomeres shorten progressively with every cell division, thereby reducing the number of tandem repeat sequences that occur.[8] Eventually, the

TABLE 30-2
Pathobiology of Aging

Theory	Definition	Cause	Genetics (G)/ Environment (E)
PROGRAMMED THEORIES			
Programmed senescence	Aging results from gene interference with the ability of the cells to reproduce	Master clock	G
Hormonal	Biologic clock alters hormone secretion, resulting in tissue changes	Decrease in levels of insulin-like growth factor-1 and the hormones estrogen, testosterone, testosterone, DHEA, and melatonin	G
Immunologic	T-cell function declines, increasing the chances of developing that infections and or cancer may develop	Alteration in the (cytokines) that are responsible for communication between immune cells	G
Telomere shortening	Shortening of telomeres in somatic cells lessens the ability of cells to divide	Cells cannot divide	G/E
RANDOM DAMAGE (STOCHASTIC) THEORIES			
Metabolic rate	The higher the basal metabolic rate (the rate at which the body, at rest, uses energy), the shorter the life span	Energy demands needed to maintain basal metabolism	G
Glycation	Glycation (browning) causes proteins to be joined, resulting in rigidity and decreased function	Elevated glucose	G/E
Somatic mutation	Mutations in genes occur with aging, eventually causing cells to stop functioning	Errors in the transmission of genetic messages over time	G
Wear and tear	Parts of cells wear out over time	Accumulated debris mechanically disrupts cell function	E
Oxygen free radicals	Tissue damage is caused by free radicals, such as superoxide or hydroxl radicals; this is a specific form of the wear-and-tear theory	Oxygen free radicals are unstable chemical compounds that can oxidize cell components such as DNA and proteins	E

From Minaker KL. Common clinical sequelae of aging. In Goldman L, Ausiello D (eds). Cecil Textbook of Medicine, 22nd edition. St. Louis, Elsevier, 2004, Table 23-1, p 106.
DHEA, Dehydroepiandrosterone.

chromosomes become unstable, and the cell is no longer able to replicate. This process acts in the manner of an inherent biologic clock by limiting the number of divisions that can be accomplished by the cells. In contrast, germ cells do not undergo telomeric shortening and have relatively unlimited capacities for cell division.[8]

Random damage theories include metabolic rate (the higher the rate, the shorter the life span), glycation (causes proteins to become joined, resulting in rigidity and decreased function), somatic mutation (mutations in genes associated with aging cause cells to stop functioning), wear and tear (parts of cells wear out over time), and oxygen free radicals (free radicals such as superoxide or hydroxyl cause tissue damage).[2,7]

Pathophysiology and Complications

Human aging after the age of 40 years is accompanied by physiologic deterioration. However, this decline is highly variable among older persons and within organ systems of any given individual.[2,4] Studies suggest that by main-taining good nutrition, exercise, and social activities, older adults can maintain better health.[2,4,9] For example, this approach has been reported to delay the onset of type 2 diabetes in older adults who are genetically programmed for this disease.

Certain homeostatic regulators appear to be affected by aging (Table 30-3). Muscle mass decreases, body fat increases, and total body water decreases with aging. The increase in body fat and the reduction in body water have an important impact on drug usage in older adults. The increase in fat volume affects the actions of lipophilic drugs, such as diazepam, by decreasing their initial effects and prolonging their action. Reduction in total body water has the opposite effect on water-soluble drugs, such as acetaminophen, in that it produces an exaggerated initial effect. These drugs often must be given in reduced dosage to older adults.[2,4,7,10]

Baroreflex sensitivity is impaired with aging. This leads to increased risk for orthostatic hypotension and decreased thermoregulation. Increased orthostatic

TABLE 30-3
Selected Age-Related Changes and Their Consequences*

Organ/System	Age-Related Physiologic Changes	Consequences of Age-Related Change	Consequences of Disease, Not Age
GENERAL	Increased fat	Increased volume for fat-soluble drugs	Obesity
	Decreased total body water	Decreased volume for water-soluble drugs	Anorexia
EYES/EARS	Presbyopia (cannot focus)	Decreased accommodation	
	Lens opacification	Increased susceptibility to glare	Blindness
	Decreased high-frequency acuity	Difficulty discriminating words if background noise is present	Deafness
ENDOCRINE	Impaired glucose	Increased glucose in response to illness	Diabetes mellitus
	Decreased thyroxine clearance and production	Decreased T_4 dose in hypothyroidism	Thyroid dysfunction
	Increased ADH, decreased renin, and decreased aldosterone		Decreased Na^+, increased K^+
	Decreased testosterone		Impotence
	Decreased vitamin D absorption and activation	Osteopenia	Osteomalacia, fracture
RESPIRATORY	Decreased cough reflex, decreased lung elasticity and increased chest wall stiffness	Microaspiration, ventilation/perfusion mismatch and decreased PO_2	Aspiration pneumonia, dyspnea, hypoxia
CARDIOVASCULAR	Decreased arterial compliance and increased systolic BP—left ventricular hypertrophy	Hypotensive response to increased heart rate, volume depletion, or loss of atrial contraction	Syncope
	Decreased β-adrenergic response	Decreased cardiac output and heart rate response to stress	Heart failure
	Decreased baroreceptor sensitivity and decreased SA node automaticity	Impaired BP response to standing, volume depletion	Heart block
GASTROINTESTINAL	Decreased hepatic function	Delayed metabolism of some drugs	Cirrhosis
	Decreased gastric acidity	Decreased Ca^+ absorption on empty stomach	Osteoporosis, B_{12} deficiency
	Decreased colonic motility	Constipation	Fecal impaction
	Decreased anorectal function	—	Fecal incontinence
RENAL	Decreased glomerular filtration rate	Impaired excretion of some drugs	Increased serum creatinine
	Decreased urine concentration/dilution	Delayed response to salt or fluid restriction/overload; nocturia	Increased/decreased Na^+
MUSCULOSKELETAL	Decreased lean body mass, muscle		Functional impairment
	Decreased bone density	Osteopenia	Hip fracture
NERVOUS SYSTEM	Brain atrophy	Benign forgetfulness	Dementia, delirium
	Decreased catechol synthesis		Depression
	Decreased dopaminergic synthesis	Stiffer gait	Parkinson's disease
	Decreased righting reflexes	Increased body sway	Falls
	Decreased stage 4 sleep	Early wakening, insomnia	Sleep apnea
	Impaired thermal regulation	Lower resting temperature	Hypothermia, hyperthermia

From Resnick NM. Geriatric medicine. In Fauci AS, et al (eds). Harrison's Principles of Internal Medicine. New York, McGraw-Hill, 1998, p 38.
ADH, Antidiuretic hormone; BP, blood pressure; HR, heart rate; SA, sinoatrial; T_4, Thyroxine.
*Changes generally observed in healthy elderly subjects free of symptoms and detectable disease in the organ system studies. The changes are usually important only when the system is stressed, or when other factors are added such as drugs, disease, or environmental challenge are added.

hypotension increases the risks of falls and serious injury. Also, the hypotensive effects of antidepressants, nitrates, and antihypertensives may be compounded by decreased baroreflex sensitivity. Impaired thermoregulation results in the absence of shivering, failure of the metabolic rate to rise, poor vasoconstriction, and insensitivity to low body heat. These effects increase the risk for hypothermia and heat stroke in older adults. Some drugs such as chlorpromazine and alcohol should be used with caution in these individuals because they may cause hypothermia.[2,4,7]

The level of activity of aortic and carotid chemoreceptors has been reported to decrease in older adults. The use of normal adult dosages of morphine can lead to severe respiratory depression in these individuals. Neurologic control of bowel and bladder function may be altered in older adults. Anticholinergic drugs such as antidepressants, antihistamines, antipsychotics, and many cold preparations must be used with care.[4]

Organ Systems and Functions Affected by Aging

Cardiovascular. A number of physiologic changes occur in the aging heart that may help to explain some of the more common age-associated cardiac disorders.[2,7] One of the most important is delayed left ventricular filling. Between the ages of 20 and 80, a 50% decline occurs in left ventricular filling,[7] which becomes more dependent on active filling late in diastole during atrial contraction.[7] This decline is due to thickening and stiffening of the left ventricular wall. The clinical result of these ventricular changes is diastolic heart failure.[2,7]

Resting heart rate tends to slow with advancing age, as does maximum exercise-induced heart rate.[7] Much of this change is due to loss of sinus node pacemaker cells (90% up to age 80 years).[7] The aorta dilates and its walls thicken with the calcification of medial walls; this reduces elasticity,[7] and the process tends to lead to a secondary increase in systolic blood pressure.[7]

Heart valves (particularly the mitral and aortic valves) thicken and stiffen with advancing age, and 25% of older individuals have flow murmurs.[2,7] The heart of a 65-year-old person beating at an average of 70 times per minute has opened and closed the heart valves 2,391,500,000 times. It is not surprising, therefore, that the valves show evidence of degenerative change, which is the most common cause of valve disease in these patients. Aortic and mitral valves are most often affected. Aortic stenosis in persons 50 to 59 years of age is most often caused by degeneration of a congenitally abnormal aortic valve. When it occurs for the first time in a 60-year-old or older individual, aortic stenosis usually is caused by degeneration of a normal aortic valve. Older adults with valvular heart disease are more prone to atrial fibrillation than are younger adults with similar lesions.[11]

The arrhythmia that is most commonly found in older individuals is atrial fibrillation. It may occur in about 33% of older persons who are undergoing surgery and is detected in about 4% of community-dwelling older adults.[2,7] Postural hypotension is common in older adults; about 20% are affected.[7] Sensitivity to filling volumes and impaired heart rate response to stress appear to contribute to this problem.[7] Postural hypotension is also common in older adults after large meals, severe infection (depressed salt and water intake), and volume-depleting stresses (diarrhea, diuretic therapy, bowel preparation for colonoscopy).[7] When older patients who may be prone to postural hypotension are evaluated, standing blood pressure becomes more important than sitting blood pressure.[7]

The incidence of all ventricular arrhythmias in older adults ranges from 69% to 96%. Ventricular tachycardia occurs in 2% to 13% of older adults.[2,7] The higher frequency—13%—is reported in patients with known heart disease.[12] Arrhythmias in older adults often require the use of pacemakers. In addition, many older adults are treated with warfarin (Coumadin) for prevention of thrombosis and embolism (see Chapter 25).

Endocarditis is a rare disease that has become more common among older adults. More than 50% of patients who have the first episode of endocarditis are 60 years of age or older. The clinical presentation of endocarditis in older adults is often atypical. The patient may be asymptomatic or may describe vague nonspecific symptoms such as anorexia, nausea, and vomiting. Only 50% to 70% of affected older adults will have fever. Neurologic symptoms, such as confusion, occur in about 33% of affected older adults. The diagnosis of endocarditis must be considered in any older adult with heart murmur, malaise, and fever (see Chapter 2).[11]

The annual incidence of new cases of heart failure increases from less than 1 per 1000 patient-years for individuals younger than 45 years, to 10 per 1000 patient-years for patients older than 65 years, to 30 per 1000 patient-years for those older than 85 years.[13] Prevalence figures for heart failure show a similar increase: 0.1% in those younger than 50 years of age to nearly 10% in persons older than age 80.[13] Today, about 4.8 million Americans have been given a diagnosis of heart failure, and about 75% of these individuals are 65 years of age or older.[13] Mortality rates are higher in older adults, and they are higher in older men than in older women (see Chapter 6).[13]

Arteriosclerotic heart disease (ASHD) is the most common category of heart disease in older adults, with a prevalence of 168.9 per 1000.[3,14] ASHD is the leading cause of death in all ethnic groups of older adults in the United States. The incidence of ASHD increases in men and women until age 75. By age 80, the incidence of ASHD is 20% in both men and women (see Chapter 4).[12]

Respiratory. With advancing age, the chest wall becomes stiffer as the result of thickening and calcification of cartilage; in addition, spinal ligaments become stiff, and joints become stiffer.[7] Loss of elastic recoil in the lungs occurs with aging.[7] These changes have little effect on resting lung function but decrease maximum breathing capacity by about 40%.[7] In addition, at the alveolar level, a significant reduction is seen in the capacity to exchange oxygen and carbon dioxide (decreases by about 50% between ages 30 and 65 years).[7] The major clinical impact of normal physiologic aging in the lungs is an earlier appearance of shortness of breath as a warning signal of underlying disease.[7] In addition, risk for infection of the lungs is increased. Oral organisms may contribute to pulmonary infection in older adults.[7]

Gastrointestinal. The esophagus continues to function relatively normally in older adults. However, the strength of muscular contraction declines and peristaltic waves slow. Also, the lower esophageal sphincter tends to become lax with advancing age.[7]

The gastric mucosa secretes less acid with advancing age.[2,7] This does not affect digestion in most individuals unless associated conditions such as atrophic gastritis are present; when this occurs, the absorption of nutrients and drugs is reduced.[7] Delayed gastric emptying appears to be a feature of aging that can lead to a false sense of satiety.[7]

The surface area of the small intestines is reduced with aging. This leads to a reduction in the absorption of some dietary components such as calcium. Colonic function appears to decline with advancing age, and stool frequency tends to decline, while stools become harder. Diverticula become more common; they are detected in about 50% of individuals older than 80 years.[7]

The most important age-related symptom in later life is constipation (may affect 60%).[7] Following is a list of the more common medical problems involving the gastrointestinal tract reported in older adults: gastroesophageal reflux, esophagitis, gastritis, peptic ulcer, enteritis, intestinal obstruction, diverticulitis, hemorrhoids, and colorectal carcinoma (see Chapter 12).

Renal. Kidney size declines by about 33% from 30 to 65 years of age, and blood flow through it declines by about 1% per year.[2,7] Starting in the late 30s, cortical nephrons drop out and sclerose at a higher rate than medullary nephrons. This can lead to a hyperfiltration syndrome that limits concentrating capacity. Resultant functional changes include a decreased ability to excrete a salt load, reduced glomerular filtration rate, delayed ability to regain sodium and potassium balance during deprivation states, and difficulty in conserving water under conditions of dehydration.[7] The kidney is susceptible to the effects of medications such as nonsteroidal anti-inflammatory drugs (NSAIDs) that can lead to hypertension due to sodium and fluid retention (see Chapter 13).[7]

Dehydration is common among frail older adults because of decreased fluid intake and increased fluid loss. A recent study showed that total water intake, output, and balance are maintained in healthy older adults, and an increase is noted in hydration of the fat-free mass.[15] Vomiting and diarrhea are the most common causes of isotonic dehydration and fever, and delirium is the leading cause of hypertonic dehydration.[7] Urinary concentrating defects and reduced thirst in these individuals increase the risk of dehydration during illness.

With advancing age, the bladder tends to become more irritable and to generate less power during contraction. Atrophy of vaginal and urethral tissues in postmenopausal women makes them more prone to urinary tract infection. Benign prostatic hyperplasia is common in older men and causes urinary retention; this and other factors (increased residual bladder volume and loss of protective factors) lead to an increased frequency of urinary tract infection.[2,7]

Hepatic. Liver weight declines by one third between ages 30 and 90 years because of the loss of hepatocytes. In addition, blood flow to the liver decreases by 40% to 45% with advanced age.[2,7] This results in reduced ability to process medications such as benzodiazepines, alcohol, and vitamin K–blocking agents.[7] Significant decreases in plasma albumin (seen in hospitalized or poorly nourished older adults) may result in greater amounts of free or unbound drug, which can cause greater drug effects. Doses of these drugs often must be adjusted and blood levels monitored when possible (see Chapter 11).[7]

Endocrine. Growth hormone levels fall with advancing age.[2,7] This decline appears to contribute to decreased muscle strength, thinning of bones and skin, and increased fat associated with aging.[7] Production and clearance rates of the thyroid hormones appear to remain constant with advancing age.[7] Parathyroid hormone levels increase with advancing age, and this increase is more marked in women.[7] Cortisone secretion by the adrenal glands is maintained with advancing age,[7] and renin and aldosterone secretion rates do decline.[7] The insulin content of the pancreas is increased in older adults, but its release may be blunted. Insulin resistance may increase in older adults, and glucose tolerance decreases, independent of obesity and physical inactivity. The primary cause of this decrease is insulin resistance in peripheral tissues, primarily skeletal muscle, at the postreceptor level. Glucagon secretion appears to be unchanged in older adults,[7] although a dramatic decline in estrogen and progesterone secretion by the ovaries is due to fibrosis and scarring. Menopause occurs at an average age of 51 years. Hot flashes, accelerated bone loss, and atrophy of estrogensensitive tissues may occur.[7] In men, levels of testosterone may begin to fall at about the age of 50 years; however, the potency of semen does not appear to be affected.[7]

Immune. A marked decrease in the size of the thymus gland occurs between puberty and the age of 60 years.[2,7] A corresponding drop in thymosin levels directly affects the number of functional T cells found in older adults. Also, T cells in older adults are less active in responding to foreign proteins.[7] Although antibody responses occur in older adults, these are less robust and less long lasting than those seen in younger individuals.[7] The decline in immune function in older adults results in increased morbidity and mortality with influenza and pneumonia.[7] The risk of reactivation of tuberculosis, herpes zoster, and other infections is increased in older adults because immune function is reduced.[7] In contrast, the decline in immune function reduces the risk that older adults will develop autoimmune disease.[7]

Hematopoietic. No age-related change has been noted in basal hematopoiesis.[7] However, the hematopoietic system in older adults is less able to respond to increased demand. This is demonstrated by a slower recovery from anemia and a reduced rise in hemoglobin during hypoxia.[7] In addition, the marrow in older adults is not as well stimulated by erythropoietin, as it is in younger adults.[7] Neutrophils from older adults may show less activity.[7]

Nervous. After the age of 60 years, the size of the brain is reduced by 5% to 10%, mainly as the result of decreased cerebral cortex tissue.[7] A progressive decline in the synthesis of neurotransmitters and in the number of their receptors has been observed.[2,7] Slower reaction times occur as a major functional change.[7] The lens of the eye becomes thickened and stiffens, causing the farsightedness of aging. The ability to distinguish colors (particularly blue) is reduced.[7]

Also, transmission of light through the lens may be reduced by as much as 65% between the ages of 25 and 60 years.[7] The thickened lens in older adults causes worse glare because of the scattering of light.[7] Tear production is reduced and visual acuity tends to decrease in older adults.[7]

About 25% of older adults experience hearing loss; however, this event is more common among men.[2,7] It is more difficult for these individuals to identify a voice or to understand a spoken message when background noise is present.[7] Often, the ability to hear high-frequency sounds and to distinguish high-pitched consonants is diminished.[7]

Sleep patterns change with advancing age. Older adults spend more time in bed and are more wakeful during the night.[7] Sleep-disordered breathing associated with sleep apnea (see Chapter 10) appears to increase in prevalence with advancing age.[7]

Musculoskeletal. Bone mass and density begin to decrease with age after the 20s.[7] In women, this loss may occur at a rate of about 1% per year until the time of menopause. After the onset of menopause, bone loss increases to 2% to 3% per year for 5 to 10 years, after which it returns to a rate of 1% per year[7] and may accelerate again in the late 80s. Men have greater bone mass than women and experience an annual loss of about 1% after the 20s. The clinical effects of this loss in men are not seen until they reach an advanced age.[7] The most important age-related clinical syndrome associated with advancing age is osteoporosis.[2,7] Women have increased susceptibility to osteoporosis with aging, and the major impact has been noted to occur after menopause. Microfractures of bone take longer to repair because of decreased osteoblastic cell activity. One study indicated that older adults are aware of the risk for osteoporosis but have an incomplete understanding of the causes of and ways to prevent the condition.[16]

Bisphosphonates are used to treat osteoporosis in postmenopausal women and to a lesser degree in men.[17,18] Alendronate and risedronate are bisphosphonates (Fosamax, Actonel, Boniva, Didronel, and Skelid) that have been approved by the U.S. Federal Drug Administration (FDA) for prevention of bone loss or for treatment of established osteoporosis in postmenopausal women.[17,18] The FDA has also approved alendronate for the treatment of osteoporosis in men. The bisphosphonates are given orally to treat osteoporosis and are used to prevent bone loss in patients with cancer. Several bisphosphonates (Zometa, Aredia, Didronel, and Bonefos) are given by intravenous injection. Osteonecrosis of the jaws is a significant complication that is associated with bisphosphonate therapy, particularly when treatment is given intravenously to patients with cancer. For a more detailed discussion of these agents and their uses, see Chapter 26.

With advancing age, tendons and ligaments become less elastic. This can lead to rupture of these structures, especially the Achilles tendon, in older individuals.[7] Cartilage and ligaments of the ribs and spine tend to become calcified and less elastic in older adults.[7] Flattening of the arches of the feet also occurs. Osteoarthritis is a very common problem in older adults, and many of the major joints are affected.

The ultimate size and strength of muscles is reached during the 20s and 30s. By the age of 70 years, both men and women have lost about 25% of their muscle mass, unless this was offset by exercise.[7] Loss of muscle mass continues, and by the age of 80 years, it may occur at a 30% to 40% lesser rate than in the peak years. Muscle mass in late life depends on exercise in earlier life (results in a higher early mass) and exercise late in life to stimulate muscle preservation.[7] An important complication of loss of muscle mass in older adults is a predisposition for falling. Falling is the leading cause of death at home for older individuals.[7]

Skin. In the mid-40s, subcutaneous tissue starts to thin, independent of injury from sun exposure. The epidermis and the dermis lose adherence, increasing the tendency for blistering, friction burning, and pressure ulceration.[7] These changes also lead to development of senile purpura (Figure 30-1) caused by tears in the small venules and trauma to the skin.[7] Ultraviolet sunlight, wind, and smoking can damage the subcutaneous tissues (elastin fibers) and epidermis, leading to the development

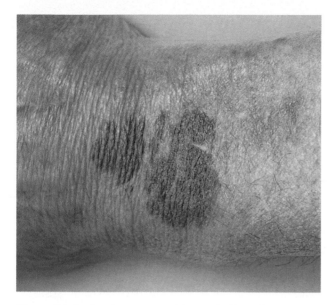

Figure 30-1. Senile purpura. (From Hoffbrand AV, Pettit JE. Color Atlas of Clinical Hematology, 3rd ed. London, Mosby, 2000.)

of wrinkles. Sun exposure can lead to slower repair of skin injuries and predisposes to the development of skin cancer (basal cell carcinoma, squamous cell carcinoma, and melanoma).[7] About 66% of older adults have at least one skin problem.[7]

Environmental exposure and age-related skin changes greatly prolong healing time for skin injuries. Skin healing takes about 50% longer in older adults than in individuals in their 30s.[7] The hair in older adults grows more slowly, and graying occurs as the result of loss of melanocytes within hair bulbs. The ability to sweat is reduced in older adults, which lessens heat loss by conduction and evaporation.[7] Older adults must protect themselves from temperature extremes.[7] Skin changes in older adults predispose to pressure sores (necrotic areas of muscle, fat, and skin) with prolonged bed rest.[7] The incidence of pressure sores among older adults in acute care hospitals is 8%, and the prevalence rate is 16%.[7] These rates are even higher for patients in intensive care and in those with hip fracture.[7]

Oral. Age-related changes in the mouth include slower production of dentine, shrinkage of the root pulp, and decreasing bone density of the jaws. Taste and smell decline progressively with advancing age, and thresholds for salt, sweets, and certain proteins are increased.[7] Food may taste more bitter, and more sugar is required. Salivary gland function usually does not change with age, and the loss of bone and tongue musculature makes the tongue appear to be enlarged.[7]

Age does not appear to play a major role in the decline of oral health. Oral cancer can lead to death by local extension or metastasis. Radiation therapy for head and neck cancer can lead to oral disorders such as mucositis, dental caries, xerostomia, or osteoradionecrosis.

Cancer elsewhere in the body can metastasize to the oral cavity (represents about 1% of cancers found in the oral cavity), and in some cases (about 20%), this may be the first sign of the presence of a distant primary cancer.[19]

Older adults underutilize dental services. Less than one third of older adults have annual dental visits, and almost one half have not seen a dentist in 5 years.[20] The primary reason for older adults to visit the dentist is to undergo a diagnostic or preventive procedure.[21] Those who are not seeking dental care do not see a need to do so, or they report that cost is a barrier.[21] A study of rural Iowa residents (65 years of age or older) found that more individuals were retaining more teeth and consequently may need and seek dental services more often than previous cohorts who were more edentulous.[22]

Dentistry should provide an aggressive educational program to get older adults to be seen and evaluated by a dentist. Other health care professionals need to provide older adult patients with an oral screening assessment and must refer to dentistry those with oral disease.[20]

Many adults 40 years ago thought that tooth loss was part of "aging." In 1957, only 40% of older adults had all or some of their natural teeth. This increased to more than 66% in 1994.[20] Tooth loss in young patients is usually due to caries or trauma. Tooth loss in adults (30 to 64 years of age) most often is caused by periodontal disease. Tooth loss in older adults is caused by periodontal disease and dental caries. Recurrent caries (involving margins of restoration) and root surface caries account for the vast majority of lesions found in older adults.[23] Older adults are predisposed to caries and tooth loss associated with aging changes. These include diminished tooth sensation, root exposure, gingival recession, compromised oral hygiene, changes in the composition of saliva, and decreased salivary flow.[20,24]

The most common age-related changes in teeth are occlusal attrition, pulpal recession, fibrosis, and decreased cellularity. Severe attrition can lead to loss of vertical dimension of occlusion. Secondary and reparative dentin leads to acellular and dehydrated dentin, and a decrease in the number of nerve fibers in the pulp of teeth occurs with aging. With aging, the teeth undergo staining, chipping, and cracking, and they become more susceptible to fracture.[24]

Older adults often feel no pain with advancing carious lesions. Acute, throbbing pain is not a common symptom of caries in the older adult, as it is in younger individuals. Older adults most often seek treatment because of food impacting within the carious lesion, or fracture of the tooth that is unsightly or lacerates oral soft tissues.[20]

Older adults show evidence of gingival recession and loss of periodontal attachment and bony support. Changes in the periodontium due to aging alone are not sufficient to cause tooth loss.[20] However, the additional effects of poor oral hygiene, systemic disease, and medication lead to increased periodontal disease and dental caries, resulting in tooth loss.

Gingival recession makes the teeth more susceptible to caries by increasing the total tooth surface that the patient must maintain and by exposing tooth surfaces not covered by enamel (e.g., cementum).[20] Results of the Health, Aging, and Body Composition cohort study, which was undertaken to determine the association between periodontal disease (6 mm or greater pocket depths) and weight loss, found that periodontal disease may be causally related to weight loss in older adults and may increase risks of morbidity and mortality.[25] Glycemic control in older patients with type 2 diabetes and periodontitis may be better controlled by effective periodontal therapy.[26]

Physical and cognitive impairment in older adults can interfere with the patient's ability to perform oral hygiene procedures. In many cases, caregivers have to take over these procedures. In cases in which no caregivers are available to assist with oral hygiene procedures, dental problems such as dental caries, tooth abscess, tooth fracture, and gingival and periodontal disease may be expected.[20]

In healthy older adults, no general diminution occurs in the volume of saliva produced.[20] Many older adults report dry mouth, and some have diminished salivary output. Systemic diseases such as diabetes mellitus can cause dry mouth. Radiation therapy for head and neck cancer can decrease salivary flow. Medications taken by older adults also can cause this problem. More than 400 drugs have been reported to cause dry mouth.[20] The following groups of drugs have been noted to cause xerostomia: tricyclic antidepressants, sedatives and tranquilizers, antihistamines, antihypertensives, cytotoxic agents, and antiparkinsonian drugs.[24]

Prolonged salivary dysfunction leads to numerous oral and pharyngeal problems in older adults. These problems include dry and friable oral mucosa, fissured tongue, decreased antimicrobial activity, diminished lubrication, caries, periodontal disease, fungal infection, burning, pain, and difficulty with mastication and swallowing.[24] Early diagnosis and treatment can prevent the problems associated with prolonged dry mouth. Diagnostic procedures may include review of the patient's history and physical findings, sialometry, sialograms, labial gland biopsy, and T99 pertechnetate scintiscans.[24] (The management of xerostomia is covered in Chapter 26.)

Changes in mastication, swallowing, and oral muscular posture occur with aging. These changes may not have adverse effects on healthy older adults. However, when compounded by systemic diseases (e.g., stroke, Parkinson's disease) and drug regimens (e.g., tardive dyskinesia associated with antipsychotic drugs), serious complications associated with chewing and swallowing, such as choking or aspiration, may occur.[24]

Older adults may report reduced food recognition and enjoyment and altered smell and taste function. Taste function undergoes few age-related changes. However, smell is dramatically diminished across the human life span.[24] Decreased smell capacity combined with changes in oral motor, salivary, and other sensory functions appears to account for the loss of flavor perception and interest in food in older adults.[24] These patients require nutritional counseling to prevent malnutrition and dehydration.[24]

The prevalence of oral mucosal lesions in U.S. adults was investigated in the Third National Health and Nutrition Examination Survey.[27] Oral examinations were performed on 17,235 individuals aged 17 years and older. Oral lesions (6003) were noted in 4801 (27.9%) persons. Denture-related lesions (8.4%) were most common. Tobacco-related lesions accounted for 4.7% of all lesions, and amalgam tattoos (3.3%) were the most prevalent lesion. Lesion prevalence increased with advancing age, wearing of dentures, and use of tobacco.[27]

An interesting association between periodontitis and oral cancer was suggested by findings from the Third National Health and Nutrition Examination Survey.[28] The severity of periodontal disease was represented by loss of clinical attachment. The independent effect of loss of clinical attachment on three separate dependent variables (tumor, precancerous lesions, and any soft tissue lesion) was assessed. Results suggested that loss of clinical attachment was related to tumors and to precancerous lesions but not to soft tissue lesions. Prospective or well-designed case control studies with histologically confirmed oral cancers are needed to confirm this possible relationship.[28]

Most oral cancers—squamous cell carcinomas—are reported in persons older than 50 years of age. Hodgkin's disease occurs in two peaks: early adulthood, and around the fifth decade of life. Non-Hodgkin's lymphoma is reported in all age groups. Benign and malignant salivary gland neoplasms are more common in older adults.

Other Considerations

Cognitive. Dementia is the loss of established intellectual ability in a way that interferes with occupational and social function. It includes impairment of memory, language, perception, calculation, abstract thinking, judgment, and executive function. Alzheimer's disease causes more than 50% of cases of dementia that is irreversible. The next most common cause of dementia is small multiple infarcts of the brain; this condition also is irreversible. Dementias are more fully discussed in Chapter 27.

Alzheimer's disease is discussed here briefly because it is the most common type of dementia. Global cognitive impairment occurs with Alzheimer's disease. Approximately 10% of older adults over 65 years of age and 45% over age 85 have Alzheimer's disease. Tacrine (Cognex) has attained short-term gain in the treatment of Alzheimer's disease, but no evidence suggests long-term benefit. Tacrine is associated with a high rate of drug toxicity.[4,29,30] Another drug, donepezil (Aricept), has shown about the same level of benefit as tacrine but without the high rate of toxicity. Tacrine and donepezil are cholinesterase inhibitors.[31] Galantamine (Reminyl) and rivastigmine (Exelon) are two other cholinesterase inhibitors that are currently used to treat mild to moderate symptoms of Alzheimer's disease.[2] The newest available drug for the treatment of Alzheimer's disease is memantine (Namenda), an NMDA (N-methyl-D-aspartate) receptor inhibitor. The FDA has approved donepezil, galantamine, rivastigmine, and memantine for the treatment of patients with mild to moderate Alzheimer's disease. Two new drugs are under investigation for the treatment of Alzheimer's disease—Alzhemed (dissolves beta-amyloid) and LY450139 (interferes with secretases and the formation of beta-amyloid). Alzhemed is under development by Neurochem Inc. of Canada, and LY450139 by Eli Lilly and Company.[32-35]

Depression. Although depression is common in older adults, age itself is not a significant risk factor. Illness and loss of a spouse or loved one are the most striking risk factors for depression. In treatment settings, the prevalence of depression in older adults is as follows: 9% to 15% in primary care practices, 15% to 25% in geriatric clinics, and 33% to 45% in hospitals and nursing homes. Medical treatment and psychotherapy both offer about the same treatment benefit, which is significant. Treatment should be offered to all older adults with depression.[4,30] Depression is more fully discussed in Chapter 29.

Suicide. Suicide rates for older men and women are higher than the average rate in the general population.[30] A decline in suicide rates has been seen in older adults of both sexes in recent years.[30] Male suicide rates increase with age, and rates in females increase until about age 60 years; they then decline from that point. Fifty to ninety percent of older adults who commit suicide have depressive illness.[30] Substance abuse or dependence is reported in about 44% of older adults who commit suicide.[30] Other important findings in older adults who commit suicide include schizophrenia, dementia, delirium, physical illness, chronic pain, and cancer.[30] With increasing age, the tendency to use more violent methods to commit suicide increases. Suicide is more fully discussed in Chapter 29.

Infectious disease. From 1981 through 2004, about 12% (114,951) of all cases of acquired immunodeficiency syndrome (AIDS) (944,306) in the United States occurred in individuals 50 years of age or older.[36] About 1.53% (14,410) of cases were reported in persons 65 years or older.[36] Severe immunosuppression was the AIDS-defining condition in more than 50% of individuals 50 years or older. The vast majority of these cases occurred in homosexual men, blood transfusion recipients, injection drug users, those who had heterosexual contact, and men who were having sex with men who were injection drug users.

The prognosis for HIV infection in individuals over age 50 years is much worse than for younger adults. HIV infection in older adults leads more quickly to subclinical immunodeficiency. Survival time after AIDS is diagnosed is inversely related to age. Leading causes of death in older adults are the same as for younger adults—opportunistic infection and bacterial infection (see Chapter 19).

Older adults are prone to develop complications when infected with the influenza virus. The aging process decreases one's ability to clear secretions and to protect the airway. Older adults with chronic illness are especially at risk for the complications of influenza, and older adults account for 80% to 90% of all influenza-related deaths. All older adults should receive an influenza vaccine each year just before the start of the flu season.[37,38]

Pneumonia is a very serious disease in older adults that often results in death. The increased risk is due to age-related deterioration of the immune system, underlying chronic illness, weakened cough reflex, decreased mobility, and the presence of oral bacteria. Older adults often do not display the classic symptoms of pneumonia (i.e., fever, chills, anorexia, and general malaise) seen in younger adults. The older adult with pneumonia often has symptoms of dehydration, confusion, and increased respiratory rate. *Streptococcus pneumoniae* is the leading cause of community-acquired pneumonia in older adults, accounting for up to 66% of cases. Nosocomial pneumonia in older adults is most often caused by *Staphylococcus aureus*. All older adults should receive the pneumococcal vaccine, starting at the age of 65 years.[38,40]

Diabetes. The prevalence of type 2 diabetes in the United States is estimated at 6% but may exceed 10% to 15% in individuals older than 50 years of age.[41] It is estimated that about 33% of cases are undiagnosed.[41] The prevalence rate for type 1 diabetes in the United States is between 0.3% and 0.4%. Incidence rises from infancy to puberty and then declines. However, in about 30% of patients, the condition is diagnosed after the age of 20 years.[41] Type 2 diabetes is much more common than type 1 diabetes in older adults. Over all ages, type 1 diabetes accounts for less than 10% of cases, and type 2 diabetes accounts for more than 90% of all cases of diabetes.[41] Patients with type 2 diabetes who are older than 65 years of age have the highest rates of comorbidity—coronary artery disease, hypertension, and osteoarthritis.[4] Diabetes mellitus is more fully discussed in Chapter 15.

Hypertension. From the age of 20 years, systolic blood pressure tends to increase with age in both men and women. In contrast, diastolic blood pressure from the age of 20 years increases until about the age of 60 years, when it begins to decrease each year.[42]

After the age of 50 years, the most common form of hypertension is isolated systolic hypertension, that is, a systolic blood pressure of 140 mm Hg or greater with a diastolic pressure less than 90 mm Hg. It is now the most common form of uncontrolled hypertension in the United States.[42] This problem was perpetuated by a past persistent focus on lowering of diastolic blood pressure, a fear of lowering blood pressure excessively in older adults, and the greater difficulty associated with lowering systolic blood pressure with available medications.[42] In older adults with isolated systolic hypertension, cardiovascular risk increases curvilinearly with increasing systolic pressure, but with an inverse relationship to diastolic pressure. For example, a blood pressure of 170/70 mm Hg carries twice the risk of coronary heart disease as a blood pressure of 170/110 mm Hg.[42] The treatment goal now with most older adults with isolated systolic hypertension is to reduce systolic blood pressure to below 140 mm Hg.[42] Hypertension is more fully discussed in Chapter 3.

Urinary incontinence. Urinary incontinence consists of the involuntary loss of urine of sufficient quantity to be a health and/or social problem.[2,7] It occurs commonly in young and middle-aged women, often in association with childbirth. It is common in middle-aged and older men with benign and malignant prostate enlargement[7] and is reported in about 33% of women and 20% of men 60 years and older who are healthy community dwellers.[7] The prevalence of urinary incontinence is about 40% in hospitalized older adults and 70% to 80% in adults living in long-term care centers.[7] Urinary incontinence causes significant physical and psychosocial problems and results in significant health care costs.[7] It contributes to skin problems and falls in older patients who rush to the bathroom.[7] It carries a social stigma and can lead to embarrassment, isolation, and depression.[7]

Medications. About 30% of all prescription medications are taken by older adults, even though they represent only about 14% of the population.[7] Nonprescription medications (herbal and over-the-counter drugs) are also used more frequently by older adults. Although gastrointestinal changes are reported in older adults, absorption of most medications does not appear to be affected[7]; however, drug distribution does change with advancing age. With declining muscle mass, fat increases as a proportion of body weight.[7] Thus, older adults are more sensitive to the effects of water-soluble drugs (i.e., a decrease in total body water concentrates water-soluble drugs) and experience prolonged but reduced initial effects with lipophilic drugs (fat-soluble drugs have longer half-lives).[7] Serum albumin levels decline with advancing age, particularly in sick older patients, resulting in a decrease in protein binding of drugs such as warfarin and phenytoin and an increase in their availability, thus enhancing drug actions. Declining renal function associated with normal aging reduces the clearance of drugs such as digoxin, aminoglycosides, and cimetidine.[7]

Hepatic metabolism of some drugs may also decline with age.[7] Oxidative reactions (phase 1) may become impaired during normal aging, although conjugation and glucuronization reactions (phase 2) do not appear to be affected.[7] Diazepam requires phase 1 and phase 2 metabolism and has a prolonged half-life in older adults,

whereas oxazepam requires only phase 2 reactions and its half-life is not affected.[7]

The brain in older adults may be more sensitive to drugs such as opiates, benzodiazepines, and neuroleptics. Doses of these medications often must be reduced when they are used in older adults. Warfarin (acts on the liver) must be used at lower doses in older adults because the liver is sensitive to blockage of vitamin K–dependent systems.[7]

Reduced compliance in taking their medications is a problem often noted in older adults. Adherence is influenced by the cost of medications, inadequate education about medications, unacceptable adverse effects, and complex medical regimens. Lower compliance is common in patients who are taking more than three prescription drugs.[7] A significant problem in older adults who are taking multiple drugs is the progressive accumulation of anticholinergic effects such as dry mouth, constipation, poor vision, urinary retention, balance disorders, and cognitive difficulties.[7] Drug classes involved include neuroleptics, antispasmodics, antianxiety agents, antihistamines, and medications used for urinary incontinence.[7]

Falls. Falls are a major age-related syndrome that results from changes in the neural, musculoskeletal, and cardiovascular systems.[2,7] Reported accidental falls usually exclude those resulting from syncope, stroke, or seizure. Approximately 33% of community-dwelling older adults fall each year.[4] In nursing homes, more than 50% fall at least once per year. Across all settings, 1 of every 6 falls produces injury, usually to soft tissue; 1 in 20 results in fracture of the hip, rib, or wrist; and 1 of every 100 leads to hospitalization.[4] Injury is the sixth leading cause of death in older adults (Table 30-4).

Intrinsic risk factors for falls in older adults consist of reductions in physical function (strength, balance, gait), neurologic disorders (stroke, dementia, parkinsonism, arthritis), sensory deficits (vision, hearing), and postural hypotension. Extrinsic risk factors for falls include poorly fitting shoes, long and loose garments, slick floors, loose rugs, obstacles, poor lighting, lack of handrails, and the number and type of medications being taken. Multiple drugs, regardless of type, increase the risk for falls in older adults.[4,7] Some drugs, however, pose a greater risk (i.e., those that affect central nervous system function and balance, such as benzodiazepines).

Laboratory Findings

Laboratory tests used to assess the older adult patient are discussed in the chapter that covers the specific illness under consideration. Little variation is noted in complete blood count, calcium, blood urea nitrogen, and cortisol or growth hormone with increasing age. Age-related decreases in levels of aldosterone, androgens, and angiotensin II are observed in older adults. In addition, age-related increases in levels of thyroid-stimulating hormone, triiodothyronine, and vasopressin may occur in these individuals.[1]

TABLE 30-4

Intrinsic Risk Factors for Falling and Possible Intervention

Risk Factor	Medical	Rehabilitative or Environmental
Reduced visual acuity, dark adaptation and perception	Refraction: Cataract extraction	Home safety assessment
Reduced hearing	Removal of cerumen: audiologic evaluation	Hearing aid if appropriate: reduction in background noise
Vestibular dysfunction	Avoidance of drugs affecting the vestibular system: neurologic or ear evaluation, if indicated	Habituation exercises
Proprioceptive dysfunction, cervical degenerative disorders, and peripheral neuropathy	Screen for vitamin B_{12} deficiency and cervical spondylosis	Balance exercises, walking aid, correctly sized footwear, home safety assessment
Dementia	Detection of reversible causes, avoidance of sedative or centrally acting drugs	Supervised exercise and ambulation, home safety assessment
Musculoskeletal	Appropriate diagnostic evaluation	Balance and gait training, muscle strengthening exercises, walking aid, home safety assessment
Foot disorders (calluses, bunions, deformities, edema)	Shaving of calluses, bunionectomy, treatment of edema	Trimming of nails, appropriate footwear
Postural hypotension	Assessment of medications, rehydration, possible alteration in situational factors such as meals, change of position	Dorsiflexion exercises, pressure-graded stockings, elevation of head of bed, use of a tilt table if condition is severe
Use of medications/ sedatives: benzodiazepines, phenothiazines, antidepressants, antihypertensives, others: (anti-arrhythmics, anticonvulsants, diuretics), alcohol	Steps to be taken: • Attempts to reduce number of medications being taken • Assessment of risks and benefits of each drug • Selection of the shortest acting medication with the least effect • Prescription of lowest effective dose • Frequent reassessment of risks and benefits	

From Tinetti ME, Speechley M: Prevention of falls among the elderly. NEJM Apr 20;320(16):1055-1059, 1989.

DENTAL MANAGEMENT

Patient Management

History. An older adult with vision loss may be unable to fill out a health questionnaire. The history of the patient should be obtained in whatever way possible; this can be done by oral interview. In cases of severe dysfunction that does not allow the patient to participate effectively, relatives or care providers will have to be involved with the medical history of the patient. The history should establish what medical problems the patient has and should uncover signs and symptoms that may indicate the presence of an undiagnosed condition.

Of particular importance are the medications older adults may be taking. Each medication that the patient is taking must be identified, including prescription, herbal, and over-the-counter drugs. Many older adults are taking multiple drugs; thus, the medication history is even more important in this group of patients. The dentist must know what drugs the patient is taking to prevent drug interactions with agents that the dentist may need to prescribe.

Clinical Examination. The clinical examination may be more difficult in some older adults. For example, patients with arthritis of the temporomandibular joint, head and neck cancer treated by surgery or radiation, neurologic disease, disorders of the musculoskeletal system, or adverse effects of antipsychotic drugs such as Parkinson-like symptoms or tardive dyskinesia may present a problem. These patients may have difficulty in opening their mouths, being able to hold still, and following the dentist's instructions regarding mouth or head positioning. The dentist may need to spend additional time and use sedative agents to complete the clinical examination. The dentist will need to speak louder, face the patient, and use shorter statements when giving directions or asking questions of patients with hearing loss or dementia. With gentle hand or finger pressure, the patient can be directed to move the head or jaws to facilitate the examination. In some patients, complex examination procedures cannot be performed. Clinical examination should include inspection of the exposed skin of the arms, legs, neck, and face and intraoral soft tissues for signs of benign and malignant lesions.

TABLE **30-5**
Selected Dental Care Problems That May Affect Older Patients

Condition	Problem	Possible Solutions
Patient easily stressed because of advanced age, systemic disease, and/or behavioral problems (anxiety)	Stress may precipitate a cardiovascular event	Short appointments, late morning or early afternoon appointments, use of sedative oral medication or nitrous oxide/oxygen
Prone to orthostatic hypotension	Syncope	Change chair position slowly, assist and support patient when getting out of chair
Dementia, physical disability, advanced illness	Difficult to follow directions, sitting still during appointment, rendering effective home care	May need to apply sedation; make short appointments; request that spouse or relatives render home care
Poor eyesight	Difficult to fill out health and dental questionnaires	Have spouse or relative fill out questionnaire, or the dentist can take an oral history from the patient
Patient taking multiple medications	Possible drug overdose, drug interactions, and potential problems with medications that the dentist may need to use	Refer patient with obvious toxic drug effects or interactions; confirm with physician that medications are current; use the lowest possible effective dose of drugs needed for dental care, and avoid drug interactions
Noncompliant patient, hypertensive patient not taking medication	Elevated blood pressure, possible risk of stroke, angina, myocardial infarction	Refer patient for reevaluation by the physician; select a drug without the adverse effects that the patient may be concerned about
Patient with signs and symptoms of systemic disease, such as leukemia, diabetes, hypertension, renal disease, and liver disease	Patient may be at great risk of for infection, bleeding, or a cardiovascular complication	Refer to physician for diagnosis and treatment, as indicated
Patients under medical treatment for cardiovascular disease	Sudden increase or decrease in blood pressure may indicate onset of complication	Monitor patient's blood pressure and pulse during dental treatment; leave blood pressure cuff on during treatment, and take the blood pressure every 10 to 15 minutes (pulse oximeter can be used to monitor the heart rate)
Patient taking an anticoagulant	Surgical procedures may cause excessive bleeding	Consult with patient's physician; surgery may be performed if INR is 3.5 or less; higher values of INR usually require reduction in the anticoagulant dosage before surgery; requires 3 to 5 days after dosage reduction for the INR to fall
Patient with prosthetic heart valve, history of endocarditis, congenital heart disease, recent open heart surgery to correct cardiovascular problem or acquired valvular heart disease	Dental bacteremias may cause bacterial endocarditis	See Chapter 2 regarding the need for antibiotic prophylaxis to prevent bacterial endocarditis
Patient taking antihypertensive, antidepressant, antipsychotic, or other medications that cause xerostomia	Increases the risk for dental caries, periodontal disease, fungal infection, and mucositis	Ask whether physician can change medication; use topical fluoride, and good home care, including brushing and flossing, saliva substitutes, and saliva stimulants (see Appendix C)

INR, International normalized ratio.

Blood pressure should be assessed on all new dental patients, including those already identified as hypertensive, and at all recall appointments. The current upper limit for normal blood pressure is 140 mm Hg for systolic and 90 mm Hg for diastolic.[43] Blood pressure should be assessed early during the first dental appointment, then again later in the appointment. The average of the two recordings should be used to record the patient's blood pressure (see Chapter 3).

Medically compromised patients may be best managed by blood pressure measurement at the start of every dental appointment and at key times during prolonged, complex dental procedures. Table 30-5 lists some of the problems the dentist may face in treating older adults.

General Guidelines. Older adults are often easily stressed by dental treatment. In general, late morning or early afternoon appointments are best for this group of patients. Medical complications are more common in these patients in the early morning as their blood pressure is rising. By late afternoon, patients may be stressed by the day's activities. The dentist should see medically compromised older adults early in the week, so that if postoperative complications develop, patients can be seen promptly. Medically compromised older adults should have their blood pressure and pulse monitored at the start of the dental appointment and several times during it (every 15 to 30 minutes; pulse oximeters are useful for this assessment). Long appointments should not be scheduled for these patients. Stress reduction[44] can be attained with the use of oral, inhalation (nitrous oxide), intramuscular, or intravenous sedation (see Chapter 28). Care must be taken to avoid overdosing with these agents.

Patients with congestive heart failure or chronic obstructive pulmonary disease may have difficulty breathing in a supine position during dental work. These patients fare much better if they are placed in an upright or semisupine position. Care should be taken when changing the chair position for older adults. The incidence of orthostatic hypotension increases with age and as an adverse effect of many drugs that these patients may be taking. A sudden change from the semisupine to the upright position may cause this type of hypotension. A matter of particular concern occurs when the older adult first gets out of the dental chair. Orthostatic hypotension at this time may lead to syncope (fainting) and a fall that could cause serious injury. Patients should be placed in an upright position slowly and should be allowed to sit for a minute; then, they should be supported by the dentist or a dental assistant when getting out of the dental chair.

Medications. A dentist who prescribes drugs for older adults should use the following guidelines: (1) The patient's medical problems should be known, (2) all drugs, including herbal and over-the-counter preparations being taken by the patient, must be identified, (3) the dentist must know the pharmacology of the drugs, (4) a new drug should be started at a small dose, and additional doses titrated on the basis of response ("start low, go slow"), (5) dosage regimens should be kept as simple as possible, and (6) visual, motor, or cognitive impairment can lead to errors or noncompliance; relatives or caregivers may have to assist with drug administration.

Sedatives and hypnotics must be used with extra care in the older adult because they may precipitate cognitive impairment. These medications should be started at the lowest dose possible, which can then be increased gradually to the minimum effective dose ("start low, go slow").[32,45] The use of short-acting agents such as triazolam (Halcion) is suggested. Nitrous oxide analgesia can be used, but care must be taken to ensure that adequate amounts of oxygen are supplied. These patients will require an escort to get home.

General anesthetics should not be used for older adults in the general dentist's office and must not be used at all for medically compromised older adults. Amide local anesthetics must be used with care or not at all in patients with advanced liver disease.

Selection of a postoperative oral analgesic requires knowledge of systemic health and medicines taken by the older adult patient. The most common adverse reaction associated with aspirin and NSAIDs is gastrointestinal upset. These agents should not be used in older adults with gastrointestinal disorders such as ulcers, gastritis, or hiatal hernia. In other older adults, these agents can be used, but care should be taken to avoid gastrointestinal irritation. This can be done by administering them with food, milk, or water (a full glass), or by having patients take a liquid antacid with aspirin or NSAIDs.

Medical Considerations

Hypertension. Any patient with a mean initial diastolic pressure of 110 mm Hg or greater should be referred at once for medical evaluation and diagnosis. Patients with initial diastolic pressures between 90 and 109 mm Hg should have their blood pressure taken again at the next dental visit. If the mean repeat diastolic pressure is greater than 90 mm Hg, the patient should be referred for medical evaluation.

Any patient with an initial mean normal diastolic pressure and a mean systolic pressure of 180 mm Hg or higher should be referred at once for medical evaluation and diagnosis. Patients with an initial normal diastolic pressure and an initial systolic pressure between 140 and 179 mm Hg should have their blood pressure taken again at the next dental visit. If the mean repeat systolic pressure is greater than 140 mm Hg, the patient should be referred for medical evaluation. Adverse effects associated with antihypertensive drugs are discussed in Chapter 3; the most common are dry mouth, orthostatic hypotension, depression, sexual dysfunction, weakness, flushing, and altered taste. Drug interactions between antihypertensive drugs and agents used by the dentist also are presented in Chapter 3. In general, only small amounts of epinephrine—maximum, 0.036 mg—should be used with these agents. NSAIDs may reduce the effectiveness of some antihypertensive drugs.

Cardiovascular. As a general guideline, no more than two cartridges of 2% lidocaine with 1:100,000 epinephrine should be used during any dental appointment for older adults with cardiovascular disease. Older adults with refractory arrhythmias, recent myocardial infarction, unstable angina, uncontrolled hyperthyroidism, recent coronary artery bypass graft, uncontrolled congestive heart failure, and uncontrolled hypertension should not receive routine dental treatment. If emergency dental treatment must be provided, a local anesthetic without a vasoconstrictor should be used (see Chapters 3, 4, 5, and 6). A pulse oximeter (Oxycount® Mini Pulse Oximeter; Weinmann, Hamburg, Germany) may be used to monitor pulse for patients with atrial fibrillation or a pacemaker.

Panoramic radiographs may reveal images of calcified atheroma in the internal carotid artery in asymptomatic patients. Lesions that cause more than 50% occlusion may be associated with increased risk for stroke.[46] In a study of panoramic radiographs of 1548 asymptomatic patients, 65 patients (4.2 %) were found to have at least one internal carotid artery atheroma.[46]

Patients in whom lesions were detected underwent Doppler ultrasonography to confirm the diagnosis and to determine the degree of stenosis. Fifteen patients were found to have an occult atheroma with greater than 50% occlusion.[46] Older dental patients with possible atheromas noted on panoramic radiographs should be referred for medical evaluation.[46]

Bleeding Problems. Anticoagulation drugs (heparin, Coumarin), antiplatelet agents (aspirin, NSAIDs), liver disease, renal disease, and cancer and the agents used to treat it are common causes of bleeding in older adults. These causes of bleeding are not related to aging itself. For example, the platelet count does not change with increasing age. Although liver mass decreases with age, this event has little or no effect on production of adequate amounts of coagulation factors for control of bleeding. Age-related renal changes, if severe, may lead to bleeding problems caused by their effects on platelet function.[47] Usually, only persons with mild forms of inherited bleeding disorders survive to old age. Dental management of the patient who may be a bleeder is discussed in Chapter 25.

Patients for whom the dosage of Coumadin was reduced before surgery (international normalized ratio [INR] greater than 3.5, or other patients whose physician has recommended a dose reduction before surgery) should be contacted within 24 to 72 hours for determination of whether postoperative bleeding is occurring.[48] The patient should then be seen at least 72 hours after surgery. If healing is progressing normally, the physician should be called and the patient returned to the normal Coumadin dosage. NSAIDs, aspirin, and acetaminophen in high doses should not be used with patients who are taking Coumadin or other anticoagulants.[48] Aspirin and NSAIDs must not be used in patients with bleeding disorders such as thrombocytopenia, hemophilia, and advanced liver disease.[10] Tylenol (acetaminophen) should not be used or should be used with care in patients who have liver or kidney disease. The combination of acetaminophen and aspirin or an NSAID must be avoided for long-term use because it increases the risk for nephropathy. (See Chapters 11, 13, and 25 for a more detailed discussion of the use of analgesics in patients with renal disease, liver failure, and bleeding disorders.)

Antibiotic Prophylaxis. Older adults with specific cardiac lesions who are at risk for bacterial endocarditis as defined by the American Heart Association should receive prophylactic antibiotics for most dental procedures (see Chapter 2). Older adults who have been given antibiotic prophylaxis to prevent endocarditis should be told to return to the dentist or to contact their physician if symptoms of anorexia, nausea and vomiting, fever, confusion, or anemia occur. These symptoms may be associated with endocarditis in older adults.

The American Dental Association and the American Academy of Orthopaedic Surgeons suggest that antibiotic prophylaxis should be considered for some older patients with joint replacements when they are about to undergo specific dental procedures (see Chapter 21).

In the past, antibiotic prophylaxis was recommended for surgical procedures performed in patients with brittle diabetes mellitus or hemophilia, in patients taking anticoagulants, and in those with other conditions. Adverse reactions associated with antibiotics (e.g., superinfection, bacterial resistance, severe allergic reaction, pseudomembranous colitis) and lack of proven benefit no longer support this type of use. If postoperative infection occurs in these older adults, treatment in the form of local and systemic agents may be provided. Older adults who are about to receive dental implants are given antibiotics at the time of surgical placement of the implant, to prevent postoperative infection and failure of the implant. This treatment is also provided for patients who are about to receive orthopaedic implants, heart valves, and other surgically placed devices.

Skin and Oral Lesions. Basal cell carcinoma (Figure 30-2) and melanoma (Figure 30-3) of the skin are lesions that are commonly found in older adults. In addition, squamous cell carcinoma of the oral cavity (lower lip), Figure 30-4, is more common in older adults (see Chapter 26). Psoriasis is a dermatologic disorder that is common in older adults (and in adolescents) (Figure 30-5). Another common skin lesion that may develop in older adults is seborrheic keratosis (Figure 30-6). Lesions of senile purpura (see Figure 30-1) on the face, legs, and arms of many older adults do not indicate an underlying bleeding problem. These lesions result from decreased fat content in the subcutaneous tissue and age changes in the connective tissue that allow for increased mobility.

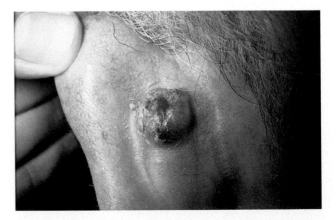

Figure 30-2. Nodular basal cell carcinoma located behind the ear. (From James WD, Berger TG, Elston DM. Andrew's Diseases of the Skin: Clinical Dermatology, 10th ed. London, WB Saunders, 2000.)

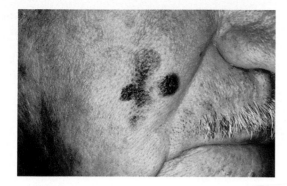

Figure 30-3. Lentigo maligna melanoma. (From James WD, Berger TG, Elston DM. Andrew's Diseases of the Skin: Clinical Dermatology, 10th ed. London, WB Saunders, 2000.)

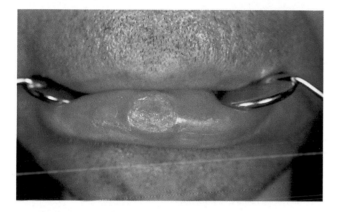

Figure 30-4. The lower lip is a common location for squamous cell carcinoma of the oral cavity.

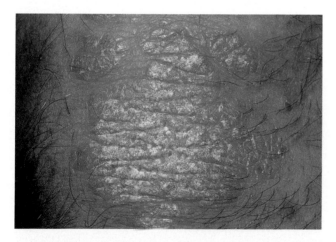

Figure 30-5. Psoriasis plaque, red plaque with silver scale on the knee. (From James WD, Berger TG, Elston DM. Andrew's Diseases of the Skin: Clinical Dermatology, 10th ed. London, WB Saunders, 2000.)

Increased mobility of the skin produces shearing forces that rupture small blood vessels. Blood lost through this bleeding takes about 1 to 3 weeks to be cleared from the skin. Senile purpura is common in older women. Platelet count and platelet function are normal in these patients;

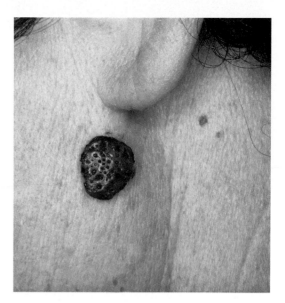

Figure 30-6. Large and disfiguring seborrheic keratosis reveals evidence of horn pearls. (From James WD, Berger TG, Elston DM. Andrew's Diseases of the Skin: Clinical Dermatology, 10th ed. London, WB Saunders, 2000.)

however, bruising may be a sign of thrombocytopenia or a bleeding tendency.

Oral lesions may be found in patients with pemphigus vulgaris, cicatricial pemphigoid, lichen planus, lupus erythematosus, erythema multiforme, leukemia, neutropenia, anemia, salivary gland tumors, cancer, and a host of other conditions. History, clinical findings, laboratory tests, cytology, and biopsy are used to establish the diagnoses of oral lesions (see Appendix C). If the dentist is unable to establish the diagnosis for a particular lesion, he or she should refer the patient to an oral medicine specialist, an oral maxillofacial surgeon, or an oral maxillofacial pathologist.

Referral and Consultation. Older adults with advanced organ disease such as liver, kidney, lung, or heart disease may be at increased risk for invasive or prolonged dental treatment. Before dental treatment is provided, the dentist should consult with the patient's physician to establish the patient's current status and to confirm all drugs that the patient is taking. Special management procedures that are being planned for the patient should be reviewed with the patient's physician for input and modification when needed.

Older adults who are found to be hypertensive should be referred to a physician for diagnosis and treatment. Patients with signs or features of oral cancer should be referred for further diagnosis and treatment. Those with signs and symptoms that suggest untreated systemic disease such as diabetes or AIDS should be referred for diagnosis and treatment.

When surgery is planned for older adults who are taking anticoagulants (Coumadin), the dentist should consult with the patient's physician to determine the

INR. Most often, dental surgery can be performed without adjustment in dosage for patients who are being maintained in therapeutic ranges of anticoagulation (INR, 1.5 to 3.5). Patients with an INR greater than 3.5 should have their dosage of Coumadin reduced by their physician 3 to 5 days before undergoing dental surgery (see Chapter 25).

When problems with the patient's medications such as signs and symptoms of overdose or drug interaction are identified, the dentist should communicate those findings to the patient's physician. Also, the older adult who is taking multiple medications and who has not seen a physician over the previous year should be directed to make an appointment, so the doctor can review the appropriateness of the patient's current medications.

The patient's physician should review the drugs being taken on a regular basis. If it has been longer than 1 year since the older adult dental patient has seen the physician, the patient should be referred for this review. The dentist and the physician must consider that new symptoms or problems could be drug induced.[29] Use of multiple drugs must be avoided whenever possible.

Individuals who report dry mouth and who are taking medications that have been reported to cause xerostomia (the dentist can measure salivary flow to determine whether it has been reduced) can best be served by the dentist's consultation with the physician to determine whether another drug without this adverse effect could be used to control the patient's systemic condition.

Patients with signs and symptoms suggestive of systemic disease should be referred for medical evaluation, diagnosis, and treatment. Patients with oral lesions that the dentist is unable to diagnose must be referred for diagnosis and treatment.

REFERENCES

1. Ferri FF, Fretwell MD, Wachtel TJ. Practical Guide to the Care of the Geriatric Patient, 2nd ed. St. Louis, Mosby–Year Book, 1997.
2. Resnick NM, Dosa D. Geriatric medicine. In Kasper DL, Braunwald E, Fauci AS, et al (eds). Harrison's Online Principles of Medicine, 16th ed. New York, McGraw-Hill, 2005, pp 43-53.
3. Fried LP. Epidemiology of aging: Implications of the aging of society. In Goldman L, Ausiello D (eds). Cecil Textbook of Medicine. Philadelphia, WB Saunders, 2004, pp 100-103.
4. Katz MS, Gerety MB. Gerontology and geriatric medicine. In Stein JH (ed). Internal Medicine, 2nd ed. St. Louis, Mosby Online, 1998, Chapter 373.
5. Landis SH, Murray T, Bolden S, Wingo PA. Cancer statistics: 1998. CA Cancer J Clin 1998;48:6-29.
6. Eliopoulos C. Manual of Gerontologic Nursing, 2nd ed. St. Louis, Mosby, 1999.
7. Minaker KL. Common clinical sequelae of aging. In Goldman L, Ausiello D (eds). Cecil Textbook of Medicine. Philadelphia, WB Saunders, 2004, pp 105-111.
8. Mera SL. The role of telomeres in ageing and cancer. Br J Biomed Sci 1998;55:221-225.
9. American Diabetes Association 57th Annual Meeting and Scientific Sessions, June 21-24, 1997, Boston, Mass. Clin Rev 1997;7:162-165.
10. Rho JP, Wong FS. Principles of prescribing medications. In Yoshikawa TT, Cobbs EL, Brummel-Smith K (eds). Practical Ambulatory Geriatrics, 2nd ed. St. Louis, Mosby–Year Book, 1998, pp 19-25.
11. Channer KS. Valvular heart disease in old age. In Tallis R, Fillit H, Brocklehurst JC (eds). Geriatric Medicine and Gerontology, 5th ed. New York, Churchill Livingstone, 1998, pp 337-349.
12. Trumble TJ, Taffet GE. Cardiac problems. In Yoshikawa TT, Cobbs EL, Brumel-Smith K (eds). Practical Ambulatory Geriatrics, 2nd ed. St. Louis, Mosby–Year Book, 1998, pp 453-464.
13. Massie BM. Heart failure: Pathophysiology and diagnosis. In Goldman L, Ausiello D (eds). Cecil Textbook of Medicine. Philadelphia, WB Saunders, 2004, pp 291-299.
14. Kannel WB, Thom TJ. Incidence, prevalence, and mortality of cardiovascular diseases. In Hurst JW (ed). The Heart, Arteries, and Veins, 7th ed. New York, McGraw-Hill, 1990, pp 627-638.
15. Bossingham MJ, Carnell NS, Campbell WW. Water balance, hydration status, and fat-free mass hydration in younger and older adults. Am J Clin Nutr 2005;81: 1342-1350.
16. Burgener M, Arnold M, Katz JN, et al. Older adults' knowledge and beliefs about osteoporosis: Results of semistructured interviews used for the development of educational materials. J Rheumatol 2005;32:673-677.
17. Finkelstein JS. Osteoporosis. In Goldman L, Ausiello D (eds). Cecil Textbook of Medicine, 22nd ed. Philadelphia, Elsevier (WB Saunders), 2004, pp 1547-1555.
18. Kanis JA. Paget's disease of bone (osteitis deformans). In Goldman L, Ausiello D (eds). Cecil Textbook of Medicine, 22nd ed. Philadelphia, Elsevier (WB Saunders), 2004, pp 1579-1582.
19. Little JW, Falace DA, Miller CS, Rhodus NL. Oral Cancer: Dental Management of the Medically Compromised Patient, 6th ed. St. Louis, Mosby, 2002, pp 387-417.
20. Lloyd PM. Oral and dental problems. In Yoshikawa TT, Cobbs EL, Brummel-Smith K (eds). Practical Ambulatory Geriatrics, 2nd ed. St. Louis, Mosby–Year Book, 1998, pp 412-422.
21. Macek MD, Cohen LA, Reid BC, Manski RJ. Dental visits among older U.S. adults, 1999: The roles of dentition status and cost. J Am Dent Assoc 2004;135:1154-1162; quiz 65.
22. Ettinger RL, Warren JJ, Levy SM, et al. Oral health: Perceptions of need in a rural Iowa county. Spec Care Dentist 2004;24:13-21.
23. Fure S. Ten-year cross-sectional and incidence study of coronal and root caries and some related factors in elderly Swedish individuals. Gerodontology 2004;21: 130-140.
24. Ship JA, Mohammad AR (eds). Clinician's Guide to Oral Health in Geriatric Patients, 1st ed. Baltimore, The American Academy of Oral Medicine, 1999.
25. Weyant RJ, Newman AB, Kritchevsky SB, et al. Periodontal disease and weight loss in older adults. J Am Geriatr Soc 2004;52:547-553.

26. Promsudthi A, Pimapansri S, Deerochanawong C, Kanchanavasita W. The effect of periodontal therapy on uncontrolled type 2 diabetes mellitus in older subjects. Oral Dis 2005;11:293-298.

27. Shulman JD, Beach MM, Rivera-Hidalgo F. The prevalence of oral mucosal lesions in U.S. adults: Data from the Third National Health and Nutrition Examination Survey, 1988-1994. J Am Dent Assoc 2004;135:1279-1286.

28. Tezal M, Grossi SG, Genco RJ. Is periodontitis associated with oral neoplasms? J Periodontol 2005;76:406-410.

29. Thornburg JE. Gerontological pharmacology. In Brody TM, Larner J, Minneman KP (eds). Human Pharmacology: Molecular to Clinical, 2nd ed. St. Louis, Mosby, 1994, p 855-861.

30. Shah A, Tovey E. Psychiatry of old age. In Wright P, Stern J, Phelan M (eds). Core Psychiatry, 2nd ed. Edinburgh, Elsevier, 2005, pp 481-493.

31. Scharre DW, Cummings JL. Dementia. In Yoshikawa TT, Cobbs EL, Brummel-Smith K (eds). Practical Ambulatory Geriatrics, 2nd ed. St. Louis, Mosby–Year Book, 1998, pp 290-301.

32. Aisen PS. The development of anti-amyloid therapy for Alzheimer's disease: From secretase modulators to polymerisation inhibitors. CNS Drugs 2005;19:989-996.

33. Geerts H. NC-531 (Neurochem). Curr Opin Investig Drugs 2004;5:95-100.

34. Siemers E, Skinner M, Dean RA, et al. Safety, tolerability, and changes in amyloid beta concentrations after administration of a gamma-secretase inhibitor in volunteers. Clin Neuropharmacol 2005;28:126-132.

35. Siemers ER, Quinn JF, Kaye J, et al. Effects of a gamma-secretase inhibitor in a randomized study of patients with Alzheimer disease. Neurology 2006;66:602-604.

36. Centers for Disease Control and Prevention. HIV/AIDS Surveillance Report, 2004, vol 16. Atlanta, U.S. Department of Health and Human Services, 2005, pp 1-46.

37. Hayden FG. Influenza. In Goldman L, Ausiello D (eds). Cecil Textbook of Medicine. Philadelphia, WB Saunders, 2004, pp 1974-1978.

38. Weltitz PB. Respiratory function. In Lueckenotte AG (ed). Gerontologic Nursing, 1st ed. St. Louis, Mosby, 1996, pp 566-605.

39. Limper AH. Overview of pneumonia. In Goldman L, Ausiello D (eds). Cecil Textbook of Medicine. Philadelphia, WB Saunders, 2004, pp 551-557.

40. Mandell L. Pneumococcal pneumonia. In Goldman L, Ausiello D (eds). Cecil Textbook of Medicine. Philadelphia, WB Saunders, 2004, pp 1764-1770.

41. Sherwin RS. Diabetes mellitus. In Goldman L, Ausiello D (eds). Cecil Textbook of Medicine. Philadelphia, WB Saunders, 2004, pp 1424-1452.

42. Victor R. Arterial hypertension. In Goldman L, Ausiello D (eds). Cecil Textbook of Medicine. Philadelphia, WB Saunders, 2004, pp 346-363.

43. Joint National Committee on Prevention, Evaluation, and Treatment of High Blood Pressure. The Sixth Report of the Joint National Committee on Prevention, Detection, Evaluation, and Treatment of High Blood Pressure. Washington DC, National Institutes of Health, National Heart, Lung, and Blood Institute, 1997.

44. Little JW. Anxiety disorders: Dental implications. J Gen Dent 2003;51:562-570.

45. Fretwell MD. Optimal pharmacotherapy. In Ferri FF, Fretwell MD, Wachtel TJ (eds). Practical Guide to the Care of the Geriatric Patient, 2nd ed. St. Louis, Mosby–Year Book, 1997, pp 359-370.

46. Friedlander AH, Garrett NR, Chin EE, Baker JD. Ultrasonographic confirmation of carotid artery atheromas diagnosed via panoramic radiography. J Am Dent Assoc 2005;136:635-640; quiz 82-3.

47. Erban JK. Hematologic problems of the elderly. In Reichel W (ed). Care of the Elderly: Clinical Aspects of Aging, 4th ed. Baltimore, Williams & Wilkins, 1995, pp 373-380.

48. Little JW, Miller CS, Henry RG, McIntosh BA. Antithrombotic agents: Implications in dentistry. Oral Surg Oral Med Oral Path Oral Radiol Endod 2002;93:544-551.

A Guide to Management of Common Medical Emergencies in the Dental Office*

APPENDIX

A

GENERAL CONSIDERATIONS

The best management of a dental office medical emergency is prevention. Dental practitioners must be prepared to treat the seemingly well but chronically ill patient whose condition is managed by a variety of drugs. Dentists and the members of their office staff must first be aware of the patient's medical condition. This knowledge provides a strong indicator of the patient's risk for having a medical emergency and also gives practitioners an opportunity to take measures that could prevent such emergencies. If an emergency does occur, an informed dentist will have a better idea of the type of medical problem the patient is experiencing. The dentist must also understand the pathophysiologic factors regulating disease processes and the pharmacodynamics of drug action and interaction.

Patients frequently experience physical reactions during treatment and this places considerable responsibility on the dentist to respond to any emergencies quickly, efficiently, and competently with adequate resuscitative procedures. Obviously one of the most important precepts of good medical emergency management is to keep a cool head, don't panic, and implement basic cardiac life support (BCLS). The health professional is responsible for knowing and using those techniques that are known, practiced, safe, and efficient. An unfamiliar or unreliable maneuver should never be attempted. The dentist must be trained in providing BCLS, and in many

cases may wish to pursue advanced cardiac life support (ACLS) training. Dental practitioners should also be aware that there were some changes in basic cardiopulmonary resuscitation (CPR) guidelines in 2005.

Although dentists should be prepared to provide resuscitative procedures in emergency situations, they should give even more consideration to preventing them. This can be accomplished by obtaining an adequate medical history of the patient, making an appropriate physical evaluation, and ensuring that the patient and environment are prepared before treatment begins. Sometimes emergencies may be prevented through the recognition of physical limitations before treatment begins.

Management of emergencies must begin long before they occur. The dentist must be prepared with a plan of action and an adequate armamentarium to meet emergencies. Presenting a plan for every situation that may arise in the dental office is impossible. No cookbook solutions exist, and hurried emotional responses are hazardous. The actions of the dental team must be based on a thorough background, continued study, and carefully prepared and rehearsed emergency procedures in which each individual has specific duties and responsibilities. This necessitates the presence of appropriate resuscitative equipment and drugs to permit the team to work calmly and precisely. This teamwork must be based on knowledge, practice, sound judgment, and confidence. Every dental office should have a written plan that spells out specific duties for each member of the office staff, covering areas such as who will call the emergency medical services (EMS) system (call 911), start CPR, begin an intravenous (IV) line, and administer drugs. A designated staff member should record every event and the time of each action.

A good medical history, appropriate physical evaluation, and proper consultation may prevent the onset of a life-threatening situation. However, unforeseen

---

*Much of the material contained herein is modified from Malamed SF: Medical Emergencies in the Dental Office, ed 4, St Louis, 2007, Mosby; the American Heart Association Guidelines for Basic Cardiac Life Support and Advanced Cardiac Life Support (Current Emergency Cardiovascular Care), Circulation, 102(8s), August 22, 2000; 2005 American Heart Association Guidelines for Cardiopulmonary Resuscitation and Emergency Cardiovascular Care, Circulation, 112(24)s, December 13, 2005.

circumstances do occur and the dentist should make every effort to prevent irreversible physiologic damage.

Physical evaluation of patients has become more important because of the introduction of more complicated and lengthy dental procedures, the increasing number of medical risk patients, the growing number of geriatric patients, and the use of conscious sedation techniques. The goal of evaluation is to determine the ability of a patient to safely tolerate a specific procedure by gathering reliable information so that intelligent decisions can be made during treatment. It is not to diagnose and treat medical conditions. This approach eliminates the element of surprise, heightens the awareness of potential risk, produces confidence, establishes rapport with the patient, and provides a basis for communication with a physician when indicated.

Consultation with the patient's physician should be made to ensure adequate knowledge of the patient's particular problem and the proposed dental treatment plan. Generally, consultation with the physician does not alter the treatment plan, though occasionally it will do so significantly. Rarely, however, will consultation delay treatment. These consultations serve only as guidelines to patient management. The dentist must make final decisions regarding dental treatment.

In most emergencies the dentist and staff should employ BCLS procedures and call the EMS 911 system phone number. Dentists should also be familiar with the use of an automated external defibrillator (AED).

Dentists with ACLS training may start an IV line and administer drugs through it as indicated. Use of the pulse oximeter and electrocardiography can be important adjuncts for monitoring a patient's vital signs.

GENERAL PRINCIPLES OF EMERGENCY CARE

Most life-threatening office emergencies are caused by the patient's inability to withstand physical or emotional stress or the patient's reaction to drugs. Emergencies also can be caused by a complication of a preexisting systemic disease. Cardiopulmonary systems can be involved, thus requiring some emergency supportive therapy.

In all emergencies, the following procedures must be performed:
1. Place the patient in the supine position if possible; if still conscious, the patient may prefer a more upright position
2. Give the patient the basics of life support (cardiopulmonary resuscitation [CPR]), which include the following:

NOTE: The American Heart association made some changes to CPR procedures in 2005.
   a. Air passage opened and cleared if necessary
   b. Breathing ensured (by artificial respiration if necessary)
   c. Carotid pulse checked as a way of ensuring circulation; CPR administered if there is no carotid pulse, and blood pressure checked if carotid pulse is present
   d. Use of automated external defibrillator (AED)

Once the emergency has been diagnosed, proper treatment in most cases includes the following:
1. Emergency medical system activated by 911 phone call.
2. Administration of oxygen (10 L/min. flow)
3. Use of IV line for rapid drug administration (with ACLS training)
4. Administration of CPR
5. Use of AED
6. Treatment with drugs (ACLS training for IV line)

Key Points

Elements essential to the successful treatment of medical emergencies include the following:
1. Quick recognition and diagnosis of signs and symptoms
2. Early response time (4 to 6 minutes without oxygen leads to irreversible brain damage)
3. Airway clearance (circulation meaningless without oxygen)
4. Proper monitoring of vital signs (e.g., carotid pulse)
5. Continued monitoring of patient status (e.g., color, ventilation, pulse, blood pressure, pupils)
6. Assurance that patient receives proper medical care

TYPES OF EMERGENCIES AND THEIR TREATMENT

Unconsciousness

Syncope and Psychogenic Shock

Cause. Cerebral hypoxia (reduced blood flow to brain)

Symptoms
1. Early
   a. Pallor
   b. Sweating
   c. Nausea
   d. Anxiety
2. Late
   a. Pupillary dilation
   b. Yawning
   c. Decreased blood pressure
   d. Bradycardia (slow pulse)
   e. Convulsive movements
   f. Unconsciousness

Treatment
1. Lower head slightly and elevate legs and arms (for pregnant women, roll on left side)
2. Administer oxygen at 10 L flow/min
3. Administer spirits of ammonia
4. Apply cold compresses to forehead
5. Monitor and record vital signs
6. Reassure patient

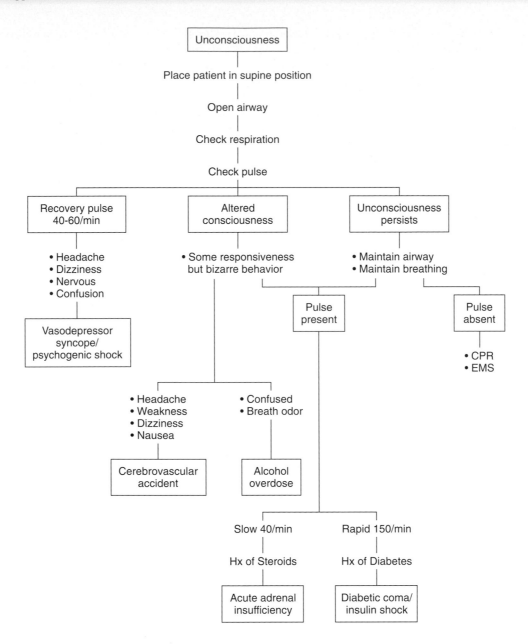

For low blood pressure or pulse (systolic is less than previous diastolic), the following procedures should be followed:

1. Low blood pressure
   a. Lower head and raise arms and legs
   b. Start 5% dextrose and lactated Ringer's IV
   c. Administer a vasopressor drug (epinephrine 0.3-0.5 mg via subcutaneous (SC) or intramuscular (IM) routes or intravenously with ACLS training)
2. Slow pulse (less than 60 beats per minute)
   a. Administer 0.4 mg atropine via IV access to increase heart rate
   b. Repeat up to a dose of 1.2 mg, then consider use of additional vasopressors

Cardiac Arrest

Signs and symptoms
1. No pulse or blood pressure
2. Sudden cessation of respiration (apnea)
3. Cyanosis
4. Dilated pupils

Treatment
1. Airway—lift chin, clear airway if necessary, and observe for breathing
2. Breathing—inflate lungs with mouth-to-mouth resuscitation, give two initial quick breaths, and perform endotracheal intubation and positive pressure oxygen
3. Circulation—check carotid pulse; if pulse is absent, compress sternum 1 to 2 inches (2 to 3) fingerwidths above xiphoid process

NOTE: The importance of technique for chest compressions cannot be over-emphasized; they must be adequate and efficient.
   a. *One operator:* 30 compressions : 2 inflations for a rate of 100 compressions/min.

NOTE: New in 2005: compression-to-ventilation ratio of 30:2 and breaths should only take 1 minute; emphasis on the efficacy of compressions.

  b. *Two operators:* 15 compressions : 2 inflations for a rate of 100 compressions/min. Continue resuscitation until spontaneous pulse returns.
4. Use automated external defibrillator (AED).
5. IV drugs—start 5% dextrose lactated ringers (with ACLS training)
  a. Epinephrine: 0.5-1.0 ml 1:1,000, repeat every 5 minutes prn.
  b. Sodium bicarbonate: 1 mEq/kg initially and additional doses every 10 minutes until circulation is restored (or as governed by arterial blood gas measurement).
  c. Atropine sulfate: Indicated if pulse is less than 60 beats/min and systolic blood pressure is below 90. Initial dose: 0.5 mg; repeat every 5 minutes, not to exceed 2.0 mg total dose.
6. Other drugs used for treatment of cardiac arrest (with ACLS training)
  a. Lidocaine (anti-arrhythmic agent)
  b. Calcium chloride (increases myocardial contractility)
  c. Morphine sulphate (for pain relief)

Monitor and record all vital signs, drug administrations, and patient responses. Call 911 for emergency medical assistance.

Diabetic Coma versus Insulin Shock

Diagnostic Factors	Diabetic Coma (no insulin)	Insulin Shock
HISTORY		
Food intake	Normal or excessive	May be insufficient
Insulin	Insufficient	Excessive
Onset	Gradual (days)	Sudden (hours)
PHYSICAL EXAM		
Appearance	Extremely ill	Very weak
Skin	Dry and flushed	Moist and pale
Infection	Frequent	Absent
Fever	Frequent	Absent
GI SYMPTOMS		
Mouth	Dry	Drooling
Thirst	Intense	Absent
Hunger	Absent	Occasional
Vomiting	Common	Rare
Abdominal pain	Frequent	Absent
BREATH	Acetone odor	Normal
BLOOD PRESSURE	Low	Normal
PULSE	Weak and rapid	Full and bounding
TREMOR	Absent	Frequent
CONVULSIONS	None	In late stages

Treatment

1. Place patient in supine position.
2. Administer oxygen.
3. If patient is conscious, give patient a high sugar–containing drink such as Glucola or orange juice.
4. If patient is unconscious, a glucose paste can be applied to the buccal mucosa. A dentist with ACLS training can start IV 5% dextrose (D5LR) and run the IV drip as fast as possible.
5. Monitor and record vital signs.
6. Activate EMS system by calling 911.
7. Transport patient to emergency room if some improvement is not fairly rapid.
   NOTE: If in doubt, treat as insulin shock.

Response to treatment

1. Insulin shock: rapid improvement after carbohydrate administration
2. Diabetic coma
   a. No improvement after carbohydrate administration
   b. Slow improvement (6-12 hours) after insulin administration

Acute Adrenal Insufficiency

Cause. Adrenal suppression (low adrenocorticotropic hormone) because exogenous steroids suppress adrenal production. The patient may be medicated with steroids for dozens of medical problem; or the cause may be primary or secondary malfunction of the adrenal cortex.

Signs and symptoms

1. Altered consciousness
2. Confusion, weakness, fatigue
3. Headache
4. Pain in abdomen, legs
5. Nausea, vomiting
6. Hypotension and syncope
7. Coma

Treatment

Management of the Patient With Acute Adrenal Insufficiency

Conscious	Unconscious
1. Position patient semireclining	1. Position patient supine
2. Monitor and record vital signs	2. BCLS
3. Administer oxygen	3. Administer oxygen
4. Administer steroids, hydrocortisone 100 mg, or dexamethasone 4 mg (IV with ACLS training)	4. Summon EMS (911 call)
5. May have to transfer to hospital for lack of fluids	5. Review patient's medical history
	6. Administer steroids hydrocortisone 100 mg, or dexamethasone 4 mg
	7. Administer vasopressor (epinephrine 0.5 ml)
	8. Rapid transfer of patient to hospital

Cerebrovascular Accident

Signs and symptoms
1. Early warning signs
   a. Dizziness (patient may fall)
   b. Vertigo and vision changes
   c. Nausea and vomiting
   d. Transient paresthesia
   e. Unilateral weakness or paralysis
2. General symptoms
   a. Headache
   b. Nausea
   c. Vomiting
   d. Convulsions, coma

NOTE: Blood pressure and pulse are generally normal. Raised blood pressure and body temperature and lowered pulse and respiration indicate increased intracranial pressure.

Treatment
1. Call EMS (911).
2. Position patient in reclining, semi-sitting position with the head elevated.
3. Provide the following support:
   a. Oxygen at 10 L/min flow
   b. No sedative use
   c. Airway and breathing maintenance
4. Monitor and record vital signs.
5. Keep patient quiet and still.
6. Ensure rapid transfer to hospital.

Convulsions

Causes
1. Syncope
2. Drug reactions
3. Insulin shock
4. Cerebrovascular accident
5. Convulsive seizure disorder

Signs and symptoms
1. Aura—flash of light or sound
2. Mental confusion
3. Excessive salivation
4. Tonic contractions and tremors
5. Convulsive movements of extremities
6. Rolling back of eyes
7. Loss of consciousness

Treatment
1. Protect patient from personal damage.
2. After convulsion, make sure airway is open.
3. Dispense oxygen at 10 L/min flow.
4. For status epilepticus, administer diazepam (Valium) 5-20 mg IV.
5. Monitor and record vital signs.
6. Support respiration (patient may have respiratory arrest).

Local Anesthesia Drug Toxicity

Causes
1. Too large a dose of local anesthetic per body weight
2. Rapid absorption of drug or inadvertent IV injection
3. Slow detoxification or elimination of drug

Signs and symptoms
1. Early
   a. Talkative, restless, apprehensive, excited manner
   b. Convulsions
   c. Increase in blood pressure and pulse rate

NOTE: The stimulation is followed by depression of the central nervous system.

2. Late signs and symptoms
   a. Convulsions followed by depression
   b. Drop in blood pressure
   c. Weak, rapid pulse or bradycardia
   d. Apnea
   e. Unconsciousness, death

NOTE: Lidocaine toxicity is documented to have occasionally exhibited only the depression without the usual prodromal of the excitatory phase.

Treatment
1. Protect patient during the convulsive period (consider administration of 5-15 mg valium IV if convulsive period is prolonged).
2. Monitor and record vital signs.
3. Provide supportive therapy.
   a. Keep patient in supine position.
   b. Maintain oxygen at 10 L flow/min.
   c. Maintain blood pressure.
   d. Treat bradycardia (0.4 mg atropine IV, with ACLS training).
   e. Transport to hospital.

NOTE: If patient becomes unconscious, maintain airway, administer CPR, and call for emergency medical service.

Respiratory Difficulty

Hyperventilation

Cause
1. Excess loss of CO_2
2. Respiratory alkalosis

Symptoms
1. Rapid, shallow breathing
2. Confusion
3. Dizziness
4. Paresthesia
5. Carpal-pedal spasms

Treatment
1. Explain the problem to the patient and reassure patient.

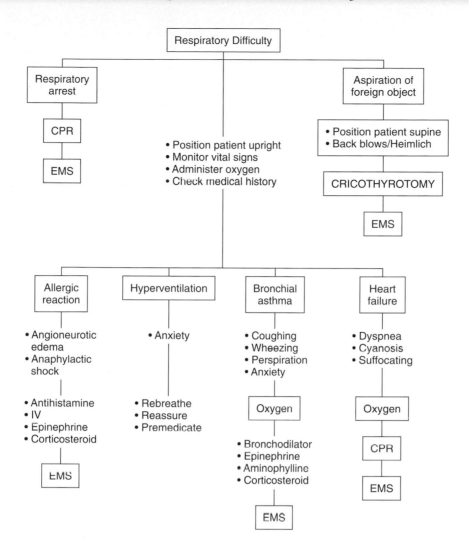

2. Instruct the patient to be calm and breathe slowly.
3. Have patient breathe slowly into a paper bag.
4. Reappoint for presedation.

Aspiration or Swallowing a Foreign Object

Cause. Foreign body in larynx or pharynx.

Signs and symptoms
1. Coughing or gagging associated with a foreign object; inability to speak.
2. Possible cyanosis from airway obstruction.
3. Violent respiratory effort.
4. Suprasternal retraction.
5. Rapid pulse.

Treatment
1. Keep patient supine if unconscious; keep standing or sitting leaning forward if conscious.
2. Establish airway (open and evaluate breathing).
3. Apply Heimlich maneuver.
NOTE: If cricothyrotomy is necessary, refer to "Cricothyroid Membrane Puncture" procedure that follows.
4. Administer oxygen.

5. Maintain the supine position and transport patient to hospital for radiographs.
   A. Posterior-anterior chest view
   B. Lateral chest view
   C. Flat plane abdominal view to establish location
NOTE: If foreign object is in GI tract, follow with x-ray examination. Foreign object in trachea or lung requires a bronchoscopy or thoracotomy. If foreign object has occluded the airway, the Heimlich maneuver may be of benefit before initiation of a cricothyrotomy.

Cricothyroid Membrane Puncture.
The approach to a patient with acute airway obstruction should be:
1. Recognition of obstruction
2. Use of nonsurgical maneuvers to relieve obstruction (i.e., back blows, Heimlich maneuver)
3. Administration of mouth-to-mouth breathing to bypass obstruction or to diagnose obstruction
4. Activation of EMS with 911 call
5. Establishment of an emergency surgical airway (cricothyrotomy) if Heimlich maneuver is unsuccessful

Cricothyrotomy
1. Place patient in head-down position with neck hyperextended,

2. Ensure that chin and sternal notch are held in median plane.
3. Perform 2-cm vertical incision through skin over cricothyroid cartilage.
4. Perform 2-cm transverse incision over cricothyroid membrane.
5. Insert small scissors or hemostats through cricothyroid membrane and into the tracheal space, or use large (8-gauge) needle.
6. Expand instrument and dilate transversely.
7. Insert tube into trachea between beaks of dilating instrument.
8. Remove scissors or hemostats.
9. Tape tube into place.
10. Use positive pressure or enriched oxygen flow if patient is breathing independently.
11. Arrange for rapid transfer of patient to the hospital.

Bronchial Asthma

Signs and symptoms
1. Sense of suffocation
2. Pressure in chest
3. Nonproductive cough
4. Expiratory wheezes
5. Prolonged expiratory phase
6. Increased respiratory effort
7. Chest distension
8. Thick, stringy mucous sputum
9. Cyanosis (in severe cases)

Treatment
1. Use Beta2-agonist inhaler (e.g., Isuprel mistometer) 1 to 2 deep inhalations
2. Activate EMS (911 call)
3. Dispense oxygen at 10L/min flow
4. If unresponsive, administer epinephrine (0.3-0.5 ml, 1:1000, SC; repeat every 20 minutes prn)
5. Dispense theophylline ethylenediamine (aminophylline) 250-500 mg IV slowly over a 10-minute period
6. Administer hydrocortisone sodium succinate (Solu-Cortef), 100 mg IV
7. Monitor and record vital signs
8. Arrange for rapid transport of patient to the hospital
NOTE: Because aminophylline may cause hypotension, it should be given with extreme caution to patients with asthma who are hypotensive.

Mild Allergic Reaction

Symptoms
1. Mild pruritus (itching)—slow appearance
2. Mild urticaria (rash)—slow appearance

Treatment
1. Administer diphenhydramine (Benadryl) 25-50 mg PO, IV, or IM (if dentist has ACLS training)

2. Repeat dose up to 50 mg every 6 hours orally for 2 days
3. If suspected allergy to medication, withdraw drug administration

Severe Allergic Reaction

Symptoms
1. Skin reactions—rapid appearance
   a. Severe pruritus (itching)
   b. Severe urticaria (rash)
2. Swelling of lips, eyelids, cheeks, pharynx, and larynx (angioneurotic edema)
3. Anaphylactic shock
   a. Cardiovascular—fall in blood pressure
   b. Respiratory—wheezing, choking, cyanosis, hoarseness
   c. Central nervous system—loss of consciousness, dilation of pupils

Treatment
1. Call EMS (through 911)
2. Administer epinephrine 0.3-0.5 mg 1:1000 SC or IM (*contraindication: severe hypertension*) or IV if dentist has ACLS training; repeat every 5-10 minutes as needed
3. Administer theophylline ethylenediamine (aminophylline) 250-500 mg IV over 10 minutes (*contraindication: hypotension*) if dentist has ACLS training
4. Dispense steroids—hydrocortisone sodium succinate (Solu-Cortef), 100 mg SC or IM or IV if dentist has ACLS training
5. Administer oxygen
6. Monitor and record vital signs
7. Perform CPR if needed (including use of Automated External Defibrillator (AED)
8. Use cricothyrotomy if needed
9. Ensure rapid transfer of patient to hospital
NOTE: Aminophylline may cause hypotension and should be given with extreme caution to patients with asthma who also are hypotensive.

Respiratory Arrest

Cause
1. Physical obstruction of airway (tongue or foreign object)
2. Drug-induced apnea

Signs and symptoms
1. Cessation of breathing
2. Cyanosis

Treatment
1. Place patient in supine position
2. Keep airway open by tilting head back and removing obstruction if possible; if not possible perform Heimlich maneuver

3. Activate EMS (911 call)
4. Ventilate patient 12 to 15 times per minute
   a. If apnea is secondary to narcotic, give 0.4 mg naloxone hydrochloride (Narcan) IV, IM, or SC and administer oxygen
   b. If apnea is secondary to sedative barbiturate or diazepam overdose, the following should be performed:
      (1) Administer oxygen or artificial respiration
      (2) Keep patient awake
      (3) Support blood pressure through position of patient, parenteral fluids, and vasopressors
      (4) Take patient to hospital if necessary

NOTE: Monitor patient carefully for the duration of action of Narcan, which may be less than that of the narcotic. No reversal agent exists for sedative and barbiturate overdose. Flumazenil is an agent that can reverse the effects of diazepam. Dentists with ACLS training may select to have this drug available.

Chest Pain

Angina Pectoris

Cause. Blood supply to the cardiac muscle is insufficient (atherosclerosis or coronary artery spasm) and precipitated by stress, anxiety, and physical activity.

Signs and symptoms
1. Substernal pain or pain referred to arms, neck, or abdomen

2. Pain lasting less than 15 minutes and possibly radiating to the left shoulder
3. Positive response to nitroglycerine
4. Patient usually has a history of the condition
   NOTE: Vital signs are normal; no hypotension, sweating, or nausea occurs.

Treatment
1. Place patient in semireclining or sitting-up position with head elevated
2. Administer nitroglycerin 0.3 mg tablet sublingual or spray amyl nitrate bud (3 tablets, 1 tablet every 5 minutes up to a total of 3 tablets)
3. Administer oxygen at 10 L/min flow
4. Put patient at rest and give reassurance
5. Monitor and record vital signs

NOTE: If any doubt exists about whether angina or myocardial infarction exists, call EMS (through 911) or transport patient to hospital emergency room. Once the nitroglycerin tablet container has been opened, the remaining tablets have a poor shelf life (30 days); a new supply should be stocked.

Myocardial Infarction

Cause. Most commonly occlusion of coronary vessels occurs. Anoxia, ischemia, and infarct are present.

Signs and symptoms
1. Crushing chest pain
   a. More severe than angina, possibly radiating to neck, shoulder, jaw

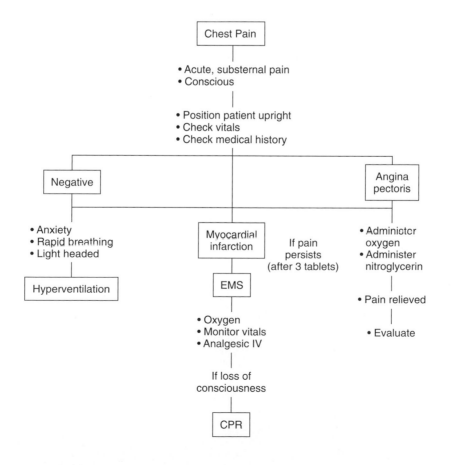

b. Longer than 15 minutes

c. Not relieved by nitroglycerin tablets

d. Squeezing or heavy feeling

2. Cyanosis, pale, or ashen appearance

3. Weakness

4. Cold sweat

5. Nausea, vomiting

6. Air hunger and fear of impending death

7. Increased, irregular pulse beat of poor quality and containing palpitations

8. Feeling of impending doom

Treatment

1. Place patient in most comfortable position

2. Administer oxygen at 10 L/min flow

3. Activate EMS (911 call)

4. Monitor and record vital signs

5. Reassure patient

NOTE: Maintain patient in most comfortable position; this may not be the supine position since the air hunger may be associated with orthopnea. Nitrous oxide-oxygen (N_2O-30%, O_2 70%), Demerol (50 mg IV), or morphine (10 mg IV) may be administered if the dentist has ACLS training. The condition may progress to cardiac arrest.

6. CPR (including use of automated external defibrillator (AED)

Other Reactions

Intraarterial Injection of Drug Into the Arm

Symptoms

1. Pain and burning sensation distal to the injection site

2. Cold and blotching hand or fingers distal to the injection site

Treatment

1. Place patient in supine position

2. Administer oxygen

3. Leave needle in place and inject 40 to 60 mg 2% lidocaine (2-3 ml), 100 mg hydrocortisone sodium succinate (Solu-Cortef) IM

4. Later, transport patient to hospital where treatment may include heparinization and brachial plexus block

Extrapyramidal Reactions

Antipsychotic drugs producing side reactions

1. Phenothiazines (Compazine, Thorazine, Phenergan, Sparine, Stelazine, Trilafon, and Mellaril)

2. Butyrophenones (Haldol and Innovar [general anesthetic])

3. Thioxanthenes (Navane and Taractan)

Signs and symptoms

1. Acute dystonic reaction (more frequent in young people, women)

   a. Rapid onset

   b. Involuntary movement of tongue, muscles of mastication, and muscles of facial expression

   c. Neck muscles affected frequently (torticollis), arms and legs less frequently

2. Akathisia (constant motion)

3. Parkinsonism

4. Tardive dyskinesia ([buccolingomasticatory triad] sucking, smacking, chewing, fly-catching movement of tongue)

Treatment

1. Position patient in semierect position

2. Administer diphenhydramine HCI (Benadryl) 25-50 mg orally, IV if dentist has ACLS training

3. Administer oxygen

4. Monitor and record patient's vital signs

5. Transfer to hospital if necessary

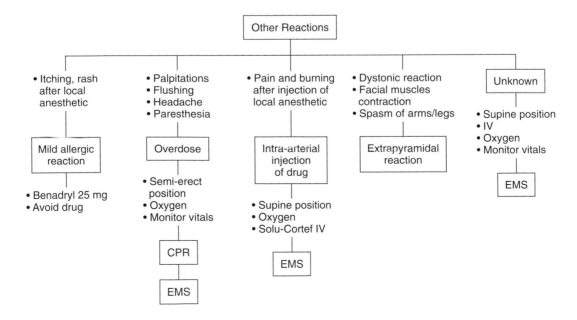

Response to Unknown Cause. When a cause for the patient's response cannot be rationally identified, a period of observation is justified.

1. Place patient in supine position
2. Activate EMS (911 call)
3. Support airway respiration and administer oxygen
4. Monitor and record vital signs
5. Start IV 5% dextrose with lactated ringers solution
6. Keep patient off all medication
7. Transfer to hospital if serious
8. Be prepared to do CPR and use the AED

Emergency Kit

Review contents, expiration date, and clarity of all drugs periodically (at least monthly). Ensure kit contains the following:

1. Oxygen setup
2. Blood pressure cuff
3. Stethoscope
4. Syringes (1, 5, 10, and 20 ml)
5. Lacrimal pocket mask
6. Disposable airway No. 2, 3, and 4
7. Butterflies No. 3, 21 gauge
8. 22-gauge needles
9. IV tubing set, Long No. 880-35
10. 250 ml dextrose, lactated ringers solution
11. Paper tape roll
12. Alcohol sponges
13. Drugs
    a. Atropine 0.4 mg ampule, 1 ml
    b. Benadryl (diphenhydramine) 50 mg tablets or 50 mg/ 1 ml syringe/22 gauge, 1-inch needle
    c. Aminophylline (theophylline ethylenediamine) 250 mg/IO ml syringe/22 gauge, 1-inch needle
    d. Hydrocortisone sodium succinate (Solu-Cortef) 100 mg/2 ml syringe/22 gauge, 1 needle
    e. Epinephrine 1:1000 1.0 ml ampule
    f. Narcan (Naloxone hydrochloride) 0.4 mg/1 ml ampule/TB syringe
    g. Amyl nitrate 0.18 ml bud
    h. Nitroglycerine 0.3 mg tabs (packed as 30/bottle)
    i. Two ammonia inhalant buds
    j. Orange juice, Glucola, glucose paste, or dextrose 50% 100 ml
    k. Sodium bicarbonate: 50 ml of 7.5% solution (44.6 mEq)—two bottles
    l. Isuprel mistometer (Isoproterenol hydrochloride)
    m. Diazepam (Valium) 5 mg/ml
    n. Lidocaine 2%, 2 ml ampules

14. Curved cricothyrotomy cannula
15. Padded tongue blade
16. Pulse oximeter/ECG (medical resources)
17. Automated external defibrillator (e.g., Heartstream FR-2, Medtronic Physio-control, Survivalink)

NOTE: Commercial medical emergency kits for dentistry are available from companies such as Banyon International and Health First.

Pediatric Drug Doses

Pediatric doses are presented on a weight basis, which can be simply multiplied. Though nomograms using weight, surface area, and other factors may be more accurate, the proposed method is suggested in an emergency situation.

1. Diphenhydramine HCL (Benadryl): 1-1.25 mg/kg up to 50 mg maximum IV, then 1-1.25 mg/kg q 6 h orally or parenteral
2. Atropine sulfate: 0.01 mg/kg up to 0.4 mg maximum IV or SC
3. Theophylline ethylenediamine (aminophylline): 3-5 mg/kg IV slowly—20 mg/min maximum
4. Epinephrine (adrenaline) 1:1,000: 0.05 mg-0.3 mg maximum SC or IM; diluted to 1:10,000 for IV administration
5. Isoproterenol sulfate 70 mEq/spray aerosol (MedVislet-Iso): 1 inhalation (70 mEq maximum
6. Amyl nitrate bud 0.3 mL: Unlikely in children—same as adult
7. Ammonia inhalants: Same as adults
8. Hydrocortisone sodium succinate. Dose: adult dose IV—50 mg, 100 mg and above
9. Sodium bicarbonate 44.6 mEq/50 ml: 1 mEq/kg IV; 0.5-1 mEq/kg q 10 mm
10. Naloxone HC1 (Narcan): No pediatric doses clearly established; 0.01 mg/kg IV (preferably) q 2-3 min for 2 to 3 doses maximum
11. 50% dextrose injection: 0.5 mg/kg or 1 ml/kg
12. Diazepam (Valium): Dose not clearly established under age 12, but in range of 0.1-0.5 mg/kg for intractable seizures

Record of Emergency Treatment				
Time Comments		BP	Pulse	Drugs

Guidelines for Infection Control in Dental Health Care Settings—2003

APPENDIX

B

Clinical Implications

The Centers for Disease Control and Prevention (CDC) believes that dental offices that follow these new recommendations will strengthen an already admirable record of safe dental practice. Patients and providers alike can be assured that oral health care can be delivered and received in a safe manner.

The recently released CDC Guidelines for Infection Control in Dental Health Care Settings—2003[1] is a major update and revision of the CDC's Recommended Infection Control Practices for Dentistry—1993.[2] As the nation's disease prevention agency, the CDC develops a broad range of guidelines intended to improve the effect and effectiveness of public health interventions and to inform key audiences, most often clinicians, public health practitioners, and the public.

Why are guidelines needed that are specific for dentistry? More than one-half million dental health care personnel (DHCP) work in the United States—approximately 168,000 dentists, 112,000 registered dental hygienists, 218,000 dental assistants,[3] and 53,000 dental laboratory technicians.[4] Most dentists are solo practitioners who work in outpatient, ambulatory care facilities. In these settings, no epidemiologists or other hospital infection control experts track possible health care–associated (i.e., nosocomial) infections or monitor and recommend safe practices. Instruments used frequently in dental practice generate spatter, mists, aerosols, or particulate matter. Unless precautions are taken, the possibility is great that patients and DHCP will be exposed to blood and other potentially pathogenic infectious material. Fortunately, by understanding certain principles of disease transmission and using infection control practices based on those principles, dental personnel can prevent disease transmission.

The CDC's first set of infection control recommendations for dentistry was published as an article in *Morbidity*

and Mortality Weekly Report, or *MMWR*, in 1986.[5] At that time, a position paper from the American Association of Public Health Dentistry commented on the state of dental infection control by noting, "Dental practitioners are virtually the only health care providers who routinely place an ungloved hand into a body cavity."[6] Reports published from 1970 through 1987 described nine clusters of patients who were believed to be infected with hepatitis B virus (HBV) through treatment by an infected DHCP.[1] However, since 1987, no transmission of HBV from dentist to patient has been reported. This good statistic possibly is the result of widespread acceptance of the hepatitis B vaccine and the adoption of universal precautions, including routine glove use. HBV seroprevalence among dentists has fallen from about 14% in 1983 to about 9% today—a proportion that is expected to decline to below that of the general population as older dentists retire (because older dentists are more likely than young dentists to be infected) (personal communication, C. Siew, PhD, American Dental Association, 2003).

In early 1988, a published report described a dentist with human immunodeficiency virus (HIV) but no admitted risk factors for HIV, which suggests the possibility of occupational transmission.[7] In addition, during the early 1990s, the health care community was shaken when six transmissions from an HIV-infected dentist to his patients were reported.[8,9] No additional reports have described HIV transmission from HIV-infected DHCP to patients, and, since the CDC began surveillance for occupationally acquired HIV, no cases of occupationally acquired HIV have been documented among DHCP.

In 1991, the U.S. Occupational Safety and Health Administration (OSHA) released the bloodborne pathogen standard that mandated certain practices for all dental offices.[10] For example, employers must provide hepatitis B vaccine for their employees, and all employees must use appropriate personal protective equipment (e.g., gloves, protective eyewear, gowns). After OSHA published its standards, the CDC published Recommended Infection Control Practices for Dentistry, 1993.[2] Those recommendations, which focused on preventing transmission of disease from bloodborne pathogens, were based primarily on health care precedent, theoretical rationale, and expert opinion. In contrast to OSHA (which is a regulatory agency), the CDC cannot mandate certain practices; it can only recommend. Nevertheless, many dental licensing boards have adopted the CDC's recommendations, or variations of them, as the infection control standard for dental practice in their states.

REFERENCES

1. Centers for Disease Control and Prevention. Guidelines for infection control in dental health-care settings—2003. MMWR Morb Mortal Wkly Rep 2003;52(No. RR-17):1-66. [Medline]

2. Centers for Disease Control and Prevention. Recommended infection control practices for dentistry, 1993. MMWR Morb Mortal Wkly Rep 1993;41(No. RR-8):1-12.

3. U.S. Census Bureau. 2001 statistical abstract of the United States: Section 12—Labor force, employment, and earnings. Available at: www.census.gov/prod/2002pubs/01statab/labor.pdf. Accessed December 2, 2003.

4. Health Resources and Services Administration. U.S. Health Work-force Personnel Factbook. Rockville, Md, Health Resources and Services Administration, 2000.

5. Centers for Disease Control and Prevention. Recommended infection control practices for dentistry. MMWR Morb Mortal Wkly Rep 1986;35:237-242. [Medline]

6. The control of transmissible disease in dental practice: A position paper of the American Association of Public Health Dentistry. J Public Health Dent 1986;46:13-22. [Medline]

7. Klein RS, Phelan JA, Freeman K, et al. Low occupational risk of human immunodeficiency virus infection among dental professionals. N Engl J Med 1988;318:86-90. [Abstract]

8. Ciesielski C, Marianos D, Ou CY, et al. Transmission of human immunodeficiency virus in a dental practice. Ann Intern Med 1992;116:798-805. [Medline]

9. U.S. Centers for Disease Control and Prevention. Epidemiologic notes and reports update: Transmission of HIV infection during invasive dental procedures—Florida. MMWR Morb Mortal Wkly Rep 1991;40;377-381. [Medline]

10. U.S. Department of Labor, Occupational Safety and Health Administration. 29 CFR Part 1910: Occupational exposure to blood-borne pathogens; needlestick and other sharps injuries; final rule. Fed Reg 2001;66:5317-5325. Available at: www.osha.gov/FedReg_osha_pdf/FED20010118A.pdf. Accessed December 2, 2003.

For more information on products and services for dental unit waterline cleaning and monitoring, visit www.ada.org, or contact the ADA Division of Science by phone at 1-800-621-8099, Extension 2878, or send an e-mail to science@ada.org.

The following updated guidelines have been modified from Kohn WG, Harte JA, et al. Guidelines for infection control in dental health care settings—2003. J Am Dent Assoc 135(1):33-47, 2004. American Dental Association.

Ten years after the 1993 recommendations, new technologies and issues have emerged; the CDC has answered thousands of questions from concerned dental providers and patients about appropriate infection control practices in dental offices. In addition, the CDC has updated or created major guidelines on specific topics such as hand hygiene, environmental infection control, *Mycobacterium tuberculosis*, disinfection and sterilization, prophylaxis after exposure to bloodborne pathogens, prevention of surgical site infection, immunization for health care workers, and infection control for health care personnel. Regulatory directives from OSHA, the U.S. Food and Drug Administration (FDA), and the U.S. Environmental Protection Agency (EPA) also affect dental practice.

This new set of CDC recommendations discusses portions of the numerous federal guidelines and regulatory mandates that are relevant to dentistry. It also consolidates previous recommendations and adds new ones specific to infection control in dental health care settings. The new dental guidelines are longer than the 1993 version, principally because they provide more background information and the scientific rationale for the recommendations.

The recommendations cover a broad range of topics and include a number of major updates and additions. Most recommendations are familiar to DHCP and already are practiced routinely. They are designed to prevent or reduce the potential for disease transmission from patient to DHCP, from DHCP to patient, and from patient to patient. The document emphasizes the use of "standard precautions" (which replaces the term "universal precautions") for the prevention of exposure to and transmission not only of bloodborne pathogens but also of other pathogens encountered in oral health care settings. Although the guidelines focus mainly on practices in outpatient, ambulatory dental health care settings, the recommended infection control practices are applicable to all settings in which dental treatment is provided.

In the recommendations, the term *DHCP* refers to all paid and unpaid personnel in dental health care who could experience occupational exposure to infectious materials, including body substances and contaminated supplies, equipment, environmental surfaces, water, or air. DHCP include dentists, dental hygienists, dental assistants, dental laboratory technicians (in-office and commercial), students and trainees, contract personnel, and other persons who are not directly involved in patient care but who could be exposed to infectious agents (such as administrative, clerical, housekeeping, maintenance, or volunteer personnel).

The guidelines have two parts. The first part provides the background and scientific evidence on which recommendations are based. More than 450 articles are referenced. From the CDC online version (www.cdc.gov/oralhealth/infectioncontrol), readers who want more information on particular topics can link to key reference documents such as the OSHA Bloodborne Pathogen Standard and other CDC infection control guidelines. The second part lists the recommendations and explains the ranking system for the level of scientific evidence for each recommendation.

Varying levels of scientific evidence support infection control practices in health care settings—and in dental settings specifically. Whenever possible, recommendations in the guidelines are based on data from well-designed scientific studies. However, only a limited number of studies have characterized the risk factors for contracting an infection in a dental office and the effectiveness of measures to prevent infection. Certain infection control practices routinely used by health care practitioners cannot be examined rigorously for ethical or logistical reasons. Because there are no scientific studies to support certain recommended practices, they are based instead on strong theoretical rationale, suggestive evidence, or the opinions of respected authorities. Those authorities base their opinions on clinical experience, descriptive studies, or committee reports. Some recommendations are derived from federal regulations. No recommendations are offered for practices for which insufficient scientific evidence exists or for which there is a lack of consensus to support their effectiveness in dental settings.

The full recommendations and ranking system follow. Reference numbers that appear in parentheses in the Recommendations section of this article relate to the first part of the full set of guidelines. Although the reference list is omitted from this article in the interest of space, reference numbers were left in the text to allow readers who copy this article to match it later with the full document.

The CDC's new guidelines for infection control in dental health care settings should provide dental practitioners with the information needed to make informed and intelligent choices when they select infection control processes, methods, and products. Although most dental practices will find that they already are carrying out most of the recommendations in the guidelines, they now will have the scientific rationale that underlies these recommendations. The practice of infection control in dentistry has made remarkable progress since the 1980s, and the CDC believes that dental offices that follow these new recommendations will strengthen an already admirable record of safe dental practice. Patients and providers alike can be assured that oral health care can be delivered and received in a safe manner.

The CDC plans to distribute these guidelines broadly to the dental community through organizational mailing lists. In addition, the guidelines will be accessible at www.cdc.gov/oralhealth. Soon, the CDC oral health website also will include a PowerPoint slide series that can be downloaded for the purpose of staff education.

Each recommendation is categorized on the basis of existing scientific data, theoretical rationale, and applicability. Rankings are based on the system used by the CDC and the Healthcare Infection Control Practices Advisory Committee (HICPAC) to categorize recommendations:

- Category IA—Strongly recommended for implementation and strongly supported by well-designed experimental, clinical, or epidemiologic studies
- Category IB—Strongly recommended for implementation and supported by experimental, clinical, or epidemiologic studies and a strong theoretical rationale
- Category IC—Required for implementation as mandated by federal or state regulations or standards. When IC is used, a second rating can be included to provide the basis of existing scientific data, theoretical rationale, and applicability. Because of state differences, readers should not assume that the absence of an IC recommendation implies the absence of any state regulations.
- Category II—Suggested for implementation and supported by suggestive clinical or epidemiologic studies or a theoretical rationale
- Unresolved Issue. No recommendation. Insufficient evidence or no consensus regarding efficacy exists.

I. PERSONNEL HEALTH ELEMENTS OF AN INFECTION CONTROL PROGRAM

A. **General Recommendations**

  1. Develop a written health program for DHCP that includes policies, procedures, and guidelines for education and training; immunizations; exposure prevention and postexposure management; medical conditions, work-related illness, and associated work restrictions; contact dermatitis and latex hypersensitivity; and maintenance of records, data management, and confidentiality (IB) (5,16-18,22).

  2. Establish referral arrangements with qualified health care professionals to ensure prompt and appropriate provision of preventive services, occupationally related medical services, and postexposure management with medical follow-up (IB, IC) (5,13,19,22).

B. **Education and Training**

  1. Provide DHCP (1) on initial employment, (2) when new tasks or procedures affect the employee's occupational exposure, and (3) at a minimum, annually, education and training regarding occupational exposure to potentially infectious agents and infection control procedures/protocols

appropriate for and specific to assigned duties (IB, IC) (5,11,13,14,16,19,22).

2. Provide educational information appropriate in content and vocabulary to the educational level, literacy, and language of DHCP (IB, IC) (5,13).

C. **Immunization Programs**

1. Develop a written comprehensive policy on immunizing DHCP, including a list of all required and recommended immunizations (IB) (5,17,18).

2. Refer DHCP to a prearranged qualified health care professional or to their own health care professional to receive all appropriate immunizations based on the latest recommendations, as well as their medical history and risk for occupational exposure (IB) (5,17).

D. **Exposure Prevention and Postexposure Management**

1. Develop a comprehensive postexposure management and medical follow-up program (IB, IC) (5,13,14,19).
   a. Include policies and procedures for prompt reporting, evaluation, counseling, treatment, and medical follow-up of occupational exposures.
   b. Establish mechanisms for referral to a qualified health care professional for medical evaluation and follow-up.
   c. Conduct a baseline tuberculin skin test (TST), preferably through a 2-step test, for all DHCP who might have contact with persons with suspected or confirmed infectious TB, regardless of the risk classification of the setting (IB) (20).

E. **Medical Conditions, Work-Related Illness, and Work Restrictions**

1. Develop and have readily available to all DHCP comprehensive written policies on work restriction and exclusion that include a statement of authority defining who can implement such policies (IB) (5,22).

2. Develop policies for work restriction and exclusion that encourage DHCP to seek appropriate preventive and curative care and report their illnesses, medical conditions, or treatments that can render them more susceptible to opportunistic infection or exposure; do not penalize DHCP with loss of wages, benefits, or job status (IB) (5,22).

3. Develop policies and procedures for evaluation, diagnosis, and management of DHCP with suspected or known occupational contact dermatitis (IB) (32).

4. Seek definitive diagnosis by a qualified health care professional for any DHCP

with suspected latex allergy to carefully determine its specific etiology and appropriate treatment, as well as work restrictions and accommodations (IB) (32).

F. **Maintenance of Records, Data Management, and Confidentiality**

1. Establish and maintain confidential medical records (e.g., immunization records, documentation of tests received as a result of occupational exposure) for all DHCP (IB, IC) (5,13).

2. Ensure that the practice complies with all applicable federal, state, and local laws regarding medical record keeping and confidentiality (IC) (13,34).

II. **PREVENTING TRANSMISSION OF BLOODBORNE PATHOGENS**

A. **HBV Vaccination**

1. Offer the HBV vaccination series to all DHCP with potential occupational exposure to blood or other potentially infectious material (IA, IC) (2,13,14,19).

2. Always follow U.S. Public Health Service/ CDC recommendations for hepatitis B vaccination, serologic testing, follow-up, and booster dosing (IA, IC) (13,14,19).

3. Test DHCP for anti-HBs 1 to 2 months after completion of the three-dose vaccination series (IA, IC) (14,19).

4. DHCP should complete a second three-dose vaccine series or be evaluated to determine if HBsAg-positive if no antibody response occurs to the primary vaccine series (IA, IC) (14,19).

5. Retest for anti-HBs at completion of the second vaccine series. If no response to the second three-dose series, nonresponders should be tested for HBsAg (IC) (14,19).

6. Counsel nonresponders to vaccination who are HBsAg negative regarding their susceptibility to HBV infection and precautions to take (IA, IC) (14,19).

7. Provide employees appropriate education regarding the risks of HBV transmission and availability of the vaccine. Employees who decline the vaccination should sign a declination form to be kept on file with the employer (IC) (13).

B. **Preventing Exposures to Blood and Other Potentially Infectious Material (OPIM)**

1. General recommendations
   a. Use standard precautions (OSHA's bloodborne pathogen standard retains the term *universal precautions*) for all patient encounters (IA,IC) (11,13,19,53).
   b. Consider sharp items (e.g., needles, scalers, burs, laboratory knives, and

wires) that are contaminated with patient blood and saliva as potentially infective, and establish engineering controls and work practices to prevent injuries (IB, IC) (6,13,113).

   c. Implement a written, comprehensive program designed to minimize and manage DHCP exposures to blood and body fluids (IB, IC) (13,14,19,97).

2. Engineering and work practice controls

   a. Identify, evaluate, and consider devices with engineered safety features at least annually and as they become available on the market (e.g., safer anesthetic syringes, blunt suture needle, retractable scalpel, or needleless IV systems) (IC) (13,97,110-112).

   b. Place used disposable syringes and needles, scalpel blades, and other sharp items in appropriate puncture-resistant containers located as close as feasible to the area in which the items are used (IA, IC) (2,7,13,19,113,115).

   c. Do not recap used needles by using both hands or any other technique that involves directing the point of a needle toward any part of the body. Do not bend, break, or remove needles before disposal (IA, IC) (2,7,8,13, 97,113).

   d. Use a one-handed scoop technique or a mechanical device designed for holding the needle cap when recapping needles (e.g., between multiple injections, before removing from a nondisposable aspirating syringe) (IA, IC) (2,7,8,13,14,113).

3. Postexposure management and prophylaxis

   a. Follow current CDC recommendations after percutaneous, mucous membrane, or nonintact skin exposure to blood or other potentially infectious material (IA, IC) (13,14,19).

III. HAND HYGIENE

  A. General Considerations

   1. Perform hand hygiene with a nonantimicrobial or antimicrobial soap and water when hands are visibly dirty or are contaminated with blood or other potentially infectious material. If hands are not visibly soiled, an alcohol-based handrub can also be used. Follow the manufacturer's instructions (IA) (123).

   2. Indications for hand hygiene include the following:

    a. When hands are visibly soiled (IA, IC)

    b. After barehanded touching of inanimate objects likely to be contaminated by blood, saliva, or respiratory secretions (IA, IC)

    c. Before and after treating each patient (IB)

    d. Before donning gloves (IB)

    e. Immediately after removing gloves (IB, IC) (7-9,11,13,113,120-123,125, 126,138).

   3. For oral surgical procedures, perform surgical hand antisepsis before donning sterile surgeon's gloves. Follow the manufacturer's instructions by using an antimicrobial soap and water, or soap and water followed by drying of hands and application of an alcohol-based surgical hand scrub product with persistent activity (IB) (121-123,127-133,137,144,145).

   4. Store liquid hand care products in disposable closed containers or closed containers that can be washed and dried before refilling. Do not add soap or lotion (i.e., top off) to a partially empty dispenser (IA) (9,120,122,149,150).

  B. Special Considerations for Hand Hygiene and Glove Usage

   1. Use hand lotions to prevent skin dryness associated with handwashing (IA) (153,154).

   2. Consider the compatibility of lotion and antiseptic products and the effects of petroleum or other oil emollients on the integrity of gloves during product selection and glove usage (IB) (2,14,122,155).

   3. Keep fingernails short with smooth, filed edges to allow thorough cleaning and to prevent glove tears (II) (122,123,156).

   4. Do not wear artificial fingernails or extenders when having direct contact with patients at high risk (e.g., those in intensive care units or operating rooms) (IA) (123,157-160).

   5. Use of artificial fingernails usually is not recommended (II) (157-160).

   6. Do not wear hand or nail jewelry if it makes donning gloves more difficult or compromises the fit and integrity of the glove (II) (123,142,143).

IV. PERSONAL PROTECTIVE EQUIPMENT (PPE)

  A. Masks, Protective Eyewear, Face Shields

   1. Wear a surgical mask and eye protection with solid side shields or a face shield to protect mucous membranes of the eyes, nose, and mouth during procedures likely to generate splashing or spattering of blood or other body fluids (IB, IC) (1,2,7,8,11,13,137).

2. Change masks between patients or during patient treatment if the mask becomes wet (IB) (2).

3. Clean with soap and water or, if visibly soiled, clean and disinfect reusable facial protective equipment (e.g., clinician and patient protective eyewear or face shields) between patients (II) (2).

B. Protective Clothing

1. Wear protective clothing such as a reusable or disposable gown, laboratory coat, or uniform that covers personal clothing and skin (e.g., forearms) likely to be soiled with blood, saliva, or OPIM (IB, IC) (7,8,11,13,137).

2. Change protective clothing if visibly soiled (134); change immediately or as soon as feasible if penetrated by blood or other potentially infectious fluids (IB, IC) (13).

3. Remove barrier protection, including gloves, mask, eyewear, and gown, before departing work area (e.g., dental patient care, instrument processing, laboratory areas) (IC) (13).

C. Gloves

1. Wear medical gloves when the potential exists for contacting blood, saliva, OPIM, or mucous membranes (IB, IC) (1,2,7,8,13).

2. Wear a new pair of medical gloves for each patient, remove them promptly after use, and wash hands immediately to avoid transfer of microorganisms to other patients or environments (IB) (1,7,8,123).

3. Remove gloves that are torn, cut, or punctured as soon as feasible, and wash hands before regloving (IB, IC) (13,210,211).

4. Do not wash surgeon's or patient examination gloves before use or wash, disinfect, or sterilize gloves for reuse (IB, IC) (13,138,177,212,213).

5. Ensure that appropriate gloves in the correct size are readily accessible (IC) (13).

6. Use appropriate gloves (e.g., puncture- and chemical-resistant utility gloves) when cleaning instruments and performing housekeeping tasks involving contact with blood or OPIM (IB, IC) (7,13,15).

7. Consult with glove manufacturers regarding the chemical compatibility of glove material and dental materials used (II).

D. Sterile Surgeon's Gloves and Double Gloving During Oral Surgical Procedures

1. Wear sterile surgeon's gloves when performing oral surgical procedures (IB) (2,8,137).

2. No recommendation is offered regarding the effectiveness of wearing two pairs of gloves to prevent disease transmission during oral surgical procedures. The majority of studies among HCP and DHCP have demonstrated a lower frequency of inner glove perforation and visible blood on the surgeon's hands when double gloves are worn; however, the effectiveness of wearing two pair of gloves in preventing disease transmission has not been demonstrated (Unresolved issue).

V. CONTACT DERMATITIS AND LATEX HYPERSENSITIVITY

A. General Recommendations

1. Educate DHCP regarding the signs, symptoms, and diagnoses of skin reactions associated with frequent hand hygiene and glove use (IB) (5,31,32).

2. Screen all patients for latex allergy (e.g., take health history) and refer for medical consultation when latex allergy is suspected (IB) (32).

3. Ensure a latex-safe environment for patients and DHCP with latex allergy (IB) (32).

4. Have emergency treatment kits with latex-free products available at all times (II) (32).

VI. STERILIZATION AND DISINFECTION OF PATIENT CARE ITEMS

A. General Recommendations

1. Use only FDA-cleared medical devices for sterilization, and follow the manufacturer's instructions for correct use (IB) (248).

2. Clean and heat sterilize critical dental instruments before each use (IA) (2,243,244,246, 249,407).

3. Clean and heat sterilize semicritical items before each use (IB) (2,249,260,407).

4. Allow packages to dry in the sterilizer before they are handled, to avoid contamination (IB) (247).

5. Use of heat-stable semicritical alternatives is encouraged (IB) (2).

6. Reprocess heat-sensitive critical and semicritical instruments by using FDA-cleared sterilant/high-level disinfectants or an FDA-cleared low-temperature sterilization method (e.g., ethylene oxide). Follow manufacturer's instructions for use of chemical sterilants/high-level disinfectants (IB) (243).

7. Single-use disposable instruments are acceptable alternatives, provided they are used only once and disposed of correctly (IB, IC) (243,383).

8. Do not use liquid chemical sterilants/ high-level disinfectants for environmental surface disinfection or as holding solutions (IB, IC) (243,245).

9. Ensure that noncritical patient care items are barrier protected or cleaned, or, if visibly soiled, cleaned and disinfected after each use with an EPA-registered hospital disinfectant with an HIV/HBV effectiveness claim (low-level disinfectant) or a tuberculocidal claim (intermediate-level disinfectant) (i.e., intermediate level if visibly contaminated with blood or OPIM) (IB) (2,243,244).

10. Inform DHCP of all OSHA guidelines for exposure to chemical agents used for disinfection and sterilization. Using this report, identify areas and tasks that have potential for exposure (IC) (15).

B. **Instrument Processing Area**

1. Designate a central processing area. Divide the instrument processing area, physically or, at a minimum, spatially, into distinct areas for (1) receiving, cleaning, and decontamination; (2) preparation and packaging; (3) sterilization; and (4) storage. Do not store instruments in an area where contaminated instruments are held or cleaned (II) (174,247,248).

2. Train DHCP to employ work practices that prevent contamination of clean areas (II).

C. **Receiving, Cleaning, and Decontaminating Work Area**

1. Minimize handling of loose contaminated instruments during transport to the instrument processing area. Use work practice controls (e.g., carry instruments in a covered container) to minimize exposure potential (II). Clean all visible blood and other contamination from dental instruments and devices before sterilization or disinfection procedures (IA) (249-252).

2. Use automated cleaning equipment (e.g., ultrasonic cleaner or washer/disinfector) to remove debris to improve cleaning effectiveness and decrease worker exposure to blood (IB) (2,253).

3. Use work practice controls that minimize contact with sharp instruments, if manual cleaning is necessary (e.g., long-handled brush) (IC) (14).

4. Wear puncture- and chemical-resistant/ heavy duty utility gloves for instrument cleaning and decontamination procedures (IB) (7).

5. Wear appropriate PPE (e.g., mask, protective eyewear and gown) when splashing or spraying is anticipated during cleaning (IC) (13).

D. **Preparation and Packaging**

1. Use an internal chemical indicator in each package. If the internal indicator cannot be seen from outside the package, also use an external indicator (II) (243,254,257).

2. Use a container system or wrapping compatible with the type of sterilization process used and that has received FDA clearance (IB) (243,247,256).

3. Before sterilization of critical and semicritical instruments, inspect instruments for cleanliness, then wrap or place them in containers designed to maintain sterility during storage (e.g., cassettes, organizing trays) (IA) (2,247,255,256).

E. **Sterilization of Unwrapped Instruments**

1. Clean and dry instruments prior to the unwrapped sterilization cycle (IB) (248).

2. Use mechanical and chemical (place an internal chemical indicator among the instruments or items to be sterilized) indicators for each unwrapped sterilization cycle (IB) (258).

3. Allow unwrapped instruments to dry and cool in the sterilizer before they are handled, to avoid contamination and thermal injury (II) (260).

4. Semicritical instruments that will be used immediately or within a short time frame can be sterilized unwrapped on a tray or in a container system, provided that the instruments are handled aseptically during removal from the sterilizer and transport to the point of use (II).

5. Critical instruments intended for immediate reuse can be sterilized unwrapped, provided that the instruments are maintained sterile during removal from the sterilizer and transport to the point of use (e.g., transported in a sterile, covered container) (IB) (258).

6. Do not sterilize implantable devices unwrapped (IB) (243,247).

7. Do not store critical instruments unwrapped (IB) (248).

F. **Sterilization Monitoring**

1. Use mechanical, chemical, and biologic monitors according to the manufacturer's instructions to ensure the effectiveness of the sterilization process (IB) (248,278, 279).

2. Monitor each load with mechanical (e.g., time, temperature, pressure) and chemical indicators (II) (243,248).

3. Place a chemical indicator on the inside of each package. If the internal indicator is not visible from the outside, also place an exterior chemical indicator on the package (II) (243,254,257).

4. Place items/packages correctly and loosely into the sterilizer, so as not to impede penetration of the sterilant (IB) (243).

5. Do not use instrument packs if mechanical or chemical indicators indicate inadequate processing (IB) (243,247,248).

6. Monitor sterilizers at least weekly by using a biologic indicator with a matching control (i.e., biologic indicator and control from the same lot number) (IB) (2,9,243,247,278,279).

7. Use a biologic indicator for every sterilizer load that contains an implantable device. Verify results before using the implantable device, whenever possible (IB) (243,248).

8. The following are recommended in the case of a positive spore test:
   a. Remove the sterilizer from service, and review sterilization procedures (e.g., work practices, use of mechanical and chemical indicators) to determine whether operator error could be responsible (II) (8)
   b. Retest the sterilizer by using biologic, mechanical, and chemical indicators after correcting any identified procedural problems (II)
   c. If the repeat spore test is negative, and mechanical and chemical indicators are within normal limits, put the sterilizer back in service (II) (9,243).

9. The following are recommended if the repeat spore test is positive:
   a. Do not use the sterilizer until it has been inspected or repaired, or the exact reason for the positive test has been determined (II) (9,243)
   b. Recall, to the extent possible, and reprocess all items processed since the last negative spore test (IB) (9,283)
   c. Before placing the sterilizer back in service, rechallenge the sterilizer with biologic indicator tests in three consecutive empty chamber sterilization cycles after the cause of sterilizer failure has been determined and corrected (II) (9,283).

10. Maintain sterilization records (i.e., mechanical, chemical, and biological) in compliance with state and local regulations (IB) (243).

G. Storage Area for Sterilized Items and Clean Dental Supplies
1. Implement practices based on date- or event-related shelf-life for the storage of wrapped, sterilized instruments and devices (IB) (243,284).
2. Even for event-related packaging, at a minimum, place the date of sterilization and, if multiple sterilizers are used in the facility, the sterilizer used on the outside of the packaging material to facilitate the retrieval of processed items in the event of a sterilization failure (IB) (243,247).
3. Examine wrapped packages of sterilized instruments before opening them, to ensure the barrier wrap has not been compromised during storage (II) (243,284).
4. Reclean, repack, and resterilize any instrument package that has been compromised (II).
5. Store sterile items and dental supplies in covered or closed cabinets, if possible (II) (285).

VII. ENVIRONMENTAL INFECTION CONTROL
A. General Recommendations
1. Follow the manufacturers' instructions for correct use of cleaning and EPA registered hospital disinfecting products (IB, IC) (243-245).
2. Do not use liquid chemical sterilants/high-level disinfectants for disinfection of environmental (clinical contact or housekeeping) surfaces (IB, IC) (243-245).
3. Use PPE, as appropriate, when cleaning and disinfecting environmental surfaces. Such equipment might include gloves (e.g., puncture- and chemical-resistant utility), protective clothing (e.g., gown, jacket, lab coat), and protective eyewear/face shield and mask (IC) (13,15).

B. Clinical Contact Surfaces
1. Use surface barriers to protect clinical contact surfaces, particularly those that are difficult to clean (e.g., switches on dental chairs), and change surface barriers between patients (II) (1,2,260,288).
2. Clean and disinfect clinical contact surfaces that are not barrier protected, by using an EPA-registered hospital low- (i.e., HIV and HBV label claims) to intermediate-level disinfectant (i.e., tuberculocidal claim). Use an intermediate-level disinfectant if visibly contaminated with blood (IB) (2,243,244).

C. Housekeeping Surfaces

1. Clean housekeeping surfaces (e.g., floors, walls, sinks) with a detergent and water or an EPA-registered hospital disinfectant/detergent on a routine basis, depending on the nature of the surface and type and degree of contamination and, as appropriate, location in the facility, and when visibly soiled (IB) (243,244).
2. Clean mops and cloths after use and allow to dry before reuse, or use single-use, disposable mopheads or cloths (II) (244).
3. Prepare fresh cleaning or EPA-registered disinfecting solutions daily and as instructed by the manufacturer (II) (243,244).
4. Clean walls, blinds, and window curtains in patient care areas when they are visibly dusty or soiled (II) (9,244).

D. Spills of Blood and Body Substances

1. Clean spills of blood or OPIM, and decontaminate surface with an EPA-registered hospital disinfectant of low (i.e., HBV and HIV label claims) to intermediate level (i.e., tuberculocidal claim), depending on the size of the spill and surface porosity (IB, IC) (13,113).

E. Carpet and Cloth Furnishings

1. Avoid using carpeting and cloth-upholstered furnishings in dental operatories, laboratories, and instrument processing areas (II) (9,293-295).

F. Regulated Medical Waste

1. General recommendations
   a. Develop a medical waste management program. Disposal of regulated medical waste must follow federal, state, and local regulations (IC) (13,301).
   b. Ensure that DHCP who handle and dispose of potentially infective wastes are trained in appropriate handling and disposal methods and informed of possible health and safety hazards (IC) (13).
2. Management of regulated medical waste in dental health care facilities
   a. Use a color-coded or labeled container that prevents leakage (e.g., biohazard bag) to contain nonsharp, regulated medical waste (IC) (13).
   b. Place sharp items (e.g., needles, scalpel blades, orthodontic bands, broken metal instruments, burs) in an appropriate sharps container (i.e., puncture resistant, color coded, and leakproof). Close container immediately before removal or replacement to prevent spillage or protrusion of contents during handling, storage, transport, or shipping (IC) (2,8,13,113,115).
   c. Pour blood, suctioned fluids, or other liquid waste into a drain connected to a sanitary sewer system, if local sewage discharge requirements are met and the state has declared this an acceptable method of disposal. Wear appropriate PPE while performing this task (IC) (7,9,13).

VIII. DENTAL UNIT WATER LINES, BIOFILM, AND WATER QUALITY

A. General Recommendations

1. Use water that meets EPA regulatory standards for drinking water (i.e., 500 CFU]/mL of heterotropic water bacteria) for routine dental treatment output water (IB, IC) (341,342).
2. Consult with the dental unit manufacturer for appropriate methods and equipment to maintain the recommended quality of dental water (II) (339).
3. Follow recommendations for monitoring water quality provided by the manufacturer of the unit or water line treatment product (II).
4. Discharge water and air for a minimum of 20-30 seconds after each patient, from any device connected to the dental water system that enters the patient's mouth (e.g., handpieces, ultrasonic scalers, air/water syringes) (II) (2,311,344).
5. Consult with the dental unit manufacturer the need for periodic maintenance of antiretraction mechanisms (IB) (2,311).

B. Boil-Water Advisories

1. The following apply while a boil-water advisory is in effect:
   a. Do not deliver water from the public water system to the patient through the dental operative unit, ultrasonic scaler, or other dental equipment that uses the public water system (IB, IC) (341,342,346,349,350).
   b. Do not use water from the public water system for dental treatment, patient rinsing, or handwashing (IC) (341,342,346,349,350).
   c. For handwashing, use antimicrobial-containing products that do not require water for use (e.g., alcohol-based handrubs). If hands are visibly contaminated, use bottled water, if available, and soap or an antiseptic towelette (IB, IC) (13,122).
2. The following apply when a boil-water advisory is cancelled:

a. Follow guidance given by the local water utility on adequate flushing of water lines. If no guidance is provided, flush dental water lines and faucets for 1 to 5 minutes before using for patient care (IC) (244,346,351,352).

b. Disinfect dental water lines as recommended by the dental unit manufacturer (II).

IX. SPECIAL CONSIDERATIONS

A. Dental Handpieces and Other Devices Attached to Air and Water Lines

1. Clean and heat sterilize handpieces and other intraoral instruments that can be removed from the air and water lines of dental units between patients (IB, IC) (2,246,275,356,357,360,407).

2. Follow the manufacturer's instructions for cleaning, lubrication, and sterilization of handpieces and other intraoral instruments that can be removed from the air and water lines of dental units (IB) (361-363).

3. Do not surface-disinfect or use liquid chemical sterilants or ethylene oxide on handpieces and other intraoral instruments that can be removed from the air and water lines of dental units (IC) (2,246,250,275).

4. Do not advise patients to close their lips tightly around the tip of the saliva ejector to evacuate oral fluids (II) (364-366).

B. Dental Radiology

1. Wear gloves when exposing radiographs and handling contaminated film packets. Use other PPE (e.g., protective eyewear, mask and gown) as appropriate if spattering of blood or other body fluids is likely (IA, IC) (11,13).

2. Use heat-tolerant or disposable intraoral devices whenever possible (e.g., film-holding and positioning devices). Clean and heat sterilize heat-tolerant devices between patients. At a minimum, use high-level disinfectant on semicritical heat-sensitive devices, according to manufacturer's instructions (IB) (243).

3. Transport and handle exposed radiographs in an aseptic manner to prevent contamination of developing equipment (II).

4. The following apply for digital radiography sensors:
   a. Use FDA-cleared barriers (IB) (243).
   b. Clean and heat-sterilize, or high-level disinfect, barrier-protected semicritical items. If the item cannot tolerate these procedures, then, at a minimum, protect with an FDA-cleared barrier, and clean and disinfect with an EPA-registered hospital disinfectant product with intermediate-level (i.e., tuberculocidal claim) activity, between patients. Consult with the manufacturer for methods of disinfection and sterilization of digital radiology sensors and for protection of associated computer hardware (IB) (243).

C. Aseptic Technique for Parenteral Medications

1. Do not administer medication from a syringe to multiple patients even if the needle on the syringe is changed (IA) (378).

2. Use single-dose vials for parenteral medications when possible (II) (376,377).

3. Do not combine the leftover contents of single-use vials for later use (IA) (376,377).

4. The following apply if multiple-dose vials are used:
   a. Clean the access diaphragm with 70% alcohol before inserting a device into the vial (IA) (380,381).
   b. Use a sterile device to access a multiple-dose vial, and avoid touching the access diaphragm. Both the needle and syringe used to access the multiple-dose vial must be sterile. Do not reuse a syringe even if the needle is changed (IA) (380,381).
   c. Keep multiple-dose vials away from the immediate patient treatment area to prevent inadvertent contamination by spray or spatter (II).
   d. Discard the multiple-dose vial if sterility is compromised (IA) (380,381).

5. Use fluid infusion and administration sets (i.e., IV bags, tubings, connections) for one patient only, and dispose of appropriately (IB) (378).

D. Single-Use (Disposable) Devices

1. Use single-use devices for one patient only, and dispose of them appropriately (IC) (383).

E. Preprocedural Mouthrinses

No recommendation is offered on using preprocedural antimicrobial mouth rinses to prevent clinical infection among DHCP or patients. Although studies have demonstrated that a preprocedural antimicrobial rinse (e.g., chlorhexidine gluconate, essential oils, povidone-iodine) can reduce the level of oral microorganisms in aerosols and spatter generated during routine dental procedures, and can decrease the number of microorganisms introduced into the patient's bloodstream during invasive dental procedures (391-399), scientific evidence is inconclusive that the use of these rinses prevents clinical infection among DHCP or patients (see discussion Special Considerations: Preprocedural Mouth Rinses) (Unresolved issue).

F. Oral Surgical Procedures

1. The following apply when performing oral surgical procedures:

   a. Perform surgical hand antisepsis by using an antimicrobial product (e.g., antimicrobial soap and water, soap and water followed by alcohol-based hand scrub with persistent activity) (IB) (127-132,137).

   b. Use sterile surgeon's gloves (IB) (2,7,121,123,137).

   c. Use sterile saline or sterile water as a coolant/irrigator when performing oral surgical procedures. Use devices specifically designed for the delivery of sterile irrigating fluids (e.g., bulb syringe, single-use disposable products, sterilizable tubing) (IB) (2,121).

G. Handling of Biopsy Specimens

1. During transport, place biopsy specimens in a sturdy, leakproof container labeled with the biohazard symbol (IC) (2,13,14).

2. If a biopsy specimen container is visibly contaminated, clean and disinfect the outside of a container, or place it in an impervious bag labeled with the biohazard symbol (IC) (2,13).

H. Handling of Extracted Teeth

1. Dispose of extracted teeth as regulated medical waste unless returned to the patient (IC) (13,14).

2. Do not dispose of extracted teeth containing amalgam in regulated medical waste intended for incineration (II).

3. Clean and place extracted teeth in a leakproof container, labeled with a biohazard symbol, and maintain hydration, for transport to educational institutions or a dental laboratory (IB, IC) (13,14).

4. Heat-sterilize teeth that do not contain amalgam, before they are used for educational purposes (IB) (403,405,406).

I. Dental Laboratory

1. Use PPE when handling items received in the laboratory, until they have been decontaminated (IA, IC) (2,7,11,13, 113).

2. Before they are handled in the laboratory, clean, disinfect and rinse all dental prostheses and prosthodontic materials (e.g., impressions, bite registrations, occlusal rims and extracted teeth) by using

an EPA-registered hospital disinfectant having at least an intermediate level of activity (i.e., tuberculocidal claim) (IB) (2,249,252,407).

3. Consult with manufacturers regarding the stability of specific materials (e.g., impression materials) relative to disinfection procedures (II).

4. Include specific information regarding disinfection techniques used (e.g., solution used and duration) when laboratory cases are sent off-site and on their return (II) (2,407,409).

5. Clean and heat sterilize heat-tolerant items used in the mouth (e.g., metal impression trays and face-bow forks) (IB) (2,407).

6. Follow manufacturers' instructions for cleaning and sterilizing or disinfecting items that become contaminated but do not normally contact the patient (e.g., burs, polishing points, rag wheels, articulators, case pans, lathes). If manufacturer instructions are not available, clean and heat sterilize heat-tolerant items, or clean and disinfect with an EPA-registered hospital disinfectant with low- (HIV/HBV effectiveness claim) to intermediate-level (i.e., tuberculocidal claim) activity, depending on the degree of contamination (II).

J. Laser/Electrosurgery Plumes/Surgical Smoke

No recommendation is offered on practices to reduce DHCP exposure to laser plumes/ surgical smoke when using lasers in dental practice. Practices to reduce HCP exposure to laser plumes/surgical smoke have been suggested, including use of (a) standard precautions (e.g., high-filtration surgical masks, possibly full face shields) (437), (b) central room suction units with in-line filters to collect particulate matter from minimal plumes, and (c) dedicated mechanical smoke exhaust systems with a high-efficiency filter to remove substantial amounts of laser plume particles. The effect of exposure (e.g., disease transmission, adverse respiratory effects) to DHCP from dental applications of lasers has not been adequately evaluated (see previous discussion, Special Considerations: Laser/ Electrosurgery Plumes or Surgical Smoke) (Unresolved issue).

K. *Mycobacterium tuberculosis*

1. General recommendations

   a. Educate all DHCP regarding the recognition of signs, symptoms, and transmission of TB (IB) (20,21).

b. Conduct a baseline tuberculin skin test (TST), preferably by using a two-step test, for all DHCP who might have contact with persons with suspected or confirmed active TB, regardless of the risk classification of the setting (IB) (20).

c. Assess each patient for a history of TB as well as symptoms suggestive of TB, and document on the medical history form (IB) (20,21).

d. Follow CDC recommendations for (1) developing, maintaining, and implementing a written TB infection control plan, (2) managing a patient with suspected or active TB, (3) completing a community risk assessment to guide employee TSTs and follow-up, and (4) managing DHCP with TB disease (IB) (2,21).

2. The following apply for patients known or suspected to have active TB:

a. Evaluate the patient away from other patients and DHCP. When not being evaluated, the patient should wear a surgical mask or be instructed to cover the mouth and nose when coughing or sneezing (IB) (20,21).

b. Defer elective dental treatment until the patient is noninfectious (IB) (20,21).

c. Refer patients requiring urgent dental treatment to a previously identified facility with TB engineering controls and a respiratory protection program (IB) (20,21).

L. Creutzfeldt-Jakob Disease and Other Prion Diseases

No recommendation is offered regarding use of special precautions, in addition to standard precautions, when treating known CJD or vCJD patients. Potential infectivity of oral tissues in CJD or vCJD patients is an unresolved issue. Scientific data indicate the risk, if any, of sporadic CJD transmission during dental and oral surgical procedures is low to nil. Until additional information exists regarding the transmissibility of CJD or vCJD during dental procedures, special precautions in addition to standard precautions might be indicated when treating known CJD or vCJD patients; a list of such precautions is provided for consideration without recommendation (see Special Considerations: Creutzfeldt-Jakob Disease and Other Prion Diseases) (Unresolved issue).

M. Program Evaluation

1. Establish routine evaluation of the infection control program, including evaluation of performance indicators, at an established frequency (II) (470-471).

HOW TO LEARN MORE

The American Dental Association (ADA) has posted on its website a "roadmap" to help guide you through the CDC guidelines and put the recommendations into practice. The roadmap will provide you with a general overview of the guidelines and the major subjects covered and provide links to existing information about them. Visit www.ada.org/prof/resources/topics/cdc/index.asp, to see what the roadmap offers.

This is an evolving document. Regular additions and updates will give you the information you need to understand and implement the new guidelines. If you have any questions, contact the ADA Division of Science at extension 2878 or at science@ada.org.

APPENDIX

C

This appendix is provided to the clinician as a guide to the management of oral lesions that may be commonly encountered in the dental practice. It is intended only as a reference and is based on correct diagnosis of the condition and background knowledge as to how the recommended therapies can be properly used. This information is also provided as a courtesy of the American Academy of Oral Medicine, which publishes a Clinician's Guide (Siegel M, Silverman S, Sollecito T. Clinician's Guide: Treatment of Common Oral Lesions. Hamilton, Ontario, Canada, BC Decker, Inc., 2006) that contains much of this same information. We, the authors (all members of the American Academy of Oral Medicine [AAOM]), acknowledge our deep appreciation for the authorization to publish this Appendix. This appendix is intended as a quick reference to the causative factors, clinical description, currently accepted therapeutic management, and patient education regarding the more common oral conditions. Some of the recommended treatments have been more thoroughly investigated than others, but all have been reported to be of clinical value.

No cure has been found for many of the oral conditions described here, but treatment modalities are available that can relieve discomfort, shorten clinical duration and frequency, and minimize recurrences.

Clinicians are reminded that an accurate diagnosis is imperative for clinical success. Every effort should be made to determine the diagnosis before treatment is initiated. Infection and malignancy must be ruled out. When signs, symptoms, and microscopic and other laboratory evidence do not support a definitive diagnosis, empiric treatment may be initiated and evaluated on a therapeutic trial basis.

Patient management should be governed by the natural history of the oral condition and whether a palliative, supportive, or curative treatment exists. A patient should be referred when his or her problems are beyond the scope of the clinical trial. Further treatment can be determined by the patient's response. However, when healing of a lesion or an expected response to treatment is not attained within an expected length of time, biopsy is recommended.

All drugs require a prescription unless they are over-the-counter (OTC) drugs. Please note that the U.S. Food and Drug Administration (FDA) has been active in recent years in allowing OTC status for drugs formerly available by prescription only. Be sure to check on dosages of newly released OTC drugs because they are usually of a different strength than those available by prescription.

SUPPORTIVE CARE

Management of oral mucosal conditions may require topical and systemic interventions. Therapy should address patient nutrition and hydration, oral discomfort, oral hygiene, management of secondary infection, and local control of the disease process. Depending on the extent, severity, and location of oral lesions, consideration should be given to obtaining a consultation from a dentist who specializes in oral medicine, oral pathology, or oral surgery. When a question arises involving a medical condition, a physician should be consulted.

Symptomatic relief of painful conditions can be provided with topical preparations such as 2% viscous lidocaine hydrochloride or 0.5% dyclonine hydrochloride. Topical anesthetic may be used as a rinse in adults but should be applied with a cotton swab in a child, so that the child does not swallow the medication. Swallowing these anesthetics is contraindicated, in part because they may interfere with the patient's gag reflex. Symptomatic relief also can be attained by mixing equal parts of diphenhydramine hydrochloride elixir and magnesium hydroxide/aluminum hydroxide. Children's formula diphenhydramine hydrochloride elixir does not contain alcohol. Sucralfate suspension also may be used before meals. The diphenhydramine mixture and the sucralfate coat the ulcerated lesions and may allow the patient to eat more comfortably.

Meticulous oral hygiene is absolutely mandatory for these patients. Mucosal lesions that contact bacterial plaque present on the dentition are more likely to become secondarily infected. Patients should be seen by the dentist or hygienist for scaling and root planing, under local anesthesia when necessary, in all cases in which oral hygiene is suboptimal. Patients must be encouraged to brush and floss their teeth after meals in a gentle yet efficient manner. This practice may be enhanced by placing a soft toothbrush under hot water to further soften the bristles. Tartar control toothpastes that contain calcium pyrophosphate should be avoided because of their caustic nature and reported involvement in circumoral dermatitis.

HERPES SIMPLEX

Infection with the herpes simplex virus produces a disease that has a primary, or acute, phase and a secondary, or recurrent, phase.

PRIMARY HERPETIC GINGIVOSTOMATITIS

Etiology

A transmissible infection with herpes simplex virus, usually type I, less commonly type II.

Clinical Description

Clear, then yellowish, vesicles develop intraorally and extraorally. These rupture within hours and form shallow, painful ulcers. Gingivae often are red, enlarged, and painful. The patient may have systemic signs and symptoms, including regional lymphadenitis, fever, and malaise. Usually, it is self-limiting and heals in 7 to 10 days.

Rationale for Treatment

Relieve symptoms, prevent secondary infection, and support general health. Supportive therapy includes forced fluids, protein, vitamin and mineral food supplements, and rest. Systemic acyclovir is effective in treating herpes in immunocompromised patients. Topical steroids should be avoided because they tend to permit spread of the viral infection on mucous membranes, particularly ocular membranes. Patients should be cautioned to avoid touching the herpetic lesions and then touching the eyes, genitals, or other body areas, because of the possibility of self-inoculation.

Topical Anesthetics and Coating Agents.

Rx (prescription).
Diphenhydramine (Benadryl) elixir 12.5 mg/5 mL
(Note: Elixir is Rx, and syrup [Benylin] is OTC),

4 oz, mixed with Kaopectate (over the counter [OTC]) 4 oz (to make a 50% mixture by volume)
Disp: 8 oz
Sig: Rinse with 1 teaspoonful every 2 hours, and spit out.

Maalox OTC can be used in place of Kaopectate. Dyclonine (Dyclone) HCl 0.5%, 1 oz, may be added to the above for greater anesthetic efficacy.

Rx.
Diphenhydramine (Benadryl) elixir 12.5 mg/5 mL
(Note: Elixir is Rx, and syrup [Benylin] is OTC)
Disp: 4-oz bottle
Sig: Rinse with 1 teaspoonful for 2 minutes every 2 hours and before each meal and spit out.
NOTE: Above Rx can be mixed with 2% viscous lidocaine or dyclonine 0.5% for additional relief.

Rx.
Lidocaine (viscous) 2.0% or 1%
Disp: 1-oz bottle
Sig: Rinse with 1 teaspoonful for 2 minutes before each meal and spit out.

Rx.
Dyclonine HCl (Dyclone) 0.5% or 1%
Disp: 1-oz bottle
Sig: Rinse with 1 teaspoonful for 2 minutes before each meal and spit out.

Systemic Antiviral Therapy. Acyclovir oral capsules may relieve and decrease the duration of symptoms.

Rx.
Acyclovir (Zovirax) capsules 200 mg
Disp: 50 (or 60) capsules
Sig: Take 1 capsule 5 times a day for 10 days (or 2 capsules 3 times a day for 10 days).
(Current FDA recommendation is that systemic acyclovir should be used to treat oral herpes only in immunocompromised patients.)

Rx.
Valacyclovir (Valtrex) caplets 500 mg
Disp: 20 caplets
Sig: Take 2 caplets twice a day for 5 days.
(Current Centers for Disease Control and Prevention [CDC] recommendation for management of genital herpes)

Systemic Antibiotics. (For secondary bacterial infection in susceptible individuals. Do not use routinely.)

Rx.
Penicillin V tablets 500 mg
Disp: 40 tablets
Sig: Take 1 tablet 4 times a day.
For patients allergic to penicillin:

Rx.
Erythromycin tablets 250 mg
Disp: 40 tablets
Sig: Take 1 tablet 4 times a day.

If nausea or stomach cramps occur, prescribe enteric-coated preparations (E-Mycin, ERYC, PCE, etc.) or a second-generation erythromycin (e.g., clarithromycin [Biaxin]).

Nutritional Supplements.
Rx.
Meritene (protein/vitamin/mineral food supplement) OTC
Disp: 1-lb can (plain vanilla, chocolate, and eggnog flavors)
Sig: Take 3 servings daily. Prepare as indicated on the label. Serve cold.

Rx.
Ensure Plus (protein/vitamin/mineral food supplement) OTC
Disp: 20 cans
Sig: Drink 3 to 5 cans in divided doses throughout the day as tolerated. Serve cold.

Analgesic.
Rx.
Acetaminophen tablets 325 mg OTC
Sig: Take 2 tablets every 4 hours as needed for pain and fever. Limit 4 g per 24 hours.
For moderate to severe pain:
Acetaminophen 300 mg with codeine 30 mg (Tylenol #3)
Sig: Take 1 or 2 tablets every 4 hours for pain (requires Drug Enforcement Agency [DEA] number).

RECURRENT (OROFACIAL) HERPES SIMPLEX

Etiology

Reactivation of the latent virus that resides in the sensory ganglion of the trigeminal nerve. Precipitating factors include fever, stress, exposure to sunlight, trauma, and hormonal alterations.

Clinical Description

Intraoral—Single or small clusters of vesicles that quickly rupture, forming painful ulcers. Lesions usually occur on the keratinized tissue of the hard palate and gingiva.
Labialis—Clusters of vesicles on the lips that rupture within hours and then crust.

Rationale for Treatment

Should be initiated as early as possible during the prodromal stage, with the objective of reducing duration and symptoms of the lesion. Oral acyclovir, given prophylactically and therapeutically, may be considered when frequent recurrent herpetic episodes interfere with daily function and nutrition.

(Current FDA recommendation is that systemic acyclovir should be used to treat oral herpes only in immunocompromised patients.)

Prevention.
Rx.
PreSun 15 sunscreen lotion (OTC)
Disp: 4 fl oz
Sig: Apply to susceptible area 1 hour before sun exposure and every hour thereafter.

Rx.
PreSun 15 lip gel (OTC)
Disp: 15 oz
Sig: Apply to lips 1 hour before sun exposure and every hour thereafter.

If recurrence on the lips usually is precipitated by exposure to sunlight, the lesion may be prevented by the application to the area of a sunscreen with a high skin protection factor (SPF 15 or higher).

Topical Antiviral Agents.
Antiviral creams and ointments are of minimal efficacy for recurrent herpes simplex. Their value may be attributable to coating of the lesion by the petrolatum vehicle, which reduces the possibility of self-inoculation. Constant or intermittent application of ice to the area for 90 minutes during the prodromal phase may result in abortion of the lesion. Cocoa butter ointment, lanolin-based lip preparations, or petrolatum (Vaseline) as an emollient may be palliative.

Rx.
Penciclovir (Denavir) topical ointment 5%
Disp: 15-g tube
Sig: Apply to the area every 2 hours during waking hours, beginning when symptoms first occur.

Rx.
Docosanol (Abbreva) cream (OTC)
Disp: 2-g tube
Sig: Dab on lesion 5 times per day during waking hours for 4 days, beginning when symptoms first occur.

Systemic Antiviral Therapy.
This is best implemented at the very onset of prodromal symptoms.

Rx.
Valacyclovir (Valtrex) caplets 500 mg
Disp: 8 caplets
Sig: Take 4 caplets at the very beginning of prodromal symptoms and 4 caplets 12 hours later.

VARICELLA ZOSTER (SHINGLES)

Etiology

Reactivation of latent herpes-varicella virus present since an original varicella infection introduced through chickenpox. Precipitating factors include thermal, inflammatory, radiologic, and mechanical trauma.

Clinical Description

Usually painful, segmental eruption of small vesicles that later rupture to form punctate or confluent ulcers. Acute zoster follows a portion of the trigeminal nerve distribution in approximately 20% of cases. It is rare in the young and more common in the elderly.

Rationale for Treatment

Promptly initiate antiviral therapy to reduce the duration and symptoms of lesions. Patients older than 60 years of age are particularly prone to postherpetic neuralgia. In the absence of specific contraindications, consideration should be given to prescribing short-term, high-dose corticosteroid prophylaxis for postherpetic neuralgia, in conjunction with oral acyclovir.

Rx.

Acyclovir (Zovirax) capsules 200 mg
Disp: 200 capsules
Sig: Take 4 capsules 5 times daily for 10 days.

Rx.

Valacyclovir (Valtrex) HCl caplets 500 mg
Disp: 42 capsules
Sig: Take 2 capsules 3 times daily for 7 days.
Use with caution in immunocompromised patients.

Rx.

Prednisone tablets 10 mg
Disp: 50 tablets
Sig: Take 6 tablets in the morning, then reduce the number by 1 on each successive day.

RECURRENT APHTHOUS STOMATITIS

Etiology

An altered local immune response is the predisposing factor. Patients with frequent recurrences should be screened for disease such as anemia, diabetes mellitus, vitamin deficiency, inflammatory bowel disease, and immunosuppression.

Precipitating factors include stress, trauma, allergies, endocrine alterations, and dietary components such as acidic foods and juices, and foods that contain gluten. Inspect the oral cavity closely for sources of trauma.

Clinical Description

Minor aphthae (canker sore), smaller than 0.6 cm— Small, shallow, painful ulceration covered by a gray membrane and surrounded by a narrow erythematous halo. They usually occur on nonkeratinized (movable) oral mucosa.

Major aphthae, greater than 0.6 cm—Large, painful ulcers. A more severe form of aphthae that may last weeks or months. They may mimic other diseases such as granulomatous or malignant lesions.

Herpetiform ulcers—Crops of small, shallow, painful ulcers. They may occur anywhere on nonkeratinized oral mucosa and resemble recurrent intraoral herpes simplex clinically but are of unknown origin.

Rationale for Treatment

Effective treatment involves barriers, amlexanox, topical or systemic corticosteroids, and immunosuppressants or combination therapy, when indicated. Treatment should be initiated as early in the course of the lesions as possible. Identification and elimination of precipitating factors may serve to minimize recurrent episodes. Medications such as mycophenolate mofetil, pentoxifylline, and thalidomide are used to treat patients with severe, persistent recurrent aphthous ulcers but should not be routinely used.

Nonsteroidal.

Rx.

Amlexanox oral paste 5%
Disp: 5-g tube
Sig: Dab on affected area 4 times a day until healed.

Rx.

Orabase Soothe-N-Seal Protective Barrier (OTC)
Disp: 1 package
Sig: Apply as per the package directions every 6 hours, when necessary.

Therapies with steroids and immunomodulating drugs are presented to inform the clinician that such modalities are available. Because of the potential for adverse effects, close collaboration with the patient's physician is recommended if these medications are prescribed. These modalities may be beyond the scope of clinical experience of general dentists, and referral to a specialist in oral medicine or to an appropriate physician may be necessary.

Topical Steroids.

Prolonged use of topical steroids (longer than 2 weeks of continuous use) may result in mucosal atrophy or secondary candidiasis, and may increase the potential for systemic absorption. It may be necessary to prescribe antifungal therapy with steroids.

Rx.

Triamcinolone acetonide (Kenalog) in Orabase 0.1%
Disp: 5-g tube
Sig: Coat the lesion with a thin film after each meal and at bedtime.

Other topical steroid preparations (cream, gel rinse, ointment) include the following:

- Ultra-Potent
  - Clobetasol propionate (Temovate) 0.05%
  - Halobetasol propionate (Ultravate) 0.05%
- Potent
  - Dexamethasone (Decadron) 0.5 mg/5 mL
- Intermediate
  - Betamethasone valerate (Valisone) 0.1%
  - Triamcinolone acetonide (Kenalog) 0.1%
- Low
  - Hydrocortisone 1%

(Mixing ointments with equal parts of Orabase B paste promotes adhesion.)

Rx.

Dexamethasone (Decadron) elixir 0.5 mg/5 mL
Disp: 100 mL
Sig: Rinse with 1 teaspoon for 2 minutes 4 times a day, and expectorate. Discontinue when lesions become asymptomatic.

Oral candidiasis may result from topical steroid therapy. The oral cavity should be monitored for emergence of fungal infection in patients who are placed on therapy. Prophylactic antifungal therapy should be initiated in patients with a history of fungal infection with previous steroid administration (see Candidiasis/Candidosis).

System Steroids and Immunosuppressants. For severe cases:

Rx.

Dexamethasone (Decadron) elixir 0.5 mg/5 mL
Disp: 320 mL
Sig:
1. For 3 days, rinse with 1 tablespoon (15 mL) 4 times a day, and swallow. Then,
2. For 3 days, rinse with 1 teaspoonful (5 mL) 4 times a day, and swallow. Then,
3. For 3 days, rinse with 1 teaspoonful (5 mL) 4 times a day, and swallow every other time. Then,
4. Rinse with 1 teaspoonful (5 mL) 4 times a day, and spit out. Discontinue medication when mouth becomes comfortable.

If mouth discomfort recurs, restart treatment at Step 3. Rinsing should be done after meals and at bedtime. Refill one time.

Rx.

Prednisone tablets 5 mg
Disp: 40 tablets
Sig: Take 5 tablets in the morning for 5 days, then 5 tablets in the morning every other day until gone.
For very severe cases:

Rx.

Prednisone tablets 10 mg
Disp: 26 tablets
Sig: Take 4 tablets in the morning for 5 days, then decrease by 1 tablet on each successive day.

Therapy with medications such as systemic steroids, immunosuppressants, and immunomodulators is presented to inform the clinician that such modalities have been reported to be effective for patients with severe, persistent, recurrent aphthous stomatitis. Medications such as azathioprine, pentoxifylline, levamisole, colchicine, dapsone, and thalidomide are used to treat patients with severe, persistent, recurrent aphthous stomatitis but should not be routinely used because of the potential for adverse effects. Close collaboration with the patient's physician is recommended when these medications are prescribed.

CHEMICAL CAUTERY

In some instances, instant cautery of the ulcer, although it is temporarily painful, diminishes overall symptoms and eliminates the ulcer.

Professionally apply the following:
Debacterol: One clinical application directly to the ulcer for 15 seconds, then rinse thoroughly.

CANDIDIASIS

Etiology

Candida albicans, a yeastlike fungus. *Candida* is an opportunistic organism that tends to proliferate with the use of broad-spectrum antibiotics, corticosteroids, medicines that reduce salivary output, and cytotoxic agents. Conditions that contribute to candidiasis include xerostomia, diabetes mellitus, poor oral hygiene, prosthetic appliances, and suppression of the immune system (i.e., acquired immunodeficiency syndrome [AIDS] or the adverse effects of some medications). It is important to determine the predisposing factors.

Clinical Description

The disease is characterized by soft, white, slightly elevated plaques that usually can be wiped away, leaving an erythematous area (pseudomembranous type). Candidiasis also may appear as generalized erythematous, sensitive areas (atrophic or erythematous type) or as confluent white areas (hypertrophic form). When the clinical diagnosis is questionable, it is advisable to culture for *C albicans* concurrent with the start of medication.

Rationale for Treatment

To reestablish a normal balance of oral flora and to improve oral hygiene. Medication should be continued for 48 hours after clinical signs have disappeared, to prevent immediate recurrence.

Topical Antifungal Agents.

Rx.

Nystatin (Mycostatin, Nilstat) oral suspension 100,000 units/mL
Disp: 60 mL

Sig: Take 2 to 5 mL 4 times a day. Rinse for 2 minutes, and swallow. Nystatin suspension has a high sugar content; therefore, good oral hygiene should be reinforced. A few drops of nystatin oral suspension can be added to the water used for soaking acrylic prostheses.

Rx.
Nystatin ointment
Disp: 15-g tube
Sig: Apply a thin coat to the inner surface of the denture and to the affected area after each meal.

Rx.
Nystatin topical powder
Disp: 15 g
Sig: Apply a thin layer under the prosthesis after each meal.

Rx (Mycostatin).
Nystatin pastilles 200,000 U
Disp: 50 pastilles
Sig: Let 1 pastille dissolve in the mouth 5 times a day.

Rx.
Nystatin vaginal suppositories 100,000 U
Disp: 40
Sig: Let suppository dissolve in the mouth 4 times a day. Do not rinse for 30 minutes.

Rx.
Clotrimazole (Mycelex) troches 10 mg
Disp: 70 troches
Sig: Let 1 troche dissolve in the mouth 5 times a day. If concern is expressed about the sugar content of nystatin and clotrimazole troches, vaginal tablets may be substituted.

Rx.
Ketoconazole (Nizoral) cream 2%
Disp: 15-g tube
Sig: Apply thin coat to inner surface of denture and affected areas after each meal.

Rx.
Clotrimazole (Gyne-Lotrimin, Mycelex-G) vaginal cream 1% (OTC)
Disp: 1 tube
Sig: Apply small dab to tissue side of denture or to infected oral mucosa 4 times a day.

Rx.
Miconazole (Monistat 7) vaginal cream 2% (OTC)
Disp: 1 tube
Sig: Apply small dab to tissue side of denture or to infected oral mucosa 4 times a day.
Systemic Antifungal Agents

NOTE: In many cases, combinations of these antifungal preparations (liquids, troches, and ointments) may be employed, depending on clinical considerations and response to therapy.

When topical therapy is not practical or is ineffective, ketoconazole (Nizoral) and fluconazole (Diflucan) are effective, well-tolerated, systemic drugs for mucocutaneous candidiasis. They should be used with caution in patients with impaired liver function (i.e., with a history of alcoholism or hepatitis). Liver function tests should be performed initially and conducted monthly when ketoconazole is prescribed for an extended period. Several drug interactions have been reported with ketoconazole.

Rx.
Ketoconazole (Nizoral) tablets 200 mg
Disp: 20 tablets
Sig: Take 1 tablet daily with a meal or with orange juice.

Rx.
Fluconazole (Diflucan) tablets 100 mg
Disp: 20 tablets
Sig: Take 2 tablets stat, then 1 tablet daily.
NOTE: Because patients are often susceptible to recurring *Candida* infection, some "burst" therapy with systemic and/or topical antifungals may be necessary, as well as ongoing maintenance therapy.

CHEILITIS AND CHEILOSIS
ANGULAR CHEILITIS AND CHEILOSIS
Etiology

Fissured lesions in the corners of the mouth are caused by a mixed infection of the microorganisms *C albicans*, staphylococci, and streptococci. Predisposing factors include local habits, drooling, a decrease in intermaxillary space, anemia, immunosuppression, and extension of oral infection.

Clinical Description

Commissures may appear wrinkled, red, fissured, cracked, or crusted.

Rationale for Treatment

Identification and correction of predisposing factors and elimination of secondary infection and inflammation

Rx.
Nystatin plus triamcinolone acetonide (Mycolog II) ointment
Disp: 15-g tube
Sig: Apply to affected area after each meal and at bedtime. Concomitant intraoral antifungal treatment may be indicated.

Rx.

Ketoconazole (Nizoral) cream 2%
Disp: 15-g tube
Sig: Apply a small dab to corners of mouth daily at
bedtime.

Rx.

Clotrimazole (Gyne-Lotrimin, Mycelex-G) vaginal
cream 1% (OTC)
Disp: 1 tube
Sig: Apply small dab to corner of mouth 4 times a
day.

Rx.

Miconazole (Monistat 7) nitrate vaginal cream 2%
(OTC)
Disp: 1 tube
Sig: Apply small dab to corner of mouth 4 times a
day.

ACTINIC CHEILITIS AND SOLAR CHEILOSIS

Etiology

Prolonged exposure to sunlight results in irreversible
degenerative changes in the vermilion of the lips, especially the everted lower lip.

Clinical Description

Normal red translucent vermilion with regular vertical
fissuring of a smooth surface is replaced by a white flat
surface that may exhibit periodic ulceration.

Rationale for Treatment

If exposure to ultraviolet light in the sun's rays is allowed
to continue, degenerative changes may progress to malignancy. Sunscreens with a high SPF (greater than 15)
should be used constantly.

Rx. Several OTC sunscreen preparations are available
(e.g., PreSun 15 lotion and lip gel). For those patients
who are allergic to para-aminobenzoic acid, non–para-
aminobenzoic acid sunscreens should be prescribed.

GEOGRAPHIC TONGUE (BENIGN MIGRATORY GLOSSITIS; ERYTHEMA MIGRANS)

Etiology

The cause is unknown. Because its histologic appearance
is similar to that of psoriasis, some have associated it with
psoriasis. This may be purely coincidental. Oral lesions
should not be associated with psoriasis if no cutaneous
signs of this disorder are evident. It also has been associated with Reiter's syndrome and atopy.

Clinical Description

Benign inflammatory condition caused by desquamation
of superficial keratin and filiform papillae. It is characterized by red, denuded, irregularly shaped patches of the
tongue dorsum and lateral borders surrounded by a raised
white-yellow border.

Rationale for Treatment

Generally, no treatment is necessary because most patients
are asymptomatic. When symptoms are present, they may
be associated with secondary infection with *C albicans* (see
Supportive Care). Topical steroids, especially when used
in combination with topical antifungal agents, are the
treatment modality of choice. Patients must be told that
this condition does not suggest a more serious disease and
is not contagious. In most cases, biopsy is not indicated
because of the pathognomonic clinical appearance.

Rx.

Nystatin-triamcinolone acetonide (Mycolog II,
Mytrex) ointment
Disp: 15-g tube
Sig: Apply to affected areas after meals and at
bedtime.

Rx.

Clotrimazole-betamethasone dipropionate
(Lotrisone) cream
Disp: 15-g tube
Sig: Apply to affected area after each meal and at
bedtime.

Rx.

Betamethasone valerate ointment 0.1%
Disp: 15-g tube
Sig: Apply to affected areas after meals and at
bedtime.

Rx.

Nystatin ointment
Disp: 15-g tube
Sig: Apply to affected areas after meals and at
bedtime.

XEROSTOMIA

Etiology

Acute or chronic reduced salivary flow may result from
drug therapy, mechanical blockage, dehydration, emotional stress, infection of the salivary glands, local surgery,
avitaminosis, diabetes, anemia, connective tissue disease,
Sjögren's syndrome, radiation therapy, and congenital
factors (e.g., ectodermal dysplasia) (see Box 26-13 in
Chapter 26).

Clinical Description

Tissues may be dry, pale, or red and atrophic. The tongue
may be devoid of papillae and may be atrophic, fissured,
and inflamed. Multiple carious lesions may be present,
especially at the gingival margin and on exposed root
surfaces.

Rationale for Treatment

Salivary stimulation or replacement therapy to keep the mouth moist, prevent caries and candidal infection, and provide palliative relief

Saliva Substitutes.

Rx.

Sodium carboxymethyl cellulose 0.5% aqueous solution (OTC)

Disp: 8 fl oz

Sig: Use as a rinse as frequently as needed.

Saliva substitutes (OTC) Oasis, MouthKote, Sage Moist Plus, Xero-Lube, MedOral, Salivart, Moi-Stir, Orex

Commercial oral moisturizing gels (OTC) Sage Mouth Moisturizer, Oral Balance

Relief from oral dryness and accompanying discomfort may be attained conservatively by sipping water frequently all day long, letting ice melt in the mouth, restricting caffeine intake, not using mouth rinses that contain alcohol, humidifying the sleeping area, and coating lips with Blistex or Vaseline.

Saliva Stimulants.
Chewing sugarless gum and sucking sugarless mints are conservative ways to temporarily stimulate salivary flow in patients with medication xerostomia or with salivary gland dysfunction. Patients should be cautioned against using products that contain sugar.

Rx.

Pilocarpine HCl solution 1 mg/mL

Disp: 100 mL

Sig: Take 1 teaspoonful 4 times a day. (Dosage should be adjusted to increase saliva while minimizing adverse effects [sweating, stomach upset].)

Rx.

Pilocarpine HCl 5-mg tablets (Salagen)

Disp: 100 tablets

Sig: Take 1 tablet 3 times a day. An extra tablet (10 mg) may be taken at bedtime.

Rx.

Cevimeline HCl (Evoxac) 30-mg tablets

Disp: 100 tablets

Sig: Take 1 tablet by mouth 3 or 4 times a day.

Rx.

Bethanechol (Urecholine) 25 mg

Disp: 21 tablets

Sig: Take 1 tablet 3 times a day.

Caries Prevention.

Rx.

Stannous fluoride gel 0.4%

Disp: 4.3 oz

Sig: Apply to the teeth daily for 5 minutes; 5 to 10 drops in a custom tray. Do not swallow the gel.

Available stannous fluoride gels include IDP Gel-Oh, Stan-Gard, Perfect Choice, Flo Gel, True Gel, Nova Gel, Omni-Gel, Control, Gel-Pro, Perfect Choice, Basic Gel, Gel-Tin, IDP Gel-Oh, Gel-Kam, Stan-Gard, Easy-Gel, and Thera-Flur.

When the taste of acidulated stannous fluoride gels is poorly tolerated, or when etching of ceramic restorations occurs, neutral pH sodium fluoride gel 1% (Thera-Flur-N) should be considered.

Rx.

Neutral NaF gel (Thera-Flur-N) 1.0% or PreviDent (Colgate) 1.1% neutral NaF

Disp: 24 mL

Sig: Place 1 drop per tooth in custom tray; apply for 5 minutes daily. Avoid rinsing or eating for 30 minutes after treatment.

FDA regulations have limited the size of bottles of fluoride because of toxicity if ingested by infants. Because most preparations do not come in childproof bottles, the sizes of topical fluoride preparations vary; 24 mL is approximately a 2-week supply for application to full dentition in custom carriers. Xerostomia provides an excellent environment for overgrowth of *C albicans*. The patient is likely to require treatment for candidiasis, along with treatment for dry mouth. In a dry oral environment, plaque control becomes more difficult. Scrupulous oral hygiene is essential.

LICHEN PLANUS

Etiology

Postulated to be a chronic mucocutaneous autoimmune disorder with a genetic predisposition that is initiated by a variety of factors, including emotional stress, hypersensitivity to drugs, dental products, or foods

Clinical Description

Lichen planus varies in clinical appearance. Oral forms of this disorder include lacy white lines that represent Wickham's striae (reticular), an erythematous form (atrophic), and an ulcerating form that is often accompanied by striae peripheral to the ulceration (ulcerative).

Lesions are commonly found on the buccal mucosa, gingiva, and tongue but may be found on the lips and palate. Lichen planus lesions are chronic and also may affect the skin.

Any refractory lesion should be considered for a biopsy, to establish a diagnosis and to rule out a malignancy.

Rationale for Treatment

To provide oral comfort if lesions are symptomatic. No known cure exists. Systemic and local relief with anti-inflammatory and immunosuppressant agents is indicated. Identification of any dietary component, dental product, or medication (lichenoid drug reaction) should be undertaken to ensure against a hypersensitivity reaction. Treatment or prevention of secondary fungal infection with a systemic antifungal agent also should be considered.

Therapies with steroids and immunomodulating drugs are presented to inform the clinician that such modalities are available. Because of the potential for adverse effects, close collaboration with the patient's physician is recommended when these medications are prescribed. These modalities may be beyond the scope of clinical experience of general dentists, and referral to a specialist in oral medicine or to an appropriate physician may be necessary.

Topical Steroids. Prolonged use of topical steroids (for a period of longer than 2 weeks of continuous use) may result in mucosal atrophy and secondary candidiasis and may increase the potential for systemic absorption. The prescribing of antifungal therapy with steroids may be necessary. Therapy with topical steroids, once the lichen planus is under control, should be tapered to alternate-day therapy or treatment given less often, depending on level of control of the disease and its tendency to recur.

Rx.

Fluocinide (Lidex) gel 0.05%
Disp: 30-g tube
Sig: Coat the lesion with a thin film after each meal and at bedtime.

Rx.

Dexamethasone (Decadron) elixir 0.5 mg/5 mL
Disp: 100 mL
Sig: Rinse with 1 teaspoonful for 2 minutes 4 times a day, and spit out. Discontinue when lesions become asymptomatic.

Other topical steroid preparations (cream, gel, ointment) include the following:
- Ultrapotent
  - Clobetasol propionate (Temovate) 0.05%
  - Halobetasol propionate (Ultravate) 0.05%
- Potent
  - Dexamethasone (Decadron) 0.5 mg/5 mL
  - Fluocinonide (Lidex) 0.05%
  - Fluticasone propionate (Cutivate) 0.05%
- Intermediate
  - Betamethasone valerate (Valisone) 0.1%
  - Alclometasone dipropionate (Aclovate) 0.05%
  - Triamcinolone acetonide (Kenalog) 0.1%
- Low
  - Hydrocortisone 1%

Oral candidiasis may result from topical steroid therapy. The oral cavity should be monitored for emergence of fungal infection in patients who are placed on therapy. Prophylactic antifungal therapy should be initiated in patients with a history of fungal infection with prior steroid administration (see Candidiasis/Candidosis).

Systemic Steroids and Immunosuppressants. For severe cases:

Rx.

Dexamethasone (Decadron) elixir 0.5 mg/5 mL
Disp: 320 mL
Sig:
1. For 3 days, rinse with 1 tablespoonful (15 mL) 4 times a day, and swallow. Then,
2. For 3 days, rinse with 1 teaspoonful (5 mL) 4 times a day, and swallow. Then,
3. For 3 days, rinse with 1 teaspoonful (5 mL) 4 times a day, and swallow every other time. Then,
4. Rinse with 1 teaspoonful (5 mL) 4 times a day, and expectorate.

Rx.

Prednisone tablets 10 mg
Disp: 26 tablets
Sig: Take 4 tablets in the morning for 5 days, then decrease by 1 tablet on each successive day.

Rx.

Prednisone tablets 5 mg
Disp: 40 tablets
Sig: Take 5 tablets in the morning for 5 days, then 5 tablets in the morning every other day until gone.

Rx.

Tacrolimus 0.03% ointment
Disp: 30-g tube
Sig: Apply to affected areas twice daily as directed.

If oral discomfort recurs, the patient should return to the clinician for reevaluation.

Many studies suggest that oral lichen planus has an intrinsic property that predisposes to malignant transformation. However, the origin is complex, and interaction between genetic factors, infectious agents, and environmental and lifestyle factors is involved in its development. Prospective studies have shown that patients with lichen planus have a slightly increased risk of developing oral squamous cell carcinoma. All patients who exhibit lichen planus intraorally, particularly those who have had the ulcerative form, should undergo periodic follow-up.

Therapy with medications such as systemic steroids, immunosuppressants, and immunomodulators is presented to inform the clinician that such modalities have been reported to be effective for patients with ulcerative lichen planus. Medications such as azathioprine, mycophenolate mofetil, tacrolimus, hydroxychloroquine sulfate, acitretin, and cyclosporin A are used to treat patients with severe, persistent, ulcerative lichen planus but should not be routinely used because of the potential for adverse effects. Close collaboration with the patient's physician is recommended when these medications are prescribed.

PEMPHIGUS AND MUCOUS MEMBRANE PEMPHIGOID

Pemphigus and mucous membrane pemphigoid are relatively uncommon lesions. These should be suspected when chronic, multiple oral ulcerations and a history of oral and skin blisters are present. Often, they occur only in the mouth. Diagnosis is based on patient history and on the histologic and immunofluorescent characteristics of a biopsy specimen of the primary lesion.

Etiology

Both are autoimmune diseases with autoantibodies against antigens that appear in different portions of the epithelium (mucosa). In pemphigus, the antigens are found within the epithelium (desmosomes), and in pemphigoid, the antigens are located at the base of the epithelium within the hemidesmosomes.

Clinical Characteristics

In pemphigus, the lesion may stay in a single location for a long time, and small, placid bullae may develop. The bullae may rupture, leaving an ulcer. Approximately 80% to 90% of patients have oral lesions. In approximately two thirds of patients, oral manifestations are the first sign of disease. All parts of the mouth may become involved. The bullae rupture almost immediately in the mouth but may stay intact for some time on the skin. One of the classic signs, Nikolsky's sign (blister formation induced by gentle rubbing of an affected mucosal site), is positive in pemphigus but is not pathognomic because it also has been found to be positive in other disorders. Because the vesicles or bullae are intraepithelial, they are often filled with clear fluid. Histologically, a cleavage (e.g., Tzanck cells, acantholytic cells) exists within the spinous layer of the epithelium.

In pemphigoid, the cleavage or split is beneath the epithelium, resulting in bullae that are usually blood filled. Mucous membrane pemphigoid is often limited to the oral cavity, but some patients have ocular lesions (e.g., symblepharon, ankyloblepharon) that must be evaluated by an ophthalmologist. Gingiva is the oral site that is most commonly involved. Pemphigoid may appear clinically as a red, nonulcerated gingival lesion.

Rationale for Treatment

Because both pemphigus and pemphigoid are autoimmune disorders, the primary treatment consists of topical or systemic steroids or other immunomodulating drugs. Custom trays may be used to localize topical steroid medications on the gingival tissues (occlusive therapy). Because they may resemble other ulcerative bullous diseases, biopsy is necessary for a definitive diagnosis. Specimens should be submitted for light microscopic, immunofluorescent, and immunologic testing. Because of the potentially serious nature of the disorder, referral to a specialist in oral medicine, dermatology, and ophthalmology must be considered. When eye lesions are present, an ophthalmologist must be consulted immediately, in an effort to prevent blindness.

Therapy with medications such as systemic steroids, immunosuppressants, and immunomodulators is presented to inform the clinician that such modalities have been reported to be effective for patients with vesiculobullous disorders such as pemphigus vulgaris and mucous membrane pemphigoid. Therapies such as dapsone, methotrexate, mycophenolate mofetil, cyclosporin A, niacinamide with tetracycline, and plasmapheresis are used to treat patients with vesiculobullous disorders such as pemphigus vulgaris and mucous membrane pemphigoid but should not be routinely used because of the potential for adverse effects. Close collaboration with the patient's physician is recommended when these medications are prescribed.

Injectable Steroids. Dexamethasone phosphate injectable, 1 ampule (4 mg/mL), may be used in the following manner. After the area is injected with lidocaine, 0.5 to 1 mL should be injected around the margins of the ulcer with a 25-gauge needle, twice a week until the ulcer heals. Therapy with systemic or injectable steroids should be coordinated with the patient's physician because of adverse effects and potential systemic complications.

ORAL ERYTHEMA MULTIFORME

Etiology

Oral erythema multiforme is believed to be an autoimmune condition that may occur at any age. Drug reactions to medications such as penicillin and sulfonamides may play a role in some cases. In a few patients who developed oral erythema multiforme, a herpetic infection occurred immediately before the onset of clinical signs.

Clinical Description

Signs of oral erythema multiforme include "blood-crusted" lips, "targetoid" or "bull's-eye" skin lesions, and a nonspecific mucosal slough. The name *multiforme* is used because its appearance may take multiple forms.

A severe form of erythema multiforme is called *Stevens-Johnson syndrome*, or *erythema multiforme major*. Erythema multiforme as a skin disease occurs most often as the result of an allergic reaction.

Rationale for Treatment

Treatment is primarily anti-inflammatory in nature. Steroids are initiated, then tapered. Because of the possible relationship of oral erythema multiforme with herpes simplex virus, suppressive antiviral therapy may be necessary before steroid therapy is initiated. Patients should be questioned carefully about a previous history of recurrent herpetic infection and prodromal symptoms that may have preceded the onset of erythema multiforme.

Dosing must be titrated to specific situations.

Steroid Therapy.

Rx.

Prednisone tablets 10 mg
Disp: 100 tablets
Sig: Take 6 tablets in the morning until lesions recede, then decrease by 1 tablet on each successive day.

Suppressive Antiviral Therapy. Renew as needed the following:

Rx.

Acyclovir (Zovirax) 400-mg capsules
Disp: 90 capsules
Sig: Take 1 tablet 3 times a day.

Rx.

Valacyclovir (Valtrex) 500-mg capsules
Disp: 30 capsules
Sig: Take 1 tablet daily.

DENTURE SORE MOUTH

Etiology

Discomfort under oral prosthetic appliances may result from combinations of candidal infection, poor denture hygiene, an occlusive syndrome, overextension, and excessive movement of the appliance. This condition may be erroneously attributed to an allergy to denture material, which is a rare occurrence. Retention and fit of the denture should be idealized, and mechanical irritation should be ruled out.

Clinical Description

The tissue covered by the appliance, especially one made of acrylic, is erythematous and smooth or granular, and the condition may be asymptomatic or associated with burning.

Rationale for Treatment

Therapy is directed toward controlling all possible origins and improving oral comfort. If therapy is ineffective, consider underlying systemic conditions such as diabetes mellitus and poor nutrition.

Treatment

1. Institute appropriate antifungal medication (see Candidiasis/Candidosis).
2. Improve oral and appliance hygiene. The patient may have to leave the appliance out for extended periods and should be instructed to leave the denture out overnight. The appliance should be soaked in a commercially available denture cleanser or soaked in a 1% sodium hypochlorite solution (1 teaspoon of sodium hypochlorite in a denture cup of water) for 15 minutes and thoroughly rinsed for at least 2 minutes under running water.
3. Reline, rebase, or construct a new appliance.
4. Apply an artificial saliva or oral lubricant gel, such as LaClede Oral Balance or Sage Gel, to the tissue contact surface of the denture, to reduce frictional trauma.

If all the above measures fail to control symptoms, biopsy or a short trial of topical steroid therapy may be used to rule out contact mucositis (an allergic reaction to denture materials). If a therapeutic trial fails to resolve the condition, a biopsy should be performed to establish the diagnosis.

BURNING MOUTH SYNDROME

Etiology

Multiple conditions have been implicated in the causation of burning mouth syndrome. Current literature favors neurogenic, vascular, and psychogenic causes. However, other conditions such as xerostomia, candidiasis, referred pain from the tongue musculature, chronic infection, reflux of gastric acid, use of medications, blood dyscrasia, nutritional deficiency, hormonal imbalance, and allergic and inflammatory disorders must be considered.

Clinical Description

Burning mouth syndrome is characterized by the absence of clinical signs.

Rationale for Treatment

To reduce discomfort by addressing possible causative factors.

Treatment

On the basis of history, physical evaluation, and specific laboratory studies, rule out all possible organic causes. Minimal blood studies should include complete blood count (CBC) and differential fasting, glucose, iron, ferritin, folic acid, B_{12}, and a thyroid profile (thyroid-stimulating hormone [TSH], triiodothyronine [T_3], and thyroxine [T_4]).

Rx.

Diphenhydramine (Children's Benadryl) elixir 12.5 mg/5 mL (OTC)
Disp: 1 bottle
Sig: Rinse with 1 teaspoon for 2 minutes before each meal, and swallow.
Children's Benadryl is alcohol free.

When burning mouth is considered psychogenic or idiopathic, a tricyclic or a benzodiazepine in low doses exhibits the properties of analgesia and sedation and are frequently successful in reducing or eliminating symptoms after several weeks or months. Dosage is adjusted according to patient reaction and clinical symptoms.

Rx.

Clonazepam (Klonopin) tablets 0.5 mg
Disp: 100 tablets

Sig: Take 1 tablet 3 times a day, then adjust dose after 3-day intervals.

This therapy is probably best managed at this time by an appropriate specialist or by the patient's physician.

Rx.

Amitriptyline (Elavil) tablets 25 mg
Disp: 50 tablets
Sig: Take 1 tablet at bedtime for 1 week, then 2 tablets at bedtime. Increase to 3 tablets at bedtime after 2 weeks, and maintain at that dosage or titrate as appropriate.

Rx.

Chlordiazepoxide (Librium) tablets 5 mg
Disp: 50 tablets
Sig: Take 1 or 2 tablets 3 times a day.

Rx.

Alprazolam (Xanax) tablets 0.25 mg
Disp: 50 tablets
Sig: Take 1 tablet 3 times a day.

Rx.

Diazepam (Valium) tablets 2 mg
Disp: 50 tablets
Sig: Take 1 or 2 tablets.

Dosage should be adjusted according to the patient's response. Anticipated adverse effects are dry mouth and morning drowsiness. The rationale for the use of tricyclic antidepressant medications and other psychotropic drugs should be thoroughly explained to the patient, and the patient's physician should be made aware of the treatment. These medications have a potential for addiction and dependence.

Rx.

Tabasco sauce (Capsaicin) (OTC)
Disp: 1 bottle
Sig: Place 1 part Tabasco sauce in 2 to 4 parts water. Rinse for 1 minute 4 times a day, and expectorate.

Rx.

Capsaicin (Zostrix) cream 0.025% (OTC)
Disp: 1 tube
Sig: Apply sparingly to affected site(s) 4 times a day. Wash hands after each application, and do not use near the eyes.

Topical capsaicin may serve to improve the burning sensation in some individuals. As with topical capsaicin, an increase in discomfort for a 2- to 3-week period should be anticipated.

CHAPPED OR CRACKED LIPS

Etiology

Alternate wetting and drying, resulting in inflammation and possible secondary infection.

Clinical Description

The surface of the vermilion is rough and peeling and may be ulcerated with crusting. Normal vertical fissuring may be lost.

Rationale for Treatment

An interrupted and chronically inflamed surface invites secondary infection. An anti-inflammatory agent in a petrolatum or adhesive base will interrupt the irritating factors and allow healing.

Rx.

Betamethasone valerate (Valisone) ointment 0.1%
Disp: 15-g tube
Sig: Apply to the lips after each meal and at bedtime.

Prolonged use of corticosteroids can result in thinning of the tissue. Their use should be closely monitored.

For maintenance, frequent application of lip care products (e.g., Blistex, Chapstick, Vaseline, cocoa butter) should be suggested.

If lesions do not resolve with treatment, consider biopsy to rule out dysplasia or malignancy.

GINGIVAL ENLARGEMENT

Etiology

Phenytoin sodium (Dilantin), calcium channel blocking agents (nifedipine and others), and cyclosporine are drugs that are known to predispose some patients to gingival enlargement. Blood dyscrasias and hereditary fibromatosis should be ruled out by history and indicated laboratory tests.

Clinical Description

Gingival tissues, especially in the anterior region, are dense, resilient, insensitive, and enlarged but essentially of normal color.

Rationale for Treatment

Local factors, such as plaque and calculus accumulation, contribute to secondary inflammation and the hyperplastic process. This further interferes with plaque control. Specific drugs tend to deplete serum folic acid levels; this results in compromised tissue integrity. Folic acid and drug serum levels should be determined every 6 months. This assessment should be coordinated with the patient's physician.

Treatment

Treatment consists of (1) meticulous plaque control, (2) gingivoplasty when indicated, and (3) folic acid oral rinse.

Rx.

Folic acid oral rinse 1 mg/mL
Disp: 16 oz
Sig: Rinse with 1 teaspoonful for 2 minutes 2 times a day, and spit out.

Rx.

Chlorhexidine gluconate (Peridex) 0.12%

Disp: 16 oz

Sig: Rinse with ½ oz 2 times a day for 30 seconds, and spit out.

TASTE DISORDERS

Etiology

Taste acuity may be affected by neurologic and physiologic changes and drugs. Diagnostic procedures should first rule out a neurologic deficiency, an olfactory deficit, and systemic influences such as malnutrition, metabolic disturbances, drugs, chemical and physical trauma, and radiation sequelae. Blood tests for trace elements should be conducted to identify any deficiencies.

Rationale for Treatment

A reduction in salivary flow may concentrate electrolytes in the saliva, resulting in a salty or metallic taste. (See Treatment for Xerostomia.) A deficiency of zinc has been associated with a loss of taste (and smell) sensation.

For zinc replacement (in patients with proven zinc deficiency):

Rx.

Orazinc capsules 220 mg (OTC)

Disp: 100 capsules

Sig: Take 1 capsule with milk 3 times a day for at least 1 month.

Rx.

Z-Bec tablets (OTC)

Disp: 60 tablets

Sig: Take 1 tablet daily with food or after meals.

MANAGEMENT OF PATIENTS RECEIVING ANTINEOPLASTIC AGENTS AND RADIATION THERAPY

Etiology

Cancer chemotherapy and radiation to the head and neck tend to reduce the volume and alter the character of the saliva. The balance of the oral flora is disrupted, allowing overgrowth of opportunistic organisms (e.g., *C albicans*). Also, anticancer therapy damages fast-growing tissues, especially in the oral mucosa.

Clinical Description

The oral mucosa becomes red and inflamed. The saliva is viscous or absent.

Rationale for Treatment

Treatment of these patients is symptomatic and supportive. Patient education, frequent monitoring, and close cooperation with the patient's physician are important. Oral discomfort may be relieved by topical anesthetics such as diphenhydramine elixir (Benadryl) and dyclonine (Dyclone). Artificial salivas (e.g., Sage Moist Plus, Moi-Stir, Salivart, Xero-Lube) reduce oral dryness. Mouth moisturizing gels (e.g., Sage Mouth Moisturizer, OralBalance Gel) also may be helpful. Nystatin and clotrimazole preparations control fungal overgrowth. Chlorhexidine rinses help control plaque and candidiasis. Fluorides are applied for caries control. A patient information sheet on this topic (Box) can be reproduced and given to the patient.

Mouth Rinses.

Rx.

Alkaline saline (salt/bicarbonate) mouth rinse (Mix ½ teaspoonful each of salt and of baking soda in a glass of water.)

Sig: Rinse with copious amounts 4 times a day.

Commercially available as Sage Salt and Soda Rinse.

Gingivitis Control.

Rx.

Chlorhexidine gluconate mouthwash (Peridex) 0.12%

Disp: 32 oz

Sig: Rinse with ½ oz 2 times a day for 30 seconds, and spit out. Avoid rinsing or eating for 30 minutes after treatment. (Rinse after breakfast and at bedtime.)

In xerostomic patients, chlorhexidine (Peridex) should be used concurrently with an artificial saliva to provide the needed protein binding agent for efficacy and substantivity.

Caries Control. (See Xerostomia.)

Rx.

Neutral NaF gel (Thera-Flur-N) 1.0%

Disp: 24 mL

Sig: Place 1 drop per tooth in the custom tray; apply for 5 minutes daily. Avoid rinsing or eating for 30 minutes after treatment.

Topical Anesthetics.

Rx.

Diphenhydramine (Benadryl) elixir 12.5 mg/5 mL (Note: Elixir is Rx, and syrup [Benylin] is OTC) 4 oz mixed with Kaopectate (OTC) 4 oz (to make a 50% mixture by volume)

Disp: 8 oz

Sig: Rinse with 1 teaspoonful every 2 hours, and spit out.

Maalox (OTC) can be used in place of Kaopectate. Dyclonine (Dyclone) HCl 0.5% 1 oz may be added to the above for greater anesthetic efficacy.

Rx.

Diphenhydramine (Benadryl) elixir 12.5 mg/5 mL (Note: Elixir is Rx, and syrup [Benylin] is OTC.)

Disp: 4-oz bottle

Sig: Rinse with 1 teaspoonful for 2 minutes before each meal, and spit out.

Rx.
Dyclonine HCl (Dyclone) 0.5% or 1%
Disp: 1-oz bottle
Sig: Rinse with 1 teaspoonful for 2 minutes before each meal, and spit out.

Antifungals. (See Candidiasis.)
Rx.
Clotrimazole (Mycelex) troches 10 mg
Disp: 70 troches
Sig: Let 1 troche dissolve in the mouth 5 times a day.

Rx.
Nystatin pastilles 200,000 U
Disp: 50 pastilles
Sig: Let 1 pastille dissolve in the mouth 5 times a day.
(See Candidiasis for additional antifungal therapy.)

KEY POINTS TO REMEMBER

- When topical anesthetics are used, patients should be warned about a reduced gag reflex and the need for caution while eating and drinking to avoid possible airway compromise. Allergies are rare but may occur.

Patient Information Sheet

The oral regimen for patients receiving chemotherapy and radiotherapy is outlined earlier in this chapter. Following are general guidelines to be individualized by your doctor. Follow your doctor's advice, or discuss any questions with your doctor if these guidelines differ from what you've been told or have heard.

A. RINSES
1. Rinse with warm, dilute solution of sodium bicarbonate (baking soda) or salt and bicarbonate every 2 hours to bathe the tissues and control oral acidity. Take 2 teaspoonfuls of bicarbonate (or 1 teaspoonful of table salt plus 1 teaspoonful of bicarbonate) per quart of water.
2. If you are experiencing pain, rinse with 1 teaspoonful of elixir of Benadryl before each meal. Be careful when eating while your mouth is numb to avoid choking.
3. If your mouth is dry, sip cool water frequently (every 10 minutes) all day long. Allowing ice chips to melt in the mouth is comforting. Artificial salivas (e.g., Moi-Stir, Salivart, Xero-Lube, Orex) can be used as frequently as needed to make the mouth moist and "slick." Keep the lips lubricated with petrolatum or a lanolin-containing lip preparation. Commercial mouth rinses with alcohol and coffee, tea, and colas should be avoided as they tend to dry the mouth.
4. If an oral yeast infection develops, antifungal medications can be prescribed.
   a. Nystatin pastille,* let 1 dissolve in the mouth 5 times a day, or
   b. Let a 10-mg clotrimazole (Mycelex)* troche dissolve in the mouth 5 times a day.

B. CARE OF TEETH AND GUMS
1. Floss your teeth after each meal. Be careful not to cut the gums.

2. Brush your teeth after each meal. Use a soft even-bristle brush and a bland toothpaste containing fluoride (e.g., Aim, Crest, Colgate). Brushing with a sodium bicarbonate/water paste is also helpful. Arm & Hammer Dental Care toothpaste and tooth powder are bicarbonate based. If a toothbrush is too irritating, cotton-tipped swabs (Q-Tips) or foam sticks (Toothettes) can provide some mechanical cleaning.
3. A pulsating water device (e.g., Water-Pik) will remove loose debris. Use warm water with a half-teaspoonful of salt and baking soda and low pressure to prevent damage to tissue.
4. Have custom, flexible vinyl trays made by your dentist for use in self-applying fluoride gel to the teeth for 5 minutes once a day after brushing.
5. Rinse with an antiplaque solution (Peridex) (if prescribed by your dentist) 2 or 3 times a day when you cannot follow other oral hygiene procedures.
6. Follow any alternative oral hygiene instructions prescribed by your dentist.

C. NUTRITION
Adequate intake of nutrition and fluid is very important for oral and general health. Use diet supplements (e.g., Carnation Instant Breakfast, Meritene, Ensure). If your mouth is sore, a blender may be used to soften food.

D. MAINTENANCE
Have your oral health status evaluated at regularly scheduled intervals by your dentist.

E. SUPPORTIVE
A humidifier in the sleeping area will alleviate or reduce nighttime oral dryness.

*Drugs that must be prescribed by your dentist or physician. The above regimen is also applicable to patients with acquired immunodeficiency syndrome (AIDS).

- In immunocompromised patients, herpes simplex virus lesions can occur on any mucosal surface and may have an atypical appearance. They may resemble major aphthae and allergic responses.
- Mixing ointments with equal parts of Orabase promotes adhesion.
- Therapy with systemic steroids and immunosuppressants is presented to inform the clinician that such modalities are available. Because of the potential for adverse effects, close collaboration with the patient's physician is recommended when these medications are prescribed.
- Although some consultants disagree with the intraoral use of vaginal creams, the efficacy of these creams has been observed clinically in selected cases in which other topical antifungal agents have failed.
- Generic carboxymethyl cellulose solutions may be prepared by a pharmacist. These cholinergics should be prescribed in consultation with a physician because of the potential for significant adverse effects.
- The rationale for use of tricyclic antidepressant medications and other psychotropic drugs should be thoroughly explained to patients, and their physician also should be made aware of the treatment. These medications have a potential for addiction and dependency.
- When testing for serum folate level, it is judicious to also check the vitamin B_{12} level because a B_{12} deficiency can be masked by the patient's use of folic acid supplement. The phenytoin level also should be assessed for future reference.

SUGGESTED READINGS

Boger J, Araujo O, Flowers F. Sunscreens: Efficacy, use and misuse. South Med J 1984;77:1421-1427.

Brooke RI, Sapp JP. Herpetiform ulceration. Oral Surg Oral Med Oral Pathol 1976;42:182-188.

Brown RS, Bottomley WK. Combination immunosuppressant and topical steroid therapy for treatment of recurrent major aphthae. Oral Surg Oral Med Oral Pathol 1990;69:42-44.

Browning S, Hislop S, Scully C, Shirlaw P. The association between burning mouth syndrome and psychosocial disorders. Oral Surg Oral Med Oral Pathol 1987;64:171-174.

Burns RA, Davis WJ. Recurrent aphthous stomatitis. Am Fam Physician 1988;32:99-104.

Bystryn JC. Adjuvant therapy of pemphigus. Arch Dermatol 1984;120:941-951.

Dilley D, Blozis G. Common oral lesions and oral manifestations of systemic illnesses and therapies. Pediatr Clin North Am 1982;29:585-611.

Drew HJ, Vogel RI, Molofsky W, et al. Effect of folate on phenytoin hyperplasia. J Clin Periodontol 1987;14:350-356.

Duxbury AJ, Hayes NF, Thakkar NS. Clinical trial of a mucin-containing artificial saliva, IRCS Med Sci 1985;13:1197-1198.

Fardal O, Turnbull RS. A review of the literature on use of chlorhexidine in dentistry. J Am Dent Assoc 1986;112:863-869.

Feinmann C. Pain relief by antidepressants: Possible modes of action. Pain 1985;23:1-8.

Fenske NA, Greenberg SS. Solar-induced skin changes. Am Fam Physician 1982;25:109-117.

Fox PC. Systemic therapy of salivary gland hypofunction. J Dent Res 1987;66:689-692 (special issue).

Gabriel SA, Jenson AB, Hartmann D, Bottomley WK. Lichen planus: Possible mechanisms of pathogenesis. J Oral Med 1985;40:56-59.

Gorsku M, Silverman S, Chinn H. Clinical characteristics and management outcome in the burning mouth syndrome. Oral Surg Oral Med Oral Pathol 1991;72:192-195.

Gorsline J, Bradlow HL, Sherman MR. Triamcinolone acetonide 21-oic acid methyl ester: A potent local anti-inflammatory steroid without detectable systemic effects. Endocrinology 1985;116:263-273.

Greenberg MS. Oral herpes simplex infections in immunosuppressed patients. Compendium 1988;9(suppl):289-291.

Grushka M. Clinical features of burning mouth syndrome. Oral Surg Oral Med Oral Pathol 1987;63:30-36.

Hay KD, Reade PC. The use of an elimination diet in the treatment of recurrent aphthous ulceration of the oral cavity. Oral Surg Oral Med Oral Pathol 1984;57:504-507.

Holst E. Natamycin and nystatin for treatment of oral candidiasis during and after radiotherapy. J Prosthet Dent 1984;51:226-231.

Huff JC, Bean B, Balfour HH Jr, et al. Therapy of herpes zoster with oral acyclovir. Am J Med 1988;85:85-89.

Hughes WT, Bartley DL, Patterson GG, Tufenkeji H. Ketoconazole and candidiasis: A controlled study. J Infect Dis 1983;147:1060-1063.

Katz S. The use of fluoride and chlorhexidine for the prevention of radiation caries. J Am Dent Assoc 1982;104:164-169.

Lamey PJ, Hammond A, Allam BF, McIntosh WB. Vitamin status of patients with burning mouth syndrome and the response to replacement therapy. Br Dent J 1986;160:81-84.

Lang NP, Brecx MC. Chlorhexidine digluconate—An agent for chemical plaque control and prevention of gingival inflammation. J Periodont Res 1986;43(suppl):74-89.

Lever WF, Schaumburg-Lever G. Treatment of pemphigus vulgaris: Results obtained in 84 patients between 1961 and 1982. Arch Dermatol 1984;120:44-47.

Lozada F, Silverman S Jr, Migliorati C. Adverse side effects associated with prednisone in the treatment of patients with oral inflammatory ulcerative diseases. J Am Dent Assoc 1984;109:269-270.

Lucatorto FM, Franker C, Hardy WD, Chafey S. Treatment of refractory oral candidiasis with fluconazole: A case report. Oral Surg Oral Med Oral Pathol 1991;71:42-44.

Lundeen RC, Langlais RP, Terezhalmy GT. Sunscreen protection for lip mucosa: A review and update. J Am Dent Assoc 1985;111:617-621.

O'Neil T, Figures K. The effects of chlorhexidine and mechanical methods of plaque control on the recurrence of gingival hyperplasia in young patients taking phenytoin. Br Dent J 1982;152:130-133.

Owens NJ, Nightingale CH, Schweizer RT, et al. Prophylaxis of oral candidiasis with clotrimazole troches. Arch Intern Med 1984;144:290-293.

Poland JM. The spectrum of HSV-1 infections in nonimmunosuppressed patients. Compendium 1988;9(suppl):310-312.

Porter SR, Sculy C, Flint S. Hematologic status in recurrent aphthous stomatitis compared with other oral disease. Oral Surg Oral Med Oral Pathol 1988;66:41-44.

Raborn GW, McGaw WT, Grace M, et al. Oral acyclovir and herpes labialis: A randomized, double-blind, placebo-controlled study. J Am Dent Assoc 1987;11:38-42.

Rhodus NL, Liljemark W, Bloomquist C, Bereuter J. *Candia albicans* levels in patients with Sjögren's syndrome before and after long-term use of pilocarpine hydrochloride. Quintessence Int 1998;29:705-710.

Rhodus NL, Schuh MJ. The effects of pilocarpine on salivary flow in patients with Sjögren's syndrome. Oral Surg Oral Med Oral Pathol 1991;72:545-549.

Rowe NJ. Diagnosis and treatment of herpes simplex virus disease. Compendium 1988;9(suppl):292-295.

Schiffman SS. Taste and smell in disease (pts a and b). N Engl J Med 1983;308:1275-1279.

Scully C, Mason DK. Therapeutic measures in oral medicine. In Jones JH, Mason DK (eds). Oral Manifestations of Systemic Disease. London, Saunders, 1980.

Sharav Y, Singer E, Schmidt E, et al. The analgesic effect of amitriptyline on chronic facial pain. Pain 1987;31:199-207.

Silverman S Jr, Gorsky M, Lozada-Nur F, Giannotti K. A prospective of findings and management in 214 patients with oral lichen planus. Oral Surg Oral Med Oral Pathol 1991;72:665-670.

Silverman S Jr, Gorsky M, Lozada-Nur F, Liu A. Oral mucous membrane pemphigoid: A study of sixty-five patients. Oral Surg Oral Med Oral Pathol 1986;61:233-237.

Sonis ST, Sonis AL, Lieberman A. Oral complications in patients receiving treatment for malignancies other than of the head and neck. JAMA 1978;97:468-471.

Straus SE. Herpes simplex virus infection: Biology, treatment, and prevention. Ann Intern Med 1985;103:404-419.

Thompson PJ, Wingfield HJ, Cosgrove RF, et al. Assessment of oral candidiasis in patients with respiratory disease and efficacy of a new nystatin formulation. Br Med J 1986;292:699-700.

Vincent SD, Fotos PG, Baker KA, Williams TP. Oral lichen planus: The clinical, historical and therapeutic features of 100 cases. Oral Surg Oral Med Oral Pathol 1990;70:165-171.

Wood MJ, Ogan PH, McKendrick MW, et al. Efficacy of oral acyclovir treatment of acute herpes zoster. Am J Med 1988;85:79-83.

Wright WE, Haller JM, Harlow SA, Pizzo PA. An oral disease prevention program for patients receiving radiation and chemotherapy. J Am Dent Assoc 1985;110:43-47.

Note: The treatment protocols included herein were adapted with permission from Siegel MA, Silverman S, Sollecito TP (eds). Clinician's Guide to Treatment of Common Oral Conditions, 5th ed. Baltimore, American Academy of Oral Medicine (AAOM), 2001, and were provided as a courtesy of the American Academy of Oral Medicine, which publishes a Clinician's Guide (Siegel M, Silverman S, Sollecito T. Clinician's Guide: Treatment of Common Oral Lesions. Hamilton, Ontario, Canada, BC Decker, Inc., 2006). This Guide contains much of this same information. We, the authors (all members of the AAOM), acknowledge our deep appreciation for the authorization to publish this Appendix. Some portions of that text are reprinted here with permission of the AAOM. For further information, or to purchase a copy of the Clinician's Guide to Treatment of Common Oral Conditions, contact:

Jane Kantor, CMP
American Academy of Oral Medicine
P.O. Box 2016
Edmonds, Washington 98020
Phone: 425.778.6162
Fax: 425.771.9588
www.aaom.com
www.jkantor@aaom.com

Drug Interactions of Significance to Dentistry

APPENDIX D

TABLE D-1

Dental Drug	Interacting Drug	Medical Condition/Situation	Effect
ANTIBIOTICS			
Antibiotics	Oral contraceptives (BCP)	Contraception	Decreased effectiveness of oral contraceptives has been suggested for several antibiotic classes because of the potential for lowering plasma levels of the contraceptive drug. However, most well-designed studies do not show any reduction in estrogen serum levels in patients taking antibiotics (except rifampin). **RECOMMENDATION: Okay to use dental antibiotics.** Provide advice to patient as to the potential risk and for consideration of additional contraceptive measures.
Beta lactams (penicillins, cephalosporins)	Allopurinol (Lopurin, Zyloprim)	Gout	Incidence of minor allergic reactions to ampicillin is increased. Other penicillins have not been implicated. **RECOMMENDATION: Avoid ampicillin.**
	Beta blockers (e.g., Tenormin, Lopressor, Inderal, Corgard)	Hypertension	Serum levels of atenolol are reduced after prolonged use of ampicillin. Anaphylactic reactions to penicillins or other drugs may be more severe in patients taking beta blockers because of increased mediator release from mast cells. **RECOMMENDATION: Use ampicillin cautiously, advise patient of potential reaction.**
	Tetracyclines and other bacteriostatic antibiotics	Infection, acne, or periodontal disease	Effectiveness of penicillins and cephalosporins may be reduced by bacteriostatic agents. **RECOMMENDATION: Avoid interaction.**
Tetracyclines Fluoroquinolones	Antacids	Dyspepsia, gastroesophageal reflux, peptic ulcer	Antacids, dairy products, and other agents containing divalent (calcium, iron) and trivalent cations will chelate these antibiotics and limit their absorption. Doxycycline is least influenced by this interaction. **RECOMMENDATION: Avoid interaction.**

TABLE D-1
cont'd

Dental Drug	Interacting Drug	Medical Condition/Situation	Effect
	Insulin	Diabetes mellitus	Doxycycline and oxytetracycline have been documented as enhancing the hypoglycemic effects of exogenously administered insulin. **RECOMMENDATION: Select a different antibiotic, or increase carbohydrate intake.**
Doxycycline	Methotrexate	Immunosuppression	In patients taking high-dose methotrexate, interaction can lead to increased methotrexate concentrations, making toxicity likely. **RECOMMENDATION: Select different antibiotic.**
Metronidazole	Ethanol	Alcohol use or abuse	Severe disulfiram-like reactions are well documented. **RECOMMENDATION: Avoid interaction.**
	Lithium	Manic depression	Inhibits renal excretion of lithium, leading to elevated/toxic levels of lithium. Lithium toxicity produces confusion, ataxia, and kidney damage. **RECOMMENDATION: Avoid interaction.**
Antibiotics/ Anti-fungals metabolized by CYP3A4 and CYP1A2 (e.g., macrolide antibiotics [erythromycin, clarithromycin], and antifungals [ketoconazole, itraconazole])	Benzodiazepines	Anxiety	Delayed metabolism of benzodiazepine, increasing the pharmacologic effects, can result in excessive sedation and irrational behavior. **RECOMMENDATION: Reduce dose of benzodiazepine.**
	Buspirone	Depression	Delayed metabolism of buspirone, increasing pharmacologic effect. **RECOMMENDATION: Avoid interaction.**
	Carbamazepine (Tegretol)	Seizure disorder	Increased blood levels of carbamazepine, leading to toxicity; symptoms include drowsiness, dizziness, nausea, headache, and blurred vision. Hospitalization has been required. **RECOMMENDATION: Avoid interaction.**
	Cisapride	Gastroesophageal reflux	Delayed metabolism of cisapride, increasing the pharmacologic effects and risk for cardiac arrhythmia and sudden death. **RECOMMENDATION: Avoid interaction.**
	Cyclosporine	Organ transplant	Enhanced immunosuppression and nephrotoxicity. **RECOMMENDATION: Avoid interaction.**
	Disopyramide, Quinidine	Cardiac arrhythmias	Inhibits CYP3A4 metabolism, resulting in large increases in antiarrhythmia drug that can lead to arrhythmias. **RECOMMENDATION: Avoid interaction.**
	Lovastatin, pravastatin, simastatin, and other statins	Hyperlipidemia	Muscle (eosinophilia) myalgia and rhabdomyolysis (muscle breakdown and pain) and acute renal failure. **RECOMMENDATION: Avoid interaction.**
	Prednisone, methylprednisolone	Autoimmune disorders, organ transplant	Increased risk of Cushing's syndrome and immunosuppression **RECOMMENDATION: Monitor patient, and shorten duration of antibiotic administration if possible.**

TABLE D-1
cont'd

Dental Drug	Interacting Drug	Medical Condition/Situation	Effect
	Theophylline (Theodur)	Asthma	Erythromycins inhibit the metabolism of theophylline, leading to toxic serum levels (symptoms of toxicity: headache, nausea, vomiting, confusion, thirst, cardiac arrhythmias, and convulsions). Conversely, theophylline reduces serum levels of erythromycin. **RECOMMENDATION: Avoid prescribing erythromycin.**
Antibiotics (especially erythromycin and tetracycline)	Digoxin (Lanoxin)	Congestive heart failure	Alters gastrointestinal flora and retards metabolism of digoxin in roughly 10% of patients, resulting in dangerously high digoxin serum levels that may persist for several weeks after discontinuation of antibiotic. Strongest documentation has been acquired for erythromycin and tetracycline. Patients should be cautioned to report any signs of digitalis toxicity (salivation, visual disturbances, and arrhythmias) during antibiotic therapy. **RECOMMENDATION: Safe in 90%, should have digoxin levels monitored during antimicrobial therapy.**
Antibiotics, cephalosporins, erythromycin, clarithromycin, metronidazole	Warfarin (Coumadin)	Atrial fibrillation, myocardial infarction, post major surgery, stroke prevention	Anticoagulant effect of warfarin may be increased by several antibiotic classes. Reduced synthesis of vitamin K by gut flora is a putative mechanism, but several antibiotics have antiplatelet and anticoagulant activity. Cephalosporins, macrolide antibiotics, and metronidazole have the most convincing documentation, monitor INR. **RECOMMENDATION: Penicillins, tetracyclines, and clindamycin would be preferred choices but must be used cautiously.**
ANALGESICS			
Acetaminophen	Alcohol	Alcohol use and abuse	Increased risk of liver toxicity, especially during fasting state or ≥4 g of acetaminophen per day. **RECOMMENDATION: Use lower dose of acetaminophen and encourage discontinuation of alcohol use.**
Acetaminophen	Warfarin (Coumadin)	Atrial fibrillation, thrombosis	Increased risk of bleeding if acetaminophen is given at a dose of >2 g/day for ≥1 week. **RECOMMENDATION: Limit acetaminophen dosing and monitor INR.**
Aspirin	Oral hypoglycemics (e.g., sulfonylureas: Glyburide, chlorpropamide, acetohexamide)	Diabetes type 2	Increased hypoglycemic effects. **RECOMMENDATION: Avoid interaction.**
Aspirin, NSAIDs	Anticoagulants (Coumarin)	Atrial fibrillation, myocardial infarction, post surgery	Increased risk of bleeding (GI, oral). **RECOMMENDATION: Avoid interaction.**
Aspirin, NSAIDs	Alcohol	Alcohol use and abuse	Increases risk of gastrointestinal bleeding. **RECOMMENDATION: Lower dose; encourage discontinuation of alcohol use.**

TABLE **D-1**
cont'd

Dental Drug	Interacting Drug	Medical Condition/Situation	Effect
Aspirin	Diltiazem	Hypertension, angina	Enhanced antiplatelet activity of aspirin. **RECOMMENDATION: Monitor for risk of prolonged bleeding with the use of PFA-100.**
NSAIDs	Beta blockers, ACE inhibitors	Hypertension, post myocardial infarction	Decreased antihypertensive effect. **RECOMMENDATION: Limit duration of NSAID dosage to about 4 days.**
NSAIDs	Lithium	Manic depression	Produces symptoms of lithium toxicity, including nausea, vomiting, slurred speech, and mental confusion. **RECOMMENDATION: NSAIDs should not be prescribed to patients who take lithium. It can result in toxic levels of lithium, or consult with physician to reduce lithium dose.**
NSAIDs (Naproxen)	Alendronate	Osteoporosis, multiple myeloma	Increased risk for gastric ulcers. **RECOMMENDATION: Use acetaminophen products.**
NSAIDs	Methotrexate (MTX)	Connective tissue disease, cancer therapy	Toxic level of methotrexate may accumulate. **RECOMMENDATION: Avoid interaction if on high-dose MTX for cancer therapy. Low-dose MTX for arthritis is not a concern.**
ANESTHETICS Lidocaine	Bupivacaine		Additive effect of these two local anesthetics increases the risk of central nervous system toxicity. **RECOMMENDATION: Limit dose of each.**
Mepivacaine	Meperidine (Demerol)		Sedation with opioids may increase risk of local anesthetic toxicity; especially in children. **RECOMMENDATION: Reduce anesthetic dose.**
SEDATIVES Barbiturates	Digoxin, theophylline, corticosteroids, oral anticoagulants	Congestive heart failure, asthma, autoimmune disease, atrial fibrillation	Barbiturates bind P450 cytochrome system in liver and enhance the metabolism of many drugs. **RECOMMENDATION: Limit dose, and observe for adverse effects.**
	Benzodiazepines, alcohol, antihistamines	Anxiety, alcohol use and abuse, seasonal allergies	Additive effects for sedation and respiratory depression. **RECOMMENDATION: Reduce dose, and administer combination of sedatives with extreme caution.**
Benzodiazepines (BZDP) (e.g., alprazolam, chlordiazepoxide, diazepam)	Cimetidine, oral contraceptives, fluoxetine, isoniazid (INH), alcohol	Peptic ulcer disease, depression, tuberculosis, alcohol use and abuse	Delayed metabolism of BZDP, increasing the pharmacologic effects, can result in excessive sedation and adverse psychomotor effects. **RECOMMENDATION: Reduce dose of benzodiazepine.**
	Digoxin (Lanoxin), phenytoin, theophylline (Theodur)	Congestive heart failure, epilepsy, asthma	Serum concentrations of digoxin and phenytoin may be increased, resulting in toxicity. Antagonize sedative effects of benzodiazepine. **RECOMMENDATION: Avoid interaction.**
	Protease inhibitors (Indinavir, Nelfinavir)	HIV and AIDS	Increased bioavailability and effects of benzodiazepines, especially triazolam and oral midazolam. **RECOMMENDATION: Avoid interaction.**

TABLE **D-1**
cont'd

Dental Drug	Interacting Drug	Medical Condition/Situation	Effect
VASOCONSTRICTOR			
Epinephrine and Levonordephrine (Neocobefrin)	Nonselective beta blockers: Propranolol (Inderal), nadolol (Corgard), penbutolol (Levatol), pindolol (Visken), sotalol (Betapace), timolol (Blocadren)	Angina pectoris, hypertension, glaucoma, migraine, headache, hyperthyroidism, panic syndromes	Unopposed effects—Increased blood pressure with secondary bradycardia. **RECOMMENDATION: Initial dose is ½ carpule containing 1:100,000 epinephrine; aspirate to avoid intravascular injection, and inject slowly. Monitor vital signs, if no adverse cardiovascular change; up to two cartridges containing a vasoconstrictor can be administered. Provide a 5-minute interval between the first and second carpules with continual monitoring. Avoid epinephrine-containing retraction cord and higher concentrations of epinephrine in the dental anesthetic.**
	Cocaine	Illicit use, topical anesthetic for mucous membrane procedures	Blocks reuptake of norepinephrine and intensifies postsynaptic response to epinephrine-like drugs. This potentiates the adrenergic effects on the heart, with the potential for a heart attack. **RECOMMENDATION: Recognize signs and symptoms of cocaine abuse; avoid use of vasoconstrictors in these patients until cocaine has been withheld for at least 24 hours.**
	Halothane	General anesthetic for surgical procedures	Stimulation of alpha and beta receptors, resulting in arrhythmia at doses that exceed 2 µg/kg. **RECOMMENDATION: Limit dose to remain below 2 µg/kg threshold, aspirate to avoid intravascular injection. Monitor vital signs. Avoid epinephrine-containing retraction cord and concentrations of epinephrine higher than 1:100,000.**
	Tricyclic antidepressants* (amitriptyline [Elavil], amoxapine, clomipramine [Anafranil], desipramine [Norpramin], doxepin [Sinequan], imipramine [Tofranil], nortriptyline [Pamelor], protriptyline [Vivactil], trimipramine [Surmontil])	Depression, severe anxiety, neuropathic pain, attention deficit disorder	Blocks reuptake of norepinephrine, resulting in unopposed effects—increased pressor response (increased blood pressure, increased heart rate)—and potential cardiac arrhythmias; effect is greater with levonordefrin. **RECOMMENDATION: Avoid levonordefrin; limit dose to 2 carpules containing 1:100,000 epinephrine (36 µg), aspirate to avoid intravascular injection. Monitor vital signs. Avoid epinephrine-containing retraction cord and higher concentrations of epinephrine in the dental anesthetic.**

TABLE **D-1**
cont'd

Dental Drug	Interacting Drug	Medical Condition/Situation	Effect
	Monoamine oxidase (MAO) inhibitors (isocarboxazid [Marplan], phenelzine [Nardil], tranylcypromine [Parnate])	Depression	Although no reports have documented the effects on blood pressure or heart rate after dental procedures, the potential for increased pressor response is present. **RECOMMENDATION: Avoid levonordefrin; limit dose to 2 carpules containing 1:100,000 epinephrine (36 μg), and aspirate to avoid intravascular injection. Monitor vital signs. Avoid epinephrine-containing retraction cord and higher concentrations of epinephrine in the dental anesthetic.**
	Peripheral adrenergic antagonists (reserpine [Serpasil], guanethidine [Ismelin], guanadrel [Hylorel])	Hypertension	Potential for increased sensitivity of adrenergic receptors to epinephrine and levonordefrin. **RECOMMENDATION: Administer cautiously. Monitor vital signs during and after administration of first carpule. Limit dose to 2 carpules containing 1:100,000 epinephrine (36 g) or less depending on vital signs and patient response. Aspirate to avoid intravascular injection. Avoid epinephrine-containing retraction cord and higher concentrations of epinephrine in the dental anesthetic.**
	Catechol-O-methyl-transferase inhibitors (tolcapone [Tasmar], entacapone [Comtan])	Parkinson's disease	Potential for increased sensitivity of adrenergic receptors to epinephrine and levonordefrin, resulting in increased heart rate, blood pressure, and arrhythmias. **RECOMMENDATION: Administer cautiously. Monitor vital signs during and after administration of first carpule. Limit dose to 2 carpules containing 1:100,000 epinephrine (36 g) or less, depending on vital signs and patient response. Aspirate to avoid intravascular injection. Avoid epinephrine-containing retraction cord and higher concentrations of epinephrine in the dental anesthetic.**

ACE, Angiotensin-converting enzyme; AIDS, acquired immunodeficiency syndrome; HIV, human immunodeficiency virus; INR, international normalized ratio; NSAIDs, nonsteroidal anti-inflammatory drugs; PFA, platelet function analyzer.
*Antidepressants, such as the serotonin reuptake inhibitors, do not interact with vasoconstrictors. However, antidepressants that block norepinephrine uptake (Venlafaxine [Effexor], Bupropion [Wellbutrin]) have the potential to interact with vasoconstrictors and result in pressor responses.

E

Alternative and Complementary Drugs

The term *alternative medicine* is used to describe practices that are used instead of mainstream medical practice.[1,2] *Complementary medicine* refers to practices that are used as adjuncts to conventional medicine.[2] These systems are divided into five major categories: alternative medical systems (traditional Chinese medicine,[3] Ayurveda medicine of India,[4,5] and Native American healing approaches[6]), biologically based therapies (natural products),[7] manipulative and body-based methods (chiropractic and osteopathic manipulation),[8] mind–body interventions (hypnosis, cognitive therapies, and biofeedback), and energy therapies (use of magnets and acupuncture[9]).[1,2] Both of these systems use treatments that often have no established efficacy. It is estimated that about 42% of Americans use alternative and complementary medicine therapies, which are supported by an estimated $30 billion industry.[2,10]

Complementary medicines are defined as herbal medicines, homoeopatic remedies, and essential oils.[11-15] The basic principle of homeopathy consists of selection of a remedy that, if given to a healthy individual, will produce a range of symptoms similar to those observed in the ill patient (like cures like).[12,16,17] Only minute amounts are given to avoid toxicity. Only one remedy is used at any one time.[12,16] Dilute tinctures are used rather than concentrated ones. In homoeopathic practice, it is common to use medication in tablet form.[16]

Standard tinctures used in Western traditional herbal medicine are very different from those used in homoeopathy.[12,13,18] Alcohol is used to dissolve the plant, and the final product is not diluted. Thus, these remedies are concentrated, highly potent preparations, and they are usually taken as the unmodified liquid tincture. Other preparations used in herbal remedies include lotions and creams for topical application. The tablet form of medication is not used very often (less than 5%).[16]

Eisenberg[19] reported that herbal remedies are most commonly used to treat patients with allergies, insomnia, lung problems, and digestive problems. They also are used for the treatment of asthma, cancer, depression, schizophrenia, bipolar disorders, heart failure, rheumatologic conditions, and others.[19-26] Both adults and children use them.[19] In the United States, the sale of herbal remedies totaled $1.6 billion in 1994 and $4.0 billion by 1998.[19] In a U.S. study, 136 (70% response rate) customers who had bought dietary supplements in one of two U.S. health food stores reported that they had used 805 supplements—84.3% were taken for disease prevention and wellness, and 15.7% were taken to treat perceived health problems. Garlic, ginseng, and *Ginkgo biloba* were the most commonly named herbal products.[19] Klepser[27] reported that the use of herbal remedies among 794 individuals studied in Iowa was 41.6%. Most of the users were white women and had been educated beyond high school.[27] Patients with cardiovascular disease in Canada were studied for their use of herbal products.[28] About 17% were found to use herbal products.[28] Products most commonly used were garlic, cayenne pepper, and ginseng.[28]

EFFICACY OF HERBAL MEDICINES

Many herbal remedies have been used for hundreds of years.[29,30] However, traditional use is not in itself a good indication of efficacy. The gold standard for testing efficacy is the randomized clinical trial (RCT).[30] This standard should apply as much to herbal medicines as to conventional medicines. Numerous RCTs of herbal medical products have been conducted. However, many of these studies differ in how they were conducted and in their findings.[30] Ernst[30] suggests that the best way to evaluate RCTs undertaken to assess the efficacy of a specific herbal medicine is to do a systematic review or meta-analysis of all RCTs for that product.

TABLE **E-1**
Claims for Herbal Actions Supported by Clinical Trials

Herb	Claimed Action	Effectiveness Supported by Clinical Trials
Kava	Used to treat anxiety	Clinical trials have shown that it reduces anxiety to a significantly greater extent than placebo.
Artichoke	Used to lower lipid levels in blood	Only one randomized clinical study shows it to moderately lower elevated total cholesterol levels when given orally for several weeks.
Feverfew	Used for women's ailments and inflammatory diseases; recently has been suggested for headache and migraine	Three studies showed greater effect than placebo in alleviating symptoms of headache or migraine.
Garlic	Used for blood pressure reduction and lowering of blood lipid levels	Data show a small but statistically significant reduction in systolic and diastolic blood pressure. No data support the claims for lipid-lowering properties of garlic.
Ginger	Used to treat nausea and vomiting	Several studies support antiemetic uses for ginger. Used to treat or prevent nausea or vomiting.
Ginkgo biloba	Used to treat cerebral insufficiency and to prevent loss of cognitive function and tinnitus	Studies have shown it to be effective in the treatment of cerebral insufficiency when given for 4 to 6 weeks. Data show that regular oral intake of *Ginkgo biloba* slows the loss of cognitive function in patients with dementia.
Hawthorn	Used to treat heart failure	In various studies, shown to be effective for the early signs of congestive heart failure.
Horse chestnut	Used to treat venous congestion	Studies have shown it to be effective in reducing signs and symptoms of chronic venous insufficiency.
Saw palmetto	Used in Europe for symptoms of prostate enlargement	Clinical trials support its use for symptoms of benign prostatic hyperplasia.
St. John's wort	Used to treat depression	Studies show that it is effective for treating mild to moderate depression. The question of its effectiveness for severe depression remains unanswered.

HERBAL MEDICINES WITH PROVEN EFFICACY

Several herbal remedies have been repeatedly tested in placebo-controlled RCTs.[30] Systematic reviews of these studies have shown that some herbal medicines are effective for particular conditions.[30] For example, *Ginkgo biloba* has been shown to be effective for the symptomatic treatment of dementia and intermittent claudication.[31,32] Table E-1 lists the more commonly used herbal medicines that have proved effective for the condition(s) listed.

HERBAL MEDICINES WITH DOUBTFUL OR NO EFFICACY

Asian ginseng, one of the most popular herbal medicines in the United States, showed no convincing evidence for efficacy as a general tonic or as a means of enhancing mental and physical performance.[33] A review of studies regarding the use of valerian as a hypnotic agent was inconclusive because of flaws in study design.[34] No evidence was found in a systematic review of RCTs that evening primrose was effective in treating women with premenstrual syndrome.[35] Garlic was not found to be effective as a cholesterol-lowering drug.[36] Table E-2 lists some of the more common herbal medicines that were found not to be effective for the conditions listed.

ADVERSE EFFECTS AND ADVERSE REACTIONS

Increased recent use of herbal remedies seems to have resulted from the public's view that natural products are harmless or at least have fewer adverse effects than regular drugs.[37] The assumption that phytomedicines (herbal medicines) have only beneficial effects has proved incorrect.[13,14,37]

Toxicity may be associated with the use of herbal remedies. These reactions may be due to accidental or deliberate contamination of the product. For example, lead, mercury, cadmium, pesticides, microorganisms, and fumigants have been found to contaminate some herbal products.[37] Substitution of animal substances such as enzymes, hormones, or organ extracts and synthetic drugs has accounted for some of the toxic reactions to herbal products.[37] Adulteration caused by the accidental or deliberate substitution of the original plant material by other plant species also has been reported to be a source of toxic reactions to herbal products.[37]

Other adverse reactions to herbal products are intrinsic or plant associated.[37]

In some cases, the manufacturer has ignored the known toxicity of a plant or constituent in the herbal product.[37] In other cases, the product contains plants for which no or insufficient data are available regarding

TABLE E-2
Claims for Herbal Actions Unsupported by Clinical Trials

Herb	Claimed Action	Effectiveness Supported by Clinical Trials
Aloe vera	Used as an adjunctive oral treatment for diabetes and skin conditions such as herpes and psoriasis	At the present time, compelling data support none of the claims made for aloe vera.
Echinacea	Used for prevention and treatment of the common cold	Overall, evidence is insufficient to suggest that Echinacea extracts are effective for the treatment or prevention of the common cold.
Evening primrose	Used for the treatment of premenstrual syndrome	Current evidence suggests uncertain value when it is used to treat this syndrome.
Ginseng	Used to treat type 2 diabetes and herpes simplex infections. Also has been used to enhance physical and psychomotor performance, as well as cognitive function	None of the 16 double-blind, randomized clinical trials supports any effective action on physical performance, psychomotor performance, and cognitive function, nor in type 2 diabetes and herpes simplex infections.
Guar gum	Used to treat obesity and overweight	Clinical trials have not supported this use.
Mistletoe	Has been suggested for the treatment of cancer	Current studies do not support these claims.
Peppermint	Used to treat irritable bowel syndrome	Studies show that it alleviates the symptoms of irritable bowel syndrome. However, many of these trials were flawed.
Valerian	Used to promote sleep	Randomized clinical studies are needed to evaluate effectiveness. Studies to date have been flawed.

safety. If a highly concentrated or a specifically processed extract is used, toxic reactions may occur. If a plant contains constituents known to affect the bioavailability and/or pharmacokinetics of other drugs, serious drug interactions may occur.[37]

Long-term users, consumers of large quantities of phytomedicines, and individuals who use many different medicinal products may be prone to adverse effects. Pregnant or nursing women, babies, the elderly, and those who are sick and undernourished also are at higher risk for adverse effects.[37,38] Some of the more common adverse effects associated with herbal remedies include bleeding with *Ginkgo biloba*; upset stomach, tiredness, dizziness, confusion, dry mouth, and photosensitivity with St. John's wort; high blood pressure, arrhythmia, nervousness, headache, heart attack, or stroke with ephedra; and feeling sleepy, rash, and motor dysfunction of skeletal muscles with kava.[39] Table E-3 lists some of the serious adverse reactions that can occur when natural products are used.

MEDICAL PROBLEMS

Some medical problems can make the taking of herbal medicines unsafe. Individuals with high blood pressure, thyroid disease, psychiatric disorders, Parkinson's disease, enlarged prostate gland, diabetes mellitus, heart disease, epilepsy, glaucoma, blood clotting problems, and a history of stroke should check with their physician before taking any herbal remedies.[39] Patients with a history of aspirin allergy may be at risk if they take an herb that contains willow bark.[40]

TABLE E-3
Selected Herbal Medicines With Potentially Serious Adverse Effects

Product	Effect
Aristolochia	Nephrotoxicity
	Carcinogenicity
Chaparral	Cholestatic hepatitis
Comfrey	Acute and chronic hepatitis
Digitalis leaf	Arrhythmia
Ephedra	Hypertension
	Stroke
	Myocardial infarction
Germander	Acute and chronic hepatitis
Kava	Hepatitis
Khat	Tachycardia
	Psychosis
Kombucha	Hepatotoxicity
	Lactic acidosis
Mistletoe	Anaphylaxis
Skullcap	Seizures
	Acute and chronic hepatitis
St. John's wort	Photosensitivity
	Possible hypertension with tyramine-containing foods

DRUG INTERACTIONS

Important drug interactions may occur between certain herbal products and conventional medications (Table E-4)[13,14] The drug most commonly involved with drug–herb interactions is warfarin.[41] The herb most commonly involved with these interactions is St. John's wort.[41]

TABLE **E-4**
Selected Natural Medicines That Potentiate or Interfere With Approved Drugs

Natural Medicine	Approved Drug
Ephedra	Theophylline (P)
	Antihypertensives (I)
	Corticosteroids (I)
Evening primrose	Anticoagulants (P)
	Antiplatelet agents (P)
	Low molecular weight heparins (P)
	Anticonvulsants (I)
Garlic	Aspirin (P)
	Clopidogrel (P)
	Ticlopidine (P)
Ginkgo leaf extract	Anticoagulants (P)
	Antiplatelet agents (P)
	Anticonvulsants (I)
Glucosamine	Antidiabetic drugs (I)
Panax ginseng	Anticoagulants (P)
	Diabetic agents (Possible P)
	Nifedipine (P)
Saw palmetto	Hormone replacement therapies (P)
Soy	Estrogenic drugs (P)
St. John's wort	Antidepressants (P)
	HIV protease inhibitors (I)
	Cyclosporine (I)
Valerian	Sedatives (P)
Yohimbe	Antihypertensives (I)

HIV, Human immunodeficiency virus; I, interferes; P, potentiates.

Markowitz,[47] in a study undertaken to evaluate the potential of St. John's wort to alter cytochrome P450 enzymes, found that a 14-day course of the herbal product significantly induced the activity of CYP 3A4, as measured by changes in alprazolam pharmacokinetics. Markowitz[42] concluded that long-term administration of St. John's wort may result in diminished clinical effectiveness or increased dosage requirements for all CYP 3A4 substrates, which represent about 50% of all marketed medications. In contrast, in another study, he found little evidence that garlic extracts would alter the disposition of coadministered medications metabolized by the CYP 3A4 pathway.[43]

Patients who take aspirin, warfarin, ticlopidine, clopidogrel, or dipyridamole should not take *Ginkgo biloba* because bleeding may occur.[39] Patients who take an antidepressant should not take St. John's wort. Patients who are taking a decongestant or a stimulant drug and individuals who drink caffeinated beverages should not take ephedra. Individuals who are taking a benzodiazepine, a barbiturate, an antipsychotic medication, or any medicine used to treat Parkinson's disease should not take kava products.[39] It is important that patients notify their general practitioner if they are taking phytomedicines concurrently with conventional drugs—especially those with cardiac, diuretic, sedative, hypotensive, or other properties.[37] Individuals who are taking a prescription

medicine should check with their physician before taking any herbal health product.[39]

DENTAL IMPLICATIONS

A limited number of recent papers describe the use of complementary and alternative medical systems for dental problems.[44-67] Two of these papers report on the use of herbal products for the treatment of periodontal disease.[44,63]

In a series of five papers, Goldstein suggests that unconventional or alternative dentistry is analogous to and conceptually inseparable from unconventional or alternative medicine.[48-52] He suggests that dentists should learn about these procedures in terms of the evidence for effectiveness and safety.[51] Dentists should accept and encompass science-based advances and should reject unproven or disproven methods.[51] Selected unconventional treatments may be incorporated with conventional dentistry in some patients for specific purposes that will be beneficial to the patient.[51]

INFORMATION FOR DENTISTS

Herbal remedies have the potential to affect the safety of invasive or prolonged dental procedures.[68] Excessive bleeding may occur with some of these medications.[68] Other herbal medicines may affect the cardiovascular system and render the patient more susceptible to cardiac arrhythmia and other cardiovascular complications.[68] Ginseng may cause hypoglycemia.[68] Chinese patients with cancer undergoing chemotherapy who were users of Chinese herbal medicine were found to have higher scores of mucositis.[69] It is important for the dentist to include a section in the patient's medical history on the taking of herbal medications and over-the-counter drugs. Because most U.S. dental schools teach very little about the use, adverse effects, toxicity, and drug interactions associated with herbal remedies, the dentist must find a way to become informed about these issues.

Important references for dentists are the *Physicians' Desk Reference for Herbal Medicines,* 3rd edition (2004) and the *Physicians' Desk Reference for Nonprescription Drugs, Dietary Supplements and Herbs* (2006), both published by Thomson. Dentists should use only treatment procedures that have been established as effective and involving minimal risk. Because clinical trials have shown some alternative and complementary treatments to be effective and safe, they may be incorporated into conventional medicine and dentistry.[70] The dentist may find that a medically compromised patient is taking an herbal remedy that is potentially harmful. This should be discussed with the patient and the patient referred to his or her physician for evaluation and treatment.

REFERENCES

1. Little JW. Complementary and alternative medicine. Oral Surg Oral Med Oral Path Oral Radiol Endod 2004;98:137-146.

2. Straus SE. Complementary and alternative medicine. In Goldman L, Ausiello D (eds). Cecil Textbook of Medicine. Philadelphia, Saunders, 2004, pp 170-174.

3. Ergil KV. Chinese medicine. In Micozzi MS (ed). Fundamentals of Complementary and Integrative Medicine, 3rd ed. St. Louis, Elsevier, 2006, pp 375-417.

4. Zysk KG, Tetlow G. Traditional Ayurveda. In Micozzi MS (ed). Fundamentals of Complementary and Integrative Medicine, 3rd ed. St. Louis, Elsevier, 2006, pp 494-507.

5. Sodhi V. Ayurveda: The science of life and mother of the healing arts. In Pizzorno JEJ, Murray MT (eds). Textbook of Natural Medicine. St. Louis, Churchill Livingstone Elsevier, 2006, pp 317-327.

6. Voss RW, Douville V, Edwards ED, Twiss G. Native American healing. In Micozzi MS (ed). Fundamentals of Complementary and Integrative Medicine, 3rd ed. St. Louis, Elsevier, 2006, pp 536-550.

7. Murray MT, Pizzorno JEJ. Nutritional medicine. In Pizzorno JEJ, Murray MT (eds). Textbook of Natural Medicine. St. Louis, Churchill Livingstone Elsevier, 2006, pp 461-475.

8. Martinez RM. Manipulation. In Pizzorno JEJ, Murray MT (eds). Textbook of Natural Medicine. St. Louis, Churchill Livingstone Elsevier, 2006, pp 417-431.

9. Nolting MH. Acupuncture. In Pizzorno JEJ, Murray MT (eds). Textbook of Natural Medicine. St. Louis, Churchill Livingstone Elsevier, 2006, pp 309-317.

10. Micozzi MS. Issues in integrative medicine. In Micozzi MS (ed). Fundamentals of Complementary and Integrative Medicine, 3rd ed. St. Louis, Churchill Livingstone Elsevier, 2006, pp 18-24.

11. Barnes J. Consumer and pharmacist perspectives. In Ernst E (ed). Herbal Medicine: A Concise Overview for Professionals. Oxford, Butterworth & Heinemann, 2000, pp 19-33.

12. Carlston M. Homeopathy. In Micozzi MS (ed). Fundamentals of Complementary and Integrative Medicine, 3rd ed. St. Louis, Churchill Livingstone Elsevier, 2006, pp 95-110.

13. Micozzi MS, Meserole L. Herbal medicine. In Micozzi MS (ed). Fundamentals of Complementary and Integrative Medicine, 3rd ed. St. Louis, Churchill Livingstone Elsevier, 2006, pp 164-180.

14. Sierpina V, Gerik S. Common herbs for integrative care. In Micozzi MS (ed). Fundamentals of Complementary and Integrative Medicine, 3rd ed. St. Louis, Churchill Livingstone Elsevier, 2006, pp 181-206.

15. Hoffman CJ. Aromatherapy. In Micozzi MS (ed). Fundamentals of Complementary and Integrative Medicine, 3rd ed. St. Louis, Churchill Livingstone Elsevier, 2006, pp 207-220.

16. Eldin S, Dunford A. Herbal Medicine in Primary Care. Oxford, Butterworth & Heinemann, 1999.

17. Lange A. Homeopathy. In Pizzorno JEJ, Murray MT (eds). Textbook of Natural Medicine. St. Louis, Churchill Livingstone Elsevier, 2006, pp 387-401.

18. Murray MT, Pizzorno JEJ. Botanical medicine—A modern perspective. In Pizzorno JEJ, Murray MT (eds). Textbook of Natural Medicine. St. Louis, Churchill Livingstone Elsevier, 2006, pp 327-339.

19. Eisenberg DM, Davis RB, Ettner SL, et al. Trends in alternative medicine use in the United States. JAMA 1998;280:1569-1575.

20. Gyorik SA, Brutsche MH. Complementary and alternative medicine for bronchial asthma: Is there new evidence? Curr Opin Pulm Med 2004;10:37-43.

21. Rathbone J, Zhang L, Zhang M, et al. Chinese herbal medicine for schizophrenia. Cochrane Database Syst Rev 2005(4):CD003444.

22. Sun A, Chia JS, Chiang CP, et al. The Chinese herbal medicine Tien-Hsien liquid inhibits cell growth and induces apoptosis in a wide variety of human cancer cells. J Altern Complement Med 2005;11:245-256.

23. Treasure J. Herbal medicine and cancer: An introductory overview. Semin Oncol Nurs 2005;21:177-183.

24. Wen MC, Wei CH, Hu ZQ, et al. Efficacy and tolerability of anti-asthma herbal medicine intervention in adult patients with moderate-severe allergic asthma. J Allergy Clin Immunol 2005;116:517-524.

25. Zhang ZJ, Kang WH, Tan QR, et al. Adjunctive herbal medicine with carbamazepine for bipolar disorders: A double-blind, randomized, placebo-controlled study. J Psychiatr Res 2007;41:360-369.

26. Zick SM, Blume A, Aaronson KD. The prevalence and pattern of complementary and alternative supplement use in individuals with chronic heart failure. J Card Fail 2005;11:586-589.

27. Klepser TB, Doucette WR, Horton MR, et al. Assessment of patients' perceptions and beliefs regarding herbal therapies. Pharmacotherapy 2000;20:83-87.

28. Pharand C, Ackman ML, Jackevicius CA, et al. Use of OTC and herbal products in patients with cardiovascular disease. Ann Pharmacother 2003;37:899-904.

29. Micozzi MS. Translation from conventional medicine. In Micozzi MS (ed). Fundamentals of Complementary and Integrative Medicine, 3rd ed. St. Louis, Churchill Livingstone Elsevier, 2006, pp 9-17.

30. Ernst E, Pittler MH. Herbal medicine. Med Clin North Am 2002;86:149-161.

31. Ernst E, Pittler MH. Ginkgo biloba for dementia: A systematic review of double-blind placebo-controlled trials. Clin Drug Invest 1999;17:301-308.

32. Pittler MH, Ernst E. Ginkgo biloba extract for the treatment of intermittent claudication: A meta-analysis of randomized trials. Am J Med 2000;108:226-281.

33. Vogler BK, Pittler MH, Ernst E. The efficacy of ginseng: A systematic review of randomised clinical trials. Eur J Clin Pharmacol 1999;55:567-575.

34. Ernst E, Pittler MH. The efficacy of herbal drugs. In Ernst E (ed). Herbal Medicine: A Concise Overview for Professionals. Oxford, Butterworth & Heinemann, 2000, pp 69-82.

35. Buderiri D, Li Won Po D, Dornan JC. Is evening primrose oil of value in the treatment of premenstrual syndrome? Controlled Clin Trials 1996;17:60-68.

36. Stevinson C, Pittler MH, Ernst E. Garlic for treating hypercholesterolemia. Ann Intern Med 2000;133:420-429.

37. Halkes SBA. Safety issues in phytotherapy. In Ernst E (ed). Herbal Medicine: A Concise Overview for Professionals. Oxford, Butterworth & Heinemann, 2000, pp 82-100.

38. Conover EA. Herbal agents and over-the-counter medications in pregnancy. Best Pract Res Clin Endocrinol Metab 2003;17:237-251.

39. Consult M. Complementary and Alternative Medicine. St. Louis, Elsevier, 2003.

40. Boullata JI, McDonnell PJ, Oliva CD. Anaphylactic reaction to a dietary supplement containing willow bark. Ann Pharmacother 2003;37:832-835.

41. Brazier NC, Levine MA. Drug–herb interaction among commonly used conventional medicines: A compendium for health care professionals. Am J Ther 2003;10:163-169.

42. Markowitz JS, Donovan JL, Devane CL, et al. Effect of St John's wort on drug metabolism by induction of cytochrome P450 3A4 enzyme. JAMA 2003;290:1500-1504.

43. Markowitz JS, Devane CL, Chavin KD, et al. Effects of garlic (*Allium sativum* L.) supplementation on cytochrome P450 2D6 and 3A4 activity in healthy volunteers. Clin Pharmacol Ther 2003;74:170-177.

44. Amrutesh S. Dentistry and Ayurveda. Indian J Dent Res 2003;14:1-5.

45. Barolet R. Acupuncture in dentistry. J Am Dent Assoc 1978;97:166-168.

46. Dougherty K, Touger-Decker R, O'Sullivan MJ. Personal and professional beliefs and practices regarding herbal medicine among the full time faculty of the Newark-based schools of the University of Medicine and Dentistry of New Jersey. Integr Med 2000;2:57-64.

47. Ferraris S. Alternative dentistry. Br Dent J 1992;173:156-157.

48. Goldstein BH. Unconventional dentistry: Part V. Professional issues, concerns and uses. J Can Dent Assoc 2000;66:608-610.

49. Goldstein BH. Unconventional dentistry: Part III. Legal and regulatory issues. J Can Dent Assoc 2000;66:503-506.

50. Goldstein BH. Unconventional dentistry: Part II. Practitioners and patients. J Can Dent Assoc 2000;66:381-383.

51. Goldstein BH. Unconventional dentistry: Part I. Introduction. J Can Dent Assoc 2000;66:323-326.

52. Goldstein BH, Epstein JB. Unconventional dentistry: Part IV. Unconventional dental practices and products. J Can Dent Assoc 2000;66:564-568.

53. Johnson NW. Complementary medicine in dentistry. Oral Dis 1998;4:69.

54. McComb D. Unconventional dentistry. J Can Dent Assoc 2001;67:190.

55. Mulrooney R. Unconventional dentistry. J Can Dent Assoc 2001;67:10-11.

56. Oepen I. A critical evaluation of unconventional diagnostic and therapeutic methods in dentistry. Fortschr Kieferorthop 1992;53:239-246.

57. Penzer V, Matsumoto K. Neuroanatomical and neurophysiological basis for use of acupuncture in dentistry. J Mass Dent Soc 1987;36:83-84.

58. Pistorius A, Willershausen B, Steinmeier EM, Kreislert M. Efficacy of subgingival irrigation using herbal extracts on gingival inflammation. J Periodontol 2003;74:616-622.

59. Romano JAJ. Acupuncture and dentistry. J Bergen Cty Dent Soc 1978;44:7-9.

60. Rosted P. Use of acupuncture in dentistry. Aust Dent J 1998;43:437.

61. Rosted P. The use of acupuncture in dentistry: A review of the scientific validity of published papers. Oral Dis 1998;4:100-104.

62. Rosted P. Introduction to acupuncture in dentistry. Br Dent J 2000;189:136-140.

63. Sastravaha G, Yotnuengnit P, Booncong P, Sangtherapitikul P. Adjunctive periodontal treatment with *Centella asiatica* and *Punica granatum* extracts: A preliminary study. J Int Acad Periodontol 2003;5:106-115.

64. Thayer T. Acupuncture in dentistry. SAAD Dig 2001;18:3-8.

65. Tobey HS. What dentists need to know about CADM: Complementary and alternative dentistry and medicine. J NJ Dent Assoc 1996;67:21-24.

66. Vachiramon A, Wang WC, Vachiramon T. The use of acupuncture in implant dentistry. Implant Dent 2004;13:58-64.

67. Wilcox CE. The practical uses of acupuncture in dentistry. CDS Rev 1982;75:25-27.

68. Ang-Lee MK, Moss J, Yuan CS. Herbal medicines and perioperative care. JAMA 2001;286:208-216.

69. Chan CW, Chang AM, Molassiotis A, Lee IY. Oral complications in Chinese cancer patients undergoing chemotherapy. Support Care Cancer 2003;11:48-55.

70. Miller FG, Emanuel EJ, Rosenstein DL, Straus SE. Ethical issues concerning research in complementary and alternative medicine. JAMA 2004;291:599-604.

INDEX

Page numbers followed by f indicate figures; t, tables, b, boxes.